Chandler and Grant's

Glaucoma

Fourth Edition

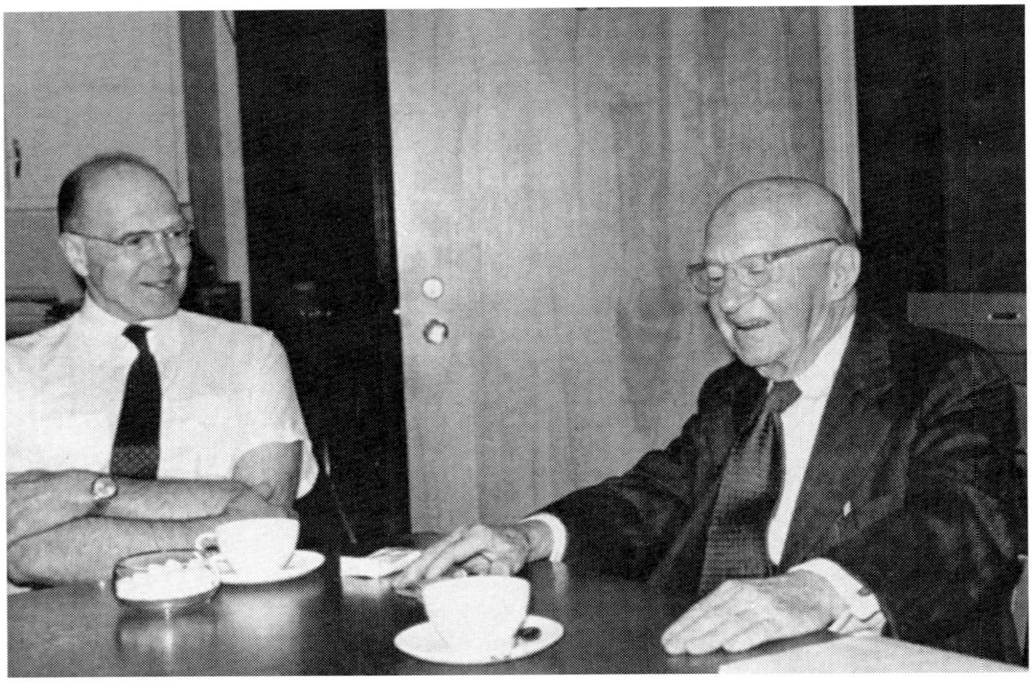

W. Morton Grant, M.D. and Paul A. Chandler, M.D. in their weekly meeting in the laboratory. (Courtesy of Marshall N. Cyrlin, M.D.)

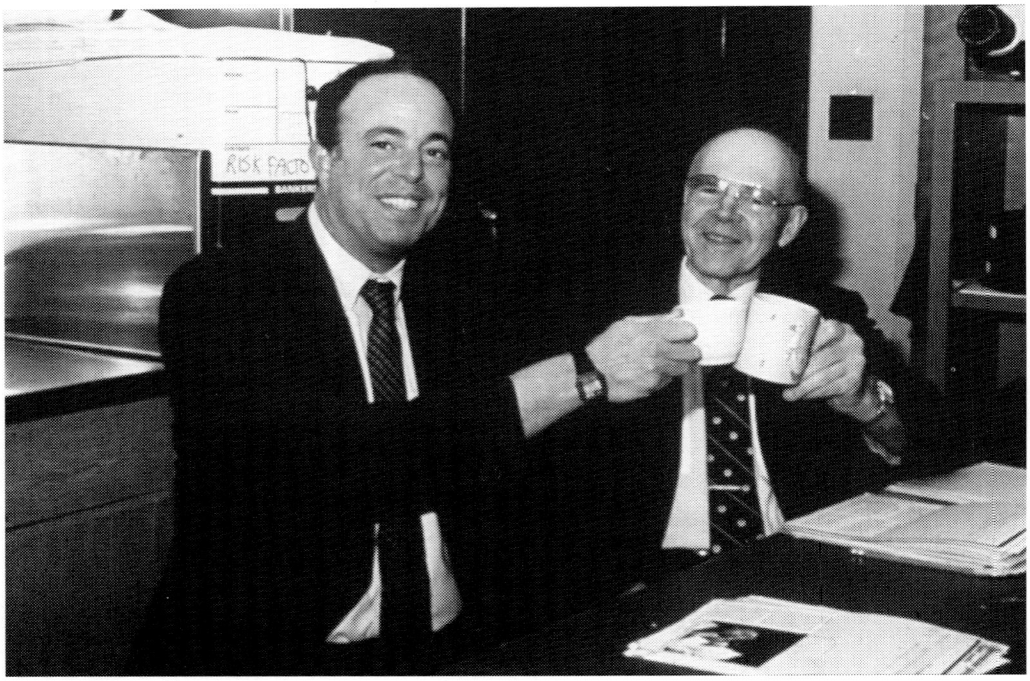

David L. Epstein, M.D. and W. Morton Grant, M.D.

Chandler and Grant's Glaucoma

Fourth Edition

David L. Epstein, M.D.
Professor and Chairman of Ophthalmology
Duke University Medical School
Duke Eye Center

with

R. Rand Allingham, M.D.
Assistant Professor of Ophthalmology
Duke University Medical School
Duke Eye Center

Joel S. Schuman, M.D.
Associate Professor of Ophthalmology
Director, Glaucoma Service
Tufts University School of Medicine
New England Eye Center

SANS TACHE

Williams & Wilkins
A WAVERLY COMPANY

BALTIMORE • PHILADELPHIA • LONDON • PARIS • BANGKOK
BUENOS AIRES • HONG KONG • MUNICH • SYDNEY • TOKYO • WROCLAW

Editor: Darlene Barela Cooke
Managing Editor: Frances M. Klass
Production Coordinator: Peter J. Carley
Book Project Editor: Kathy Gilbert
Designer: Karen Klinedinst
Illustration Planner: Peter J. Carley
Typesetter: Maryland Composition
Printer: Walsworth
Binder: Walsworth

ISBN 0-683-02808-1

9 780683 028089 90000>

351 West Camden Street
Baltimore, Maryland 21201-2436 USA

Rose Tree Corporate Center
1400 North Providence Road
Building II, Suite 5025
Media, Pennsylvania 19063-2043 USA

Accurate indications, adverse reactions, and dosage schedules for drugs are provided in this book, but it is possible that they may change. The reader is urged to review the package information data of the manufacturers of the medications mentioned.

Printed in the United States of America

Library of Congress Cataloging in Publication Data

Chandler and Grant's glaucoma.—4th ed. / [edited by] David L. Epstein; with R. Rand Allingham, Joel Schuman.
p. cm.
Rev. ed of: Chandler and Grant's glaucoma / David L. Epstein. 3rd ed. 1986.
Includes bibliographical references and index.
ISBN 0-683-02808-1
1. Glaucoma. I. Chandler, Paul A. (Paul Austin), 1896– II. Grant, W. Morton (Walter Morton), 1915– . III. Epstein, David L. IV. Allingham, R. Rand. V. Schuman, Joel S.
[DNLM: 1. Glaucoma. WW 290 C455 1996]
RE871.C45 1996
617.7′41—dc20
DNLM.DLC
for Library of Congress 96-11484
CIP

The Publishers have made every effort to trace the copyright holders for borrowed material. If they have inadvertently overlooked any, they will be pleased to make the necessary arrangements at the first opportunity

96 97 98 99
1 2 3 4 5 6 7 8 9 10

Dedication

I am grateful to my wife Susan and son, Michael, and to Duke University for their support during this special undertaking. I am indebted to Jean Odem for her thoughtful organization and assembly of the components of the text. The book is dedicated to Dr. Grant and Dr. Chandler, who taught us all to be not only good clinical observers, but to be inquisitive, and to remain humble with the realized inadequacies of our understanding of the very treacherous diseases of glaucoma.

David L. Epstein
Durham, North Carolina

Preface

Almost ten years has passed since the last edition of Chandler and Grant's Glaucoma, and much has changed in the interval, not only in glaucoma but also in the lives of the editors. Sadly Dr. Chandler has passed away, although with dignity and grace. Dr. Grant "retired" and left Mass. Eye and Ear Infirmary to go to Tufts to complete his definitive text on Toxicology of the Eye with Joel Schuman. He has now retired again! I left Boston, initially to join my close friend and scientific colleague, Jorge Alvarado, M.D. at the University of California, San Francisco, and then subsequently to Duke to join M. Bruce Shields, M.D., another good colleague and friend. Rand Allingham, M.D. and Joel Schuman, M.D., whom I had trained as fellows and with much gratitude on my part retained as colleagues on the Harvard faculty with the expectation (among many) that we would write this edition together, also left Mass. Eye and Ear Infirmary.

Thus, when I was approached about writing this edition of this book, I was initially very hesitant because I had always viewed this book as appropriately being somewhat "Bostonocentric," of which I was really no longer a part. However, on further reflection I realized that there were many glaucoma colleagues across the nation and internationally who had trained with Drs. Chandler and Grant, and who were now, like me, building upon this heritage with further experience and knowledge obtained at their new location. Clinical and scientific interchange with other colleagues "not trained in Boston" contributed to this enrichment globally, and this progression was, in fact, an appropriate part of the "Chandler-Grant tradition."

The goals of this book are explained in the first chapter. In brief, I wanted to try to write a book on glaucoma that would give practical clinical information to the clinician dealing with an individual patient, and yet at the same time, stimulate us all to ask "why," i.e., what is the mechanism for the clinical observation, and how might we be better able to treat the condition in the future. Drs. Chandler and Grant had taught me to strive to think this way. Glaucoma is a discipline commonly of subtleties and nuances with the detailed clinical observation of an individual patient quite important. To me many texts of a review type often had come up wanting, with inadequate specific information on how to treat the individual patient of concern, who might well be right now sitting in the physician's office. I also wanted to format the text with the expectation that the busy practitioner would not be able to read every word in the chapters when confronted with a puzzling patient. Hopefully the bolding and highlighted areas will thus help make this edition more reader friendly, and will not offend. I still urge students, residents, and fellows to read every word!

In this book there are many observations and "constructs" that are personally mine, which many former fellows and residents might recognize as "teaching tools" and strategies that I utilized in their clinical conferences during their training. As a teacher I often wondered how much good, if any, I was doing, but so many former trainees who are now glaucoma experts of their own have commented favorably on this material and approach from our "Monday night conferences" and which they claim to still remember, that I wanted to include this in the current edition. This material represents clinical observations over two decades of how I learned from my glaucoma patients, and how I wished to organize the thinking about glaucoma in the minds of the rising "next generation." Glaucoma is really the "thinking person's" discipline! But I also wanted to include in this book chapters written by other renowned colleagues and, who building commonly upon a Chandler-Grant heritage of detailed observation and inquisitiveness, have become true international glaucoma experts by virtue of their own unique subsequent clinical and research skills. They are an impressive group who I cherish as colleagues and realize may well have expertise far beyond my own. Finally, it is a source of great pride that I have been reunited with both Rand Allingham and Joel Schuman through this book by their expertise in integrating and amplifying the contents. A special joy to us all is the fact that Dr. Grant has reviewed the entire text! He continues to inspire—I hope "he unretires" again soon!

Collaborators

R. Rand Allingham, M.D.
Assistant Professor
Duke University Eye Center
Durham, North Carolina

Jorge A. Alvarado, M.D.
Professor of Ophthalmology
University of California—San Francisco
San Francisco, California

C. Davis Belcher, III, M.D.
Ophthalmic Consultants of Boston
Boston, Massachusetts

A. Robert Bellows, M.D.
Assistant Clinical Professor of Ophthalmology
Harvard Medical School
Surgeon in Ophthalmology
Massachusetts Eye and Ear Infirmary
Ophthalmic Consultants of Boston
Boston, Massachusetts

David P. Berry, M.D.
Assistant Consulting Professor of Ophthalmology
Duke University Eye Center
Durham, North Carolina
Piedmont Eye Associates
Spartanburg, South Carolina

Edward G. Buckley, M.D.
Professor of Ophthalmology
Associate Professor of Pediatrics
Pediatric Ophthalmology and Strabismus, Neuro-Ophthalmology
Duke University Eye Center
Durham, North Carolina

Marshall N. Cyrlin, M.D.
Clinical Associate Professor
Oakland University Eye Research Institute
Rochester, Michigan
Director, Glaucoma Service, Sinai Hospital
Detroit, Michigan
Director, Glaucoma Service, Beaumont Eye Institute
Royal Oak, Michigan

Evan B. Dreyer, M.D., Ph.D.
Director, Glaucoma Consultation Service
Massachusetts Eye and Ear Infirmary
Boston, Massachusetts

David K. Dueker, M.D.
Chief, Glaucoma Division
King Khaled Eye Specialist Hospital
Associate Clinical Professor
King Saud University
Riyadh, Saudi Arabia

Jay S. Duker, M.D.
Director, Vitreoretinal Service
New England Eye Center
Associate Professor of Ophthalmology
Tufts University School of Medicine
Boston, Massachusetts

David L. Epstein, M.D.
Professor and Chairman
Department of Ophthalmology
Duke University Eye Center
Durham, North Carolina

Sharon Fridovich Freedman, M.D.
Assistant Professor of Ophthalmology
Duke University Eye Center
Durham, North Carolina

Morton F. Goldberg, M.D.
William Holland Wilmer Professor and Director, The Wilmer Eye Institute
Johns Hopkins Medical Institutions
Baltimore, Maryland

W. Morton Grant, M.D.
Professor of Ophthalmology, Emeritus
Harvard Medical School
Massachusetts Eye and Ear Infirmary
Visiting Professor of Ophthalmology
Tufts University School of Medicine
New England Eye Center
Boston, Massachusetts

Fredric J. Gross, M.D.
Assistant Professor of Ophthalmology
Eastern Virginia Medical School
Norfolk, Virginia

Eve J. Higginbotham, M.D.
Professor and Chair
Department of Ophthalmology
University of Maryland at Baltimore
Baltimore, Maryland

Douglas H. Johnson, M.D.
Consultant, Department of Ophthalmology
Mayo Clinic and Mayo Foundation
Associate Professor of Ophthalmology
Mayo Medical School
Rochester, Minnesota

Murray A. Johnstone, M.D.
Swedish Hospital Medical Center
Clinical Instructor
University of Washington
Seattle, Washington

Mark C. Kuperwaser, M.D.
Associate Surgeon in Ophthalmology
Beth Israel Hospital
Boston, Massachusetts
Instructor in Ophthalmology
Harvard Medical School
Boston, Massachusetts

Mark A. Latina, M.D.
Associate Professor of Ophthalmology
Chief of Glaucoma Service
UMADNJ-New Jersey Medical School
Newark, New Jersey
Clinical Instructor in Ophthalmology
Harvard Medical School
Boston, Massachusetts

David Anson Lee, M.D., M.S., M.B.A.
Chief, Glaucoma Division
Professor of Ophthalmology
Director, UCLA Mobile Eye Clinic
Jules Stein Eye Institute
UCLA School of Medicine
Los Angeles, California

Paul P. Lee, M.D.
Associate Professor of Ophthalmology
University of Southern California School of Medicine
Doheny Eye Institute
Los Angeles, California

Cynthia Mattox, M.D.
Assistant Professor of Ophthalmology
Tufts University School of Medicine
New England Eye Center
Boston, Massachusetts

Shlomo Melamed, M.D.
Associate Professor of Ophthalmology
Sackler School of Medicine
Tel Aviv University
Director of the Sam Rothberg Glaucoma Center
Goldschleger Eye Institute
Tel Hashomer, Israel

Peter A. Netland, M.D., Ph.D.
Assistant Professor of Ophthalmology
Harvard Medical School
Assistant Surgeon in Ophthalmology
Associate Director, Glaucoma Consultation Services
Massachusetts Eye and Ear Infirmary
Boston, Massachusetts

Claudia U. Richter, M.D.
Clinical Assistant in Ophthalmology
Harvard Medical School
Boston, Massachusetts

Joel S. Schuman, M.D.
Associate Professor of Ophthalmology
Tufts University School of Medicine
Director, Glaucoma Service
Director, Residency Training
New England Eye Center
Boston, Massachusetts

M. Bruce Shields, M.D.
Professor of Ophthalmology
Department of Ophthalmology
Duke University Eye Center
Durham, North Carolina

Bradford J. Shingleton, M.D.
Assistant Clinical Professor of Ophthalmology
Harvard Medical School
Boston, Massachusetts

Richard J. Simmons, M.D.
Simmons Eye Associates of Boston
Associate Clinical Professor of Ophthalmology
Harvard Medical School
Surgeon in Ophthalmology
Massachusetts Eye and Ear Infirmary
Boston, Massachusetts

Ruthanne B. Simmons, M.D.
Simmons Eye Associates of Boston
Clinical Instructor of Ophthalmology
Harvard Medical School
Assistant Surgeon, Massachusetts Eye and Ear Infirmary
Boston, Massachusetts

David P. Tingey, M.D.
Ivey Institute of Ophthalmology
Assistant Professor of Ophthalmology
University of Western Ontario
London, Ontario, CANADA

E. Michael Van Buskirk, M.D.
Chief, Department of Ophthalmology
Legacy Portland Hospitals
Director, Devers Eye Institute
Clinical Professor of Ophthalmology
Oregon Health Sciences University
Portland, Oregon

David S. Walton, M.D.
Surgeon, Massachusetts Eye and Ear Infirmary
Associate Clinical Professor, Ophthalmology
Harvard Medical School
Boston, Massachusetts

Martin Wand, M.D.
Associate Clinical Professor of Ophthalmology
University of Connecticut Medical School
Farmington, Connecticut
Senior Surgeon
Hartford Hospital
Hartford, Connecticut

Janey L. Wiggs, M.D., Ph.D.
Assistant Professor, Department of Ophthalmology and Division of Genetics
Tufts University School of Medicine
New England Medical Center
Boston, Massachusetts

M. Roy Wilson, M.D., M.S.
Professor of Ophthalmology
UCLA School of Medicine
Jules Stein Eye Institute
Dean, College of Medicine
Charles R. Drew University
Los Angeles, California

Contents

VI Combined Mechanisms

VII Secondary Open Angle Glaucoma

VIII Laser Methods in Glaucoma

The Basics

I

Introduction

1

David L. Epstein

THE PROBLEM

The study of glaucoma can be both clinically satisfying and intellectually stimulating. Yet it is also the most humbling of disciplines, both because of our clinical failures but even more, our lack of real understanding. In truth, if one looks at ophthalmic knowledge in the last century, the field of glaucoma has shown the least progress.

Why is this? The chronic glaucomas are, in general, slowly progressive diseases over time. This **time factor** creates substantial difficulties in achieving meaningful clinical deductions and insight. One of the major reasons for this book is the fact that long-term clinical observations can provide a basis for meaningful knowledge. This is the true "Chandler-Grant tradition."

Those caring for glaucoma patients bear the "curse of long-term follow-up." However, such a perspective is important both for practical patient care and as a template for new knowledge, but this clinical experience does require long periods of clinical observation. Experienced clinicians do have a great deal to contribute to our knowledge in glaucoma. The fields of glaucoma are littered with relics of short-term enthusiasms for certain procedures and techniques.

OUR METHODS

However, in addition to the **time** factor, our **methods** in glaucoma are very crude and provide inadequate information. The measurement of intraocular pressure (IOP) is accurate, yet it indicates the IOP at only one instant of time. We know there is both a diurnal and seasonal variation in IOP (1). Patients often only take their antiglaucoma medication before coming to the ophthalmologist's office. Each of us measures the IOP, and because it is the only data we have, we generalize that this must be the representative IOP for that patient during the entire time interval since we have last seen the patient. This is often not true. Our office IOP measurement is a single "snapshot."

This often contributes to "fuzzy thinking" about primary open angle glaucoma (POAG). There are many population survey studies in which patients who demonstrate POAG related field loss do not have elevated IOP at the time of sampling (2–4). This has led to avenues of thought, especially abroad, that IOP is not involved in the glaucomatous optic neuropathy, even though most studies have shown that the "risk" for field loss in POAG increases linearly with the level of IOP (5). Much effort has been spent in pursuing these non-IOP related glaucoma hypotheses, even though at the same time, early filtration surgery for patients with glaucoma has been simultaneously proposed by many of the same investigators (presumably the only known efficacy of filtration surgery for glaucoma is to **consistently** lower the IOP). Some insight into possible pathogenic mechanisms in glaucoma has come from recent population studies in which a second IOP has been measured (6): the prevalence of at least one increased IOP measurement is substantially higher; that is, discovered glaucoma patients with "normal" IOP at the time of initial evaluation, may demonstrate an "elevated" IOP at a subsequent visit. What this means to one of us (DLE), is that although IOP can be accurately measured, we have vast expanses of missing data points for evaluation of glaucoma patients. A "Holter monitor" or "glycosylated hemoglobin" approach, if possible, might revolutionize understanding.

All this does not detract from the clinical fact from **long-term** clinical observations that there is varying susceptibility of the optic nerve to given levels of IOP. But what is the quality of data about this "end organ," the optic nerve, concerning damage in glaucoma? Again, methods of clinical analysis are crude. Descriptions of optic discs, cup/disc ratios, **and** disc drawings are notoriously inaccurate. The best advice one could give the beginning ophthalmic resident is to make drawings of optic nerves on all glaucoma patients and then later compare these to actual disc photographs. Stereo disc photographs should be obtained on all glaucoma patients, especially as a baseline, if at all feasible. Although there are artifacts if a true stereo image is not photographed, the newer cameras can perform this adequately (7). Regardless, a photograph, even if nonstereo, is the most objective way to obtain this "snapshot" of the optic nerve **at one point in time**.

It is still another matter to detect a **change** in appearance of the optic nerve. Direct meticulous comparison by the clinician of two photographs performed on the same camera at different points in time, or comparison by clinical examination techniques of the current appearance with the previous baseline photograph are the best that we can currently do. And, it is difficult with our subjective evaluation of such objective data to be sure of progression. We thus currently have gross methods to try to accurately assess progressive axonal death. Although computer image analysis techniques provide hope for the future, at the present time these methods are inferior to the clinician's (subjective) analysis.

What of visual fields? Although great strides have been made in the reproducibility of data with modern automated perimeter machines, these still remain subjective tests that depend on a patient pressing a button in response to a stimulus. These are subjective data. The system cries out for objective measurements. An objective visual field, perhaps made by recording an optic nerve response to a light stimulus placed on the retina, would yield more accurate and more sensitive data.

OUR BASIS OF UNDERSTANDING OF GLAUCOMA

What of glaucoma science? When one looks at all the wonderful progress in the understanding of diseases in general on a cellular and molecular level, it is humbling to see how little true progress has been made in glaucoma. Investigators do not even agree on what should be studied. There are many problems; it is a small scientific field that is fragmented both as to the areas of study (trabecular meshwork (TM), ciliary body, or optic nerve) and what to study. The tissues involved are difficult to study experimentally either because of their size or complexity. **There is no true animal model of the disease**. The clinical debate in glaucoma between an "IOP disease" **or** an "optic neuropathy" (rather than involvement of **both**) has added to the confusion.

A Concept

In the glaucoma field "the questions remain the same, but the answers keep on changing." One cannot be dogmatic, especially with so little real data. But at our current level of understanding one of us (DLE) would frame the chronic glaucomas this way:

> In almost all cases an abnormality in drainage of aqueous humor through the outflow pathway tissue, potentially at many sites in the trabecular meshwork, that leads to elevation of IOP and causes damage to the optic nerve end organ, which demonstrates varying susceptibility to different levels of IOP (including statistically "normal' IOP). The two main scientific questions are: (1) in the open angle glaucomas what is the cause of obstruction to trabecular outflow and how can this **trabecular glaucoma** be best treated?; (2) what is the cause of the optic nerve damage and especially its varying **susceptibility** (a feature which can appropriately be termed an "optic neuropathy"), and are there any specific remedies for the optic nerve beyond consistently lowering the IOP? **Both** of these questions are very important. These two schools of scientific inquiry should be complementary rather than competitive.

Clinical Implications of These Basic Concepts

For the student of glaucoma framing these concepts this way is not an academic exercise. **It does have clinical relevance**. One should strive to understand **why the IOP is elevated** (why there is the obstruction to outflow), especially on comparative examinations, and **why is the optic nerve cupping** occurring at a specific IOP?

Elevated IOP is due to impaired drainage through the TM and probably never due to above normal aqueous humor formation. When one does gonioscopy, one is looking at the diseased tissue involved in the hydrodynamic component of glaucoma. If one only understood what was going on in the tissue that one was looking at, much advancement might be possible. And although for POAG, one can detect nothing unusual in the open angle, a "sleuth-like" style in glaucoma sometimes does provide insight. Are there occult inflammatory precipitates?; Exfoliation material? Abnormal vessels? Partial angle closure? When a patient with "open angle glaucoma" returns for follow-up and an even higher IOP is measured, one should approach the problem from the "point-of-view" of the trabecular meshwork and always through repeat gonioscopy, strive to answer why is the IOP now further elevated.

This tissue-oriented approach may also help conceptually in understanding certain clinical phenomena. For example, the term "steroid responder" (Chapter 44) refers to a steroid-induced **decrease** in facility of aqueous humor drainage by the TM. It may indicate "latent POAG." In acute uveitides, when steroids are used and there is prompt subsequent elevation of IOP, this most often is **not** due to a steroid-induced **further** decrease in TM function (which is impaired due to inflammation in the TM), but rather due to the steroid **restoring** aqueous humor formation back towards normal, by suppressing inflammation in the ciliary body. Trabecular meshwork function may not, in fact, have worsened from the steroid; therefore, from a clinical point-of-view, the patient should not be labeled as a "steroid responder." In fact, steroids may not need to be discontinued, and continued steroid therapy might actually improve the impairment in TM function caused by the inflammation (Chapter 42). Similarly, by trying to explain a late onset IOP elevation after penetrating keratoplasty (Chapter 37) from the "point-of-view" of the TM, a diagnosis of steroid induced secondary open angle glaucoma may be identified that was not at first appreciated. (It is surprising how often this diagnosis is not correctly made because of the usual very low dosage of topical steroids which, however, have a cumulative effect).

There is also clearly more to optic nerve cupping than IOP alone. What are the factors that contribute to this varying susceptibility? Are they local or systemic?

Could certain systemic medications prescribed for non-ophthalmologic purposes increase the susceptibility of the optic nerve to glaucomatous cupping? When one looks at the optic nerve of a patient who is progressing despite reasonable IOP, one should step back, take a look at the whole patient, and consider whether there are any systemic or other local influences. At the present time, we really do not have such understanding, but one of us (DLE) predicts that when we eventually do, it will have originated with a clinical observation by an ophthalmologist, who was attempting to answer these questions. (For example, if there truly is increased susceptibility to optic nerve cupping in exfoliation syndrome (Chapter 20) and in systemic amyloidosis (Chapter 48), then such a clinical observation might represent this type of important clinical insight.)

The latter possibility is what makes clinical glaucoma so exciting and often so satisfying. It is a real clinical disease, where clinicians can make meaningful observations, that even in this new high-tech era can be original and unique. There is room for tremendous advancement in understanding, starting with clinical observation, especially as methods of examination will hopefully improve in the future years. These new clinical observations and unique insights can lead to specific new hypotheses that can be tested by both clinical and laboratory investigation. Medical doctors can be both clinicians and scientists in the discipline of glaucoma and, in the end, make a difference to patients with this treacherous, chronic progressive disease.

Glaucoma is a wonderful field for the young ophthalmologist to enter. It is both an intellectual and a practical clinical challenge. We are on the threshold of much new knowledge and change, with bright new talent and evolving science that can finally bring new methods of cellular and molecular inquiry to the discipline.

In some ways then, the glaucoma field today is both the "worst" and "best" of times.

GOAL OF THIS BOOK

The goal of this book is to provide practical clinical information about the management of all patients with glaucoma. We have tried to frame the current understanding in such a way as to stimulate the reader and the editors to ask, why is this glaucoma occurrence happening in this patient, and how might I be able to treat this better.

References

1. Epstein DL, Krug Jr JH, Hertzmark E, et al: A long-term clinical trial of timolol therapy versus no treatment in the management of glaucoma suspects. Ophthalmology 1989;96:1460–1467.
2. Hollows FC, Graham PA: Intra-ocular pressure glaucoma and glaucoma suspects in a defined population. Br J Ophthalmol 1966;50:570–586.
3. Bengtsson B: The prevalence of glaucoma. Br J Ophthalmol 1981;65: 46–49.
4. Dielemans I, Vingerling JR, Wolfs RCW, et al: The prevalence of primary open angle glaucoma in a population-based study in the Netherlands. Ophthalmology 1994;101:1851–1855.
5. American Academy of Ophthalmology Quality of Care Committee Glaucoma Panel. Preferred Practice Patterns: Primary Open Angle Glaucoma. San Francisco: The Academy, 1992.
6. Sommer A, Tielsch JM, Katz J, et al: Relationship between intraocular pressure and prmary oen angle glaucoma among white and black Americans: the Baltimore Eye Survey. Arch Ophthalmol 1991;109:1090–1095.
7. Greenfield DS, Zacharia PT, Schuman JS: Comparison of Nidek 3DX vs. Donaldson simultaneous stereoscopic disc photography. Am J Ophthalmol 1993;116:741–747.

Anatomy

2

E. Michael Van Buskirk

The human ocular globe is bound by three concentric, virtually spherical, layers or coats: the outer fibrous layer, the cornea and sclera; the middle vascular layer, the uveal tract; and the inner neurosensory layer, the retina. The interior of the globe is divided into three compartments: the anterior chamber between iris and cornea, the posterior chamber between lens and posterior iris, and the vitreous cavity, posterior to the lens, comprising most of the ocular volume. The aqueous humor is contained by the posterior chamber and the anterior chamber and has a volume about 200 microliters (1). Aqueous humor flows from the ciliary processes at about 2–2.5 microliters per minute (1).

The uveal tract attaches to the sclera at three sites; the optic nerve, the vortex veins, and the chamber angle. This latter consists of an inward roll of collagenous tissue, the scleral spur, which serves as the partial insertion of the ciliary muscle fibers, which are important for maintenance of aqueous humor outflow and accommodation. These attachments can become clinically relevant especially after blunt trauma when shear forces between the ocular layers tear the ciliary muscle and uvea away from the scleral spur leading to cyclodialysis, iridodialysis, or angle recession and secondary glaucoma.

AQUEOUS HUMOR OUTFLOW PATHWAYS

Aqueous humor leaves the eye primarily through the so-called conventional outflow pathways—the trabecular meshwork, Schlemm's canal, the aqueous humor collector channels, and the aqueous veins, to the episcleral veins, orbital veins, and the intracranial cavernous venous sinus. A substantial portion, up to 10% in the normal human eye, leaves by means of the uveoscleral outflow pathways, through the anterior chamber angle, the anterior extreme of the ciliary muscle, the posterior uvea, the suprachoroidal space, the sclera (perhaps along perforations for veins and nerves), and into the orbital tissues (2,3). Under normal circumstances, uveoscleral outflow probably is of little physiologic or clinical significance in the human eye, but can become important in some clinical situations. In contrast to conventional outflow, which is dependent upon the intraocular pressure, uveoscleral outflow is relatively pressure independent. It is enhanced by certain prostaglandins and can become significant in the inflamed eye possibly contributing to the low intraocular pressure sometimes seen in uveitis. In addition, new pharmacologic prostaglandin compounds, administered topically, appear to stimulate uveoscleral outflow and reduce intraocular pressure in glaucomatous eyes, even in those typically resistant to outflow stimulating drugs such as cholinergic cyclotonic agents. In addition, some absorption takes place through the iris, but it is not physiologically or clinically significant.

CONVENTIONAL AQUEOUS HUMOR OUTFLOW PATHWAYS

A thorough understanding of the anatomy of the anterior chamber angle is essential for any clinician treating glaucoma as well as for scientists investigating this tiny but complex region. The precise proportions and relations of the various structures of the chamber angle are dependent on anatomic characteristics such as size of the globe, the refractive error, the size and position of the lens, and on physiologic factors associated with aqueous secretion, accommodative tone, venous pressure, and postural position. The peripheral iris, or iris root, blends with the anterior and medial fibers of the ciliary muscle to form the apex of the anterior chamber angle, posterior to the true trabecular meshwork and scleral spur (Fig. 2.1). The ciliary muscle fibers then pass anteriorly to insert into scleral spur and trabecular meshwork to complete the angle. **Thus, the anterior chamber angle typically subtends about 30°** with the iris making one arm, the scleral spur, trabecular meshwork, and cornea comprising the other. The iris plane may vary from flat to slightly concave or convex, but typically is convex, with a smooth transition from the mid iris to the angle apex.

THE TRABECULAR MESHWORK

The trabecular meshwork lies in the corneoscleral arm of the chamber angle, just anterior to the angle apex. It extends between the scleral spur posteriorly and the peripheral cornea or Schwalbe's line anteriorly. Functionally, the scleral spur, ciliary muscle, trabecular meshwork, and Schlemm's canal work as a single unit to comprise the conventional aqueous outflow pathways. The trabecular meshwork in cross section is triangular in shape, its apex at the corneal periphery, suspended, in effect, from the peripheral extreme of Decemet's membrane, the line of Schwalbe. The base of the triangular mesh is then formed by the scleral spur and the inner fibers of the ciliary muscle.

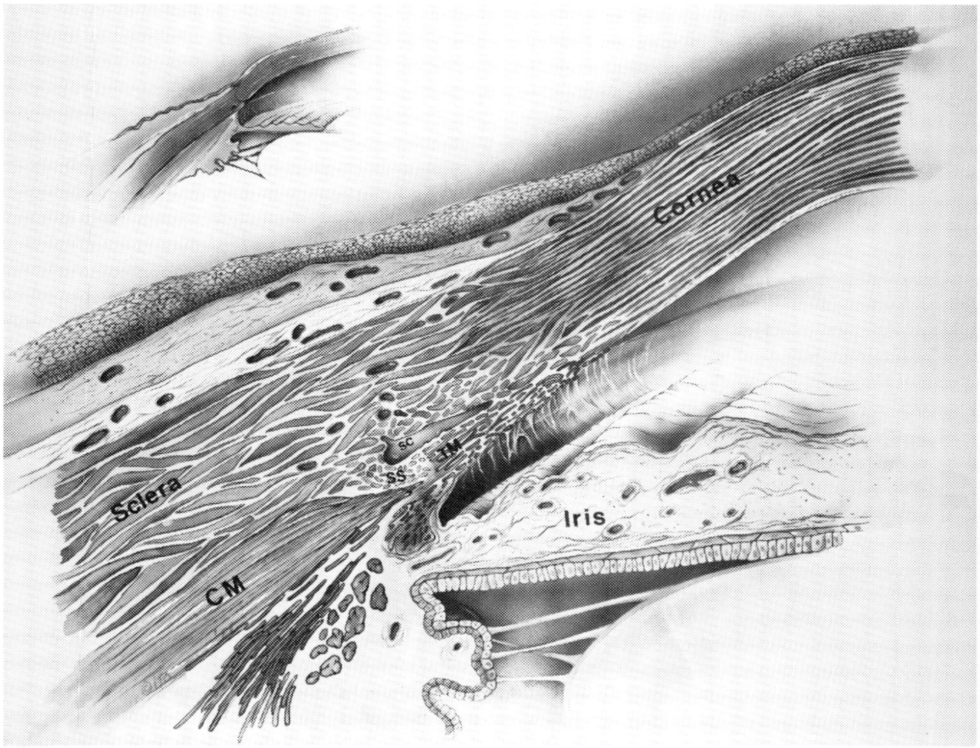

Figure 2.1. Drawing of the anterior chamber angle, bounded superiorly by the cornea, inferiorly by the iris with the trabecular meshwork (TM), scleral spur (SS) and ciliary muscle (CM) at the apex. Schlemm's canal (SC) lies within the apex of the angle, just external to the trabecular meshwork, its inner wall contiguous with the outer wall of the meshwork. From the anatomy of the limbus. Eye 1989;3:101–108.

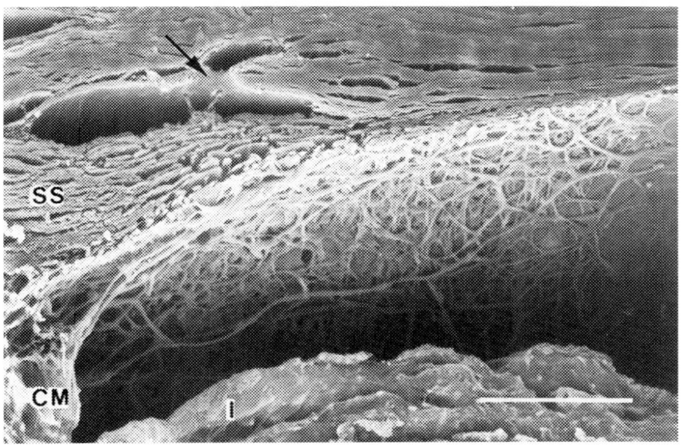

Figure 2.2. Scanning electron micrograph of the trabecular meshwork and Schlemm's canal showing the inner uveal meshwork surface, the central lamellar corneo-scleral meshwork, and the outer, juxtacanalicular meshwork adjacent to the inner wall of Schlemm's canal. Aqueous humor collector channels drain the outer wall (Arrow) to the aqueous and episcleral veins. From Van Buskirk EM. Clinical atlas of glaucoma. Philadelphia: WB Saunders, 1986:7.

The inner wall of the meshwork faces the anterior chamber and the outer, comprises the inner wall of the canal of Schlemm.

The trabecular meshwork may be divided into three histologically identifiable components: the most inner aspect, the uveal meshwork; the central component, the corneo-scleral meshwork; and the outer aspect, the juxtacanalicular tissue-inner wall of Schlemm's canal (Figs. 2.1, 2.2). Outgoing aqueous humor passes through each element sequentially, from the uveal meshwork, through the corneoscleral meshwork and then the juxtacanalicular tissue to enter the canal of Schlemm.

The uveal meshwork is perhaps most variable from eye to eye and hence, most difficult to define. During fetal development an intact tissue layer extends from cornea over the angle to the iris surface. During the final trimester this layer undergoes a dissolution process as the remainder of the trabecular meshwork matures to accommodate aqueous outflow (4). The **uveal meshwork** contains large spaces between tissue lamellae and, thus, typically contributes little if any significant resistance to aqueous humor outflow. When the **iridocorneal fetal tissue layer** fails to undergo normal developmental dissolution in the final gestational trimester, this tissue, anomalous uveal meshwork, can block aqueous humor outflow leading to so-called **primary congenital glaucoma**. Such membranes can be incised surgically to restore physiologic aqueous outflow. In other unusual circumstances such persistent tissue layers apparently are sufficiently permeable to permit adequate intraocular pressure in early childhood but become clinically significant in adolescence with a visible uveal tissue layer covering the normal trabecular meshwork. The remaining uveal tissue remnants become the uveal meshwork, and typically consist of strands of uveal tissue from peripheral iris to the mid or anterior corneoscleral meshwork. These are sometimes called **iris processes,** may contain melanin, and can be variably pigmented. In some cases uveal meshwork strands extend all the way to Schwalbe's line. Prominent uveal meshwork with iris processes are not particularly associated with glaucoma but are sometimes seen with various forms of congenital glaucoma. In other subjects, the uveal meshwork has a diaphanous membranous quality. Usually, the uveal meshwork does not form a significant component to aqueous humor outflow resistance, but, when substantial, probably can contribute, for example in some congenital or juvenile onset glaucomas.

The bulk of the trabecular meshwork consists of the corneo-scleral portion. This consists of about 10 to 15 perforated collagenous sheets, or layers, suspended between Schwalbe's line or the peripheral cornea anteriorly and ciliary muscle or scleral spur posteriorly. The outer layers arise directly from scleral spur, but the inner layers directly arise from the insertions of the inner fibers of the ciliary muscle. Each lamella consists of a central collagen "core," overlain by basement membrane, and endothelial type trabecular cells and a complex extracellular macromolecular interstitium. Trabecular cells form a variably intact monolayer to line the interstices of the meshwork. They are multipotential cells with great phagocytic and migratory capabilities in response to physiologic, pathologic, and injurious stimuli (5). The trabecular cells gradually diminish in density throughout life (6). This trabecular depopulation is accelerated in primary open angle glaucoma (6). Stimulation of the trabeculum with some forms of mild injury, such as laser trabeculoplasty, appear (5) to enhance trabecular cell division and migration, temporarily repopulating the tissue with newly formed cells (7,8). The relative mechanical tension of the ciliary muscle fibers on the corneo-scleral lamella plays a major role in modulating resistance to aqueous humor outflow but the exact mechanism of this modulation is not well understood. The insertion of the longitudinal ciliary muscle fibers into the scleral spur and corneoscleral sheets is vital for maintenance and modulation of aqueous humor outflow. Shearing forces associated with the global distortion during blunt ocular trauma can disrupt the ciliary muscle insertion leading to collapse of the trabecular meshwork against the scleral wall, increased trabecular outflow resistance and severe glaucoma, known as **angle recession.** Because of the disinsertion of the ciliary muscle, conventional cyclotonic therapy with cholinergic stimulating agents like pilocarpine become ineffective with angle recession.

The juxtacanalicular tissue (or cribriform meshwork) comprises the most outer portion of the trabeculum and lies between the most outer corneo-scleral lamella and Schlemm's canal. This tissue is a more loosely organized, reticulated connective tissue comprised of variable amounts of collagen, proteoglycans, glycoproteins, and hyaluronic acid (9). It is hypocellular compared to the corneoscleral meshwork. The outer aspect of the juxtacanalicular tissue consists of the endothelial cells lining the inner wall of Schlemm's canal. These are joined by tight junctions but appear to be highly distendable forming giant vacuoles in response to a pressure gradient across the trabecular meshwork (Fig. 2.3) (10–13). The exact route by which aqueous humor passes from the interstices of the corneoscleral meshwork to the lumen of Schlemm's canal is unknown. Convincing arguments have been advanced that pores develop between or through endothelial cells (11,12). Some believe the formation and collapse of the giant vacuoles to be important to maintenance of aqueous humor outflow (10,13). In the juxtacanalicular tissue, the outflowing aqueous humor directly encounters an extracellular tissue barrier through which it must percolate without access to open spaces. Thus, anatomically, this tissue, with the inner wall endothelial lining of Schlemm's canal, appears to account for the principal component of aqueous humor outflow resistance, and experimental studies in monkeys and eyebank eyes confirms its primary importance (14). Moreover, accumulation in this juxtacanalicular tissue of extracellular material, appearing as "plaques" in electron microscopic sections, is associated with open angle glaucoma (15). **Thus, the precise site of resistance to outflow in the normal and glaucomatous eye is not completely understood, but the peripheral juxtacanalicular connective tissue and Schlemm's canal inner wall appear to be the most likely location.** Many of the

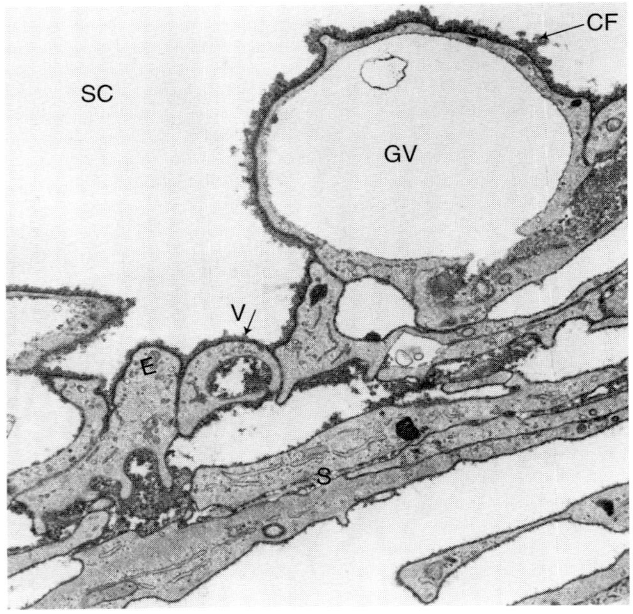

Figure 2.3. Inner wall of Schlemm's canal in a cynomolgus monkey after cationized ferritin perfusion at 15 mm Hg IOP (sagittal section, electron micrograph, original magnification x21,000). E = endothelial lining of Schlemm's canal (SC); CF = cationized ferritin labeling of cell membranes, GV = giant vacuole, V = vacuole filled with CF. From Epstein DL, Robert JW. Morphology of the trabecular meshwork and inner-wall endothelium after cationized ferritin perfusion in the monkey eye. Invest Ophthalmol Vis Sci 1991;32:160–171.

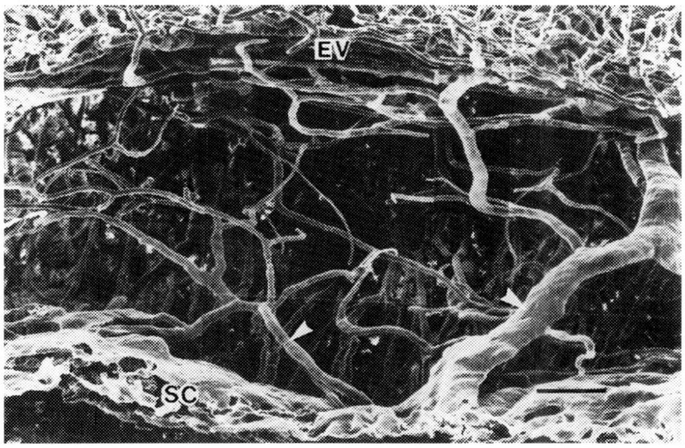

Figure 2.4. Methacrylate Luminal Casting of Schlemm's canal, showing draining collector channels (arrowheads) and the episcleral veins (EV). The limbal collagenous tissue has been digested away. From Van Buskirk EM. Clinical atlas of glaucoma. Philadelphia: WB Saunders, 1986:9.

pathophysiologic mechanisms cited, for example, cellular depopulation and plaque accumulation, also are associated with aging, but are accelerated and exaggerated in the glaucomatous eye.

Schlemm's canal is an endothelial lined aqueous conducting channel lying circumferentially parallel to, and contiguous with, the outer aspect of the trabecular meshwork; its inner wall endothelium comprises the outer lining of the juxtacanalicular tissue (Figs. 2.1, 2.2, and 2.4). The canal is oval in shape cross-sectionally, its posterior aspect determined by the scleral sulcus, lying within the scleral spur internally and posteriorly and with the scleral wall externally. Most of the inner aspect lies adjacent to the trabecular meshwork and anteriorly is bordered by the junction of the anterior meshwork and the cornea. Although the canal usually forms an intact circumferential channel, it is crossed by numerous septae from inner to outer wall, and branches to multiple lumens in some locations. The outer wall is perforated by about 30 to 35 collector channels whose endothelium is contiguous with that of intrascleral veins (Fig. 2.4). Although one can commonly observe retrograde flow of blood from these veins into the lumen of Schlemm's canal, in the adult eye most aqueous humor appears to travel radially across the lumen of the canal with little circumferential flow in the canal lumen (16).

CILIARY BODY ANATOMY

The ciliary body lies posterior to the iris and comprises the ciliary muscle and ciliary processes (Fig. 2.1). Both structures possess unique morphologic features that are essential to their specialized functions for accommodation, outflow facility regulation, and aqueous humor formation.

The ciliary muscle subtends a triangular cross-sectional profile with its apex pointing posteriorly, ending at the ora serrata. The outermost longitudinal fibers insert as tendinous bands into the corneoscleral trabecular meshwork and scleral spur, whereas the middle radial and inner circular fibers are only loosely adherent to the adjacent sclera via sparse collagen fibers. Ciliary muscle contraction decreases the resistance to outflow of aqueous humor, apparently through mechanical tension on the trabecular meshwork.

Lying internal to the ciliary muscle, the ciliary processes form the pars plicata, which, along with the more posterior pars plana, constitute the lateral wall of the posterior chamber (Fig. 2.1). Approximately 70 radially arrayed major ciliary processes project into the posterior chamber (Fig. 2.5). Their anterior borders arise from the iris root, sweeping behind the iris to form the ciliary sulcus (Fig. 2.1). These major processes measure approximately 2 mm long, 0.5 mm wide, and 1 mm high and possess an irregular surface. Smaller minor ciliary processes lie between the major processes and do not project as far into the posterior chamber.

In cross section, the major ciliary processes manifest three components (Fig. 2.6): an inner capillary core, a surrounding loose stroma, and a double-layered epithelium continuous with that of the pars plana. These components each possess unique morphologic features that underpin their contribution to aqueous humor formation, a two-stage process that begins with passive ultrafiltration of plasma from the capillaries into the stroma followed by movement through the ciliary epithelium into the posterior chamber. Because the aqueous humor derives from the ciliary processes, reduction of intraocular pressure can be accomplished by disturbing the ciliary body pharmacologically or surgically. Many drugs block aqueous humor inflow by interfering with the normal secretory process in the epithelium or by reducing arteriolar perfusion of regional

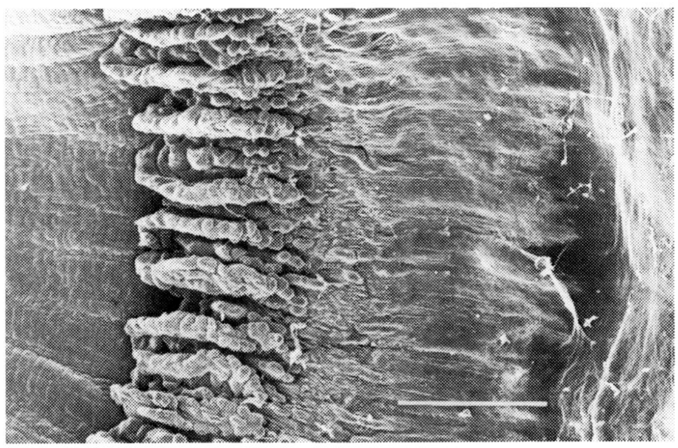

Figure 2.5. Scanning electron micrograph of the ciliary body showing the ciliary processes with alternate major process with the smaller minor processes between them. The posterior surface of the iris lies to the left side of the photograph, the pars plana of the ciliary body to the right. From Van Buskirk EM. Clinical atlas of glaucoma. Philadelphia: WB Saunders, 1986:5.

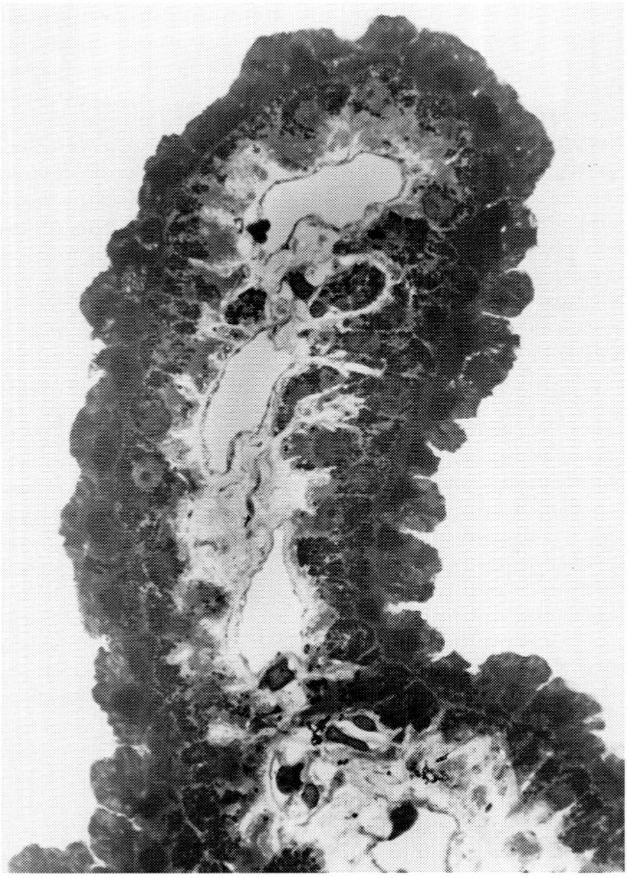

Figure 2.6. Cross sectional profile of the primate ciliary process showing the capillary core, stromal connective tissue and the bilayer ciliary epithelium. From Ritch R, Shields MB, Krupin T, eds. The glaucomas. St. Louis: CV Mosby, 1989:77.

ciliary processes. Most of the pharmacologic agents such as carbonic anhydrase inhibitors, beta adrenergic antagonists, or alpha-2 adrenergic agonists, appear in this manner to act directly on the ciliary epithelium. Some of the vasoactive adrenergic agents also can induce localized arteriolar constriction in the anterior ciliary processes (17).

Aqueous humor inflow can also be inhibited by destruction of some or all of the ciliary processes with cryotherapy or laser photocoagulation. The treating clinician must be aware of the anatomic location of the processes at the anterior portion of the ciliary body, about 1.5 to 2 mm posterior to the corneoscleral limbus, to achieve the most effective result with the least tissue destruction.

CILIARY BODY MICROVASCULATURE

The ciliary body receives blood from two sources: the anterior ciliary arteries and the long posterior ciliary arteries. Branches from all of these arteries anastomose freely with each other to produce a complex, redundant system characterized by numerous collateral channels that ensure consistent anterior segment perfusion even after partial interruption of its arterial supply, such as following strabismus and retinal detachment surgery (18). Derived from the ophthalmic artery, two anterior ciliary arteries approach the limbus from the border of each rectus muscle with the exception of the lateral rectus, which contributes only one. Within the episclera, these arteries commonly branch and then interconnect, often forming a nearly complete anastomotic vascular ring, which occasionally can be observed clinically.

At the limbus several branches from each anterior ciliary artery turn inward, perforating the limbal sclera to enter the capillary bed of the ciliary muscle. These branches arborize within the ciliary muscle and interconnect with each other and with branches from the nasal and temporal long posterior ciliary arteries (18). These interconnections form a second anastomotic vascular ring, the intramuscular circle, which represents the major source of collateral blood flow to the ciliary body between the anterior and long posterior ciliary arterial systems.

Branches from the intramuscular arterial circle supply capillaries to the ciliary muscle, which are densely packed and oriented parallel to the muscle fibers. Venous blood from the ciliary muscle drains primarily to the choroidal veins.

Other branches from the intramuscular circle pass anteriorly to the root of the iris, where they bend and branch at right angles to form the major arterial circle, which lies tangential to the limbus. The major arterial circle is often discontinuous and may constitute the only minor contributor to anterior segment collateral blood flow (Fig. 2.7).

The ciliary processes receive their arterial supply from two types of arterioles, anterior and posterior, that emanate from the major arterial circle (19). Anterior arterioles arise in tufts and often show focal constrictions as they span the ciliary sulcus (Fig. 2.8). As they enter the processes, they rapidly dilate into irregular, large, vein-like capillaries that initially are directed anteriorly toward the ciliary process tip. These capillaries then turn and pass posteriorly within the internal margin of the process to empty into the choroidal veins. The posterior arterioles, generally less numerous and less constricted than the anterior, enter the basal regions of the ciliary processes, apparently to serve the basal and posterior regions of the ciliary processes. These capillaries also travel in a posterior direction, concentric to those from the anterior arterioles. Thus capillaries derived from anterior arterioles serve the margins of the ciliary process and those arising more posteriorly are situated within the base of the process. Interprocess connections also arise from the posterior arterioles and serve the minor ciliary processes on either side and the basal regions of neighboring major processes.

THE CILIARY EPITHELIUM

The ciliary epithelium actively secretes some components of aqueous humor and provides the barrier that prevents

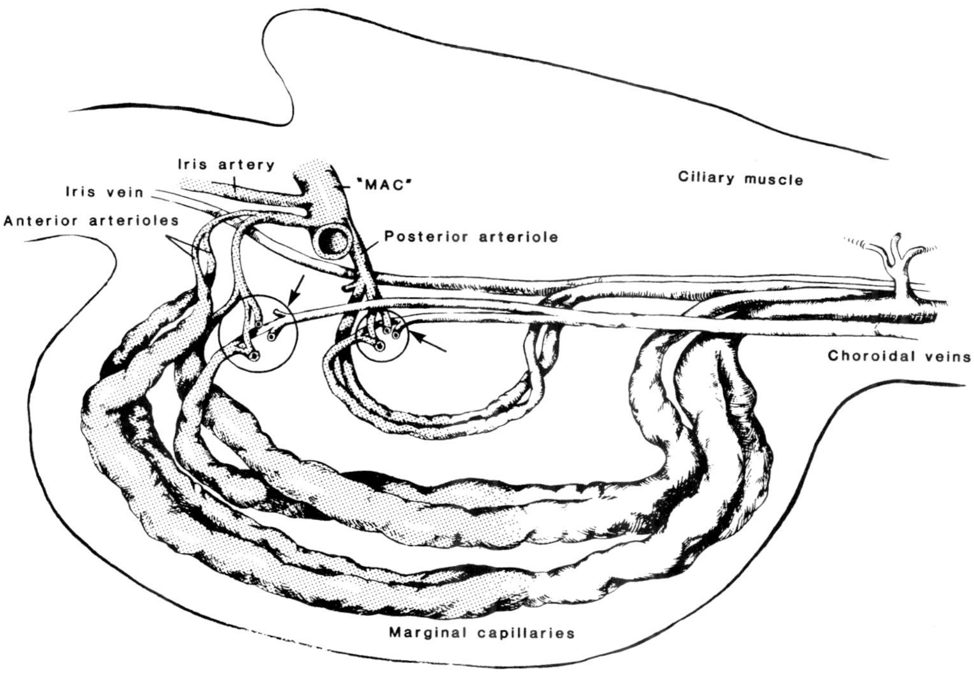

Figure 2.7. Schematic drawing of the vasculature of the major ciliary processes in profile showing the anterior and posterior arterioles arising from the discontinuous major arterial circle (MAC). From Morrison JC, Van Buskirk EM: Ciliary process microvasculature of the primate eye. Am J Ophthalmol 1984;97(3):381.

macromolecules from reaching the posterior chamber. The ciliary epithelium consists of two layers of cells, the outer pigmented and the inner nonpigmented, facing the posterior chamber. Despite its bilayered structure, the ciliary epithelium is not compound but consists of two simple epithelia joined apex to apex with the basal lamina of the pigmented layer resting on the stroma of the ciliary body and that of the nonpigmented layer lining the posterior chamber. This unusual arrangement results from invagination of the optic vesicle to form the optic cup during embryonic development.

The inner nonpigmented ciliary epithelium is continuous anteriorly with the pigment epithelium of the iris and posteriorly with the neurosensory retina at the ora serrata. The pigmented epithelium continues anteriorly as the anterior myoepithelium of the iris and posteriorly as the retinal pigment epithelium. The nonpigmented ciliary epithelial cells lack melanin and, compared with the cells of the pigmented epithelium, have more and larger mitochondria and rough endoplasmic reticulum, indicating a greater metabolic capacity. These features are amplified in the cells of the nonpigmented layer that lie in the anterior pars plicata whence derives the greater contribution overall to the production of aqueous humor (20).

Both the pigmented and nonpigmented epithelial cells are interconnected by specialized intercellular junctions that control the passage of water, ions and macromolecules into the aqueous humor (21,22). Desmosomes and gap junctions lie within and between both layers of the ciliary epithelium and the desmosomes appear to maintain adjacent cells, approximately 17 nm apart. The resulting intercellular cleft is spanned by branching filaments connecting

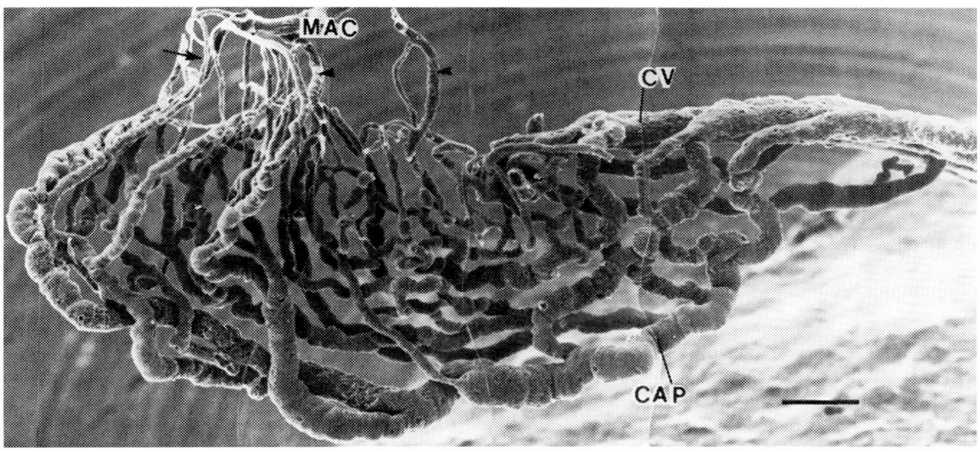

Figure 2.8. Scanning electron micrograph of a luminal methacrylate casting of the microvasculature of a single ciliary process in profile showing the anterior constricted arterioles (arrows) and posterior arterioles (arrowheads), the distended marginal capillaries (CAP), and the posterior choroidal veins (CV). From Morrison JC, Van Buskirk EM: Ciliary process microvasculature of the primate eye. Am J Ophthalmol 1984;97(3):374.

the cytoplasmic surfaces of the adjoining cells. Near their apical surfaces, nonpigmented ciliary epithelial cells are joined by zonulae occludens, or tight junctions, which constitute the **blood-aqueous barrier** of the ciliary body (15,20). Zonulae occludens appear as one or more areas of direct contact between intramembranous proteins of the adjacent plasma membranes, to block the intercellular spaces between adjacent plasma membranes, thus occluding the intercellular cleft.

The tight junctions located between the nonpigmented epithelial cells represent a selective barrier that allows diffusion of water and small molecules into the posterior chamber, while maintaining the osmotic and electrical gradients across the ciliary epithelium that are required for the final, active step in aqueous humor production. These junctions permit and modulate electrical and metabolic coupling of ciliary epithelial cells, permitting the two layers to operate as a functional unit for aqueous humor production.

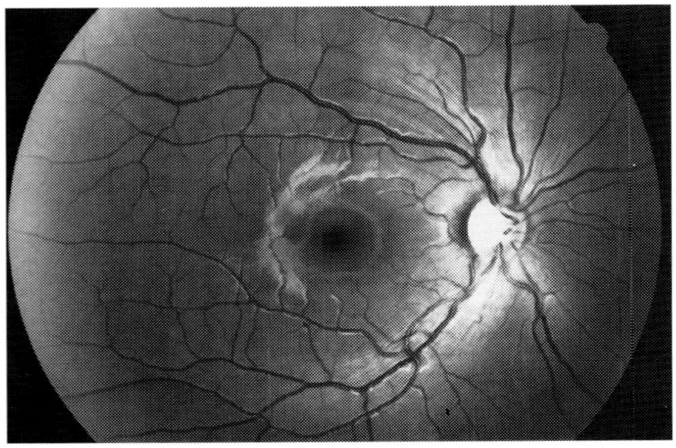

Figure 2.9. Photograph of the ocular fundus taken with red free light to accentuate the retinal nerve fiber layer, shown as prominent striations radiating from the optic disc. Slit-like defects in the nerve fiber layer are visible inferiorly emanating from the 11:30 o'clock position on the optic nerve head. From Van Buskirk EM: Clinical atlas of glaucoma. Philadelphia: WB Saunders, 1986:29.

THE OPTIC NERVE

The optic nerve transmits visual and other photopic stimuli between the neurosensory retina and the lateral geniculate body and the cerebral visual pathways. The nerve is primarily composed of neural fibers (the retinal ganglion cell axons), glial cells, extracellular matrix supportive tissue, and vascular elements (23–27). The optic nerve "head" refers to the anterior surface of the optic nerve which is seen "en face" during clinical funduscopic examination. When viewed stereoscopically in clinical examination, the nervehead assumes a bagel-like configuration, convex in the periphery, as the nerve fibers bend from the axis of the nerve to comprise the nerve fiber layer of the retina. This neural component manifests an orange-pink tint on funduscopy. Because the fibers so abruptly change direction, bending centrifugally, a central concavity, or optic nerve "cup" is created, the base of which appears more yellow because of the collagenous fibers of the lamina cribrosa underlying the supporting tissue. The central cupped zone typically occupies about 30% of the diameter of the nerve head but the proportions are highly dependent on the size of the eye and the diameter of the scleral canal. Glaucomatous eyes that lose nerve fiber tissue gradually develop progressively larger cup size until virtually no neural tissue persists in the final stages of the disease.

The neural component of the optic nerve is composed of approximately **1.2 to 1.5 million axons**. The intraorbital optic nerve is divided into the anterior and the posterior components. The anterior optic nerve extends from the retinal surface to the retrolaminar region just as the nerve exits the posterior aspect of the globe. The posterior optic nerve transits the orbit from the globe to the optic canal. The diameter of the optic nerve head and anterior portion of the optic nerve is approximately 1.5 mm (28). The optic nerve expands to approximately 3 to 4 mm in diameter upon exiting the globe, with the glial tissue, the leptomeninges (optic nerve sheath) and the beginning of the axonal myelination.

Retinal ganglion cell axons, comprised of retinal nerve fiber layers, converge radially to form the optic nerve as they abruptly turn posteriorly to exit the eye through the lamina cribrosa. The nerve fibers enter the optic nerve from the retina in a characteristic anatomic pattern (Fig. 2.9). Fibers entering the superior and inferior temporal aspects of the optic nerve arise from the peripheral temporal retina (29,30). These "arcuate" nerve fibers originate either superior to or inferior to the medial raphe of the temporal neurofiber layer, and assume an arcuate course around, above or below, the fovea. These are the fibers most susceptible to damage in early glaucomatous optic neuropathy. Careful well focused funduscopic examination of the posterior pole of the human eye will permit visualization of the striations of the retinal nerve fiber layer in the clinical situation, especially when the striations are enhanced by red free illumination. Loss of neural fibers as in glaucoma can also be seen clinically by the loss of striations in the affected location (Fig. 2.9). When sufficient fibers are lost from a specific location, **the clinician expects to correlate the location of visual field defects with the anatomic findings in the fundus**. Hence, loss of superior arcuate neural fibers leads to an inferior defect in the visual field, also subscribing an arcuate pattern corresponding to the zone of reduced retinal function. Since the arcuate neural fibers terminate along an anatomically defined raphe in the temporal retina, such arcuate visual field defects also respect the anatomy and produce a nasal stepped defect ending along the horizonal axis. Fibers originating from the macular region, or the "papillomacular fibers," occupy approximately ⅓ of the temporal optic nerve head. Papillomacular fibers take a more direct course from the macular and perimacular region to the optic nerve. Other nerve fibers from the superior, inferior and nasal retina radially converge at the nerve as shown in the figure.

The anterior optic nerve conveniently divides into four anatomic regions (Fig. 2.10) (26,31,32). The most anterior zone is the superficial nerve fiber layer region which is continuous with the nerve fiber layer of the retina. This region is primarily composed of the axons of the retinal ganglion cells in transition from the superficial retina to the neuronal component of the optic nerve. Immediately posterior to the nerve fiber layer is the pre-laminar region, which lies contiguous with the peripapillary choroid. Next posteriorly, the laminar region is adjacent to the sclera, where the axons pass out of the eye through the lamina cribrosa. This complex, collagenous, relatively elastic structure consists of fenestrated, connective tissue lamellae which allow the transit of neural fibers through the scleral coat (Fig. 2.11) (23,26,31,32). The lamina cribrosa is composed of a series of fenestrated sheets of connective tissue and provides the main support for the optic nerve as it exits the eye and penetrates the scleral coat. Between the optic nerve and the adjacent peripapillary tissue lies a rim of connective tissue, the border tissue of Elschnig (33). The connective tissue beams of the lamina cribrosa extend from this surrounding connective tissue border and are arranged in a series of parallel stacked plates. The beams of connective tissue are composed primarily of collagen and other extracellular matrix components, including elastin, laminin, and fibronectin. These connective tissue layers are perforated by various size fenestrations through which the neural elements of the optic nerve pass. Central, larger fenestrae allow transit of the central retinal artery and central retinal vein. **The neural fenestrations within the lamina are, histologically, larger superiorly and inferiorly as compared to the temporal and nasal aspects of the optic nerve.** These differences have been suggested to play a role in the development of glaucomatous optic neuropathy. Alteration of the shape of the optic nerve head, enlargement of the physiologic cup both peripherally and posteriorly, most characterizes the neuropathy of glaucoma. Thus, not only is neural tissue lost, but also the connective tissue becomes distorted with posterior bowing of the lamina. Whether this shape change causes or derives from the glaucomatous damage is uncertain, but clearly, alterations in the connective tissue in this region seems a likely contributor to the pathophysiology of this unique neuropathy (31). The fenestrations of the lamina cribrosa can be seen clinically in the base of the optic nerve head cup on ophthalmoscopic examination. The retro-laminar region lies posterior to the lamina cribrosa, is marked by the beginning of axonal myelination, and is surrounded by the leptomeninges of the central nervous system.

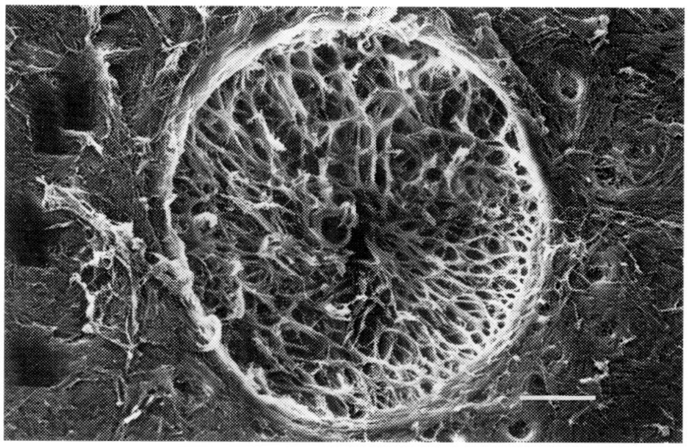

Figure 2.11. En face view of the lamina cribrosa of the human optic nerve prepared by trypsin digestion of the neural tissue leaving only the collagenous lamellae, showing the perforations to allow penetration of the nerve fiber bundles. From Van Buskirk EM: Clinical atlas of glaucoma. Philadelphia: WB Saunders, 1986:23.

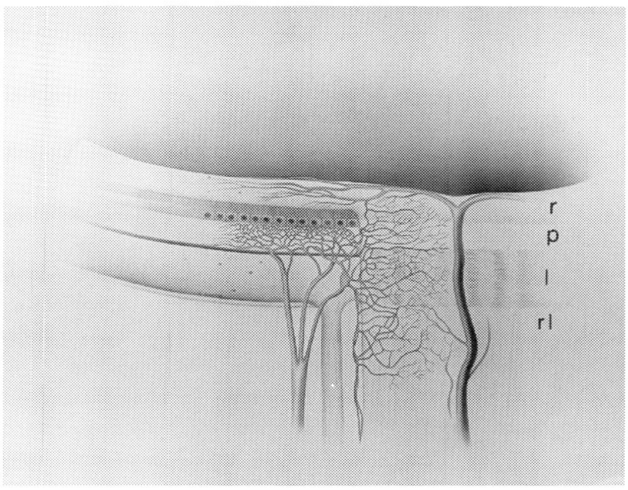

Figure 2.10. Schematic drawing of the anterior optic nerve head showing the arterial blood supply and the four anatomic layers, the retinal (r), prelaminar (p), laminar (l) (lamina cribrosa), and the retrolaminar (rl) zones. From Ritch R, Shields MB, Krupin T: The glaucomas, basic sciences. Volume I, 2nd ed. St. Louis: Mosby, 1996.

VASCULATURE OF THE OPTIC NERVE

The arterial supply of the anterior optic nerve derives entirely from branches of the ophthalmic artery. One to five posterior ciliary arteries divide in the posterior orbit from the ophthalmic artery, itself a branch of the internal carotid artery (26,27,34,35). Typically, between two and four posterior ciliary arteries course anteriorly before dividing into approximately ten to twenty short posterior ciliary arteries, just prior to entering the globe posteriorly. Often, the posterior ciliary arteries separate into a medial and a lateral group before branching into the short posterior ciliary arteries. In addition, the long posterior ciliary arteries, which are also branches of the posterior ciliary arteries, course anteriorly along the outside of the globe before penetrating

PERIPAPILLARY ATROPHY

Joel S. Schuman

A significant controversy exists with regard to peripapillary atrophy and its relationship to glaucomatous optic neuropathy. These atrophic areas, which often take the form of crescents, sometimes correlate with areas of nerve fiber layer atrophy and cupping, as well as with visual field loss (1–4). Peripapillary atrophy may progress, and may precede the development of cupping and visual field loss in a given region (5).

Peripapillary atrophy may be related to impaired optic nerve or choroidal circulation, and this has spurred speculation with regard to the relationship between this phenomenon and damage to the optic nerve (2,3,6). Should vascular factors play a significant role in glaucomatous optic neuropathy, as well as in the development of peripapillary atrophy, regions of peripapillary atrophy could be used as predictors of future optic nerve damage.

References

1. Wilensky JT, Kolker AE: Peripapillary changes in glaucoma. Am J Ophthalmol 1976;81:341.
2. Anderson DR: Correlation of the peripapillary anatomy with the disc damage and field abnormalities in glaucoma. In: Greve EL, Heijl A, eds. Fifth international visual field symposium. The Netherlands: Dr. W Junk Publishers, 1983.
3. Anderson DR: Relationship of peripapillary haloes and crescents to glaucomatous cupping. In: Krieglstein GK, ed. Glaucoma update III. Berlin: Springer-Verlag, 1987.
4. Heijl A, Samander C: Peripapillary atrophy and glaucomatous visual field defects. In: Greve EL, Heijl A, editors. Sixth international visual field symposium. The Netherlands: Dr. W Junk Publishers, 1985.
5. Airaksinen PJ, et al: Change of peripapillary atrophy in glaucoma. In: Krieglstein GK, ed. Glaucoma update III. Berlin: Springer-Verlag, 1987.
6. Airaksinen PJ, Tuulonen A, Werner EB: Clinical evaluation of the optic disc and retinal nerve fiber layer. In: Ritch R, Shields MB, Krupin T, eds. The glaucomas. St Louis: CV Mosby Co., 1989: 467–494.

the sclera to supply the iris, ciliary body and the anterior region of the choroid.

The short posterior ciliary arteries penetrate the sclera surrounding the optic nerve to supply the peripapillary choroid and the majority of anterior optic nerve. Some short posterior ciliary arteries course, without branching, through the sclera directly into the choroid; others divide within the sclera to provide branches to both the choroid and the optic nerve. Often a noncontinuous, arterial circle exists within the perineural sclera, known as the circle of Zinn-Haller (36). This structure is formed by the confluence of branches of the short posterior ciliary arteries. This arterial circle may completely encircle the optic nerve, and often is, or may be interrupted along its course. Multiple branches from this arterial circle penetrate the various regions of the anterior optic nerve, to the peripapillary choroid, and to the pial arterial system. The central retinal artery, also a posterior orbital branch of the ophthalmic artery, penetrates the optic nerve approximately 10 to 15 mm behind the globe, but has few if any intraneural branches the exception being an occasional small branch within the retro-laminar region.

MICROVASCULATURE OF SPECIFIC OPTIC NEURAL REGIONS

The superficial nerve fiber layer is supplied principally by recurrent retinal arterioles branching from the central retinal artery. As the central retinal artery emerges from within the optic nerve, it branches into a superior and an inferior trunk. From these major trunks, as well as from more distal branches, small arterioles emerge to supply the superficial nerve fiber layer of the optic nerve and peripapillary retina (Figs. 2.12, 2.13, 2.14). The capillary branches from these vessels are continuous with the retinal capillaries at the disk margin, but they also have posterior anastomoses with the prelaminar capillaries of the optic nerve.

The prelaminar region is principally supplied by direct branches of the short posterior ciliary arteries and by branches of the circle of Zinn-Haller, when it is present (Figs. 2.12, 2.13). In eyes with a well developed circle of Zinn-Haller (Fig 2.12), fine arterial branches supply both the prelaminar and laminar regions. Most of these vessels do not arise from the choroid but merely pass through it from this short posterior ciliary arterial origin. Branches from the circle of Zinn-Haller and from the short posterior ciliary arteries course through the choroid and ultimately supply the optic nerve in this region. Occasional small centripetal arteries or arterioles do branch from the larger vessels of the peripapillary choroid, but direct arterial supply to the prelaminar region arising from the choroidal vasculature is minimal. No direct connection exists between the peripapillary choriocapillaris and the prelaminar region.

The lamina cribrosa region also receives its blood supply from branches of the short posterior ciliary arteries or from branches of the circle of Zinn-Haller and is similar to the prelaminar region (Figs. 2.12, 2.13, 2.14). These precapillary branches perforate the outer aspects of the lamina cri-

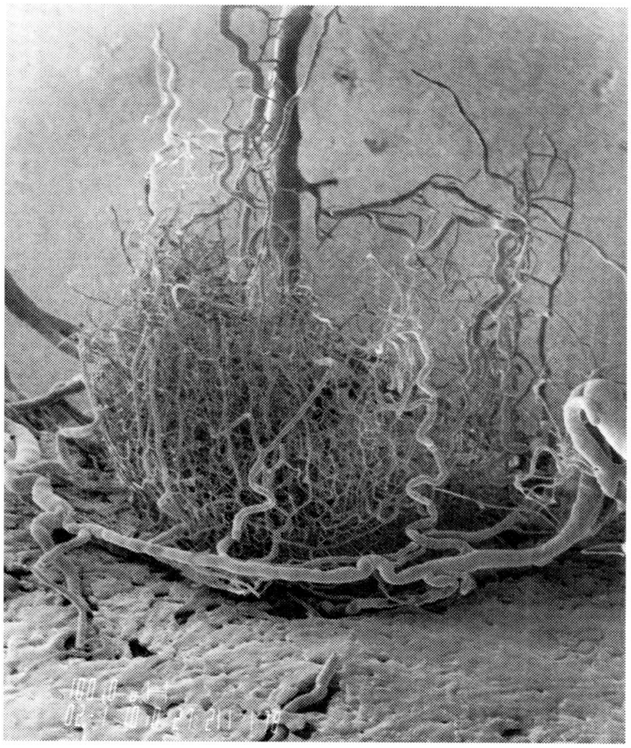

Figure 2.12. Scanning electron micrograph of a methacrylate luminal casting of the human eyebank optic nerve microvasculature showing the arterial circle of Zinn-Haller encircling the base of the optic nerve as it exits the globe. Arteriolar branches supply the anterior portions of the optic nervehead. The circle of Zinn-Haller is a terminal confluence of short posterior ciliary arteries and is variable in extent from being absent to quite prominent as in this photograph. From Onda E, George CA, Bacon DR, Van Buskirk EM: Microvasculature of the human optic nerve. Am J Ophthalmol 1995;120:95.

brosa before branching into an intra-septal capillary network. As in the prelaminar region, the larger vessels of the peripapillary choroid may contribute occasional small arterioles to this region, although there is no connection between the peripapillary choriocapillaris and the capillaries of the optic nerve.

The retro-laminar region is also supplied by branches from the short posterior ciliary arteries, but also by pial arterial branches (Fig. 2.14). The pial arteries originate from both the central retinal artery, before it pierces the retrobulbar optic nerve, and branches of the short posterior ciliary arteries more anteriorly.

Thus, with the exceptions of the superficial nerve fiber layer branches of the central retinal artery, the occasional retro-laminar branches of the central retinal artery, and the small contribution of the choroidal vasculature to the prelaminar and laminar regions, the principal arterial supply to the anterior optic nerve is derived from the short posterior ciliary arteries.

The rich capillary beds of each of the four anatomic regions within the anterior optic nerve are anatomically confluent. These capillary interconnections anatomically unite the microvasculature along the length of the anterior optic nerve, but appear to be such fine resistent capillaries that there is probably little physiologic confluence among them. Capillaries in the nerve fiber layer region are continuous with the retinal capillaries at the disk margin. More posteriorly, the capillaries of the nerve fiber layer region form a complicated plexus which interconnects with the capillaries of the pre-laminar regions. The capillaries of the laminar region conform to the pattern of the connective tissue septae which compose the laminar supportive architecture. Capillaries in the laminar region are organized in the polygonal pattern of the laminar septae.

The arterioles along the periphery of the optic nerve have a limited smooth muscle layer surrounding the endothelial layer. The capillary network of the anterior optic nerve is composed of non-fenestrated vessels, similar to the capillaries of the retina. These capillaries are comprised of a single layer of tight-junctioned endothelial cells surrounded by supportive glial tissue and intermittent pericytes.

The venous drainage of the anterior optic nerve is almost

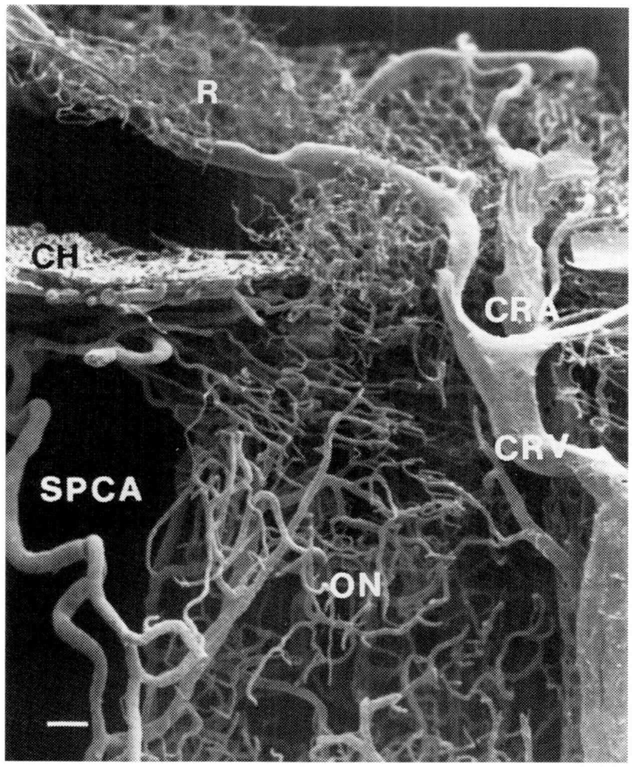

Figure 2.13. Scanning electron micrograph of a methacrylate luminal casting of the anterior optic nerve head of the cynomolgus monkey (similar to human), but in cross section showing the prelaminar, laminar and retrolaminar portions. R = retina, CRA = central retinal artery, CRV = central retinal vein, CH = choroid, SPCA = short posterior ciliary artery, ON = optic nerve. From George CA, Van Buskirk EM: Microvasculature of the anterior optic nerve. Surv Ophthalmol 1994;38S:S110.

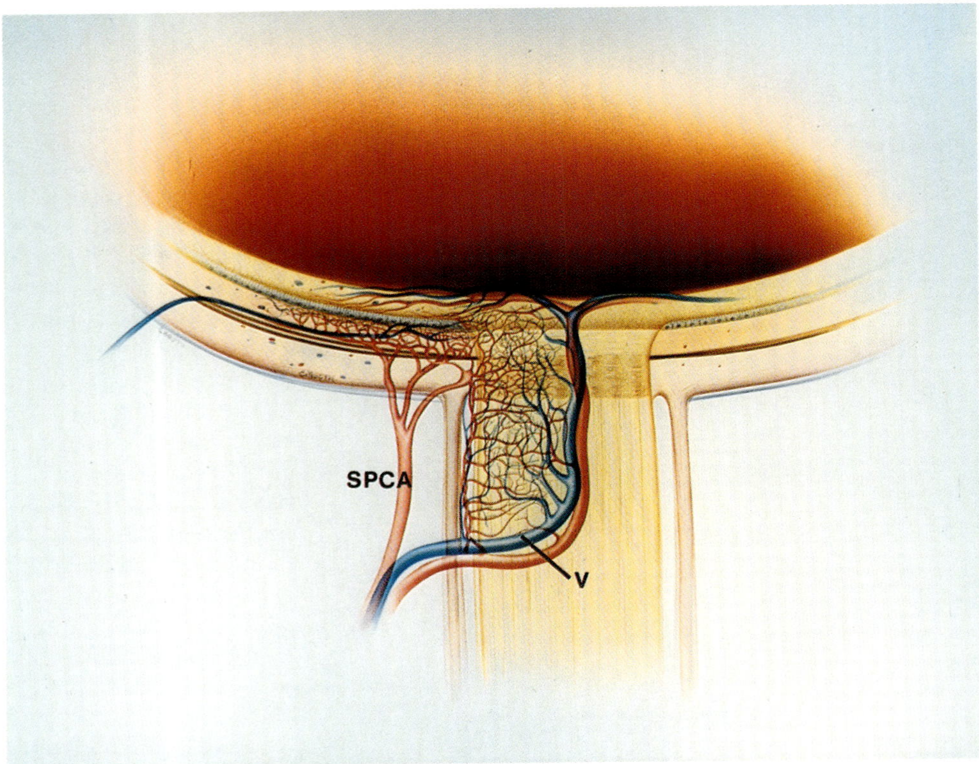

Figure 2.14. Schematic drawing of the microvasculature of the optic nerve head showing the arterial supply primarily derived from branches of the short posterior ciliary arteries (SPCA) and the venous drainage by way of the central retinal vein (V). From Cioff, GA, Van Buskirk EM: Glaucoma section. In: Wright K, ed. Ophthalmology: A comprehensive text. Baltimore: Williams & Wilkins. In press.

exclusively via the central retinal vein (Figs. 2.13, 2.14). In the nerve fiber layer, blood is drained directly into the retinal veins which then join to form the central retinal vein. In the pre-laminar, laminar and retro-laminar regions, venous drainage also occurs via the central retinal vein or axial tributaries to the central retinal vein. Occasionally, small venules connecting the optic nerve and the peripapillary choroid can be identified, mainly within the prelaminar region.

VARIABILITY OF VASCULAR PATTERNS

There is marked inter-individual variation in the precise vascular patterns of the anterior optic nerve and peripapillary region. Among individuals, the predominant variability is observed in the arterial supply. The posterior ciliary arteries vary in number, distribution, and caliber. These arteries may be distributed only medially and laterally, or a third superior grouping may be present (35,36,37,38,39). The grouping of these vessels into lateral and medial groups could play a role in the clinical presentations subsequent to an ischemic event. The distribution of the posterior ciliary arteries may explain the altitudinal visual field defects seen following anterior ischemic optic neuropathy, the nasal visual field loss seen in glaucoma, and the arcuate field loss seen in acute optic nerve infarction (40,41). These hypotheses rely heavily on physiologic inference from anatomic findings and thus remain unproven, if attractive, speculations.

References

1. Brubaker RF: The flow of aqueous humor in the human eye. Trans Am Oph Soc 1982;80:391–474.
2. Bill A, Phillips S: Uveoscleral drainage of aqueous humor in human eyes. Exp Eye Research 1971;12:275.
3. Pederson JE, Gaasterland DE, MacLellan HM: Uveoscleral aqueous outflow in the rhesus monkey: Importance of uveal reabsorption. Invest Ophthal Vis Sci 1977;16:1008–1017.
4. Van Buskirk EM: Clinical implications of iridocorneal angle development. Ophthalmology 1981;88:361–367.
5. Rohen JW, van der Zypen E: The phagocytic activity of the trabecular meshwork endothelium: An electron microscopic study of the verve (Cercopithesus aethiops). V Graefe's Arch Klin Exp Ophthalmol 1968; 175:143.
6. Alvarado J, Murphy C, Polansky J, Juster R: Trabecular meshwork cellularity in primary open-angle glaucoma and nonglaucomatous normals. Ophthalmology 1984;91:564.
7. Acott TS, Samples JR, Bradley JMB, et al: Trabecular repopulation following laser trabeculoplasty by anterior trabecular meshwork cells. Am J Ophthalmol. In Press.
8. Acott TS, Samples JR, Bradley BS, Bacon DR, et al: Trabecular repopulation by anterior trabecular meshwork cells after laser trabeculoplasty. Am J Ophthalmol 1989;107:1.
9. Acott, TS: Biochemistry of aqueous humor outflow. In: Textbook of Ophthalmology, Podos, Steven M and Yanoff, Myron (Editors) Volume 7 Glaucoma, Kaufmann, Paul I. and Mittag, TW (Associate Editors) Mosby, 1991.

10. Tripathi RC: The functional morphology of the outflow systems of the ocular and cerebrospinal fluids. Exp Eye Res 25 (suppl) 1977;65–116.
11. Bill A, Svedbergh B: Scanning electron microscopic studies of the trabecular meshwork and the canal of Schlemm. An attempt to localize the main resistance to outflow of aqueous humor in man. Act Ophthalmol 1972;50:295–320.
12. Epstein DL, Rohen JW: Morphology of the trabecular meshwork and inner wall endothelium after cationized ferritin perfusion in the monkey eye. Invest Ophthal Vis Sci 1991;32:160–171.
13. Fink AL, Feliz MD, Fletcher RC: Schlemm's canal and adjacent structures in glaucomatous patients. Am J Ophthalmol 1972;74:893–906.
14. Maepea O, Bill A: The pressure in the episcleral veins, Schlemm's canal and the trabecular meshwork in monkeys: Effects of changes in intraocular pressure. Exp Eye Res 1989;49:645–663.
15. Rohen, JW, Witmer, R: Electron microscope studies on the trabecular meshwork in glaucoma simplex. Graefes Arch Clin Exp Ophthalmol 1972;83:251–266.
16. Van Buskirk, EM: Trabeculotomy in the immature, enucleated human eye. Invest Ophthal Vis Sci 1977;16:63–66.
17. Van Buskirk EM, Bacon DR, Fahrenbach WH: Replication of ciliary vasomotor effects with controlled intravascular corrosion casting. Trans Am Ophthalmol Soc 1990;87:124–142.
18. Morrison JC, Van Buskirk EM: Anterior collateral circulation in the primate eye. Ophthalmology 1983;90:707.
19. Morrison JC, Van Buskirk EM: Ciliary process microvasculature of the primate eye. Am J Ophthalmol 1984;97:372.
20. Hara K, Lütjen-Drecoll E, Prestle H, Rohen JW: Structural differences between regions of the ciliary body in primates. Invest Ophthalmol Vis Sci 1977;16:912.
21. Raviola G: The structural basis of the blood-ocular barriers. Exp Eye Res (Suppl) 1977;25:27.
22. Raviola G, Raviola E: Intercellular junctions in the ciliary epithelium. Invest Ophthalmol Vis Sci 1978;17:958.
23. Hernandez MR, Lua XX, Igoe F, Neufeld AH: Extracellular matrix of the human lamina cribrosa. Am J Ophthalmol 1987;104:567.
24. Kronfeld PC: Normal variations of the optic disc as observed by conventional ophthalmoscopy and their anatomic correlations. Trans Am Acad Ophthalm Otol 1976;81:214.
25. Hayreh SS: Anatomy and physiology of the optic nerve head. Trans Am Acad Ophthal Otol 1974;78:240.
26. Anderson DR: Ultrastructure of human and monkey lamina cribrosa and optic nerve head. Arch Ophthal 1969;82:800.
27. Liebermann MF, Maumenee AE, Green WR: Histologic studies of the vasculature of the anterior optic nerve. Am J Ophthal 1976;82:405.
28. Jonas JB, Gusek GC, Guggenmoos-Holtzmann I, Naumann GOH: Size of the optic nerve scleral canal and comparison with intravitreal determination of optic disc dimensions. Graefe's Arch Ophthal 1988;226:213.
29. Radius RL, Anderson DR: The histology of retinal nerve fiber layer bundles and bundle defects. Arch Ophthal 1979;97:948.
30. Radius, RL, Anderson DR: The course of axons through the retina and optic nerve head. Arch Ophthal 1979;97:115.
31. Quigley HA, Addicks EM: Regional differences in the structure of the lamina cribrosa and their relation to glaucomatous optic nerve damage. Arch Ophthalmol 1981;99:137.
32. Radius RL, Gonzales M: Anatomy at the lamina cribrosa in human eyes. Arch Ophthalmol 1981;99:2159.
33. Elschnig A: Der normal Sehnerveneintritt des menschlichen Auges, Denkschriften der Mathematisch-Naturwissenschaftliche Classe der Kaiserlichen Akademie der Wissenschaften in Wien 1901;70:219–303.
34. Hayreh SS: Blood supply of the optic nerve head and its role in optic atrophy, glaucoma and oedema of the optic disc. Br J Ophthalmol 1969; 53:721.
35. Cioffi GA, Van Buskirk EM: Vasculature anatomy of the optic nerve. In: Ritch R, Shields MR, Krupin T, eds. The glaucomas. St. Louis: CV Mosby, 1994;8.
36. Zinn IGL. Descriptio Anatomica Ocuoli Humani. Ist ed. Gottingen. Abrami Vandenhoeck 216–217, 1755.
37. Hayreh SS: Inter-individual variation in blood supply of the optic nerve head. Its importance in various ischemic disorders of the nerve head, and glaucoma, low-tension glaucoma and allied disorders. Doc Ophthalmol 1985;59:217.
38. Hayreh SS: Anterior ischemic optic neuropathy. Arch Neurol 1981;38: 675.
39. Geijssen HC: Studies on normal pressure glaucoma. New York: Kugler, 1991:8–31.
40. Lichter PR, Henderson JW: Optic nerve infarction. Am J Ophthalmol 1978;85:302.
41. Olver JM, Spalton DJ, McCartney ACE: Microvascular study of the retrolaminar optic nerve in man; the possible significance in anterior ischemic optic neuropathy. Eye 1990;4:7.

Practical Aqueous Humor Dynamics

3

David L. Epstein

CLINICAL RELEVANCE

Aqueous Humor Formation

Aqueous humor is produced by the ciliary body and flows into the posterior chamber at a rate of approximately 2 to 3 microliters per minute (1). It is believed that at least a majority of this aqueous humor production derives from active secretion of the ciliary epithelium bilayer, which is in continuity posteriorly with the adjacent retinal and, anteriorly, iris epithelia (see Fig. 2.5). The outer (sclerad) pigmented ciliary epithelial cell layer lies apex to apex to the inner (vitread) nonpigmented ciliary epithelial cell layer (Chapter 2). The base of the latter cells faces the posterior chamber. (Exfoliation material may occur on the base of this cell layer.)

The stroma of the ciliary body (sclerad to the pigmented ciliary epithelium) contains numerous capillaries (see Fig. 2.6). Potentially both this blood supply area (see Fig. 2.8) as well as the secreting ciliary epithelia cells, themselves, may be sites of drug or laser obliterative actions. Although the nonpigmented ciliary epithelium has frequently been identified as containing the enzymatic machinery involved in active aqueous humor secretion (2–4), the actual process may require the coupling of both the nonpigmented and pigmented cell layers (5).

It is believed that bicarbonate is actively secreted into the posterior chamber by the ciliary epithelium, carrying water with it and thus representing part of the active secretion of aqueous humor (6). This is under the control of the enzyme, carbonic anhydrase, in the ciliary epithelium (presumably non-pigmented). Thus **carbonic anhydrase inhibitors** can reduce aqueous humor formation (up to 40 to 50%).

Beta-adrenergic agonist activity has been believed to be involved in active secretion of aqueous humor (1), such that beta blockade will result in a decrease in this secretion (Chapter 12). Many investigators have thought that the site of beta blocker activity is at the level of the ciliary epithelium, but a vascular site has not been totally ruled out. The effects of beta blockade and carbonic anhydrase inhibition are not fully additive, suggesting that there is some linkage and interrelated effects (7).

Apraclonidine, an **alpha-2 agonist**, reduces aqueous humor formation (8), and is also partially additive to both carbonic anhydrase inhibitors and beta blockers, but it is not certain whether the site of action is ciliary epithelial or vascular. (The vasoconstriction that the drug produces [Chapter 12] might suggest the latter.)

The part of aqueous humor formation that is not active transport has in previous times been called "ultrafiltration." However, whether this is a passive pressure driven process (presumably under vascular control) or some other ciliary epithelial cell process (for example, uncatalyzed hydration of CO_2) is unclear.

Aqueous humor moves from the ciliary epithelium into the posterior chamber, and then through the pupil into the anterior chamber (Fig. 3.1). Because there is usually some pupillary resistance to forward fluid flow (which is termed relative pupillary block), the pressure is slightly higher in the posterior chamber than the anterior chamber, resulting in forward iris convexity. In the extreme, this can cause the peripheral iris to move over the front of the trabecular meshwork and thus cause angle closure glaucoma (usually due to pupillary block) (Chapter 22). **Iris convexity or concavity is thus a useful indicator of relative pressures in the posterior and anterior chambers.** (See later discussions of iris concavity in pigmentary glaucoma (Chapter 21) and also various iris retraction syndromes where, for example, there is posterior movement of fluid out of the eye through a retinal hole.)

The amount of aqueous humor in the posterior chamber acts as a force (vector) to move the iris forward in a convex configuration. **Agents that decrease aqueous humor formation can by themselves act to decrease this iris convexity** (Chapter 22). These agents thus are effective in treating the process of angle closure glaucoma due to pupillary block (independent of the obvious IOP effect itself), but just as importantly, can lead to confusion in evaluating (usually asymptomatic) narrow angled eyes by lessening this posterior chamber vector and thereby deepening the angle.

The aqueous humor in the posterior chamber is likely in equilibrium with fluid in the vitreous cavity (Chapter 29). With retinal tears and detachments, the resulting hypotony most likely occurs because there is net fluid movement out of the eye through the retinal hole. The hyaloid is involved in this fluid exchange between vitreous and posterior chamber. In malignant glaucoma, fluid is retained in an expanded vitreous chamber, and it is commonly required to disrupt the hyaloid barrier (with a YAG laser or surgically), in order to restore the normal anatomy, and allow fluid exchange between the posterior and anterior segments (Chapter 29).

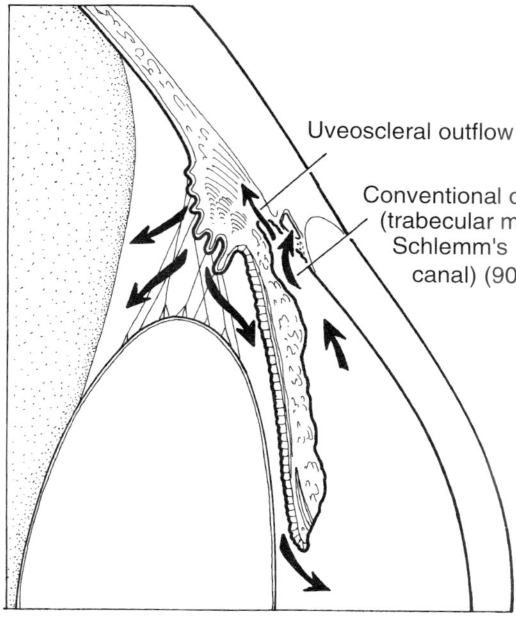

Figure 3.1. Aqueous humor is actively secreted by the ciliary epithelium into the posterior chamber, flows through the pupil into the anterior chamber and drains through the conventional and unconventional pathways.

Diurnal Variation of IOP

We know that there is a diurnal variation in IOP which is believed to be mostly or entirely due to changes in the rate of aqueous humor formation (1). Although the studies of Kronfeld suggested that there might be a small fluctuation in tonographic outflow facility as well (9,10), we believe that such possible changes are small and may be explained, at least in part, by the "noise" in the tonographic technique. There is also a small seasonal variation in IOP (11), but the mechanism behind this has not been determined. IOP tends to be higher in winter and lower in summer.

What causes the varying rate of aqueous humor production during the day has not been fully determined. It is most common for the highest IOP to occur in the morning, and, in fact, an IOP spike upon awakening is believed to occur commonly in primary open angle glaucoma (POAG). On the other hand, the literature describes many patients with other diurnal patterns, and there is much individual variation. The systemic catecholamine burst upon awakening might be implicated in the morning IOP elevation because beta-adrenergic agonists are believed to slightly stimulate aqueous humor formation (1) (Chapter 12) (and thus beta blockers interfere with this, and therefore act to diminish aqueous humor production), but this has not been unequivocally resolved. Although systemic cortisol levels have been proposed to relate to the diurnal variation of aqueous humor production, recent evidence does not support this (12).

The lowest IOP is believed to occur during sleep, again due to decreased aqueous humor formation (1,13). One might over-simplify this and conceptualize that the pumps in the ciliary body have similarly "gone to sleep."

Some investigators have proposed that patients with glaucoma can show elevated "spikes" of IOP at odd hours, including while asleep. One of the problems with these data is that it is possible that the act of performing these measurements, by waking people up to take their IOP, may not accurately reflect their "true" IOP steady state while asleep. There is a need for new noninvasive measurements of IOP during the course of a day or during several days in order to provide this important information. As discussed in Chapter 1, our IOP measurements, although extremely accurate, are only one "snapshot" in time, and the field of glaucoma would benefit from a "Holter monitor" equivalent for IOP measurements.

Another problem with such diurnal IOP data is that the common technique used to obtain it is to do a "diurnal curve;" that is, to have the patient come to the office (or worse, inpatient setting) for these measurements. It really has not been established that these measurements reflect the patient's "true" diurnal curve during the patient's normal "active" day's schedule. (The senior editor (DLE) rarely performs "diurnal curves"; instead uses tonography to gain an estimate of outflow function, with the expectation/assumption that with severe impairments of outflow, small variations in aqueous humor production which might normally be expected during the course of the day, should be reflected in larger fluctuation of IOP (to higher levels) (Table 3.1). On the other hand, the two associate editors frequently use office "diurnal curve" measurements.)

Conventional Outflow Pathway (Trabecular Meshwork-Schlemm's canal)

In humans, more than 90% of the aqueous humor fluid in the anterior chamber exits the eye via the trabecular meshwork—Schlemm's canal system (the conventional outflow pathway) (see Fig. 2.2) (14,15). Schlemm's canal communicates via a series of collector channels (see Fig. 2.4) with the aqueous veins, part of the venous system, which are apparent on the outside of the eye (aqueous veins are much less frequently observed in eyes with glaucoma than in normal eyes) (16). There is a resistance and a pressure decrease across the inner wall of Schlemm's canal (see Fig. 2.3) (either at or just proximal to the inner wall in the juxtacanalicular tissue) (17–21) such that the pressure in the trabecular meshwork (TM) just proximal to the canal (towards the anterior chamber (AC)) is higher than that in the canal. Thus at elevated IOP, the TM distends and the inner wall moves towards the outer wall of Schlemm's canal (22,23). The locus of abnormal resistance in POAG is believed to be at the same general location (juxtacanalicular-inner wall Schlemm's

AN INTERESTING QUESTION

David L. Epstein

An interesting question is as follows: If one wishes to use a topical beta blocker only once a day, and we assume, what is likely true, that the maximum effect of such therapy on aqueous humor production extends for less than a full 24 hours, what time of day should the solitary drop be administered? If what seems true for the vast majority of patients that aqueous humor production (and hence IOP) is diminished during sleep, it would seem logical to administer the beta blocker first thing in the morning (so that the less than maximal IOP effect would coincide with sleep). On the other hand, if one believes that the morning "spike" in IOP, which curiously in some studies lasts for less than 30 minutes, is the greatest risk for optic nerve damage, then one might do the opposite (assuming that the glaucoma patient is a morning IOP "spiker"). The data are not clear, but one of us (DLE) prefers to administer the once a day beta blocker therapy in the morning.

canal) (17) as a normal eye, but theoretically abnormal resistance in the various glaucomas can be added at any place along the aqueous humor outflow pathway.

Relation of Episcleral Venous Pressure to IOP

In conditions with elevated episcleral venous pressure (e.g., dural shunt or some cases of Sturge-Weber syndrome), this elevated venous pressure is transmitted back to Schlemm's canal and then into the anterior chamber (and therefore the whole eye) (Chapter 46). Although IOP is elevated, the resistance across the inner wall of Schlemm's canal may be unchanged, and tonographic outflow facility may thus be normal (in fact, normal outflow facility is observed in "fresh" cases of dural shunt quite commonly). Put another way, if the "draining back pressure" is elevated, the pressure at all proximal points in the system are elevated without need for any change in coefficient of outflow across the normal resistance site. (Outflow facility ("C" value) is the inverse of resistance.)

Segmental Nature of Outflow: Implications for Angle Closure Glaucoma

Although Schlemm's canal extends for 360 degrees inside the limbus, there is considerable resistance to circumferential flow in Schlemm's canal, at least in adult eyes. It has been calculated that aqueous humor exiting through 1 hour of the Schlemm's canal circumference effectively has access to only approximately 1 additional hour of circumference of Schlemm's canal on either side (24). **The TM-Schlemm's canal aqueous drainage system behaves as several separate segmental outflow pathways rather than a freely communicating single circumferential entity.** Thus, in progressive chronic angle closure glaucoma (due to relative pupillary block), the amount of IOP elevation is roughly proportional (in a progressive way) to the amount of angle closure. Aqueous humor moving through the open portions of the angle cannot move freely into the entire circumference of Schlemm's canal. (Although irreversible changes in the TM and Schlemm's canal can occur as a consequence of PAS formation in this condition or possibly after chronic iris "touch" to the TM without synechia formation, most commonly after pupillary block is alleviated, areas of prior appositional closure which now become "open," once again segmentally drain a portion of aqueous humor, and IOP can thereby be normalized. In fact, with fresh PAS formation, using an argon laser to break the synechias (gonioplasty), can restore normal outflow function (Chapter 60).

Thus by evaluating the amount of open functional angle (full width TM) in narrow angled eyes with partial appositional or synechial closure, one can relate the number of presumably functionally closed hours of angle to the magnitude of the IOP elevation (Table 3.1).

For example, if 6 of 12 hours of the angle are functionally closed, one would expect the outflow (and thus outflow facility) to be halved (the resistance to be doubled). From the Goldmann equation, one can estimate the expected IOP elevation.

For example, assume F (flow) = 2 microliters (ul)/minute; C (outflow facility) = 0.2 ul/min/mm Hg; and Pe (episcleral venous pressure) = 8 mm Hg. Then

$$P \text{ (pressure)} = F/C + Pe$$

$$P = 2/0.2 + 8 = 18$$

$$P = 18 \text{ mm Hg}$$

If half of the angle becomes closed, then outflow facility is halved, and

$$P = 2/0.1 + 8 = 28 \text{ mm Hg}$$

That is, in this example, closure of 6 hours of the angle results in a 10 mm Hg IOP elevation.

TESTING OF NEW GLAUCOMA DRUGS

David L. Epstein

An important implication of this usual diurnal variation in IOP relates to the testing of potentially new antiglaucoma agents for efficacy. The best studies are those where a baseline diurnal curve is obtained without active drug first. Then, on another day, over the same time interval, the experimental medication is applied to one eye only, and IOP effects are determined in relation to the baseline visit, comparing similar hours of the two days.

A common, potentially fallacious technique instead is to put the drop in one (or sometimes both) eyes and measure the IOP several hours later, and then compare the measurements to the baseline "time zero" measurement on the single testing day, thus ignoring the endogenous diurnal rhythm of IOP in the patient. The fellow eye in a unilateral administration trial does have some utility as a "control" (the diurnal change in aqueous humor formation under systemic influence is likely very similar for the two eyes). However, the outflow status in patients with POAG may not be symmetrical in both eyes, and thus the magnitude of the observed IOP change may be different, although in the same direction, in the two eyes during the course of a single day. Regardless, many medications have contralateral effects through undefined mechanisms that can obscure these drug effects. Thus a "single drop, then look and see" protocol is really justified only in the very first such human applications, especially when evaluating safety.

Obviously the initial inherent outflow facility of the 12 hours of open TM-Schlemm's canal may vary among different individuals and will influence this calculation, as will the rate of aqueous humor formation and the true value of Pe (which may possibly be lower than 8 mm Hg). Nevertheless, in patients without any "open angle glaucoma disease," one would, for example, most likely not expect IOP levels into the 30's with only 3 hours of the angle functionally closed. On the other hand, patients with exfoliation open angle glaucoma not uncommonly can develop an additional angle closure component to their glaucoma (as, in fact, Paul Chandler, M.D. did). If the open portions of the angle have impaired outflow (reduced C value), then lesser amounts of superimposed functional angle closure can result in more substantial IOP elevation.

For example, let C = 0.08 ul/min/mm Hg for 12 hours of open angle due to exfoliation. Then

$$P = 2/0.08 + 8 = 33 \text{ mm Hg}$$

If 3 of 12 hours subsequently become functionally closed, C = 0.06. Then

$$P = 2/0.06 + 8 = 41.3 \text{ mm Hg}$$

In contrast if 12 hours of open angle had normal outflow facility (C = 0.20), then 3 hours of closure would result only in an IOP elevation from 18 to 21.3 mm Hg.

Another clinical implication from this type of analysis is that **for greater amounts of angle closure beyond 6**

Table 3.1
Examples of Difference in the Degree to Which the Intraocular Pressure (P) is Calculated to Be Affected by Changes in Flow (F) and Facility of Outflow (C) in Different Types of Eyes, Assuming Constant Episcleral Venous Pressure (Pe)

	(mm Hg) Pe	+	(μl/min) (F	÷	(μl/min/mm Hg) C)	=	(mm Hg) P
Normal =	9		1.5		0.25		15
	9		1 to 2		0.25		13 to 17
	9		1.5		0.30		14
Glaucoma =	9		1.5		0.05		39
	9		1 to 2		0.05		29 to 49
	9		1.5		0.10		24
Good normal =	9		1.5		0.30		14
½ angle closed =	9		1.5		0.15		19
¾ angle closed =	9		1.5		0.075		29
Poor normal =	9		1.5		0.15		19
½ angle closed =	9		1.5		0.075		29
¾ angle closed =	9		1.5		0.0375		49

hours, the amount of IOP elevation expected for each additional hour of closure dramatically increases. For example for C = 0.20 ul/min/mm Hg and the above parameters:

$$P = 2/0.2 + 18 = 18 \text{ mm Hg}$$

For 6 hours of closure: P = 2/0.10 + 8 = 28 mm Hg. That is, there is an increase of 10 mm Hg for the 6 hours that are closed. But assume now that an additional 3 hours become closed:

$$P = 2/0.05 + 8 = 48 \text{ mm Hg}$$

That is, there is an additional increase in IOP of 20 mm Hg for the 3 additional hours of closure (now totaling 9 hours of closure), whereas the initial 6 hours of closure only resulted in a 10 mm Hg IOP elevation.

Thus knowledge of Goldmann's equation and the segmental nature of aqueous outflow through the TM-Schlemm's canal pathway allows one to make reasonable predictions from gonioscopic observations (as well as allows reasonable information for the patient and physician about the chances for "residual OAG" after iridectomy-Chapter 38). This important subject is further discussed in Chapter 7.

Ciliary Muscle Tension

The longitudinal part of the ciliary muscle inserts not only on the scleral spur (see Fig. 2.1) but also sends extensions of the tendons into the trabecular meshwork and juxtacanalicular tissue (25). Thus, the outflow pathway tissue is under mechanical tension normally. Under the influence of a cycloplegic drug, this tension is diminished, and in fact, approximately one third of primary open angle glaucoma (POAG) patients (not on pilocarpine therapy) will show an increase in IOP (26) (and a decrease in tonographic outflow facility) after cycloplegic drug administration. This cycloplegic IOP rise by an open angle mechanism is rare in the normal population (27) (approximately one percent). It raises the question as to whether ciliary muscle tone might be involved in the mechanism of POAG. Is POAG really a disease of the ciliary muscle instead of the TM-Schlemm's canal?

The onset of increased prevalence of POAG is similar to that of presbyopia. Yet, in the majority of patients with POAG (not on pilocarpine therapy) there is no worsening of outflow facility after instillation of a cycloplegic, and although pilocarpine, a cholinergic agonist that causes ciliary muscle contraction, is a useful drug for glaucoma and improves outflow facility, the disease process of POAG nevertheless continues.

One might hypothesize instead that with a primary abnormality in the TM-Schlemm's canal system in POAG, ciliary muscle tension becomes even more important as a factor to increase outflow (e.g., by "widening" the spaces in the outflow pathway that are somehow partially compromised by the POAG process). Still we should not dismiss the importance of ciliary muscle tension normally for the proper function of the outflow pathway (28), and there may be more of a role for ciliary muscle dysfunction in POAG than we perhaps now realize. For example, contraction of cells in the outflow pathway may be important in outflow regulation (29), and the tethering of cells by their mechanical suspension to extensions of ciliary muscle tendons thus may be a critical phenomenon. Perhaps if plasma-derived proteins are constantly seeping into the TM from the root of the iris (30,31), ciliary muscle tension, perhaps intermittent, might be important in "stirring" functions to prevent protein aggregation and deposition.

As mentioned, the cholinergic drug, pilocarpine, works to decrease the IOP by an outflow effect that is mediated by the ciliary muscle. No direct effects of cholinergic drugs on the TM-Schlemm's canal cells have been demonstrated. Disinserting the ciliary muscle from the scleral spur in experimental animals prevents pilocarpine's effects on outflow (32). Morphologically, pilocarpine leads to widening of the spaces in the JCT and TM (33), and this is believed to occur by the increase in mechanical tension that is transmitted through the extensions of the ciliary muscle tendons into the TM (25).

Unfortunately, so far it has not proven possible to separate pharmacologically the contraction of only selected portions of the ciliary muscle. Therefore, pilocarpine and other direct cholinergic antiglaucomatous agents such as carbachol necessarily can cause in addition, an increase in accommodation as well as pupillary sphincter contraction and thus miosis (Chapter 13). It would be advantageous if a cholinergic drug could be developed that could cause selective contraction of the longitudinal portion of the ciliary muscle, and thus have an isolated outflow effect by this mechanism. The main limitation in the use of pilocarpine clinically are the presence of these additional cholinergic side effects (as well as a need for relatively frequent instillation as with most eye drop formulations).

There is much merit conceptually in treating POAG with an outflow drug (34), even perhaps a mechanical one such as pilocarpine, but there is no evidence that pilocarpine alters the natural history of progressive impairment in outflow facility with time that characterizes the disease of POAG. The latter is presumably due to the slowly progressive changes that occur as a primary event within the outflow pathway.

POTENTIALLY NEW OUTFLOW DRUGS

These are discussed in more detail in Chapter 16, but are included here because of their relationship to aqueous humor dynamics.

Uveo-Scleral Outflow (Nonconventional Outflow)

There is reportedly a steady low level "seepage" of aqueous humor out from the anterior chamber through the face of the ciliary body, through the ciliary muscle and ultimately leaving the eye either through the sclera or uveal blood vessels (Chapter 2). This has been termed either uveoscleral outflow or uveovascular-scleral outflow, the latter to indicate the ultimate fluid movement, which is believed by some to be into the uveal vasculature (35). **Although this unconventional outflow pathway may represent up to 40% of outflow in certain species such as sub-human primates (36), in humans it is believed to represent no more than 10% of total outflow (14,15,35).** Contraction of the ciliary muscle by cholinergic agents is believed to decrease outflow by this pathway (37,38), whereas cycloplegics can act, by relaxing the ciliary muscle, to increase such outflow (38,39). Although there are isolated anecdotal case reports where this pathway through such pharmacological manipulation may have had important effects on IOP (where trabecular-Schlemm's canal outflow was impaired), it is still difficult to be certain that the usual normal "seepage" of aqueous humor through this pathway has clinically important effects on IOP.

In contrast, when the barriers to this nonconventional outflow pathway are diminished either in ocular disease, such as uveitis, or under the influence of certain drugs such as prostaglandins (40–42), IOP can be lowered substantially, sometimes to near hypotonous levels. It previously has been taught that IOP is low in uveitis because of inflammation in the ciliary body which diminishes active aqueous humor secretion. Although this is still believed to be true, an additional mechanism likely is enhanced uveovascular-scleral outflow. Although theoretically there might be much concern about prostaglandin-like drugs that would similarly increase fluid movement through this pathway, there have been encouraging preliminary reports that such medications can be both safe and effective (43,44). As with most drugs the benefit/risk ratio is dose dependent, and it is possible that low, submaximal dosages of these agents may prove clinically useful. However, we still have much to learn about this pathway, which in some ways is an "internal lymph" pathway for the eye with possible immunological relevance. For example, one of us (DLE) is fairly convinced that treatment with prostaglandin antagonists, such as the synthetase inhibitor, indomethacin, topically, presumably by an anterior effect can reverse post-surgical cystoid macular edema. Although the opposite implication is not necessarily true, the clinician should be alert for possible adverse effects from drugs that might break down the normal barrier to such uveal fluid, and possibly cellular, movement.

Classically, it has been described that this pathway is pressure-independent (and more recently, minimally pressure dependent (35)). That is, at elevated IOP such seepage in terms of volume of fluid movement minimally increases. Conceptually, it is as if it were a constant seepage. Thus tonography, in which the IOP is experimentally elevated and the decay curve measured, does not appreciably measure such pressure independent (or minimally pressure dependent) outflow.

In cyclodialysis, a communication is created either surgically or as a result of trauma from the anterior chamber posterior to the scleral spur into the suprachoroidal space (Chapter 66). Classically, it was believed that this detachment of the ciliary body resulted in impaired aqueous humor production. However, an additional mechanism for the decreased IOP might be enhanced uveovascular-scleral outflow as a result of this new pathway into the suprachoroidal space.

Trabecular Outflow Drugs

Because the locus of abnormal resistance to aqueous humor outflow in POAG resides in the trabecular meshwork, drug therapy specifically targeted at this tissue makes a great deal of sense. It is rational medicine to try to intervene within the diseased tissue and attempt to reverse the abnormality in aqueous humor outflow (34). This is an area of exciting active investigation, with the potential for many novel "trabecular drugs" that could be developed to treat glaucoma (Chapter 16).

References

1. Brubaker RF: Flow of aqueous humor in humans: the Friedenwald lecture. Invest Ophthalmol Vis Sci 1991;32:3145–3166.
2. Lütjen-Drecoll E, Lonnerholm G, Eichhorn M: Carbonic anhydrase distribution in the human and monkey eye by light and electron microscopy. Graefe's Arch Clin Exp Ophthalmol 1983;220:285–291.
3. Lütjen-Drecoll E, Eichhorn M: Morphologische Grundlagen des Kammerwassersekretionssystems und seine Veranderungen durch antiglaukomatose Pharmaka. Fortschr Ophthalmol 1988;85:25–32.
4. Polansky JR, Lui GM, Alvarado JA, et al: Receptor characterization of cultured human non-pigmented and pigmented ciliary epithelial cells using cyclic nucleotide responses. In: Basic Aspects of Glaucoma Research III. Edited by E. Lutjen-Drecoll. New York, Schattauer, 1993: 243–256.
5. Chen J, Lui G, Wood I, et al: Localization of the "blood-aqueous barrier" in cultured human ciliary epithelial cells. Invest Ophthalmol Vis Sci (Suppl) 1994;35:1849.
6. Maren TH: The rates of movement of Na, Cl, and HCO_3 from plasma to posterior chamber: Effect of acetazolamide and relation to the treatment of glaucoma. Invest Ophthalmol 1976;15:356–364.
7. Berson FG, Epstein DL: Separate and combined effects of timolol maleate and acetazolamide in open angle glaucoma. Am J Ophthalmol 1981; 92:788–791.
8. Gharagozloo NZ, Relf SJ, Brubaker RF: Aqueous flow is reduced by the alpha-adrenergic agonist, apraclonidine hydrochloride (ALO 2145). Ophthalmology 1988;95:1217.
9. Kronfeld PC: Tonography. Arch Ophthalmol 1952;48:393–404.
10. Kronfeld PC: Some basic statistics of clinical tonography. Invest Ophthalmol 1968;7:319–327.
11. Epstein DL, Krug Jr JH, Hertzmark E, et al: A long-term clinical trial of timolol therapy versus no treatment in the management of glaucoma suspects. Ophthalmology 1989;96:1460–1767.

12. Sheridan PT, Brubaker RF, Larsson L-I, et al: The effect of oral dexamethasone on the circadian rhythm of aqueous humor flow in humans. Invest Ophthalmol Vis Sci 1994;35:1150–1156.
13. Larsson L-I, Rettig ES, Brubaker RF: Aqueous flow in open angle glaucoma. Arch Ophthalmol 1995;113:283–286.
14. Bill A, Phillips CI: Uveoscleral drainage of aqueous humour in human eyes. Exp Eye Res 1971;12:275.
15. Bill A: The drainage of aqueous humor via Schlemm's canal and uveoscleral routes. Ophthal Res 1980;12:130.
16. Ascher KW: The aqueous veins. Springfield, Illinois, Thomas 1961: 269.
17. Grant WM: Experimental aqueous perfusion in enucleated human eyes. Arch Ophthalmol 1963;69:783–801.
18. Ellingsen BA, Grant WM: Trabeculotomy and sinusotomy in enucleated human eyes. Invest Ophthalmol 1972;11:21–28.
19. Ellingsen BA, Grant WM: Influences in intraocular pressure and trabeculotomy on aqueous outflow in enucleated monkey eyes. Invest Ophthalmol 1971;10:705–709.
20. Peterson WS, Jocson VL, Sears ML: Resistance to aqueous outflow in the rhesus monkey eye. Am J Ophthalmol 1971;72:445–451.
21. Maepa O, Bill A: Pressures in the juxtacanalicular tissue and Schlemm's canal in monkeys. Exp Eye Res 1992;54:879–883.
22. Johnstone MA, Grant WM: Pressure dependent changes in structures of the outflow system of human and monkey eyes. Am J Ophthalmol 1973;75:365–383.
23. Grierson I, Lee WR: Pressure-induced changes in the ultrastructure of the endothelium lining Schlemm's canal. Am J Ophthalmol 1975;80: 863–884.
24. Van Buskirk EM, Grant WM: Lens depression and aqueous outflow in enucleated primate eyes. Am J Ophthalmol 1973;76:632–640.
25. Rohen JW: Why is intraocular pressure elevated in chronic simple glaucoma? Anatomical considerations. Ophthalmology 1983;90:758–765.
26. Harris LS, Galin MA: Cycloplegic provocative testing. Arch Ophthalmol 1969:81:544–547.
27. Harris LS, Galin MA, Mittag TW: Cycloplegic provocative testing and topical administration of steroids. Arch Ophthalmol 1971;86:12–14.
28. Kaufman PL, Gabelt BT: Aging, accommodation and outflow facility. In: Basic Aspects of Glaucoma Research III. Edited by E Lutjen-Drecoll. New York, Schattauer, 1993:257–274.
29. Epstein DL, de Kater AW, Erickson-Lamy K, et al: The search for a sulfhydryl drug for glaucoma: From chemistry to the cytoskeleton. In: Basic Aspects of Glaucoma Research III. Edited by E Lütjen-Drecoll. New York, Schattauer, 1993:345–354.
30. Barsotti M, Bartels SP, Freddo TF, et al: The source of proteins in the aqueous humor of the normal monkey eye. Invest Ophthalmol Vis Sci 1992;33:581–595.
31. Johnson M, Gong H, Freddo TF, et al: Serum proteins and aqueous outflow resistance in bovine eyes. Invest Ophthalmol Vis Sci 1993;34: 3549–3557.
32. Kaufman PL, Bárány EH: Loss of acute pilocarpine effect on outflow facility following surgical disinsertion and retrodisplacement of the ciliary muscle from the scleral spur in the cynomolgus monkey. Invest Ophthalmol 1977;15:793–807.
33. Grierson I, Lee WR, Abraham S: The effects of pilocarpine on the morphology of the human outflow apparatus. Br J Ophthalmol 1978;62: 302–313.
34. Epstein DL: Will there be a remedy to reverse the changes in the trabecular meshwork and the optic nerve? A personal point-of-view on glaucoma therapy. J Glaucoma 1993;2:138–140.
35. Pederson JE, Gaasterland DE, MacLellan HM: Uveoscleral aqueous outflow in the rhesus monkey: Importance of uveal reabsorption. Invest Ophthalmol Vis Sci 1977;16:1008–1017.
36. Bill A: Aqueous humor dynamics in monkeys. Exp Eye Res 1971;11: 195–206.
37. Bill A: Effect of atropine and pilocarpine on aqueous humor dynamics in cynomolgus monkeys (Macaca irus). Exp Eye Res 1967;6:120–125.
38. Bill A, Wålinder P-E: The effects of pilocarpine on the dynamics of aqueous humor in a primate (Macaca irus). Invest Ophthalmol 1966;5: 170–175.
39. Bill A: Effects of atropine on aqueous humor dynamics in the vervet monkey (Cercopithecus ethiops). Exp Eye Res 1969;8:284–291.
40. Toris CB, Camras CB, Yablonski ME: Effects of PhXA41, a new prostaglandin F_{2a} analog, on aqueous humor dynamics in human eyes. Ophthalmology 1993;100:1297–304.
41. Racz P, Ruzsonyi MR, Nagy ZT, et al: Maintained intraocular pressure reduction with once-a-day application of a new prostaglandin F_{2a} analogue (PhXA41). An in hospital, placebo-controlled study. Arch Ophthalmol 1993;111:657–661.
42. Ziai N, Dolan JW, Kacere RD, et al: The effects on aqueous dynamics of PhXA41, a new prostaglandin F_{2a} analogue, after topical application in normal and ocular hypertensive human eyes. Arch Ophthalmol 1993; 111:1351–1358.
43. Alm A, Villumsen J, Törnquist P, et al: Intraocular pressure-reducing effect of PhXA41 in patients with increased eye pressure. A one-month study. Ophthalmology 1993;100:1312–1317.
44. Alm A, Widengård I, Kjellgren D, et al: Latanoprost administered once daily caused a maintained reduction of intraocular pressure in glaucoma patients treated concomitantly with timolol. Br J Ophthalmol 1995; 79:12–16.

The Patient's History; Symptoms of Glaucoma

4

David L. Epstein

SYMPTOMS

Blurred Vision with Haloes

When intraocular pressure (IOP) is suddenly elevated from any cause, fluid may move into the cornea exceeding the capacity of the corneal endothelial pumps to remove it. Resulting corneal epithelial edema can produce symptoms of blurred vision and the perception of colored haloes around lights. (The presence of colored haloes is important, for noncolored haloes around lights are a common symptom of myopia, astigmatism, and other refractive problems with no IOP implication.) Colored haloes are also common symptoms of patients with nuclear sclerotic lens changes, especially early, without any elevation of IOP. Although such symptoms are more common in various forms of angle closure glaucoma (especially subacute forms) in which there is rapid elevation of IOP when the iris moves into apposition with the surface of the TM, colored haloes can also be seen in open angle forms of glaucoma with similarly rapid elevation of IOP, such as with glaucomatocyclitic crisis, post-cataract surgery, pigmentary glaucoma, juvenile open angle glaucoma, etc. However, in primary open angle glaucoma (POAG), except for cases with very high IOP, there are usually no such symptoms. This is what makes the disease so treacherous. Most patients with POAG are unaware of any symptoms until there is substantial visual field loss, at which time visual function is compromised.

Colored haloes with blurred vision in the morning upon arising is a common symptom in patients with Chandler's syndrome, an ICE syndrome variant. It can be seen also in patients with non-glaucomatous primary corneal disease in which edema accumulates in the corneal epithelium overnight because of the lack of helpful evaporation when the eyelids are closed.

Pain

Rapid elevation of IOP can also be accompanied by pain. Although some of this pain may be due to corneal edema or irregularity of the epithelial surface, it characteristically behaves as if it were more global in origin, as perhaps from stretching of the ocular coats. Topical anesthetics typically do not totally alleviate this symptom. With long-standing elevation of IOP, the corneal endothelium may be able to prevent corneal epithelial edema presumably due to the compensatory pump action of the endothelium. Nevertheless, patients with sustained elevation of IOP to levels of 50 mm Hg or greater often complain of pain even in the absence of corneal edema. Ocular pain may accompanied by nausea and vomiting.

Blurred Vision (Without Haloes)

In some forms of secondary angle closure glaucoma such as malignant glaucoma or uveal effusion syndromes in which there is a forward shift of the crystalline lens, symptoms of myopia can occur. A fascinating entity in this category is the myopia due to sensitivity to systemic sulfonamides and other medications (Chapter 36), in which either forward shift of the crystalline lens and/or lens swelling (or at least increased anterior-posterior lens thickness) can result in temporary myopia.

Rarely if the retina and choroid are elevated due to suprachoroidal fluid, such as may occur after filtration surgery or in certain uveal effusion syndromes (usually when there is minimal change in position of the crystalline lens), a hyperopic shift can be observed.

Subjective Visual Field Defects

Since the chronic open angle glaucomas usually produce peripheral visual field loss (without regular symmetry between the two eyes), most patients are unaware of their visual field defects and do not demonstrate symptoms until the disease is far advanced. However, in certain forms of glaucoma such as low tension glaucoma or open angle glaucoma associated with myopia, early field defects of considerable density can occur close to fixation and may be symptomatic to the patient. Because loss of visual acuity in glaucoma is especially debilitating, **patients with field loss close to fixation need to be monitored closely with central field programs that measure actual sensitivity levels around fixation**. When patients have little or no margin to follow in remaining central points of their visual field, one is justified to move to filtration surgery without documented further field progression (unless medical or laser therapy results in target IOPs close to or at what one might expect with filtration surgery).

Sometimes patients with open angle glaucoma (POAG, low tension, exfoliation, etc.) give a reliable history of a sudden onset of a subjective paracentral scotoma. It makes the clinician contemplate whether some acute "mini-event" has occurred in the chronic progressive natural history of the open angle glaucoma. One wonders about small vascular events occurring at the level of the optic nerve (1).

Subjective Loss of Vision (Acuity)

With high, sustained IOP in angle closure glaucoma but also in certain forms of open angle glaucoma, optic atrophy can develop with accompanying loss of visual acuity and pallor of the optic nerve without the contour changes in the disc rim that characterize the "cupping" that is more commonly seen in chronic glaucoma (Chapter 8).

However, when a patient reports a subjective loss of acuity and has advanced glaucomatous field loss or dense field loss above and below close to fixation, as commonly is seen in low tension glaucoma or OAG associated simply with myopia, this is a dangerous warning sign that, at a minimum, indicates the need to advance therapy to further reduce IOP. As mentioned, this is often an indication for urgent filtration surgery. In patients with such visual field changes, it is often useful to have the patient test their subjective acuity at home between visits by viewing objects on the wall, etc., or by using an **Amsler grid.**

Loss of Color Vision

Subjective loss of color vision is not uncommon in patients with long-standing POAG, and objective measures of color vision often demonstrate abnormalities in such patients. Clinically, though it is difficult to relate progression of the disease with measured progressive changes in color vision. It is intriguing that there are some encouraging reports about using colored stimuli on different colored backgrounds in testing visual field when evaluating follow-up patients with POAG (Chapter 10).

Patient's Sense of (Painless) "Pressure" in the Eye

Many patients insist that they can sense what the pressure is in their eyes. These are notoriously inaccurate except in some patients with acute, intermittent secondary glaucomas with wide fluctuations of IOP. Yet one of us (DLE) has been impressed over the decades how many of glaucoma patients' questions and queries that were initially quickly dismissed, later proved to have some merit (for example, the relationship of POAG to systemic hypertension which is now (2), but not a decade ago, well accepted). (Similarly there does now seem to be a relationship between POAG and thyroid disease (3); a question that has been asked by numerous patients over the past decades.) Therefore we should listen to our glaucoma patients for potential new insights, and although we still do not really believe that patients can sense their IOP (except for perhaps the acute secondary elevations), there may be some subgroup or some heretofore unappreciated mechanism for this symptom in certain patients.

What also needs to be emphasized is the obligation of the clinician to take the time to talk to all patients with glaucoma, fully explaining their conditions, and listening to their concerns, and especially to be sensitive to how their diseases and our treatments affect the quality of their lives. The glaucomas are one of only a few chronic eye conditions that are usually slowly progressive with time, requiring repetitive visits with usually only our nonspecific therapies to offer. Most glaucoma patients "bond" to their glaucoma practitioner, and such communication is an obligation of our profession. Sometimes all that can be done for a patient is to talk to them and honestly explain their condition. It is humbling how many second opinions are requested by glaucoma patients, in truth only to find a clinician who will take the time to talk to them.

Blackouts

With high levels of IOP in the 50 mm Hg range or greater whether due to acute or chronic causes, patients may experience blackouts, presumably because the elevated IOP is interfering with vascular perfusion of the optic nerve or retina. In patients with more moderate elevation of IOP, blackouts should suggest the possibility of underlying carotid disease, where presumably ocular hypoperfusion is being exacerbated by the elevated IOP. Glaucoma patients with this symptom should have a neuro-ophthalmologic evaluation.

Systemic Diseases

In response to the constant queries of glaucoma patients as to whether there was some relationship between their systemic hypertension and their glaucoma, it used to be taught that such a relationship did not exist. We know now there is epidemiologic evidence documenting the association between systemic hypertension and POAG (2,4), likely both in terms of elevated IOP and optic nerve damage. Why had this association not been uncovered previously? The truth is that properly controlled epidemiologic studies had not been performed. For this chronic progressive disease of aging, epidemiologic studies could be revealing in providing insights into mechanisms of the disease and of potential new therapies. We could be on the threshold of important new information from application of such standard clinical investigative techniques (Chapter 72).

Epidemiologic studies are becoming increasingly important in ophthalmology, and because glaucoma represents a common progressive chronic disease of the eye, there is a special need for such studies in glaucoma patients. There are tantalizing leads that deserve more extensive evaluation.

How might one explain the relationship between systemic hypertension and trabecular and optic nerve pathology in POAG? Perhaps they share aging connective tissue on the one hand, but abnormal "vascular" structures on the other hand. (Schlemm's canal can be considered a vessel of sorts, perhaps related to venules or lymph channels, with adjacent contractile cells and adventitia).

There is preliminary evidence that thyroid disease may be associated with POAG (3), and anecdotal experience (that we share) that correction of thyroid status may result in lowering of IOP (5).

Diabetes has sometimes been associated with POAG (6–8) but the mechanism has not been established.

There are no other recognized common systemic diseases that have been unequivocally associated with POAG, but have we performed the appropriate inquiries?

There are many secondary glaucomas that are associated with systemic disease and they will be detailed in further chapters. For example, increased episcleral venous pressure due to dural shunts or Sturge-Weber syndrome, cortisone-secreting pituitary tumors, various forms of secondary angle closure from tumors, neovascular glaucomas from diabetes or carotid ischemic disease, etc. One might suspect that formation of exfoliation material should be part of some systemic disease. In fact, there is some evidence of systemic deposition of similar material (9,10).

ACTIVITIES

There is no evidence that a patient with POAG or truly any other form of glaucoma should alter his or her daily life activity. Some patients with pigmentary glaucoma (Chapter 21) episodically liberate pigment into the anterior chamber sometimes after vigorous exercise of certain types usually involving head movement (11,12). In the absence of more specific management, treatment is given like that for POAG to prevent acute damage to the optic nerve from the transient IOP elevation. It is unclear whether it might even be desirable to shed this pigment earlier and acutely rather than later and more chronically.

Exercise both acutely (13) and chronically (14) may actually lower IOP in POAG patients. **Vigorous exercise by patients just before their ophthalmologic visits should be discouraged to avoid spuriously low IOP readings.**

Some have claimed that a supine position at night results in "spikes" of IOP elevation and optic nerve damage. It is true that in both normal and glaucoma patients, the IOP is slightly (1–2 mm Hg) higher in the supine position (15). This likely relates to changes in venous pressure influencing the eye pressure. There are likely compensatory vascular responses. Although this area, like most in glaucoma, deserves further evaluation, it seems quite premature to instruct patients to significantly alter their life style, sleeping postures, etc., without a firm understanding of the implications of this normal postural change in IOP.

One study demonstrated elevated IOP to substantially high levels in patients sleeping prone with firm eye pressure against a pillow (16). This should also be evaluated further; any change in recommended behavior for glaucoma patients seems premature.

A question in all these studies is how long the elevation in IOP is sustained. For example, if one pushes on one's eye, one can substantially elevate IOP initially, but then changes in ocular vascular volume and enhanced outflow from the eye as in tonography may provide compensation. One might imagine that sustained levels of high IOP might induce pain or some discomfort to either awaken the patient or change head position (which is likely changing spontaneously regardless).

Reading and close work, if anything, by increasing mechanical traction on the scleral spur and TM from contraction of the ciliary muscle, similar to pilocarpine, would be expected to lower IOP in patients with open angle glaucoma.

Theoretically, close work might be thought to potentially increase relative pupillary block in a patient with a predisposed narrow angle, but if ever a factor, it would be in those patients who had not yet been diagnosed. Those with known angle closure glaucoma who have had an iridectomy would not be at risk. (Spontaneous angle closure attacks precipitated by close work must be very rare, perhaps for the same reason that very weak concentrations of pilocarpine usually similarly do not precipitate such attacks, and more commonly can actually be used to treat an attack. [See Chapter 22 for discussion of vectors involved in acute angle closure glaucoma due to pupillary block.]

EMOTIONS

Many patients with POAG will inquire whether their emotions have affected their IOP, and rarely a patient is encountered whose IOP seems better controlled when tranquilizers are prescribed. (Some patients get apprehensive having their IOP measured, especially at the slit lamp, and may hold their breath or contract their eye muscles to give spurious readings (see Chapter 6 for techniques to avoid such artifacts, e.g., use the Perkins hand held applanation tonometer). Yet there still is a rare patient in whom tranquilizers seem to cause modest though real IOP lowering. However, except for this rare seemingly real occurrence, in general, the answer to this question is that there is no such known relationship. One hopes that time will not prove this to be a premature incorrect answer based on insufficient data, similar to past patient queries about such conditions as systemic hypertension.

In contrast, in patients with unsuspected narrow angles,

emotion (presumably from sympathetic discharge resulting in pupillary dilatation) can precipitate an attack of angle closure glaucoma. Numerous cases have been observed where emotion was believed to have been involved. Of course, patients with known angle closure who have had iridectomies will not be at risk (except perhaps for some rare cases of plateau iris, see Chapter 26). A common situation in which emotion-induced glaucoma may occur is in the fellow eye of an eye with acute angle closure glaucoma (which often from the acute pain, etc. has much emotional effect on the patient), as well as strong emotional events such as death of a close relative, or severe physical injury or illness.

FOOD AND DRINK

In the patient's diet, we know of no food that influences glaucoma one way or another, although some transient osmotic influences might be detectable. Large volumes of water consumed rapidly do cause a transient increase in IOP in many glaucomatous eyes, and this is the basis of the so-called water drinking test. However, the fluid intake in ordinary living, if it has any deleterious effect on glaucoma at all, must be so insignificant in the overall picture that it has not seemed to us necessary to advise a patient with glaucoma to change his usual intake of fluid in any way. In the case of tea and coffee, we think the same advice applies.

Rarely, very high levels of caffeine intake in patients with POAG have been associated with some IOP elevation, but attempts to study this systematically in POAG patients have commonly yielded negative results (17). This must be a rare phenomenon. Regardless, patients with POAG under poor control with vastly excessive caffeine intake (usually from coffee) should prudently be counseled to try to decrease this, for general medical health reasons, if not also for some possible beneficial effect on IOP.

Argemone oil has been an occasional toxic contaminant of edible cooking oils. It has been of interest for many years, principally in India, because it has been suspected of causing "epidemic dropsy glaucoma." This glaucoma is described as a reversible, noninflammatory, open angle glaucoma, occurring in epidemics of toxic dropsy. The IOP is raised, and in the most severe cases there is glaucomatous damage to the optic nerves. The elevation of IOP is spontaneously reversible, but the damage to the optic nerves is not. Alkaloids that are found in argemone oil, particularly sanguinarine and dihydrosanguinarine, have been suspected to be the active toxic components of argemone oil. A more detailed review of observations on argemone oil has been made in 1993 by Grant and Schuman (18).

Alcoholic beverages need not be avoided by glaucomatous patients. In fact, the intraocular pressure is nearly always temporarily lowered by strong alcoholic drinks, and it may be lowered even by wine and beer (19,20). **Patients, however, should be asked not to imbibe on the day of an office visit simply because it may result in a falsely low intraocular pressure level that is not sustained.** Lowering of pressure by alcohol is slight in normal eyes, but in glaucomatous eyes it is occasionally sufficient to cause a transitory decrease from pressure levels of 30 or 40 mm Hg to normal. When the equivalent of 50 ml of ethyl alcohol is consumed rapidly, the intraocular pressure may be lowered for several hours, returning to its previous level in 4 or 5 hours. The condition of the intraocular pressure in so-called hangover has not been investigated. In exceptional instances, before the prolonged lowering of intraocular pressure, there has been a brief rise of a few millimeters of intraocular pressure a few minutes after drinking whiskey.

The duration of lowering of pressure is longer than we would expect from the theoretical osmotic action of ethyl alcohol, which is known to pass from blood to aqueous humor only a little less rapidly than water. Alcohol taken in a dilute form such as beer can induce essentially the same changes in intraocular pressure as an equal amount of alcohol in concentrated form such as whiskey.

It is most intriguing that the duration of diuresis induced by alcohol is similar to the duration of effect on intraocular pressure. Since alcohol is believed to induce diuresis principally through suppression of release of antidiuretic hormone from the hypophysis, it would be interesting to learn whether the change in concentration of the hormone in the circulation is involved in the lowering of intraocular pressure.

SYSTEMIC MEDICATIONS

Atropine and many drugs having anticholinergic, atropine-like properties are reputed to be dangerous for patients who have glaucoma. For this reason, a considerable proportion of drugs that have been introduced in recent years, including many psychopharmacologic agents, antihistaminics, antispasmodics, and medications for parkinsonism, have been labeled with warnings against their use in the presence of glaucoma. Actually, only in eyes that are anatomically predisposed to angle-closure glaucoma do atropine-like drugs present a significant hazard, and these eyes constitute a small proportion of all glaucomatous eyes in the Western Hemisphere. In eyes that have the anatomic peculiarity of a very shallow anterior chamber with precarious narrowing in the periphery, the angle can be caused to close and an attack of acute angle closure glaucoma can be provoked by dilation of the pupil with atropine-like medicines given systemically. Eyes of this special type are subject to angle-closure glaucoma from many other influences, including sympathomimetic agents and mydriasis in response to darkness (Chapter 22).

Ironically, patients who have precariously narrowed angles, in whom an acute attack of angle-closure glaucoma

SPECIAL POINTS IN THE PATIENT HISTORY

David L. Epstein

A complete medical and ocular history including current and past medications should be routine, but the following are points of potential special interest.

Use of Corticosteroids

Sustained periods of corticosteroid use whether by ocular, systemic, nasal spray (1,2) or dermatologic use about the eyes may have caused past periods of elevated IOP and disc cupping, which now may present as an apparent "low tension glaucoma-like" condition.

Past History of Trauma

Angle recession (Chapter 43) from trauma may be subtle, but typically leads to glaucoma years to decades later. These past episodes are often forgotten by the patient. (Any truly unilateral case of open angle glaucoma needs to be explained as something other than POAG.)

Systemic Diseases

There is a known association of POAG with systemic hypertension (3,4), diabetes (5–7), and thyroid disease (8,9) (and likely other diseases that have so far been unappreciated but may only be detected by compulsive documentation). Systemic diseases may require use of medications such as corticosteroids or beta blockers with direct relationships to IOP.

It is also very important to probe the patient about cardiovascular disease and especially any respiratory disease that might influence one's choice of antiglaucoma therapy. The presence of respiratory "allergies" or "childhood asthma" even though no longer present, should be "warning flags" against the potential use of topical beta blockers. It is shocking how it is not rare for topical beta blockers to precipitate respiratory symptoms only after chronic use (Chapter 12), and only then do patients sometimes recall asthmatic symptoms in childhood or adolescence. Topical beta adrenergic agonists can also have cardiac side effects. Systemic carbonic anhydrase inhibitors are relatively contraindicated in patients with respiratory or renal disease (Chapter 14).

Systemic Medications

Corticosteroids have been mentioned. Patients on systemic beta blockers can show some reduction of IOP (which is individually variable), and this can lead to a confusing picture of a seeming low tension glaucoma "equivalent" (Chapter 19). Calcium-channel blockers are important to document as some observers have felt they might be protective of the optic nerve in low tension glaucoma, and some preparations may have some IOP lowering effects (Chapter 19).

Family History

There is a genetic component to many of the glaucomas, and in the future, genetic analyses will likely identify different subtypes with different prognoses. However, the presence of family members who are "blind" from glaucoma or take medications, have had surgery or laser for glaucoma, etc., should be a true warning signal to the clinician. Even if the patient in question has elevated IOP with no end organ damage, the presence of a family history of such "real" glaucoma should serve to make the clinician more aggressive about this patient's disease with regard to closeness of follow-up and the need for treatment.

Symptoms of Secondary Disease

Many such symptoms were discussed. However, one always probes for symptoms of past uveitis perhaps associated with systemic disease, but also perhaps just ocular, such as in glaucomatocyclitic crisis. Past episodes of red eyes, photophobia, corneal epithelial edema, etc. are searched for in the history.

Exercise-induced symptoms are routinely queried with particular relevance to pigmentary glaucoma (Chapter 21). Neurological queries (headaches, weakness, ischemic symptoms) should also be routine (glaucoma, in the end, is an optic neuropathy). Neurological symptoms in the presence of low tension glaucoma are an indication for neurological referral. Migraine and Raynaurd's phenomenon have been associated with low tension glaucoma (10). Dural shunts can cause increased episcleral venous pressure and secondary open angle glaucoma (Chapter 46).

Retinal tears and detachments, often subtle, can cause puzzling forms of glaucoma (11) (Schwartz Syndrome-Chapter 42). Histories of seeing flashes, floaters, etc. should be solicited. Miotics, particularly indirect acting agents, can cause posterior vitreous detachment and retinal tears (12).

Sudden Loss of Vision

Rarely, patients with apparent progressive low tension glaucoma symptomatically and with follow-up behave as if there had occurred some type of acute, non-progressive optic nerve event. This is very uncommon, and since low tension glaucoma is characteristically slowly progressive, the burden is on the ophthalmologist to be sure such a diagnosis is, in fact, accurate (Chapter 19). As mentioned, some patients with low tension glaucoma or myopia notice the sudden onset of a paracentral scotoma close to fixation, but global loss of vision is unusual and is more often due to an acute event such as a vascular occlusion.

Loss of Consciousness; Massive Blood Loss

A history of loss of consciousness and massive blood loss can be associated with a non-progressive form of low-tension glaucoma (13). Although there seem to be some rare cases where this is true, the overwhelming majority of cases of low-tension glaucoma even with such a history are, in fact, progressive, and all non-progressive forms of low-tension glaucoma place an extreme burden on the ophthalmologist for accurate diagnosis.

Recent Myocardial Infarction or Hypotension

Cases have been well documented in which with seemingly well controlled OAG, a recent myocardial infarction has led to unexpected disc and field progression. Patients with recent myocardial infarcts deserve special evaluation with this possibility in mind, as do patients with substantial hypotensive episodes from other causes. Unfortunately, such patients can continue to show further progression of their disease without any other (obvious) acute episodes.

References

1. Dreyer EB: Inhaled steroid use and glaucoma [letter]. N Engl J Med 1993;329:1822.
2. Opatowsky I, Feldman RM, Gross R, et al: Intraocular pressure elevation associated with inhalation and nasal corticosteroids. Ophthalmology 1995;102:177–179.
3. Wilson MR, Hertzmark E, Walker AM, et al: A case control study of risk factors in open angle glaucoma. Arch Ophthalmol 1987; 105:1066–1071.
4. Dielemans I, Vingerling JR, Algra D, et al: Primary open-angle glaucoma, intraocular pressure, and systemic blood pressure in the general elderly population. Ophthalmology 1995;102:54–60.
5. Becker B: Diabetes mellitus and primary open-angle glaucoma. The XXVII Edward Jackson Memorial Lecture. Am J Ophthalmol 1971;71:1–16.
6. Klein BEK, Klein R, Jensen SC: Open-angle glaucoma and older-onset diabetes. Ophthalmology 1994;101:1173–1177.
7. Tielsch JM, Katz J, Quigley HA, et al: Diabetes, intraocular pressure, and primary open-angle glaucoma in the Baltimore Eye Survey. Ophthalmology 1995;102:48–53.
8. Smith KD, Arthurs BP, Saheb N: An association between hypothyroidism and primary open angle glaucoma. Ophthalmology 1993; 100:1580–1584.
9. Smith KD, Tevaarwerk GJM, Allen LH: Reversal of poorly controlled glaucoma upon diagnosis and treatment of hypothyroidism. Can J Ophthalmol 1992;27:345–347.
10. Corbett JJ, Phelps CD, Eslinger P, et al: The neurologic evaluation of patients with low tension glaucoma. Invest Ophthalmol Vis Sci 1985;8:1101–1104.
11. Netland PA, Mukai S, Covington HI: Elevated intraocular pressure secondary to rhegmatogenous retinal detachment. Surv Ophtahlmol 1994;39:234–240.
12. Schuman JS, Hersh P, Kylstra J: Vitreous hemorrhage associated with pilocarpine. Am J Ophthalmol 1989;108:333–334.
13. Drance SM, Morgan RW, Sweeney VP: Shock-induced optic neuropathy: a cause of non-progressive glaucoma. N Engl J Med 1973; 288:392–395.

may be precipitated by an atropine-like drug, are rarely aware of any threat of imminent glaucoma in their eyes; whereas patients in whom chronic open-angle glaucoma has been diagnosed and who are under proper treatment stand in little or no danger from systemic use of drugs having atropine-like effects. In other words, the atropine-like drugs pose a threat to people who are unaware of the possibility of glaucoma, whereas these drugs present little or no problem to people in whom glaucoma is already diagnosed and under proper treatment. On the warning labels of drugs having atropine-like effects it is appropriate to advise that one should be alert to the possibility of precipitating acute glaucoma in patients who have abnormally shallow anterior chambers.

Simple inspection with a flashlight is useful and effective to detect abnormal shallowness of the anterior chamber. With a little practice, every physician can easily learn to identify eyes in which the iris is situated hazardously close to the cornea and to distinguish these from eyes in which there is a safe, wide space separating iris and cornea. Eyes that appear to have abnormally shallow anterior chambers by this simple method of inspection should be examined further with slit-lamp and gonioscope. If the angle then proves to be precariously narrow, one should be prepared to diagnose and treat angle-closure glaucoma, in case it develops. In detecting eyes that are prone to trouble from dilation, simple inspection with a flashlight is more effective than routine tonometry, because in most susceptible eyes the IOP is normal until the angle closes and glaucoma actually develops.

In eyes that have open angle glaucoma, the dimensions of the anterior chamber are usually near normal and closure of the angle is not induced by dilation of the pupil. However, paralysis of accommodation in open-angle glaucoma can, as mentioned in Chapter 3, in some cases cause IOP to increase. If the patient is already under treatment for chronic open-angle glaucoma, the effect of locally applied miotic drugs is expected to outweigh the effect of the small concentration of parasympatholytic, atropine-like compounds that may reach the eye via the systemic circulation.

In patients under treatment for open angle glaucoma, we have found that the simplest answer to the question of

STEROID-INDUCED ELEVATION OF IOP

David L. Epstein

Although classically believed to require 6 or so weeks of topical corticosteroid therapy to produce an IOP elevation in patients predisposed to POAG, this "dogma" actually reflects one particular dosage regimen of one particular strength of drug. The steroid-induced increase in aqueous outflow resistance is a dose-response phenomenon perhaps in all individuals, with an increased sensitivity in patients "predisposed" to POAG. Thus, very frequent, e.g. hourly dosages of a strong topical corticosteroid can cause some IOP elevation within a day or two (and commonly some contralateral effect). On the other hand, reported weaker topical corticosteroids that supposedly do not usually elevate IOP, may still, in fact, do so with longer periods of continued therapy and observation. Systemic corticosteroids, presumably because they yield lower intraocular drug levels than topical preparations, may similarly require a longer time to produce elevation of IOP. By derivation, but also based on some clinical evidence, "normal" patients without a pre-disposition to POAG may still possibly show IOP elevation with long enough duration of therapy of high enough dosage.

Thus the ophthalmologist and the general medical doctor need to understand these dose response relationships in arranging follow-up for such patients. The bottom line: with long-term use of either systemic or topical corticosteroids, potential IOP effects need to be monitored, even if shorter term observations do not detect IOP elevation.

Systemically administered corticosteroids thus can cause elevation of IOP in patients with POAG, although less so than topical corticosteroids. There is usually a considerable latency for this action, usually more than several weeks. Therefore, in any urgent situation corticosteroids can be given to patients with POAG, and ophthalmological evaluation routinely scheduled at a later time. Although probably prudent to evaluate such patients initially and after a few weeks of continued systemic corticosteroid therapy, likely the greater risk is after several months (to years) of such treatment, and it is important for the ophthalmologist to arrange such longer term surveillance, even if there is no short-term elevation of IOP.

whether it is safe to administer an anticholinergic drug systemically is to go ahead and try it and base the conclusion on a comparison of IOPs measured before and after the drug is administered. As a rule, standard antiglaucoma treatment is adequate to prevent appreciable rise of IOP.

In patients who have open angles of safe width and moderately elevated IOP, but who because of entirely normal optic discs, are not being treated for glaucoma, the question of whether it is safe to administer an anticholinergic drug systemically can be answered differently. One can test for tendency to increase IOP by applying two drops of cyclopentolate to one eye and measuring the IOP every half hour during the next 2 hours. If the topical anticholinergic cyclopentolate cycloplegia does not cause IOP to increase, we believe there will also be no increase from a systemic anticholinergic drug. If the topical cyclopentolate does cause an increase, then one needs to test the systemic drug in the same manner as in patients under treatment for open-angle glaucoma. If much of an increase is produced by the systemically administered drug, one should weigh whether to accept this as a justifiable additional risk to the optic disc or whether to start some antiglaucoma treatment to counteract the influence of the drug on the IOP.

Vasodilator drugs administered systemically are safe in both open angle glaucoma and in eyes with narrow angles, according to our experience and what has been published by others. Inhalation of 10% CO_2 causes a brief, small increase of IOP that disappears in minutes even if the inhalation is continued. We see no reason to withhold systemic vasodilators from glaucoma patients when vasodilators are indicated for systemic disease.

References

1. Tuulonen A: Asymptomatic miniocclusions of the optic disc veins in glaucoma. Arch Ophthalmol 1989;107:1475–1480.
2. Wilson MR, Hertzmark E, Walker AM, et al: A case control study of risk factors in open angle glaucoma. Arch Ophthalmol 1987;105: 1066–1071.
3. Smith KD, Arthurs BP, Saheb N: An association between hypothyroidism and primary open angle glaucoma. Ophthalmology 1993;100: 1580–1584.
4. Dielemans I, Vingerling JR, Algra D, et al: Primary open-angle glaucoma, intraocular pressure, and systemic blood pressure in the general elderly population. Ophthalmology 1995;102:54–60.
5. Smith KD, Tevaarwerk GJM, Allen LH: Reversal of poorly controlled glaucoma upon diagnosis and treatment of hypothyroidism. Can J Ophthalmol 1992;27:345–347.
6. Becker B: Diabetes mellitus and primary open-angle glaucoma. The XXVII Edward Jackson Memorial Lecture. Am J Ophthalmol 1971;71: 1–16.
7. Klein BEK, Klein R, Jensen SC: Open-angle glaucoma and older-onset diabetes. Ophthalmology 1994;101:1173–1177.
8. Tielsch JM, Katz J, Quigley HA, et al: Diabetes, intraocular pressure, and primary open-angle glaucoma in the Baltimore Eye Survey. Ophthalmology 1995;102:48–53.

9. Schlotzer-Schrehardt UM, Koca MR, Naumann GOH, et al: Pseudoexfoliation syndrome. Ocular manifestation of a systemic disorder? Arch Ophthalmol 1992;110:1752–1756.
10. Streeten BW, Li Z-Y, Wallace RN, et al: Pseudoexfoliative fibrillopathy in visceral organs of a patient with pseudoexfoliation syndrome. Arch Ophthalmol 1992;110:1757–1762.
11. Epstein DL, Boger WP, Grant WM: Phenylephrine provocative testing in the pigmentary dispersion syndrome. Am J Ophthalmol 1978;85: 43–50.
12. Schenker HI, Luntz MH, Kels B, et al: Exercise-induced increase of intraocular pressure in the pigmentary disperson syndrome. Am J Ophthalmol 1980;89:598.
13. Harris A, Malinovsky V, Martin B: Correlates of acute exercise-induced ocular hypotension. Invest Ophthalmol Vis Sci 1994;35:3852–3857.
14. Passo MS, Goldberg L, Eliott DL, et al: Exercise training reduces intraocular pressure among subjects suspected of having glaucoma. Arch Ophthalmol 1991;109:1096–1098.
15. Anderson DR, Grant WM: The influence of position on intraocular pressure. Invest Ophthalmol 1973;12:204–212.
16. Kornefeld MS, Dueker DK: Occult intraocular pressure elevations and optic cup asymmetry: sleep posture may be a risk factor. Invest Ophthalmol Vis Sci 1994(Suppl.);34:994.
17. Higginbotham EJ, Kilimanjaro HA, Wilensky JT, et al: The effect of caffeine on intraocular pressure in glaucoma patients. Ophthalmology 1989;96:624–626.
18. Grant WM, Schuman JS: Toxicology of the Eye, 4th ed. Springfield, Thomas, 1993.
19. Peczon JD, Grant WM: Glaucoma, alcohol, and intraocular pressure. Arch Ophthalmol 1965;73:495–501.
20. Houle RE, Grant WM: Alcohol, vasopressin, and intraocular pressure. Invest Ophthalmol 1967;6:145–154.

Examination of the Eye

5

David L. Epstein

It is very important to perform a complete ophthalmological examination including dilated slit lamp examination, peripheral retinal examination, etc., in addition to the specific glaucoma evaluation in *all* patients with glaucoma. **For the most common cause of glaucoma, primary open angle glaucoma (POAG), there are no other apparent ocular signs; therefore, a diagnosis of POAG is really a diagnosis of exclusion.** The ophthalmologist should view him or herself as a diagnostic sleuth, looking for unusual causes and looking for new insights into mechanisms of the disease, including POAG. It is really astounding how little we understand about the various glaucomas. Even more importantly, glaucoma, because it likely involves interconnection of more than one pathogenic mechanism, offers the opportunity to the observant and inquisitive clinician to make important new discoveries about known and new forms of glaucoma. This can only happen as a result of a complete and meticulously documented full ophthalmological examination.

In design of a patient chart, one of us (DLE) recommends that the initial full comprehensive examination be set apart in an always easily accessible place for constant reference. One frequently wants to know what the patient's examination showed at baseline.

One should develop a routine for approaching the patient. Obviously as long as a truly complete ophthalmological examination is performed, the sequence can vary. But one approach is as follows.

REFRACTION

Patients should be refracted first for their best distant and near acuity. As detailed, measurement and assessment of visual acuity (which can be adversely affected by the glaucoma disease process itself) are very important in the glaucoma patient evaluation. The proper refraction should be determined, and this information used for visual field testing, which is best performed before any ocular diagnostic manipulation.

PENLIGHT EXAMINATION

There is a tendency to "hone in" right away on the slit lamp examination and optic nerve evaluation, especially in the follow-up of glaucoma patients in continuing care. However, glaucoma patients can develop basal cell carcinomas, neurologic motility abnormalities, etc., as much as any other patient. It is useful therefore to first approach the patient with a penlight: examine the lids and conjunctiva grossly initially. Topical allergies to glaucoma medications and diseases of the conjunctiva are often more apparent on penlight examination than on slit lamp examination, especially if high magnification for the latter is routinely chosen. Note the position of the upper lids: this can be very important in planning where to perform a laser iridectomy or a filtration procedure in the future, so that the lid will naturally cover the manipulated site (even slight exposure of such sites can produce monocular diplopia and unrelenting patient unhappiness).

Ptosis can develop after filtration or cataract surgery due to uncertain mechanisms (lid or superior rectus surgical trauma or possible filtration surgery fluid movement) that needs to be discriminated from neurological causes.

Next the pupils should be examined both as to size and reactivity with the penlight. The swinging flashlight test should be performed, looking for an afferent pupillary defect (Marcus-Gunn pupillary phenomenom). The latter is obviously important to potentially diagnose other neuro-ophthalmologic disease that may be masquerading as glaucoma, and also as baseline for future examinations when, e.g., new neurologic symptoms might develop from other causes and complicate the clinical situation and diagnosis. This is also an example of what was mentioned above about clinician sleuths making new and important observations, even in POAG. It used to be believed that a positive swinging flashlight test (Marcus-Gunn pupillary phenomenon) was indicative of non-glaucomatous optic nerve disease, but there have been numerous observations by clinicians documenting that this can occur as a result of glaucoma alone. Patients with extensive glaucomatous damage, if asymmetrical between the two eyes, or even more importantly, glaucoma patients with field loss close to fixation can demonstrate an afferent pupillary defect (as can patients with unilateral macular disease). (The pupillary light reflex is relatively macular driven.)

Heterochromia (e.g., in Fuch's heterochromic iridocyclitis) can often be best appreciated on penlight examination (or even better with bright room lights or sunlight).

Binocular eye position (cover test) and extraocular movements should also be routinely evaluated. Although one can correctly argue that these probably relate the least to glaucoma, nevertheless most patients with glaucoma

THE RULE OF FIVE PERCENT

David L. Epstein

Some may think that this emphasis on compulsive thorough ocular examination in glaucoma patients is not that necessary. Although likely less true in glaucoma than other ocular conditions, the eye is a wonderful self-healing and self-correcting organ. In fact, one of us (DLE) teaches ophthalmic residents that for most issues, 95% of the time things turn out satisfactorily, even if non-optimal methods or treatments are used. But the whole point of a residency or fellowship training or, in truth, a book such as this, is to learn what to do for that other 5% of patients who will truly suffer if imprecise methods of understanding are implemented. In treating the glaucomas we must aim for "100%" (realizing that even "100%" today, with so little true understanding, will not be satisfactory in the future).

For example, about 90% of the time slit lamp examination alone can identify narrow occludable angles. Because in POAG one sees nothing definitely abnormal in the angle, and causes of secondary open angle glaucoma are rare, then why do gonioscopy? The answer is that 90% is not good enough, especially for skilled professionals who have undergone 3 or more years of ophthalmologic training. One can only hope that with ever-expanding managed care health systems we still will not be satisfied with less than 100%.

will "bond" to one clinician for life, and glaucoma patients may develop other ocular and systemic diseases in the course of their routine glaucoma follow-up. Examples of these include exophorias and tropias in patients who develop unilateral cataracts (not uncommon in patients with previous filtration surgery, especially with long term follow-up), ocular muscle restrictions following "tube" type implants, diabetic nerve palsies, and ocular myasthenia.

Documenting the actual size of the pupils in patients on cholinergic miotic therapy may help the clinician gain insight into issues of medication compliance over time (Chapter 13).

SLIT LAMP EXAMINATION

One should always use at least two levels of magnification on slit lamp examination. Some observations are actually easier to make with lower magnification (conjunctival disease, iris transillumination defects). Start with low power and examine the lids and conjunctiva. Note whether the punctum is in proper position. Many patients with glaucoma complain of epiphora, which may be a sign of drug allergy, but more commonly results from non-related abnormalities of lid position, meibomitis, punctal stenosis, or "dry eyes." Patients with underlying external ocular disease may complain of excessive "stinging" and irritation (and thus intolerance) of antiglaucoma agents. Initial treatment of a coincident chronic external ocular disease might allow subsequent acceptance of topical antiglaucomatous therapy (or at least a more accurate assessment of the side effects of the latter).

Note palpebral conjunctival injection or follicle formation (Fig. 5.1). The latter are common side effects from adrenergic agonists such as epinephrine and dipivalylepinephrine (and more recently apraclonidine), and the "redness" from these agents are often not correctly interpreted by the patient because they are commonly a delayed response (since the initial conjunctival response to the adrenergic agonist may be vasoconstriction, patients often feel these drugs help their red eye, and many patients do not inform their "glaucoma doctor" about their red eye, attributing it to general "allergies"). Thus, the ophthalmologist may not be the first to correctly identify that there is a problem.

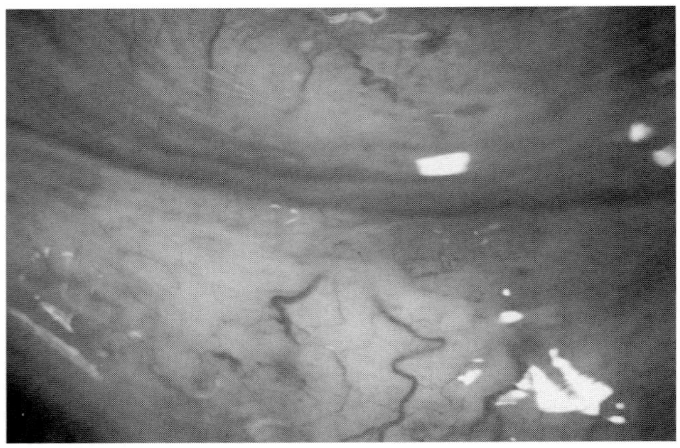

Figure 5.1. Conjunctival follicles from apraclonidine allergy.

Patients may develop **follicles** from other causes, e.g., benign lymphoid hyperplasia or lymphoma, and such entities are often best appreciated under lower magnification.

Always pull down the lower lid and look for possible early **symblepharon** formation, which might indicate early pemphigoid type disease (Fig. 5.2). Although uncommon, miotics, especially anticholinesterase inhibitors

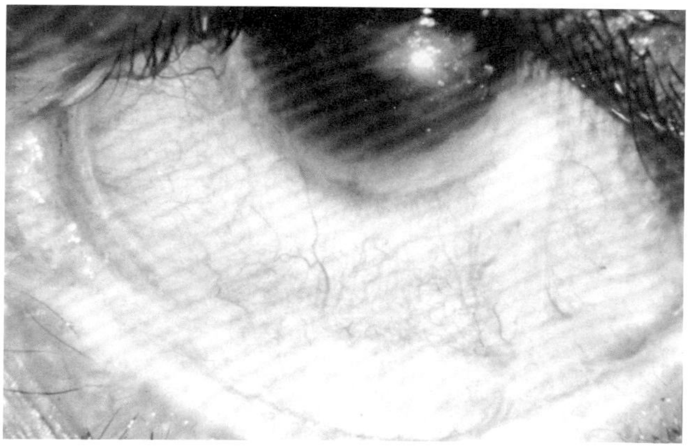

Figure 5.2. Fornix shortening and fibrosis in ocular cicatricial pemphigoid.

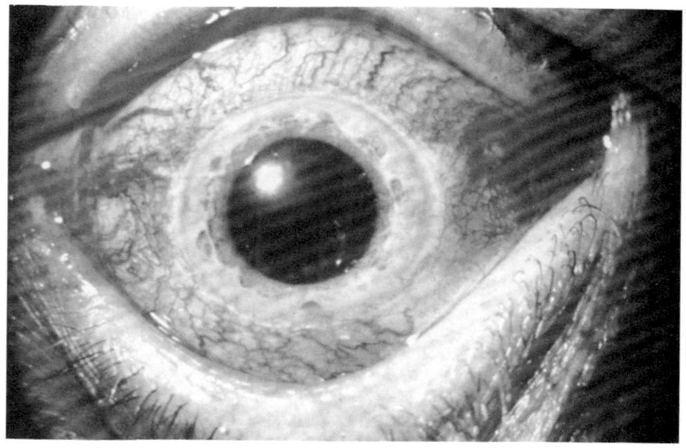

Figure 5.4. Dilated episcleral vessels in patient with dural sinus fistula.

but also direct cholinergic drugs such as pilocarpine, can cause a pemphigoid type syndrome (1), which can be progressive (and indicate the need to discontinue the medication). Here again one finds extremely useful and important one's baseline, compulsively thorough, comprehensive ophthalmologic examination. Patients with primary ocular pemphigoid can develop POAG as a separate unrelated entity (2), and the frequent lack of baseline data may obscure a proper interpretation of the exact incidence of miotic (or other anti-glaucoma agent)-induced ocular pemphigoid and confuse the choice of appropriate glaucoma therapy.

As a routine it is useful to test conjunctival mobility superiorly, in case filtration surgery is required in the future. The presence of conjunctival scarring from previous ocular surgery (most commonly cataract surgery but also perhaps childhood motility surgery that might not be recalled by the patient), from early yet undiagnosed pemphigoid syndromes, or previous inflammatory disease is important for one's therapeutic plan, prognosis, and discussions with the patient.

Look at the episcleral vessels on the bulbar conjunctiva. Increased episcleral venous pressure (Chapter 46) is not a rare cause of secondary open angle glaucoma. The prominent usually dilated episcleral veins are the signature of this entity and can sometimes be missed (Fig. 5.3). (This glaucoma with "red eyes" is sometimes attributed incorrectly to ocular injection as a side effect of topical medication.) The anterior ciliary arteries in the episclera usually can be distinguished from episcleral veins as the arteries extend forward from the recti muscles and usually penetrate deep into the sclera, often in pairs, and disappear a few millimeters from the limbus. (Some have described the anterior ciliary arteries as being more attenuated in POAG than normals.) Episcleral veins may be thin and inconspicuous in normals, but with increased episcleral

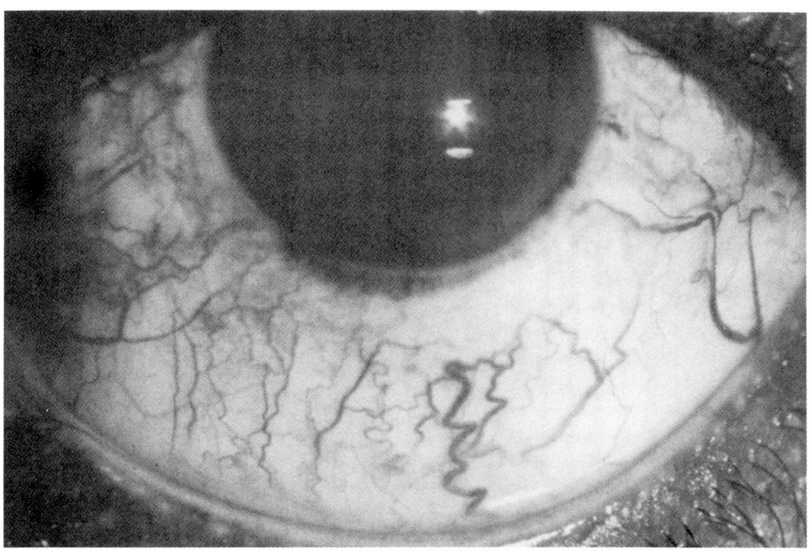

Figure 5.3. Abnormally prominent episcleral veins in a patient with elevated episcleral venous pressure.

venous pressure they become quite prominent and dilated and seemingly more numerous (Fig. 5.4). The pressure in these episcleral veins can be measured with a special device (Chapter 46).

If there is any confusion between conjunctival blood vessels that may be dilated due to topical allergy or inflammation and dilated episcleral veins, one should place a drop of a topical vasoconstrictor, such as weak phenylephrine, on the eye that will blanch the conjunctival but not the episcleral vessels.

In normal eyes one can sometimes identify clear channels within a millimeter of the limbus which are carrying aqueous humor to the surface of the eye. These aqueous veins (of Ascher) merge into episcleral veins, and at the junction of the two a laminated appearance where aqueous is mixing with blood is often apparent. Curiously such aqueous veins are only rarely seen in eyes with POAG.

CORNEA

One examines the corneal epithelium looking for corneal edema, and the corneal stroma looking for ghost vessels (old interstitial keratitis) or increased thickness (some have reported that abnormal stromal thickness may substantially alter IOP measurements (3)). One routinely examines the corneal endothelium for signs of Fuchs corneal endothelial dystrophy, which possibly may be associated with POAG, but which also has implications for possible future glaucoma surgery (shallow post-operative chambers create potential additional problems in patients with pre-existing corneal endothelial disease-even iris touch can be damaging). In the various ICE (irido-corneal endothelial) syndromes abnormalities (a beaten metal "mini-guttata" appearance) occur in the corneal endothelium. Posterior polymorphous dystrophy can also seemingly be associated with open angle glaucoma (Fig. 5.5). One should always look for the presence of peripheral anterior synechias that extend onto the peripheral cornea, e.g., in ICE syndrome

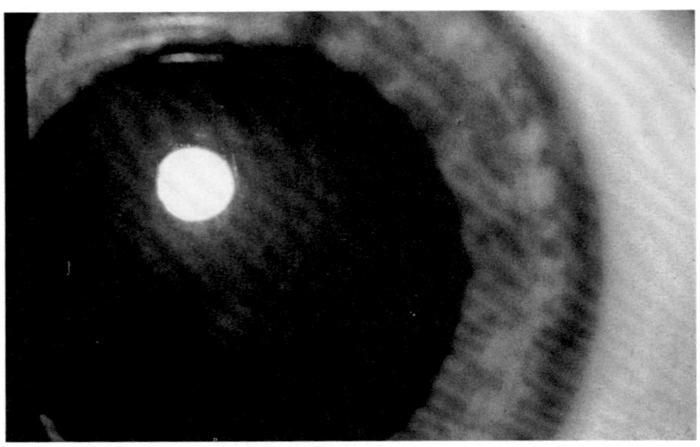

Figure 5.5. Cornea in patient with posterior polymorphous dystrophy.

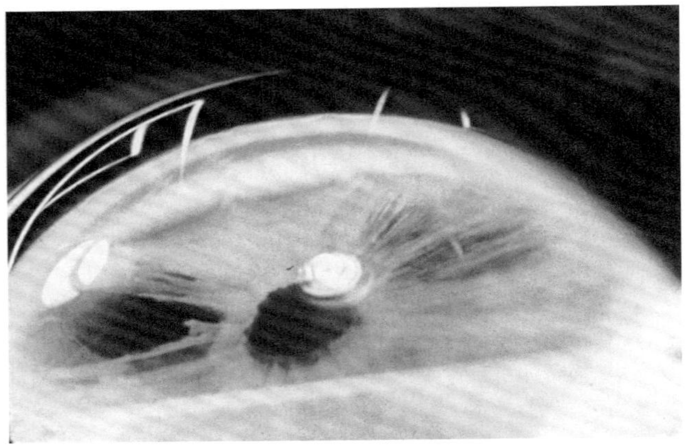

Figure 5.6. Iris changes with synechial angle closure in patient with essential iris atrophy.

(Fig. 5.6) or after a post-operative flat chamber. Various anterior segment cleavage syndromes such as Rieger's syndrome contains bridging iris processes to a prominent posterior embryotoxon (anterior end of Descemet's membrane).

In ICE syndrome there may be a peculiar yellow deposit at the level of the corneal endothelium just anterior to the synechia.

One should critically examine the corneal endothelium looking for deposits from the aqueous humor. Pigment deposition may not form a true Krukenberg spindle, but might be a sign of pigmentary dispersion, exfoliation, iris and ciliary body cysts, or past inflammation. A very small amount of corneal endothelial pigmentation can occur as a normal aging change, perhaps commonly in post-partum women, or accompany changes of Fuchs' corneal endothelial dystrophy, but pigment on the corneal endothelium always needs to be explained.

Inflammatory deposits on the corneal endothelium (KP) are a sign of ocular inflammatory disease that may explain certain puzzling cases of glaucoma (Fig. 5.7). **However, such KP can be subtle, often no more than a single "smudge" or two, in cases of occult trabeculitis (occult KP in the angle).** (Glassy, stellate KP with indiscreet margins are commonly seen in Fuchs' heterochromic iridocyclitis.) One should attempt to explain all corneal endothelial deposits or abnormalities.

ANTERIOR CHAMBER DEPTH

The clinician should routinely record the anterior chamber depth both axially and peripherally in all patients. The easiest way to do this is to estimate the number of corneal thicknesses that one can place between the back of the cornea and the anterior surface of the crystalline lens (axial depth) and between the back of the peripheral cornea and the surface of the peripheral iris (peripheral depth).

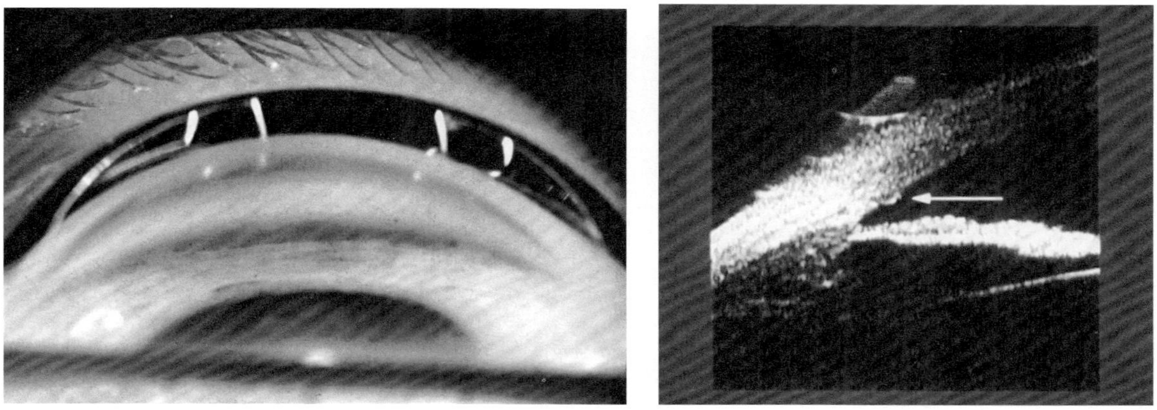

Figure 5.7. **A,** Note subtle KP (arrow) in inferior angle of patient with uveitis. **B,** KP (arrow) in the angle of a patient imaged using ultrasonic biomicroscopy (Courtesy of Joel S. Schuman, M.D.).

In estimating peripheral chamber depth one needs to construct one's own "standard curve" and standardize one's technique on normal patients. Different slit lamps may give slightly different "normal values." In general, one directs the beam 45 to 60 degrees at the far peripheral cornea, and the observation of one quarter corneal thickness or less for this peripheral anterior chamber depth is suspicious of a narrow, occludable angle (Von Herick's Rule).

Because of relative pupillary block in most elderly eyes, the pressure is higher in the posterior chamber than the anterior chamber and the peripheral iris is ballooned convex forward towards the peripheral cornea (Chapter 22). (In myopic eyes without this iris convexity and without such relative pupillary block the peripheral anterior chamber depth may, in contrast, be one full corneal thickness or greater). After laser iridectomy for eyes with narrow angles, with pressure now equalized in the posterior and anterior chambers, peripheral chamber depth should deepen, but usually just to $\frac{1}{4}$ to $\frac{1}{2}$ corneal thickness.

Although the peripheral anterior chamber depth deepens after laser iridectomy, the axial depth remains unchanged.

The axial depth reflects the position of the crystalline lens. In hyperopic eyes where the middle segment of the eye is "short", the crystalline lens is normally closer to the corneal endothelium than in an emmetropic or myopic eye. Using a similar technique as for measuring peripheral anterior chamber depth, axial anterior chamber depths of 3 corneal thicknesses or less are suggestive of a narrow angle. After iridectomy and alleviation of relative pupillary block, the crystalline lens position does not change. That is, there is no change in the axial anterior chamber depth. In fact, conditions where axial anterior chamber depth does change are indicative of other pathological processes such as postoperative malignant glaucoma or other causes of increased posterior segment volume (Chapter 28). In these situations, it is very important to appreciate the fact that the crystalline lens has shifted forward to diagnose and appropriately treat the disease. For example, with axial anterior chamber depth shallowing associated with elevated IOP after filtration surgery the diagnosis must be malignant glaucoma (or suprachoroidal hemorrhage) until proven otherwise. Similarly in other clinical settings, sequential changes in axial depth are important in the management of the patient. For example, progressive deepening in a post-filtration surgery patient with choroidal detachment may indicate that the condition is spontaneously improving and surgical drainage may not be required. **A patient with normal axial anterior chamber depth but shallow peripheral depth should be suspected of having plateau iris** (Chapter 26). It is thus essential to accurately estimate both axial and peripheral anterior chamber depth. These considerations are further amplified in Chapter 22.

IRIS

Trans-pupillary iris transillumination should be a routine part of every slit lamp examination. The slit lamp beam should be narrowed vertically and placed coaxial with the oculars and the width adjusted to fill the pupil, and the transillumination pattern viewed under low magnification. Peripupillary defects are frequently observed in exfoliation syndrome and mid-peripheral radial slits in pigmentary dispersion syndrome (with or without glaucoma). In addition to transpupillary retroillumination iris transillumination can be performed using a fiberoptic light source (Chapter 21).

The pupillary collarette should be carefully examined. Loss of pupillary ruff can occur in exfoliation (Fig. 5.8). Rubeosis is often first seen in the pupillary area. Ectropion uveae occurs in neovascular glaucoma. Pupillary sphincter tears are indicative of past blunt trauma. Slight eccentricity of the pupil can be seen in ICE syndrome. Vertical extension of the pupil postoperatively should suggest iris incarcerated in the surgical wound.

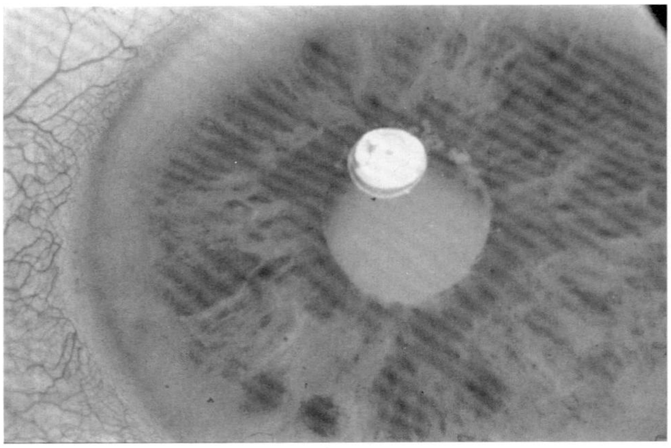

Figure 5.8. Note accumulation of exfoliative material on pupillary margin.

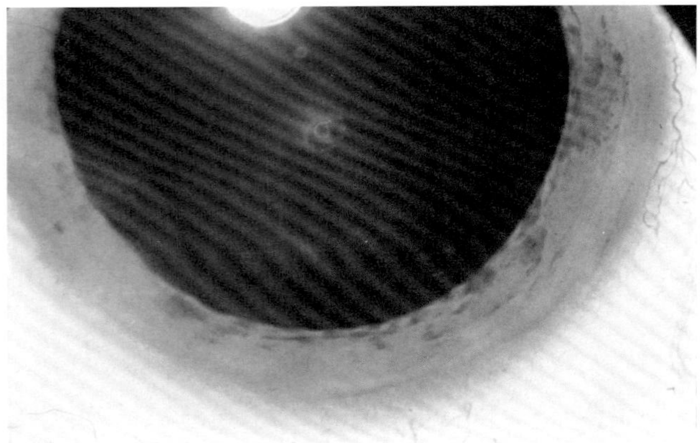

Figure 5.10. Pigmented iris cyst in a patient observed after dilation.

The texture of the iris should be commented on, nevi noted and drawn in the chart. Iris nodules can be seen in certain manifestations of the ICE syndrome, in neurofibromatosis, and with inflammatory deposits in various uveitides.

Sometimes it is easy to miss mass lesions on the iris, e.g., early iris melanoma or juvenile xanthogranuloma, unless iris texture is carefully examined.

Gray areas of iris stromal atrophy are usually indicative of past episodes of angle closure (Chapter 23), although they can also be observed from severe episodes of past iritis, especially due to herpes zoster. Iris stromal atrophy leading to hole formation can be seen in ICE syndrome.

Iridoschisis is associated with (usually chronic) angle closure glaucoma.

Membranes may occur on the surface of the iris or extending into the anterior chamber, e.g., in epithelial cysts (Fig. 5.9) or, if localized, with fibrous ingrowth. Membranes are also histologically associated with ICE syndrome, angle recession, or certain post-inflammatory conditions. In neovascular glaucoma the meandering blood vessels on the iris surface are accompanied histologically by a fibrous membrane that is not apparent clinically except perhaps by a subtle loss of iris surface texture.

Iris pigment epithelial cysts (Chapter 34) on the posterior surface of the iris cannot be directly visualized except occasionally after pupillary dilation or if there is an iridectomy (Fig. 5.10). However, such cysts often produce a bumpy peripheral iris contour which may be better appreciated on gonioscopy.

CRYSTALLINE LENS

The anterior surface of the lens should be examined looking for changes of exfoliation (Fig. 5.11). Through an undilated pupil the changes of exfoliation can be subtle and easily missed. Most commonly the central pupillary area of the lens demonstrates a matted, translucent disc of exfoliation. **After pupillary dilation, slit lamp examination should be repeated** with a drawing of existing lens opac-

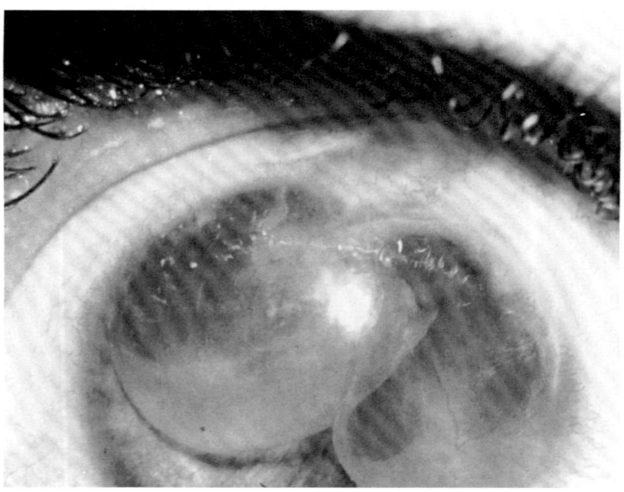

Figure 5.9. Post surgical epithelial inclusion cyst.

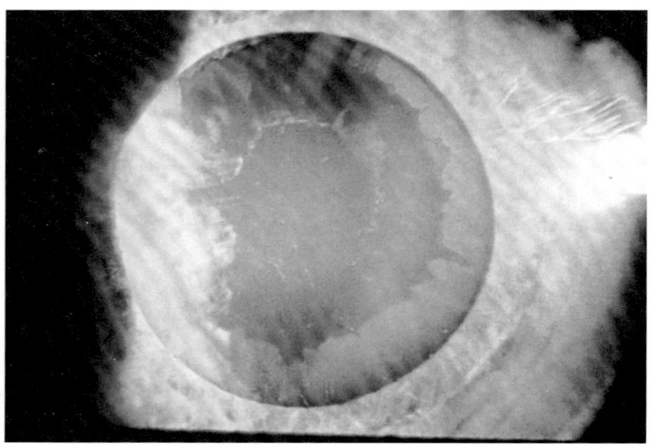

Figure 5.11. Marked exfoliation on anterior lens surface. Exfoliation is often subtle and easily overlooked, especially if the patient is not reexamined at the slit lamp after dilation.

ities both by angled slit view but also retroillumination. Exfoliation or pigment on the zonules, partial subluxations, and other abnormalities should be noted. In exfoliation there is commonly a clear area on the anterior capsule that separates the central matted disc from more peripheral scallops of white material. In pigmentary dispersion syndrome there is commonly pigment deposited in a peripheral "pocket" between posterior lens surface, zonules, and hyaloid that can only be appreciated following pupillary dilation. In patients who have had acute angle closure in the past Glaukomflecken may be present within the anterior lens cortex (Chapter 23).

VITREOUS

During the slit lamp examination the anterior vitreous should be examined for cells or pigment. Pigment particles in the vitreous may be seen with inflammation but also with certain glaucoma syndromes associated with retinal detachment (Schwartz's syndrome). The presence of a posterior vitreous detachment, if present, should be recorded.

IOP

The above has detailed pen-light examination and then slit lamp examination, but has so far not mentioned IOP measurement (Chapter 6). Although it seems common to perhaps first measure the IOP and then do the slit lamp examination, this is not recommended. Slit lamp examination should be performed first if for no other reason to rule out infection or corneal epithelial abnormalities. Also the act of taking the IOP first can cause a fine corneal epithelial irregularity (and fluorescein staining) that can interfere with the clarity of the subsequent examination and also can produce artifacts on visual field measurements. It is recommended therefore that the visual field be performed first prior to ocular manipulation.

HOW MUCH VISUAL ACUITY DECREASE DOES THE MEDIA EXPLAIN?

In all patients with decreased visual acuity, the ophthalmologist must try to explain the reason for this on the basis of the clinical examination. **The best way to assess the contribution of ocular media to diminished visual acuity is with the direct ophthalmoscope to compare the patient's visual acuity with the clarity of one's own view of the patient's fundus.** If one has a clear view of the disc and posterior pole, then this is a "20/20 view." If the disc can only hazily be seen, then this is commonly a 20/200 view. One quickly learns the range in between. For example, in patients with best corrected visual acuity of 20/70, one can be very definitive that the media either does or does not explain the visual acuity.

It is best to perform this important evaluation with the direct ophthalmoscope before anesthetic drops are applied to the eye or other examination manipulations occur, such as gonioscopy. Therefore, a usual routine is to perform the pen-light and slit lamp examinations (which also might help orient the clinician as to the cause of the media changes) and then perform direct ophthalmoscopic examination of the posterior pole (drawing the disc cupping) and media through the patient's undilated pupil (this is the aperture through which the patient is looking, so the clinician should look in through the same opening to assess media clarity). Visual acuity and media assessment can be repeated after dilation for supplemental data, but the patient has usually experienced tonometry, gonioscopy, and application of various topical agents which might complicate the interpretation. Always record the estimate of the visual acuity that the patient's media accounts for along with the examination technique that was used.

With long-term follow-up of glaucoma patients, it is not rare for there to be uncertainty as to whether the vision is decreased on the basis of cataract or glaucoma. For example, a not uncommon scenario is that a patient with 20/60 visual acuity but no documentation as to the cause undergoes possibly successful filtration surgery, but over the years there is further visual acuity decrease. Should the cataract be removed? What visual acuity does the current media explain? What were the findings at the time of filtration surgery? A glaucoma patient with advanced disease may have filtration surgery to "save" his or her vision, but then with the passage of time and cataract formation there is a tendency to "write off the eye because of severe" damage from glaucoma. The commonly occurring fact that the eye did not see well from the time of filtration surgery (which may have been due to early cataract formation or progression of the pre-existing cataract and was not documented) may thus, not be appreciated and, therefore erroneously, appropriate cataract surgery may not be performed.

Thus **assessing the effect of the media on visual acuity should be a routine part of every glaucoma examination, and it should be performed before there is other manipulation of the eye.**

Another clinically important point is that for an eye with advanced glaucoma field loss close to fixation, lesser amounts of cataract formation may explain a disproportionately larger effect on visual acuity. It is as if with existing scotoma present adjacent to fixation, small amounts of added distortion can produce larger decreases in visual acuity than without such paracentral scotoma. With experience and the routine use of this method of assessing media clarity, the glaucoma clinician learns to appropriately assess such patients.

OPTIC NERVE EVALUATIONS

It is frequently useful even with an undilated pupil to perform 90 diopter lens evaluation of the optic nerve. As will be commented on in an upcoming chapter (Chapter 8), we need to take every opportunity to examine the optic nerve for changes of glaucoma with multiple different techniques of examination (which frequently seem to highlight different aspects of disc cupping). We are critically examining the **contour** of the remaining rim of tissue of the optic nerve, and our methods are somewhat "gross", likely not detecting very early changes, and thus there is merit to multiple methods of examination including direct ophthalmoscopy.

Obviously at the time of direct ophthalmoscopy, an assessment and drawing of the optic disc as far as the contour changes of cupping (Chapter 8) should be made through the undilated pupil, even if the patient will subsequently be dilated (when this then should be repeated). In many follow-up visits, the pupil will not be dilated, and therefore it is useful to have this baseline information as viewed through the undilated pupil.

After pen-light, slit lamp, and then direct ophthalmoscopic examination, IOP should next be measured as detailed in the next chapter (Chapter 6). After this gonioscopy should be performed (Chapter 7), and then pupillary dilation. (During the latter the patient should be instructed to keep their eyes closed to prevent corneal drying from infrequent blinking, resulting from the use of topical anesthetics for the IOP measurement and gonioscopy.)

Dilated slit lamp examination with description and drawing of crystalline lens changes should then be made along with examination of the vitreous for pigment and cells, as well as evaluation of the optic nerve with the 90 diopter lens, as will be detailed later. Then it is useful to repeat direct ophthalmoscopy of the disc (and macula). Although a non-stereo view, use of parallax in direct ophthalmoscopy can complement contour information from direct stereo methods. The disc cupping and rim contour should be drawn.

Indirect ophthalmoscopy with retinal drawing with attention to the retinal periphery for possible occult tears (that might explain certain unusual secondary glaucomas such as Schwartz's syndrome), or areas of peripheral retinal pathology that might contraindicate miotic therapy, should be performed. The status of the macula (because this also influences visual acuity assessment) should next be evaluated and drawn.

Baseline stereo disc photographs should be performed on all patients with glaucoma or risk of glaucoma for future reference (thus constituting a true baseline standard to assess future change). Such photographs should be repeated every year or two, depending on disease severity.

The examination is not complete until the impressions are listed with an assessment of the glaucoma status and **target IOP**, and then the plan of action is laid out in the medical record.

Finally, it is very important to talk to the patient and fully explain the condition, the plan, and the areas of uncertainty. If one can relate the plan to the patient in terms of what one would do if the clinician's own eye were so affected, then this is the highest level of care. Especially for new patients, adequate time to talk to the patient must be scheduled.

References

1. Patten JT, Cavanagh HD, Allansmith MR: Induced ocular pseudopemphigoid. Am J Ophthalmol 1976;82:272–276.
2. Tauber J, Melamed S, Foster CS: Glaucoma in patients with ocular cicatricial pemphigoid. Ophthalmology 1989;96:33–37.
3. Johnson M, Kass MA, Moses RA, et al: Increased corneal thickness simulating elevated intraocular pressure. Arch Ophthalmol 1978;95:664–665.

Tonometry & Tonography

6

W. Morton Grant
Joel S. Schuman

EXAMINATION OF THE EYE IN GLAUCOMA

Intraocular Pressure

TONOMETRY

The Goldmann applanation tonometer has become a standard of reference in clinical tonometry (Fig. 6.1). The principle of applanation tonometry is old. It is based on the physical relationship that applies to the flat end of a piston at rest: The pressure against the piston is calculated from the force applied to the piston divided by the area of the face of the piston. This principle has been used in the Russian Maklakov applanation tonometer since the nineteenth century, but it was never applied with great precision until the advent of the Goldmann applanation tonometer. In the Goldmann instrument, the force is measured with a sensitive spring or counterpoise balance, and the area is precisely established by an accurate split-field device.

Simple as the principle of applanation tonometry may appear to be, seeming only to require measurements of the applied force and of the resulting flattened area of cornea for determination of the pressure, in actual development of a practical and accurate instrument, a number of additional complicating factors had to be considered. These factors include the effect of capillary attraction between the face of the applanation tonometer and the cornea, the stiffness of the cornea itself, the translation of the force and area on the outer surface of the cornea to intraocular pressure at the inner surface of the cornea, the influence of varying corneal curvatures, the influence of corneal astigmatism, the influence of varying amounts of fluid on the cornea, and the influence of varying scleral rigidity. The Goldmann applanation tonometer actually permits measurement of intraocular pressure with very little disturbance of this pressure and with insignificant error from variation of scleral rigidity. It also has a well-defined range of insensitivity to the other factors listed (1).

In the Goldmann applanation tonometer, the end-point diameter of applanation is fixed by the construction of the plastic prisms within the instrument to be suitable especially for the human eye. The diameter of applanation has been selected to give a balance between the capillary attractive force of the tear film and the opposing resistive force of the cornea, while producing essentially the same area of flattening of the endothelial suface of the cornea. For the human eye, the diameter of flattening employed is 3.06 mm. The same diameter is not suitable for use on animal eyes, presumably due to differences in structures of the corneas. For each species, Goldmann found that it is necessary to use a different specific diameter of flattening, usually larger than that which is best for the human eye.

A portable adaptation of the spring-type Goldmann applanation tonometer (Fig. 6.2), available as the Perkins applanation tonometer, is well suited to measurements on patients in either the seated or the supine position. The Perkins applanation tonometer is particularly useful in measuring the IOP in young children, permitting accurate measurement without having to position the child at a slit lamp, which can be both inconvenient and alarming to the child. The Perkins tonometer has made tonometry on awake children so much easier than formerly that the need for general anesthesia has been reduced; however, this tonometer is also convenient and well suited for measurements on children in the supine position under general anesthesia.

The Perkins applanation tonometer allows the accurate measurement of IOP in individuals in whom the Goldmann tonometer produces a falsely elevated IOP. The IOP can be measured more accurately with the Perkins than the Goldmann tonometer in persons who hold their breath during Goldmann tonometry, obese individuals, extremely large breasted women, patients with tight collars, or patients with great anxiety at the slit lamp. By permitting applanation tonometry outside the confines of the slit lamp, the Perkins tonometer enables precise assessment of the IOP in a more relaxed setting for the patient.

For topical anesthesia for Goldmann applanation tonometry use is made of a drop of a preparation (Fluress, Pilkington Barnes Hind, Sunnyvale, CA) containing both a topical anesthetic (benoxinate) and 1/4% fluorescein, stabilized by polyvinylpyrrolidone, or of proparacaine 0.5% and a fluoresceinated paper strip. The resulting flourescent tear film is more suitable than a colorless film for observing and measuring flattening of the cornea by the applanation device. To enhance fluorescence, a blue light is used to illuminate the eye and its tear film. Looking with a slit-lamp microscope, one sees at the moment of contact of the tonometer with the eye a bright yellow-green spot that breaks into two bright yellow-green semicircular arcs as the tonometer is moved slightly farther forward. The arcs should then be seen in sharp focus. By suitable adjustment of a graduated drum, which varies the force applied to the cornea, **the arcs can be made to overlap so that the inner edge of the upper can be aligned with the inner edge of the lower.** This is the desired end point at which a reading is taken from the graduated drum. The numerical reading on the drum indicates grams of force applied by the tonometer and equivalent mm Hg intraocular pressure. Thus, number 1 on the drum is equal to 10 mm Hg and 2 is equal to 20 mm Hg.

The precision with which the inner edges of the overlapping upper and lower arcs can be lined up is limited because of the ocular pulse, which causes the edges to keep swinging back and forth. The best that can be done is to adjust the alignment to a mean position in which there is equal swing to either side of the aligned position.

Measurement is made first on one eye and then the other, alternating back and forth, repeating measurements until reasonably constant values are obtained. This is important because, particularly with apprehensive patients, the initial reading may be several mm Hg higher than the readings obtained when the patient has become relaxed and accustomed to the procedure. Usually, three measurements on each eye suffice, but if the last two measurements do not agree within 1 mm Hg, more measurements should be made. Presumably, when initial measurement is higher than the later steady-state measurement, the initial measurement is erroneous.

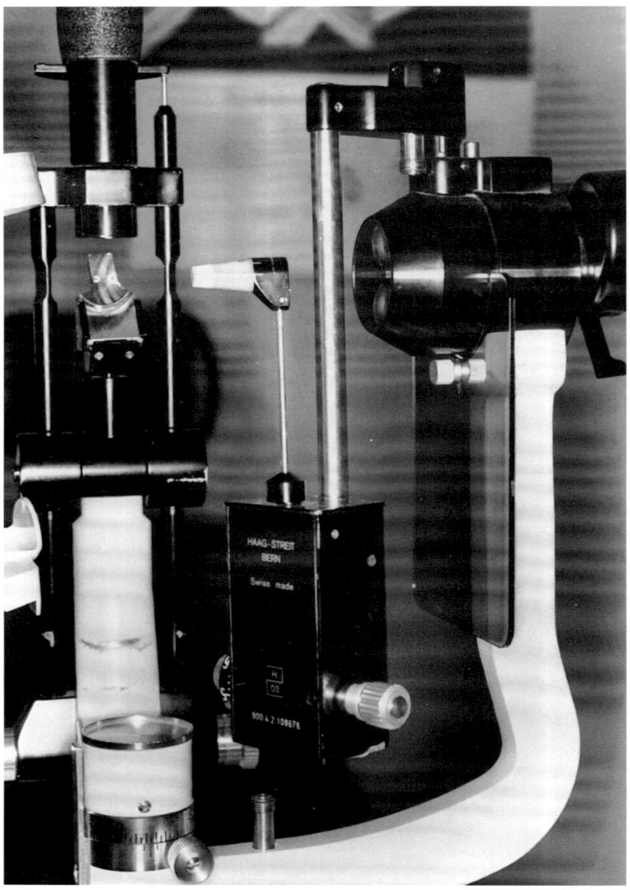

Figure 6.1. The Goldmann applanation tonometer, the "gold standard" instrument for the measurement of intraocular pressure.

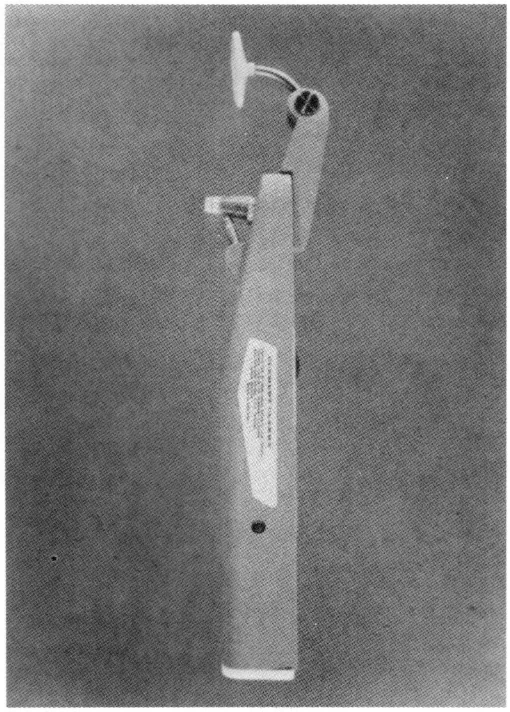

Figure 6.2. The Perkins applanation tonometer is portable and allows accurate IOP measurement without the use of a slit lamp. It is useful in applanation on children and elderly patients. Occasionally, patients (particularly if they are obese) demonstrate breathholding and presumed increased venous pressure when IOP is measured with the slit lamp with false elevation of IOP; these elevations are not confirmed when the Perkins instrument is used.

The significance of readings obtained with the Goldmann applanation tonometer when the patient is relaxed may be generalized as follows: reliable and repeated measurements of 22 or more mm Hg pressure suggest that the eye is abnormal.

In practically all eyes that have a definite pressure of 22 mm Hg or higher, the tonographic P_0/C ratio is 100 or higher, which indicates possible glaucoma. The higher the pressure, the more definite is the indication. How dangerous a given pressure may be to a given eye depends on how many additional factors, such as the nature of the optic nerve head, the height and duration of IOP elevation, and possibly the blood pressure, all of which are discussed elsewhere.

An IOP of 21 mm Hg by applanation should be regarded as borderline. IOP from 18 to 20 mm Hg does not rule out glaucoma if these are single samplings at a single time of day. It is not uncommon for the intraocular pressure in eyes having definite glaucoma to vary during the course of 24 hours from the high teens to the high twenties, thirties, or even forties. Thus, a single measurement, be it ever so accurate at the moment, may give a completely misleading impression, if by chance it happens to be obtained at the low point of the daily fluctuation.

The Goldmann applanation tonometer can be modified for use on the eyes of infants with small palpebral fissures as well as on eyes of adult patients who have had penetrating keratoplasty and are suspected of developing glaucoma. The end of the cylindrical plastic cone of the tonometer can be reduced in diameter by turning down in a lathe, leaving just enough of the flat applanating surface to still give accurate pressure measurements (2,3).

The **Schiotz tonometer** continues to be a widely used instrument for estimation of intraocular pressure because it offers a reasonable combination of convenience and reliability. It is subject to more error than the Goldmann applanation tonometer, but the Schiotz tonometer has advantages in portability, availability, ease of use, and lower price.

In the customary manner of using the Schiotz tonometer, the patient is recumbent with gaze vertical and corneas anesthesized by a drop of topical anesthetic. The tonometer is allowed to rest on the patient's cornea, and the extent to which the weighted plunger of the tonometer indents the cornea is shown on a scale by a simple lever arm indicator. The lever arm system magnifies the motion of the plunger 20-fold so that a 0.05-mm movement of the plunger is represented by a 1 mm space between units on the tonometer scale. Thus the scale readings merely indicate the depth to which the plunger indents the eye. The softer the eye, the greater is the depth of the indentation. A reference point is provided by a convex test block resembling the cornea but made of steel, plastic, or glass, which does not indent. On a suitable test block of this sort the tonometer should give a reading of zero.

A conversion table or graph is required to convert from scale readings obtained when the Schiotz tonometer is resting on the cornea to the corresponding mm Hg intraocular pressure (Fig. 6.3). The precision with which the scale reading can be ascertained from the tonometer is limited by oscillation of the indicator needle caused by the ocular pulse and by other physiologic moment-to-moment variations in intraocular pressure. The accuracy with which intraocular pressure can be estimated is further limited by variability of elastic properties of the eye and by variation in curvature of the cornea. In common clinical pratice, the mechanical Schiotz tonometer is read to the nearest quarter scale unit, but it is sometimes difficult to read to the nearest half scale unit. More precise readings, estimating to the nearest tenth of a scale unit, can be made with electronic Schiotz tonometers, in which the scale of the instrument is expanded by the use of electronic amplification in place of the simple lever arm.

Chart for Tonometer No. ....

Approved by the Committee on Standardization of Tonometers of the American Academy of Ophthalmology and Otolarynogology. **1955**

R Tonometer Reading	5.5 gm.	7.5 gm.	10 gm.	15 gm.
	Load, gm. Pressure, mm. Hg.			
0.0	41.5	59.1	81.7	127.5
0.5	37.8	54.2	75.1	117.9
1.0	34.5	49.8	69.3	109.3
1.5	31.6	45.8	64.0	101.4
2.0	29.0	42.1	59.1	94.3
2.5	26.6	38.8	54.7	88.0
3.0	24.4	35.8	50.6	81.8
3.5	22.4	33.0	46.9	76.2
4.0	20.6	30.4	43.4	71.0
4.5	18.9	28.0	40.2	66.2
5.0	17.3	25.8	37.2	61.8
5.5	15.9	23.8	34.4	57.6
6.0	14.6	21.9	31.8	53.6
6.5	13.4	20.1	29.4	49.9
7.0	12.2	18.5	27.2	46.5
7.5	11.2	17.0	25.1	43.2
8.0	10.2	15.6	23.1	40.2
8.5	9.4	14.3	21.3	38.1
9.0	8.5	13.1	19.6	34.6
9.5	7.8	12.0	18.0	32.0
10.0	7.1	10.9	16.5	29.6
10.5	6.5	10.0	15.1	27.4
11.0	5.9	9.0	13.8	25.8
11.5	5.3	8.3	12.6	23.3
12.0	4.9	7.5	11.5	21.4
12.5	4.4	6.8	10.5	19.7
13.0	4.0	6.2	9.5	18.1
13.5		5.6	8.6	16.5
14.0		5.0	7.8	15.1
14.5		4.5	7.1	13.7
15.0		4.0	6.4	12.6
15.5			5.8	11.4
16.0			5.2	10.4
16.5			4.7	9.4
17.0			4.2	8.5
17.5				7.7
18.0				6.9
18.5				6.2
19.0				5.6
19.5				4.9
20.0				4.5

R. O. GULDEN & CO., INC.
225 Cadwalader Ave., Elkins Park, Pa. 19117

Figure 6.3. The Schiotz tonometry calibration scale, revised in 1955. This table converts the scale reading of the Schiotz tonometer to the intraocular pressure in millimeters of mercury. Each weight is indicated by a separate column; the scale reading corresponds to an intraocular pressure dependent on the weight used.

In interpreting the scale readings obtained when the Schiotz tonometer is applied to the patient's eye, it can be said that most normal eyes give readings from 5 to 8 units on the scale and that when readings of 4 or less units on the scale are obtained, the eye should be suspected of being glaucomatous and should be subjected to additional testing.

If the IOPs indicated by the Schiotz tonometer on any type of eye are near borderline between normal and glaucomatous, the IOP should also be measured with the Goldmann applanation tonometer. In the myopic eye in particular, the IOP should be checked by an applanation tonometer, even though it is apparently normal by Schiotz tonometer. There is little need to resort to the applanation tonometer in cases in which the Schiotz tonometer gives measurements well in the glaucoma range in eyes of ordinary size and shape. There is, however, an advantage to comparing the Schiotz and applanation tonometer to determine whether the values indicated by the Schiotz tonometer are accurately applicable to a given eye or whether a correction factor is needed.

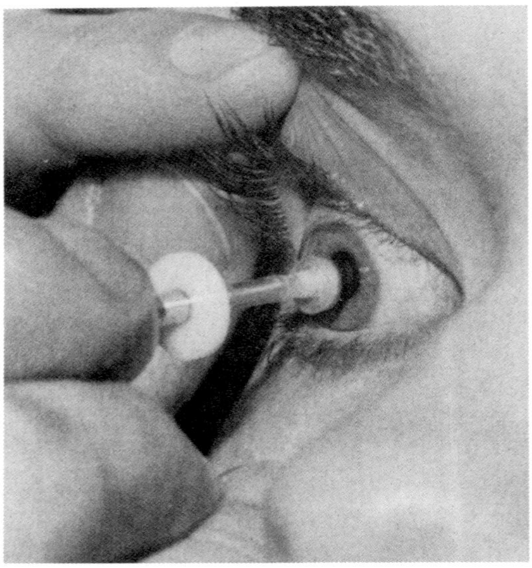

Figure 6.4. The pneumotonometer is useful in measuring IOP in patients with abnormal corneas in whom regular mires with the Goldmann applanation tonometer cannot be obtained, or in children or patients with limited ability to cooperate for Goldmann applanation tonometry. Machines, however, vary in calibration. It is best to construct "a standard curve" for a particular machine, comparing its readings to those of the Goldmann instrument in routine glaucoma patients who have normal corneas.

Patients with abnormal corneas may present difficulty in measurement of intraocular pressure. After penetrating keratoplasty, if irregular mires are observed, Goldmann applanation tonometry should be performed. **It is often useful to rotate the applanation prism into more than one meridian to check the reliability of the measurement.** If distorted mires are observed due to the presence of an abnormal cornea, the pneumotonometer (Fig. 6.4) or Mackay-Marg tonometer (Fig. 6.5) have proven useful in estimating intraocular pressure.

The **pneumotonometer** measures IOP by calculating the force required to flatten an area of cornea using an elastic membrane inflated with gas or air. The newer models use compressed air rather than fluorocarbon gas. This device is extremely useful and accurate, especially in the setting of an irregular corneal surface. Additionally, the pneumotonometer can be used against the sclera near the limbus, with IOP results nearly identical to those achieved by contact with the cornea. Pneumotonometry also produces a tracing of the IOP during measurement; this gives the examiner the ability to determine the quality of the examination. A good measurement will produce a flat tracing, with the presence of ocular pulsations evident. During the examination, there is a high-pitched, whining noise. Absence of the pulsations or of this sound indicates an error in measurement. The pneumotonometer handpiece has two lines, one black and one red, on the metal rod which moves within the handpiece and to which the elastic membrane is attached.

The **Tono-Pen** can be used for intraocular pressure measurement both as a screening tool and in eyes with irregular surfaces (Fig. 6.6) (4–6). This tonometer, however, may overestimate the intraocular pressure in eyes with low intraocular pressure, and underestimate the intraocular pressure in eyes with high intraocular pressure (6–8). The Tono-Pen also has poor reproducibility of measurements (9).

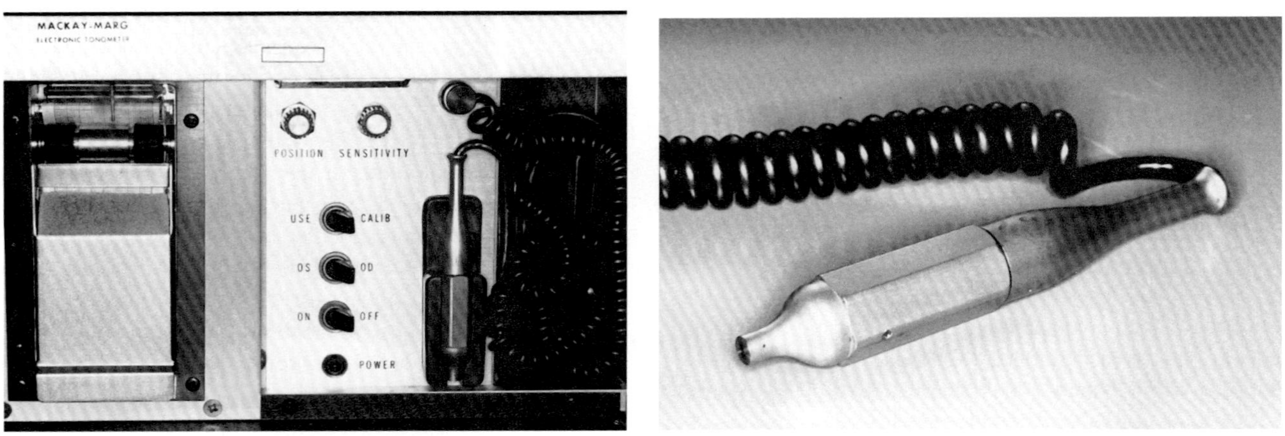

Figure 6.5. The McKay-Marg tonometer, like the pneumotonometer, is particularly valuable for intraocular pressure measurement in the setting of corneal irregularity.

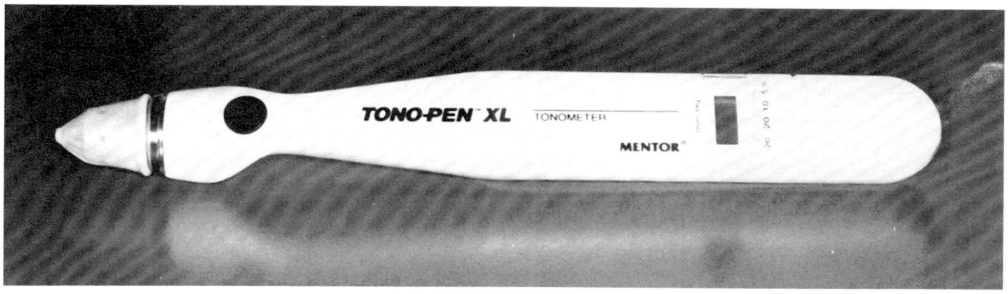

Figure 6.6. The Tonopen is a small, portable device that can be used with ease even by technicians.

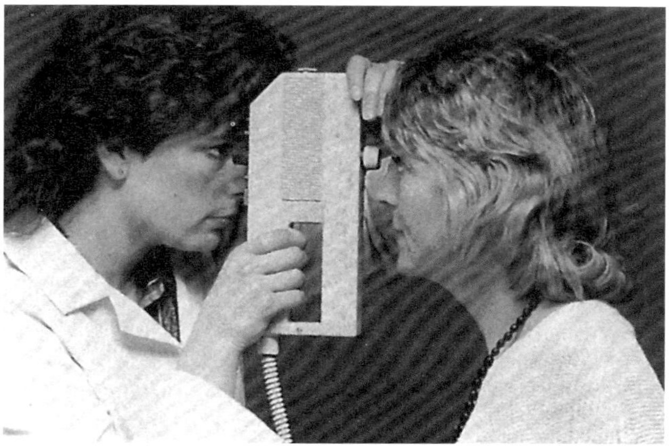

Figure 6.7. The noncontact air-puff tonometer has the advantage of minimizing the risk of transmission of communicable disease, but suffers from lack of accuracy.

Despite the problems with early models of the instrument, the Tono-Pen has improved over the years, and is in frequent use, especially by non-glaucoma specialists. The Tono-Pen's ease of use, and the fact that it can measure IOP even in the presence of corneal irregularity, have enabled technicians and other support personnel to aid in the evaluation of patients by recording IOP taken with this device. Additionally, its portability allows the use of the Tono-Pen in examination of IOP in remote locations and in screenings. Nevertheless, the Goldmann tonometer remains the "gold standard," and if available, is preferred to the Tono-Pen in the measurement of IOP.

Non-contact, **air-puff tonometers** have been used for screening of intraocular pressures, especially in optometry (Fig. 6.7). No anesthesia is required for measurement with this device. Unfortunately, reproducibility of measurements is poor (9). Additionally, a microaerosolized mist of tear film is created on use of air-puff tonometers, introducing the risk of dispersion of infectious material, particularly viral particles (10).

The estimation of IOP by palpation of the globe is notoriously inaccurate. This technique can be relied on only to determine whether the eye is hard or soft and can be depended on to distinguish an IOP greater than 30 mm Hg (11).

The following section deals with TONOGRAPHY, a technique by which the actual facility of aqueous outflow is measured in living patients. While it is the only clinical measure of trabecular meshwork function available to ophthalmologists, it is exceedingly difficult to perform and interpret, and requires the resources of a skilled technician to perform the test and a trained ophthalmologist to interpret it. Additionally, results can be variable, as well as technician dependent. For these reasons, tonography is relegated to the status of "research tool." We continue to find this a valuable clinical resource, but recognize the difficulty involved in bringing this technology to the community.

Tonography

Tonography, in ophthalmology, means recording IOP during several minutes while the eye is subjected to the weight of the Schiotz tonometer, the purpose being to determine how rapidly the pressure drops under this load, and from this to calculate the facility of aqueous outflow (12,13).

Clinically, the principal reason for resorting to tonography is that tonometry alone may not give enough information about the eye unless it is repeated several times in the course of 24 hours; the intraocular pressure may be found normal by tonometry during some portions of the day even though the facility of aqueous outflow is all the while much less than normal. In eyes with subnormal facility of aqueous outflow, significant elevation of intraocular pressure may be detectable by ordinary tonometry only if by chance the tonometry is performed at a time when the pressure happens to be elevated. Although in most cases, frequent careful tonometry can make it unnecessary for one to resort to tonography, tonography is in some ways more convenient and in certain cases can provide valuable warning of the danger of pressure rise before such a rise is actually detectable by regular tonometry. For example, one might expect that the patient with compromised outflow will experience wider swings in intraocular pressure related to variations in aqueous production than the patient with normal outflow facility. This aids the clinician in the assessment of patients, especially those with borderline intraocular pressures in the 24 to 29 mm Hg range, as these patients are likely to experience greater intraocular pressures throughout the day. The clinician sees only a snapshot of the intraocular pressure in time; tonography permits extrapolation to the intraocular pressures the patient may experience when not in the office.

Another situation in which tonography can provide a warning of potential rise of IOP before it is detectable by regular tonometry is after operation or after intraocular inflammation, which may be followed by days, weeks, or months of low IOP. If in these conditions the facility of aqueous outflow remains subnormal, eventually the IOP is likely to rise to glaucomatous levels. Tonography can provide warning of this possibilty.

In pure "primary" open-angle glaucoma, there is chronically subnormal facility of outflow, with the angle of the anterior chamber open at all times, whereas in pure angle-closure glaucoma the facility of outflow is impaired in direct proportion to the extent of closure of the angle and is entirely normal when the angle is open. Tonography in association with gonioscopy has been instrumental in establishing this fundamental difference between open-angle and angle-closure glaucoma (14,15).

Tonography has been useful not only in evaluating physiologic, pathologic and surgical influences on the hydrodynamics of the eye, but also has helped in analyzing the mode of action of drugs on the hydrodynamics of the eye. Tonographic measurements have, for instance, shown that drugs related to pilocarpine reduce intraocular pressure by enhancing facility of aqueous outflow, and have shown that drugs related to acetazolamide reduce IOP by reducing the rate of formation of aqueous humor.

The equipment needed for tonography consists of an electronic Schiotz (V. Mueller, Chicago, IL) tonometer and a recorder to make a record of the movement of the plunger of the tonometer. When an electronic Schiotz tonometer is not available, use can be made of a pneumotonometer; the procedure can then be called pneumotonography (16,17).

The technique of carrying out tonography on patients has been described in detail in the third edition of this book, but in the present edition is only briefly outlined.

With the patient comfortably recumbent, a drop of topical anesthetic is applied to each eye, and the tonometer is allowed to rest on the cornea as in ordinary tonometry. However, instead of the tonometer being applied only momentarily, it is allowed to rest on the cornea of each eye for at least 4 minutes. During this time, the tonometer and recorder will show that the IOP has been gradually falling. The aim is to obtain a smooth tonographic curve with a superimposed ocular pulse. The tonographic curve may be interpreted as follows.

Before the Schiotz tonometer is applied, the eye is in a steady state, with steady IOP, steady rate of formation of aqueous, and steady outflow of aqueous, but when the tonometer is placed on the eye the IOP is immediately artificially raised, as a result of indentation of the cornea. Raising IOP raises the rate of outflow of aqueous, with little or no influence on formation of aqueous. As soon as aqueous outflow exceeds inflow, the IOP begins to fall, gradually approaching the pressure of the original steady state. In performance of tonography the recording shows the IOP immediately raised at the start, then gradually falling. The rate of fall depends on the facility of aqueous outflow and the height to which the IOP was initially raised above steady state. Data from the first 4 to 5 minutes of recording are used for calculation of the facility of aqueous outflow (C).

For numerical evaluation of the data supplied by the tonographic curve, the initial tonometer scale reading provides, by way of standard tables, knowledge of the IOP in the steady state before application of the tonometer, and IOP with the tonometer applied to the eye. (These parameters are known as P_0 and P_T (in mm Hg), respectively.) The volume of aqueous humor expressed from the eye in excess of steady state, or as a function of time, can be obtained from standard tables relating ocular pressure (in mm Hg) to volume (in microliters). A simple nomogram can be used to determine C from scale readings at the initial peak and at 4 minutes (Fig. 6.8). Essentially the same results can be obtained from tonographic curves more quickly and conveniently by computer (18–22). The C value is expressed in microliters per minute per millimeter Hg of intraocular pressure, based on calculations for eyes of supposedly average physical characteristics. We have established by comparison of results from a large number of tonograms that the C value, obtained by means of a nomogram from scale readings at the start and at 4 minutes from a smoothed curve carefully drawn through acceptable recordings, is in good agreement with the value obtainable by more laborious calculation from a great many points on the original recordings.

For clinical detection of glaucoma, the ratio of P_0 to C is considerably more useful than either P_0 or C individually. In the absence of all forms of treatment, both local and systemic, a P_0/C ratio less than 100 is characteristic of normal eyes, while a P_0/C ratio greater than 100 is characteristic of glaucomatous eyes.

For purposes other than diagnosis, such as for evaluating effectiveness and mechanism of action of medical and surgical treatment for glaucoma, individual variations of P_0 and C are interpreted according to the belief that steady-state intraocular pressure is governed by only three variables: the net rate of flow of aqueous humor through the eye, the facility of aqueous outflow, and the back-pressure

Initial Reading		5.5 gm wt (change in scale reading)										
Po	ISR	0	.50	1.00	1.50	2.00	2.50	3.00	3.50	4.00	4.50	5.00
38	.50	0	.06	.14	.24	.39	.61	.94				
36	.75	0	.06	.13	.22	.35	.53	.78				
35	1.00	0	.05	.12	.21	.32	.47	.66	.94			
33	1.25	0	.05	.12	.19	.29	.42	.59	.81			
32	1.50	0	.05	.11	.18	.27	.38	.53	.71	.94		
30	1.75	0	.05	.11	.17	.25	.35	.48	.64	.83		
29	2.00	0	.05	.10	.16	.24	.33	.44	.58	.74	.93	
28	2.25	0	.05	.10	.16	.23	.31	.41	.53	.68	.84	
27	2.50	0	.04	.09	.15	.22	.30	.39	.49	.62	.76	.92
25	2.75	0	.04	.09	.15	.21	.28	.37	.46	.58	.70	.84
24	3.00	0	.04	.09	.14	.20	.27	.35	.44	.54	.65	.78
23	3.25	0	.04	.09	.14	.20	.26	.33	.42	.51	.62	.74
22	3.50	0	.04	.08	.13	.19	.25	.32	.40	.49	.59	.70
22	3.75	0	.04	.08	.13	.19	.25	.31	.38	.47	.56	.66
21	4.00	0	.04	.08	.13	.18	.24	.30	.37	.45	.54	.63
20	4.25	0	.04	.08	.13	.18	.24	.30	.36	.43	.52	.60
19	4.50	0	.04	.08	.12	.17	.23	.29	.35	.42	.50	.58
18	4.75	0	.04	.08	.12	.17	.23	.28	.34	.41	.48	.56
17	5.00	0	.04	.08	.12	.17	.22	.27	.33	.40	.47	.54
17	5.25	0	.04	.08	.12	.17	.22	.27	.33	.39	.46	.53
16	5.50	0	.04	.08	.12	.16	.21	.26	.32	.38	.45	.52
15	5.75	0	.04	.08	.12	.16	.21	.26	.32	.38	.44	.50
15	6.00	0	.03	.07	.11	.15	.20	.25	.31	.37	.43	.49
14	6.25	0	.03	.07	.11	.15	.20	.25	.31	.37	.43	.49
13	6.50	0	.03	.07	.11	.15	.20	.25	.30	.36	.42	.48
13	6.75	0	.03	.07	.11	.15	.20	.24	.30	.36	.41	.47
12	7.00	0	.03	.07	.11	.15	.20	.24	.29	.35	.40	.46
11	7.50	0	.03	.07	.11	.15	.19	.24	.29	.34	.39	.45
10	8.00	0	.03	.07	.11	.15	.19	.24	.29	.34	.39	.45
9	8.50	0	.03	.07	.11	.15	.19	.23	.28	.33	.39	
9	9.00	0	.03	.07	.11	.15	.19	.23	.28	.33		
8	9.50	0	.03	.07	.11	.15	.19	.23	.28			
7	10.00	0	.03	.07	.11	.15	.19	.23				
6	11.00	0	.03	.07	.11	.15						

Initial Reading		7.5 gm. wt. (Change In Scale Reading)										
Po	ISR	0	.50	1.00	1.50	2.00	2.50	3.00	3.50	4.00	4.50	5.00
54	.50	0	.05	.12	.23	.41	.76					
52	.75	0	.05	.12	.21	.36	.63					
50	1.00	0	.04	.11	.19	.32	.50	.79				
48	1.25	0	.04	.10	.17	.29	.44	.65				
46	1.50	0	.04	.09	.16	.26	.38	.55	.79			
44	1.75	0	.04	.09	.15	.24	.34	.48	.67			
42	2.00	0	.04	.09	.14	.22	.31	.43	.58	.78		
41	2.25	0	.04	.09	.14	.20	.29	.39	.52	.68		
39	2.50	0	.04	.08	.13	.19	.27	.36	.47	.60	.77	
37	2.75	0	.04	.08	.13	.18	.25	.33	.43	.54	.68	
36	3.00	0	.03	.07	.12	.17	.23	.31	.40	.50	.62	.76
34	3.25	0	.03	.07	.12	.17	.22	.29	.37	.46	.57	.69
33	3.50	0	.03	.07	.11	.16	.21	.28	.35	.43	.53	.63
32	3.75	0	.03	.07	.11	.15	.21	.26	.33	.41	.49	.59
30	4.00	0	.03	.06	.10	.15	.20	.25	.32	.39	.46	.55
29	4.25	0	.03	.06	.10	.15	.19	.25	.30	.37	.44	.52
28	4.50	0	.03	.06	.10	.14	.18	.24	.29	.35	.42	.50
27	4.75	0	.03	.06	.10	.14	.18	.23	.28	.34	.40	.47
26	5.00	0	.03	.06	.10	.13	.17	.22	.27	.33	.39	.45
25	5.25	0	.03	.06	.10	.13	.17	.22	.27	.32	.38	.43
24	5.50	0	.03	.06	.09	.13	.16	.21	.26	.31	.37	.42
23	5.75	0	.03	.06	.09	.13	.16	.21	.26	.31	.36	.41
22	6.00	0	.03	.06	.09	.12	.16	.20	.25	.30	.35	.40
21	6.25	0	.03	.06	.09	.12	.16	.20	.25	.29	.34	.39
20	6.50	0	.03	.05	.09	.12	.15	.19	.24	.28	.33	.39
19	6.75	0	.03	.05	.09	.12	.15	.19	.24	.28	.33	.38
18	7.00	0	.03	.05	.08	.12	.15	.19	.23	.27	.32	.37
17	7.50	0	.03	.05	.08	.12	.15	.19	.23	.27	.31	.36
16	8.00	0	.03	.05	.08	.11	.15	.18	.22	.26	.30	.35
14	8.50	0	.03	.05	.08	.11	.15	.18	.22	.26	.30	
13	9.00	0	.03	.05	.08	.11	.15	.18	.22	.25		
12	9.50	0	.03	.05	.08	.11	.15	.18	.22			
11	10.00	0	.03	.05	.08	.11	.14	.18				
10	11.00	0	.03	.05	.08	.11	.14					

Figure 6.8. The 1955 nomogram for estimation of outflow facility by tonography. Three columns are present, as in Schiotz tonometry, for correlation of scale value to outflow facility dependent on the weight used during testing.

in the recipient veins. Since the recipient venous pressure seldom varies, except in unusual conditions, the steady-state intraocular pressure is considered to be governed principally by the other two variables, the net rate of aqueous flow and the facility of aqueous outflow. Thus, at levels of intraocular pressure above the normal recipient venous pressure of about 10 mm Hg, any lack of correlation between measured variation in P_0 and C is blamed on variation in rate of aqueous formation.

However, there has been increasing recognition that variation in uveosceral outflow needs also to be taken into consideration, particularly in studies of mechanism of action of drugs that influence intraocular pressure (23).

The possibility of error in evaluating P_0 and C because of abnormalities of the physical characteristics of individual eyes is quite real when the conversion from Schiotz scale readings to P_0 and C values is based on data for average normal eyes. At present, the most sensitive and reliable means for detecting significant abnormalities in the elastic properties of individual eyes is based on comparison of the P_0 value given by the Goldmann applanation tonometer and the P_0 value given by the Schiotz tonometer.

Table 6.1 contains typical data derived from tonographic measurements to illustrate how the basic parameters of episcleral venous pressure (P_e), flow rate or rate of formation of aqueous humor (F), facility of outflow (C), and intraocular pressure relate to one another in various types of eyes (Table 6.1). Not included in this table are data for "pseudofacility," i.e., suppression of aqueous formation by intraocular pressure. Also not included are data for change in facility of outflow by intraocular pressure, and data for uveoscleral outflow. However, the data that are presented suffice to illustrate some general conceptual principles concerning the manner in which normal and glaucomatous eyes differ from each other clinically, in the behavior of their intraocular pressure.

In this table, the episcleral venous pressure (P_e) has been assumed to be constant at 9 mm Hg under all the illustrated clinical circumstances. This is probably a valid approximation according to most of what has been published on the subject, but there are conditions in which P_e is significantly different. These special conditions will be considered elsewhere. This table is intended to illustrate only the most common clinical conditions and concepts.

In the first section of this table, which exemplifies "normal" parameters, **a twofold change in the rate of aqueous formation can be expected to cause a change in intraocular pressure of only 4 mm Hg, and a change in facility of outflow of 0.05 μl/min/mm Hg is expected to produce a change of intraocular pressure of only 1 mm Hg in a normal eye.**

Table 6.1
Examples of Difference in the Degree to Which the Intraocular Pressure (P) is Calculated to Be Affected by Changes in Flow (F) and Facility of Outflow (C) in Different Types of Eyes, Assuming Constant Episcleral Venous Pressure (Pe)

	(mm Hg) Pe	+	(μl/min) (F	÷	(μl/min/mm Hg) C)	=	(mm Hg) P
Normal =	9		1.5		0.25		15
	9		1 to 2		0.25		13 to 17
	9		1.5		0.30		14
Glaucoma =	9		1.5		0.05		39
	9		1 to 2		0.05		29 to 49
	9		1.5		0.10		24
Good normal =	9		1.5		0.30		14
½ angle closed =	9		1.5		0.15		19
¾ angle closed =	9		1.5		0.075		29
Poor normal =	9		1.5		0.15		19
½ angle closed =	9		1.5		0.075		29
¾ angle closed =	9		1.5		0.0375		49

In the second section of the table, exemplifying "glaucoma," the noteworthy differences from the normal include the low facility of outflow and the elevated intraocular pressure, and in particular, the fact that **a twofold change in the rate of aqueous formation can be expected to cause a change in intraocular pressure of 20 mm Hg instead of the 4 mm Hg change seen in the "normal" eye.** Furthermore, in the "glaucoma" example, a change in facility of outflow of 0.05 μl/min/mm Hg is expected to produce a change in intraocular pressure of 15 mm Hg, in contrast to the 1 mm Hg change seen in the normal eye. The main concept to be derived from this comparison is that **glaucomatous eyes have reason to exhibit greater variability of pressure than normal eyes in response to changes in aqueous formation and in facility of outflow.** This helps explain to us why a glaucomatous eye (with open angles) can show spontaneous diurnal variations of pressure considerably greater than normal and why various drugs that influence facility of outflow or aqueous formation tend to cause greater changes in pressure in glaucomatous than in normal eyes.

The data presented in the lower half of Table 6.1 exemplify relationships between the extent of closure of the filtration angle (by synechia or by apposition of the iris to the trabecular meshwork) and the intraocular pressure, as influenced also by the underlying characteristics of a given eye when its angle is normally open. It will be noted that in the lower half of the table, we are concerned with a "good normal" eye and a "poor normal" eye. This distinction is based on the fact that among normal human eyes there is a wide range of normal pressures (e.g., 10–20 mm Hg) and a range of normal values of facility of outflow (e.g., 0.15–0.60). Thus some eyes are naturally far from glaucomatous, for instance the "good normal" eye in the table with facility of outflow of 0.30 μl/min/mm Hg and intraocular pressure of 14 mm Hg. Other eyes are not so far from the end of the normal range where it begins to border on glaucomatous, for instance the "poor normal" eye with facility of outflow of 0.15 μl/min/mm Hg and intraocular pressure of 19 mm Hg.

The next conceptually and practically important point is to note the effects of obstructing aqueous outflow through the angle of the anterior chamber in either one-half or three-quarters of its circumference (such as by peripheral anterior synechias or by appositional angle closure). Obstruction of half the circumference reduces the facility of outflow by 50% and obstruction of three-quarters reduces facility of outflow by 75%. The practical clinical consequence of this upon the intraocular pressure is different for the "good normal" eye with its angle completely open than for the "poor normal" eye with its angle open. Closing or otherwise obstructing the filtration angle in half of the circumference raises the pressure in both eyes; only to 19 mm Hg (still within the normal range) in the "good normal" eye, but to 29 mm Hg in the "poor normal" eye. With closure of three-quarters of the angle, the difference between the eyes in resultant elevation of intraocular pressure is still more drastic, 29 mm Hg compared with 49 mm Hg.

We conclude from these considerations, derived from our clinical tonographic and gonioscopic observations, that it is useful to take into account the original facility of outflow and intraocular pressure of a given eye when attempting to assess how much of a therapeutic problem a given extent of PAS may pose for that eye. This may have a decisive influence on the choice of operation, and will be considered further in Chapter 23, where it is pointed out that angle-closure glaucoma often develops in one eye before the other and that comparing tonographic and gonioscopic data from the eye with closure of part of its angle compared with data from the contralateral eye with its open angle can be utilized to advantage in deciding on the type of treatment.

Diurnal Variations

In normal eyes, the intraocular pressure varies not more than 2 or 3 mm Hg throughout the day and night. Also, in some glaucomatous eyes, the pressure shows little variation and remains elevated at all times. However, more characteristically in glaucomatous eyes, the pressure varies up and down in a diurnal pattern that seems to be an exaggeration of the slight variation detectable in normal eyes. This variation can be studied best in eyes in which there is a constant obstruction to aqueous outflow, such as in glaucoma due to peripheral anterior synechias, to traumatic recession of the angle, to the innate changes in the aqueous outflow channels in well-established primary open-angle glaucoma, in open-angle glaucoma associated with exfoliation, or in pigmentary glaucoma. (One cannot identify the diurnal variation of pressure so well in intermittent angle-closure glaucoma because of additional and confusing variation attributable to opening and closing of the angle.)

From tonographic measurements in eyes having various forms of open-angle glaucoma uncomplicated by intraocular inflammation, the facility of aqueous outflow is usually at almost the same subnormal value at both the high and low points in the diurnal curves of variation of intraocular pressure. The pressure in the aqueous veins has been reported to remain essentially constant. Therefore, we conclude that the fluctuation of intraocular pressure is attributable mainly to a varying rate of formation of aqueous humor.

Observations on patients having different severity of open-angle glaucoma in the two eyes or having one normal and one glaucomatous eye show that the spontaneous diurnal variations of pressure usually run parallel in the two eyes but that in the eye having the greater obstruction to aqueous outflow, the variation in pressure characteristically exceeds the variation in the more nearly normal eye. There may be a striking difference in the two eyes in the amplitude of fluctuation, but usually not in the timing.

The range of diurnal variation of intraocular pressure for a given severity of glaucoma varies greatly from patient to patient and seems to be more closely related to some special characteristic of the individual patient than to the absolute degree of obstruction of aqueous outflow. One cannot predict with certainty from the fact that the tonographic facility of outflow is low that there will be significant diurnal fluctuation of IOP, but the likelihood of large fluctuation is slight in eyes with normal or near-normal facility of outflow.

These observations strongly suggest that the variation in the rate of aqueous formation that is manifest in both eyes simultaneously must result from some systemic controlling influence reaching both eyes simultaneously. One can be reasonably sure that this influence does not reach the eyes via the ocular nerves. Clinical observations on patients who have various defective innervations of the eye and experimental studies on animals involving either stimulation or interruption of nerves to the eye have not as yet provided evidence for neural influence on diurnal variation of aqueous formation or intraocular pressure of the magnitude that is observed clinically. The only other way in which systemic influences might reach the eye would be through variations in composition of the blood or through variations in circulating hormones. Hormonal control seems to us to be the most attractive probability.

When investigating the mechanism of diurnal variation of intraocular pressure, it is attractive to attempt to relate this to diurnal variations in other physiologic functions, such as kidney function, and this may ultimately prove fruitful. A peculiarity of the diurnal variation of intraocular pressure is that in most glaucomatous patients it results in rise of pressure to a maximum early in the morning before the patient gets out of bed, but in another considerable proportion of patients, the maximum occurs at a different time, such as late afternoon or evening. The reason for these differences is unknown. However, these individual differences may well prove to be a valuable feature when attempts are made to correlate this phenomenon with other systemic variables.

No investigator has provided a greater understanding of aqueous humor flow than Brubaker and his coworkers. Brubaker has demonstrated through fluorophotometry, a technique (24,25) that demonstrates aqueous humor production by diffusion of fluorescein into the anterior chamber and then dilution of that fluorescein concentration over time, that **the rate of aqueous humor production is lowest during sleep and it increases dramatically just before waking** (26). The cycle of aqueous production corresponds to the diurnal variation in intraocular pressure. Further, Brubaker's most recent studies indicate that circulating catecholamines, specifically epinephrine, may be responsible for the diurnal variation in aqueous production (26).

One feature of diurnal IOP variation that deserves particular thought is that the fundamental problem seems to be not so much to explain the high phase of IOP as it is to explain the low phase of the IOP. When the IOP is high, it appears from tonographic measurements that aqueous humor is being formed at a normal rate and that when the IOP decreases spontaneously to a lower level, with facility of outflow still subnormal, this decrease of pressure is attributable to a decrease in aqueous formation to a subnormal rate. An explanation is needed for this decrease in aqueous formation. If we understood it, we might be able to exploit it therapeutically.

Practically, measurement of the intraocular pressure at intervals of 2 to 4 hours around the clock is a valuable procedure, not only in establishing the diagnosis of glaucoma, but in the management of cases of established open-angle glaucoma. If IOP is measured in the office at approximately the same time at each visit, we may be measuring

IOP at the time of the lowest level of diurnal variation and thus have a false sense of security, whereas if the IOP had been measured at a different time of day we might have found a considerably elevated IOP and then would have realized that things were not going as well as we had thought. With hospital costs so high, it is impractical in most cases to admit a patient to the hospital for IOP studies around the clock. Furthermore, the necessarily "artificial" inpatient environment seems in some patients to alter the magnitude of the diurnal variation. A possible alternative is to see the patient in the office at intervals from early morning until late in the afternoon for measurement of IOP. However, the amplitude of the IOP variation from day to day may not be constant, and it may be necessary to make repeated IOP measurements during three or more cycles to obtain a fair understanding of the degree and timing of the variation.

An even better way is to furnish the patient with a Schiotz, Tono-Pen or other home tonometer and teach a member of the family to measure the IOP at various times during the day and night. We have found this valuable in a number of instances, although this is not suitable for many patients.

References

1. Goldmann H: Applanation tonometry. In: Symposium on Glaucoma. Transactions of the Second Conference. New York: Josiah Macy Jr. Foundation, 1957.
2. Menage MJ, Kaufman PL, Croft MA, et al: Intraocular pressure measurement after penetrating keratoplasty: Minified Goldmann applanation tonometer, pneumatonometer, and Tono-Pen versus manometry. Br J Ophthalmol 1994;78:671–676.
3. O'Donoghue E: The minified Goldmann applanation tonometer. Br J Ophthalmol 1994;78:671–676.
4. Christoffersen T, Fors T, Ringberg U, et al: Tonometry in the general practice setting (I): Tono-Pen compared to Goldmann applanation tonometry. Acta Ophthalmologica 1993;71:103–108.
5. Denis P, Normann JP, Bertin V, et al: Evaluation of the Tono-Pen 2 and the X-Pert noncontact tonometers in cataract surgery. Ophthalmologica 1993;207:155–161.
6. Geyer O, Mayron Y, Loewenstein A, et al: Tono-Pen tonometry in normal and in post-keratoplasty eyes. Br J Ophthalmol 1992;76:538–540.
7. Moore CG, Milne ST, Morrison JC: Noninvasive measurement of rat intraocular pressure with the Tono-Pen. Invest Ophthalmol Vis Sci 1993;34:363–369.
8. Zimmerman TJ, Gupte RK, Wall JL: Tonometry comparison: Goldmann versus Tono-Pen. Ann Ophthalmol 1992;24:29–36.
9. Wilson MR, Baker RS, Mohammadi P, et al: Reproducibility of postural changes in intraocular pressure with the Tono-Pen and Pulsair tonometers. Am J Ophthalmol 1993;116:479–483.
10. Britt JM, Clifton BC, Barnebey HS, et al: Microaerosol formation in noncontact air-puff; tonometry. Arch Ophthalmol 1991;109:225–228.
11. Baum J, Chaturvedi N, Netland PA, et al: Assessment of intraocular pressure by palpation. Am J Ophthalmol 1995;119:650–651.
12. Grant WM: Past, present, and future. Ophthalmology 1978;85: 252–258.
13. Grant WM: A tonographic method for measuring the facility and rate of aqueous flow in human eyes. Arch Ophthalmol 1950;44:204–314.
14. Chandler PA: Narrow angle glaucoma. Arch Ophthalmol 1952;47: 695–716.
15. Grant WM: Clinical measurements of aqueous outflow. Arch Ophthalmol 1951;46:113–131.
16. Feghali JG, Azar DT, Kaufman PL: Comparative aqueous outflow facility measurements by pneumotonography and Schiotz tonography. Invest Ophthalmol Vis Sci 1986;27:1776–80.
17. Langham ME, Leydhecker W, Krieglstein G, et al: Pneumotonographic studies on normal and glaucomatus eyes. Adv Ophthalmol 1976;32: 108–33.
18. Woodhouse DF: A computer evaluation on tonography. Exp Eye Res 1969:127–142.
19. Dallow RL, Adler A, Weihrer AL, et al: Tonogram reading by digital computer. Am J Ophthalmol 1970;70:922–928.
20. Brennen M: Tonography Software and Hardware Interface. Ann Ophthalmol 1984;16:1133–1135.
21. Eisenberg DL, Schuman JL, Wang N: An ultra-sensitive ocular perfusion system. Invest Ophthalmol Vis Sci ARVO Suppl 1984.
22. Teitelbaum CS, Podos SM, Lustgarden JS: Comparison of standard and computerized tonography instruments on human eyes. Am J Ophthalmol 1985;99:403–410.
23. Crawford K, Kaufman PL, Gabelt BT: Effects of topical PGF2 alpha on aqueous humor dynamics in cynomolgus monkeys. Curr Eye Res 1987; 6:1035–44.
24. Maurice DM: The movement of fluorescein and water in the cornea. Am J Ophthalmol 1960;49:1011–1016.
25. Jones RF, Maurice DM: New methods of measuring the rate of aqueous flow in man with fluorescein. Exp Eye Res 1966;5:208–220.
26. Brubaker RF: Flow of aqueous humor in humans. Invest Ophthalmol Vis Sci 1991;32:3145–3166.

The Angle of the Anterior Chamber

7

W. Morton Grant
Joel S. Schuman

The angle of the anterior chamber normally provides the main outflow system for aqueous humor. In most of the glaucomas, it is here that aqueous outflow is obstructed. Gonioscopy is our clinical means for looking into the angle and identifying the cause of obstruction in many cases.

GONIOSCOPY (PROCEDURE)

Gonioscopy is one of the most important tools in the management of glaucoma. Of course, many cases of glaucoma have been and are being treated successfully without gonioscopy, but in many other cases gonioscopy may be the sole means of arriving at the correct diagnosis, leading to the correct treatment. Inaccurate gonioscopy may not only be unhelpful, it may actually be misleading. Whereas accurate gonioscopy can give one the correct diagnosis and can point to the most appropriate treatment, an incorrect interpretation of the gonioscopic findings may lead the ophthalmologist far astray. It is certainly worth the time and effort to learn gonioscopy well and to make the best use of it in every case of glaucoma.

In this chapter, we will describe methods that in our hands have been most satisfactory for learning gonioscopic anatomy and for performing gonioscopy on patients. Throughout the text, frequent consideration will be given to gonioscopic findings. Peculiarities of the angle in infants and children, as well as congenital abnormalities of the angle, are discussed in Chapters 68–71.

LEARNING GONIOSCOPY

The most effective and valuable step in learning gonioscopy makes use of enucleated human eyes, such as used as donors in corneal transplanting procedures. By studying the angle of the anterior chamber with the binocular microscope and by performing simple dissections, one can obtain the best understanding of the identity and anatomical relationship of the structures seen in the eyes of patients.

To obtain the most instructive view of the anatomy of the angle, one makes a cut with a razor blade perpendicularly through the center of the cornea, bisecting the anterior segment, cutting smoothly through the angle structures and the anterior 2 or 3 mm of sclera on both sides. Then, with scissors, one-half of the bisected anterior segment is removed by cutting the sclera circumferentially, parallel to the limbus. This leaves half the circumference of angle open to direct viewing as in clinical gonioscopy and, at the same time, provides a cross-sectional display of the angle where the structures have been cut by the razor blade at both sides of the hemisphere.

The eyes prepared in this manner can be examined with a slit-lamp microscope or a dissecting microscope; or one can use the hand-held gonioscopy microscope and a focal illuminator, as in clinical Koeppe gonioscopy. In this arrangement there is, of course, no need for a gonioscopic contact lens, as there is no cornea in the line of view.

One should first identify the structures of the cross-sectioned angles, since this will be the most readily recognizable aspect, because it is similar to the cross-sectional type of view that is so familiar in microscopic histology slides used in the study of ocular pathology. One should have no trouble in identifying ciliary muscle, ciliary processes, and iris, as well as sclera and cornea. Finer details may require considerable study to recognize, and it is helpful to have a stained microscopic section to refer to for comparison.

In the dissected unstained eye there is a conspicuous continuous dark brown, almost black, pigmented layer on the back surface of the iris and on the processes and pars plana of the ciliary body, but beneath this pigmented layer the ciliary body and the ciliary muscle are remarkably pale and colorless. In bisected eyes the ciliary muscle is often separated from the sclera by an artifactual "anterior choroidal separation" except at its most anterior extremity where it attaches like a fine tendon to the scleral spur and corneoscleral trabecular meshwork. Just anterior and close to the scleral spur, a fine slit can be identified as Schlemm's canal, cut in cross section. For easier identification, the lumen of Schlemm's canal may be caused to open slightly by gentle traction applied to the ciliary muscle or to the iris.

Angle structures that are seen in frontal view of the angle can be identified with the same structures in the cross-sectional view, by following each structure from its perpendicularly cut surface to the farthest recess of the open anterior chamber. In this way, one should be able to identify the corneoscleral trabecular meshwork, Schlemm's canal, scleral spur, and ciliary band.

On further study, one can see that the corneoscleral

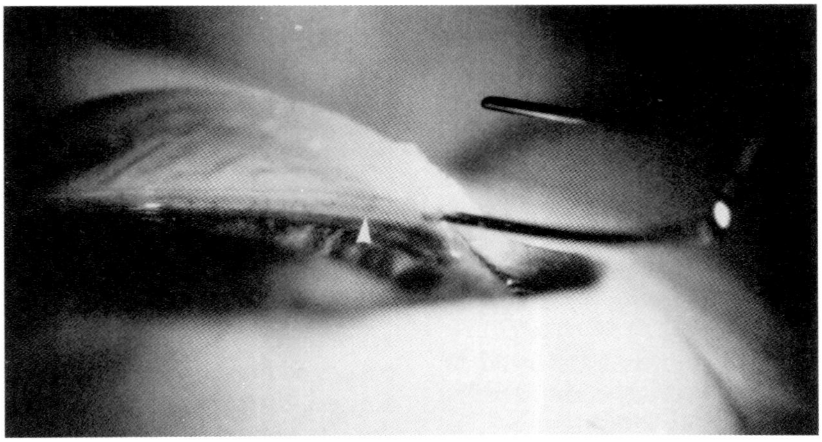

Figure 7.1. A dissected human eye with trabeculotomy probe inserted into Schlemm's canal. The latter lies sclerad to the posterior half of the trabecular meshwork (the filtration portion), which is just above the scleral spur (arrowhead). (Courtesy of Robert Rosenquist, MD, and Jean Pei, MD).

trabecular meshwork and the scleral spur have a special whiteness that is attributable to a background of white sclera. A transition from the white of the scleral spur to the slight gray shade of the ciliary band can be seen. Posterior to the scleral spur the sclera curves away with a greater radius of curvature so that it is more tangential to the gonioscopic line of view than is the scleral background of the corneoscleral trabecular meshwork and therefore reflects the gonioscopic light less efficiently. Furthermore, the anterior end of translucent ciliary muscle is attached to the scleral spur and this also reduces the amount of light reflected from the sclera posterior to the spur. In white races, there is little or no pigment in the anterior sclera or ciliary muscle to influence the color of the ciliary band. Only in darkly pigmented races is pigmentation in these structures sometimes enough to make the ciliary band appear slate gray, with or without distinguishable brown infiltration.

Schlemm's canal (Fig. 7.1) and the filtration portion of the trabecular meshwork, just anterior to scleral spur, are often demarcated in eyes of elderly people by a finely granular collection of pigmented particles within the portion of the trabecular meshwork overlying Schlemm's canal. This pigment is visible as a narrow, finely granular, brown band just anterior to the white of scleral spur within that portion of the trabecular meshwork which separates Schlemm's canal and anterior chamber, through which aqueous humor passes to reach Schlemm's canal.

Once the principal anatomical features of the angle have been learned in enucleated eyes, it is easy to proceed to examination of patients, to become familiar with features that are not otherwise readily appreciated, particularly the variable character of anterior chamber depth, contour of iris, distribution and texture of uveal meshwork, and presence of blood vessels in iris and angle. Variations of details in the gonioscopic findings and abnormalities in the angle will be discussed later on in this chapter.

CLINICAL PROCEDURE

For clinical gonioscopy, the equipment that proved most satisfactory to us in the 1950s to 1990s included: (1) the

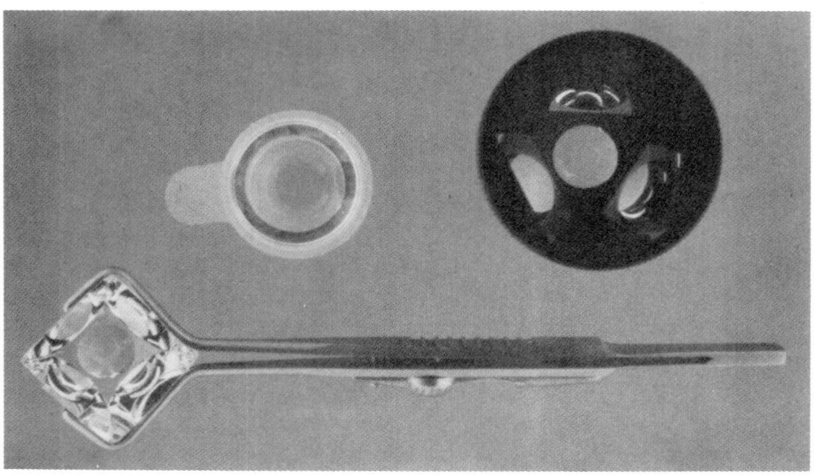

Figure 7.2. Three types of gonioscopic lenses: Koeppe (top left), Goldmann (top right), and Zeiss four-mirror (bottom).

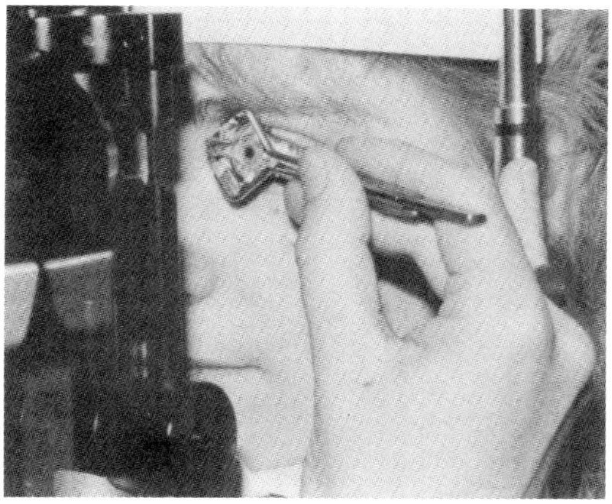

Figure 7.3. A Zeiss lens is in use at the slit lamp. This lens is useful for rapidly viewing the angle without the need for gonioscopic fluid. Indentation with this lens allows identification of peripheral anterior synechias.

Koeppe gonioscopy contact lens, (2) the Barkan hand-held focal illuminator, or alternately, a transilluminator or muscle light and (3) a hand-held binocular microscope.

In more recent times, other gonioscopic equipment has become more popular, particularly to meet requirements of new procedures, such as laser treatment of the angle (Figs. 7.2, 7.3).

Modern systems of gonioscopy employ mirrored contact lenses, such as the Goldmann lens and the slit-lamp biomicroscope, and require the patient to be sitting up. **These lenses provide a reversed image, but the image is not crossed.** In other words, if one were looking at the inferior angle through a Goldmann lens, with the goniomirror centered at 12:00, the 7:00 angle would be seen at the 11:00 position, the 6:00 angle at the 12:00 position, and the 5:00 angle at the 1:00 position (Fig. 7.4).

The lens and light source must be manipulated to alter the angle of view over peripheral convex iris or to examine successive portions of the circumference. The need for these manipulations may result in a false interpretation of angle depth. For example, in eyes having convex irides, the angle may appear to be partially closed with a mirrored contact lens due to the inability to vary the angle of view so as to look down into the crack between iris and angle wall. We have seen numerous examples in which such angles that were judged to be closed by use of a mirrored lens have in fact been observed to be open to the full width of trabecular meshwork, scleral spur, and occasionally, even narrow ciliary body band with use of a Koeppe lens system.

On the other hand, corneal distortion and indentation with the use of a mirrored contact lens can actually open an angle that is appositionally occluded. The angle is opened by posterior displacement of aqueous humor against the iris, consequent to the corneal indentation. This phenomenon is actually put to good use with the Zeiss indentation gonioscopy lens, popularized by Max Forbes, (1) in which such displacement can be used to identify peripheral anterior synechias (PAS). Because differentiating open-angle from angle-closure glaucoma is perhaps the most important question asked during clinical gonioscopy, **we routinely employ the Koeppe system as the first method of gonioscopy, particularly in new patients,** for it allows a direct view into the angle over a convex iris without corneal distortion (2). Additionally, it permits

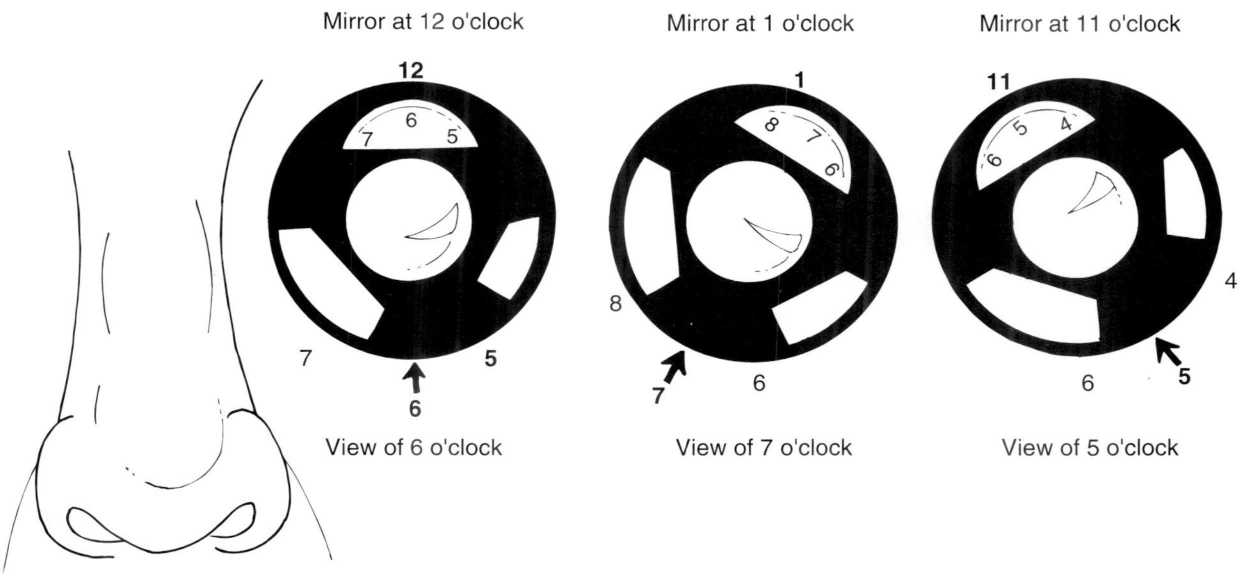

Figure 7.4. The mirrored goniolens does not invert the image of the angle. If the mirror is centered at 12:00, the 12:00 position of the mirror represents 6:00, the 11:00 position of the mirror represents 7:00, and the 1:00 position of the mirror represents 5:00. Knowledge of the position in the angle relative to the image in the mirror is essential, particularly in laser treatment of the angle.

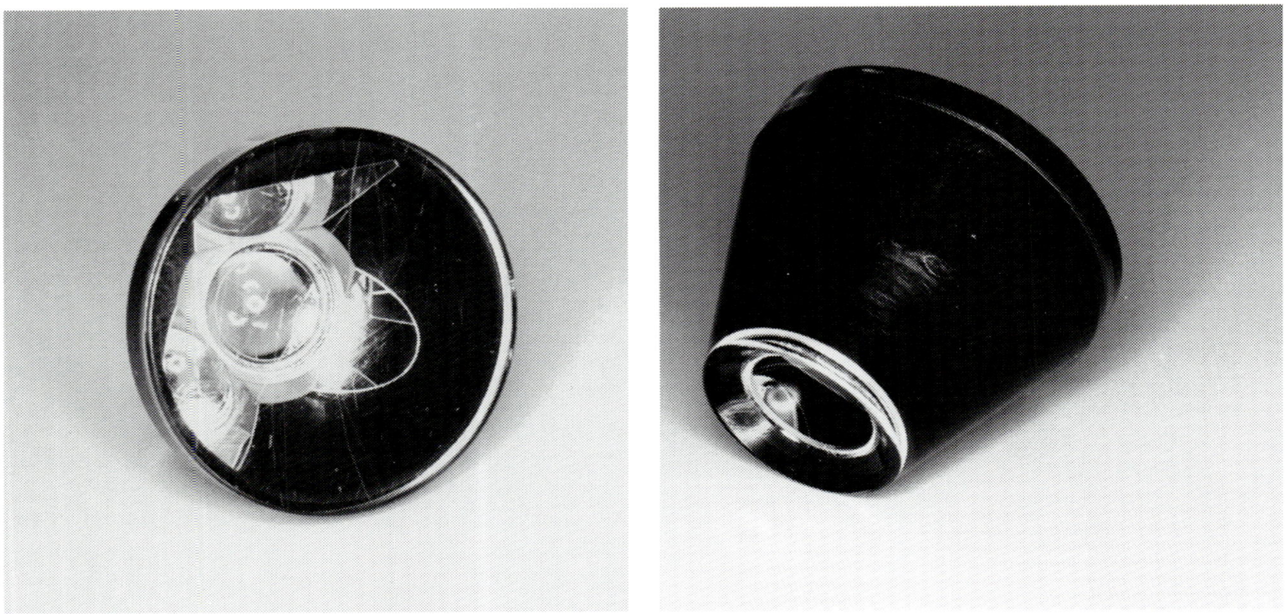

Figure 7.5. Goldmann 3-mirror lens gonioscopy. The Goldmann lens allows high magnification examination of angle structures. The rounded, parabola shaped mirror is used for gonioscopy.

bilateral, simultaneous gonioscopy, as well as examination of the angle by multiple observers without removal and replacement of contact lenses. In cases of suspected angle closure, this can then be followed by indentation gonioscopy with the Zeiss lens, to evaluate the angle for the presence of PAS.

We recommend that the beginner learn to perform gonioscopy with the single, simple, universally applicable system of direct examination with the Koeppe lens, and then to use the various mirrored indirect lenses (Figs. 7.5 and 7.6). For example, the Goldmann gonioscopic lens provides an excellent high-magnification view of certain angle details, such as new blood vessels, and inflammatory deposits. Use of this gonioscopic lens is required when performing laser treatment to the angle and it needs to be mastered by the ophthalmologist. The Zeiss indentation gonioscopy lens is invaluable in identifying peripheral anterior synechias during indentation and can be used to rapidly view an angle at the slit lamp in a postoperative patient.

GOLDMANN THREE-MIRRORED GONIOSCOPY

The Goldmann three-mirror lens is an invaluable tool, and is the utility player of the gonioscopist's roster. It is useful in quick evaluation of the angle, as well as for intense, high-powered scrutiny, laser trabeculoplasty or gonioplasty, examination of the peripheral retina or even ste-

A 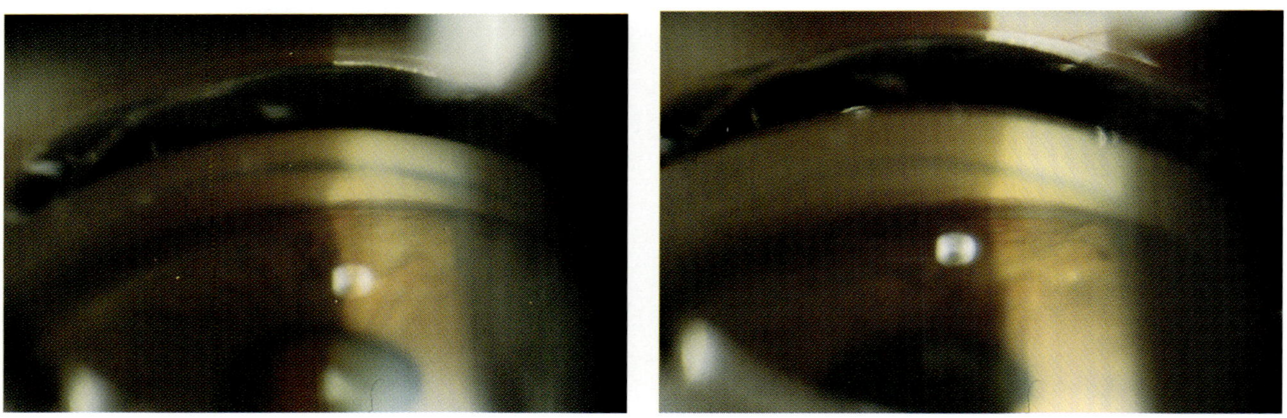 B

Figure 7.6. Zeiss indentation gonioscopy. **A,** Zeiss gonioscopy view of closed angle. **B,** Indentation gonioscopy reveals appositional closure, with absence of peripheral anterior synechias.

reoscopic study of the optic nerve head. The student of gonioscopy must become a master with this lens to succeed at the task, but such mastery is not difficult.

The lens is applied using methylcellulose as a coupling agent. The patient's lids are spread wide, and the lens is fitted into the palpebral fissure by using one edge to push down the lower lid from the bulbar side, then inserting the upper portion of the lens beneath the upper lid, while lifting that lid with the other hand. Performing this procedure gently is essential in order to maintain the patient's confidence.

Once the lens is in place, the angle is studied using the goniomirror, the parabola shaped mirror of the three, which reflects the trabecular meshwork and other structures. The slit lamp biomicroscope is used at high power, and the slit beam is adjusted so as to distinguish the structures in the angle. The slit beam can be narrowed to give the parallelopiped effect, in which the beam reflected from the anterior cornea, and that portion reflected from the posterior cornea, come together at Schwalbe's line. This can be used in poorly pigmented angles to determine whether the angle is open or not, if the landmarks of the trabecular meshwork are indistinguishable due to pallor. The techniques of gonioscopy are described below, but some mention should be made first of the Zeiss goniolens.

ZEISS FOUR-MIRRORRED GONIOSCOPY

The Zeiss four-mirror goniolens is every gonioscopist's friend, handy for a quick assessment of the angle or for indentation gonioscopy to determine if closure is appositional or synechial. This lens requires only the natural tears for coupling, and of course, topical anesthetic for the patient. While the lens is useful, one can easily be mislead with the Zeiss lens, such as by a convex iris in which the angle structures cannot be seen due to a steep approach to the angle (the goniscopist with a Zeiss lens would call this angle appositionally closed, as the trabecular meshwork can be seen only with indentation, when in reality it can by seen to be open with a narrow inlet by Koeppe gonioscopy). **The Zeiss lens can also readily fool the gonioscopist into thinking that an appositionally closed angle is open, due to unintentional pressure placed on the lens,** the diameter of which, unlike the Koeppe or Goldmann, is less than that of the cornea, although the radius of curvature is greater than that of the cornea. This diameter and radius of curvature are what allow indentation gonioscopy. The same is true for the Sussman lens, a Zeiss lens without a handle, or the Posner lens, which is a Zeiss lens with a screw-in handle. All these lenses can cause unintentional compression; however, the gonioscopist has clues that compression is occurring. Folds are seen in Descemet's membrane, and gentle, partial removal of the lens results in lens-iris diaphragm movement anteriorly.

INDENTATION GONIOSCOPY

When indentation gonioscopy is intentionally sought, the Zeiss four-mirrorred lens is applied, and the angle is carefully examined using the slit-lamp biomicroscope at high magnification. While observing the angle, the lens is moved slightly posteriorly, indenting the cornea and forcing the lens-iris diaphragm posteriorly in cases of relative pupillary block. The lens-iris diaphragm will not move in the presence of a patent surgical iridectomy, but generally will be forced back even with a patent laser iridectomy, due to its small size. Indentation gonioscopy is useful in evaluating the angle for appositional closure or peripheral anterior synechia, as well as for iridodialysis or cyclodialysis clefts.

For Koeppe gonioscopy, a hand-held microscope can be used, such as is salvageable from old slit-lamp microscopes or is manufactured in lighter weight expressly for gonioscopy by Haag Streit. The size of Koeppe lens suitable for most eyes is 18 mm in diameter (measured from the outer edges of the flange that fits under the lids against the eye); but occasionally, for eyes having an abnormally small palpebral fissure and for children, a 16-mm diameter lens is useful. This combination of equipment, which is to be used with the patient recumbent, provides a direct panoramic magnified view of the angle in a simple manner, requiring the patient to do nothing but to lie relaxed. This same simple arrangement for direct gonioscopy is practical in the operating room for examination of patients on the operating table, such as for immediate preoperative evaluation of the extent of opening of the angle by intensive medication in angle-closure glaucoma and for examination of babies under general anesthesia, particularly in relation to congenital glaucoma.

Another favorable factor is observed in examination of eyes having convex irides and narrow or possibly closed angles, in which it is necessary to **vary the angle of view to look down into the crack between iris and angle wall as far as possible in attempting to determine whether the filtration portion of the trabecular meshwork is occluded by the periphery of the iris.** Using the Koeppe lens and hand-held microscope, the examiner can vary his direction and angle of view with ease to select the most suitable position for seeing into the slit between convex iris and angle wall, without having to make any change of position of the lens. Also, one can quickly compare one portion of the angle with another, or the angle of one eye with that of the the other (Fig. 7.7).

In certain conditions, such as in suspected traumatic recession of the angle and in congenital glaucoma, comparison of one eye with the other is partic-

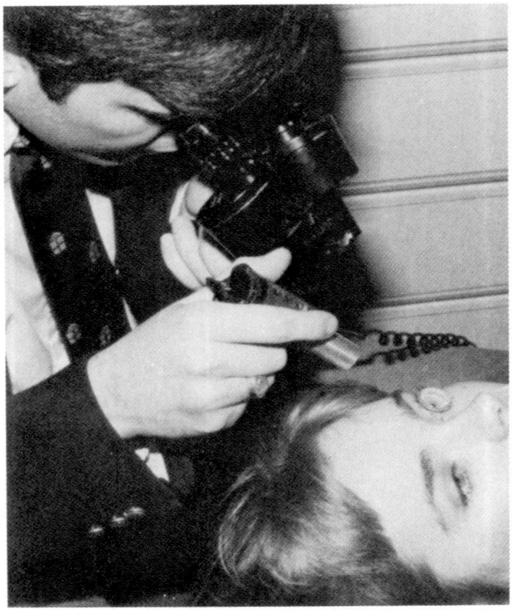

Figure 7.7. The examiner uses hand-held oculars and a Barkan focal illuminator to view the angle directly through the Koeppe lens. By allowing variation in the examiner's ocular viewing position and placement of the illumination in the angle, this system allows the best (and least distorted) view of a narrow angled eye.

ularly helpful. This is conveniently accomplished with Koeppe lenses on both eyes, alternating the view with the hand-held microscope easily back and forth from one eye to the other.

It is convenient to have the examiner's stool or chair freely sliding or rolling on casters so that the examiner can swing around from one side of the recumbent patient to the other to obtain a panoramic view of the whole circumference. If the patient is recumbent in an examining chair, the examiner may conveniently use a typist's chair on casters, with the chair turned backward, so that the examiner sits straddling the back of the chair, using its back for a support for his elbows, or he may steady his arms on the side of the back if the patient's head is lower. In this way, a continuous inspection of the whole angle is easily made as the examiner rolls in an orbit around the head of the patient. Only to examine the 12 o'clock portion of the angle is it necessary to lean forward somewhat over the patient's chest. When the Koeppe gonioscope lens is used, air bubbles can be displaced from the small space between cornea and the back of the lens with a few drops of a suitable solution, such as sterile 0.9 to 1.4% sodium chloride solution. The solution must contain no chlorobutanol preservative, however, because this preservative, when held in contact with the epithelium for several minutes, can produce a keratitis epithelialis that can make the patient uncomfortable for many hours, or until the epithelium heals spontaneously in a day or two. Methylcellulose may also be used to provide an excellent interface between the cornea and contact lens, and its viscosity limits the entry of air bubbles into the field of view.

If a lens is chosen to have a radius of inside curvature of 7.8 to 8.0 mm instead of the more common 7.4 mm, the space between lens and cornea is so small that it can be filled by the patient's tears. However, one should avoid an excessively shallow lens that actually presses on the cornea, because this can distort the cornea, inducing corrugations of the posterior surface of the cornea, which interfere with a view of the angle.

The lens should be centered on the cornea and not allowed to become displaced into an eccentric position, because if the rim of the lens encroaches on the cornea excessively in one quadrant, it tends to indent the limbus and to cause artificial narrowing of the angle. This is most likely to occur if the patient's head is elevated on a thick pillow, which causes the neck to be flexed forward. In this position, when the gaze is vertical, as it should be for gonioscopy, the upper lid presses excessively on the Koeppe lens and may make the upper angle appear closed. As a sign warning of this artifact, the gonioscopist may observe that a ridge paralleling the limbus is protruding inward at the periphery of the cornea superiorly and that on the inner surface of the cornea there are abnormal rugae or wrinkles running radially over the ridge, due to wrinkling of Descemet's membrane. Correction of this condition is simple. One merely removes the excessively thick pillow or has the patient raise the chin and extend the neck, so that the excess pressure of the upper lid on the lens is relieved. The gonioscopist then sees that the artificial ridge disappears, and what may have been thought to be a sector of closed angle may be seen actually to be open. Unwanted indentation of the limbus due to eccentricity and uneven pressure on the lens can be induced in other quadrants if the head is turned or if one holds the lens forcefully against the eye. With a cooperative patient and proper lens, there is no need for the lens to be malpositioned or to be held by hand.

Modifications that have been occasionally suggested in the direct gonioscopy method consist of suspension of the microscope to lessen its weight and fixation of the light to the microscope to make it a one-handed affair. A simple suspension system consisting of a cord from the hand-held binocular microscope going up over a couple of pulleys to a counterweight is simple, practical, and greatly favored by some expert gonioscopists, but is not essential, since

GONIOSCOPY DURING OPERATION

W. Morton Grant and Joel S. Schuman

In certain cases of angle-closure glaucoma, e.g., when a laser iridectomy cannot be performed or its patency is uncertain, it is impossible to tell by regular gonioscopy how much of the closure is due to permanent synechial adhesion of iris to corneoscleral trabecular meshwork and how much is due to a simple pressing of the iris against the meshwork without actual attachment. If extensive closure of the angle is present, it is very important in deciding the type of operation that will be most suitable to determine accurately how much of the closure is permanent and how much is functional and reversible. This is most clearly and conclusively accomplished in the operating room as a preliminary to the antiglaucoma operation itself. Under sterile conditions, a corneal paracentesis is performed and the aqueous is drained completely, allowing sufficient time for emptying of the aqueous from the posterior chamber, through the pupil to the anterior chamber, as well as for evacuation of the anterior chamber. Then, sterile saline solution is injected through the paracentesis wound into the anterior chamber. The iris acts as a check valve against the crystalline lens to prevent saline solution from going behind the iris into the posterior chamber. The result is that the iris no longer is ballooned forward in the periphery by fluid in the posterior chamber, and the angle can become greatly widened as the anterior chamber is filled with saline solution. By gonioscopy under sterile conditions, one sees that the iris becomes closely applied to the entire front of the crystalline lens and dips into a distinct sulcus at the equator of the lens. In portions of the angle in which there are no synechias, the angle wall is displayed in full width, with all structures clearly identifiable; but where there are peripheral anterior synechias, the attachment of iris overlying the scleral spur and corneoscleral trabecular meshwork appears distinct and in unmistakable contrast. The procedure for deepening the anterior chamber and the interpretation of findings are discussed in detail in Chapters 23 and 25.

one can readily learn to rest the elbows on the examining table, the back of a chair, or on one's knees for support and stability. It is best not to have the light attached to the microscope, in the interests of flexibility and variability of illumination. It is preferable to hold the microscope in one hand and the light in the other with the two hands partially interlocked (see Fig. 7.7) and the elbows resting on some support. While looking at the angle, it is useful to be able to vary the path of illumination, particularly when the cornea is not clear, and to be able to change from a sharp focal line in the angle to various degrees of indirect illumination by simple small changes in the position of the hand-held light.

GONIOSCOPY (FINDINGS)

In this section we will discuss variations and abnormalities that are found by gonioscopy. Details concerning congenital abnormalities are given in Chapters 68–71.

IRIS CONTOUR AND CHARACTER

At the start of the gonioscopic examination, one can decide whether the contour of the iris is to be characterized as slightly convex, very convex, flat, or concave (Table 7.1).

A slight convexity of the iris is seen in the majority of normal adult eyes, due to a pushing forward of the pupillary portion of the iris by the anterior surface of the lens and

Table 7.1
Conditions Involving Iris Contour and Character

Findings	Conditions
Slight convexity	Normal, physiologic
Excessive convexity	Hypermetropia
	Angle-closure glaucoma
Plateau iris	Angle-closure glaucoma
Flat iris	Pigmentary glaucoma
	Myopia, aphakia
Concave iris	Cyclitic membrane
	Pigmentary glaucoma
	Peripheral anterior synechias in aphakia
Irregularity of contour	Dislocation of lens
	Cyst or tumor
	Pupillary block in aphakia
	Segmental atrophy
Segmental atrophy of iris	Previous acute glaucoma
	Herpes zoster
Pigment sprinkling	Exfoliation
	Pigmentary glaucoma
	Malignant melanoma
	Tumors or cysts of iris or ciliary body
Pigmentation abnormality	Nevus
	Heterochromic cyclitis
	Glaucomatocyclitic crises
	Hemangioma
	Neurofibroma
	Siderosis or chalcosis

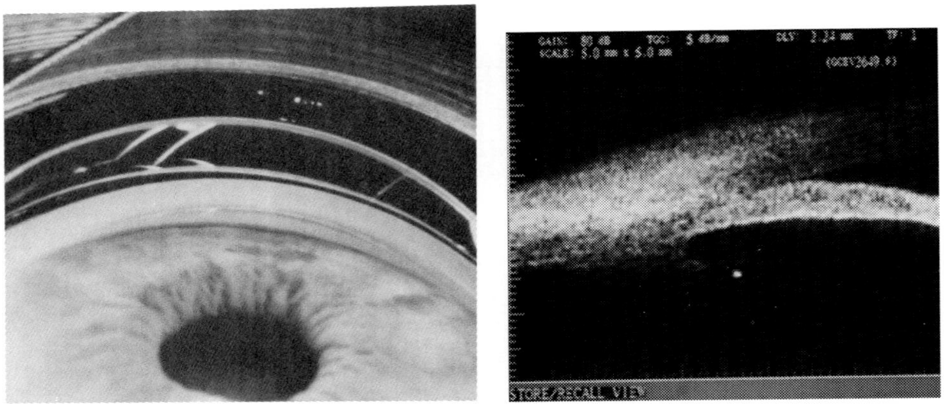

A B

Figure 7.8. Convex iris and narrow angle in a hyperopic patient. Only midtrabecular meshwork is visible and the angle is judged to be potentially occludable. **A,** Goniophotograph. **B,** Ultrasound biomicrograph of convex iris and narrow angle. Ultrasound biomicroscopy allows high resolution (20–50 microns) imaging of the anterior segment in cross-section, to a depth of approximately 4 mm. (Goniophotograph courtesy of David D. Donaldson, MD).

a slight, physiologic ballooning forward of the periphery of the iris caused by a physiologic difference in pressure between posterior chamber and anterior chamber. The pressure in the posterior chamber ordinarily is slightly greater than that in the anterior chamber because of a small resistance that the aqueous encounters in flowing forward through the area of contact of iris and lens *en route* to the pupil and anterior chamber. We have often noted that the peripheral convexity of the iris in the average eye is lost when a hole is made in the periphery of the iris. This allows aqueous to go freely from posterior to anterior chamber. The convexity also is lost when the pupil is widely dilated or when the crystalline lens is removed. A **convex iris contour** is seen typically in hypermetropic eyes, which have a small anterior segment (Fig. 7.8). If the lens is relatively large and positioned forward, shallowing the anterior chamber axially, the resistance to flow of aqueous forward from posterior to anterior chamber is greater than normal, and this may cause the periphery of the iris to bulge forward so as to narrow or even close the angle (Fig. 7.9), as described in Chapter 22. Beyond the central convex portion of the iris, in many eyes, a peripheral furrow or sulcus is found. The farther back the root of the iris is attached on the ciliary muscle and the shallower the axial depth of the anterior chamber, the more likely there is to be a peripheral sulcus. The peripheral sulcus develops gradually during childhood and later life, as the lens grows. No sulcus is found in infants' eyes.

A **flat iris contour**, and in exceptional cases, even a slight concavity, is most characteristically observed in myopia and aphakia. When the iris is flat, one should note where the plane of the iris lies in relation to the structures in the angle. In myopic and aphakic eyes, this plane generally lies well back of the level of the scleral spur. However, in other types of eyes, the plane of the iris is sometimes quite differently situated. Particularly, in the peculiar condition known as **plateau iris**, the root of the iris is attached close behind the scleral spur and the plane of the iris is even further forward, sometimes at the level of the anterior trabecular meshwork or Schwalbe's line. This brings the peripheral iris almost against the filtration portion of the trabecular meshwork with little or no assistance from excess pressure of aqueous in the posterior chamber. This is the rare type of eye in which, even after an iridectomy has been performed, dilation of the pupil can cause closure of the angle, and glaucoma. In such eyes, the ciliary processes can be abnormally rotated forward, in contact with the back of the iris, seemingly holding the iris forward in the periphery (Fig. 7.10). In normal eyes, the ciliary processes are not in contact with the back surface of the iris.

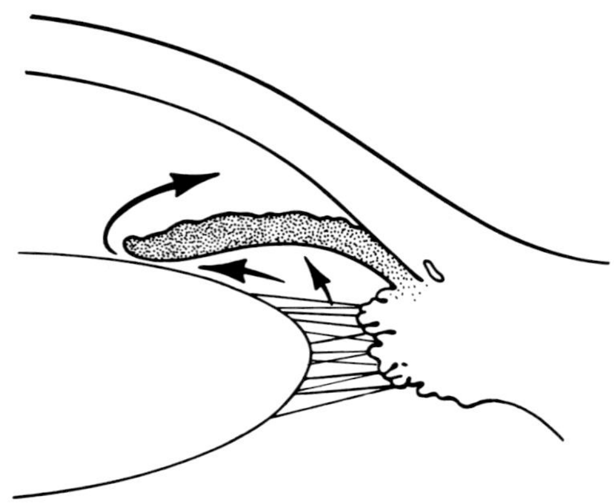

Figure 7.9. Aqueous humor is formed by the ciliary epithelium and moves between posterior iris surface and lens through the pupil, and into the anterior chamber. In small hyperopic eyes, some resistance is present to flow through the pupil (relative pupillary block) that results in a slightly greater pressure in the posterior chamber than in the anterior. The result is forward iris convexity.

Most emmetropic eyes demonstrate a slight iris convexity (forward) due to slight relative pupillary block. When

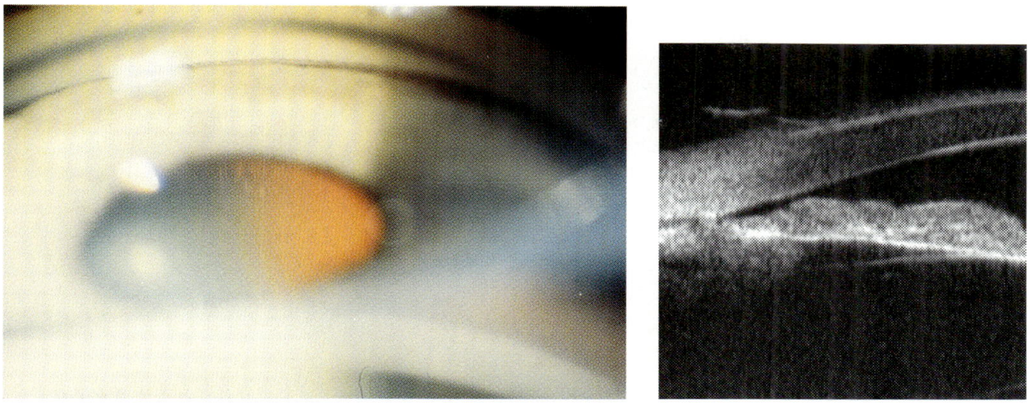

A B

Figure 7.10. Plateau iris configuration. **A,** Goniophotograph. **B,** Ultrasound biomicrograph. Iris is pushed into angle by anteriorly rotated ciliary processes, causing angle closure with dilation despite the presence of a patent peripheral iridectomy in plateau iris syndrome.

a high degree of relative pupillary block is present, angle-closure glaucoma can ensue from the resulting forward movement of the iris into the angle.

Concavity in the iris contour may be associated with pigment dispersion syndrome and pigmentary glaucoma (Fig. 7.11); old posterior uveitis, from contraction of inflammatory tissue behind the iris; or it may be associated with peripheral anterior synechias in aphakic eyes.

Irregularity of iris contour in moderate degree is not necessarily abnormal. Eyes having a coarse or lacy stromal structure are particularly likely to have wave-like billows or prominences at various places in the angle, without pathologic significance or threat of angle closure. However, a large, rounded, mound-like elevation of one portion of the iris can signify a dislocation and forward tilting of the lens in that area, or the presence of cyst or benign or malignant tumor of ciliary body or posterior layer of the iris. A cyst may be solitary and present in only one eye, but more characteristically cysts are multiple and present in both eyes. If a single isolated cyst is present, it is usually situated temporally. Often, the spaces in the iris stroma over a cyst are slightly spread apart by the stretching over the bulge, so that some of the front surface of the pigment layer can be seen. Further details of identification after wide dilation of the pupil, and treatment, are described in Chapter 34.

Segmental atrophy of the iris with localized flattening, contrasting with a general convexity of the rest of the iris, is seen most typically in eyes that have suffered an attack of acute glaucoma with high IOP. In this condition, the atrophic, thinned area of iris has a grayish appearance. Previous herpes zoster with iritis can also cause atrophic areas in the iris but with less characteristic segmental character and gray appearance.

Pigment sprinkling on the anterior surface of the iris is recognizable and not uncommon in association with pig-

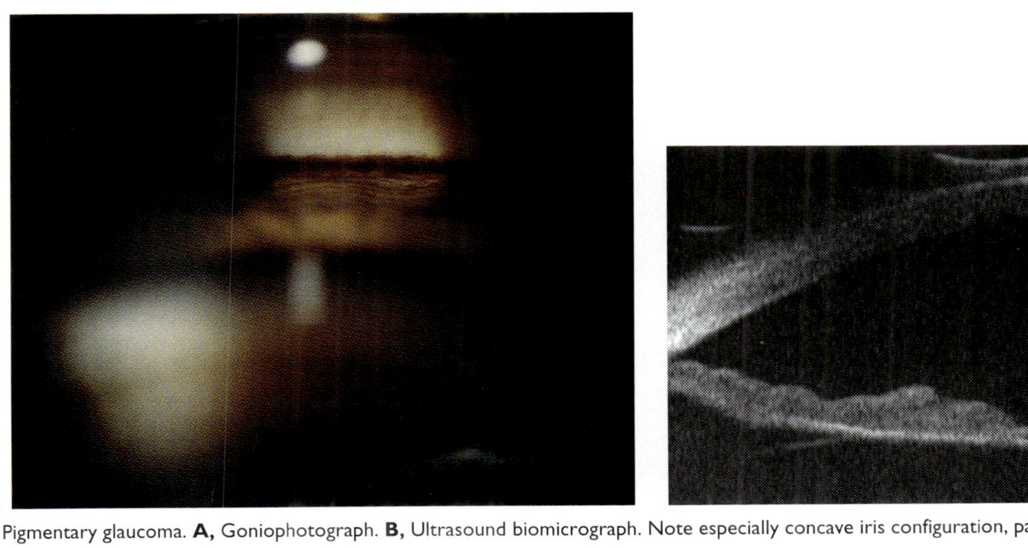

A B

Figure 7.11. Pigmentary glaucoma. **A,** Goniophotograph. **B,** Ultrasound biomicrograph. Note especially concave iris configuration, particularly evident in ultrasound biomicrograph.

mentary glaucoma and exfoliation, also with malignant melanoma (Chapter 41) and other tumors and cysts of the ciliary body. Pigment sprinkling on the surface of the iris is less definite and less readily noticeable than pigmentation of the angle, which will be discussed separately.

Abnormal pigmentation of the iris also occurs with nevi and heterochromia. Nevi are not of much significance unless they extend forward over the trabecular meshwork. Heterochromia of the iris is an accompaniment of heterochromic cyclitis, glaucomatocyclitic crises, hemangiomatosis, neurofibromatosis, and discoloration from intraocular copper or iron. Abnormalities of vessels of the iris and adhesions of iris to other structures are discussed later on in this chapter. Iridodonesis is easily detectable during gonioscopy with the patient recumbent. It is common in myopia, in pigmentary glaucoma, and after rupture of lens zonules.

ANGLE WIDTH

After noting the contour and character of the iris, one may estimate the width of the angle by examining the distance between Schwalbe's line and the nearest part of the iris. The angle may be described as wide, intermediate, narrow, excessively narrow, or closed (Table 7.2). Simple descriptive words are more explicitly and more widely understood than arbitrary classifications by numbers. The angle tends to be wide in normal, myopic, and aphakic eyes, but narrower in hypermetropic eyes.

Table 7.2
Conditions Reflecting Angle Width

Findings	Conditions
Wide	Normal, myopia and aphakia
Intermediate width	Normal
Narrow	Hypermetropia
Excessively narrow	Angle-closure glaucoma
Closed	Angle-closure glaucoma
Irregular narrowing	Anatomical narrowing superiorly
	Subacute angle-closure glaucoma
	Dislocation of lens
	Cysts
	Posterior adhesions plus pupillary block
Irregular widening	Traumatic recession of angle
	Dislocation of lens
	Cyclodialysis

The width of the angle normally varies about the circumference, anatomically usually narrowest at the 12 o'clock portion. An uncommon unevenness in width of the angle may be caused by cysts of the posterior layer of the iris or of the ciliary body (Fig. 7.12), by dislocation of the lens, by tumors of the ciliary body (Fig. 7.13), or by pupillary block accompanied by extensive posterior adhesions to the lens, to the vitreous, or to membranes in aphakic eyes. One sees excessive narrowing of the angle in eyes subject to angle-closure glaucoma. The angle is uniformly narrowed in eyes subject to severe acute attacks of angle-closure glaucoma, whereas it is narrowed less uniformly in eyes subject to subacute or chronic angle-closure glaucoma. The angle is seen to be closed in the whole circumference in an acute attack, in a part of the circumference in a subacute episode. This is discussed in more detail in Chapters 22, 23, and 24.

SCLERAL SPUR

After the examiner has formed his opinion of the contour of the iris and the width of the angle, he should attempt to identify the scleral spur, because this is helpful for orientation in an open angle and also valuable in narrow angles to determine whether the angle is open back beyond the filtration portion of the trabecular meshwork (Table 7.3, Fig. 7.14). In closed or extremely narrow angles, the scleral spur is hidden by the peripheral iris. Even in an open angle, the scleral spur is not always readily visible, for it is often covered and obscured by uveal meshwork. In a wide and open angle, the scleral spur is obscured in this way most commonly in the nasal quadrant, where the uveal mesh-

A

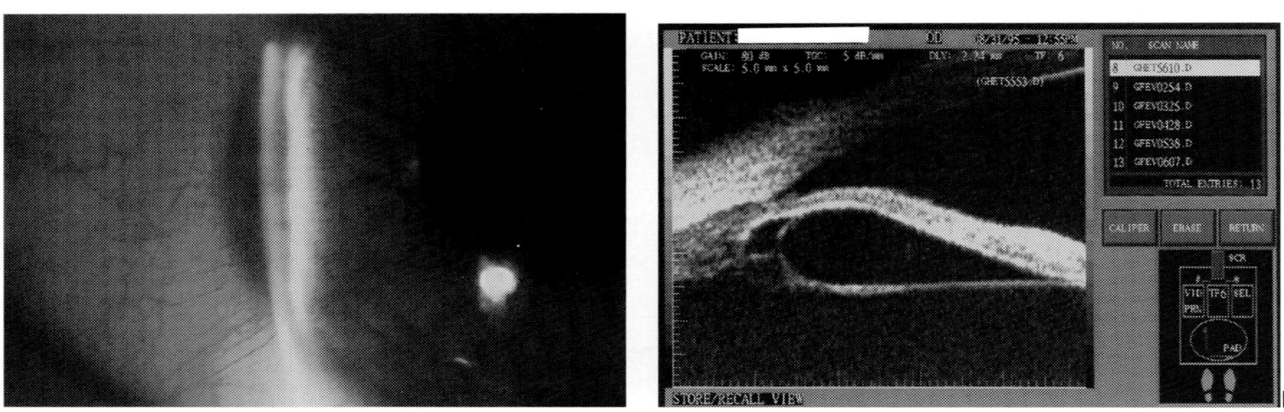

B

Figure 7.12. Cysts (not visible in slit lamp or goniophotograph) of the posterior iris surface and ciliary body that result in an irregular bumpy contour to the peripheral iris and in focal narrowing of the angle. **A,** Slit-lamp photograph. **B,** Ultrasound biomicrograph.

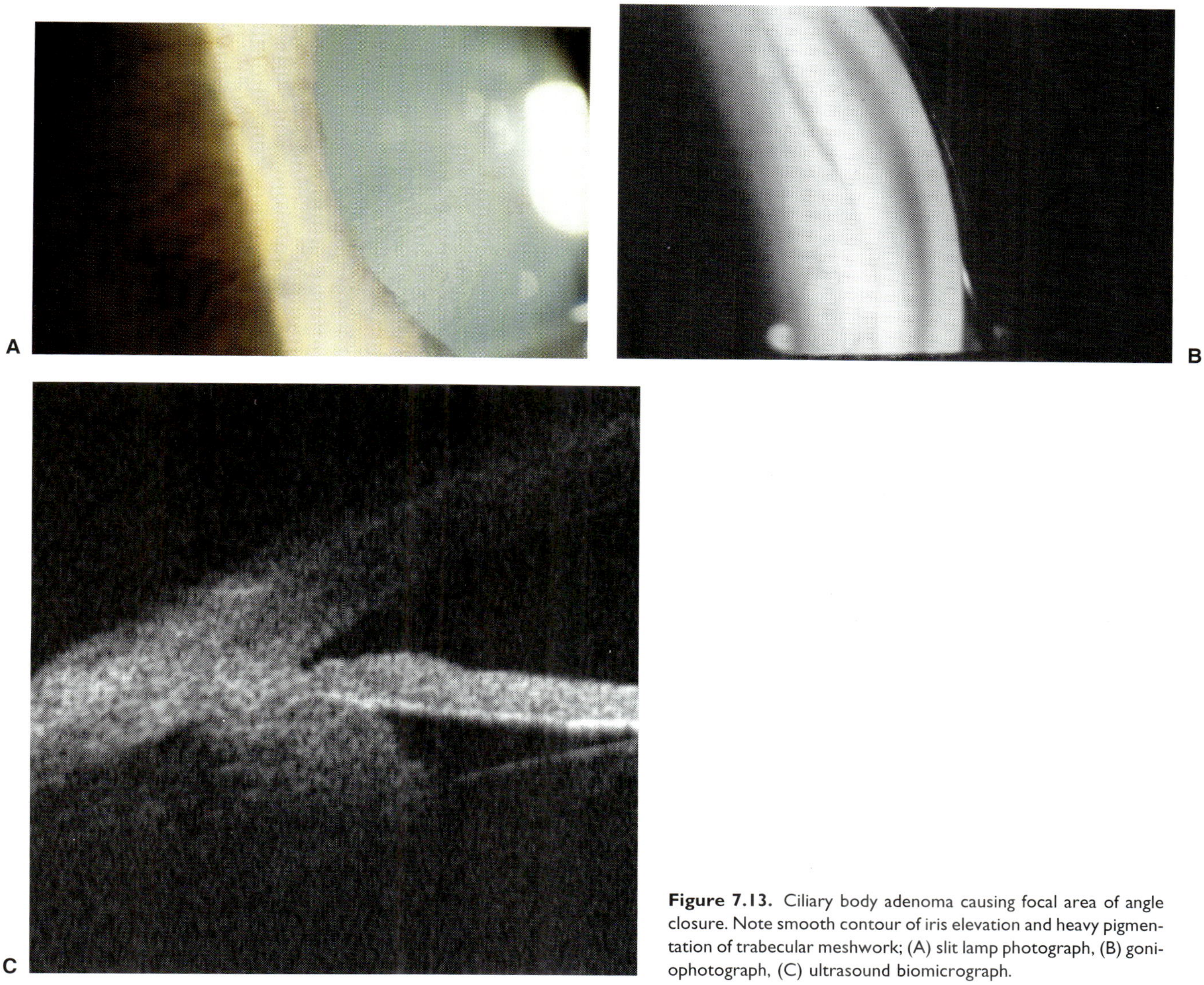

Figure 7.13. Ciliary body adenoma causing focal area of angle closure. Note smooth contour of iris elevation and heavy pigmentation of trabecular meshwork; (A) slit lamp photograph, (B) goniophotograph, (C) ultrasound biomicrograph.

work is usually most abundant. Sometimes, the uveal meshwork is abundant in the whole circumference, but there is almost always some area or portion of the angle in which uveal meshwork is thin enough and the scleral spur is sufficiently distinct so that it can be identified. Once identified, the spur can usually be traced around even

Table 7.3
Conditions Involving the Scleral Spur

Findings	Conditions
Spur all visible	Angle open
Spur hidden	Uveal meshwork
	Excessively narrow angle
	Closed angle
	Synechias
	Inflammatory exudates
Spur unusually prominent and white	Uveal meshwork torn
	Ciliary muscle torn
	Cyclodialysis cleft

in the areas in which uveal meshwork is thickest. When the scleral spur can be seen, it is recognizable as the posterior edge of the corneoscleral trabecular meshwork. It is of the same whiteness as the trabecular meshwork and whiter than the ciliary band that extends posteriorly from the scleral spur.

If the scleral spur can be positively identified in the whole circumference at a time when the intraocular pressure is elevated or the facility of outflow is subnormal, one can be sure that some form of open-angle glaucoma rather than angle-closure is responsible for the obstruction to outflow and elevated pressure. Rarely, the scleral spur inferiorly can be hidden by inflammatory exudates.

An abnormal whiteness, distinctness, and protrusion of the scleral spur may result from disruption of the uveal meshwork and detachment of the ciliary muscle from the scleral spur, such as is caused by blunt trauma to the eye

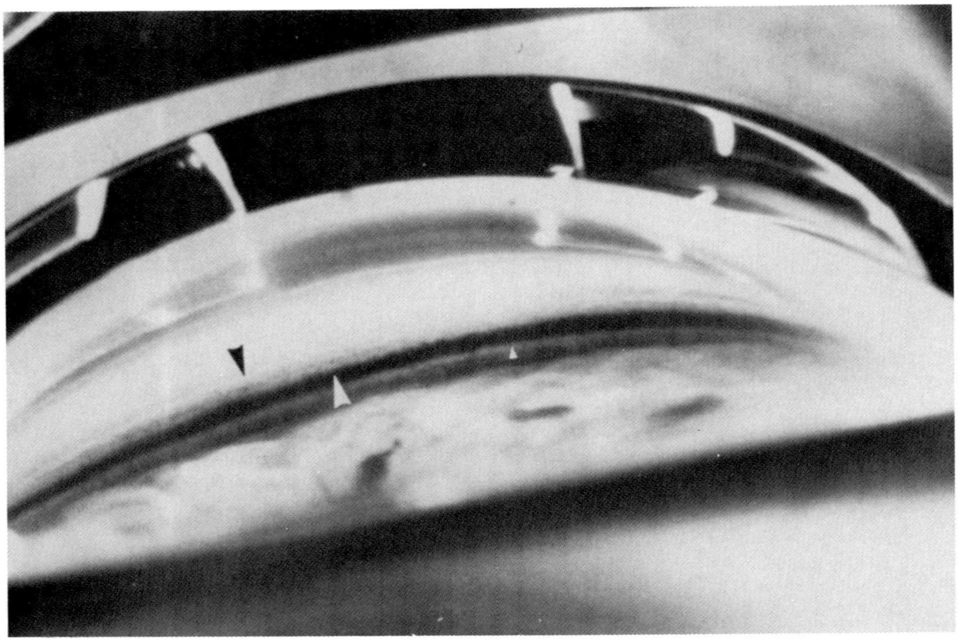

Figure 7.14. Patient with pigmentary glaucoma demonstrates angle landmarks well. The aqueous humor drains through the posterior aspect of the trabecular meshwork in which the pigment band lies (large white arrowhead). Anterior trabecular meshwork contains much less pigment. Schwalbe's line (black arrow head) and the scleral spur (small white arrow head) are easily defined (From Donaldson, DD: Atlas of External Diseases of the Eye, Vol IV: Anterior Chamber, Iris, and Ciliary Body. St. Louis, C.V. Mosby Co., 1973.)

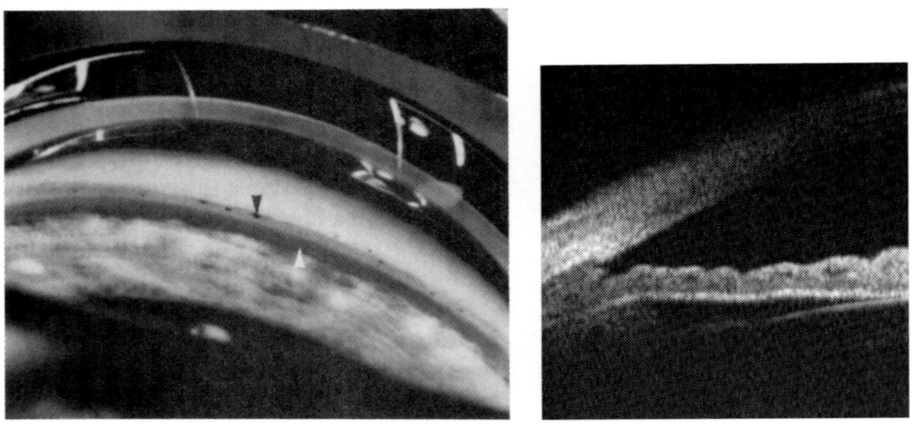

A B

Figure 7.15. 360-degree angle recession. Posterior displacement of the root of the iris is present with a widening of the ciliary body band. The gray veil-like tissue in the ciliary body band represents a probable previous tear into the ciliary muscle. The round black deposits on the trabecular meshwork represent degenerated blood elements from the original injury. **A,** Goniophotograph. **B,** Ultrasound biomicrograph.

or by surgical cyclodialysis. This is discussed further in Chapter 43.

CILIARY BAND

The ciliary band is composed of the anterior end of the ciliary muscle where it is within gonioscopic view, extending from the root of the iris to the scleral spur, plus a variable layer of uveal meshwork and occasional strands of iris stroma overlying the muscle. The overlying uveal meshwork varies greatly in texture, density, and pigmentation; in some eyes scarcely veiling the muscle, whereas in other eyes completely hiding it behind a dense forest of brown strands. These variations are discussed further under "Uveal Meshwork." Almost always, even with the most abundant uveal meshwork, one can find some chinks or thinner places somewhere in the circumference through which to identify ciliary muscle, provided that the angle is not too narrow and that the iris is not attached abnormally far forward.

When the ciliary muscle can be seen, its color has some racial variations dependent upon presence or absence of pigment among the muscle fibers (Table 7.4). Characteristically in white races, with either blue or brown eyes, the ciliary muscle itself is unpigmented and appears only slightly less white than the corneoscleral trabecular meshwork. In darkly pigmented races, the ciliary muscle usually contains an appreciable amount of melanin and has a gray

Table 7.4
Conditions Involving the Ciliary Band

Findings	Conditions
Very light gray	Normal in white race
Darker gray, traces of brown	Normal in dark races
Darker, slate gray	Melanoma
Whitish, cobwebby	Tear into the muscle
Scleral whiteness, cleft behind the spur	Tear through the muscle, or cyclodialysis

appearance or may even show traces of brown deep within the tissue.

An abnormal amount of pigment in the ciliary muscle gives the ciliary band a slate-gray or dark-brown appearance that may be a clue to malignant melanoma in the ciliary body. When present in only part of the circumference, the discoloration contrasts with the color of the normal portions.

An abnormally light-gray appearance with a fine, loose, cobwebby texture, lacking the customary structure of uveal meshwork, is characteristic of a tear into the ciliary muscle. The intact muscle is nearly colorless or very slightly gray in white races, and when the muscle has been torn, the lighter appearance is presumably due to the white of sclera showing through the thinned layer of tissue.

A scleral whiteness of the ciliary band results when the full thickness of ciliary muscle has been torn off the scleral spur, exposing the sclera to gonioscopic view. Sclera may be identified not only by its color, but sometimes by the presence of penetrating branches of short anterior ciliary arteries on its inner surface. These vessels emerge from the sclera a variably short distance behind the scleral spur and run directly posteriorly out of sight behind the ciliary body.

Defects in the ciliary band after blunt trauma to the eye (Fig. 7.15) often consist of a tearing apart of the ciliary muscle and the overlying uveal meshwork, sometimes associated with tearing or indirect damage to the trabecular meshwork, leading to glaucoma. A defect in the ciliary band is also found after surgical cyclodialysis that leaves a cleft just behind the scleral spur. The cleft following successful cyclodialysis is a bottomless tunnel going back as far as one can see; but when the operation has failed, the cleft can usually be seen to have a definite bottom where the tissues have healed together.

The level of attachment of the periphery of the iris on the ciliary muscle has a wide range of anatomic variation, and this influences the width of the ciliary band. Unusual narrowness of the ciliary band is common in congenital glaucoma; this will be discussed further in the chapter on that subject. Abnormal synechial attachment of the iris to scleral spur or to corneoscleral trabecular meshwork can narrow or completely hide the ciliary band. Abnormal widening of the ciliary band is usually caused by tearing of the ciliary muscle by blunt trauma or by surgical cyclodialysis. Irregularity or unevenness in width of the ciliary band that is noted as one scans the whole circumference is often a clue to abnormality, such as a tear, in the ciliary muscle, which can be discerned by close inspection.

Blood vessels and pigment on the ciliary band are discussed later in more detail under "Blood Vessels in the Angle" and "Pigment in the Angle:" and involvement in "Peripheral Anterior Synechias" is described under that heading.

UVEAL MESHWORK

The uveal meshwork deserves considerable attention, not because of any known functional significance, but because proper recognition and appreciation of the character of the uveal meshwork helps one to avoid errors in identification of normal structures in the angle and particularly helps to avoid confusion with peripheral anterior synechias that sometimes look misleadingly similar.

The uveal meshwork lines the angle from peripheral iris over ciliary band, scleral spur, and part of the trabecular meshwork in all eyes, but it varies greatly in thickness, pigmentation, texture, and extent from patient to patient. It also varies remarkably with age, developing from an inconspicuous and colorless, fine, homogeneous structure in the infant to a coarse, lacy forest of brown strands in some adult eyes or to an unpigmented, fine fibrillar layer in others (Table 7.5).

In addition to the uveal meshwork, which essentially lines the angle, in some eyes there are occasional separate, distinctive **iris processes**. The iris processes are long, slender isolated strands that stand out away from the uveal meshwork and bridge the angle from the periphery of the iris to the anterior half of the corneoscleral trabecular meshwork (Fig. 7.16). These strands may have a remote relationship to the pectinate ligaments of animal eyes. In adults, the iris processes are pigmented or unpigmented, corresponding to the stroma of the iris. In infants, the iris

Table 7.5
Conditions Involving the Uveal Meshwork

Findings	Conditions
Homogeneous, transparent, glittering, unpigmented	Infantile
Network of grayish strands, variable amount	In blue-eyed adults
Network of brown strands, variable amount	In brown-eyed adults
Uneven pigmentation	Corresponding to uneven iris pigmentation and nevi
Greater amount nasally	Common normal finding
Disruption or defects, baring underlying structures	Result of tear by blunt trauma or cyclodialysis
Separation of sheet or shelf	Result of blunt trauma

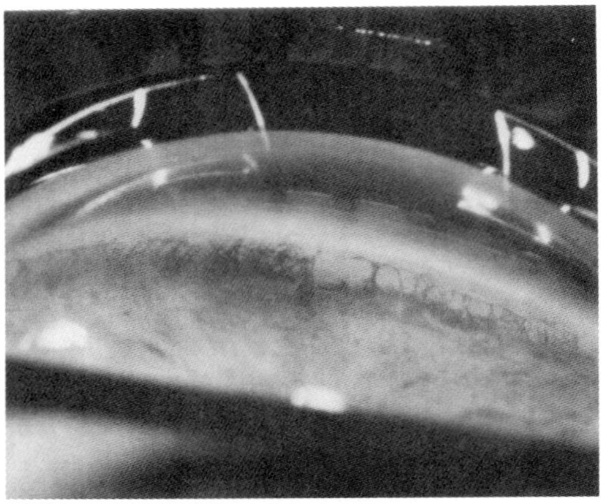

Figure 7.16. Patient with Axenfeld's syndrome, demonstrating abnormally prominent and thick uveal meshwork (iris processes). These processes are not peripheral anterior synechias. (Courtesy of David D. Donaldson, MD).

processes may be present at a time when the uveal meshwork is a homogeneous undifferentiated sheet (by gonioscopy), but iris processes are usually colorless and inconspicuous at that stage. The distribution of iris processes seems to be haphazard from eye to eye and from one part of the circumference to another. The iris processes seem to have little diagnostic or pathologic significance, except that one may note that they are ruptured in association with traumatic recession of the angle, and one might speculate that they could provide the initial bridge for development of the strange iridocorneal adhesions of essential atrophy of the iris. We will say no more about iris processes, and in the rest of this section will discuss only the uveal meshwork proper.

Incidentally, we avoid using the term "pectinate ligaments" in describing structures of the human angle, because we feel that this term is properly restricted to a specific type of structure characteristically present in the eyes of certain animals, but not present in any closely related form in human eyes.

A good appreciation of the nature of the uveal meshwork is obtained by considering its development. At birth and during the first few months of life, in normal human eyes, the uveal meshwork can be discerned, by careful focusing of the goniomicroscope, as a smooth, delicate, homogeneous layer extending from iris periphery toward the anterior part of the trabecular meshwork. The infantile uveal meshwork is situated in front of the ciliary band, scleral spur, and filtration portion of the trabecular meshwork, but distinctly separated from them. It comes into focus a little closer to the observer than the other structures of the wall of the angle. The infant's uveal meshwork has a finely granular texture with a surface luster or glitter suggestive of ice or fine ground glass. It has no discernible holes or coarse strands in its structure, but is so delicate and transparent that the anatomical landmarks on the wall of the angle beyond are clearly seen through it. In fact, one can easily fail to notice the uveal meshwork in the infant's eye unless examining with special care.

Toward the end of the first year of life, in eyes having brown irides there commonly develops a fine fringe of brown strands or tendrils extending from the iris forward on the face of the uveal meshwork. In eyes of darkly pigmented individuals, fine brown strands appear also at a deeper layer, at the level of the ciliary muscle.

Gradually, during childhood, the uveal meshwork loses its homogeneous sheetlike appearance and changes to a more lacy, open structure that appears to be composed of fibrils or strands. Through childhood, the surface generally maintains a more lustrous reflecting quality than is observed in the adult. There is wide variation in the final form into which the uveal meshwork develops in different types of adult eyes. In blue eyes, the layer of uveal meshwork that lines the angle, overlying ciliary band, scleral spur, and trabecular meshwork, most commonly becomes a delicate grayish or colorless structure of fine strands that interferes little with the visibility of ciliary band, scleral spur, or trabecular meshwork. In brown eyes, it may become much more conspicuous, owing to the development of brown pigmentation of the same color as the iris stroma. The amount of pigmentation and the coarseness and density of the tissue vary even among brown eyes, in some being only a fine lacy brown network overlying the ciliary body, but in others consisting of a dense forest of coarse interlacing brown strands extending from peripheral iris to various levels on the trabecular meshwork, hiding ciliary band, scleral spur, and posterior portion of the trabecular meshwork. Most commonly in eyes having moderate pigmentation of the iris stroma, the pigmented uveal meshwork consists of a lacy open-textured network of strands extending from iris periphery and terminating on the trabecular meshwork over the filtration area.

Typically, the spaces between strands of uveal meshwork in adults are coarse enough to permit the ciliary band and scleral spur to be discerned behind this meshwork. The most common form of pigmented uveal meshwork might be likened to ivy on a wall. Typically, its anterior edge on the trabecular meshwork has many fine branching terminations like the tendrils that hold a vine to a wall, often with darker tiny clusters of pigment where the tendrils attach to the wall.

Appreciation of normal variations in uveal meshwork can be obtained occasionally in eyes in which pigmentation is splotchy or in which portions of the iris are blue and portions are pigmented. In such eyes, parts of the angle show the in conspicuous fine grayish uveal meshwork characteristic of the blue eye, while adjacent portions of the circumference show the more conspicuous brown pigmented uveal meshwork of brown eyes.

The uveal meshwork is normally avascular at all stages. However, normal vessels of ciliary body and iris are occasionally seen on the ciliary band, and pathologic new vessels sometimes grow over the angle. This is discussed in the section "Blood Vessels in the Angle."

A satisfactory firsthand examination of variations in character of uveal meshwork can be obtained in enucleated human eyes in which a 5- or 6-mm porthole has been cut out of the center of the cornea with a trephine to permit direct inspection of the angle structures. In brown eyes with extensive brown uveal meshwork extending up onto the trabecular meshwork, it is easy by means of a goniotomy knife to peel the uveal meshwork from its forward edge backward toward the iris. The uveal meshwork separates easily and cleanly, leaving the trabecular meshwork and the scleral spur unnaturally distinct. **Measurement of facility of aqueous outflow by aqueous perfusion before and after coarse pigmented uveal meshwork has been dissected off the trabecular meshwork has shown no significant influence on facility of outflow.**

Also in blue eyes the uveal meshwork can be dissected off as a definite, although inconspicuous, veil of tissue and this, as in brown eyes, makes the corneoscleral trabecular meshwork and its scleral spur appear strikingly white and distinctly contrasting with the off-white shade of the adjacent ciliary muscle. This simulates what one sometimes sees in an eye after blunt trauma has caused tearing apart of uveal meshwork, but little disruption of ciliary muscle.

The greatest practical problem that the uveal meshwork presents is that it often misleads those who are learning gonioscopy into a mistaken diagnosis of peripheral anterior synechias. We have seen many patients who have been referred with a description of synechias in the angle, when the angle presented only an unusually abundant or extensive uveal meshwork. It is very important to make the correct identification, because, as will be discussed in more detail under "Peripheral Anterior Synechias," the presence of synechias can be a crucial factor in identifying the type of glaucoma and in determining the appropriate treatment. Experience in looking at many angles is the most valuable and effective means of gaining familiarity with the fundamental characteristics and the great variations of the uveal meshwork.

The feature that seems to be most significant in distinguishing normal tissue from acquired synechias is a difference in apparent solidity of the tissue. The uveal meshwork in normal adult eyes regularly has the lacy, open character of a meshwork made up of many interconnected strands, with spaces and holes between, whereas peripheral anterior synechias regularly have a more uniform, solid, and imperforate character.

Another feature that can help in distinguishing uveal meshwork from peripheral anterior synechias is the location of radial iris blood vessels. The radial blood vessels of the iris are normally never attached forward anterior to the scleral spur, but iris vessels may be drawn abnormally forward in formation of synechias. One must carefully distinguish dragged radial iris vessels from new-formed vessels and from loops or knuckles of large circumferentially arranged blood vessels that are not uncommonly seen on the ciliary band in the uveal meshwork, and from certain other vessels to be described under "Blood Vessels in the Angle."

Defects in the uveal meshwork are seen after blunt trauma to the eye even in cases in which no tear of the ciliary muscle is observable. These defects are noticeable in two forms. In one, the ciliary band has an uncommonly blank or bare appearance. If one makes a careful comparison with the other eye, especially by using gonioscopic lenses on both eyes at the same time, or if one compares various portions of the circumference, one may see that in the damaged portion there are broken iris processes and that the lacy uveal meshwork has been disrupted and characteristically has contracted into little clumps where its ends have remained attached. The bared ciliary muscle appears unusually pale and clean, and the scleral spur may look white and more prominent than normal. In the other form **of defect in uveal meshwork from trauma,** the most notable feature is a lamina or shelf of uveal meshwork stretching as a cord across one sector of the angle, with only one free edge detached and separated from the wall of the angle. This lamina may hang down in front of the ciliary band, revealing an unusually white and glistening scleral spur above and beyond it.

Finding defects in the angle that can be attributed to trauma may help to establish the cause of an otherwise puzzling monocular glaucoma, or in cases of bilateral but asymmetrical chronic open-angle glaucoma may help to explain why the glaucoma has been so much more severe in one eye than in the other.

TRABECULAR MESHWORK

The corneoscleral trabecular meshwork extends from scleral spur to Schwalbe's line. How well it can be seen and identified depends largely on how much uveal meshwork overlies and hides the scleral spur and the posterior portion of the trabecular meshwork (Table 7.6). Identification of the anterior edge of the trabecular meshwork depends upon the distinctness of Schwalbe's line. Identification is easy if scleral spur has little covering and is well developed and distinct. Also, identification is easy if Schwalbe's line happens to be present as a prominent refractile ridge at the termination of Descemet's membrane. Otherwise one may recognize **a characteristic grayish, finely granular texture, or sometimes a narrow band of pigment granules in the filtration portion of the trabecular meshwork,** between the middle and posterior thirds, just anterior to the scleral spur. Even when free of pigment, the corneoscleral trabecular meshwork is not as white as its scleral background. It is distinguishable from sclera not only by its characteristic finely granular texture, but by a slightly

Table 7.6
Variations in the Trabecular Meshwork

Findings	Conditions
Normal variables	Covering by uveal meshwork
	Distinctness of scleral spur
	Distinctness of Schwalbe's line
	Blood in Schlemm's canal
Characteristic feature	Filtration area finely granular, translucent, with or without pigment
Acquired abnormalities	Excessive pigment
	Inflammatory deposits
	Blood vessels
	Synechias
	Loss of normal texture
	Traumatic rupture
Congenital abnormalities	Posterior embryotoxon
	Iridocorneal malformations

translucent quality unlike solid sclera. As an additional aid in identification, during gonioscopy one occasionally sees blood in Schlemm's canal (Fig. 7.17). One sees it as a red line or band showing through the filtration portion of the trabecular meshwork just anterior to scleral spur, in a part or all of the circumference. The translucent filtration portion of the trabecular meshwork veils the line of blood slightly but does not hide its bright redness. This has such a distinctive appearance that from it one can feel sure of one's orientation. Entrance of blood into Schlemm's canal is favored by low intraocular pressure and local congestion of the episcleral circulation when the pressure of the rim of the gonioscopic lens is uneven. It is common to see the blood come and go or shift into different quadrants during the examination. So far, little significance has been attached to variations in appearance of blood in the canal, except perhaps in connection with hemangioma of the lid and glaucoma.

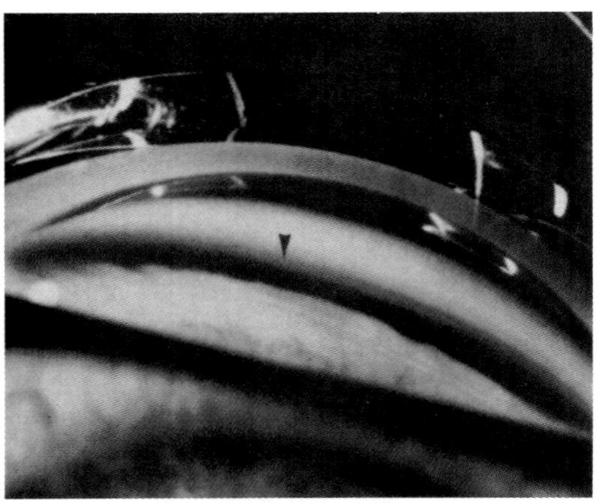

Figure 7.17. Blood reflux into Schlemm's canal *(arrowhead)*. Note the position in the posterior aspect of the trabecular meshwork just above the scleral spur. Such blood reflux is common in normal eyes but uncommon in eyes with glaucoma, except those with elevated episcleral venous pressure. (Courtesy of David D. Donaldson, MD).

Having identified the corneoscleral trabecular meshwork, one examines it particulary to assess the amount of pigment accumulated in it, and the presence on it of inflammatory exudates, blood vessels, or synechias. Each of these is of great significance in the diagnosis of different types of glaucoma and each often also involves adjacent tissues, in addition to the trabecular meshwork. However, there is a rule applying specifically to the trabecular meshwork that pigment and peripheral anterior synechias cause glaucoma only when they obstruct the filtration portion of this tissue. It is, therefore, important in the gonioscopic examination to establish accurately the degree and extent to which the filtration area is involved. As we have already mentioned, **the filtration area is just anterior to the scleral spur, overlying Schlemm's canal,** and constitutes approximately the middle third of the trabecular meshwork, appearing normally to have a slightly granular and translucent character by gonioscopic observation. It is through this portion that the aqueous humor passes on its way out. From clinical observations and experiments on enucleated eyes, we believe very little goes through the anterior third of the trabecular meshwork, and very little goes through the scleral spur or through the ciliary band. In primary open-angle glaucoma and in glaucoma attributable to abnormal accumulation of pigment filtered out of the aqueous in the filtration portion of the trabecular meshwork, quantitative aqueous perfusion measurements and dissections post mortem have indicated that the principal glaucomatous obstruction lies in the filtration portion of the corneoscleral trabecular meshwork.

Trauma occasionally causes a splitting or circumferential rupture of trabecular meshwork, as though it was ripped by a momentary strong pull by the ciliary muscle on the scleral spur. When fresh, the split in the filtration portion of the trabecular meshwork has sharp or distinct edges, gaping slightly, but in the course of months the edges of the tear become rounded and less distinct. Eventually, a small trough-like depression in the meshwork is all that remains (Fig. 7.18).

Congenital abnormalities affecting portions of the trabecular meshwork, such as posterior embryotoxon and Rieger's syndrome, are discussed principally in Chapters 68 and 71. However, these abnormalities are also seen in adults. They consist of abnormalities in the development of the periphery of the cornea, sometimes associated with abnormal connections between the iris and cornea. The peripheral rim of Descemet's membrane is particularly involved. This rim forms the so-called line of Schwalbe at the anterior edge of the corneoscleral trabecular meshwork. Occasionally, it is thickened, beaded, and prominent, conspicuous both on gonioscopy and on slit-lamp examination. This condition, known as "posterior embryotoxon," when it occurs alone is compatible with normal functioning of the eye. However, when the iris is also involved, glaucoma may result. One finds in glaucoma from Rieger's

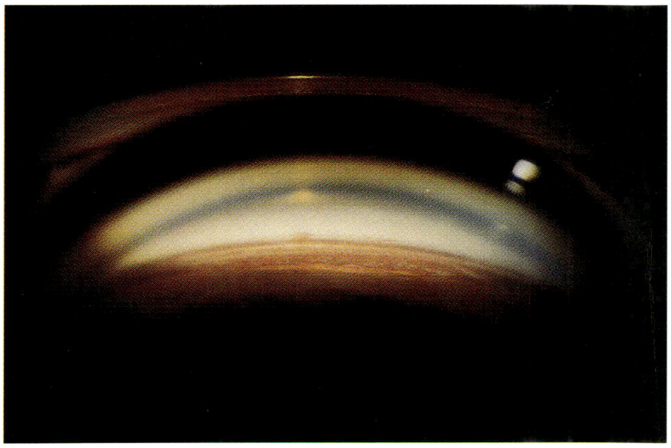

Figure 7.18. Tear in trabecular meshwork, an occasional result of blunt trauma to the globe. Note bright white band, the outer wall of Schlemm's canal, visible through torn trabecular meshwork.

syndrome that, along with posterior embryotoxon, the peripheral iris may be congenitally irregularly attached in sheets or strands to Schwalbe's line or that coarse ropes of refractile material bridge across the angle from the region of Schwalbe's line to the iris. The angle may in part appear to be obstructed or blanketed by the tissues that extend across the angle, and this could account for the associated glaucoma; but, even in the open portions of the angle the trabecular meshwork usually does not seem to have normal texture, and the other angle structures are difficult to recognize.

PUPIL AND LENS

Through the gonioscopic contact lens and microscope one can occasionally discover abnormalities of the pupil and lens that may be difficult or impossible to see from a frontal view with the slit-lamp biomicroscope.

Exfoliation often can be diagnosed by looking just behind the border of the pupil where the iris touches the lens. Not uncommonly, one can discover the pathognomonic, fine dandruff-like material hidden in this little niche, although none may be evident by frontal view on the anterior edge of the pupillary margin or on the front surface of the lens, unless the pupil is dilated. Discovery of the material of exfoliation can be a great help in establishing what type of glaucoma one is dealing with (Chapter 20).

Posterior synechias, between iris and lens, occasionally can be identified more definitely by looking behind the pupillary border through the gonioscopic apparatus than by viewing from in front with the slit lamp.

Cysts of the iris at the pupillary border, such as are induced by strong miotics, are usually seen as easily by ordinary frontal view as from the gonioscopic viewpoint, because they tend principally to project into the pupil. However, occasionally the type of cyst that develops spontaneously in the posterior pigment layer of the iris extends from the periphery to close behind the pupillary margin and is seen only with the gonioscopic apparatus. The cysts of ciliary body and posterior layer of iris that are located more peripherally usually elevate the peripheral iris in rounded mounds without disturbing the pupil. To see and positively identify this type of cyst, one must dilate the pupil widely and look in back of the iris. Typically, one or more smooth, rounded dark-brown masses are seen between iris and lens, holding the iris forward and sometimes indenting the lens. Characteristically, a slightly glistening reflex is evident through the layer of dark brown pigment. The relationship of cysts of this type to glaucoma is discussed in Chapter 34.

Atrophy of the pupillary border, both the diffuse patchy type associated with old age and with exfoliation and the type associated with segmental grey atrophy of the iris from previous very high IOP, are about as well determined by ordinary slit-lamp biomicroscopic view as by gonioscopic view. In exceptional instances, when there is some difficulty in distinguishing between tiny pale patches of pupillary atrophy and possible exfoliation material, the decision is relatively easy from the gonioscopic view. Also, in those rare instances after a severe attack of acute angle-closure glaucoma in which the pupil is irregularly and permanently dilated in association with segmental grey atrophy of the iris, it is sometimes possible by means of the gonioscopic apparatus to find a space where the iris has actually become lifted away from the lens, providing an unimpeded path for aqueous from posterior to anterior chamber, and thus making impossible any further attacks of angle closure, as discussed in Chapter 23.

Ectropion of the pupillary margin sometimes is correlated most conveniently during gonioscopic examination with abnormalities in the angle, particularly with peripheral anterior synechias. Peripheral anterior synechias and slight ectropion of the pupillary margin in the same sector are observable with all types of peripheral anterior synechias, most strikingly with those of neovascular glaucoma and essential atrophy of the iris, suggesting that the iris stroma is pulled peripherally to the area of synechia, causing the pupillary margin to roll out slightly in the same direction.

Pigment behind the equator of the lens, where the posterior zonules attach to the lens, is well seen in many cases of pigmentary glaucoma, if one looks through the pupil and examines this region, making use of the gonioscopic apparatus.

Dislocation of the lens in cases in which the lens has returned to an axial position may be revealed by inspection with the gonioscopic apparatus. A different level or convexity of the iris on one side compared with the other is a clue to tilting of the lens, and this may be noted when the pupil is small. When the pupil is intermediate in size, one may find in addition a slight tilting of the pupil and front surface of the lens. If the pupil is dilated, one may look through the pupil behind the iris. On the side on which the lens is tilted backward, one may see a rounded bulge of vitreous herniating anterior to the equator of the lens where zonules and hyaloid have been ruptured. The vitreous may hold the dilated pupil away from the lens without actually reaching the pupil where it would be visible by frontal slit-lamp view.

CILIARY PROCESSES

One can see and examine the ciliary processes by means of gonioscopic equipment in several special conditions (Table 7.7). Sometimes the tips of the processes can be seen when the pupil is extremely dilated, but they are more readily seen when a cyst, tumor, or a dislocated lens holds a portion of the iris forward. They are most easily and most commonly seen through a surgical coloboma of the iris. In congenital aniridia, one sees the full extent of ciliary processes. In general, the ciliary processes have a brown irregular surface, not as dark brown as the posterior pigment layer of the iris. Normally, the processes are uniform in size and do not hold the periphery of the iris forward.

The abnormalities that may be discovered by means of gonioscopy include cysts, tumors, discoloration, distortion, atrophy, and abnormal positioning.

Cysts of the posterior iris and ciliary body can cause a special variety of angle-closure glaucoma, and these cysts also can be a source of abnormal pigment deposition in the trabecular meshwork. Cysts originating in the iris have a smooth, dark brown, rounded surface. Cysts involving the ciliary processes at times convert several adjacent processes into grotesquely enlarged structures that may push against and indent the lens, as well as push the iris forward to close the angle. Cysts of the ciliary processes are usually brown, smooth, and slightly glinting, but in some instances, they may be unpigmented and clear.

Table 7.7
Conditions Involving Ciliary Processes

Findings	Conditions
Visible gonioscopically	In extreme mydriasis
	With cyst or tumor behind iris
	With dislocated lens
	In surgical coloboma
	In aniridia
Enlargements	Cysts, tumor
Lateral displacements	By epithelial implantation cysts
	By tumors of ciliary body
Gray covering or discoloration	Exfoliation
	Epithelialization
	Cyclitic membrane
Shrinkage and pallor	Postinflammatory atrophy
Elongated or sheet-like	Buphthalmos
Anteriorly rotated	Plateau iris, angle-closure
	Anterior choroidal separation
	After scleral buckling operation
	From adherence to limbal scar

Cysts originating in the ciliary processes and iris are readily distinguishable from implantation cysts of epithelium introduced by a penetrating traumatic or surgical wound from the outside. Both types may push aside ciliary processes as they grow and they may involve the iris extensively, but implantation cysts have thin gray or translucent walls without surface pigmentation. Also, characteristically, inside an implantation cyst one may see gray particulate debris, which is partially suspended and floating about in a fluid, showing a considerable flare in a focused beam of light. Implantation cysts are accompanied by evidences of previous penetrating injury or operation, usually including injury to the lens with loss of all or a large part of the lens.

Tumors such as malignant melanoma of the ciliary body and choroid usually do not involve the ciliary processes primarily, but by growing and expanding from locations closer to the sclera, may push a row of ciliary processes and the adjacent pars plana inward toward the lens.

Powdery, light gray material clinging to otherwise normal-appearing ciliary processes is sometimes seen in eyes having exfoliation.

Envelopment of ciliary processes in a grayish, cobwebby cocoon may be seen in epithelialization of the anterior chamber in aphakic eyes. The epithelial membrane can be seen to have spread from a limbal wound over contiguous iris and vitreous face, often extending circumferentially in the posterior chamber on the vitreous behind the pillars of a coloboma in the iris.

Shrinkage and whitening of the ciliary processes can occur as a result of inflammation or cyclodestructive treatment. With protracted iridocyclitis, the ciliary processes may become remarkably shrunken, in extreme cases practically disappearing. At the same time they may become whitish from a covering of cyclitic membrane. Only a low, whitish ridge may remain with no discernible individual processes. In eyes having this degree of atrophy of the ciliary body, the formation of aqueous humor is far below normal. In some such eyes, even if there is extensive obstruction of the angle by postinflammatory synechias, the intraocular pressure may not be elevated, or, if it is elevated, it is subject to erratic variation because of precarious and uncertain balance between the effects of damage to the mechanisms of both inflow and outflow.

In babies' eyes in which the diameters of the cornea and anterior chamber have greatly enlarged as a result of abnormally high intraocular pressure, the ciliary processes tend to become elongated radially, with the rest of the ciliary body extending from them peripherally in a flattened sheet. The lens remains of normal size in buphthalmos, but the ring of ciliary body increases in diameter as the cornea and sclera stretch. Since the ciliary body is attached by the zonules to the lens, it seems that the deformed, drawn-out appearance of the processes is probably a mechanical result of the disproportion between the size of lens and the size of anterior segment.

Anterior rotation of the ciliary processes is observed infrequently and only in rather special conditions. We have seen certain instances of angle-closure glaucoma in which the iris had a plateau form, instead of the common general convexity. Even after good iridectomies were performed, angle-closure glaucoma recurred spontaneously or under the influence of a mydriatic. These angles could be reopened by miosis induced by light or medication. After iridectomy, the periphery of the iris appeared to be raised in a uniform roll or hump above the central plain of the iris, making the angle precariously narrow. The position of the ciliary processes seen through the surgical coloboma was abnormally rotated forward in a position to hold the periphery of the iris forward. Nothing else was seen to explain the peripheral elevation of the iris. The posterior chamber was otherwise ample, and the equator of the lens was well separated from ciliary processes and iris. The condition has tended to be binocular, and is an anatomical peculiarity. More recently, ultrasound biomicroscopy has confirmed the anatomic position of the ciliary processes in many additional cases of plateau iris configuration (Fig. 7.10).

Anterior rotation of ciliary processes and narrowing or closure of the angle similarly are seen in association with anterior separation of choroid and ciliary body or as a consequence of scleral buckling.

We have reproduced this condition experimentally in enucleated human eyes (3–8) and have determined by quantitative aqueous perfusion that, as the ciliary processes are made to rotate forward, the resistance to aqueous outflow increases. We have found that this effect can be induced without closure of the angle, and even after the whole iris has been removed. However, with the iris intact, if the ciliary processes are made to rotate far enough forward to push the iris against the trabecular meshwork, this does produce angle closure with severe obstruction of aqueous outflow.

Forward rotation of the ciliary processes with obstruction of the mid and posterior trabecular meshwork can have a profound effect on outflow facility, as aqueous is drained primarily through the mid to posterior trabecular meshwork, with little outflow through the anterior trabecular meshwork. This holds true in primary angle closure glaucoma as well. If only the anterior trabecular meshwork remains unobstructed, the effect on outflow facility (and intraocular pressure) can be nearly as pronounced as if the angle were closed completely.

The influence of inducing forward rotation of ciliary processes on facility of outflow is opposite to that which results when the ciliary processes are forced backward, such as by artificial deepening of the anterior chamber (3–8), in which case the facility of outflow is increased. We postulate that in both conditions the abnormal position of the ciliary body exerts forces on the trabecular meshwork that influence the facility of flow through this tissue. In support of this belief, we find that detachment of the ciliary body from the trabecular meshwork or an incision made from the anterior chamber to Schlemm's canal, abolishes the effect of artificial deepening of the anterior chamber.

A local distortion of ciliary processes with adhesion to a surgical scar or an amputation of ciliary processes at the site of operation, are common gonioscopic findings. These have little significance except in cases in which ciliary processes may be seen to be plugging an intended filtration fistula, which can explain the failure of an antiglaucoma filtration operation.

VITREOUS FACE

The view that one can obtain of the face of the vitreous with gonioscopic equipment is often much more informative than that obtained from a frontal view with the slit-lamp biomicroscope (Table 7.8). This is so because the most significant portions are often hidden from direct frontal view, in the angle, or behind the iris, or behind an area of corneal edema.

In phakic eyes, rupture of the hyaloid commonly occurs when the eye has been hit hard enough to rupture some of the zonules of the lens. The lens may remain in the pupil, but it is usually tilted. By looking through the gonioscopic lens under the pupillary border of the iris in the space between the back of the iris and the backward-tilted lens, one may identify a rounded colorless mass of vitreous herniating in front of the equator of the lens, showing the hyaloid, as well as the zonules, to have been ruptured. The significance of this condition is discussed in Chapter 43.

Vitreous in an antiglaucoma filtration fistula is found occasionally by gonioscopy in phakic eyes in which the zonules of the lens and the hyaloid were inadvertently injured during surgery. A column of colorless vitreous may be seen extending forward, attached to the surgical fistula on the inside of the eye, sometimes apparently filling the opening.

In aphakic eyes, vitreous block of the pupil and iridectomy can be established only by gonioscopy. Of course, if

Table 7.8
Findings Involving the Vitreous Face

Findings in phakic eyes
Rupture of peripheral hyaloid with dislocation of lens Vitreous in antiglaucoma filtration fistula
Findings in aphakic eyes:
Adhesion of vitreous to cornea underlying bullous keratopathy Vitreous block of pupil and iridectomy Adhesion of vitreous to surgical wound Epithelialization

no iridectomies were performed, the presence of pupillary block can be established by ordinary slit-lamp examination on the basis of complete filling of the pupil by bulging hyaloid associated with shallowing of the anterior chamber. If iridectomies were performed, one can reasonably infer that the iridectomies as well as the pupil are blocked, if, in addition to forward bulging of hyaloid and iris, the IOP is even slightly elevated. If there is any question of pupillary block from findings at slit-lamp examination, or from other indications described in Chapter 22, a gonioscopic examination is indicated. If complete iridectomy has been performed, one can examine the most peripheral portions of the coloboma and can ascertain whether the hyaloid is in a position to block the whole opening.

Often, a supposedly complete iridectomy can be seen to be not truly basal, but merely an upward enlargement of the pupil. One can see the hyaloid filling the opening completely in contact with the borders of pupil and iridectomy all around, leaving no place for unobstructed flow of aqueous from posterior to anterior chamber, and establishing pupillary block.

One can establish that an eye does not have pupillary block if one can see that the vitreous face, although in contact with the lower portion of the pupil, is distinctly separated peripherally from one or both pillars of the coloboma. When one can see that the hyaloid curves normally backward behind the ciliary processes, with a definite space separating the hyaloid from one or both edges of the coloboma in the iris, one can be sure that there is an unobstructed opening for flow of aqueous from the posterior to the anterior chamber. This is what is usually found when iridectomy is truly basal.

If surgical peripheral iridectomy has been performed, and vitreous is blocking the iridectomy as well as the pupil, one can identify the slightly glistening hyaloid filling the peripheral hole in the iris, provided that the anterior chamber is not too shallow at the time of examination. Normally, without block, when one examines a peripheral iridectomy, the hole in the iris appears completely unobstructed. If the hole is large enough, one may see normal ciliary processes and may be able to identify the hyaloid further posteriorly.

In aphakic eyes, adhesion of vitreous to the surgical wound may or may not be associated with pupillary block or with edema of the adjacent cornea. Most commonly, a slightly gray and sometimes glistening thin sheet of hyaloid, obviously continuous with the hyaloid in the pupillary portion of a surgical coloboma of the iris, extends forward to where it is caught in the inner lips of the wound. This does not necessarily cause trouble. Exceptionally, one sees a broad sheet of hyaloid and the adjacent pillars of the surgical coloboma of the iris caught and held in the wound, usually because of loss of vitreous at surgery. If the whole pupil and coloboma are sealed by the sheet of hyaloid, and there is no patent peripheral iridectomy, pupillary block is almost certain. In these particular circumstances, with pupil and hyaloid updrawn, the anterior chamber may not become so conspicuously shallowed axially as in other forms of pupillary block; but interiorly, the angle may be seen to be closed, and as usual, glaucoma results.

Epithelial invasion of the eye is seen advantageously with gonioscopic equipment. With rare exceptions, it occurs in eyes with all or most of the lens missing. Epithelium enters the eye by way of a surgical or traumatic wound, usually in the angle of the anterior chamber. By slit lamp, the ingrowing epithelium appears as a thin gray membrane resembling ground glass, extending onto the hyaloid and iris and usually onto the back surface of the cornea from the region of the wound. Epithelialization has to be differentiated from the following abnormalities: corneal scar, which is stationary; remnants of capsule, which have a characteristic coiled and refractile appearance; from corneal edema caused by pupillary block and adhesion of vitreous to cornea, which can be identified gonioscopically; and inflammatory membranes, which tend to be more opaque. An epithelial sheet tends to be more homogeneous than other membranes. No confusion with fibrovascular or neovascular membranes is likely, since the membrane of epithelialization is avascular.

In epithelialization, the membrane is very thin, translucent, and gray. By transillumination with the slit lamp, it has a finely granular appearance resembling ground glass. The advancing edge on the back of the cornea is usually slightly thickened and forms a slight ridge. By gonioscopy, the epithelial sheet may be seen to extend from the wound indiscriminately onto all contiguous structures of the anterior segment. If the hyaloid and iris pillars have been caught in the surgical scar, the epithelial membrane may be observed to grow down, sealing the face of vitreous and iris together, and causing pupillary block when the pupil has been sealed completely. On the surface of the iris, the advancing edge of epithelium is less obvious than it is on the hyaloid, but one can distinguish the epithelial membrane on the face of the iris by an appearance of smoothness and slight glistening of the surface not seen in the unaffected normal areas. If hyaloid and iris are not caught in the wound, the pupil is not so readily blocked by spread of the sheet of epithelium, which may develop into a thicker, grayer membrane on iris and hyaloid before it causes glaucoma by obstructing the angle itself. With an open coloboma of the iris, the epithelium may extend posteriorly to form a gray cocoon, enveloping the ciliary processes, with delicate cobwebby gray sheets on the adjacent vitreous face.

Gonioscopic distinction of epithelialization from inflammatory membrane involving remnants of hyaloid or lens remnants presents the greatest difficulty, and one may have to rely upon observing characteristic progressive spread to identify epithelialization. If a leaking fistula in the wound and hypotony are present, these strongly favor the diagnosis of epithelialization.

BLOOD VESSELS IN THE ANGLE

Normal vessels in the angle vary greatly from eye to eye in different individuals, but certain characteristics permit one to distinguish the normal from the abnormal with reasonable certainty. To become familiar with the characteristics and identity of the vessels visible by clinical gonioscopy in normal eyes, it is worthwhile to review the anatomy of the blood supply of the anterior segment.

In the human eye, the principal arterial source for the structures of the angle is the arterial circle of the ciliary body. This "circle" is formed by the joining of long posterior ciliary arteries and anterior ciliary arteries, mostly within the ciliary muscle. The long posterior ciliary arteries come forward on the inner surface of the sclera, one nasally and one temporally. These each divide in the anterior segment of the globe into branches that arch and run circumferentially in the ciliary body. The anterior ciliary arteries enter the globe anteriorly from the outer surface. The anterior ciliary arteries have a distinctive, conspicuously sinuous or serpentine form on the outer surface of the sclera, and they typically enter the globe abruptly via small pits in the sclera known misleadingly as "emissaries." These entrances are scattered at varying distances from the limbus, usually between 1 and 4 mm. The anterior ciliary arteries penetrate the sclera to the ciliary muscle and there join the arching branches of the long posterior ciliary arteries.

The arterial circle (Fig. 2.7) in the ciliary muscle is actually irregular, rarely a true uniform circle. The segments of which the circle is formed are wandering and usually not continuous in the circumference. The nasal and the temporal halves in particular tend to be separate. From this arterial "circle," and from its tributary posterior and anterior ciliary arteries, arise fine branches that supply the ciliary muscle and larger branches, which become the radial arteries of the iris.

The arterial circle of the ciliary body, as a rule, is posterior to the periphery of the iris. The radial arteries of the iris generally extend forward a short distance from their origin in the arterial circle to the peripheral fold or knuckle of the pigment layer of the iris. There they turn and extend in the stroma of the iris in the direction of the pupil. The radial arteries in the stroma of the iris appear by gonioscopic view much as they do by slit lamp, their visibility being influenced by the thickness and degree of pigmentation of the stroma. They have a variable corkscrew form, influenced by the size of the pupil. They tend to go directly to the region of the pupil, and the returning veins tend to radiate similarly directly to the periphery, where they turn posteriorly around the peripheral fold or knuckle of the pigment layer of the iris to pass into the ciliary processes and back to choroid and vortex veins.

Normal radial iris vessels can be seen to have a covering of iris stroma and characteristically conform to a radial pattern, with little tendency to branch, anastomose, or wander diagonally. When the eye is inflamed or the intraocular pressure is elevated, the normal radial vessels tend to enlarge and become more noticeable.

In the human eye, there is no arterial circle of the iris; and in most eyes, the arterial circle of the ciliary body is not visible by gonioscopy. Occasionally, however, portions of the arterial circle of the ciliary body are situated uncommonly far forward on the surface of the ciliary muscle and may be seen anterior to the root of the iris on the ciliary band. Sometimes, the artery encroaches on the root of the iris at its juncture with the ciliary band.

Characteristically, only short segments of the artery come into gonioscopic view in this way, and these always have an obviously circumferential direction. Typically, such circumferential vessels are seen in profile and suggest in appearance a sea serpent with an undulating form, the anterior portion of some of the loops being in view and the posterior portions out of view below the level of attachment of iris on the ciliary muscle. The extent to which anteriorly wandering loops of circumferential artery are visible gonioscopically is affected in part by the thickness and degree of pigmentation of the uveal meshwork and iris stroma. Vessels of this type tend to be most conspicuous in eyes in which the superficial tissues are thin and unpigmented and are least noticeable when the covering tissues are thick and dark brown.

Normal circumferential vessels on the ciliary band never attach anterior to the scleral spur. However, a knuckle of vessel carrying uveal meshwork or strands of iris stroma occasionally protrudes from the surface of the angle sufficiently far forward in the angle to stand in front of the scleral spur and trabecular meshwork, locally obscuring these from direct gonioscopic view, but not in contact with the trabecular meshwork, as can be determined by viewing the angle slightly tangentially.

In addition to the normal radial vessels of the iris and wandering portions of the circumferential artery of the ciliary body, a third type of vessel is seen occasionally in normal human angles, i.e., vertical vessels deep in the ciliary band, probably the anterior ciliary arteries, extending from the interior surface of the sclera, from an "emissary" passage, to the arterial circle in the ciliary muscle. These deep vertical vessels against the sclera are visible in the ciliary band in eyes that are lightly pigmented and have thin, fairly transparent uveal meshwork. One must look through the uveal meshwork and ciliary muscle to see them. These same vessels are sometimes laid bare to gonioscopic view as a result of traumatic disruption of the overlying uveal meshwork and ciliary muscle, the so-called traumatic recession of the angle. They are not normally bare or near the inner surface of the angle.

In rare instances in normal eyes, we have seen what appeared to be an anterior ciliary artery on the inner surface of the ciliary band extending straight forward, without branching, to disappear abruptly into the sclera, usually just behind the scleral spur, but once or twice into or just anterior to the spur, with no evidence of connection with Schlemm's canal (i.e., no blood in the canal).

Two varieties of abnormal, newly formed vessels are distinguishable in the angle:

1. Neovascularization associated with vascular retinopathy secondary to occlusion of the central retinal vein or artery, diabetes, Eales' disease, or extraocular arteriovenous fistula.
2. Neovascularization associated with chronic iridocyclitis or cyclitis, especially with heterochromic cyclitis.

The vessels of neovascularization of the angle that are associated with vascular retinopathy appear to be of the same sort in the several different types of retinopathy, but to differ appreciably from the new vessels of chronic iridocyclitis. In association with the retinal vascular diseases listed above, new vessels grow from the circumferential artery of the ciliary body onto the surface of the iris and onto the surface of the wall of the angle. **On the iris, these vessels are seen to take an erratic, meandering course, without either the distinct radial or the circumferential direction that is characteristic of the normal vessels** (Fig. 7.19). The new vessels also are distinguished from the normal by the fact that they grow on the surface of the iris, not within the stroma. They usually are not connected with the normal stromal vessels.

Neovascularization of the iris in some cases conspicuously involves the portions of the iris visible by slit lamp, producing so-called rubeosis. Less frequently new vessels extend in the form of a fibrovascular membrane onto the pupil itself, onto the surface of the lens, or onto pupillary membranes of other sorts.

In some cases, neovascularization is restricted to the angle, at least at an early stage, and is detectable only by gonioscopy. In the angle, one sees vessels extending from the juncture of iris and ciliary band onto the periphery of the iris and up the wall of the angle. On the wall, the vessels grow vertically forward over the ciliary band and scleral spur onto corneoscleral trabecular meshwork, where they arborize and often appear to dip into the filtration portion of the meshwork as though to Schlemm's canal (Fig. 7.20). Usually there are multiple arborizing vessels.

Newly formed vessels are readily distinguishable from the rare solitary, unbranching anomalous vessel from ciliary band to trabecular meshwork that we describe in the following section on "Anomalous Vessels." New vessels are also different from vessels associated with congenital abnormalities of the angle, which consist of knuckles or hairpin loops of radial iris vessels, tented forward and unbranching.

New blood vessels on the angle wall, and also those on the iris, are accompanied by a transparent sheet of fibrous tissue that cannot be seen by gonioscopy or by slit lamp biomicroscopy. The fibrous sheet does not noticeably hide underlying angle structures from view, yet presumably, it is this transparent sheet between the vessels, rather than the slender vessels themselves which obstructs the filtration portion of the trabecular meshwork and interferes severely with aqueous outflow, causing the disastrous form of glaucoma known as "neovascular" or "hemorrhagic" glaucoma. In this type of glaucoma, the intraocular pressure can become greatly elevated when nothing is visible by gonioscopy on the trabecular meshwork but the arborizing new vessels. The fibrovascular membrane is demonstrable only histologically.

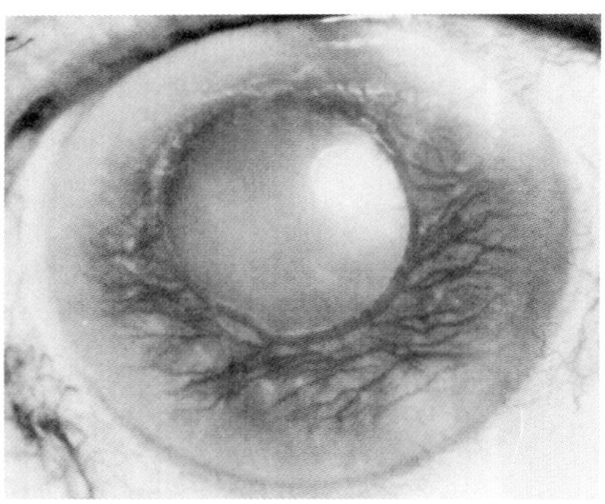

Figure 7.19. Florid neovascularization of the iris. Reprinted with permission from Donaldson DD: Atlas of External Diseases of the Eye. Vol. IV. Anterior Chamber, Iris, and Ciliary Body. St. Louis: C.V. Mosby Co., 1973.

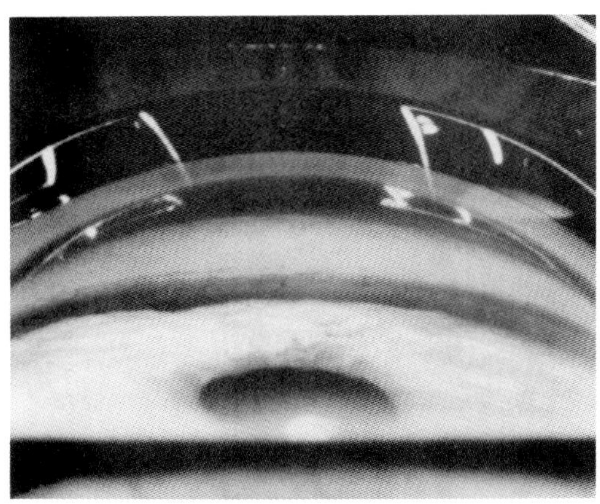

Figure 7.20. Neovascularization of the angle. Note arborization of vessels. Glaucoma can be present with the angle still open at this stage, before synechial formation occurs. (Courtesy of David D. Donaldson, MD).

The neovascularized angle associated with vascular retinopathy usually does not long remain as described above, but tends to go through the following stages. Some of the vertical, newly formed vessel trunks lining the wall of the angle from iris root to trabecular meshwork tend to enlarge and to stand out from the angle wall as stout columns. Along the sides of these vascular columns, the iris appears to be pulled forward until tents of iris stroma reach the trabecular meshwork. From these initial points of attachment, the iris becomes progressively more widely adherent to the trabecular meshwork, both circumferentially and anteriorly, until the whole angle may be closed far forward by peripheral anterior synechias. The layer of fibrovascular tissue that first grew on the angle wall becomes sandwiched in the adhesion between iris and wall of the angle. At this stage, the vessels on the surface of the iris can be seen to enter and disappear at the point of juncture of iris and angle wall. Later, the membrane on the front of the iris may contract and cause extensive ectropion uveae at the pupil.

The character of vascularization of the angle in neovascular glaucoma associated with retinopathy appears to be the same whether it is associated with diabetic retinopathy or is secondary to occlusion of the central retinal artery or vein or other vascular retinopathy.

The other type of neovascularization of the angle, which is associated with heterochromic or other chronic iridocyclitis, appears to differ in some fundamental way. Both types of neovascularization cause obstruction of the trabecular meshwork and induce glaucoma that is resistant to medical treatment, owing to formation of a membrane over the trabecular meshwork, but **the membrane associated with vascular retinopathy has a great tendency to induce peripheral anterior synechias or synechial closure of the angle, whereas the membrane associated with neovascularization of chronic iridocyclitis does not.** Both types of membranes are transparent and not ordinarily discernible by gonioscopy, although they are demonstrable histologically. Occasionally, however, in eyes that have a cuticular membrane covering the angle, comparison made with a contralateral normal eye produces the impression that the angle structures have a less distinct appearance in the affected eye than in the normal.

In Fuchs' heterochromic cyclitis the vessels appear to be finer, fewer, more solitary and have less tendency to arborize on the trabecular meshwork than vessels associated with neovascular glaucoma secondary to vascular retinopathy. The fine solitary vessels found in the angle in heterochromic cyclitis have a tendency to wander apparently aimlessly over all the angle structures, circumferentially as well as radially, whereas those associated with vascular retinopathy cross the angle only in a direct radial manner. The vessels in heterochromic cyclitis have a characteristic tendency to bleed easily, either spontaneously or as a consequence of abrupt lowering of the intraocular pressure by paracentesis or other operation. The amount of bleeding typically is small, detectable by microscopic examination of a sample of aqueous, or visible gonioscopically as a fine line of blood squirting from the vessel on the angle wall to form a tiny hyphema, which may be visible only gonioscopically. In heterochromic cyclitis, abnormal vessels may also be found in eyes that do not develop glaucoma.

In rare instances in otherwise normal eyes, a solitary vessel is seen extending from the ciliary band forward, crossing the scleral spur, and disappearing into the corneoscleral trabecular meshwork just anterior to the scleral spur. Although the vessel disappears in the region of Schlemm's canal, no blood has been observed in the canal in such eyes. Such vessels may possibly be aberrant anterior ciliary arteries. They have no branchings on the trabecular meshwork or on the ciliary band.

Normally, all vessels in the angle are restricted to the ciliary band and iris and do not go as far forward as the scleral spur or trabecular meshwork.

Congenitally abnormal vessels are seen in cases of congenital glaucoma, in which the iris stroma is abnormally knuckled forward in the periphery. Exceptionally, there is also a forward bend or knuckling of the radial vessels of the iris, which may go anterior to the level of the scleral spur. In cases of embryotoxon and of Axenfeld's syndrome, such vascular loops sometimes extend even as far forward as Schwalbe's line. The arch or loop form of the vessels, which may approximate the shape of a hairpin, and the accompanying iris stroma serves to distinguish these congenital abnormally placed vessels from those of neovascularization. The vessels of neovascularization typically have one end at the root of the iris and the other ending in fine branches on the trabecular meshwork; whereas the congenitally looped vessels have both ends in the iris, and they do not arborize on the angle wall.

In association with persistent hyperplastic primary vitreous in infants, one may see a vessel taking a bizzare course from behind the iris through the pupil, bending sharply around the pupillary border, and extending across the surface of the iris to the ciliary band.

In conclusion, one can make the following generalizations concerning vessels in the angle. No pathologic significance is attached to radial vessels seen within the iris stroma, sea-serpent type circumferential vessels seen in the angle in the periphery of the iris or against the ciliary band, or short, straight vessels seen deep in the ciliary muscle and disappearing below the scleral spur. However, vessels that have an erratic course on the surface of the iris without either distinct radial or circumferential direction, and vessels that extend up the angle wall beyond the scleral spur to the trabecular meshwork are, with rare exceptions, pathologic.

PIGMENT IN THE ANGLE

In evaluating pigment in the angle, one must distinguish pigment that is deposited in the angle from the brown uveal meshwork that is normally present in many eyes. This distinction is readily made on the basis of the location, form, and color of the pigment. Brown uveal meshwork typically occurs in the form of strands or a network of strands, often extending across the ciliary band and scleral spur onto the posterior half of the corneoscleral trabecular meshwork. Deposited pigment, which has been carried by the aqueous to the trabecular meshwork, is characteristically located in a band overlying Schlemm's canal in the filtration portion of the meshwork, roughly in its middle third. Occasionally, pigment may also be indiscriminately scattered on the back of the cornea, on Schwalbe's line, and on other structures, particularly in the lower angle. Deposited pigment, either that in the filtration portion of the trabecular meshwork or that which is indiscriminately scattered, characteristically has a finely granular appearance and is brown or black, like the pigment of the posterior pigment layer of the iris, distinctly darker than the brown of the iris stroma (Table 7.9).

Through infancy and childhood, the trabecular meshwork remains completely clean of pigment deposits; but during adult life there is commonly a gradual, slight accumulation of pigment in the trabecular meshwork, faintly delineating the filtration area overlying Schlemm's canal. In advanced years, a distinct, fine, granular brown band of pigment commonly accumulates in the trabecular meshwork. **The slender band of deposited pigment in elderly people is usually most evident in the nasal quadrant,** where also the uveal meshwork tends to be most pronounced. In some such normal eyes, the faint but definite band extends also into the lower and upper nasal quadrants. However, with rare exceptions, the temporal quadrant remains clean in normal eyes.

Table 7.9
Conditions Involving Pigment in the Angle

Pigment in the Angle	Conditions
None	Normal in young
Band nasally and inferiorly	Normal in elderly
Faint band, whole circumference	Normal in elderly
Dense band, whole circumference, both eyes	Exfoliation
	Pigmentary glaucoma
	Pigment dispersion syndrome
Dense band, whole circumference, one eye	Exfoliation
	Malignant melanoma
	Cysts or tumors of iris or ciliary body
Scattered, mostly in lower angle	Previous intraocular surgery
	Previous inflammation
	Previous hyphema
Patchy band, whole circumference	Occasional in open-angle glaucoma
Dense isolated patch	Nevus
Light-brown, very fine pigment	From brown iris stroma
Dark-brown fine granular pigment	From posterior pigment layers
Black, fine and coarse, balls and granules	Old blood

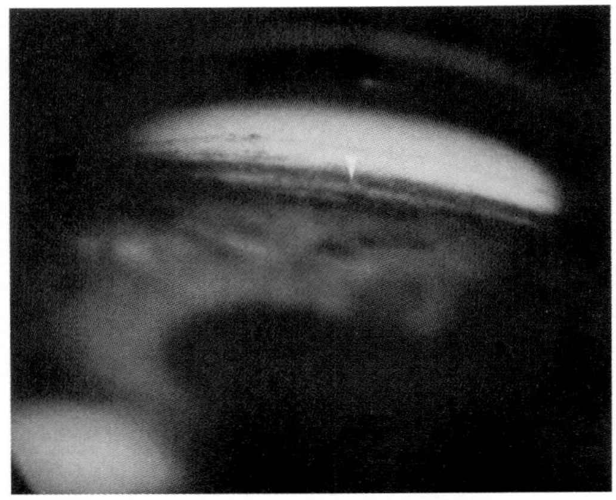

Figure 7.21. Increased pigmentation and exfoliation material (arrowhead) in the angle of a patient with exfoliation glaucoma.

Pigment deposition in a solid band in the whole circumference is, in almost all instances, pathologic. The denser and broader the band, the more likely it is to be pathologic. In an elderly patient, when excessive pigment deposition is seen in the angle, the first suspicion is **exfoliation** (Fig. 7.21), which can readily be looked for under the pupillary border where the gonioscope reveals fine light-gray flecks of material that look like dandruff.

In young individuals, before the age of nuclear sclerosis, excessive pigment in the trabecular meshwork first suggests **pigmentary glaucoma**, in which there is degeneration of the posterior pigment layer of the iris toward the mid-periphery, and no dandruff-like exfoliation. This occurs most commonly in association with myopia in young males and is usually, but not always, accompanied by abnormal deposition of pigment on the back of the cornea. In this condition, transillumination of the globe typically shows abnormal transillumination of the pigment layer of the iris in a patchy annulus in the midperiphery, with no discernible abnormality of the stroma of the iris (Chapter 21).

Although excessive pigment deposition in the trabecular meshwork seems both clinically and experimentally to obstruct aqueous outflow and cause glaucoma, not every eye having excessive pigment in the angle is glaucomatous. One sees occasional instances of Krukenberg's spindle pigment on the back of the cornea, with heavy deposition of pigment in the whole angle, with normal pressure and normal facility of outflow. It may be that the size of pigment particles can differ enough and be sufficiently critical to influence significantly the degree of obstruction. We suppose that if the particles are large enough they may stay on the surface rather than penetrate into the deeper portion of the trabecular meshwork and may therefore fail to plug the channels in the presumably most critical endothelial layer next to Schlemm's canal. Differences in trabecular endothelial cell response to the pigment may also be important. Presumably, phagocytosis of the pigment by trabecular endothelium can "unplug" the outflow channel. We have perfused homologous pigment into the outflow pathways of living monkeys and produced the expected temporary obstruction to aqueous outflow. Despite repeated pigment perfusions, however, outflow facility always returned to normal values in these monkeys (9). Thus it seems that, in pigmentary glaucoma, there must be other abnormalities in addition to pigment particle liberation, and that it may be the trabecular cell response to pigment, rather than the pigment itself, which results in the reduction of outflow facility.

When excessive pigmentation of the filtration portion of the angle occurs in only one eye of a patient, this suggests exfoliation as a first possibility. The pigmentation in exfoliation tends to be coarser, and more of a salt and pepper pattern, than the uniform, fine pigmentation seen in pigment dispersion. This may relate to the mechanism of pigment release, with pigment dispersion syndrome typically resulting from ballotment of the posterior iris against the zonules, and pigment release in pseudoexfoliation coming from rubbing of the iris against the abnormally roughened anterior lens capsule. Otherwise, asymmetrical pigmentation suggests **cysts of iris or ciliary body**, or **malignant melanoma** in the ciliary body or iris, which can cause shedding of pigment that comes forward and becomes enmeshed in the trabecular meshwork, sometimes enough to cause glaucoma.

Pigment that is coarser and scattered indiscriminately in tiny clumps of varied sizes in the dependent portion of the angle, concentrated along Schwalbe's line, and rather diffusely dirtying the trabecular meshwork without selective concentration in the filtration portion, is a common finding after intraocular surgery or inflammation, and does not necessarily produce glaucoma. Similar indiscriminately scattered pigment that is black, varying from fine to coarse, and especially in the form of small balls is characteristic of previous hyphema and presumably consists of the decomposition products of blood (Fig. 7.22).

In eyes having open-angle glaucoma, we have occasionally seen a small amount of pigment in the filtration portion of the trabecular meshwork in a conspicuously patchy distribution in the whole circumference, but we have not seen this in completely normal eyes. The appearance suggests to us that, in such eyes, this patchy distribution may be caused by irregular pathologic alteration of the trabecular meshwork. This is possibly a manifestation of increased resistance and less than normal flow of aqueous through those areas that are white, with most of the flow restricted to the adjacent areas in which the accumulation of pigment indicates that aqueous has been undergoing filtration. A number of alternate explanations occur to us, but all are conjectural, not worth detailing at this time.

After laser trabeculoplasty, the trabecular meshwork may take on a variegated appearance, with intermittent areas of pigmentation and whitening. It is not known whether the white areas represent laser damaged tissue that is no longer filtering, or areas stimulated by the laser treatment to be cleared of pigment.

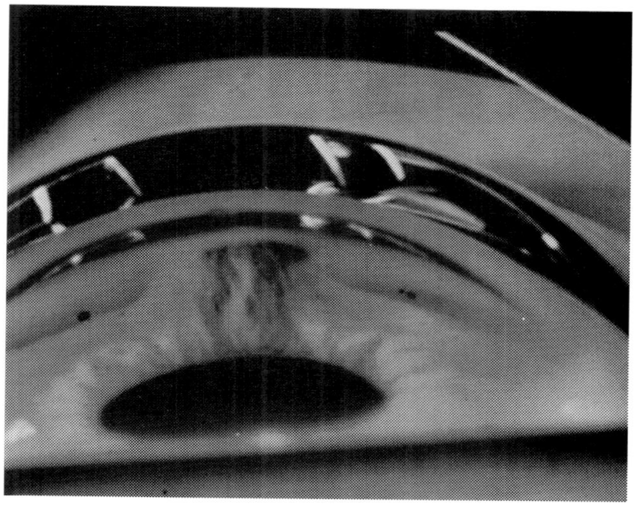

Figure 7.22. Round black balls in angle represent old blood, most likely secondary to blunt trauma.

INFLAMMATORY DEPOSITS IN THE ANGLE

In association with intraocular infection, inflammation, or rarely, tumor (10), *hypopyon* is commonly detectable by ordinary examination with a flashlight or slit lamp, but occasionally a hypopyon is so small and so peripherally situated that it is detectable only by gonioscopy. When one inspects a hypopyon with the gonioscope, one sees a blanket of whitish inflammatory exudate extending from peripheral iris over the angle structures (Fig. 7.23), filling

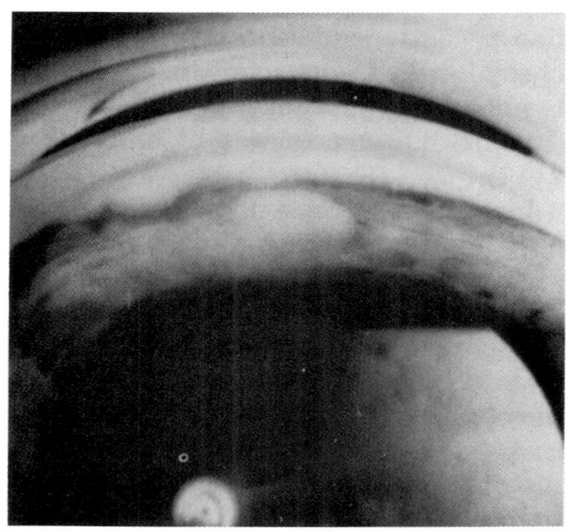

Figure 7.23. "Hypopyon" in the angle due to retinoblastoma. Reprinted with permission from Donaldson DD: Atlas of External Diseases of the Eye. Vol IV. Anterior Chamber, Iris, and Ciliary Body. St. Louis: C. V. Mosby Co., 1973.

in the angle and hiding the angle structures to a variable degree, with considerable resemblance to a snowdrift. A hypopyon characteristically is associated with obvious cellular reaction in the aqueous, and most commonly is restricted to the lower quadrant of the angle, as a result of the cells settling to the lowest portion. This is often the case in intraocular infections, more rarely in simplex keratitis, occasionally in spontaneous lysis and leakage of hypermature cataracts, and in cases of retained cortex after extracapsular extraction or traumatic cataract. In such cases, inflammatory cells may be present and demonstrable histologically in the trabecular meshwork in the whole circumference in sufficient quantity to obstruct aqueous outflow and cause glaucoma, yet not of sufficient density to be discernible gonioscopically except in the lower quadrant. However, in rare instances, we have seen a complete blanketing of the angle in the whole circumference by inflammatory exudate accompanied by severe glaucoma. In one patient, who a short time later died of acute pneumococcal septicemia, the angle of each eye was completely blanketed, and IOPs were in the eighties. Histologically, the trabecular meshwork was densely infiltrated, as well as completely covered by inflammatory cells. There were no synechias.

Inflammatory precipitates on the trabecular meshwork in the form of keratic precipitates (KP) are far less obvious than hypopyon in the angle and are easily overlooked, unless one has them specifically in mind during examination of the angle. KP on the trabecular meshwork are apparently the same as KP on the back of the cornea, consisting of discrete clumps of inflammatory cells; but in certain cases, KP are detectable in the angle when none are found on the cornea and when there is no evidence of inflammation by slit lamp. This condition occurs especially in sarcoidosis. **The discovery of KP by careful gonioscopy can provide the most important clue for explaining the basis for a puzzling case of glaucoma.**

KP on the trabecular meshwork are sometimes very inconspicuous. They consist of small gelatinous-looking, colorless mounds, projecting into the anterior chamber from the surface of the trabecular meshwork. They resemble KP seen on the cornea, but generally are broader and flatter. They may be confluent, making a continuous line of exudate over 2, 3, or 4 hours of the clock. Their presence is most readily revealed by their projection from the surface, which is notable because, by gonioscopic view, they are seen mainly in profile (Fig. 7.24). Inflammatory deposits in the angle are discussed further in Chapter 42.

Occult KP in the angle can simulate primary open angle glaucoma if not properly diagnosed. Proper detection and treatment are essential, as a paradoxical response to treatment can result if KP on the trabecular meshwork are not suspected. For example, in this setting, pilocarpine can cause a dramatic elevation in intraocular pressure, while topical steroid therapy can be curative.

PERIPHERAL ANTERIOR SYNECHIAS

The term peripheral anterior synechia (PAS) signifies a condition in which the iris has become attached further forward in the angle than normal. The abnormal forward attachment may extend to anterior portions of the ciliary band, to the scleral spur, to corneoscleral trabecular meshwork, to Schwalbe's line, or, in some instances, even to the cornea. Peripheral anterior synechias are a complication of many ocular conditions and may develop in various ways (Table 7.10). Their presence and special characteristics are significant in differential diagnosis in certain instances, but their principal importance is that they can interfere with aqueous outflow if they obstruct a significant portion of the trabecular meshwork and can cause intraocular pressure to become elevated.

In open-angle glaucoma that is not associated with intraocular inflammation, PAS do not occur, unless the origi-

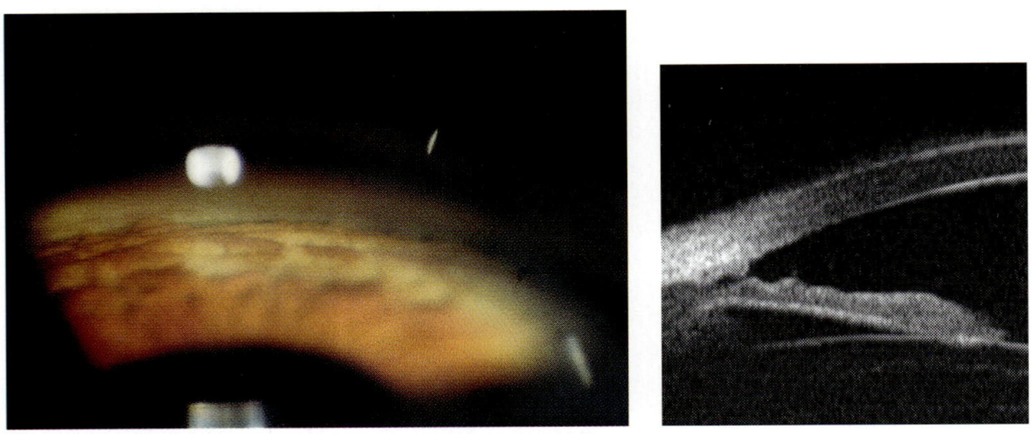

A B

Figure 7.24. Inflammatory precipitates in angle. **A,** Goniophotograph. **B,** Ultrasound biomicrograph. Precipitates are gelatinous and amorphous in appearance, and can be very difficult to distinguish. Ultrasound biomicroscopy enables quantification of precipitate dimensions, and facilitates follow-up. Typically, such precipitates are exquisitely sensitive to topical steroid therapy.

Table 7.10
Variations in Peripheral Anterior Synechias

Conditions	Findings
Primary open-angle glaucoma	Never synechias in these glaucomas, so long as uncomplicated by other disease or by operation
Exfoliation with glaucoma	
Pigmentary glaucoma	
Heterochromic cyclitis with glaucoma	Synechias to all levels, but not to cornea, and not bridging angle structures
Angle-closure glaucoma	
Absence or excessive shallowing of the anterior chamber after surgery	Synechias to all levels, sometimes to cornea, after surgery sometimes bridging angle
Iris bombé in phakic or aphakic eyes	Same as above
Glaucoma secondary to iridocyclitis or KP on the trabecular meshwork	Typically tents and columns to all levels, but not to cornea
Neovascular glaucoma	Broad synechias to full width of angle, with new vessels
Essential atrophy of the iris	Synechias advancing on the cornea, sometimes obstructing trabecular meshwork
Chandler's syndrome of atrophy of stroma of iris with corneal endothelial dystrophy and edema	Synechias advancing irregularly on corneoscleral meshwork, later to cornea
After laser trabeculoplasty	Small irregular synechias to scleral spur, occasionally to posterior trabecular meshwork

nal disease is complicated by some additional disease, such as occlusion of the central retinal vein, or by surgery or laser therapy. Following laser trabeculoplasty, it is not uncommon to see small, irregular PAS to the level of scleral spur and occasionally to posterior trabecular meshwork in the areas of treatment. Rarely, extensive PAS with accompanying significant obstruction to outflow may be observed.

We have seen no exception to the rule that PAS are never found in uncomplicated primary open-angle glaucoma, in open-angle glaucoma associated with exfoliation, or in "pigmentary glaucoma" (except after laser therapy).

If a definite PAS is seen in a case of supposedly primary open-angle glaucoma, it most commonly is the result of previous surgery or is a manifestation of neovascular glaucoma due to occlusion of the central retinal vein. **If a definite PAS is present but there is no supporting evidence of neovascular glaucoma or previous operation, then the diagnosis must be changed to some form of secondary glaucoma, most often due to KP in the angle.**

The most common mistake leading to an erroneous diagnosis of PAS is to confuse normal uveal meshwork with acquired synechial attachment of iris to angle wall. Both normal uveal meshwork, pigmented or unpigmented, and peripheral anterior synechias are found in similar locations, overlying ciliary band, scleral spur, and corneoscleral trabecular meshwork, but uveal meshwork and PAS have definite distinguishing characteristics that one can recognize gonioscopically. As already described in a previous section on "Uveal Meshwork," this tissue in adult eyes is present normally in the angle in amounts and densities varying from a thin, delicate, colorless veil in some blue eyes to a thick brown forest of strands in some brown eyes, but it always has a lacy structure composed of a network of strands with discernible openings and is porous in appearance. The strands may extend individually vertically up the wall of the angle or they may be part of a lacy sheet extending from peripheral iris to the angle wall. Transillumination, with the light turned just to one side or other of the field of view, so that it illuminates the white scleral background and displays pigmented structures in the angle contrastingly dark against the bright background, can be utilized in some brown eyes to demonstrate the porosity of the uveal meshwork especially well. Not uncommonly in brown eyes, the uveal meshwork presents a network of fine strands that is more extensive where it overlies the midportion of the trabecular meshwork than where it crosses the ciliary muscle band. Tiny feet or dots of darker brown are often evident at the anterior edge of a fringe of brown lacy uveal meshwork on the trabecular meshwork.

True PAS differ from uveal meshwork in being more solid and in being definitely composed of iris stroma. Synechias take numerous characteristic forms, ranging from tiny tent-like adhesions to complete closure of the angle. The type of PAS is related to the variety of disease that has caused the formation of the adhesion. This is worth special attention as an aid in differential diagnosis.

True acquired PAS are seen in the following conditions: angle-closure glaucoma; after prolonged absence of the anterior chamber after intraocular surgery; after laser trabeculoplasty; after iris bombé in both phakic and aphakic eyes; in certain forms of glaucoma due to intraocular inflammation; in iridocorneal endothelial (ICE) syndromes (Chapter 32); and after injury to the eye.

In instances in which PAS are attached to the cornea anterior to Schwalbe's line, as in certain cases of ICE syndrome or after iris bombé either in phakic or aphakic eyes, the PAS may be readily detected by slit-lamp examination. In other cases, the diagnosis must be made by gonioscopy.

One of the most significant features to determine gonioscopically is whether the PAS are in a position to obstruct the filtration portion of the trabecular meshwork, just anterior to the scleral spur, approximately the central third of the trabecular meshwork directly overlying Schlemm's canal, the portion in which pigment particles become trapped as the aqueous is filtered on its way out of the eye. Extension of PAS onto the anterior third of the trabecular meshwork is of little additional significance. Probably very little aqueous goes through the anterior third of the trabecular meshwork.

In angle-closure glaucoma, identification of peripheral anterior synechias is important. If the angle is examined between attacks and is found to be hazardously narrow, but open, the diagnosis may remain uncertain, but if true residual synechias are identifiable, this strongly substantiates the diagnosis. However, in angle-closure glaucoma it may be very difficult to be sure in the unoperated eye whether an area of closure represents simple contact of iris with trabecular meshwork or is actual synechial closure. If, in surveying the angle, one finds an abrupt transition from clearly open angle to adjacent definitely closed angle, there is a strong probability that the closure is synechial, but one cannot be certain. In eyes in which there is no pigment line delineating the filtration portion of the corneoscleral meshwork and the angle is so narrow that the scleral spur cannot be seen, it may be difficult to estimate how much of the filtration area is covered and whether it is by simple contact or by synechias.

In these situations, use of the Zeiss lens (Fig. 7.6) for indentation gonioscopy is most informative. As mentioned previously, simple placement of the Zeiss lens on the cornea commonly indents the cornea and displaces aqueous humor posteriorly; this can be accentuated by deliberate posterior movement of the lens on the cornea. The iris is observed to be bowed posteriorly and areas of previous iris-angle appositional closure can be observed to open under the influence of the indentation lens. Alternatively, definite peripheral anterior synechias can be identified as areas of continued adherence of iris to angle wall despite the indentation. However, for the latter, substantial displacement of the iris should be observed during the indentation process. Often, good indentation cannot be performed when the intraocular pressure is high. One can be more certain of PAS with this method when there is an abrupt transition from deep open angle to localized synechias. It is often easier to diagnose the absence rather than the presence of PAS with this technique. The absence of PAS with indentation gonioscopy does not rule out chronic appositional angle-closure glaucoma.

In angle-closure glaucoma, episodes of closure of the angle by contact eventually lead to synechial closure. The duration of closure by contact necessary to cause synechial closure appears to vary greatly from patient to patient. The congested eye appears to form synechias more quickly than the quiet eye. However, there are exceptions to this rule. Eyes have been observed in which the angle opened completely after an acute attack of many days' duration. In other eyes, an acute attack of not more than 48-hours' duration has been known to result in extensive synechial closure. One extraordinary patient whom we have seen had a history of repeated attacks of angle closure over a period of 8 years, yet after peripheral iridectomy, only a small fraction of the angle was found to be closed by PAS.

Primary angle-closure typically causes adhesion of the iris to the wall of the angle from its deepest portion forward to various levels on the trabecular meshwork, forming no bridges and sparing no structures in the advance of the iris forward, but never extending anterior to Schwalbe's line. The synechias characteristically consist of bands of adhesion, rather than narrow tents or columns such as produced by inflammation. The bands of PAS are often broad and, in the worst cases, involve the whole circumference. How far forward the iris is adherent is important because obstruction to aqueous outflow is caused only by synechias that cover the filtration portion of the trabecular meshwork, not by attachments posterior to this special area.

Prolonged absence of the anterior chamber after surgery for glaucoma or cataract also is a well-known cause of PAS, which are usually in the form of broad bands of adhesion of iris to various levels on the angle wall similar to those that occur in primary angle-closure glaucoma. Sometimes, however, after postoperative flat anterior chamber, a row of fine tent-like synechias results. More rarely, the iris appears to become adherent anterior to the filtration portion of the trabecular meshwork, forming a bridge, with an open tunnel between the iris and the filtration zone. In such instances, gonioscopy may suggest that there is extensive synechial closure of the angle, but the IOP is much easier to control, and the facility of outflow is much better than one would expect if the angle were actually closed so extensively. On close inspection of the lateral edges of the bands of synechia, one may be able to see the open end of a tunnel running behind the synechia, although it is not possible to say how far. This has to be inferred from measurement of the IOP and the facility of outflow.

When pupillary block develops after surgery for congenital cataract in childhood, it is prone to cause disastrous PAS. In children, the PAS acquired in this way often extend onto clear cornea. Once extensive PAS develop in such cases, treatment becomes very difficult and unsatisfactory.

After filtering operations for glaucoma, absence of the anterior chamber is not unusual and may lead to the formation of PAS. PAS formation is usually not extensive. If one is fortunate enough to obtain an excellent filtering scar, the IOP may be controlled despite extensive PAS, but if the filtering scar is less than adequate or fails to develop entirely, extensive PAS from prolonged absence of the anterior chamber may make the glaucoma much worse than it was before operation.

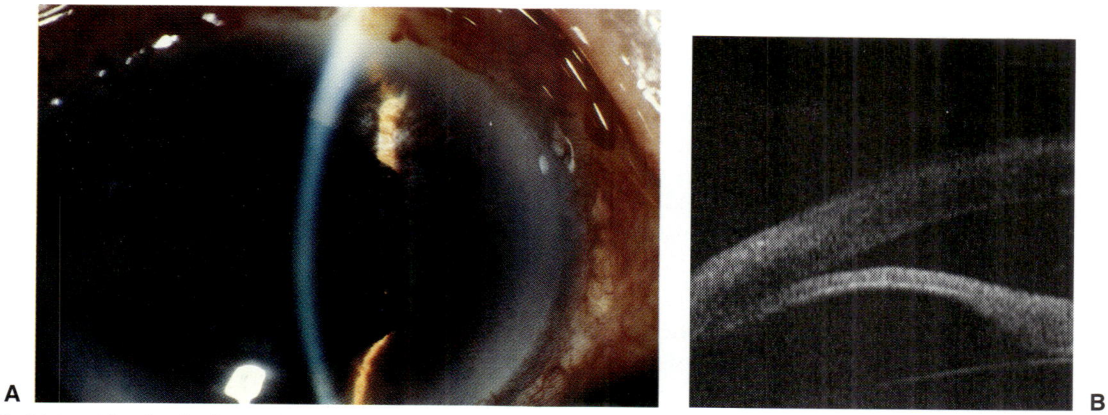

Figure 7.25. Iris bombé and angle-closure glaucoma due to posterior synechias from chronic uveitis. A, Slit lamp photograph. B, Ultrasound biomicrograph.

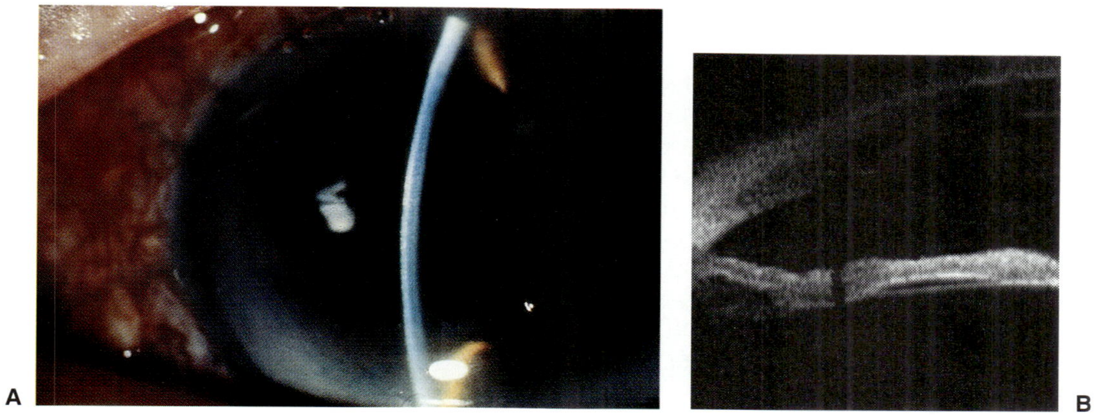

Figure 7.26. Same eye shown in Figure 7.25, following laser peripheral iridectomy. Note resolution of iris bombé, but persistence of posterior synechias. A, Slit lamp photograph. B, Ultrasound biomicrograph.

Iris bombé (Figs. 7.25 and 7-26) from posterior synechias in phakic eyes can quickly lead to PAS that may extend onto the cornea and may cause severe glaucoma. The bombé should be relieved as promptly as possible by laser iridectomy with the aim of preventing further formation of PAS.

Acute iritis and uveitis rarely cause PAS and probably do so only in eyes having anatomically narrow angles in which the edematous peripheral iris may actually come in contact with the trabecular wall. However, in a form of chronic iridocyclitis characterized by exudates on the corneoscleral meshwork similar to KP, PAS frequently form (Fig. 7.27). Gonioscopically, one can observe these exudates in all stages of organization forming synechias.

When a collection of inflammatory cells protrudes far enough from the surface of the trabecular meshwork to touch the periphery of the iris, a junction is formed. The space between the projecting mound of inflammatory cells and the periphery of the iris may be narrowed by inflammatory thickening of the iris and by a layer of inflammatory exudate on the surface of the iris. When the space is bridged and contact is made, the iris adheres and it may

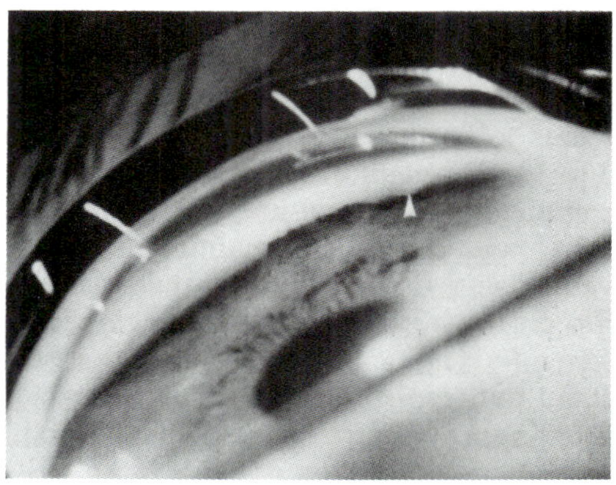

Figure 7.27. Localized peripheral anterior synechia in an otherwise wide open angle in a patient with uveitis. Resolving KP on trabecular meshwork is present (arrowhead). (Courtesy of David D. Donaldson, MD).

be pulled further forward when KP organize. A tent of iris then remains fastened by a scar to the trabecular meshwork. **Organization of KP on the trabecular meshwork in uveitis most characteristically forms columnar or pyramidal synechias.**

In **neovascular glaucoma,** after the angle has become lined by a fibrovascular membrane, PAS are formed, as described in the section "Blood Vessels in the Angle." Severe glaucoma is usually present both before and after PAS develop. The formation of PAS in this condition seems to be caused by contracture of the fibrovascular membrane, which can completely close an angle that was formerly wide open. The membrane of new vessels and fibrous tissue grows initially flat on the surface of all the angle structures, then, some of the vessels stand out from the surface, bridging from the iris to the corneoscleral meshwork. Contraction of these bridging vessels pulls the iris forward until it is in complete contact with the angle wall as far forward as Schwalbe's line. This process usually goes on in several regions of the angle simultaneously, forming broad columns and bands of PAS that may close the entire angle, sandwiching new vessels and fibrous tissue between iris and angle wall, as far forward as Schwalbe's line.

In ICE syndrome, special types of PAS develop, associated with spread of a transparent cellular and basement membrane. In these conditions, PAS can be observed gonioscopically in all stages of development, without any evidence of inflammation. Typically, in the essential atrophy of the iris form of ICE syndrome, the PAS are gross, and they may extend anterior to Schwalbe's line onto the cornea. A little yellowish amorphous material may be noted at the juncture of synechias with the cornea. The synechias tend to spread circumferentially with distortion of the pupil and atrophy and partial disappearance of all layers of the iris. If synechias obstruct the filtration portion of the corneoscleral meshwork, intraocular pressure may rise dangerously. Where the angle wall is visible between synechias, it may function normally, or it may be obstructed by overgrowth of a membrane.

Synechial attachments of iris, extending farther forward than Schwalbe's line, actually onto the back of the cornea, are found not only in ICE syndrome, but also in the following conditions; after neglected postoperative flat anterior chamber; with epithelialization of the anterior chamber; with iris bombé either in phakic, pseudophakic or aphakic eyes; occasionally in neovascular glaucoma; and with pupillary block, especially after congenital cataract operation.

In certain cases of essential atrophy of the iris, a considerable extent of the angle may be hidden by synechias but there may be no proportional elevation of IOP, and facility of aqueous outflow may be surprisingly good. This is analogous to the condition occasionally observed when there has been prolonged absence of the anterior chamber after cataract extraction. A large portion of the angle may appear closed on gonioscopic examination, yet the IOP may be readily controlled by medical means. **In such cases, the iris root appears actually to bridge the corneoscleral meshwork and attach only to Schwalbe's line and cornea, leaving the filtration portion of the meshwork uninvolved.**

Attachments between peripheral iris and Schwalbe's line that bridge the angle, with an open tunnel behind the bridge, may be seen not only with essential atrophy of the iris and following flat anterior chamber after cataract operation, but also as congenital anomalies in association with posterior embryotoxon, in which Schwalbe's line is characteristically abnormally coarse, thickened, and beaded. No such bridging of the meshwork seems to occur in primary angle-closure or as a result of intraocular inflammation. In these conditions, the iris becomes firmly attached to all structures beneath, and if the filtration portion of the corneoscleral meshwork is covered, there is a proportionate interference with aqueous outflow.

Treatment of PAS, with the aim of removing obstruction to aqueous outflow, appears to be ineffectual except in the case of very fresh and tenuous adhesions. Experimental dissection of peripheral anterior synechias from the trabecular meshwork and evaluation of facility of outflow by perfusion post mortem show that synechialysis is of no benefit once synechias have become well established. Microscopy of cross sections shows disorganization or scarring of the corneoscleral trabecular meshwork in areas underlying old synechias, and it is understandable that, even with the synechias freed, the meshwork itself does not function normally. However, it is likely that freeing very recently formed PAS may be of some value. Experimentally, significant improvement in facility of outflow was obtained by synechialysis post mortem in one eye that had very recently formed PAS.

Gonioplasty (Chapter 60) with the argon laser has proven efficacious in freeing recently formed PAS. With the pupil made miotic with pilocarpine, treating the peripheral iris with large spot diameter, low-energy laser burns through a goniolens can cause prompt lysis of the iris adhesion. We have observed improvement in intraocular pressure and tonographic outflow facility in cases treated with iridogonioplasty as long as 6 months after angle closure and formation of PAS.

If gonioplasty is ineffective, it is occasionally valuable to perform the procedure of deepening the anterior chamber and goniosynechiolysis. This is accomplished by paracentesis and release of aqueous, allowing sufficient time for escape of aqueous from the posterior as well as from the anterior chamber, after which saline solution is injected through the paracentesis opening to deepen the anterior chamber at the expense of evacuated posterior chamber, and thus to spread the angle wide and display to direct gonioscopic examination the extent of actual attachment of iris onto the angle wall. Old PAS can be freed surgically with a spatula; however, we have abandoned this procedure because of lack of evidence of benefit to the glaucoma although others have reported success with this operation (11).

In practice, the principle stands that the most desirable and effective countermeasures against PAS are those designed to prevent their formation.

BLOOD IN THE ANGLE

When fresh and red, blood in the angle presents no problem in recognition, appearing much as it does by ordinary slit-lamp examination, but in some cases the amount is so small that it is discoverable only by gonioscopy. Old, degenerated blood characteristically consists of black deposits, varying from fine granules to coarse balls, scattered indiscriminately on all angle structures, but most densely in the lower angle (Fig. 7.22). A blood clot that has persisted extraordinarily long in the angle can become fibrosed and produce synechial obstruction of the angle (Table 7.11).

Spontaneous hyphema, without history or evidence of trauma, most often comes from the abnormal new vessels that develop in the angle in association with the vascular retinopathy from diabetes or in association with occlusion of the central retinal vein or artery. Gonioscopic search for neovascularization in the angle is necessary to establish the diagnosis, unless rubeosis of the iris is already evident by slit-lamp examination. Glaucoma is usually already present when hyphema develops from neovascularization.

In rare instances, we have seen sudden small spontaneous hemorrhage develop in eyes that have been otherwise normal to all examination, including gonioscopy, and we have not discovered the source. Intraocular pressure has become moderately elevated within a half hour because of measurable obstruction to outflow, but within a few hours there has been spontaneous improvement. Within a day or two the blood has gone, and the pressure and facility of outflow have returned to normal. Rarely, we have seen eyes with subtly abnormal iris vascular tufts at the pupillary margin present with this clinical picture.

In rare instances, in normal eyes during gonioscopy, we have seen blood dribble into the angle from some indifferent-looking site in the trabecular meshwork, from blood that has been caused to reflux into Schlemm's canal by the pressure of the rim of the contact lens. This has been transient and of no special significance that we are aware of.

Bleeding in the angle is occasionally induced by a sudden fall of intraocular pressure, resulting from the escape of aqueous humor from the eye during diagnostic aspiration of the aqueous. This occurs rarely in normal eyes. However, in eyes that have heterochromic iridocyclitis, acute hypotony characteristically causes slight, inconsequential bleeding into the anterior chamber from the special type of new blood vessels that form in the angle in this disease. (These vessels have been described in the section Blood Vessels in the Angle.)

Blood rarely refluxes from Schlemm's canal through normal trabecular meshwork into the anterior chamber when the intraocular pressure is rapidly lowered; but after a goniotomy has been performed, blood often refluxes into the anterior chamber while the goniotomy knife is being withdrawn from the eye and the aqueous is escaping from the wound in the cornea. Anatomically, it appears that the junctions between the endothelial cells of the inner wall of Schlemm's canal ordinarily prevent blood reflux back from the canal into the eye (12), but that this can be altered in certain abnormal conditions.

Vascularization of the inner aspect of a cataract wound can cause repeated hyphema. This has been well described by Swan (13). Treatment of the abnormal vessels with the argon laser can be effective. Rarely, a similar chronic vascularization process can occur on the inner aspect of a trabeculectomy (scleral flap filter) wound. Occasionally also in the immediate postoperative situation, hyphema can occur, ostensibly originating from the cut edge of Schlemm's canal. This is rarely a chronic problem, although we have observed recurrent hyphema for as long as 3 weeks after trabeculectomy.

Blunt trauma to the eye is probably the most common cause of hyphema. The blood comes from torn vessels in the angle. Gonioscopy most commonly reveals a tear or disruption of the uveal meshwork and ciliary muscle. Anterior ciliary arteries entering the ciliary muscle from the sclera seem to be in a particularly vulnerable position. Less commonly, dialysis of the iris is found in the periphery; the associated rupture of radial arteries of the iris near their origin from the circumferential ciliary artery is a potential source of bleeding.

Table 7.11
Conditions Involving Blood in the Angle

Conditions	Findings
Fresh blood	Bright red puddle, sheet or clot
Old, degenerated blood	Black particles and balls scattered in the angle
Organized persistent clot	Synechias filling the angle
Spontaneous hyphema	From new vessles in angle or iris associated with neovascular glaucoma
	From microhemangiomas of iris
	From blood in Schlemm's canal
	From vessels on inner surface of cataract wound
	In infants: Xanthogranuloma
Hyphema from sudden hypotony	From new vessels in the angle in heterochromic cyclitis
	From blood in Schlemm's canal
Hyphema from blunt trauma	From rupture of vessels in angle or iris

PARTICLES IN THE ANGLE

In the angle of the anterior chamber, it is not uncommon to see one or more particles that are obviously sitting on the surface of the angle structures and are not a part of them. Particles are most often seen after intraocular surgery or injury. One should distinguish these surface particles from diffusely deposited pigment granules infiltrating the trabecular meshwork, and from inflammatory precipitates in the angle, which appear cemented in intimate contact with the trabecular meshwork (Table 7.12).

Brown chunks, strands, or fragments of pigmented tissue in the dependent angle or on the back of the cornea are usually small pieces of iris left in the anterior chamber after operations involving the iris and have no special significance except to be distinguished from pigmented masses such as nevi and melanomas and from pigmented KP and PAS.

Black balls in the angle typically are from degenerated blood, as described under Blood in the Angle. These may remain for many years.

Gray flakes or particles, sometimes fluffy, sometimes resembling dandruff, and usually inconspicuous, are characteristic of exfoliation (Fig. 7.21). Typically, the material is more obvious at or under the pupillary border, and very few flakes are seen in the angle. Further details are given in Chapter 20. There may or may not be an associated abnormal deposition of pigment in the corneoscleral trabecular meshwork. Usually there is when glaucoma is present.

Refractile scrolls in the angle, resembling coiled or curved small pieces of thin, shiny, or glassy plastic are most characteristic of pieces of Descemet's membrane that have been inadvertently torn from the back of the cornea by a knife tip, cyclodialysis spatula, or iris repositor during intraocular surgery, or that, in one case we have seen, were blasted off the back of a portion of the cornea by a firecracker. The lens capsule has a similar refractile appearance and could be mistaken for Descemet's membrane if a piece were loose in the angle; but almost always, when remnants of capsule are left in an eye, they seem to be held in a wound or in a pupillary membrane rather than being completely detached. In time, pieces of either material may adhere to the iris if they are in contact with it. In themselves, sheets of Descemet's membrane or lens capsule have no tendency to cause glaucoma.

Table 7.12
Conditions Involving Particles in the Angle

Findings	Conditions
Brown chunks	Tissue remnants from surgery
Black balls	Old blood
Gray flakes or particles	Exfoliation
Refractile scrolls	Descemet's membrane
Refractile solid particles	Glass, plastic
Light gray fibers	Cotton fibers
Bright red specks	Rubber
Silvery particles	Aluminum
Chalk-white particles	Congenital cataract remnants

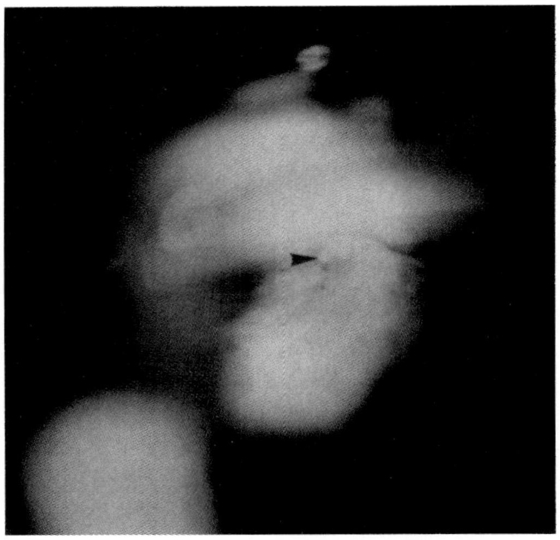

Figure 7.28. Foreign body (arrowhead) in the angle with a localized synechia formation.

Table 7.13
Common Errors in Gonioscopy

Error	Solution
Angle closed	Insure that view is good, that maximal angle is seen. If using a mirrored lens, have patient look toward mirror to maximize view. Still, if the angle has a narrow approach, but is actually open, a mirrored goniolens, even with the best viewing technique, may give the appearance of angle closure, particularly if the iris is excessively convex. A Koeppe lens is the best solution to this problem; to maximize the view, move into position to obtain best view of the angle.
Angle excessively deep	This problem occurs most commonly with the Zeiss, Posner or Sussman lens, and is due to the small diameter of the lens allowing the lens to rest on the cornea only, without extending onto the sclera, as the other goniolenses do. This property, which permits indentation gonioscopy, can also result in the appearance of an excessively deep angle, or **can make an appositionally closed angle appear open.** The solution is to **apply less pressure to the goniolens.** A clue that this problem is occurring is the presence of **folds in Descemet's membrane.**
Angle recession	This can easily be missed, especially if subtle. The optimal solution is to perform bilateral simultaneous Koeppe gonioscopy, and to switch back and forth between eyes to compare for asymmetry. Other clues are an abnormally bright whiteness of the scleral spur and absence or tearing of iris processes and uveal meshwork.
Appositional versus synechial angle closure	The Zeiss, Posner, or Sussman lens allows indentation gonioscopy, permitting differentiation between appositional and synechial angle closure.

Refractile solid particles (Fig. 7.28) that are flat, with sharp irregular edges, and varying thickness, rather than the uniform thickness of sheets of Descemet's membrane or lens capsule, are usually foreign bodies of glass or solid plastic. If these particles are free to move in the anterior chamber, they sometimes injure the corneal endothelium and cause edema, usually in the lower third or half of the cornea. If one is unaware of the foreign body, which frequently can be discovered only by gonioscopy, one may suspect glaucoma to be the cause of the edema, but glaucoma is seldom induced by this type of foreign body, unless the irritation also gives rise to iritis, which in rare instances, may be accompanied by glaucoma.

Light gray fibers in the angle and on the surface of the iris are ordinarily cotton fibers introduced inadvertently during intraocular surgery. Usually, they are solitary and seem to excite no reaction. Fragments of cellulose microsponges used during intraocular surgery have rarely been observed in the angle, occasionally associated with a mild inflammatory reaction.

Bright red specks, usually with a slightly granular or irregular surface, typically are of red rubber, coming from rubber bulbs used to irrigate the anterior chamber during intraocular surgery. These particles in the angle or on the surface of the iris have not been seen to excite an appreciable reaction, and are now rare due to modifications in surgical equipment and technique.

Chalk-white particles in the angle are seen after extracapsular operations for congenital cataract. These particles are characterized particularly by their whiteness and opaque appearance, which is suggestive of calcification. Usually, very few or just a single particle is seen, and the sizes vary widely. They appear to excite no reaction and may persist for 20 or 30 years, or possibly longer, in the angle. Presumably, these are pieces of the original dense white plaques that are seen in some congenitally cataractous lenses, and which may be released into the anterior chamber after the capsule is opened. These do not appear to be a cause of glaucoma. We have seen them in one eye of a middle-aged woman who was developing open-angle glaucoma in both eyes many years after uncomplicated operations for congenital cataracts in childhood; no particles were present in the other eye, and we think the glaucoma was the primary hereditary variety, unrelated to the earlier cataracts and surgery.

Common errors in performing gonioscopy are presented in Table 7.13.

References

1. Forbes M: Indentation gonioscopy and efficacy of iridectomy in angle-closure glaucoma. Trans Am Ophthalmol 1974;72:488–515.
2. Campbell DG: A comparison of diagnostic techniques in angle-closure glaucoma. Am J Ophthalmol 1979;88:197–204.
3. Rosenquist RC Jr, Melamed S, Epstein DL: Anterior and posterior axial lens displacement and human aqueous outflow facility. Invest Ophthalmol Vis Sci 1988;29:1159–1164.
4. Van Buskirk EM, Grant WM: Lens depression and aqueous outflow in enucleated primate eyes. Am J Ophthalmol 1973;76:632.
5. Van Buskirk EM: Changes in the facility of aqueous outflow induced by lens depression and intraocular pressure in excised human eyes. Am J Ophthalmol 1976;82:736.
6. Van Buskirk EM: Anatomic correlates of changing aqueous outflow facility in excised human eyes. Invest Ophthalmol Vis Sci 1982;22:625.
7. Barany E: On the mechanism by which chamber depth affects outflow resistance in excised eyes. Doc Ophthalmol 1959;13:84.
8. Grant WM: Experimental aqueous perfusion in enucleated human eyes. Arch Ophthalmol 1963;69:783–801.
9. Epstein DL, Freddo TF, Anderson PJ, et al. Experimental obstruction to aqueous outflow by pigment particles in living monkeys. Invest Ophthalmol Vis Sci 1986;27:387–395.
10. Donaldson DD: Atlas of External Diseases of the Eye. St. Louis: Mosby, Co., 1966;I–III.
11. Campbell DG, Vela A: Modern goniosynechialysis for the treatment of synechial angle-closure glaucoma. Ophthalmology 1984;91:1052.
12. Raviola G: Effects of a paracentesis on the blood-aqueous barrier: An electron microscope study on Macaca mulatta using horseradish peroxidase as a tracer. Invest Ophthalmol 1974;13:28–858.
13. Swan KC: Late hyphema due to wound vascularization. Trans Am Acad Ophthalmol Otol 1976;81:138–144.

Examination of the Optic Nerve 8

David L. Epstein

METHODS OF EXAMINATION

The clinician should use all available techniques to examine and draw the optic nerves in patients with glaucoma, and repeat these during the examination and after pupillary dilatation. It is curious how the "cupping" contour can look different with different tools, and one is striving to make very subtle, yet anatomically correct drawings and interpretations. Having observed residents in training, one of us (DLE) has concluded that it is only after hundreds of disc evaluations/drawings that one becomes sensitive to the changes in glaucoma and can accurately depict this in drawings.

There are essentially three tools: the direct ophthalmoscope, the 90 diopter lens at the slit lamp, and stereophotographs. As indicated in Chapter 5, even if the patient is being dilated subsequently, one should assess the disc appearance (and the clarity of the media) undilated, for, on the one hand, the patient will not be dilated at every follow-up visit and therefore the undilated appearance of the disc is important for future reference; and on the other hand, comparison of the undilated interpretation with the later dilated appearance will improve the clinician's skills in optic nerve evaluation.

Although the direct ophthalmoscope provides a nonstereo view, the use of parallax and the attention to the bend of small vessels after they cross the disc margin provide remarkably accurate assessment (confirmed by subsequent comparison to stereo disc photographs) of **the contour of the rim tissue, which is the key parameter that is being assessed.** If one chooses general ophthalmology practice, ophthalmoscopy with the direct ophthalmoscope must be mastered because this is a major tool. The ophthalmology resident must realize that it is much easier to evaluate optic disc cupping in a referral glaucoma center during training, when the pupils of all patients are dilated (and the diagnosis of a possible glaucoma entity has already been made). In the real world, the general ophthalmologist must evaluate many patients through undilated pupils and for the first time detect possible glaucoma-like changes. The general ophthalmologist must be a true "disc sleuth" and deserves all of our praise for detecting glaucomatous changes in the optic nerve (usually initially through an undilated pupil).

Unfortunately many have observed that recent residency graduates are not as skilled with the direct ophthalmoscope as the previous generation: our newer techniques should supplement but not totally replace previous valid methods. The truth is that we need all the "help" we can get in this difficult assessment, which unfortunately represents damage to the optic nerve at a later stage than we ultimately aspire to detect it.

The 90 D lens at the slit lamp is a very important technique to master, in addition to direct ophthalmoscopy. For this technique the slit beam of the slit lamp is made coaxial with the oculars, and the 90 D lens is placed in front of the patient's eye perpendicular to the beam, and antero-postero movements are made to bring the optic nerve into focus. This technique is easiest to perform with a dilated pupil, but sometimes it is surprising how good a view is obtained with an undilated pupil. It is important to draw what one sees, and later compare this to actual stereo-photographs. It is curious how contour changes sometimes are accentuated with the 90 D lens, and sometimes not as easily appreciated as with direct ophthalmoscopy. We therefore need to master all techniques to properly assess these contour changes.

One should draw (at least once) the appearance of the optic nerve based on the above methods, but with the pupil dilated, stereo disc photographs should be obtained and later compared to the drawings. **If stereo photographs cannot be obtained, a non-stereo photo should be obtained, especially for a baseline.** Disc drawings are notoriously inaccurate. All subsequent evaluations will be asking the question: has there been progression in the optic nerve cupping and visual field? Evaluation of the visual field alone, which is a subjective technique, is not sufficient. Detailed baseline information, as indicated in Chapter 5, is crucial to optimal patient management.

Some "stereo" disc cameras do not obtain true simultaneous stereo photographs, and some artifact from the resulting two photographic angles is possible. But, it is an imperfect world, and our 90 D drawings and direct ophthalmoscopic views also have their artifacts. This is why it is important to assess the appearance of the optic nerve with all available methods. When one thinks about it, the optic nerve is "staring us in the face" and thus should be available to provide us with objective data about the progress of the glaucomatous process, if we could only design the proper detection instrument. In the future, the evolving optical/computer evaluation techniques will make this possible, but at the present time we must rely on the above three clinical methods. When we evaluate cupping, we are looking at the actual "signature" of the disease process, and we must strive repetitively and compulsively to depict it accurately.

Therefore, stereo or other disc photographs must be reviewed when they become available and compared with the physician's disc drawings. This is a learning process for all clinicians. One of us (DLE) strongly recommends that residents in training have "disc drawing rounds."

Indirect ophthalmoscopy provides notoriously inaccurate assessment of the contour changes in glaucoma and should be avoided in glaucoma evaluation (although it is important in all glaucoma patients to examine the peripheral retina with indirect ophthalmoscopy).

We have found determination of "cup/disc ratio" to be practically useless in the management of any individual patient. The glaucomatous changes in the contour of the rim tissue rarely are exactly symmetrical, and thus do not lend themselves to such a general measurement. This term could be used in verbal discussions dealing with generalities, but otherwise should be avoided.

The process of glaucoma affects the contour of the rim tissue between the edge of the physiological cup and the edge of the disc (Fig. 8.1). **The glaucoma process causes a backward bowing of this rim tissue that may result in a fairly discreet (deep) extension of the cup in one meridian, or a gentler sloping backward which may be termed saucerization.** With this loss of substance of the optic nerve there is a change in color, presumably due to the accompanying loss of small blood vessels. However, the key parameter is the change in the **contour** of the rim tissue.

In nonglaucomatous optic atrophy there is loss of color, hence atrophy, but there is usually no contour change in the rim tissue. For example, after vascular occlusion the disc is pale, but there is usually no increase in size of the "cup," i.e., no contour change (Fig. 8.2). However, there

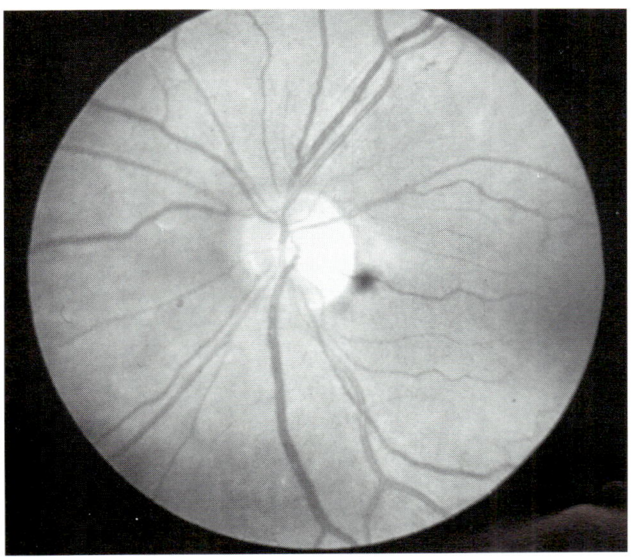

Figure 8.1. Normal optic nerve.

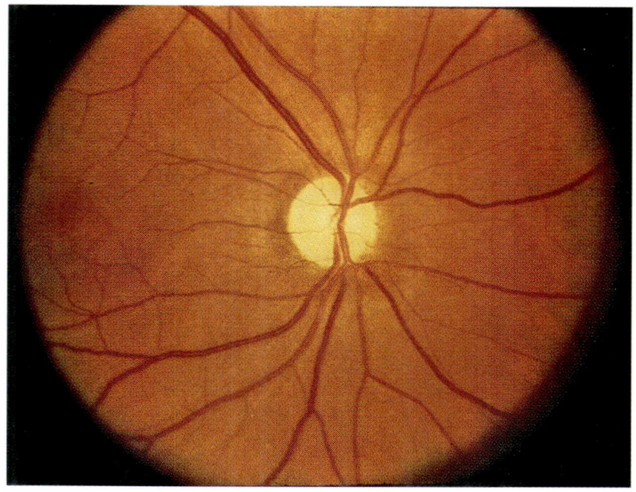

Figure 8.2. Anterior ischemic optic neuropathy. Note optic nerve pallor without associated cupping.

are certain optic atrophies that can be accompanied by contour changes, and these occasionally present diagnostic puzzles: temporal arteritis, other ischemic optic neuropathies, intracranial neoplasms, methanol intoxication, hereditary optic atrophies, and lues, and of course optic cup pits or colobomas. These are unusual (except perhaps for temporal arteritis and certain dominant hereditary optic neuropathies such as Kjer's). Some of these have been called pseudo-glaucomatous because of the contour change. **What often proves helpful in diagnosing pseudoglaucomatous contour changes is to assess the color of the intact rim tissue in the other quadrents of the disk.** In pseudoglaucomatous cases, the color of the intact rim tissue is often pale, unlike glaucoma where normal color is observed.

The assessment of the contour of the remaining optic nerve rim tissue throughout its entire circumference is crucial both to the detection of glaucoma, and also its progression. We use all the above three diagnostic evaluation methods, which include true stereo viewing, as well as parallax and clues such as the course of small vessels which cross the disc margin, to make this crucial assessment.

Figure 8.3 through Figures 8.13 portray the "Chandler-Grant" interpretation of the changes in rim contour that occur in the progression of the glaucomatous process, based on their long term clinical observations. The cross sectional views in these figures help clarify what is observed and we have used these in patient charts. Beginning residents in ophthalmology are encouraged to draw these cross sectional diagrams.

The key is the detection of the backward bowing and the extent of this in relation to the edge of the disc, and the apparent depth of this change. The following terms have been used to characterize the apparent depth of the contour change: saucerization (as in a saucer plate) connoting a mild change in depth, shelving an intermediate change in

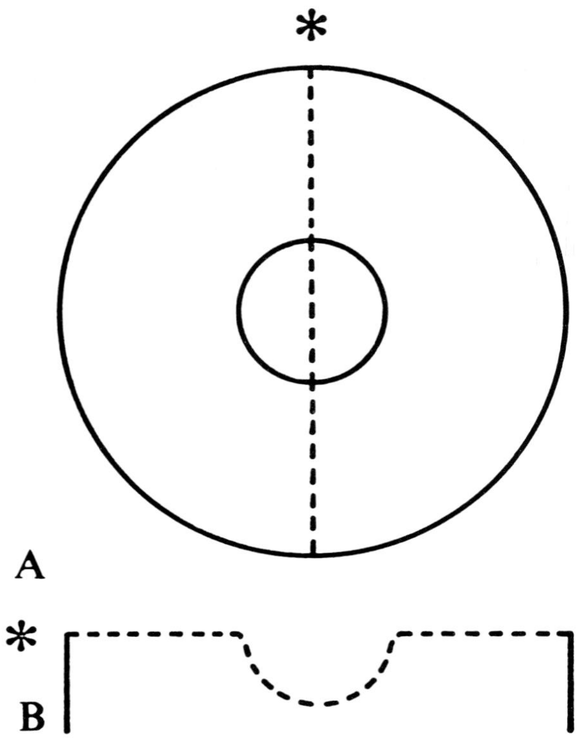

Figure 8.3. A, Frontal view of central physiologic cup. **B,** Cross-sectional view of central physiologic cup.

depth, and excavation a precipitous change in depth "like the north wall of the Grand Canyon," or like the edge of the normal central cup. Chandler and Grant intended the term "saucerization" to indicate an uncommon more generalized backward bowing like a saucer plate (see Figs. 8.8, 8.12) to contrast this with the more common excavated change of a "tea cup," but the term **saucerization** has evolved to indicate a common subtle change in disc rim contour that appears to be an early acquired change.

For practical purposes, the terminology is not as important as the detection of the contour change of shallow or deep backward bowing of disc rim tissue. The deeper changes, whether shelving or excavation, are difficult to fully differentiate from each other, but the more subtle posterior bowing of rim tissue commonly called "saucerization" and its progression to deeper and/or more extensive changes has become an important part of "disc sleuthing."

Thus, although the disease process does produce glaucomatous optic atrophy and thereby a color change in the disc, as in other cases of optic atrophy, it is the contour changes that distinguish the changes in glaucoma from these other conditions. The clinician needs to be able to assess and record these contour changes to diagnose and evaluate follow-up in patients with glaucoma.

In assessing the contour of the rim tissue of the optic nerve special attention should be placed on the straight temporal portion of the optic disc, which receives the papillomacular bundle fibers. **In POAG associated with myopia and in low tension glaucoma there can be preferential early cupping in this area with corresponding field loss that can extend into or actually involve central fixation.** Therefore the amount of rim tissue and its "healthiness" in terms of contour changes in this straight temporal area are important factors in glaucoma decision making.

As discussed in Chapters 18 and 19, in patients with advanced disease it is crucial to know how much margin there is that can be followed further should the target IOP be incorrect. Although this "margin" can be expressed as the amount of remaining field and the actual sensitivity measurements close to fixation, another factor is the contour condition of the straight temporal optic disc rim tissue that corresponds to these central points in the visual field. For example, sometimes fixation is split in glaucoma, but in addition to assessing the actual sensitivities in the central field in the remaining half (e.g. the inferior field), evaluating the extent of contour changes in the corresponding (superior) portion of the straight temporal rim tissue of the optic nerve provides additional information about how much "margin" there is left to follow.

The myopic disc is notoriously difficult to evaluate for early glaucomatous changes because of its usual generalized sloping contour. Nevertheless, in POAG associated with myopia one needs to carefully examine the straight temporal margin of rim tissue for early glaucomatous contour changes because of the possibility that the initial field loss might involve central fixation (Chapter 18). This uncertainty in detecting the earliest possible disc cupping change in myopic eyes legitimately suggests the need to potentially treat elevated IOP somewhat more vigorously in these eyes.

Chandler and Grant were excellent observers of the optic nerve and emphasized the importance of asymmetry and "verticalization" of the cup, as well as the predictive value of the optic nerve changes for visual field changes. They wrote:

> In nearly every type of glaucoma, we are greatly concerned with the condition of the optic disc (optic nerve head). In the diagnosis of glaucoma, the appearance of the optic disc often provides us with valuable clues. In decisions concerning the necessity for and in evaluation of the adequacy of treatment of glaucoma, we can often obtain essential guidance from the appearance of the optic disc and evaluation of the field of vision.

It is true that in certain varieties of glaucoma a decision that treatment is urgently needed can be made mainly on the basis of very high intraocular pressure, but in many more cases the character of both the optic disc and visual field greatly influences the decision.

Change in the optic disc can forewarn of change in the visual field in some cases, and usually the nature of the abnormality of the optic disc can be valuably correlated with abnormality of the visual field, to help establish whether a given field defect is correctly attributable to glaucoma or to some other cause.

We will first describe the changes in appearance of the optic disc that are characteristic in glaucoma and their correlation with abnormalities in the visual field.

OPHTHALMOSCOPIC FINDINGS

Nearly all of the observations to be described were made originally with the direct ophthalmoscope, which, though monocular, permits valuable appreciation of depth and contour, confirmed by comparison with stereophotographs. However, considerable practice is required to learn how to make use of a number of monocular clues to depth perception.

ASYMMETRY OF THE OPTIC CUPS

A simple enlargement of the physiologic cup in all directions is not infrequently a sign of early glaucoma (see Fig. 8.14). **Asymmetry of the physiologic cups in the two eyes is seldom seen in normal eyes and, until proven otherwise, must be considered a sign of early glaucoma** (see Fig. 8.15). When the asymmetry of the physiologic cups is first noted, the IOP is usually slightly higher in the eye with the wider cup, but this is not invariably the case. In one of us (PAC), an asymmetry of the physiologic cups was first discovered when the IOP was normal and equal in both eyes. It was only after 4 or 5 years that an elevated IOP was found in the eye with the wider cup.

The size of the physiologic cup in normal eyes varies considerably from person to person, and if the cups are equal in size one cannot tell in an individual case from a single examination whether the cups are larger than they were previously. The only way the ophthalmologist can say that the cups are becoming larger, i.e., due to bilateral early glaucomatous change, is to compare the results of this examination with previous stereophotographs of the discs or very accurate, previously prepared drawings. The photographs are much to be preferred. Since previous stereophotographs or accurate drawings are seldom available to the practicing ophthalmologist, if the cups are symmetric and equal in size, one cannot be sure from the first examination whether the size of the physiologic cups is normal for this individual.

However, if the physiologic cups are asymmetric, that is, if the cup in one eye, although physiologic when considered by itself, is definitely wider than the cup in the fellow eye, this must be considered very likely to be an early glaucomatous change. A difference in the size of the cups in the two eyes is a common finding in early glaucoma.

There has been considerable discussion in the ophthalmic literature concerning cup/disc ratio. We know that the size and depth of the physiologic cup vary greatly among different individuals. We feel that the significant factor is not the cup/disc ratio, but the shape of the cup and its comparison to that of the cup in the fellow eye (Figs. 8.3, 8.4).

ABNORMAL CUPPING

In most patients in whom glaucomatous changes develop in the optic disc, the physiologic cup enlarges to reach the margin downward and temporally. This is a definite glaucomatous change; but at first the cup is shelving and is not an excavation, and there may not be a field defect (Fig. 8.4).

The shelving of the cup to the lower temporal margin gradually becomes deeper, not yet a real excavation. Gradually the cup becomes deeper at the margin, and a real excavation becomes evident (Fig. 8.5). It is now usually possible to find an upper field defect—an upper Bjerrum scotoma, or nasal step or both—but there may be none if there is as yet no atrophy of nerve fibers. At first, such pathologic cupping extends only to the major inferior vessels, but later may involve the whole lower pole of the disc.

Excavation, as we use the term, indicates that the wall of the cup is precipitous. It does not necessarily imply undermining of the edge or a disappearance of blood vessels from view.

In certain cases, the physiologic cup first enlarges upward. As the disease progresses, the upwardly enlarged cup comes closer to the disc margin and is seen to be excavated

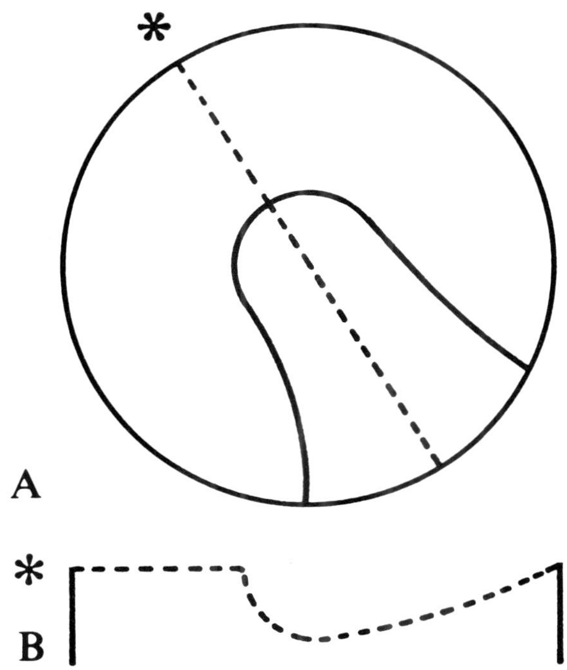

Figure 8.4. A, Frontal view of cup extending to the margin below and temporally (left eye). **B,** Cross-sectional view. The cup is shelving. It is not an excavation. There is no field defect.

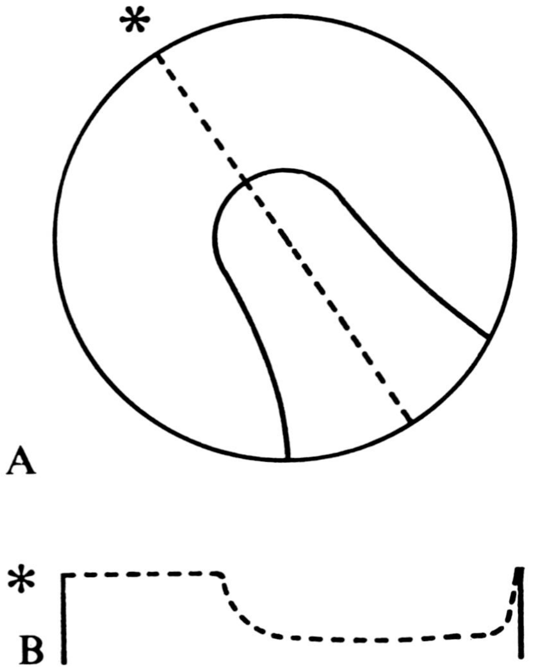

Figure 8.5. A, Similar frontal view of cup extending to the margin below and temporally (left eye). **B,** Cross-sectional view. The cup is now an excavation. There is an upper field defect.

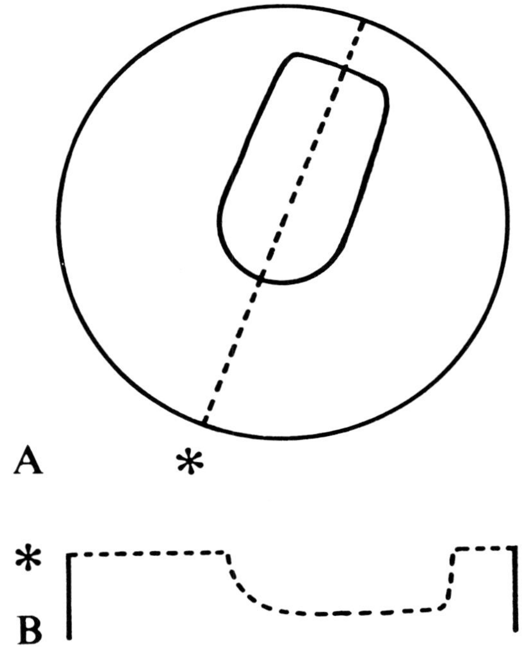

Figure 8.6. A, Frontal view of enlargement of the cup above and temporally. It does not reach the margin (left eye). **B,** Cross-sectional view. The upper border of the cup is an excavation. There is a lower field defect.

at its upper border (Fig. 8.6). At this stage, although the cup still does not quite reach the upper outer margin, there is usually a lower field defect—a lower Bjerrum scotoma, or a lower nasal step, or both.

In some cases, the cup may enlarge toward both the upper and lower borders simultaneously (Fig. 8.7); and it is in this type of glaucomatous change that we eventually find both an upper and lower Bjerrum scotoma, isolating a central island of vision, varying in size from patient to patient, with variable degree of loss in the peripheral field.

Eventually, the excavation reaches the margin above as well as below, and the disc may become totally cupped to the margins everywhere: however, in some such cases, there is still a rim of normal tissue on the nasal side.

Not all visual field defects in a patient with elevated intraocular pressure are necessarily due to glaucoma. **It is important to correlate the optic cup appearance with the visual field. Dense field defects are to be regarded with suspicion if they are not explainable by the optic disc appearance.**

We wish therefore to emphasize the importance of excavation in determining whether there is a field defect. This seems clear enough when the cupping is lower temporal and the excavation extends to the margin, but it is not so obvious when the cupping extends upward. We have seen that even when the cup has not reached the margin above and temporally, there may be a lower field defect. This may seem surprising, but when we analyze such an upward

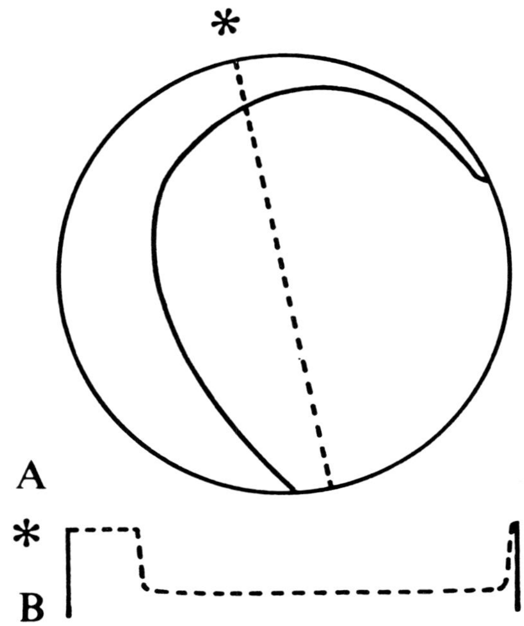

Figure 8.7. A, Frontal view of cup reaching the margin below and temporally, not quite to the margin above (left eye). **B,** Cross-sectional view. There is an excavation both above and below. There is both an upper and a lower field defect.

and temporally enlarged cup, we note that this often represents an excavation rather than a shelving from the very beginning; whereas when the cup reaches the margin below and temporally, it is for some time commonly a shelving cup, not an excavation, and we may find no field defect. It is only when the lower outer enlargement becomes an excavation that we almost always find a field defect. Thus, we see that the contour of the pathologic cup appears to be the most important factor in determining whether a field defect will be found and where it will be found. With a lower excavation, the excavation may in some cases at first be narrow, and it is not unusual to find a narrow upper Bjerrum scotoma. As the lower excavation becomes broader, the Bjerrum scotoma becomes wider.

In an upper excavation, the excavation is wider from the beginning, and we usually do not find a very narrow lower Bjerrum scotoma similar to the narrow upper scotoma that sometimes is seen superiorly. The lower Bjerrum scotoma, even at an early stage, is wider. This might suggest that, from a clinical standpoint, there is a mechanical (anatomical) factor in the pathologic cupping that causes field defects in glaucoma. We will leave it to others to provide a scientific explanation of these clinical findings.

SAUCERIZATION

Uncommonly, the first pathologic change in the disc may be a slight backward bowing in the periphery of a portion of the disc or of the whole disc, in a form that we have called "saucerization" (Fig. 8.8): The contour of such a

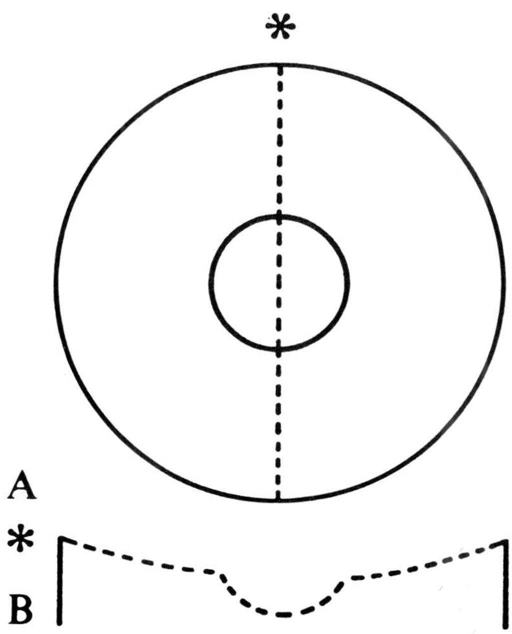

Figure 8.8. A, Frontal view of a disc with saucerization. The physiologic cup is not enlarged. **B,** There is backward bowing of the entire disc, but the physiologic cup is unchanged.

disc closely resembles the contour of an ordinary saucer, in contrast to an excavation, in which the contour of the disc more closely resembles the contour of a teacup. The early shelving cup to the lower outer margin we do not call "saucerization." Saucerization has a different appearance that is difficult to describe. It involves not less than a quadrant of the disc and may involve any portion of the disc, sometimes even the nasal portion or the entire disc. In some cases, one may see pathologic cupping at one border of the disc and saucerization at the other. Whether the saucerization involves the entire disc or only a portion of it, it represents a definite glaucomatous change and must be taken into account along with the other signs in the management of the case.

In some cases, there is saucerization of the entire disc, but there still may be no field defect until the saucerization becomes considerably deeper. Eventually, we find loss of field; with advanced saucerization of the whole disc, however, this may not be the typical nerve fiber bundle defect, but rather a concentric contraction of the field. Such cases are much more difficult to follow by perimetry than those characterized by the ordinary type of cupping.

Saucerization of the disc is a relatively rare form of glaucomatous cupping. We find ordinary glaucomatous cupping in 9 out of 10 cases. Its importance seems to be that if we recognize saucerization of a portion or of the whole disc, even if there is no loss of field whatsoever, we can make a positive diagnosis of glaucoma no matter what level of IOP is found at the moment.

In some eyes, we find a crescent all around the disc, sometimes called a halo (see Fig. 8.16). In such cases, it may be difficult to determine just where the border of the disc is. If we consider the crescent as the disc border, we may conclude that the cup, although large, does not reach the margin anywhere; whereas with a more critical examination, we may conclude that the cup does in fact reach the margin of the disc, which is well inside the borders of the crescent.

The importance of observing contour changes in the optic cup and other aspects of the glaucomatous cup are further illustrated in Figures 8.9 through 8.13 and Figures 8.17 through 8-21.

ATROPHY

Thus far, we have spoken mainly of the changes in contour of the optic disc that occur in glaucoma and have only incidentally mentioned atrophy. We must remember that the ultimate cause of irreversible loss of function in glaucoma is atrophy of nerve fibers, whether or not there is pathologic cupping.

With the exception of cases of high IOP or acute glaucoma in which atrophy and loss of vision may develop with little or no pathologic cupping, and about which we will say more later, in most cases of chronic glaucoma without

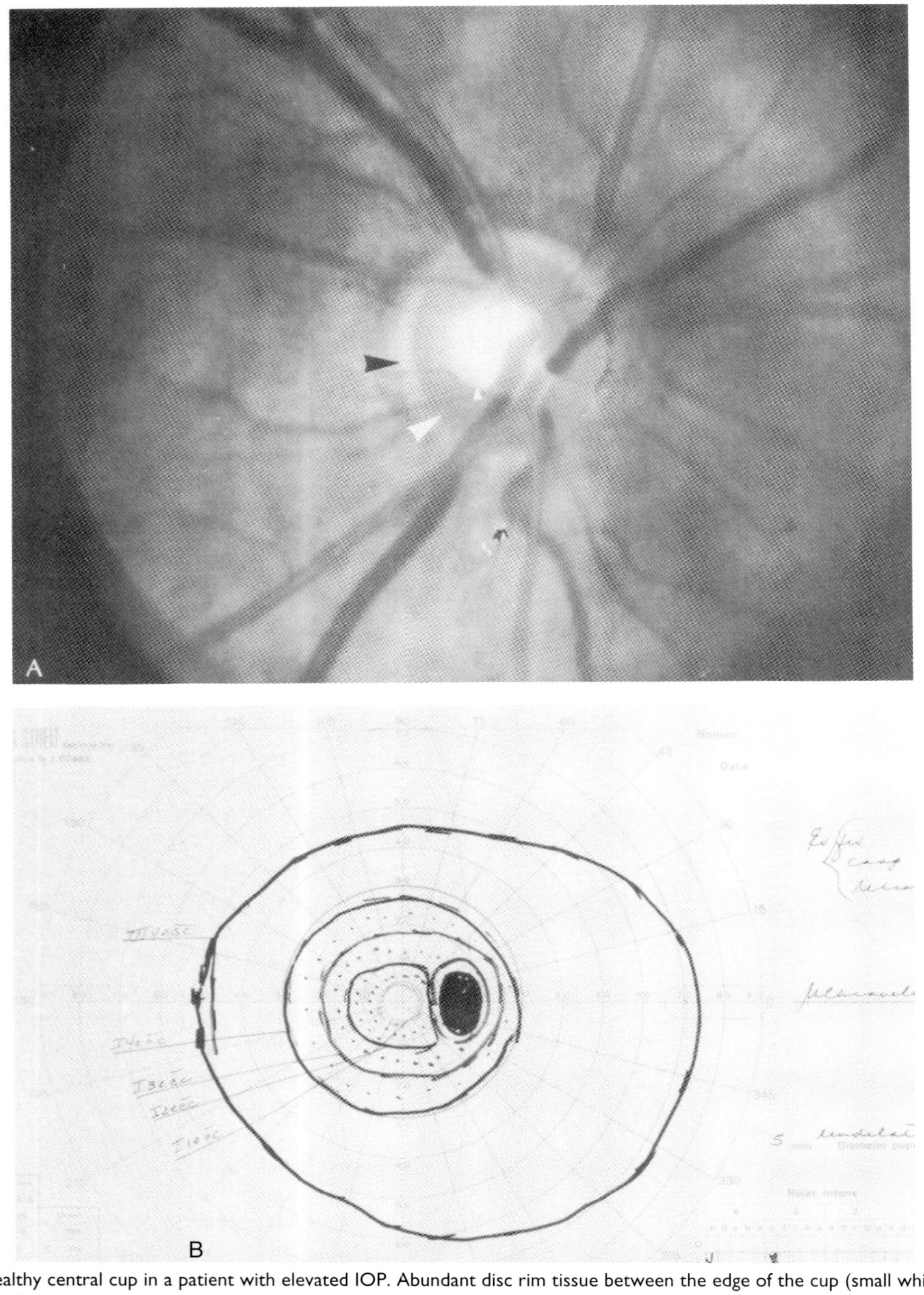

Figure 8.9. A, Healthy central cup in a patient with elevated IOP. Abundant disc rim tissue between the edge of the cup (small white arrowhead) and the edge of the disc (large white arrowhead) is present. The rim tissue is of normal contour and is on a plane with the retina (compare Fig. 8.3). **B,** No field loss would be expected with such a disc appearance. The scleral crescent (black arrowhead) should not be mistaken for the edge of the disc.

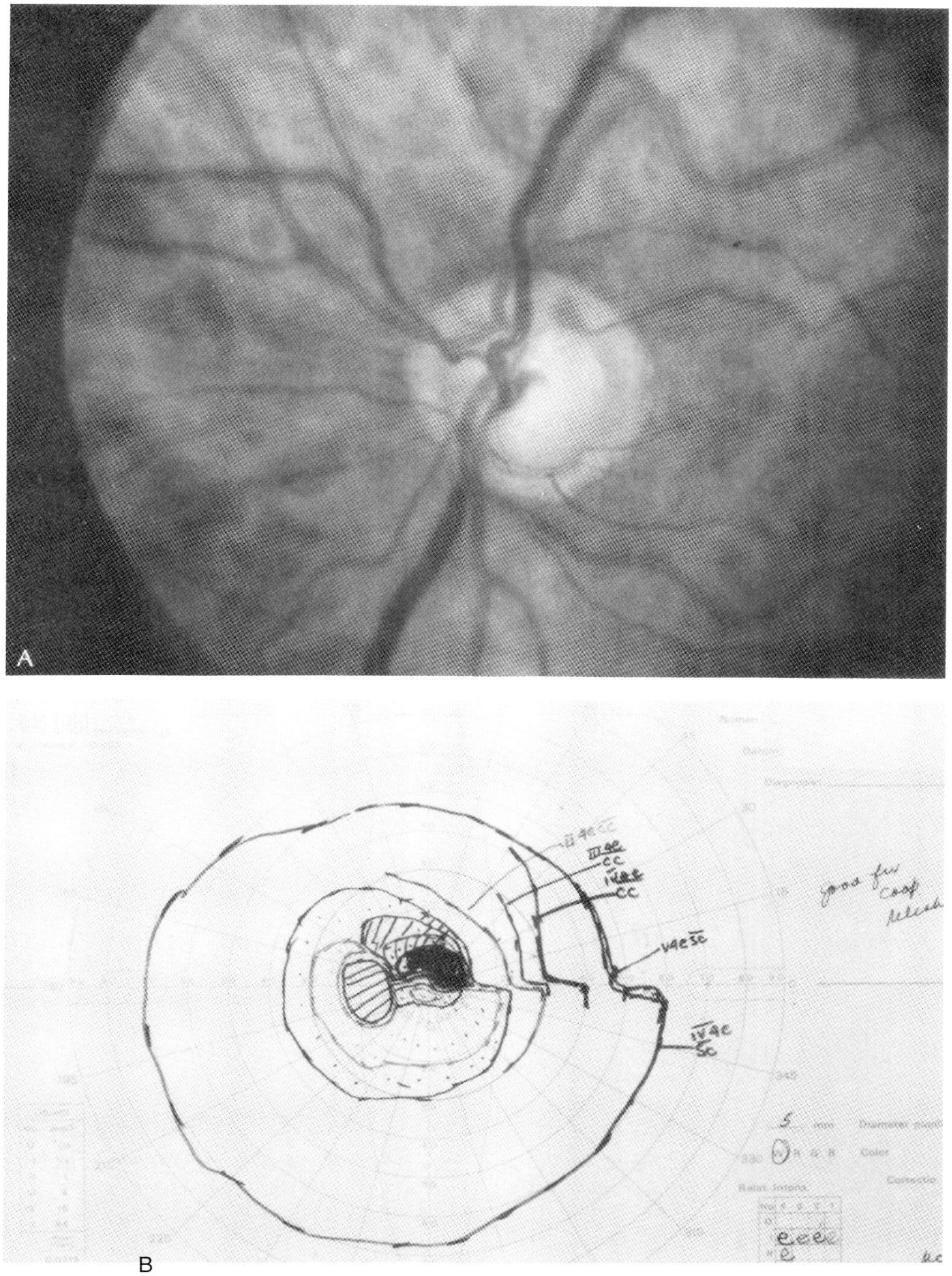

B

Figure 8.10. A, Cupping extending to the inferior rim (left eye). **B,** Associated with superior field loss (compare Fig. 8.5). Note the bending of the inferior disc vessels over the edge of the cup. (Courtesy of Robert Rosenquist, MD).

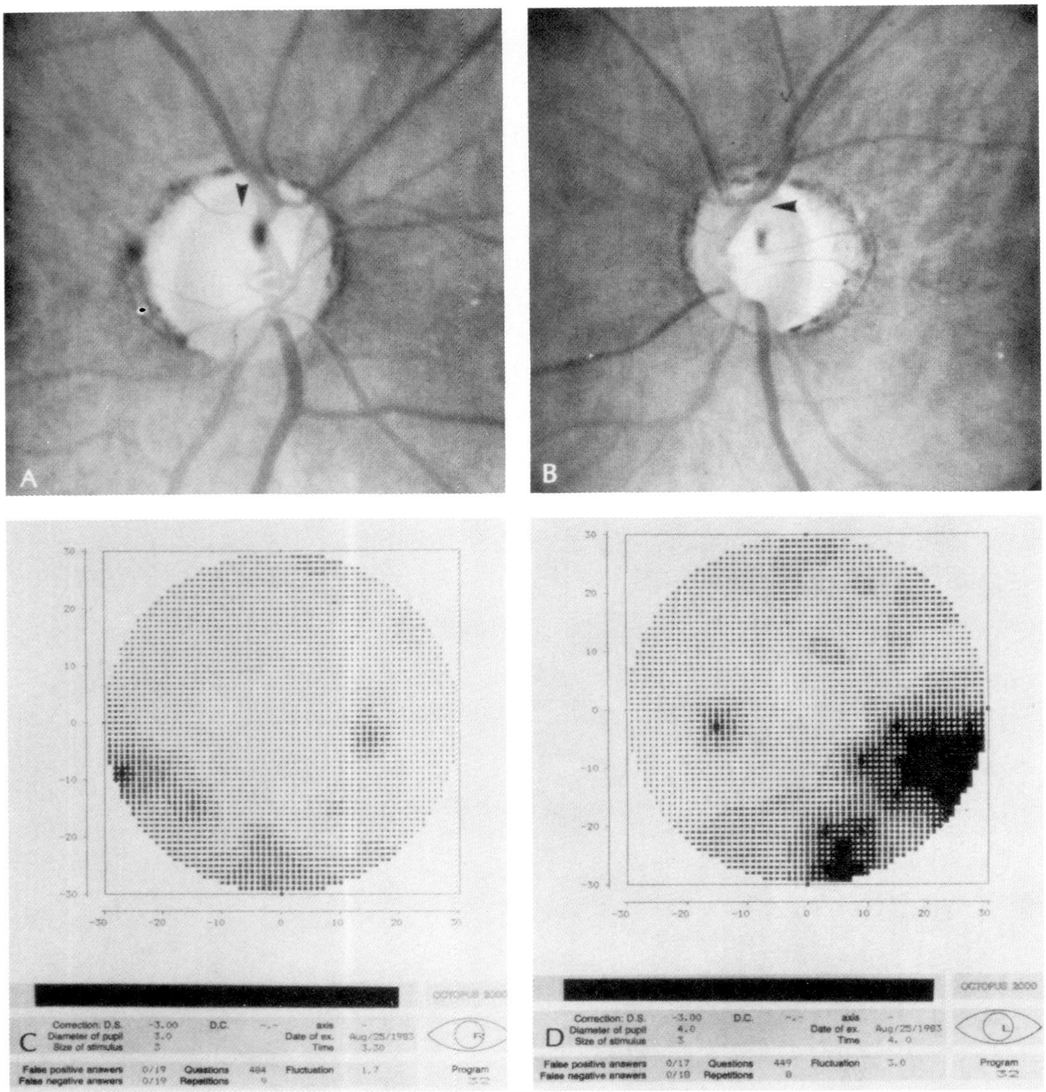

Figure 8.11. A, B. Superior extension of the cup (black arrowheads) in each eye in association with inferior field loss OU (C,D) (compare Fig. 8.12). The left disc shows the greater attenuation of the superior rim, and correspondingly denser field loss is present in this eye. Of interest, the previous field performed with the Goldmann perimeter demonstrated field loss only in OS.

very high IOP, the first change in the optic disc is a change in the cupping that conforms to the various patterns described in the foregoing pages. As already stated, **abnormal changes in the contour of the optic disc are characteristically recognized before there is an irreversible abnormality in the visual field detectable by ordinary clinical means.** It is when atrophy of nerve fibers develops in association with cupping that characteristic changes in the visual field appear, corresponding anatomically to the location of visibly affected portions of the optic disc. In exceptional cases, there may be typical glaucomatous visual field defects that do not correspond to visible changes in the optic disc if the fields are measured when the intraocular pressure is considerably elevated, but these are functional changes that are reversible when the IOP is reduced. Reversible field defects can be induced in normal eyes and in glaucomatous eyes by raising the intraocular pressure, such as by pressing on the eye.

Our prime concern is with the irreversible loss of visual field, and it is here that ophthalmoscopic recognition of atrophy can be helpful in validating results of visual field testing. When atrophy and field loss are extensive, it is generally easy to recognize the degree of atrophy by the whiteness and lack of fine vessels in the optic disc; but when atrophy is partial or limited to a small portion of the disc, it may be difficult to be sure. Characteristically, when there is localized pathologic cupping and corresponding field defect, one can appreciate that the affected

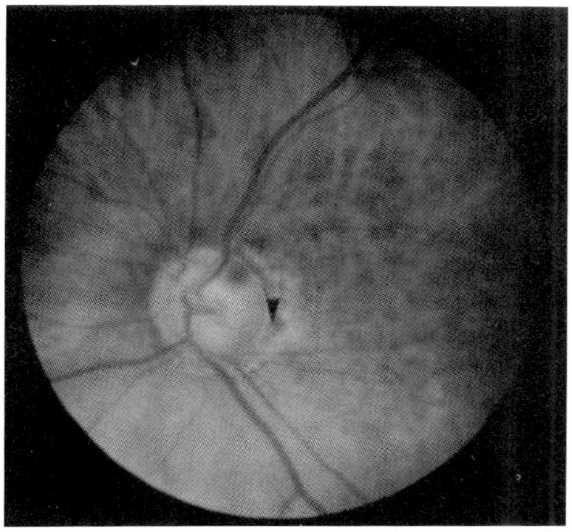

Figure 8.12. "Saucerization" of the disc. Note the path centrally on the disc of a vessel (arrowhead) that crosses the disc margin and that is at the retinal level just inside the disc margin. It then immediately moves posteriorly on the surface of the proximal disc substance, which is bowed posteriorly as in a saucer. Observation of the course of the smaller disc vessels can aid in detection of subtle changes in the shape of the cup. The observation of such contour changes (rather than color; cup/disc ratio) is a key factor in glaucoma patient management. (Courtesy of David D. Donaldson, MD).

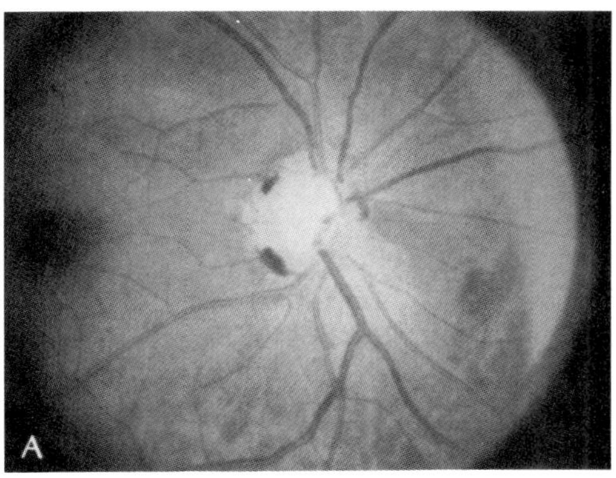

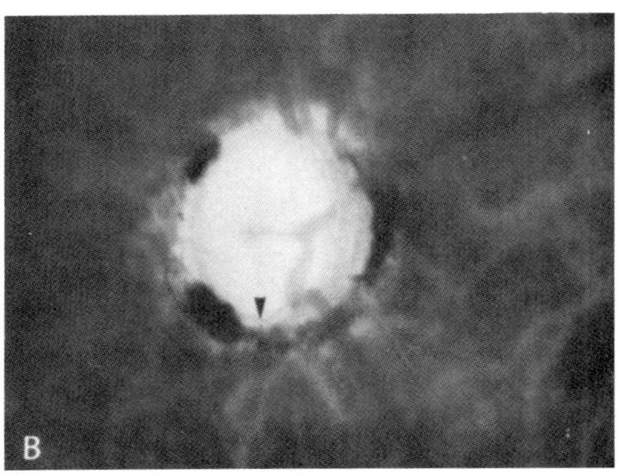

Figure 8.13. Loss of disc rim tissue over a 10-year period in a patient with uncontrolled glaucoma. Note the change in location of the inferior disc vessel (arrowhead) that accompanied the loss of disc rim substance.

portion of the disc is atrophic by its relative lack of pink color compared with the more normal portions of the disc. The affected area may appear slightly gray.

One can be misled in evaluating atrophy of the optic disc with the ophthalmoscope and fail to appreciate the characteristic whitening of the disc if the patient's crystalline lens has yellow nuclear sclerosis. This yellow lens can act as a filter, altering the apparent color of the disc. Examination of the lens with the slit lamp biomicroscope helps to evaluate how much yellowing of the nucleus is present. One can also be misled and fail to appreciate the whiteness of an atrophic optic disc if the incandescent bulb of the ophthalmoscope is operated at subnormal voltage, since this provides a yellowish light.

In the eyes with considerable hyperopia, optic disc atrophy may have a special ophthalmoscopic appearance. Eyes that are very hyperopic tend normally to have rosy-appearing discs, with small physiologic cups. In such eyes, partial optic atrophy may not cause the optic disc to appear white, but may only cause it to lose some of its previous pink or rosy appearance.

VIEWING THE DISC THROUGH THE KOEPPE LENS

Ophthalmoscopic examination of the optic disc is extraordinarily difficult in some patients, but there are several circumstances in which the examination can be greatly facilitated by the use of the same type of Koeppe contact lens that is used for gonioscopy (Fig. 8.22).

The Koeppe goniolens can be applied in the same manner as it is for regular gonioscopy, with the patient supine, and the space between lens and cornea can be filled with sterile saline solution. This is particularly convenient if one is planning to perform both gonioscopy and ophthalmoscopy. However, if gonioscopy has been performed at some other time, and one merely wishes to utilize the lens to facilitate direct ophthalmoscopy, this can be done easily with the patient sitting up, as for ordinary direct ophthalmoscopy. For use sitting up, the concavity of the goniolens is filled with clear goniogel, and the lens is applied to the patient's eye just as though he were lying down, with the flange under the upper and lower lids. The lens is best held in place with thumb and forefinger while ophthalmoscopy is carried out in the normal manner.

Looking through the Koeppe goniolens at the central fundus, one needs several more diopters of plus lens in the ophthalmoscope than when one looks at the fundus without the Koeppe lens. The optic disc appears smaller when seen through the Koeppe lens, but it may be seen with striking clarity. One of the advantages of fundoscopy through the Koeppe lens is that, when holding the lens against the eye with thumb and forefinger, the examiner can steady the eye during the examination and can easily

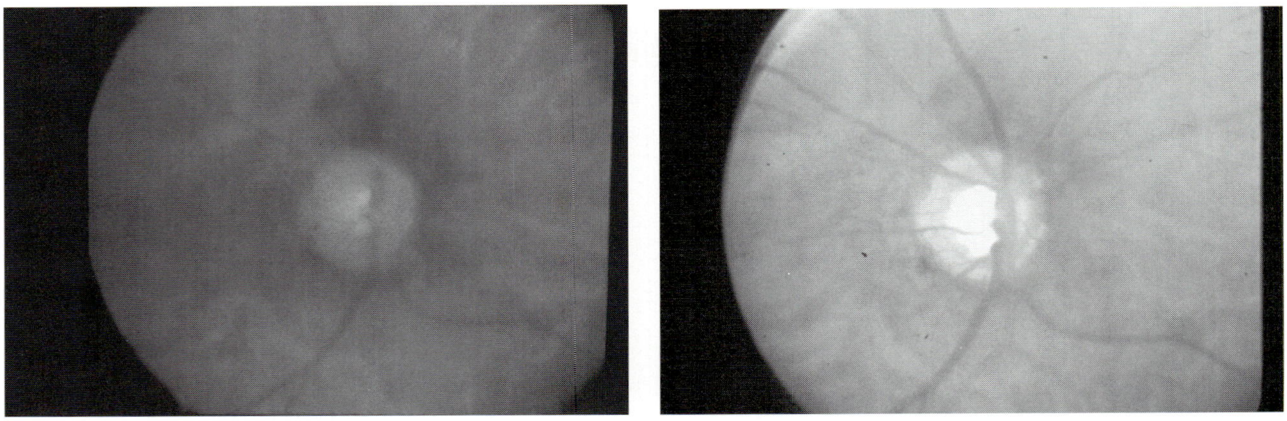

Figure 8.14. Progressive enlargement of the optic cup in this patient with glaucoma.

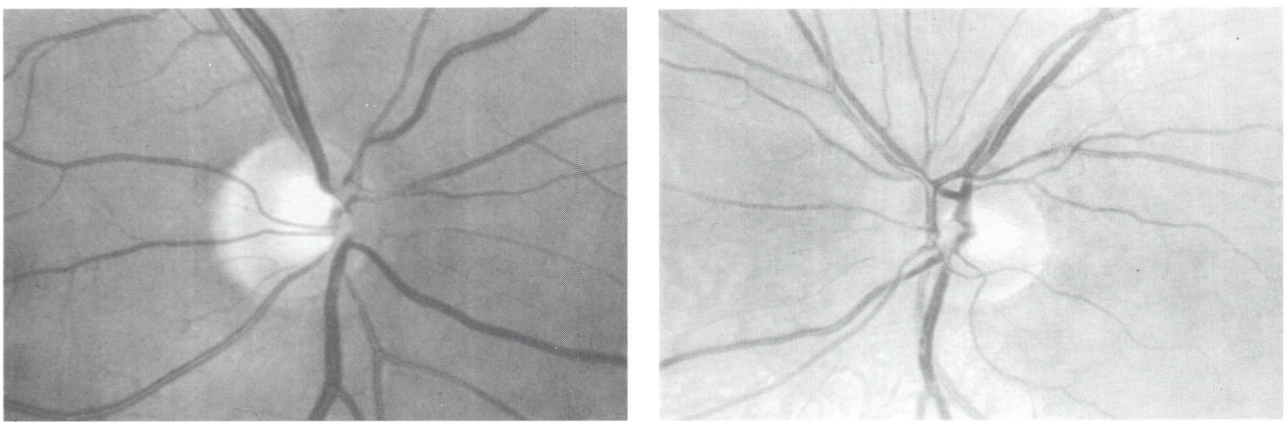

Figure 8.15. Asymmetry of optic nerve cupping in this patient. This degree of asymmetry is unusual in the normal population.

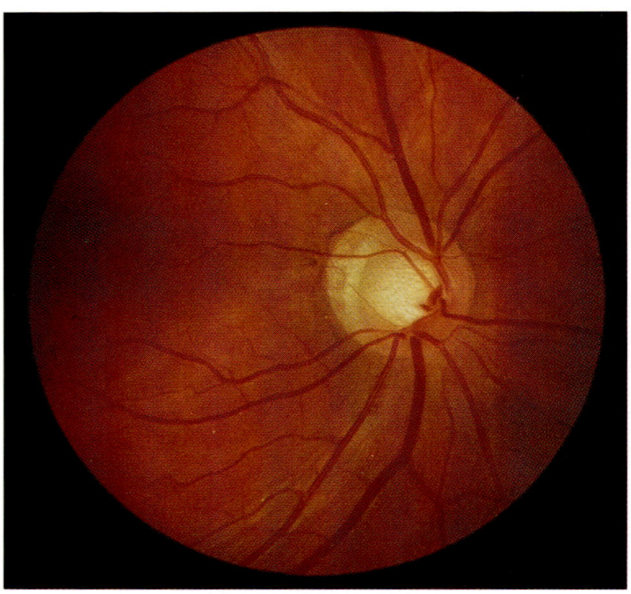

Figure 8.16. Peripapillary halo in this patient with glaucoma.

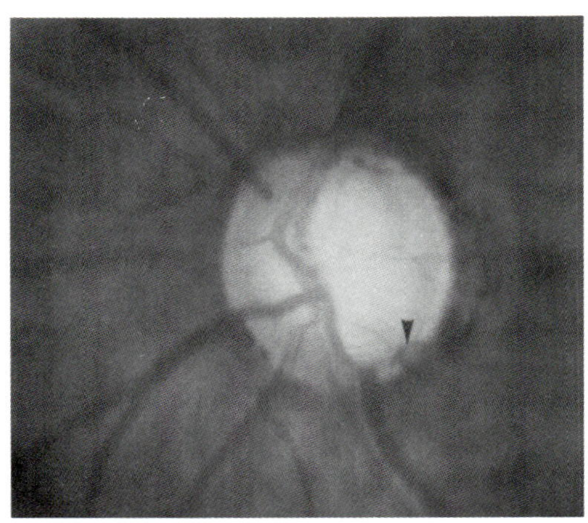

Figure 8.17. Large optic disc hemorrhage (arrowhead) in a patient who has advanced glaucomatous disc cupping.

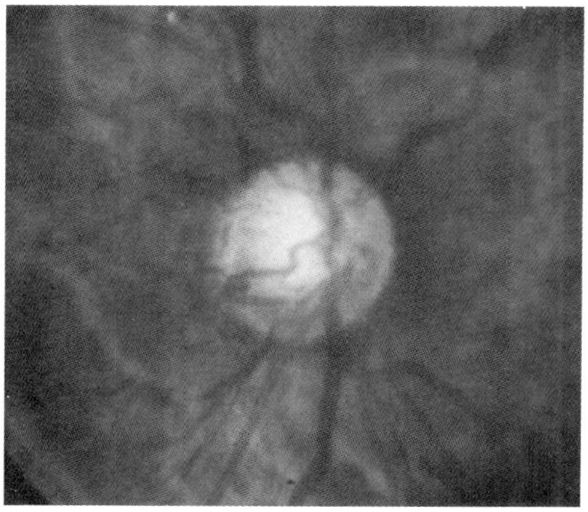

Figure 8.18. Abnormal appearing disc vessels are sometimes seen in patients who have chronic open angle glaucoma. Whether they represent sequelae of unsuspected partial vein occlusions or other effects of elevated intraocular pressure is not certain.

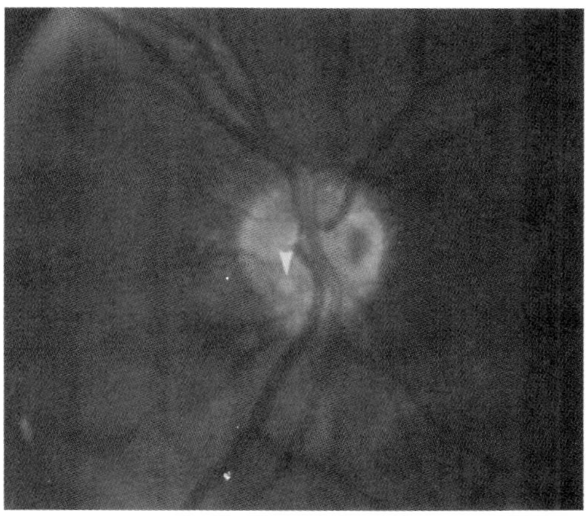

Figure 8.19. Multiple drusen of the optic disc in a patient who has open-angle glaucoma. Such drusen (arrowhead) themselves can produce various field defects and should be searched for (among other possibilities) when the disc appearance does not explain the field defect.

move the eye to bring the disc or macula conveniently into view.

We have found ophthalmoscopy through the Koeppe goniolens to have real advantages in the following situations:

In babies and adults with irregularity of the surface of the cornea, either from drying or from epithelial edema, one can usually obtain a clearer view of the fundus by using the lens.

In children with aniridia and nystagmus, or with nystagmus from other causes, the rubber-flanged Koeppe lens permits one to hold the eye still and to examine the fundus with most of the motion eliminated.

In older people with small pupils that one cannot dilate or does not wish to dilate, or in people who seem unable to keep their eyes still, application of the Koeppe lens permits easier viewing of the central fundus. Also, in older patients who have immature cataracts, it is sometimes surprising how well the optic disc and central fundus can be seen through the Koeppe lens, even though it is almost impossible to see them without this aid.

A wider, more panoramic view of the fundus is obtained more easily with the direct ophthalmoscope through a pupil of moderate size when the Koeppe lens is used than by the direct ophthalmoscope unaided.

RELATION OF OPTIC DISC TO VISUAL FIELD

The extent and location of field defects from cupping and atrophy in glaucoma correspond to changes that are visible in the optic disc with the ophthalmoscope. For instance, if the pathologic cupping and atrophy are confined to the lower outer pole of the disc, as they are in the majority of early glaucomas, the only possible field defect due to glaucoma is an upper nasal step, or an upper Bjerrum scotoma, or both.

If, on the other hand, the physiologic cup enlarges upward and the lower pole of the disc is still normal, any glaucomatous field defect will be a lower Bjerrum scotoma, or lower nasal step, or both. If the pathologic cupping involves the whole temporal side of the disc, then there may be an upper or lower Bjerrum scotoma, or both. With an inverse-type disc in which the principal vessels leave the disc on the temporal rather than on the nasal side, the first cupping may be nasal and the field defect temporal.

In cases of total cupping and atrophy or excavation to the margin of the temporal half or two-thirds of the disc, one cannot tell from the appearance of the optic disc what the location or the type of field defect may be. Also, in highly myopic eyes, the appearance of the disc is notoriously hard to interpret from the standpoint of glaucoma.

We believe that in most eyes (not highly myopic) there can be no field defects due to glaucoma if the disc is normal, unless the IOP is high at the time of the examination or has been high a short time previously. If the IOP is elevated at the time of examination, glaucomatous field defects may be found. Such defects may disappear if IOP is promptly reduced to normal. If such field defects are permanent, then within a few weeks, atrophy is evident. In the type of case in which the IOP is high at the time of examination, or has been high in the recent past, treatment is generally planned on the basis of IOP alone. Measurement of the field is of limited value in management of such a case.

In exceptional cases, one may find glaucomatous-type field defects such as a Bjerrum-type scotoma or a Ronne step with the IOP and the disc completely normal, but these field defects we know cannot be due to glaucoma. We have seen many patients who had glaucoma and were alleged to be losing field, or who had lost field despite good IOP control, but the appearance of the disc did not correlate with the field defect. The inconsistencies were

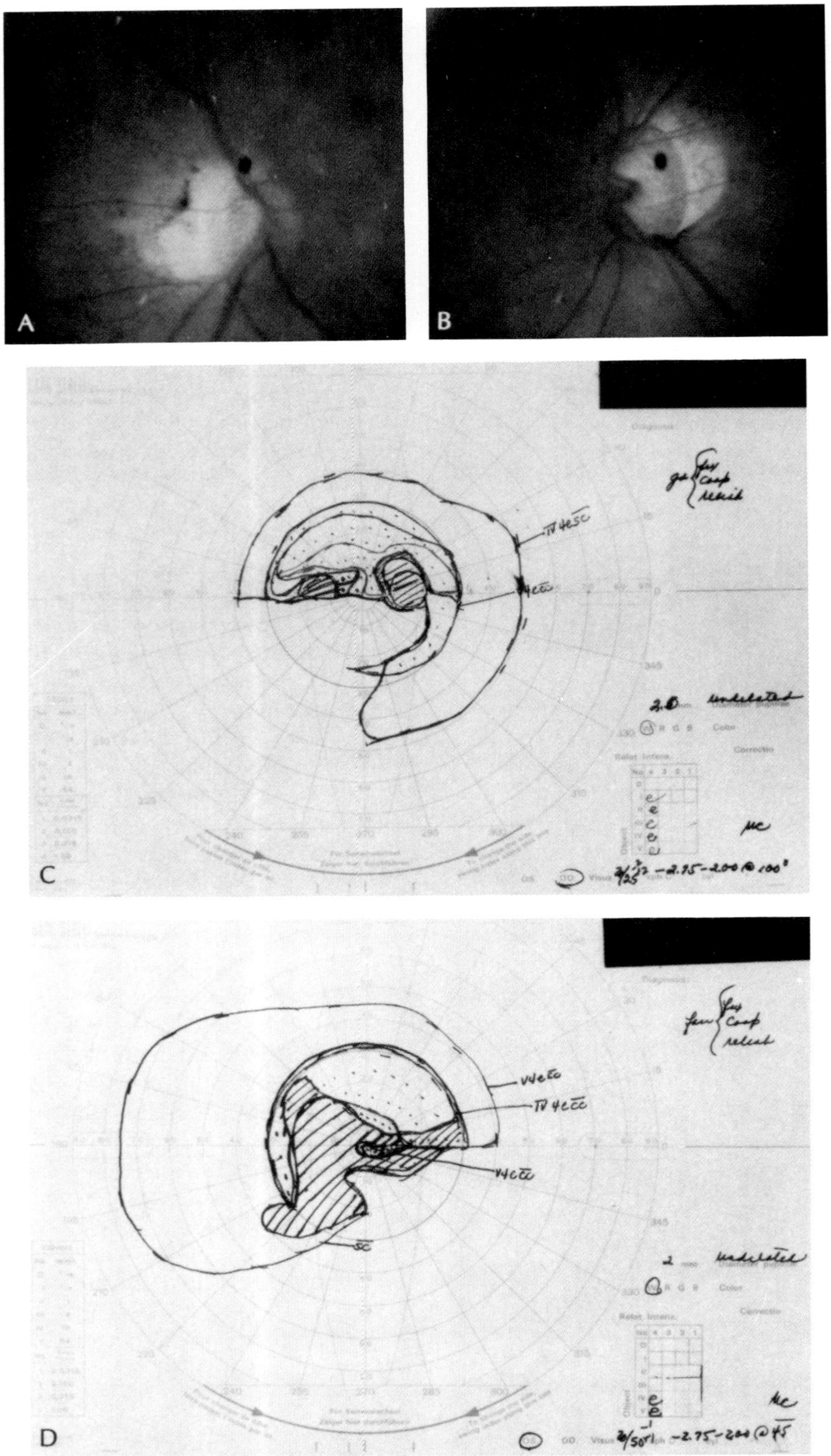

Figure 8.20.

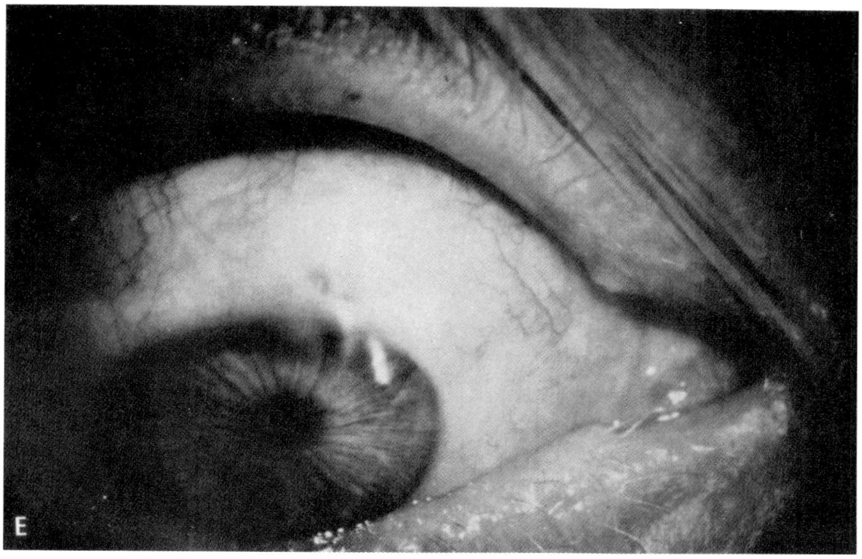

Figure 8.20. Myopic sloping discs (**A, B**) that are difficult to evaluate in a 61-year-old patient who has well-defined exfoliation glaucoma and field loss (C,D) that involves fixation in the left eye. Bilateral full-thickness filters were performed with resulting IOP of 5 OD (E) and 8 OS with maintenance of good visual acuity (20/25 OD; 20/50 OS) and with stable fields over a 3-year period.

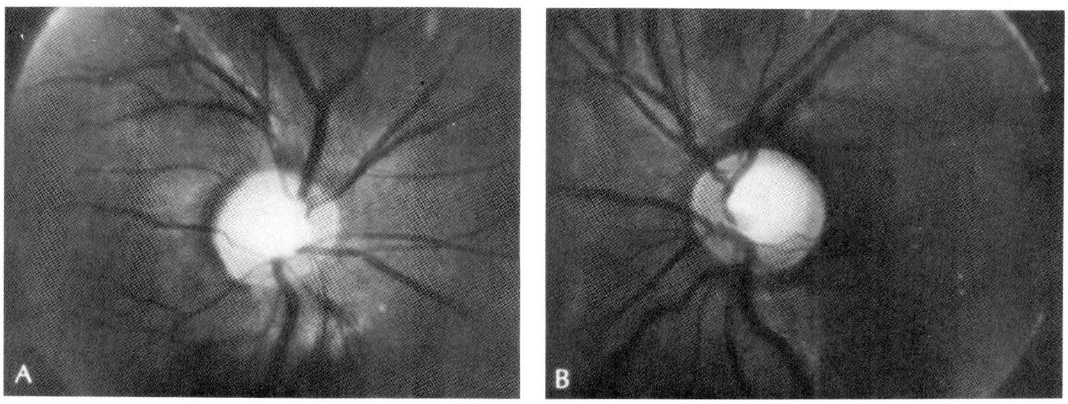

Figure 8.21. Asymmetrical size of the optic disc cups (A,B) in a patient who has early open angle glaucoma. The left disc (B) shows enlargement of the cup superiorly.

resolved by the findings of vascular occlusions, old chorioretinitis, drusen on the optic disc, or neurologic disorders, including brain tumors, retinitis pigmentosa, retinal detachment, or retinoschisis.

Local indentations of the peripheral fields that do not correspond to what would be expected from the appearance of the disc indicate in particular a search for retinoschisis or retinal cyst. A dense arcuate scotoma extending from the blind spot can be produced by Jensen's juxtapapillary choroiditis, by drusen in the optic disc, by occlusion of a macular artery, or by pituitary tumor. A ring scotoma simulating a double Bjerrum scotoma can be produced by retinitis pigmentosa.

Any disparity between the visual field and the character of glaucomatous changes in the optic disc should raise one's suspicions of an intraocular or extraocular cause of the defect other than glaucoma. Of course, one is most easily misled if the patient does have glaucoma and does have some cupping, atrophy, and field loss from glaucoma, but also has homonymous hemianopsia from cerebrovascular occlusion or bitemporal constriction from pituitary tumor. These can be detected by their lack of conformity to the types of changes in the optic nerve and visual field produced by glaucoma.

The following case illustrates field loss in a glaucomatous eye that was actually due to retinal detachment.

Case 8-1. A 56-year-old man was referred with a history of IOP right 41 and left 31, but, under pilocarpine, right and left 18; corrected vision right 6/9 +, left 6/6; angles wide and open. The cups were physiologic, but the cup was wider in the left eye than in the right. The fields were full. A year and a half later he was referred back. IOP was right and left 19. Fields were full. One year later he was referred back because of loss of all of the upper field in the right eye. However, this could not be explained by the glaucoma because the discs were unchanged. Examination indicated detach-

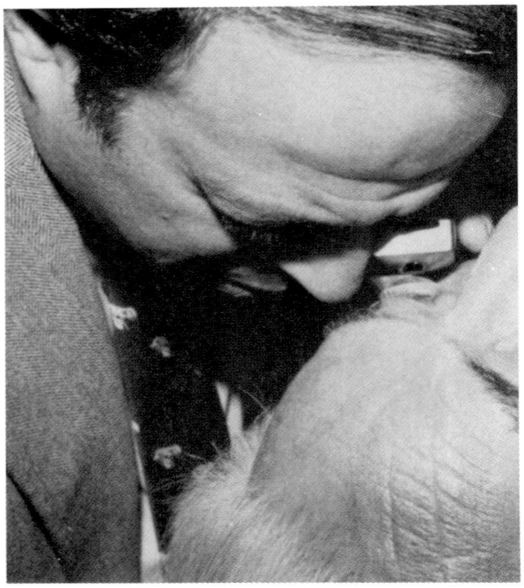

Figure 8.22. An excellent view of the optic disc is obtained through the Koeppe lens with a direct ophthalmoscope. This is especially useful in patients who have small pupils and media opacities.

ment of approximately the lower half of the right retina. A retinal operation was done, and the retina was reattached. Seven years later when last seen, corrected vision was right 6/12, left 6/6; there were increased reflexes in the macula of the right eye; fields were normal.

INTRAOCULAR PRESSURE AND CHANGES IN THE OPTIC DISC

An important factor in pathologic cupping of the optic disc, regardless of type, might be called susceptibility. It has not been explained to our satisfaction why some eyes develop pathologic cupping and field loss with IOP a little above normal, or even in the normal range, and other eyes sustain a much higher IOP over a long period of time without developing pathologic cupping. It is, however, a fact of life. Whatever level of IOP is found, if there is pathologic cupping we must strive with all the means at our disposal, both medical and surgical, to bring the IOP to a lower level.

The degree of glaucomatous cupping and atrophy of the disc is a particularly important consideration in estimating how low one may need to reduce the intraocular pressure in the treatment of individual cases of glaucoma. Thus if the disc is normal when the diagnosis of glaucoma is first made, one finds that the eye tends to withstand elevated IOP relatively well. In an eye with a completely normal disc, especially if the physiologic cup is small and the color rosy, an IOP as high as 30 mm Hg may cause little or no loss of function over a period of many years. **Where there is already marked acquired glaucomatous cupping when the diagnosis of glaucoma is first made, to prevent further loss of function, a much lower IOP is required than in a case in which the disc shows minimal cupping.** If excavation of the disc is severe, an IOP as high as 18 mm Hg usually causes loss of function over a period of years. In cases of limited cupping, the eye tolerates increased IOP less well than in cases in which the disc is normal, but better than in cases of total cupping. Thus, the greater the extent and depth of glaucomatous cupping, the lower the IOP must be maintained to prevent further loss of vision.

The types of cupping, atrophy, and field loss that develop in primary open angle glaucoma, progressing in some eyes even after the IOP is reduced to the high normal range and stopping only when a low IOP is achieved, appear clinically identical with the changes that are found in patients who have never been known to have had abnormally elevated IOP (low tension glaucoma). These circumstances, sometimes termed "low tension glaucoma equivalent," are discussed further in Chapter 19.

It has been suspected that the blood pressure and the

A

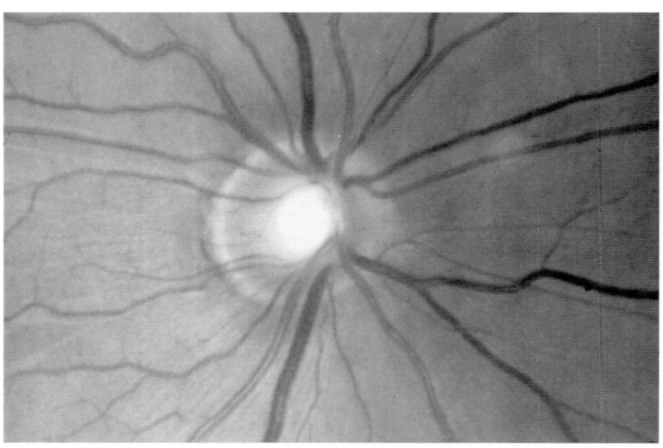

B

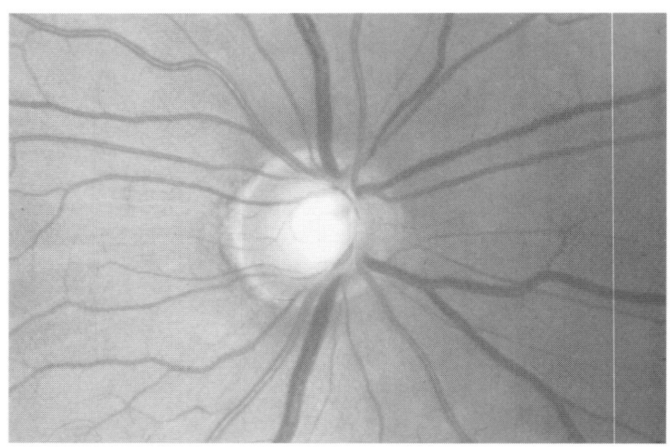

Figure 8.23. Optic disc of a 25-year-old patient with juvenile open angle glaucoma. Note enlargement of optic cup from baseline when IOP was 16 mm Hg (A) and when IOP was 47 mm Hg (B). The optic nerve returned to its original appearance once IOP was reduced by medical therapy. (Courtesy of William N. White, II, MD).

circulation of the optic nerve head may have significant influence on its vulnerability in these circumstances. This possibility is discussed further later on in this chapter under the heading Blood Pressure and the Optic Disc.

When the intraocular pressure is elevated, we know that the higher the IOP the greater is the danger to the optic disc, but we should also be aware that the height of the IOP significantly influences the type of damage that is done to the optic nerve. In fact, highly elevated IOP alone can sometimes, especially in young patients, acutely enlarge the optic cup. This change is reversible if the IOP is reduced within a few days or weeks (Fig. 8.23).

A moderate elevation of IOP produces the common varieties of glaucomatous pathologic cupping, followed by atrophy, whereas **a high IOP can cause a predominance of atrophy with less pathologic cupping in a shorter period** (Fig. 8.24). **Thus, an IOP of 40, 50, or 60 mm Hg maintained over several weeks may cause atrophy, with minimal pathologic cupping.**

With persistent or repeated IOP of 40 or 50 mm Hg or higher, one should rely more on the visual fields than on ophthalmoscopy to warn of increasing damage to the optic nerve head, since at these pressures, loss of vision may occur before there is appreciable increase in cupping and before atrophy of the optic disc is visible.

In neglected acute angle closure glaucoma, where the IOP is characteristically very high, the end result may be pure atrophy with virtually no pathologic cupping.

We have called attention to the clinical observation that optic discs with acquired glaucomatous cupping are more susceptible than normal discs to damage by intraocular pressure, but clinical observation suggests that atrophy apart from cupping does not make the disc abnormally susceptible to further damage by intraocular pressure. It seems that an optic nerve head that has been made pale or whitish by partial optic atrophy with little or no cupping after acute high intraocular pressure or due to some other cause is not abnormally susceptible to injury by subsequent moderate pressure elevation. Thus, after acute glaucoma and partial disc atrophy, when IOP has been reduced by surgery and medicine, it seems that, to prevent further loss of vision, the control of IOP needs to be no more strict than for other discs that have the same type of cup. However, these clinical situations need further evaluation.

Returning to discussion of differences in vulnerability among optic discs that ostensibly are not yet pathologically cupped and are not atrophic, we also need to consider whether eyes with unusually large physiologic cups are extraordinarily vulnerable.

In some eyes, the physiologic cups are exceptionally wide and deep; in some, the rim of normal tissue at the border of the disc may be no more than the width of one or two major vessels on the disc. Eyes with such wide and deep cups withstand increased IOP more poorly than eyes in which the physiologic cup is considerably smaller.

It has been stated by us and others that highly myopic eyes withstand increased IOP less well than eyes with low-grade myopia or those with hyperopia. Further observations are required. However, there are two other important factors in myopic eyes with POAG. It may be difficult to detect early cupping because of the sloped nature of the myopic disc, and such eyes may demonstrate initial field loss due to glaucoma close to or actually involving fixation. Therefore myopic eyes with POAG require special attention and likely earlier treatment (Chapter 18).

BLOOD PRESSURE AND THE OPTIC DISC

There is an important and debated question concerning whether the level of the arterial blood pressure influences the susceptibility of the optic disc to damage by intraocular pressure. The question is, does elevated arterial blood pressure tend to protect the optic disc from elevated intraocular pressure, and conversely, does low blood pressure render the disc more vulnerable? There are two conditions in which this question has great practical relevance. First, in patients who have both glaucoma and systemic hypertension, is there risk of an increase in damage to the optic discs if the systemic hypertension is treated and the blood pressure is reduced? Second, in patients with so-called low tension glaucoma, or its equivalent (Chapter 19) can cupping, atrophy, and loss of vision be caused by subnormal arterial blood pressure while the intraocular pressure is within the normal range? The most fundamental question underlying these practical clinical questions is to what extent ischemia is involved in damage of the optic disc in chronic glaucoma. The answer is not known, but opinions are not lacking.

Several approaches have been taken to try to answer both the fundamental and the practical clinical questions. Numerous studies have been made of the vascular anatomy of the disc and its surroundings, measurements have been made of variation in flow in the vessels, and decreases in vision have been demonstrated to occur acutely when intraocular pressure is artificially raised; but as analyzed by Maumenee, the relevance of these studies to the gradual cupping, atrophy, and field loss that occur in chronic glaucoma has not been shown (1).

We will examine clinical information concerning influences on the optic disc, first from systemic blood pressure and then from arterial occlusive disease affecting the blood supply to the eye.

SYSTEMIC BLOOD PRESSURE

Clinical comparisons have been made between groups of glaucomatous patients with similar intraocular pressures but different blood pressures, looking for differences in the prevalence of visual field defects. Such studies have lead

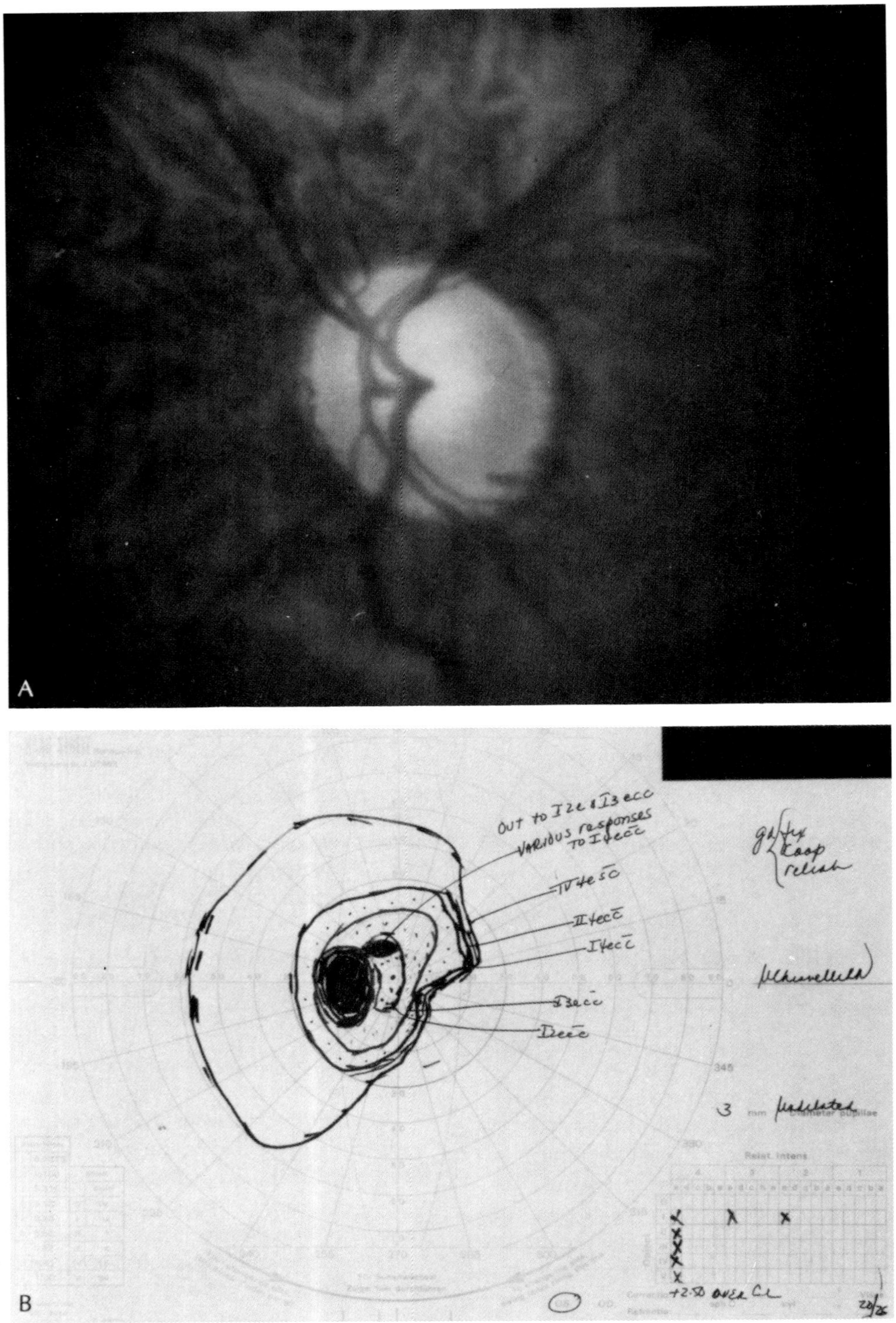

Figure 8.24. Optic atrophy (A) and dense nasal field loss (B) was believed to be due to temporary high IOP after cataract surgery. The predominate feature of the disc is pallor (atrophy) with only slight contour changes in the shape of the cup. Findings have been stable for 10 years. Visual acuity is 20/25.

Reese and McGavic (2), Sachsenweger (3), Lobstein (4), Ebner (5), and Said et al. (6) to believe that elevated blood pressure had an unfavorable influence. Fruhauf (7), Tuovinen et al. (8), and Simonett (9) in similar studies found no evidence of influence of arterial blood pressure. There are great difficulties in making meaningful comparisons in this way, because in addition to the blood pressure, the intraocular pressure, the extent of pathologic cupping, and the visual fields at the time of testing, there are many other variables to be taken into consideration.

Some clinicians who have written about the influence of blood pressure seem to have been most impressed with individual case reports in which rapid deterioration of visual field was observed when elevated blood pressure was drastically reduced in patients who had glaucoma that previously had been considered to be adequately regulated. However, there are many people who have both chronic glaucoma and systemic hypertension, and a large number of these people have been given treatment to reduce their blood pressure. In view of this, the small number of cases of apparent adverse effect actually reported is remarkable. The cases most often cited are those of Harrington, who described three patients who had high blood pressure and who had been under treatment with pilocarpine for glaucoma, with IOPs not normalized, but stable visual fields for 3 years, 2 years, and a shorter period, when reserpine, with or without hydralazine, was started (10). These patients had large decreases in blood pressure and distinct increases in visual field defects within a few days to 4 weeks, without change in intraocular pressure or in appearance of the discs. Cessation of systemic medications was followed by partial recovery of lost field in only one case.

McLean mentioned, without further details, one patient whom he had seen "lose field at the same IOP level on which he previously maintained it when his internist succeeded in drastically controlling his hypertension." (11)

Francois and Neetens have given brief case reports (with no information on time relationships) of seven instances of increase in loss of visual field after medical treatment for systemic hypertension while intraocular pressure was thought to be adequately controlled (12).

In these few suggestive case reports, there has been no way to be sure that the changes in visual fields after antihypertensive treatment were caused by reduction of blood pressure or were coincidental. The need is evident for a large-scale prospective clinical study, extending over many years, to ascertain whether elevated systemic blood pressure is in fact protective against the damaging effect of elevated intraocular pressure on the optic disc and whether treating systemic hypertension in glaucomatous patients significantly increases the risk of damage to the optic disc.

Kolker et al. have used corticosteroids (13), Heilmann has used acetazolamide and clonidine (14), and Phelps and Phelps have used phenylephrine in acute experiments to alter relationships between intraocular pressure and blood pressure and to examine the influence on visual fields in glaucoma (15), indicating that reduced blood pressure is disadvantageous. Such short-term experiments on visual fields, however intriguing and suggestive, do leave the question unsettled as to whether there are corresponding long-term relationships, and what relationship there may be to the cupping of the optic disc.

There have been several recent reports calling attention to the potential adverse influence of nocturnal hypotension on the course of glaucomatous optic nerve damage (16–19).

While the role of blood pressure and the mechanism of glaucomatous cupping and atrophy are being investigated in clinical and experimental research centers, and while we are waiting for the answers, it seems reasonable from a practical clinical standpoint that, whenever medication for systemic hypertension is given to a patient who has glaucoma that is not very well controlled, the frequency of examination of the optic disc and visual fields should be increased. In patients who demonstrate unexpected progression of their glaucoma disease, the possibility of nocturnal hypotension needs to be contemplated and internal medicine consultation obtained.

ARTERIAL OCCLUSIVE DISEASE

In questioning the possible relationship of blood pressure and vulnerability of the optic disc in glaucoma, it is relevant to note that interference with arterial blood supply by extraocular vasculopathy has not thus far been shown to have significant influence. One would think that there must be many patients who have carotid obstructive disease, often unilateral, as well as glaucoma, and that if a normal arterial supply was critically important for the fate of the optic disc in glaucoma, we would see evidence of it.

The literature on ocular effects associated with occlusion of carotid arteries and with the aortic arch syndrome, or pulseless disease, contains many example in which the influences on intraocular pressure and on ocular pulse are described. Acute common and internal carotid occlusions are known to produce an acute decrease of intraocular pressure by a few mm Hg, as repeatedly demonstrated during carotid compression tonography. During chronic occlusion, the ocular pulse, recorded by tonography or by measurement of the corneal pulse, and the orbital pulse, recorded by ophthalmodynamography, are reduced, and pressure in the central retinal arteries can be shown by ophthalmodynamometry to be reduced. However, rarely is mention made of influence on cupping or atrophy of the optic disc or changes in the visual field such as are associated with glaucoma. It might be postulated that the optic nerve may be protected from reduced arterial supply by a simultaneous reduction of intraocular pressure. However, only severe reduction of arterial blood supply, such as produced by bilateral carotid disease or by the aortic arch

CLINICAL ASSESSMENT OF THE NERVE FIBER LAYER

Joel S. Schuman

Examination of the nerve fiber layer (NFL) is a challenging portion of the ophthalmologic evaluation. It requires patience and practice, and is not easily mastered. The NFL, because of its structure of parallel tubular fibers, reflects light differently than the remainder of the retina. The absence of these fibers results in decreased reflectance.

The NFL is most easily visualized using red-free light. It can be examined using a direct ophthalmoscope, but is better appreciated with a dilated pupil and a 78 D lens in stereoscopic biomicroscopy at the slit lamp. The beam is widened slightly from that used for anterior segment evaluation, to provide an adequate field of view, but not so wide as to cause discomfort to the patient. In younger patients with clear media, a gleam can sometimes be seen from the internal limiting membrane. The NFL appears as a series of striations radiating in an arcuate fashion from (really toward) the optic nerve head (ONH) over and under the macula, not crossing the horizontal meridian. Since the NFL is thickest at the superior and inferior poles, the reflectance is greatest in these areas, and they appear more white.

When examining the NFL, one looks for areas of focal loss, which appear as dark bands fanning out from the ONH, with a bright-dark-bright pattern or areas of diffuse loss. Diffuse loss is seen as a decrease in reflection from the tissue, and the underlying vasculature can then be differentiated more easily. In the peripapillary region, less than tone disc diameter from the ONH, secondary, tertiary and quaternary vessel branches are poorly seen, and do not have sharp borders, with a healthy NFL. As the NFL thins, the vessels, and vessel borders, become more distinct. This is most clearly evident in advanced glaucoma, when all vessel branches are easily distinguished.

Documentation of NFL appearance by photography is probably the best way to examine this structure, but the technique is difficult to perform, and requires a willingness on the part of the photographer. Photographs, in black and white, can be studied for NFL appearance, and provide an excellent record to use for future visits.

Several methods have been devised for grading the degree of NFL loss quantitatively, but they are difficult to learn and to use. Simple qualitative assessment of NFL status seems the best option for examination of this tissue, with descriptive terms such as normal, thin or absent, or description of which vessels are visible, and to what level of branching, in a given area.

Because clinical examination of the NFL is qualitative and difficult, technology is currently under development, with some already available, for actual quantitation of NFL thickness, as described in Chapter 9. No technology, however, can replace the ophthalmologist's study of the patient's eye, and evaluation of the NFL clinically is an essential part of that examination.

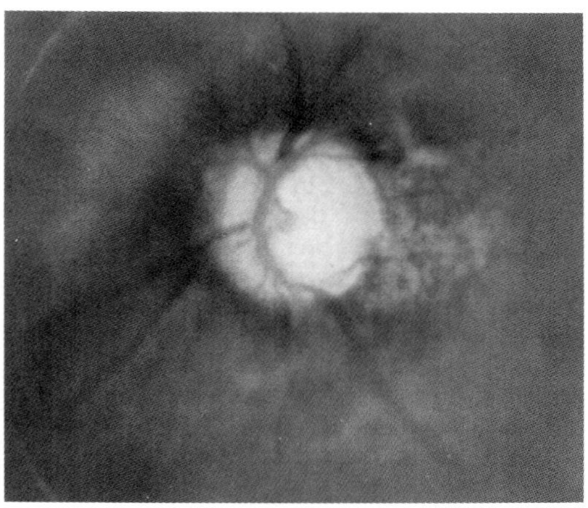

Figure 8.25. The patient was observed with acute ischemic optic neuropathy due to temporal arteritis. When the disc edema resolved, the disc appeared to be totally cupped with contour changes that were indistinguishable from those of glaucoma. (No evidence existed for any abnormality in intraocular pressure.)

syndrome, produces much chronic decrease in intraocular pressure.

When the arterial supply to the eye is so severely insufficient that it causes marked reduction of intraocular pressure, meaningful long-term studies of the influence of the blood supply on the optic disc are practically precluded by degenerative changes in the eye, such as secondary neovascularization of the iris and anterior chamber angle, necrosis of the anterior segment, hypoxic retinopathy, and retinal degeneration.

A long-term study and comparison of the optic discs and visual fields in patients with moderate reduction of blood supply to one eye and constantly, equally elevated intraocular pressure in both eyes, would be most informative. One eye would serve as a control for the other, the difference in arterial supply being the principal variable. It is remarkable how little information of this sort is available.

Ignoring for the moment cases of temporal or giant cell arteritis because they tend to be complicated by intraocular vascular disease, which would confuse the study of the influence of blood supply alone, there is one report in which patients with normal IOPs but with reduced ocular blood supply due to so-called subclavian steal have had atrophic changes and cupping in the disc, with visual field change in the periphery, sometimes with an upper nasal defect, usually bilateral (20). The nature of the cupping and any anatomic relationship to loss of visual field are not described in this study, so it is unclear whether there is significant analogy to the changes in glaucoma or in progressive low-tension glaucoma.

Another study concerns 13 patients with IOPs in the normal range who had their retinal arterial pressure reduced 20 to 25% in one eye for several years after unilateral carotid ligation. In these patients the optic nerves and all visual functions remained intact (21).

Coming closer to the desired controlled study of bilaterally glaucomatous eyes with asymmetric arterial supplies is a report on 5 patients with elevated intraocular pressure, but bilateral severe artery disease, who developed no glaucomatous disc or field changes during observation for 3 to 12 years (22). This is interesting, but the definitive controlled investigation is yet to be done.

The reported effects of temporal or giant cell arteritis on the optic nerve head are mentioned here because they are interesting in their own right, indicating a relationship of intraocular vascular disease to cupping of the optic disc (Fig. 8.25). However, we do not know what relationship this may have to the main topic of "blood pressure and the optic disc."

Hayreh and Miller have reported that when ischemic optic neuropathy has developed from occlusion of posterior ciliary arteries in temporal arteritis, there has been loss of central vision with pale edema of the optic disc, followed 2 to 3 months later by cupping and atrophy of the optic disc, becoming deep after 4 to 5 months (23,24). This has occurred in eyes that have been thought to have had normal intraocular pressure throughout. Hayreh noted relatively slight cupping in eyes with occlusion of posterior ciliary arteries due to arteriosclerosis. We have observed at least five cases of anterior ischemic optic neuropathy secondary to biopsy proven giant cell arteritis where optic nerve changes indistinguishable from glaucomatous cupping were observed (25). After non-arteritic ischemic optic neuropathy we have only rarely observed any suspicious glaucoma-like changes involving the optic nerve.

References

1. Maumenee AE: The pathogenesis of visual field loss in glaucoma. In: Controversy in Ophthalmology. Philadelphia: W.B. Saunders Co., 1977.
2. Reese AB, McGavic JS: Relation of field contraction to blood pressure in chronic primary glaucoma. Arch Ophthalmol 1942;27:845–850.
3. Sachsenweger R: Der Einluss des Bluthochdruckes auf die Prognose des Glaukoms. Klin Monatsbl Augenheilkd 1963;142:625–633.
4. Lobstein A: Factors affecting the susceptibility of the glaucomatous eye to raised intraocular pressure. In: Modern Problems in Ophthalmology. Edited by R. Sampaolesi. New York: Karger, 1968.
5. Ebner R: Die Prognose des Glaukoms im Hinblick auf den arteriellen Blutdruck. Wien Med Wochenschr 1967;117:1024–1026.
6. Said A, Labib MAM, Abboud I, et al: The relationship between systemic hypertension and chronic simple glaucoma. Bull Ophthalmol Soc Egypt 1967;60:71–81.
7. Fruhauf A: Untesuchungen über den Einfluss des arteriellen Blutdrucks auf den Verlauf des Glaucoma simplex. Dtsch Gesundh Wes 1971;26: 273–275.
8. Tuovinen E, Jägerroos P, Vänttinen S: Die Bedeutung des arteriellen Blutdruckes für die Prognose des Glaucoma simplex. Wiss Z Univ Rostock, Math.-nat, Reihe, 1965;14:131–137.
9. Simonett B: Der Brachialisblutdruck und seine Beziehung zum Verlauf des Glaucoma simplex. Klin Monatsbl Augenheilkd 1959;135: 196–205.
10. Harrington DO: The pathogenesis of the glaucoma field. Clinical evidence that circulatory insufficiency in the optic nerve is the primary cause of visual field loss in glaucoma. Am J Ophthalmol 1959;47:177–185.
11. McLean JM: Management of the primary glaucomas. Am J Ophthalmol 1957;44:323–334.
12. Francois J, Neetens A: The deterioration of the visual field in glaucoma and the blood pressure. Doc Ophthalmol 1970;28:70–132.
13. Kolker AE, Becker B, Mills DW: Intraocular pressure and visual fields: Effects of corticosteroids. Arch Ophthalmol 1965;72:772–782.
14. Heilmann K: Augendruck, Blutdruck und Glaukomschaden. Bucherei des Augenartes. 1972;61:1–82.
15. Phelps GK, Phelps CD: Blood pressure and pressure amaurosis. Invest Ophthalmol 1975;14:237–240.
16. Kaiser HJ, Flammer J: Systemic hypotension: a risk factor for glaucomatous damage? Ophthalmologica 1994;203:105–108.
17. Hayreh SS, Zimmerman MB, Podhajsky P, et al: Nocturnal arterial hypotension and its role in optic nerve head ischaemic disorders. Am J Ophthalmol 1994;117:603–624.
18. Béchetoille A, Bresson-Dumont H: Diurnal and nocturnal blood pressure drops in patients with focal ischemic glaucoma. Clin Invest 1994;232: 675–679.
19. Stuart LG, et al: Ambulatory blood pressure monitoring in glaucoma, the nocturnal dip. Ophthalmology 1995;102:61–69.
20. Dwyer-Joyce P: The fields in subclavian steal. Trans Ophthalmol Soc UK 1972;92:819–824.
21. Cristiansson J: On the late effect of carotid ligation upon the human eye. Acta Ophthalmol 1962;40:271–280.
22. Jampol LM, Miller NR: Carotid artery disease and glaucoma. Br J Ophthalmol 1978;6:324–326.
23. Hayreh SS: Pathogenesis of cupping of the optic disc. Br J Ophthalmol 1974;58:863–876.
24. Miller S: The enigma of glaucoma simplex. Optic disc cupping in normal eyes. Trans Ophthalmol Soc UK 1972;92:563–584.
25. Sebag J, Thomas JV, Epstein DL, et al: Optic disc cupping in arteritic anterior ischemic optic neuropathy resembles glaucomatous cupping. Ophthalmology 1986;93:357–361.

Imaging of the Optic Nerve Head and Nerve Fiber Layer in Glaucoma

9

Joel S. Schuman

INTRODUCTION

The objective of devices designed for imaging the optic nerve head (ONH) and nerve fiber layer (NFL) is to provide a quantitative assessment of the structure of these tissues. In this way, ONH parameters, such as degree of cupping, area of neuroretinal rim, diameter of disc, and others, as well as NFL thickness, may be assessed objectively and with a high degree of precision and accuracy. Such instrumentation is required since clinical examination of the ONH and NFL is limited and subjective (1,2). Quigley determined that up to 40% of nerve fibers may be lost before detection by conventional clinical means (3,4). When using these methods, the threshold for detection of damage in glaucoma is high. These machines aim to reduce that threshold dramatically.

Historical Perspective

The optic nerve was not visualized in living humans until the invention of the ophthalmoscope by Helmholtz in 1851 (5). In 1855, von Graefe described optic atrophy in glaucoma as "amaurosis with excavation of the optic nerve" (6). Schnabel found nerve fiber loss with formation of cavities in glaucoma (7), but it was not until the work of Fuchs and Elliot that glaucomatous changes in the optic nerve were described. Fuchs noted disappearance of the anterior glial fibers, followed by the deeper glial fibers, with bending backward and thinning of the lamina cribrosa as the result of elevated intraocular pressure (IOP). Fuchs thought that the changes found in the ONH were significant and preceded visual field loss (8).

Interpretation of ONH cupping is subjective; significant variation has been noted between observers and between examinations by the same observer (1,2). Despite this, ONH examination alone with IOP measurement and visual field assessment are used to diagnose glaucoma and determine progression. Because ONH evaluation is largely subjective and visual field testing results may be difficult to interpret, and because IOP, while the prime risk factor for glaucoma, in and of itself is not diagnostic, it is essential that new objective tools be created to permit the early diagnosis of the disease and the early detection of its progression. In response to this demand, technologies have been developed to allow objective measurement of the ONH and NFL.

ASSESSMENT OF THE OPTIC NERVE HEAD

Fundus Photography

The first significant advance toward the goal of objective ONH assessment came with the development of fundus photography. The Nordenson camera was introduced in the early 20th century; stereoscopic fundus cameras soon followed. Stereoscopic fundus photography allowed the objective documentation of the appearance of the ONH and retina over time (9); however, the interpretations of these pictures were still subjective. Even experts presented with a series of stereoscopic ONH photographs are unable to agree in the discrimination between glaucomatous and normal ONHs (1). This limits the utility of stereoscopic ONH photography for detecting the presence or progression of glaucoma.

To further increase the value of ONH photography, manual and automated mapping techniques have been attempted, but these require an experienced observer and produce variable results (10).

Optic Nerve Head Analyzers

Optic nerve head analyzers were introduced to quantitate cupping, measure neuroretinal rim area and provide measurements of other ONH parameters. These instruments are automated and use standard fundus camera optics. The first of these units was the PAR IS 2000 (now Topcon IMAGEnet, Topcon Instruments, Paramus, NJ), which could capture simultaneous digital stereoscopic fundus images, or could digitize images from 35 mm slides (11). The instrument created a three-dimensional map of the ONH, using computer algorithms for image registration and cross-correlation to calculate depth values at corresponding points. There was an element of subjectivity in the analysis, as the user was required to define the disc margin by selecting four points in the image. The instrument determined the cup margin as 120 μm posterior to the disc margin. From these points, the device created a statistical profile of the ONH.

The Humphrey Retinal Analyzer (Humphrey Instru-

THE GLAUCOMA-SCOPE

M. Bruce Shields

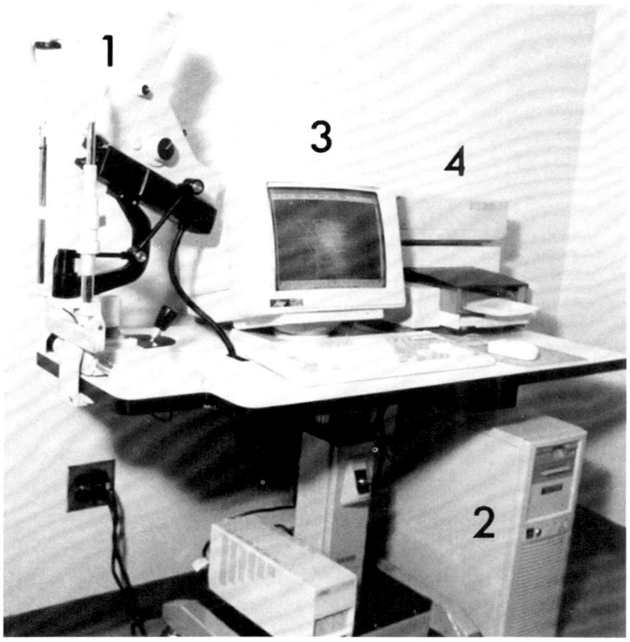

Figure. The Glaucoma-Scope for computerized topographic image analysis of the optic nerve head, showing basic components: Optical head for image acquisition (1); microprocessor (2); monitor (3); printer (4).

The Glaucoma-Scope is one of several types of computerized instruments that provides detailed topographic maps of the optic nerve head and peripapillary retina. The basic principle of the instrument has been referred to as rasterstereography (the term "raster" simply referring to a scanning pattern from side-to-side in lines from top-to-bottom). The instrument consists of two main parts: the optical head for image acquisition and a microprocessor for image analysis. (Figure) The optic nerve head is illuminated with approximately 25 horizontal lines, the deflections of which are proportional to the extent of papillary excavation. A video image of the disc and projected lines is captured and stored in digital form on a disc drive or an optical disc drive in the image analyzer. The horizontal lines are scanned in raster fashion, and quantitative topographic depth measurements of the optic nerve head are generated by an algorithm which converts the line data into corresponding depth values. Each line has a reference plane that is defined by the retinal surface located approximately 350 microns nasal and temporal to the disc.

The depth or elevation of the disc and surrounding retina are computed at approximately 8,750 data points, from which approximately 760 values in microns are provided in both numeric and gray scale printouts. In the initial study, the printout provides actual depth values at each point, while subsequent measurements are automatically compared with the first and printed to show any changes in depth values of 50 microns or greater. More recent software printouts also provide a three-dimensional grid map, disc and cup outlines with a battery of related data, and horizontal and vertical cross sections of the optic nerve head.

The reproducibility of topographic measurements with the Glaucoma-Scope has been studied in normal subjects and glaucoma patients (1,2). The results have been favorable, with 95% confidence intervals that are well within the 50 micron limit. Preliminary studies with a plastic eye model also suggest that the data being reproduced is an accurate representation of the actual ocular structures (unpublished data). Limitations of the instrument include the need for pupillary dilation of approximately 5 mm, clear media, and an experienced technician. As with all computerized image analyzers of the optic nerve head, the remaining question is whether the information provided will allow the clinician to detect true progression of glaucomatous optic atrophy sooner than is possible with current clinical measures. Long-term studies are currently under way to answer this question.

References

1. Hoskins HD, Hetherington J, Glenday M, et al. Repeatability of the Glaucoma-Scope measurements of the optic nerve head topography. J Glauc 1994;3:17–27.
2. Pendergast SD, Shields MB. Reproducibility of optic nerve head topographic measurements with the Glaucoma-Scope. J Glauc 1995;4:170–176.

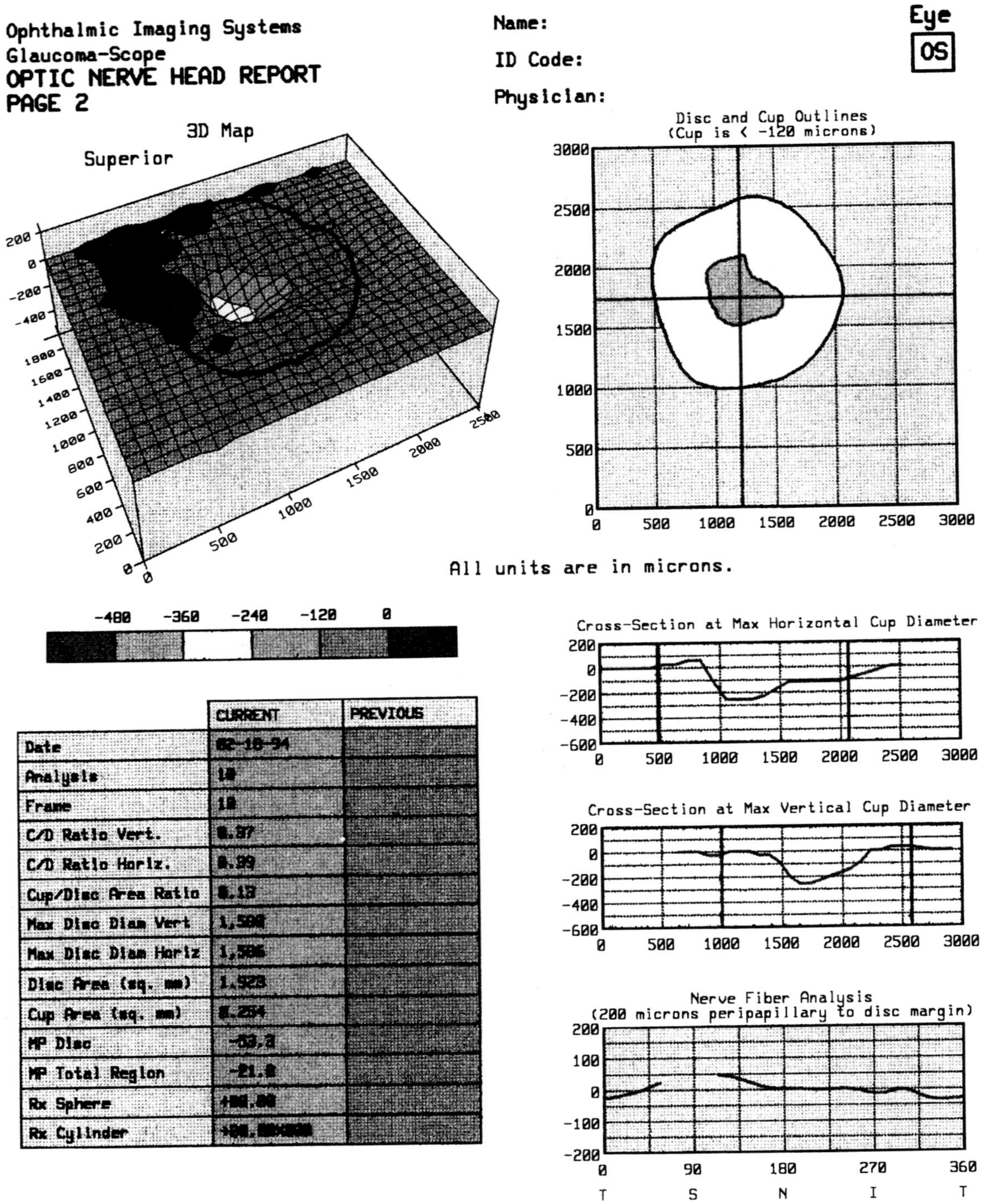

Figure 9.1. Glaucoma-Scope™ report on an eye with a normal appearing optic nerve head and normal visual field. Note vertical and horizontal cross-sectional analyses of optic nerve head, which vary dramatically with small shifts in positioning of the patient. "Nerve Fiber Analysis" is an adaptation of Caprioli's technique for assessment of NFL height; change analysis requires a stable, unchanging reference point. From Schuman JS, Noecker RJ: Imaging of the optic nerve and nerve fiber layer in glaucoma. Ophthalmol Clin North Am 1995;8:259–279.

ments, Inc., San Leandro, CA) was similar to the PAR, but used a red-free stereoscopic video camera, and required the user to select eight points in order to define the disc margin. The disc calculated by this instrument was oval, rather than round (12).

The Rodenstock Optic Nerve Head Analyzer (Rodenstock Instruments, Danbury, CT) was also similar to the PAR, but defined the cup as 150 μm posterior to the disc margin. A simultaneous stereoscopic video camera could capture images directly, while two sets of seven evenly spaced lines were projected on the ONH. One hundred forty depth values were calculated along the 14 stripes (13).

The technique of defining the cup as some distance below the disc margin overestimates small cups and underestimates large ones (14). Magnification error occurrs, in part due to refractive error. Variability of measurements are high, especially when multiple observers are introduced, but can be reduced by the use of simultaneous stereoscopic ONH photographs (15). These instruments require a constant plane of reference from which to calculate cup depth; of course, none exists. Although the use of three points outside the peripapillary area has been suggested as a stable reference plane, this is still a troublesome issue for the optic nerve head analyzers.

The latest of this type of device is the Glaucoma-Scope (Ophthalmic Imaging Systems, Inc., Sacramento, CA). This instrument, based on the principle of raster stereography, projects lines onto the ONH using an infrared light source; deflection is proportional to the depth of the reflecting surface. Depth is measured at 8750 points, while a reference plane is calculated from two vertical lines 350 μm on either side of the ONH (16–18). This device relies on the operator to select a reference point and outline the disc margin; on subsequent examinations, the operator simply identifies the reference point and the computer analyzes the data. The depth values are reported on a printout, with each number representing a cell 75 μm by 100 μm in size (Figs. 9.1–9.4). The reproducibility of measurements made with the Glaucoma-Scope is 46.56 μm for healthy ONHs, and 52.64 μm for glaucomatous ONHs. The average individual cell standard deviation from one exam to the next is 11.64 μm in healthy eyes and 13.16 μm in glaucomatous ones. Patient re-alignment and instrument adjustment is the largest source of between-visit variability, while the inherent variability of the instrument and computer analysis is the main source of image-to-image variation (19).

Although promising, ONH analyzers are unable to differentiate normal from glaucomatous ONHs, and are limited in their ability to detect glaucomatous progression over time (20–28). The parameter measured most reliably by these instruments is the neuroretinal rim area (26), but overall measurement variation for ONH topography is approximately 165 μm (12,29). Measurements made with these instruments remain subjective, in that most of the variability is attributable to the operator (12,22,26–28).

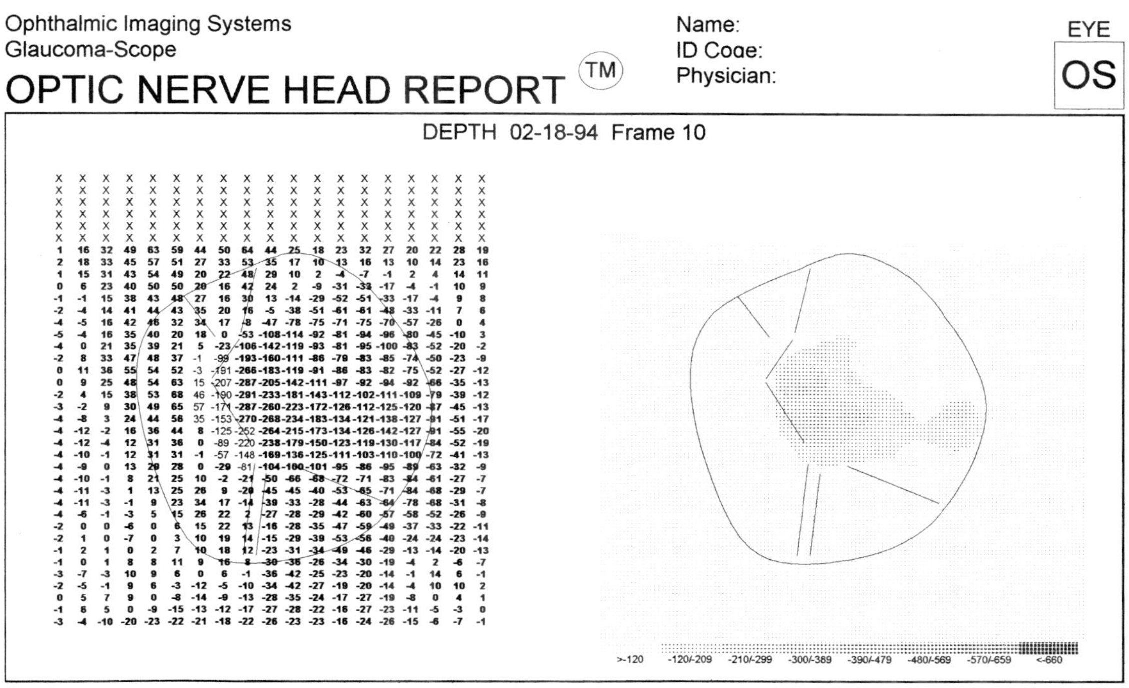

Figure 9.2. Glaucoma-Scope™ gray-scale and numerical displays in an eye with a normal appearing optic nerve head and normal visual field. From Schuman JS, Noecker RJ: Imaging of the optic nerve and nerve fiber layer in glaucoma. Ophthalmol Clin North Am 1995;8:259–279.

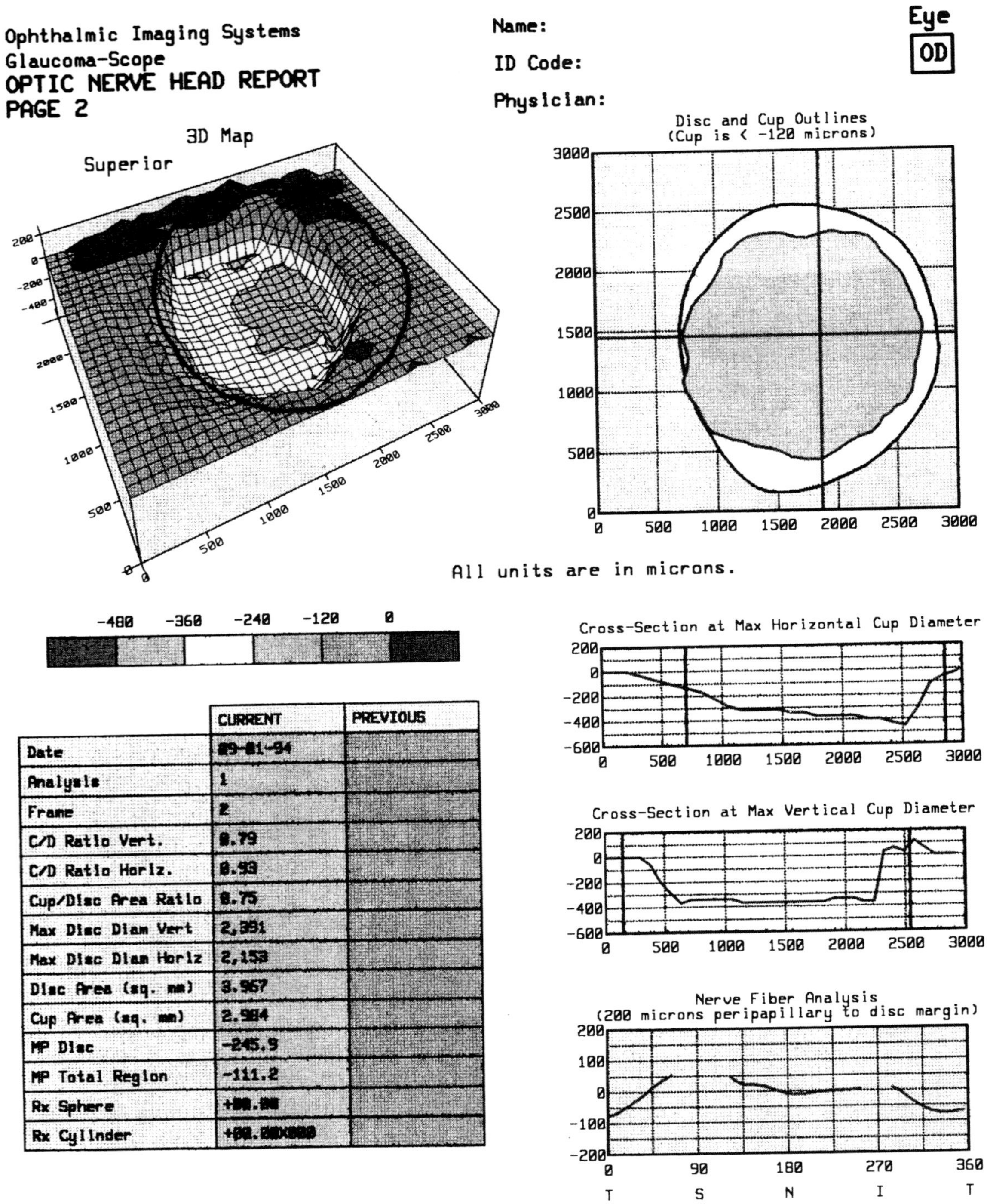

	CURRENT	PREVIOUS
Date	09-01-94	
Analysis	1	
Frame	2	
C/D Ratio Vert.	0.79	
C/D Ratio Horiz.	0.93	
Cup/Disc Area Ratio	0.75	
Max Disc Diam Vert	2,391	
Max Disc Diam Horiz	2,153	
Disc Area (sq. mm)	3.967	
Cup Area (sq. mm)	2.984	
MP Disc	-245.9	
MP Total Region	-111.2	
Rx Sphere	+00.00	
Rx Cylinder	+00.00X000	

Figure 9.3. Glaucoma-Scope™ report on an eye with advanced cupping. From Schuman JS, Noecker RJ: Imaging of the optic nerve and nerve fiber layer in glaucoma. Ophthalmol Clin North Am 1995;8:259–279.

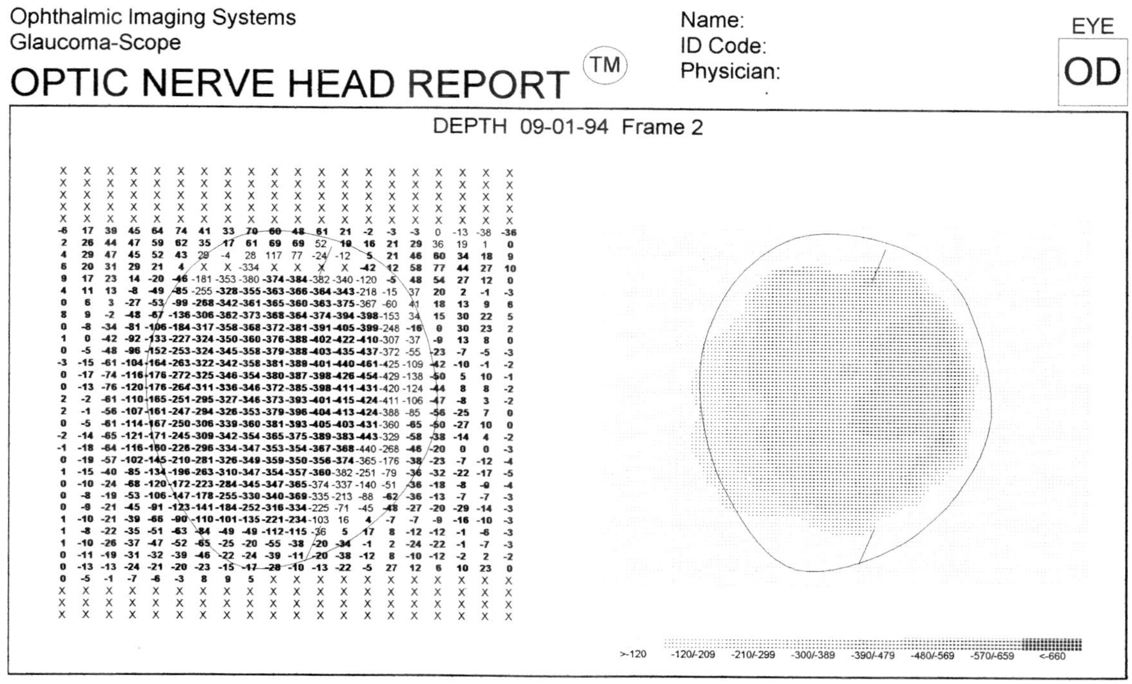

Figure 9.4. Glaucoma-Scope™ gray scale and numerical displays in an eye with advanced cupping. From Schuman JS, Noecker RJ: Imaging of the optic nerve and nerve fiber layer in glaucoma. Ophthalmol Clin North Am 1995;8:259–279.

ONH analyzers are an attempt to provide automatically an objective measurement of the ONH, but accuracy and reproducibility of measurements remain limited by the optics of the system, and these devices still rely heavily on operator control and interpretation.

Scanning Laser Ophthalmoscopes

Compared with OHN analyzers, axial resolution is improved, and variability reduced, by measuring ONH topography with confocal laser scanning ophthalmoscopy. This technology produces coronal optical sections of the retina and ONH. The earliest scanning light ophthalmoscope was developed in Boston and used rectangular line patterns on the retina (30). Systems now use point sources of laser light, and are either confocal or non-confocal.

NON-CONFOCAL SYSTEMS

Initially, scanning laser ophthalmoscopy used non-confocal optics. A 10–20 μm diameter laser beam is focused onto the retina, scanned linearly, and reflected back to a detector. The detected signal is videographically displayed. The illumination and detection apertures are separate and inverted compared with conventional fundus photography (31). Much less illumination is required for this type of imaging than for fundus photography, increasing patient comfort. However, corneal reflections are a significant problem (32,33).

CONFOCAL IMAGING

Contemporary scanning laser ophthalmoscopes use a double scanning confocal optical system (34), wherein the incident laser is scanned across the retina together with the detector system. Only a single spot on the retina is illuminated at any one time, using a pinhole aperture; a second pinhole then receives the reflected light, allowing only that light from the illuminated retinal area to be detected, and blocking all other light (35-37). Only the plane of interest is in focus, as reflections from out of focus planes are blocked by the pinhole. This results in high contrast imaging as compared to non-confocal systems, and the ability to optically section the retina coronally. Light scattering from tissues outside the area of focus is negligible, as the imaging pinhole excludes light reflected outside the focal plane (30,32,34).

The Rodenstock Confocal Scanning Laser Ophthalmoscope

The Rodenstock confocal scanning laser ophthalmoscope uses a He-Ne or argon laser of 0.1 mW power, 30 Hz repetition rate with 100 ns interval between pulses, 10 J energy per image, to scan a retinal plane in 1/30 second with a field of view of 20 to 40 degrees. The plane is 300 μm thick, and is displayed as a 525 horizontal line analog video signal (32–34,36). The image is displayed in real-time and can be stored on video tape (30). Reflectometry is used to perform image analysis of differences in wavelength-dependent reflection. Three dimensional reconstruction is possible (38). Monochromatic viewing permits coronal optical retinal sectioning, with the focal plane adjusted by motorized movement of the objective lens.

This system can display images on the patient's retina at precise locations, and can be used for functional retinal evaluation.

Because the laser scans point by point, a registration strategy is necessary to adjust the image for movement artifact that occurs during scanning. The device creates a composite image of the scanned structure, for example, the ONH, by scanning the ONH surface one focal plane at a time, and then bringing the images into register.

As noted, illumination levels during confocal imaging are low as compared to fundus photography or ophthalmoscopy, since a laser is used to scan one spot at a time. While this increases patient comfort, the fact that the laser beam diameter is small also allows scanning through a small, undilated pupil, using the remainder of the pupil for light collection from the fundus. The intensity of the incident laser light is well within safety standards (30,39).

Resolution is dependent on laser spot size and the diameter of the imaging pinhole. Vertical resolution is dependent on the distance between focal planes. Reflection from deeper tissues is attenuated by overlying structures, but there is less than 50% reduction from peak value in the optical sections (30,32).

The Rodenstock confocal scanning laser ophthalmoscope produces high quality optical tissue sections and can measure three-dimensional structures with good reproducibility (40).

The Heidelberg Laser Tomographic Scanner

The Heidelberg Laser Tomographic Scanner (Heidelberg Instruments, Heidelberg, Germany) uses a He-Ne laser to image up to a 20 degree field of view, scanning line by line in a pointwise fashion (41). A single plane contains 256 by 256 pixels for analysis. The operator defines the thickness of the area to be studied. From this 32 evenly spaced consecutive coronal sections are obtained. For example, in studying the ONH, the anteriormost plane is directly above the first retinal reflection, while the posteriormost plane is just below the bottom of the cup. With a typical topographic depth of 1550 μm, the distance between focal planes is 50 μm (41), focal plane half-thickness is 20-60 μm (42), the depth resolution is 300 μm, and each image contains 2,097,152 pixels (43). Scan time is approximately 4 seconds.

The Zeiss Laser Tomographic Scanner, The Topographic Scanning System and The Heidelberg Retinal Tomograph

The Zeiss Laser Tomographic Scanner (LTS, Zeiss Instruments, Thornwood, NJ) uses a He-Ne laser, while the Topographic Scanning System (TopSS, Laser Diagnostic Technologies, Inc., San Diego, CA) and the Retinal Tomograph (HRT, Heidelberg Engineering GmbH, Heidelberg, Germany) use diode lasers at 670 nm wavelength (44,45). These systems are similar to other confocal scanning laser microscopes, achieving high lateral resolution through the use of a small pinhole. Reproducibility of measurements is on the order of 50 μm (41). Coronal sections of the retina and ONH can be taken and analyzed (Figs. 9.5, 9.6). However, due to limited depth resolution, the substructure of the retina cannot be resolved, and only mean depth measurements can be made accurately. Nerve fiber layer thickness cannot be determined with precision, as the posterior margin of the NFL is not easily detected using this instrumentation.

In contrast to ONH analyzers, confocal scanning laser ophthalmoscopes offer higher axial resolution and greater reproducibility in evaluating ONH topography. The variability of the HRT measurements in vitro, in a model eye, is 31–56 μm (41), whereas in vivo the variability on a

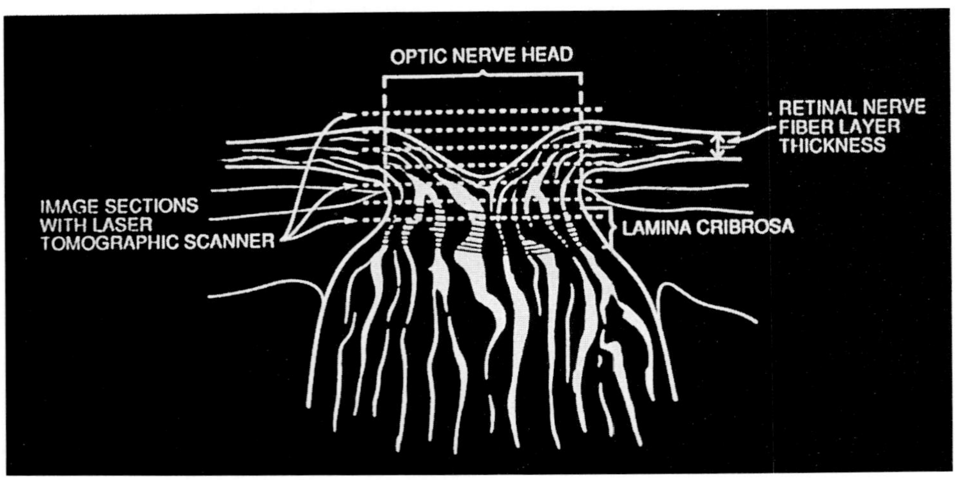

Figure 9.5. Plane of section of laser tomographic scanners (coronal). From Schuman JS, Noecker RJ: Imaging of the optic nerve and nerve fiber layer in glaucoma. Ophthalmol Clin North Am 1995;8:259–279.

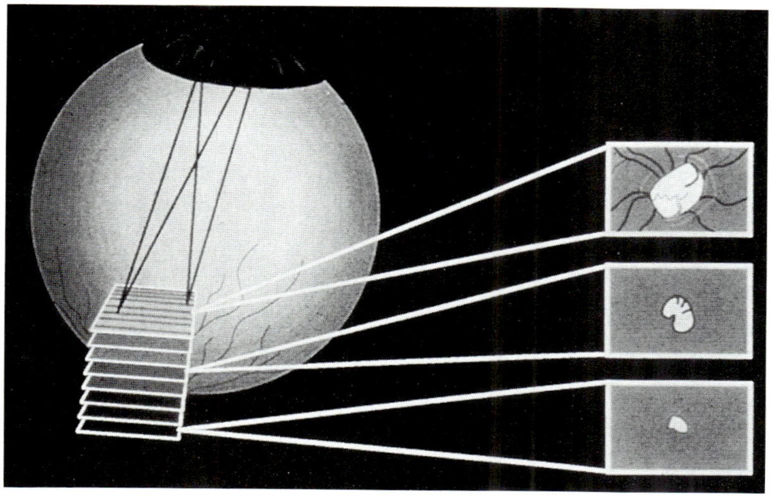

Figure 9.6. Schematic depiction of coronal planes of section taken by laser tomographic scanners. From Schuman JS, Noecker RJ: Imaging of the optic nerve and nerve fiber layer in glaucoma. Ophthalmol Clin North Am 1995;8: 259–279.

single scan is 25–40 μm (44,45). A series of three or more repeated scans may improve reproducibility (45). In comparison, the confocal laser scanning ophthalmoscopes have a variability of 100 μm in vivo (29). ONH analyzers can measure neuroretinal rim area and cupping and are able to provide good structural data (Fig. 9.7), but are unable to differentiate between normal and glaucomatous ONHs, and cannot be used to detect change over time. Because the axial resolution is only 300 μm (41), cross-sectional imaging of the fundus with confocal scanning laser ophthalmoscopes and tomographs is not feasible.

NERVE FIBER LAYER ANALYSIS

Evaluation of the optic nerve head has been the "gold standard" in the examination of eyes for glaucoma since the time of Hermann von Helmholtz. However, the optic nerve is a conglomeration of axons from all of the ganglion cells in the retina, together with structural and vasculature tissues. The goal for diagnosis of glaucoma and early detection of glaucomatous progression is to note the earliest abnormalities possible. Conventional techniques, such as examination of the optic nerve, stereoscopic ONH photography, and even the ONH analyzers and laser scanning ophthalmoscopes and tomographs described above, lack sufficient sensitivity and reproducibility to detect the earliest signs of glaucomatous damage or progression (1,2). As noted, nearly half of the axons in an eye must be lost before an abnormality is noted by conventional means, such as ONH cupping and visual field loss (3,4,46). Even a reduction in NFL thickness of 10–20 μm may be a significant sign of impending visual field loss (3). **It is ganglion cell death that produces visual loss in glaucoma, and the NFL and ONH are composed of the axons of these ganglion cells.** Because these axons are more readily evident, and less compacted, in the NFL, the newest technologies have focused on the quantitation of NFL thickness as a means by which to detect glaucomatous damage.

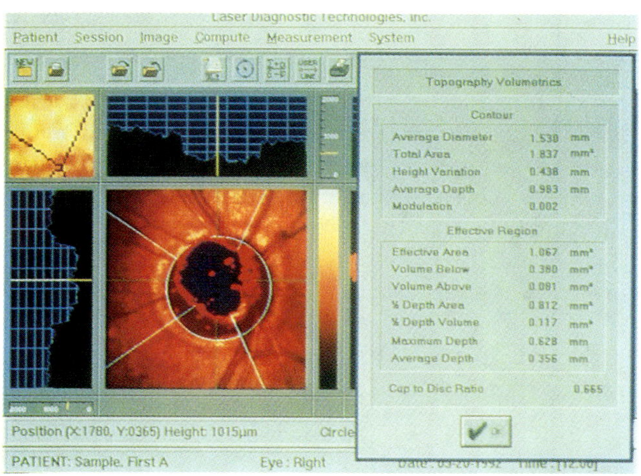

Figure 9.7. Display of TopSS, similar to HRT. Note the possibility for computer analysis of multiple ONH parameters. From Schuman JS, Noecker RJ: Imaging of the optic nerve and nerve fiber layer in glaucoma. Ophthalmol Clin North Am 1995;8:259–279.

Nerve fiber layer examination is difficult at best. Clinical examination of the NFL, using a red free light with an ophthalmoscope or slit lamp biomicroscope, is a subjective and qualitative process, as is NFL photography (2). Still, NFL defects can be the earliest sign of glaucomatous damage (47), and NFL defects can precede the development of visual field defects (48,49). The ONH analyzer described can be used to map peripapillary NFL contour, detecting depressions in areas of NFL loss, corresponding to cupping and visual field loss (24,50), but this technique depends on a stable floor from which to measure contour, and there is no reference plane in the retina which does not change over time.

The Nerve Fiber Analyzer

Attempts to quantitate NFL thickness with the scanning laser ophthalmoscopes described have been unsuccessful.

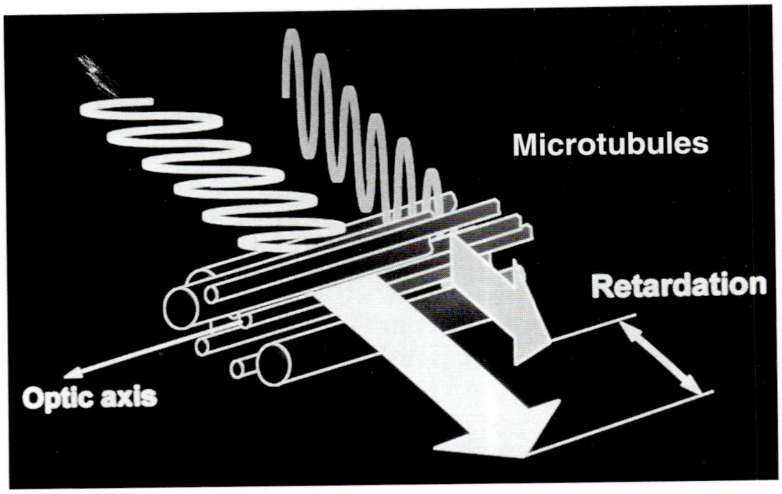

Figure 9.8. Graphic depiction of "retardance," the delay of polarized light by birefringent fibers. From Schuman JS, Noecker RJ: Imaging of the optic nerve and nerve fiber layer in glaucoma. Ophthalmol Clin North Am 1995;8:259–279.

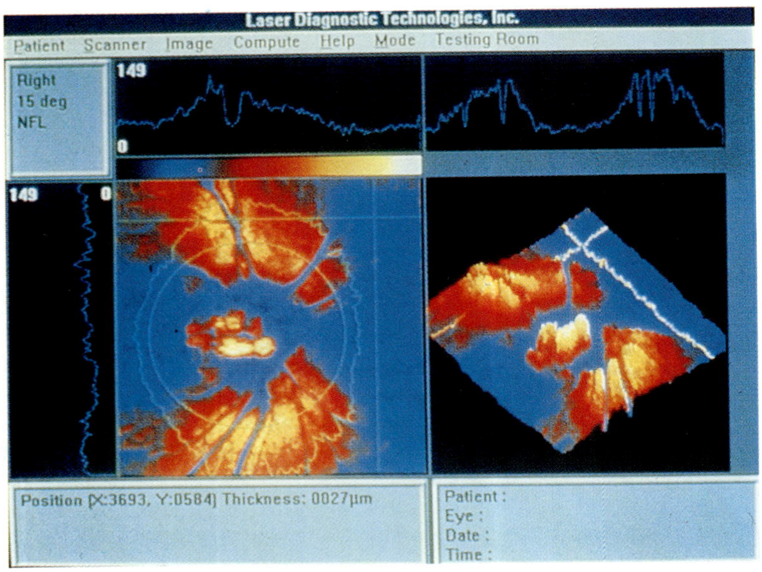

Figure 9.9. Display of NFA. Note thicker NFL superiorly and inferiorly. From Schuman JS, Noecker RJ: Imaging of the optic nerve and nerve fiber layer in glaucoma. Ophthalmol Clin North Am 1995;8:259–279.

The Nerve Fiber Analyzer (NFA, Laser Diagnostic Technologies, Inc., San Diego, CA) measures the rotation of polarized light reflected from the retina to determine NFL thickness, using the birefringence of the NFL to change the polarization (51). The NFL birefringence, similar to that found in Henle fibers, causes a change in polarization called "retardance" (Figs. 9.8, 9.9). The assumption used by the NFA is that the polarized light rotation is in proportion to NFL thickness, and this retardance is measured using Fourier ellipsometry (52–54).

Because the measurement depends on assumptions about the optical properties of the retina, and the eye as a whole, rather than a physical property of the device itself, the measurement of NFL thickness made by the NFA is indirect. The NFL collects light returning from all depths of the retina, and NFL thickness is determined from the polarization rotation of the reflected light. The assumptions are as follows: that the NFL is the main source of retinal birefringence, that most of the light is reflected from the outer retina, and therefore passes through the full thickness of the NFL, and that the birefringence of the NFL is homogeneous. Additionally, there may be other birefringent structures in the eye, such as the lens and cornea, and their effects on polarized light may change over time, independent of that of the NFL.

Preliminary in vitro studies show a positive correlation between NFA measurements and NFL thickness (54,55). However, preliminary in vivo work indicates difficulty in detecting areas of NFL thinning using the NFA (56). The resolution in vitro is approximately 13 μm (51).

Scanning Laser Ophthalmoscopes

Digital image processing can be used to enhance the contrast of the NFL using confocal scanning laser ophthalmos-

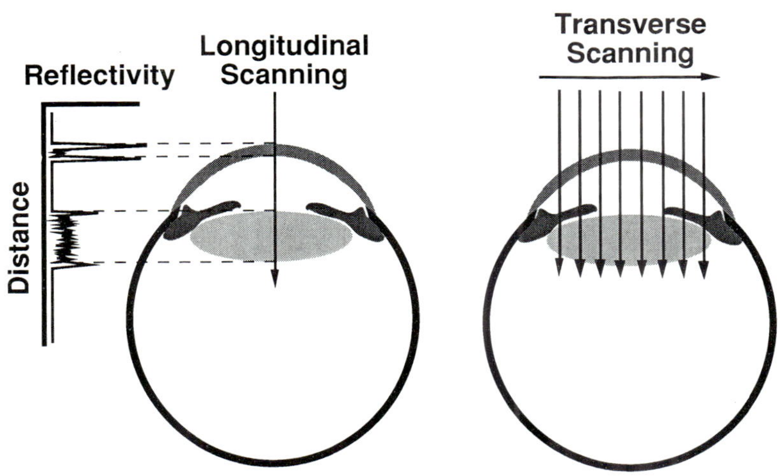

Figure 9.10. Analogous to ultrasound B-mode, cross-sectional tomographic images are created from a series of axial reflectance profiles obtained while scanning the probe beam across the tissue. From Schuman JS, Noecker RJ: Imaging of the optic nerve and nerve fiber layer in glaucoma. Ophthalmol Clin North Am 1995;8:259–279.

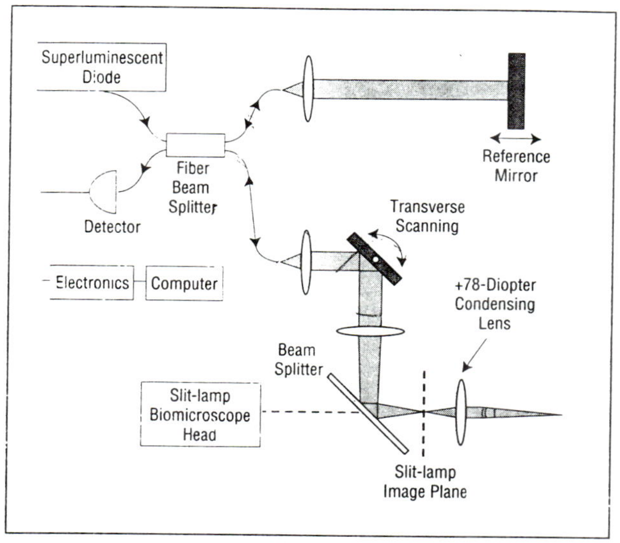

Figure 9.11. Schematic diagram of the high-speed, fiber-optic OCT scanner. Axial profiles of backscattering within biological tissue are measured by translating the reference mirror and recording the interferometric signal. The axial resolution is determined by the coherence length of the superluminescent diode (SLD) source and is 10 μm (FWHM) inside the eye. From Schuman JS, Hee MR, Puliafito CA, et al. Quantification of nerve fiber layer thickness in normal and glaucomatous eyes using optical coherence tomography: A pilot study. Arch Ophthalmol 1995;113: 586–596.

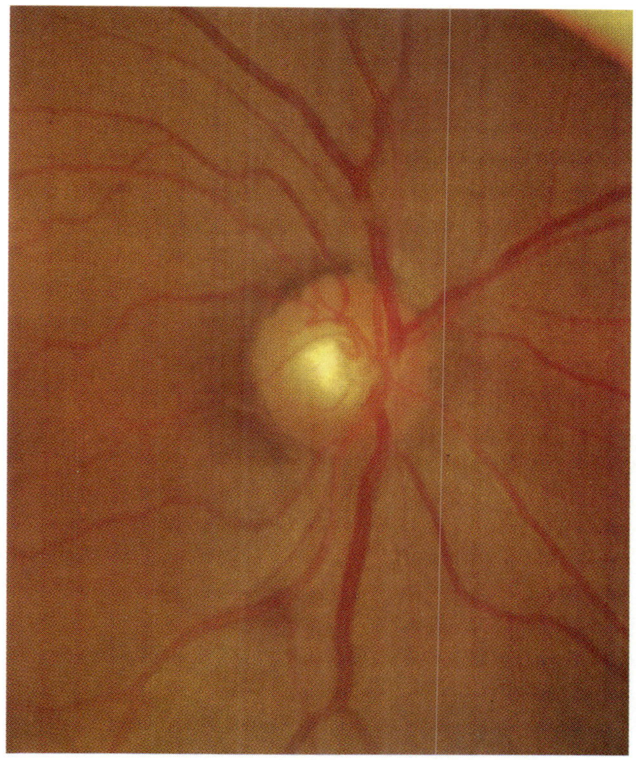

Figure 9.12. Stereo ONH photograph (Nidek 3Dx, Nidek Technologies, Inc., Pasadena, CA) from a normal eye. From Schuman JS, Hee MR, Puliafito CA, et al. Quantification of nerve fiber layer thickness in normal and glaucomatous eyes using optical coherence tomography: A pilot study. Arch Ophthalmol 1995;113:586–596.

copy (51,52). NFL striations can be seen with high lateral resolution and contrast, and as described above, this type of imaging is less dependent on pupil size and media clarity than conventional fundus photography. Birefringence is used in the imaging of the NFL by using simultaneously obtained images with orthogonal polarization (57).

Optical Coherence Tomography

Optical Coherence Tomography (OCT) is a new optical diagnostic technology that performs high resolution cross-sectional imaging utilizing low coherence light (58–67). It is a non-contact, noninvasive means for tomographic imaging of the ONH and NFL (59,61,62,65,67). Resolution with OCT is on the order of 10 μm, and reproducibility of measurements of NFL thickness is approximately 15 μm, near the theoretical limit of the device (59). Measurements of NFL thickness with OCT correlate with histological measurements of the same tissue (61).

Although OCT is a confocal imaging system, unlike the scanning laser ophthalmoscopes and tomographs described, it produces cross-sectional optical sections, rather than imaging in coronal planes; additionally, the optical sectioning capability is not limited by pupil aperture or ocular optical aberrations (33,40). It differs from the NFA in providing high resolution cross-sectional images of the retina from which the NFL may be viewed and quantitated directly (65).

OCT is analogous to B-mode ultrasound, except that it uses light instead of sound waves to create images with much higher resolution both axially and laterally (Fig. 9.10). Unlike ultrasound, OCT does not require contact with the eye or immersion in saline. Image contrast is dependent on differences in optical reflectivity rather than acoustic backscatter.

OCT is a low cost fiber-optic based interferometer which may be used for either anterior or posterior segment imaging (Fig. 9.11) (62,63,67). The cross-sectional information produced by OCT is derived from time of flight of reflected or backscattered light. High resolution is obtained by using a broad bandwidth, low coherence light source from a superluminescent diode coupled to a fiber-optic Michelson interferometer. Near-infrared light, 830-843 nm, is divided by a 50-50 beam-splitter to reference and sample arm paths, and both beams are reflected back to a detector. The reference mirror oscillates at 40 Hz, and only when the light reflected from the reference mirror and the optical path of the light reflected from the eye are within the coherence length of the light is a signal sensed at the detector. This limits the resolution to the coherence length of the source light, approximately 10-20 μm (61).

A single OCT probe produces a signal similar to an ultrasound A-scan, with an axial profile of reflectivity versus depth. By rapidly taking a series of scans, and interpolating between signals, a cross-sectional image of the retina is obtained. Axial resolution is determined by the coherence properties of the light source, and is independent of numerical aperture or quality of beam focus, unlike confocal scanning laser ophthalmoscopes and tomographs (61). As with these other systems, however, lateral resolution is dependent on the optical quality and entrance pupil of the eye (30).

OCT is delivered using a conventional slit-lamp biomicroscope via fiberoptic. Two galvanometrically driven mirrors translate the beam into any desired geometric pattern, typically a line or a circle. The beam is projected into the eye through a 78 D lens, and infrared videography replaces conventional viewing optics. This reduces light incident upon the retina, increases patient comfort, and decreases the need for pupillary dilation. The OCT beam is in the near infrared range, is not visible to the patient, and is well within safety standards.

A single OCT scan, consists of 100 to 200 axial scans that requires 2.5 seconds to acquire. Both the OCT and

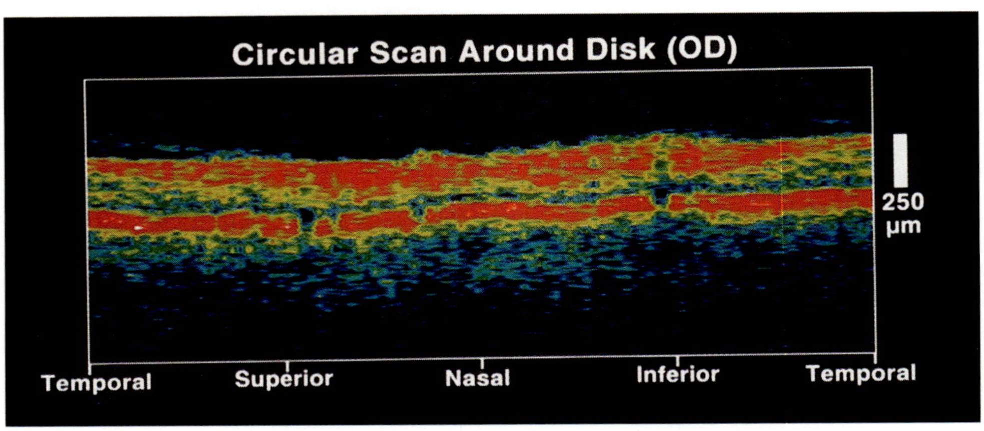

Figure 9.13. Circular OCT tomograph in normal eye (Fig. 9.12) taken in cylindrical section of tissue surrounding the optic nerve head, with scan at 3.37 mm diameter, centered on optic nerve head. The vertical scale has been expanded by a factor of three to accentuate axial depth information. Note thicker NFL, the anteriormost red reflection in the false color image, superiorly and inferiorly. A number of layers may be distinguished in the OCT, including the NFL, the inner and outer plexiform layers (yellow), the photoreceptor layer (dark on OCT), and a red reflection of the retinal pigment epithelium, choroid and sclera. From Schuman JS, Hee MR, Puliafito CA, et al. Quantification of nerve fiber layer thickness in normal and glaucomatous eyes using optical coherence tomography: A pilot study. Arch Ophthalmol 1995;113: 586–596.

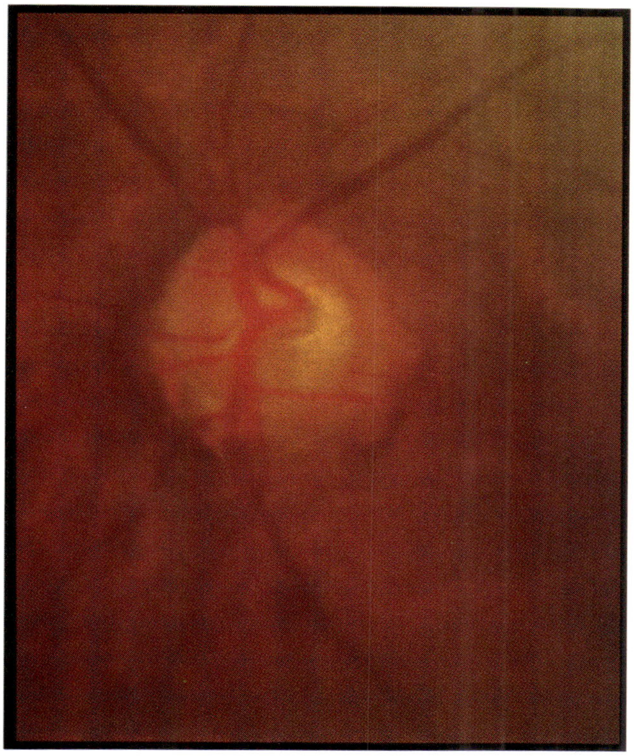

A

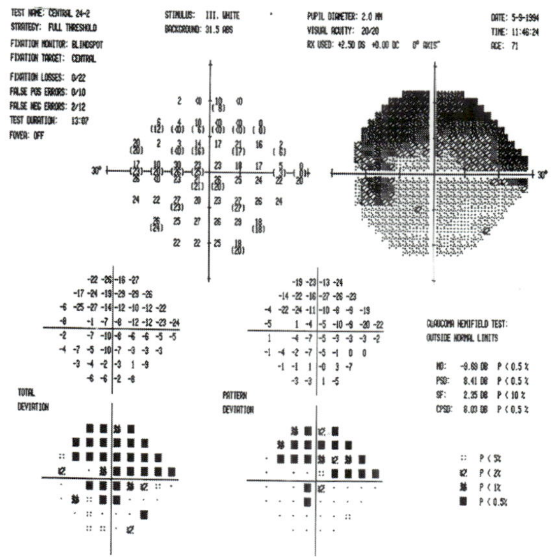

Circular Scan Around Disc (OS)

B

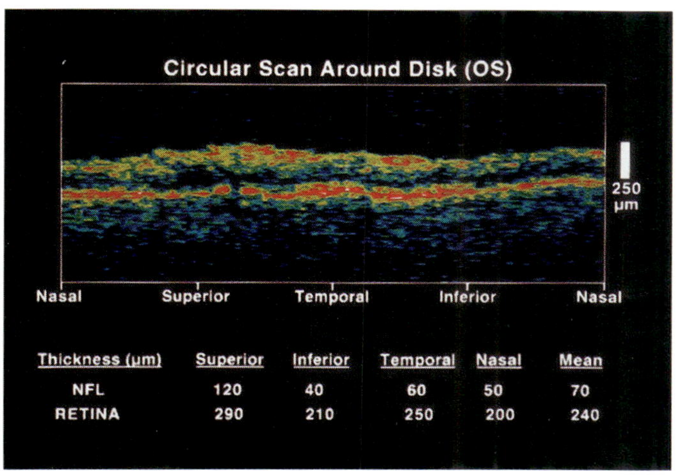

C

Figure 9.14. A. Stereo optic disc photograph of subject with glaucoma. Moderate to marked cupping of the optic nerve head is seen, particularly inferiorly. B. Humphrey 24-2 visual field. Subject has dense superior arcuate scotoma. C. OCT of same eye shown in Figure 9.14A. Note thinning of NFL inferiorly, corresponding to superior visual field loss. From Schuman JS, Hee MR, Puliafito CA, et al. Quantification of nerve fiber layer thickness in normal and glaucomatous eyes using optical coherence tomography: A pilot study. Arch Ophthalmol 1995;113:586–596.

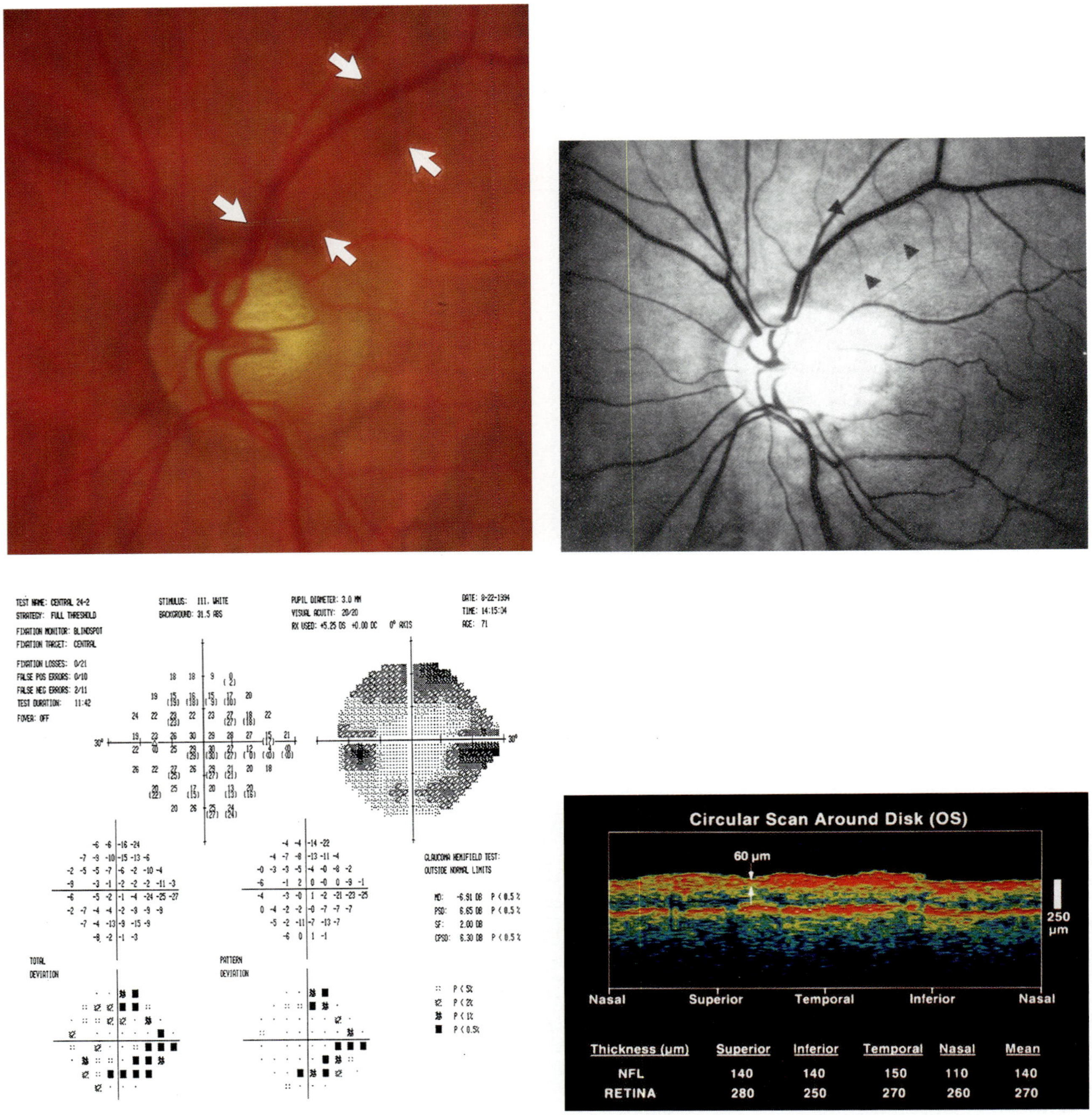

Figure 9.15. A. Stereo optic disc photograph of left eye of subject with a localized arcuate NFL defect superotemporally. B. Red-free NFL photograph demonstrates the localized arcuate NFL defect superotemporally (arrows). C. Humphrey 24-2 visual field shows an inferonasal step corresponding to superotemporal NFL defect. D. OCT illustrates NFL defect superotemporally in cross-section. Note especially thinning of the nerve fiber layer in the region of the defect from both above and below. From Schuman JS, Hee MR, Puliafito CA, et al. Quantification of nerve fiber layer thickness in normal and glaucomatous eyes using optical coherence tomography: A pilot study. Arch Ophthalmol 1995;113:586–596.

Table 9.1
Comparison of Features of Currently Available Optic Nerve Head and Nerve Fiber Layer Imaging Devices

Instrument	Target	Imaging Principle	Price ($)	Min Pupil Size (mm)	Measurement Time
IMAGEnet	ONH	Stereoscopic videographic imaging	79,000	7	2 seconds
Glaucomascope	ONH/NFL	Raster stereography	24,900	4.5	2 minutes
Retinal Tomograph	ONH/NFL	Confocal laser scanning	45,900	1	1.5 seconds
TopSS	ONH/NFL	Confocal laser scanning	From 34,500	1	0.9 seconds
Nerve Fiber Analyzer	NFL	Laser scanning polarimetry	54,000	1	0.7 seconds
Optical Coherence Tomography	NFL	Optical coherence	75,000	4	2.5 seconds

Instrument	Resolution	Reference plane?	Advantages	Disadvantages
	Lateral/Axial			
IMAGEnet	100/300μ	yes	Works with existing fundus camera	Pupil dilation, long processing times
Glaucomascope	50/300μ	yes	Relatively inexpensive	Long imaging times
Retinal Tomograph	20/300μ	yes	No dilation	Complicated software, uses reference plane
TopSS	20/300μ	yes	No dilation, easy software	Measures only optic nerve head topography and NFL height currently
Nerve Fiber Analyzer	20/13μ	no	High resolution of NFL measurement	Calculates NFL thickness using birefringence
Optical Coherence Tomography	20/10μ	no	Direct cross sectional imaging with highest resolution of NFL	

From Schuman JSS, Noecker RJ: Imaging of the optic nerve head and nerve fiber layer in glaucoma. Ophthalmol Clin North Am 1995;8:259-279.

infrared videography are displayed in real-time. The axial depth of the scan is typically 3 mm. Digital processing is used to remove artifacts due to subject motion. Quantitation of NFL thickness is automated, and displayed by quadrant, clock-hour, and as an overall mean (65). Manual measurements can be made as well.

Although OCT can be used for both anterior and posterior segment imaging, it is a powerful tool for quantitative evaluation of the NFL (Figs. 9.12, 9.13). OCT measurements correlate with visual field findings, demonstrating, for example, thinning of the NFL inferiorly in eyes with superior visual field defects (Fig. 9.14). Small, focal NFL defects can be detected with OCT (Fig. 9.15). OCT can demonstrate significantly thinner NFL in glaucomatous eyes as compared to normal eyes, particularly in the inferior quadrant (Fig. 9.16) (65). Glaucomatous progression can be seen by sequential OCT scans, both experimentally, in the glaucomatous monkey model, and in humans where the disease has progressed.

OCT is the first technology to reveal the NFL and retinal profile in cross-section. While there is still a great deal to be learned regarding the behavior of the NFL in both normal and glaucomatous eyes, OCT has demonstrated thinning of the NFL with normal aging, although there is no significant relationship between cupping of the ONH or neuroretinal rim area. OCT supports the contention that NFL thickness bears a closer relationship to glaucoma status and visual function than does the appearance of the ONH (65).

OCT offers the promise of an objective, quantitative measurement of NFL thickness. With the development of a normative database of NFL thickness stratified by age, OCT measurements of NFL thickness could aid in the early detection of the presence of glaucoma, perhaps prior to the development of visual field defects, and of glaucomatous progression, with minimal functional loss.

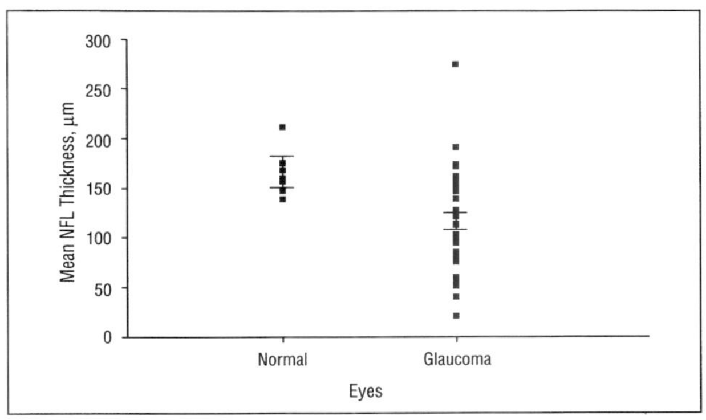

Figure 9.16. Mean inferior-quadrant nerve fiber layer (NFL) thickness in normal and glaucomatous eyes. Mean NFL thickness was 165.0 ± 16.2 microns in normal eyes (n = 7) and 125.7 ± 6.4 microns in glaucomatous eyes (n = 44) (P = 0.04). The inferior quadrant (the 4:30 to 7:30 positions) proved most sensitive to the difference in NFL thickness between normal and glaucomatous eyes. From Schuman JS, Hee MR, Puliafito CA, et al. Quantification of nerve fiber layer thickness in normal and glaucomatous eyes using optical coherence tomography: A pilot study. Arch Ophthalmol 1995;113:586–596.

CONCLUSIONS

We have come far since the earliest descriptions of the optic nerve nearly 150 years ago, yet our goal remains unchanged. Ophthalmologists strive to detect glaucoma at its initial stages, at the first possible sign of the disease, and to catch the just noticeable difference that occurs with glaucomatous progression. While clinical examination affords the assessment of the ONH and NFL qualitatively, technological advances have allowed the characterization of the ONH with higher precision than previously possible, and current instrumentation enables quantitative analysis of the NFL. These and future developments may let us ascertain the presence of glaucoma, and the progression of glaucomatous changes, before significant functional damage has occurred, enabling the earliest possible introduction of treatment to preserve sight and prevent visual loss.

References

1. Tielsch JM, Katz J, Quigley HA. Intraobserver and interobserver agreement in measurement of optic disc characteristics. Ophthalmology 1988; 95:350.
2. Lichter PR. Variability of expert observers in evaluating the optic disc. Trans Am Ophthalmol Soc 1976;74:532.
3. Quigley HA, Addicks EM, Green WR. Optic nerve damage in human glaucoma. Arch Ophthalmol 1982;100:135.
4. Quigley HA, Miller NR, George T. Clinical evaluation of nerve fiber layer atrophy as an indicator of glaucomatous optic nerve damage. Arch Ophthalmol 1980;98:1564-1571.
5. Helmholtz H. Beschreiburg eines Augenspiegels zur Untersuchung der Netzhaut in lebenden Augi. Berlin: A Forstner, 1851.
6. Von Graefe A. Ueber die Wirkug der Iridectomie bei Glaucom. Arch Ophthalmol 1857;3:456.
7. Schnabel I. Die Entwicklungsgeschichte der glaukomatosen Exkavation Z Augenheilkd. 1905;14:1.
8. Elliot RU. Treatise on Glaucoma. London: Henry Fraude and Hodder & Stroughton LTD, 1922:195–218.
9. Drance SM, Fairclugh M, Butler DM, et al. The importance of disc hemorrhage in the prognosis of chronic open angle glaucoma. Arch Ophthalmol 1977;95:226.
10. Takamoto T, Schwartz B. Reproducibility of photogrammetric optic disc cup measurements. Invest Ophthalmol Vis Sci 1985;26:814.
11. Varma R, Spaeth GL. The PAR IS 2000: A new system for retinal digital analysis. Ophthalmic Surg 1988;19:1183.
12. Dandona L, Quigley HA, Jampel HD. Reliability of optic nerve head topographic measurements with computerized image analysis. Am J Ophthalmol 1989;108:414.
13. Bishop KI, Werner EB, Krupin T, et al. Variability and reproducibility of optic disk topographic measurements with the Rodenstock Optic Nerve Head Analyzer. Am J Ophthalmol 1988;106:696.
14. Echelman DA, Shields MB. Optic nerve head imaging. In: Principles and practice of ophthalmology. DA Albert, FJ Jakobiec, eds. Philadelphia: W.B. Saunders, 1993.
15. Nicholl JE, Katz LJ, Steinmann WC, et al. Optic disk computerized analysis comparing three photographic techniques. Invest Ophthalmol Vis Sci 1989;30(Suppl):174.
16. Belyea DA, Dan JA, Lieberman MF, et al. The Glaucoma-scope: reproducibility and accuracy of results. Invest Ophthalmol Vis Sci 1994;(Suppl)35:429.
17. Hamzavis S, Stewart WC, Thompson TL. Inter-and intraobserver variation of the optic nerve head in cadaver eyes using the Glaucoma-scope. Invest Ophthalmol Vis Sci 1994;(Suppl)35:427.
18. Takamoto T, Netland PA, Schwartz B. Comparison of measurements of optic disc cup by glaucoma-scope and stereophotogrammetry. Invest Ophthalmol Vis Sci 1994;35(suppl):433.
19. Hoskins HD, Hetherington J, Glenday M, et al. Repeatability of the Glaucoma-scope measurements of optic nerve head topography. Glaucoma 1994;3:177–185.
20. Airaksinen PF, Drance SM, Schulzer M. Neuroretinal rim area in early glaucoma. Am J Ophthalmol 1985;l(99):1.
21. Balazsi GA, Drance SM, Schulzer M, et al. Neuroretinal rim area in suspected glaucoma and early chronic open-angle glaucoma. Arch Ophthalmol 1984;102:1011.
22. Caprioli J, Klingbeil U, Sears M, et al. Reproducibility of optic disc measurements with computerized analysis of stereoscopic video images. Arch Ophthalmol 1986;104:1035.
23. Caprioli J, Miller JM. Videographic measurements of optic nerve topography in glaucoma. Invest Ophthalmol Vis Sci 1988;29:1294.
24. Caprioli J, Ortiz-Colberg R, Miller JM, et al. Measurements of peripapillary nerve fiber layer contour in glaucoma. Am J Ophthalmol 1989; 108:404.
25. Mikelberg FS, Airaksinen PJ, Douglas GR, et al. The correlation between optic disk topography measured by the video-ophthalmograph (Rodenstock analyzer) and clinical measurement. Am J Ophthalmol 1985;100:417.
26. Shields MB, Martone JF, Shelton AR, et al. Reproducibility of topographic measurements with the optic nerve head analyzer. Am J Ophthalmol 1987;104:581.
27. Shields MB. The future of computerized image analysis in the management of glaucoma. Am J Ophthalmol 1989;108:319.
28. Shields MB, Tiedeman JS, Miller KN, et al. Accuracy of topographic measurements with the optic nerve head analyzer. Am J Ophthalmol 1989;107:273.
29. Cioffi GA, Robin AL, Eastman RD, et al. Confocal laser scanning ophthalmoscope. Reproducibility of optic nerve head topographic measurements with the confocal laser scanning ophthalmoscope. Ophthalmology 1993;100:57-62.
30. Webb RH. Scanning laser ophthalmoscope. In: Noninvasive diagnostic techniques in ophthalmology. BR Masters, ed. New York: Springer-Verlag, 1990:438–450.
31. Plesch A, Klingbeil U. Optical characteristics of a scanning laser ophthalmoscopy. SPIE Ophthalmic Imaging, San Diego, CA, 1980.
32. Plesch A, Klingbeil U, Rappl W, et al. Scanning ophthalmic imaging. In: Scanning laser ophthalmoscopy and tomography. JE Nasmann, ROW Burk, eds. Munchen: Quintessenz, 1990.
33. Webb RH, Hughes GW, Delori FC. Confocal scanning laser ophthalmoscope. Applied Optics 1987;26:1492.
34. Peli E. Electro-optic fundus imaging. Surv Ophthalmol 1989;34:113.
35. Kino GS, Corle TR. Confocal scanning optical microscopy. Physics Today 1989;42:55.
36. Masters BR, Kino GS. Confocal microscopy of the eye. In: Noninvasive diagnostic techniques in ophthalmology. BR Masters, ed. New York: Springer-Verlag, 1990:152–171.
37. Shuman H, Murray JM, DiLullo C. Confocal microscopy: An overview. Biol Techniques 1989;7:154.
38. Weinreb RN, Dreher AW, Bille JF. Quantitative assessment of the optic nerve head with the laser tomographic scanner. Int Ophthalmol 1989; 13:25–29.
39. Institute ANS. Safe use of lasers. New York: American National Standards Institute, 1986:34.
40. Bille J, Dreher G, Zinser G. Scanning laser tomography of the living human eye. In: Noninvasive diagnostic techniques in ophthalmology. BR Masters, ed. New York: Springer-Verlag, 1990:528–547.
41. Dreher AW, Tso PC, Weinreb RN. Reproducibility of topographic measurements of the normal and glaucomatous optic nerve head with the laser tomographic scanner. Am J Ophthalmol 1991;111:221.
42. Bartsch DU, Intaglietta M, Bille JF, et al. Confocal laser tomographic analysis of the retina in eyes with macular hole formation and other focal macular diseases. Am J Ophthalmol 1989;108:277.
43. Burk ROW, Rohrshneider K, Volcker HE, et al. Scanning laser tomogra-

phy. In: Scanning laser ophthalmoscopy and tomography. JE Nasmann, ROW Burk, eds. Munchen: Quintessenz, 1990.
44. Kruse FE, Burk RO, Volcker HE, et al. Reproducibility of topographic measurements of the optic nerve head with laser tomographic scanning. Ophthalmology 1989;96:1320–1324.
45. Weinreb RN, Lusky M, Bartsch DU, et al. Effect of repetitive imaging on topographic measurements of the optic nerve head. Arch Ophthalmol 1993;111(5):636-638.
46. Quigley HA, Addicks EM. Quantitative studies of retinal nerve fiber layer defects. Arch Ophthalmol 1982;100:807–814.
47. Hoyt WF, Newman NM. The earliest observable defect in glaucoma? Lancet 1972;1:692–693.
48. Sommer A, Miller NR, Pollack I, et al. The nerve fiber layer in the diagnosis of glaucoma. Arch Ophthalmol 1977;95:2149–2156.
49. Sommer A, Katz J, Quigley HA, et al. Clinically detectable nerve fiber atrophy preceded the onset of glaucomatous field loss. Arch Ophthalmol 1991;109:77.
50. Caprioli J. The contour of the juxtapapillary nerve fiber layer in glaucoma. Ophthalmology 1990;97:358.
51. Weinreb RN, Dreher AW, Coleman A, et al. Histopathologic validation of Fourier-ellipsometry measurements of retinal nerve fiber layer thickness. Arch Ophthalmol 1990;108:557.
52. Dreher AW, Reiter K, Weinreb RN. Spatially resolved birefringence of the retinal nerve fiber layer assessed with a retinal laser ellipsometer. Appl Optics 1992;31:3730–3735.
53. Dreher AW, Reiter K. Retinal laser ellipsometry: A new method for measuring the retinal nerve fiber layer thickness distribution? Clin Vision Sci 1992;7:481–488.
54. Dreher AW, Reiter K, Weinreb RN. Measurement of the circumpapillary nerve fiber layer thickness distribution by polarimetry. Invest Ophthalmol Vis Sci 1991;32(Suppl):811.
55. Reiter K, Dreher AW, Weinreb RN. Accuracy and reproducibility of a retinal laser ellipsometer. Invest Ophthalmol Vis Sci 1991;32(Suppl): 812.
56. Airaksinen PJ, Vihanninjoki K, Tuulonen A. Polarimetric measurements of the retinal nerve fiber layer in glaucoma. Ophthalmology 1994; 101(suppl):107.
57. Morsman CD, Karwatowski WSS, Weinreb RN. Reproducibility of retinal nerve fiber layer thickness measurements by scanning laser polarimetry and correlation with red free photography in normal eyes. Invest Ophthalmol Vis Sci 1993;34 (Suppl):1507.
58. Hee MR, Izatt JA, Swanson EA, et al. Optical coherence tomography for ophthalmic imaging. IEEE Engineer Med Biol 1995;14:67–75.
59. Hee MR, Izatt JA, Swanson EA, et al. Optical coherence tomography of the human retina. Arch Ophthalmol 1995;113:325–332.
60. Huang D, Stinson WG, Schuman JS, et al. High-resolution measurement of retinal thickness using optical coherence domain reflectometry. Invest Ophthalmol Vis Sci 1991;32 (Suppl):1019.
61. Huang D, Swanson EA, Lin CP. Optical coherence tomography. Science 1991;254:1178–1181.
62. Izatt JA, Hee MR, Huang D, et al Ophthalmic diagnostics using optical coherence tomography. Ophthalmic Technologies III, Ren Q, Pavel J-M, Eds., Proc SPIE, 1993:1877.
63. Izatt JA, Hee MR, Swanson EA et al. Micron-resolution imaging of the anterior eye with optical coherence tomography. Arch Ophthalmol 1994;112:1584–1589.
64. Puliafito CA, Hee MR, Lin CP et al. Imaging of Macular Diseases with Optical Coherence Tomography (OCT). Ophthalmology 1995;102: 217–229.
65. Schuman JS, Hee MR, Puliafito CA, et al. Quantification of nerve fiber layer thickness in normal and glaucomatous eyes using optical coherence tomography: A pilot study. Arch Ophthalmol 1995;113:586–596.
66. Swanson EA, Huang D, Hee MR, et al. High-speed optical coherence domain reflectometry. Opt Lett 1992;17:151–153.
67. Swanson EA, Izatt JA, Hee MR, et al. In vivo retinal imaging by optical coherence tomography. Opt Lett 1993;18:1864–1866.

Visual Fields and Their Relationship to the Optic Nerve

10

R. Rand Allingham

GENERAL CONSIDERATIONS

In glaucoma, we are concerned about the status and function of the optic nerve. If there was no optic nerve damage in glaucoma, it would cease to exist as a disease entity. Although in certain cases the need to treat urgently can be determined mainly on the basis of very high intraocular pressure, in most cases the character of both the optic disc and visual field are the major factors considered during management decisions. Therefore, to make the diagnosis of glaucoma, the appearance of the optic disc often provides us with essential information about the existence and course of the disease (Chapter 8). In addition to optic nerve appearance, it is highly useful to assess optic nerve function. Most commonly this is done by evaluating the visual field, although other methods are being investigated. Correlating the information obtained by careful examination of the optic nerve with its function is far superior to using either piece of information alone.

THE VISUAL FIELD

The Normal Visual Field

The visual field can be defined as that area of vision seen with eyes open. The dimensions of the field of vision are defined relative to fixation. The normal visual field extends approximately 60 nasal and superior, 70 inferior, and 90–100 temporal to fixation. The blind spot occupies the area defined by the optic nerve head and is typically located 15 temporal to fixation. It varies in size according to optic disc size and extent of peripapillary retino-choroidal atrophy.

Traquair described the visual field in three dimensions, describing it as "an island of vision surrounded by a sea of blindness." This important concept reflects the addition of retinal sensitivity to the two-dimensional area of visual field. The most sensitive region in the normal visual field is that relative to the fovea. The retinal sensitivity drops rapidly within 15 of the foveal peak. From this point there is a gradual reduction in retinal sensitivity which extends to the periphery where it abruptly drops off. In cross section the blindspot appears as a "well" with steep sides.

The size and contour of a visual field can be influenced by a multitude of factors in addition to glaucomatous or neuroophthalmic conditions that include facial structure, eyelid anatomy, pupil size, ocular media (corneal and lens status), refraction, testing artifact, as well as patient experience, reliability, and fatigue.

The Glaucomatous Visual Field

Glaucomatous optic nerve damage produces characteristic changes in the contour and shape of the visual field.

Generalized depression of the visual field is considered the most common change noted in glaucoma (1). However, this finding is non-specific and can be produced by a variety of conditions including cataract, corneal disease, fatigue, incorrect refractive correction, among others.

Nerve fiber bundle defects as a result of glaucomatous optic nerve damage produce visual field changes that are considered to be characteristic of glaucoma. These changes reflect retinal and optic nerve anatomy. Retinal nerve fibers radiate from the optic nerve head and are distributed in an arcuate manner around the foveal region (Fig. 10.1). **Therefore glaucomatous damage at the optic nerve head produces visual field defects in the region subserved by the affected nerve fibers.** The visual field defects produced from retinal nerve fiber bundle defects include localized paracentral scotomas, arcuate defects, nasal steps, and temporal defects (Fig. 10.2). The most common location of visual field defects occurs within an arcuate area commonly referred to as Bjerrum's area (or region) which includes that portion of the arcuate region that extends from the blind spot to the median raphe, where it extends 10-20 nasally from fixation (2).

Paracentral scotomas are discrete defects in the visual field caused by localized reduction in retinal sensitivity. These may be relative or absolute and are frequently found in Bjerrum's region (3). Initially, these may appear intermittently as one or more shallow depressions detected sporadically on repeat examination prior to developing into permanent visual field defects (4–6). **With progression, paracentral scotomas become deeper and larger and may gradually coalesce forming an arcuate or Bjerrum scotoma.**

A **nasal step** occurs when there is a difference in the rate or location of visual field loss above and below the horizontal raphe nasal to fixation. This produces a distinct

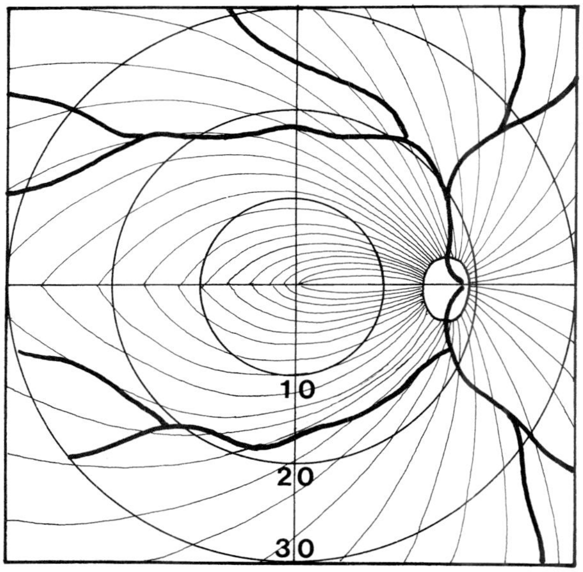

Fig. 10.1. Superotemperol and inferotemporal retinal nerve fibers follow an arcuate path around the fovea meeting at median raphe. Damage to this portion of the nerve fiber layer is responsible for arcuate field defects seen in glaucoma. Modified from Shields MB: Textbook of Glaucoma, 3rd ed. Baltimore: Williams & Wilkins, 1992.

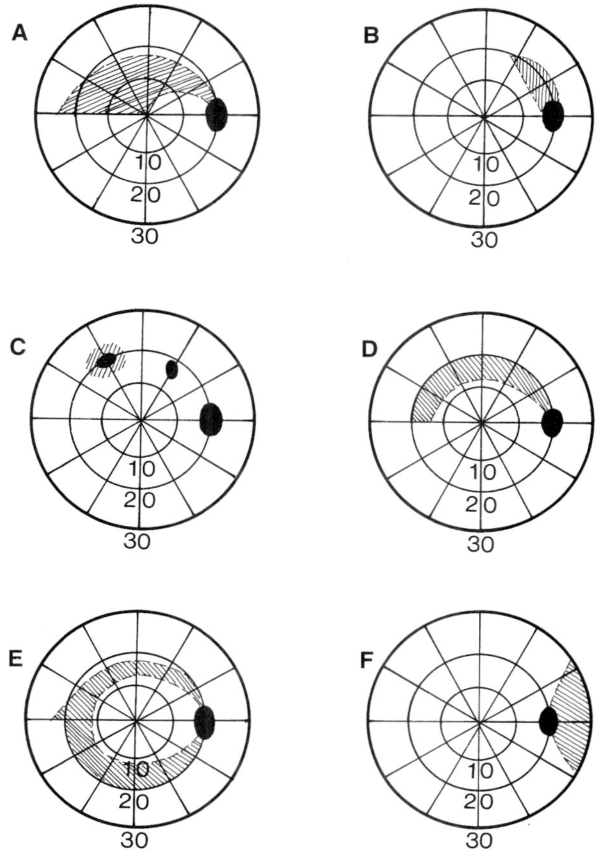

Fig. 10.2. Arcuate visual field defects. Bjerrum's region extends from the blind spot to the median raphe in an arcuate path which encompasses 10–20 degrees nasally from fixation (a). Seidel scotoma (b). Paracentral scotomas (c). Arcuate or Bjerrum scotoma (d). Double arcuate scotoma (e). Temporal wedge defects are produced by damage to the nasal neuroretinal rim and are not arcuate in nature (f). Modified from Shields MB: Textbook of Glaucoma, 3rd ed. Baltimore: Williams & Wilkins, 1992.

"step" which may occur along any, but not necessarily all isopters (7,8).

Temporal visual field defects are produced by damage to the nasal neuroretinal rim. Nerve fibers radiate without deviation from the nasal optic nerve; therefore, wedge defects develop. Temporal defects are usually found as a late manifestation of glaucomatous visual field loss (9).

METHODS OF PERIMETRY

Representation of the Visual Field

Typically the results of visual field testing are represented in two dimensions. The actual features of the field are determined by the method of testing.

Kinetic visual field testing is performed, as the name implies, with a moving test object. The object, usually a light of variable size and intensity projected on an evenly illuminated surface, is moved from a non-seeing area toward a seeing area. The location is recorded when the patient sees the object. The process is repeated until a boundary of seeing and non-seeing is determined. This boundary line is called an isopter (Fig. 10.3). Several isopters are usually obtained using test objects of different size and/or intensity.

Static visual field testing involves the use of non-moving test objects. Test objects are presented for a short period of time. A record of the patient response is then made (seen or not seen) at the specific location. A suprathreshold test employs test objects with an intensity which are higher than that normally seen at specific locations within the visual field. Threshold testing uses test objects of increasing or decreasing intensity at each location, which are used to determine the threshold stimulus, or that stimulus that is seen 50% of the time. The result is typically recorded as a symbol, numeric value, or graphically in greyscale (Fig. 10.4).

CONFRONTATIONAL VISUAL FIELDS

In a new case, a confrontation field should always be performed as a first step. A confrontation field can often be performed even with the most uncooperative patient in whom one can quickly demonstrate gross field defects. The confrontation field may be of great value and the only practical method for patients who have dense media opacities such as cataracts or corneal disease. It is also of considerable practical value in determining the location and approximate size of a small residual field in advanced glaucoma. In some cases a visual field has been recorded as a central island in patients in whom visual acuity was less than 6/60, due not to media opacity or macular change,

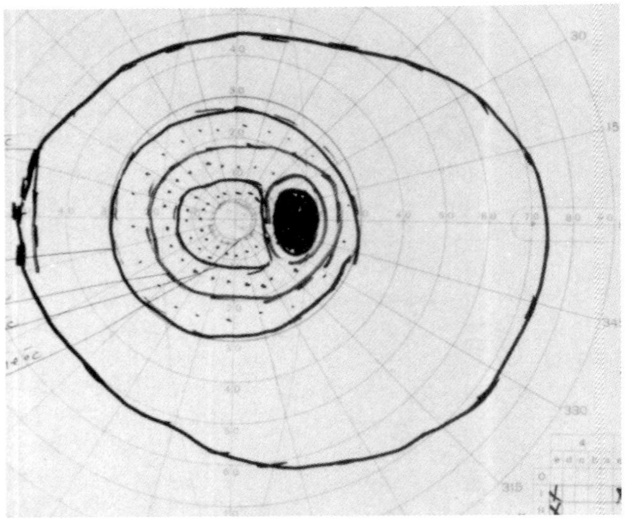

Fig. 10.3. Normal kinetic and static visual field (Courtesy of Mary Chiavelli).

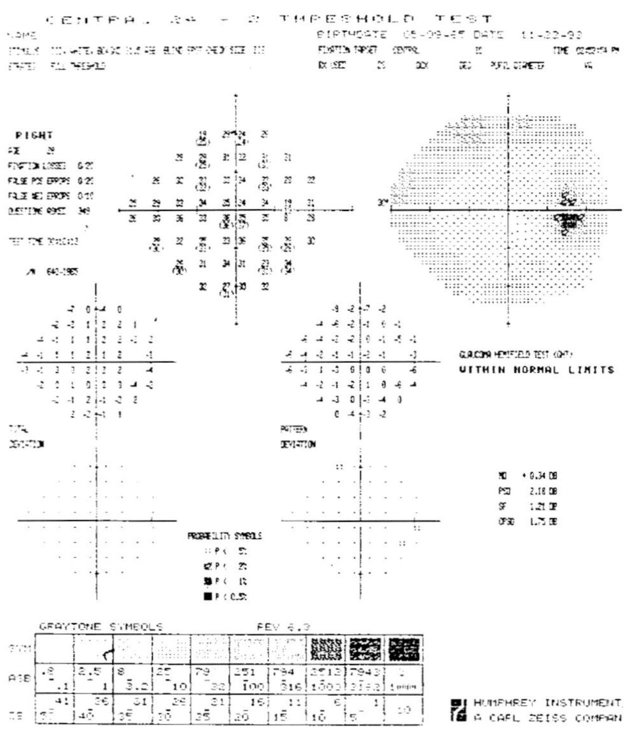

Fig. 10.4. Normal (static) automated full threshold visual field (Humphrey Field Analyzer, Central 24-2).

but to glaucoma itself. In these cases the true temporal location of the field defect has been quickly determined.

Manual Perimetry

Manual perimetry involves the use of a perimetrist, an individual skilled in the science (and art) of performing perimetry, and an instrument used by a perimetrist to perform and usually record the result. Several different instruments are available, although some are primarily of historical interest.

Tangent Screen

This device consists of an evenly illuminated flat black screen with a central fixation target mounted on a wall. The patient is seated facing the screen 1 or 2 meters away. The central 30 of the visual field can be tested using both kinetic and static methods employing test objects of different size or color.

Although infrequently used today, the tangent screen, when used in experienced hands can be an extremely valuable method to detect the relative size and location of visual field defects in glaucomatous and neuroophthalmic disorders. However, similar to confrontation fields, it is difficult if not impossible to detect small progressive changes in the visual field which is required in order to manage glaucoma.

Manual Bowl Perimetry

The prototype instrument used in some manner for most modern perimetry is the Goldmann perimeter. It consists of an evenly illuminated bowl (31.6 apostilbs) with a radius of approximately 300 mm. A chin rest supports the patient's head. A lens holder is used to provide correct refraction for central visual field testing.

The Goldmann perimeter is used to record the central and peripheral visual field by using an illuminated bowl and employing illuminated test objects of variable size, intensity, and transmission. This instrument can be used for kinetic and static perimetry.

The Harms or Tübingen perimeter is another manually operated bowl perimeter, which was designed for static perimetry. This perimeter can provide a representational static cut through the visual field at selected locations. It is no longer in common use.

Automated Perimetry

Because the results of manual perimetry can be heavily influenced by the skill of the perimetrist, a great deal of effort has been expended to reduce this variable by automating perimetry. Currently, a number of computer-driven automated instruments are available.

Most automated perimeters use static targets and employ suprathreshold and/or threshold strategies. Test targets can be projected onto the bowl or are integrally placed in the bowl as LEDs or with fiberoptics. Fixation can be monitored with a telescope, verified by periodically testing the blind spot, or by monitoring the corneal light reflex. Testing strategies are controlled by a computer, and the results are recorded on a computer printout.

Despite the implication that these units are "fully automated" there is still a critical need for skilled technical support before and during visual field testing with these units (Table 10.1). In addition to proper pupil dilation, refraction and positioning, patients require careful instruction regarding the process and rationale of the test. The importance of fixation throughout the test should be stressed. Simple encouragement can be very helpful for patients performing a test which is often protracted, tiring, and anxiety provoking. Ultimately, the usefulness of the test result is dependent on the manner in which the test was conducted.

Reliability indices help the clinician evaluate patient performance. Those indices most commonly used are short-term fluctuation, false positive responses, false negative responses, and fixation losses.

Short-term fluctuation represents intratest variability. During the test, several locations are re-tested and the differences in threshold values at these locations are determined. Short-term fluctuation is the square route of the variance obtained from the re-test values. Some short-term fluctuation is expected. However, when this value is abnormally high it may represent a lack of attention or reliability on the part of the patient, or may occur as a result of extensive visual field damage.

False positive errors occur when patients give a response when no target is presented (though a sound may be made by the machine). **False negative errors** occur when the patient fails to respond to a stimulus that is of greater intensity than one seen previously in the same location. False positives may result from "trigger happy" patients or those who are trying to "help" the test. The anxiety of "not seeing" stimuli that are infrathreshold can be substantial. Patients may feel that their condition may be getting worse. Reassuring the patient that it is normal not to see many of the targets can reduce this problem. False negatives may represent inattentiveness, a shift in head position, or may be a byproduct of searching for targets. Careful reinstruction often remedies this problem.

Fixation losses reduce reliability of visual field testing. Patients may alter fixation as a natural response to stimuli in the peripheral field, a desire to "help" the examiner, or in some cases, due to vision loss, the patient is unable to see the fixation target. Generally, careful instruction will remedy the first two. Some perimeters have a group of fixation targets surrounding central fixation, which help the patient center their gaze where loss of central vision is the primary problem. For patients who are unable to suppress their desire to look about, manual perimetry with constant observation by the perimetrist may be required.

Table 10.1
Common Causes of Visual Field Artifact

Source	Comment
Refractive error	Check refraction
Improper near correction	Always use full correction according to perimeter manual for patients with pseudophakia, aphakia, and after cycloplegia
Lid artifact	May need to gently elevate lid with tape
Lens rim artifact	Reposition patient or corrective lens
Fatigue or stress	Patient reassurance, rest between visual fields
Patient movement	Reposition patient

TESTING STRATEGIES AND PATTERNS

Automated perimeters present stimuli randomly within a fixed pattern. This eliminates the patient's ability to anticipate the location of the next stimulus and may help reduce fixation losses from this source. Stimulus intensity is adjusted to "fit" the visual field contour, which helps reduce testing time.

As stated previously, **suprathreshold testing** involves the use of stimuli which are of greater intensity than the presumed threshold at each location, thus suprathreshold. Some instruments present a second high intensity stimulus at locations where the first stimulus is not detected to

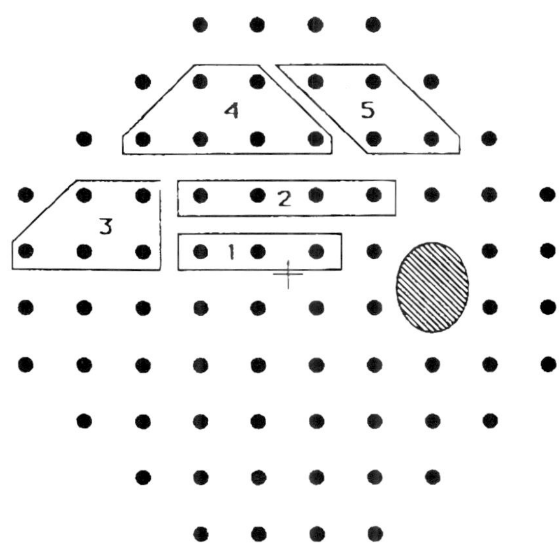

Fig. 10.5. Superior visual field zones used in the glaucoma hemifield test. Summated test scores (in decibels) within each zone are compared with the mirror zone below the horizontal meridian.

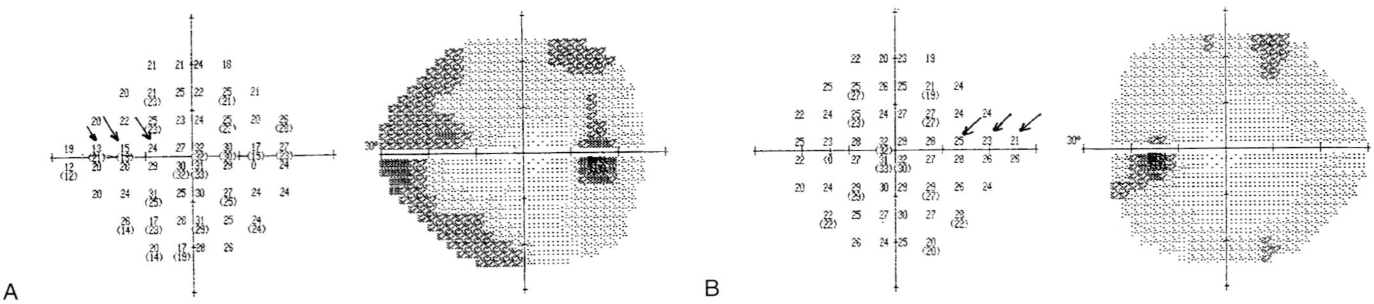

Fig. 10.6. Patient with inferotemporal optic nerve cupping from POAG. The right eye demonstrates an early scotoma superior to the nasal horizontal meridian (arrows) which was identified by the Glaucoma Hemifield Test (A). Interestingly, the left eye has what appears to be an early depression in the same region which was not identified by this computer strategy (B).

differentiate between relative and absolute visual field defects. Suprathreshold testing may be useful for glaucoma screening; however, this test strategy does not precisely delineate the depth of visual field abnormalities and is therefore not suitable for baseline or follow-up examinations.

In **threshold perimetry**, the patient's retinal threshold is determined at each test location. The visual field pattern typically consists of 70 or more test locations distributed within the central 24–30 . A stimulus is presented and increased or decreased till it crosses the patient's retinal threshold. The process may then be repeated using stimuli with smaller intensity increments to further define the threshold value measured in decibels.

Glaucoma hemifield testing has been introduced recently as an additional test strategy that incorporates the comparison of specified regions of the visual field above and below the horizontal midline (Fig. 10.5). This approach has a high degree of specificity and sensitivity when compared with other test strategies (10–12). Regardless of whether this specific test strategy is present in the automated visual field unit in use, the clinician can use this concept when evaluating whether a visual field may demonstrate early damage (Fig. 10.6).

BLUE-ON-YELLOW PERIMETRY

The loss of short wavelength sensitivity is greater in glaucomatous than normal eyes (13–15). This has led to the development of perimetry using a blue stimulus on a yellow background (blue-on-yellow). In comparisons between standard white-on-white with blue-on-yellow perimetry, visual field defects are identified earlier and appear to be larger with blue-on-yellow perimetry (16–19). The development of hardware and software for widespread use of blue-on-yellow perimetry in the office setting is progressing rapidly. The ability to perform quantitative analysis of blue-on-yellow perimetry using a large population database for reference is being developed (16).

CORRELATING THE OPTIC NERVE WITH THE VISUAL FIELD

Change in the optic disc from glaucoma often predates change in the visual field (20–22). Additionally, the location of the abnormality of the optic disc typically correlates with abnormality of the visual field.

In most patients in whom glaucomatous changes in the optic disc develop, the physiologic cup enlarges to reach the disc margin downward and temporally. This is a definite glaucomatous change; but at first the cup becomes shelved rather than excavated. A visual field defect may not be present at this early stage. As the cup becomes deeper at the inferior disc margin a real excavation becomes evident which may then produce a superior visual field defect (see Fig. 8.10).

Similarly, in other cases, the physiologic cup may enlarge superiorly. As the disease progresses, the cup comes closer to the superior disc margin and becomes excavated. At this stage, although the cup still does not quite reach the upper outer margin, there is usually a lower field defect—a lower Bjerrum scotoma, or a lower nasal step, or both (Fig. 10.7).

The cup may enlarge toward both the upper and lower borders simultaneously. It is in this type of glaucomatous change that we eventually find both an upper and lower Bjerrum scotoma, isolating a central island of vision, varying in size from patient to patient, with variable degree of loss in the peripheral field (see Fig. 8.20).

Eventually, the excavation may reach the margin above as well as below, and the disc may become totally cupped to all margins. In these cases, the central visual field may be lost or consist of a small central island. Usually the nasal neuroretinal rim clings on to the last leaving only a temporal island of vision. Ultimately, in the absence of effective intervention, all vision is lost.

We believe a valuable axiom is that in ordinary eyes (not those which are highly myopic) there can be no field defects due to glaucoma if the disc appearance is normal, unless the IOP is high at the time of the exami-

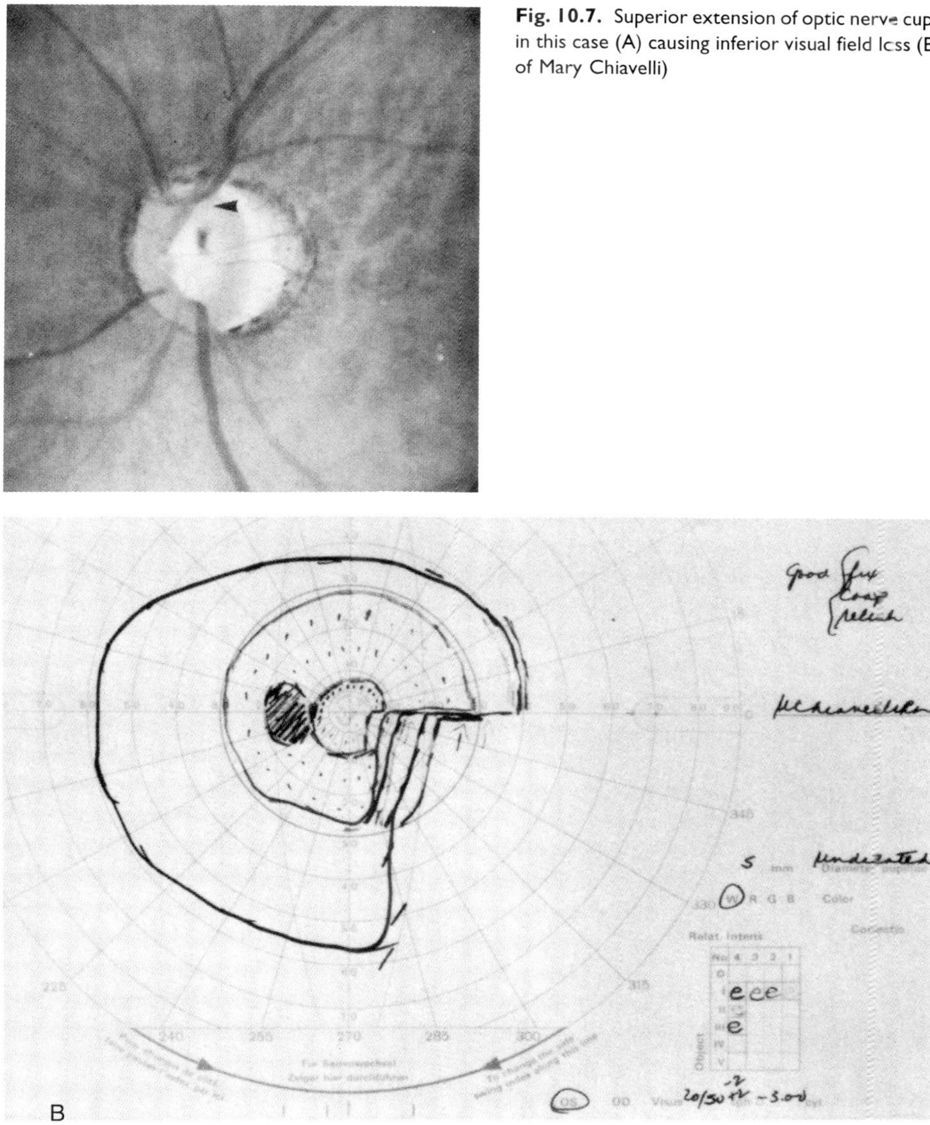

A

B

Fig. 10.7. Superior extension of optic nerve cupping (arrow) in this case (A) causing inferior visual field loss (B). (Courtesy of Mary Chiavelli)

nation or has been high a short time previously. If the IOP is elevated at the time of examination, glaucomatous field defects may be found. Such defects may reverse if the IOP is promptly reduced to normal. If such field defects are permanent, then within a few weeks, evidence of optic atrophy usually becomes evident.

In cases in which glaucoma-like visual field defects occur where the IOP and the disc appear completely normal another explanation should be sought out. We have seen many patients who had glaucoma and were alleged to be losing field or who had lost field despite good IOP control where the appearance of the optic nerve did not correlate with the field defect. In the vast majority of cases these inconsistencies were explained by the presence of optic nerve head drusen, retinal vascular occlusions, chorioretinal lesions, retinal degeneration, retinal detachment, retinoschisis or neurologic disorders such as brain tumors, stroke, or head trauma (Fig. 10.8) (Table 10.2).

ADVANCED VISUAL FIELD LOSS

Central and Temporal Islands

Patients who have a central island of vision remaining often require more frequent assessment of their visual field. Additionally, the intact portion of the patient's visual field may represent only a small portion of that which is being tested. If automated perimetry is being used, **assessing only the central 10 degrees with a finer grid pattern can improve resolution of the remaining visual field** and reduce test time (Fig. 10.9).

Where there is little or no remaining central vision but a temporal island remains, Goldmann perimetry may be

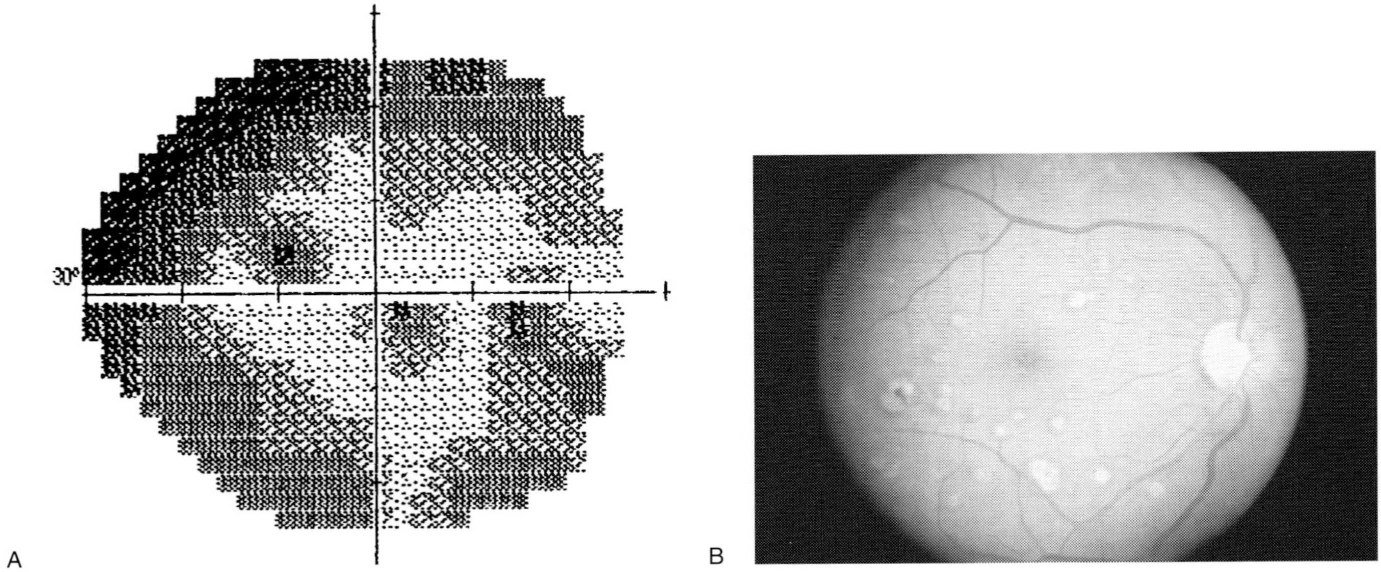

Fig. 10.8. Patient with ocular hypertension whose visual field loss (A) is explained by previous laser treatment for diabetic retinopathy (B).

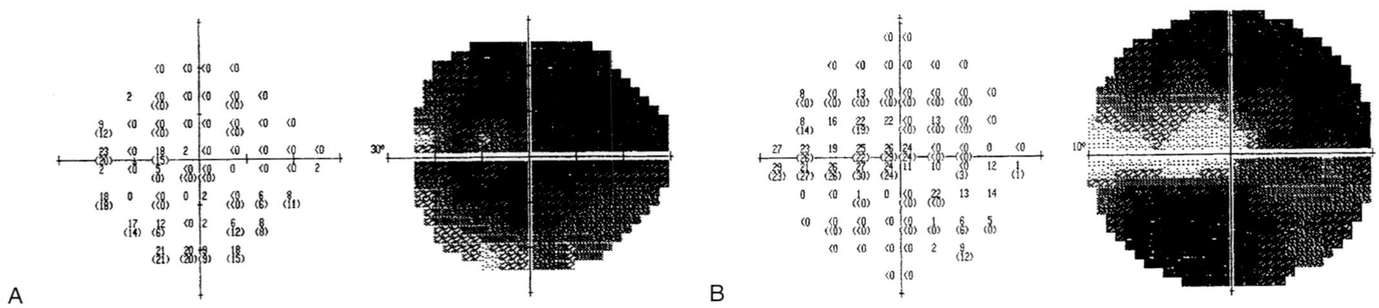

Fig. 10.9. Patient with 20-20 visual acuity and severe optic nerve damage OS. The automated full threshold central 24 visual field is virtually extinguished (A). The finer grid pattern of the central 10 visual field (B) increases definition of the small remaining central island, reduces test time, and is easier to follow for progression.

Table 10.2
Causes of Glaucoma-like Visual Field Defects

Chorioretinal lesions
Chorioretinal scars
Retinal vascular occlusions
Retinal detachment
Retinoschisis
Myelinization of NFL
Status post retinal laser treatment
Optic nerve head lesions
Optic nerve head drusen
Optic nerve coloboma or pit
Chronic papilledema
Anterior ischemic optic neuropathy
Lesions posterior to optic nerve head
Chiasmal lesions (e.g. pituitary adenoma)
Optic foramen or peri-sellar tumor (e.g. meningioma)
Cerebrovascular disease

used to follow the residual visual field. Where the central field is severely depressed but not completely lost a larger target size, for example size V, can be substituted for the standard target size (III).

FREQUENCY OF VISUAL FIELD TESTING

The baseline visual field will, in most cases, be referred to for comparison after each subsequent visual field. Due to a well described "learning curve," initial visual field tests should not be relied on as baseline examinations. Two or more examinations may be required before visual field test results are consistent, reliable, and can be used for future reference. These tests should be spaced within a few months of each other to promote the learning process. As stated above, glaucoma patient follow up should only employ quantitative threshold rather than suprathreshold testing; the latter strategy does not quantitate defects and is only suitable for screening purposes.

In patients who require periodic visual field assessment testing may be repeated in weeks, months, or years depending on specific clinical circumstances. In cases where IOP, optic nerve status, and visual fields have been stable for years (e.g., glaucoma suspects) annual or even biannual visual field assessment may suffice (ophthalmic examinations may be required more often).

In most cases in which IOP is well controlled, visual fields should be repeated every 9 to 15 months. However, when an interim change is detected in a visual field, a repeat examination should be performed within weeks or months to confirm the findings. Since intertest (long-term) fluctuation is common, **it is wise not to undertake a major therapeutic intervention based on a single examination.**

Relatively frequent visual field assessment (e.g., every 2-4 months) may be required in cases where there is advanced visual field loss. In these situations surgical intervention may be considered for small degrees of progressive visual field loss.

PROGRESSION OF VISUAL FIELD LOSS

Determining whether visual fields are stable or, in fact, whether progressive visual field loss has occurred can be challenging. A multitude of factors should be considered before one can conclude that visual field loss is glaucomatous (23).

The process of comparing visual fields is best done in a methodical manner. Comparison of new fields should be made to a reliable and stable baseline examination along with a representative sample (preferably all) of the intervening visual fields. **A common error is to compare visual fields to only those obtained most recently since they are often the most readily located in the medical record.** In this manner, small changes can easily be explained away as "long-term fluctuation" and the recognition of significant visual field loss may go unnoticed for long periods of time. It is best to have all visual fields for each eye placed sequentially in one location in the chart for easier reference and comparison.

It is important to consider visual field reliability, pupil size, the perimetrist's comments regarding patient performance, and other factors for each examination. Discard early pre-baseline and unreliable visual fields.

The most common patterns of field loss should be considered. Not only is the superior hemifield the region most likely to demonstrate early visual field loss, but it is also the region where loss is most rapidly progressive (24,25). For this reason, one should be cautious about explaining the cause of superior visual field loss as a "droopy eyelid." More often than not field loss remains confined to one hemifield for extended periods of time (26,27). Additionally, **areas of existing damage are far more likely to demonstrate progressive loss, either by scotomatous enlargement or deepening, than undamaged areas** (27). Therefore, it is useful to examine these areas more carefully when examining a series of visual fields.

It is difficult if not counterproductive to give specific decibel "cut offs" for progression vs long-term fluctuation when examining intertest changes. The more eccentric the test location from fixation, the greater the long-term fluctuation (28). Additionally, progression may have occurred if two or more test locations are depressed versus a single point, especially if these are within or adjacent to a region of previous field loss.

Finally, if new visual field loss is suspected, it is necessary to repeat the visual field examination and perform a corroborative optic nerve and fundus evaluation before reaching a firm conclusion or recommending a change in therapy.

References

1. Anctil JL, Anderson DR. Early foveal involvement and generalized depression of the visual field in glaucoma. Arch Ophthal 1984;102:363.
2. Harrington DO. The Bjerrum scotoma. Am J Ophthal 1965;59:646.
3. Hart WM, Becker B. The onset and evolution of glaucomatous visual field defects. Ophthalmology 1982;89:268.
4. Harrington DO. The pathogenesis of the glaucomatous visual field. Am J Ophthalmol 1958;47:177.
5. Drance SM. The early field defect in glaucoma. Invest Ophthalmol 1969; 8:84.
6. Werner EB, Drance SM. Early visual field disturbances in glaucoma. Arch Ophthalmol 1977;95:1173.
7. LaBlanc RP, Becker B. Peripheral nasal field defects. Am J Ophthal 1971;72:415.
8. Drance SM. The glaucomatous visual field. Br J Ophthal 1972;56:186.
9. Brais P, Drance SM. The temporal field in chronic simple glaucoma. Arch Ophthalmol 1976;88:518.
10. Asman P, Heijl A. Glaucoma Hemifield test. Automated visual field evaluation. Arch Ophthalmol 1992;110:812–819.
11. Asman P, Heijl A. Evaluation of methods for automated hemifield analysis in perimetry. Arch Ophthalmol 1992;110:820-826.
12. Asman P. Computer-assisted interpretation of visual fields in glaucoma. Acta Ophthalmol Suppl 1992;(206):1-47.
13. Drance SM, Lakowski R, Schulzer M, et al. Acquired color vision changes in glaucoma: use of 100 Hue Test and Pickford anomaloscope as predictors of glaucomatous field change. Arch Ophthalmol 1981;99:829–831.
14. Adams AJ, Rodie R, Husted R, et al. Spectral sensitivity and color discrimination changes in glaucoma and glaucoma-suspects. Invest Ophthalmol Vis Sci 1982;23:516–524.
15. Sample PA, Weinreb RN, Boynton RM. Acquired dyschromatopsia in glaucoma. Surv Ophthalmol 1986;31:54–64.
16. Johnson CA, Adams AJ, Casson EJ, et al. Progression of early glaucomatous visual field loss as detected by blue-on-yellow and standard white-on-white automated perimetry. Arch Ophthalmol 1993;111:651–656.
17. Sample PA, Weinreb RN. Progressive color visual field loss in glaucoma. Invest Ophthalmol Vis Sci 1992;33:2068–2071.
18. Sample PA, Taylor JD, Martinez GA, et al. Short-wavelength color visual fields in glaucoma suspects at risk. Am J Ophthalmol 1993;115: 225–233.
19. Johnson CA, Adams AJ, Casson EJ, et al. Blue-on-yellow perimetry can predict the development of glaucomatous visual field loss. Arch Ophthalmol 1993;111:645–650.
20. Zeyen TG, Caprioli J. Progression of disc and field damage in early glaucoma. Arch Ophthalmol 1993;111:62–65.
21. Pederson JE, Anderson DR. The mode of progressive disc cupping in

ocular hypertension and glaucoma. Arch Ophthalmol 1980;98: 490–495.
22. Odberg T, Riise D. Early diagnosis of glaucoma: the value of successive stereophotography of the optic disc. Acta Ophthalmol 1985;63: 257–263.
23. Zulauf M, Caprioli J. What constitutes progression of glaucomatous visual field defects? Sem Ophthalmol 1992;7:130–146.
24. Heijl A, Lundqvist L. The location of earliest glaucomatous visual field defects documented by automated perimetry. Doc Ophthalmol Proc Series 1983;35:153–158.
25. O'Brien C, Schwartz B. the visual field in chronic open angle glaucoma: The rate of change in different regions of the field. Eye 1990;4:557–562.
26. Hart WM, Becker B. The onset and evolution of glaucomatous visual field defects. Am J Ophthalmol 1989;89:268–279.
27. Mikelberg FS, Drance SM. The mode of progression of visual fields in glaucoma. Am J Ophthalmol 1983;98:443–445.
28. Heijl A, Lindgren G, Olsson J. Normal variability of static perimetric threshold values across the central visual field. Arch Ophthalmol 1987; 105:1544–1549.

The Visual Evoked Response (VER) in Glaucoma

11

Mark C. Kuperwaser

RATIONALE

The visual evoked response (VER) is a measurement of the electrical activity of the visual cortex in response to a visual stimulus. The measurement is made by applying one or more pairs of electrodes to certain areas of the scalp and using signal amplification and recovery techniques to extract the tiny portion of electroencephalographic activity, which bears a temporal relationship to the visual stimulus presented—hence the visual evoked response. **The VER signal represents summated electrical activity arriving to the visual cortex from the anterior visual pathways.** Measuring from the anatomic midline in a normal individual the contributions to the VER signal from either eye should be equal. If, in the absence of other neural pathway disease or lesions, an individual is tested one eye at a time (partner eye occluded), then the VER can be used as a means of comparing electrical conduction activity of the two optic nerves. One would expect, for example, that an optic nerve that had suffered loss of axons as a result of glaucomatous atrophy would yield a smaller or possibly delayed VER response when compared with a healthier partner nerve (1). The VER can thus be used as an objective means of assessing and longitudinally following optic nerve function in glaucoma.

PRACTICAL CONSIDERATIONS

Generating the VER

Visual evoked responses are produced by two types of visual stimuli: unpatterned bright flashes of light (strobe lamp), or reversal of high-contrast checkerboard patterns of various sizes (computer-driven video monitor). Each stimulus type has certain practical advantages (Fig. 11.1).

The flash VER represents electrical activity in response to a net change in overall luminance striking the retina and does not depend too much on precise optical focus. It can be used as a means of assessing optic nerve function in the presence of media opacity such as cataract. The flash VER suffers from a wide variation in morphology between normal individuals which limits its usefulness in establishing population based norms. One can, however, make valid interocular comparisons and longitudinal comparisons in one individual using the flash VER.

The pattern VER generates electrical activity by stimulating anatomically organized receptor fields of the retina (excitatory "on" centers, inhibitory "off" surrounds) and in the process of reversing the checkerboard pattern stimulates ganglion cells, which are attuned to these receptor fields without changing the overall luminance striking the retina. This obviously requires a well-focused image upon the retina but offers the advantage of a more uniform morphology in the generated signal which allows interindividual comparisons of VERs and the establishment of population based norms.

Analyzing the VER

Different signal processing techniques can be used to analyze VER responses. Individual VER responses to infrequent stimuli are called "transient" responses and differ in character from the "steady state" VER response obtained to a constantly repeating stimulus.

The transient VER is obtained by spacing the stimuli far enough apart so that an individual VER response is generated, sampled for its entire duration, and allowed to extinguish before re-stimulating. Typically the electrical response is sampled for a period of 250 msec after a stimulus and stimuli are spaced 400 msec apart to allow for total extinction of the signal between stimuli. Multiple transient responses are averaged together yielding a relatively well-defined VER waveform in the time domain which represents an average of approximately 100 samples obtained at a rate of about 2 per second which takes about 1 minute. Conventional signal averaging generates an easily interpreted real-time VER waveform; however, the technique is limited to low stimulus rates that may not be sensitive to early disease pathology.

If one shortens the inter-stimulus interval and advances the stimulus rate to much higher temporal frequencies, the individual VER responses blend into a sort of oscillatory waveform which reflects the rate of stimulus repetition. This is the steady state VER for a given stimulus frequency. A variety of different frequencies can be tested and the amplitude and phase lag of the VER response plotted as a function of stimulus frequency. This results in a frequency-domain

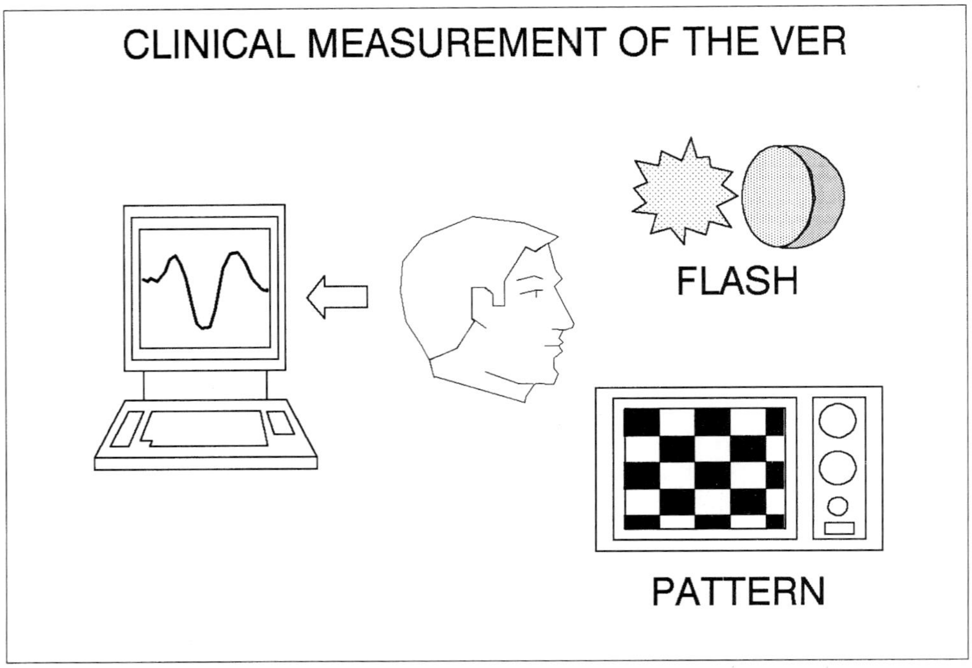

Figure 11.1. The VER is produced by two types of visual stimuli, unpatterned bright flashes of light (flash) or the reversal of a high contrast checkerboard pattern (pattern).

plot (Fourier analysis), which while not as intuitively simple to interpret, does free one from the constraint of low frequency testing. This type of technique has yielded increased sensitivity to glaucomatous changes in the VER (2).

A novel third approach that combines the benefits of transient signal averaging (easily interpreted time-domain waveform) and steady-state Fourier analysis (ability to test at higher temporal frequencies) is the use of randomly timed stimuli and cross-correlation signal analysis. This technique is under investigation (3).

Regardless of the method of signal analysis, it is useful to establish each test trial at about 1 minute so that total testing session, which would include a number of different types of stimuli for each eye, should not exceed about 10 to 15 minutes. The amount of patient cooperation required is small, namely the ability to keep the appropriate eye open and to fixate the stimulus for about one minute at a time. It is helpful to have an alert patient. There are fewer subjective judgement artefacts than in a comparable conventional perimetry test. The VER thus emerges as a potentially powerful objective correlate of optic nerve function and progression in glaucoma.

PHYSIOLOGIC CORRELATES OF THE VER IN GLAUCOMA

Ganglion Cell Characterization

Research spanning over 50 years has resulted in identification of multiple subtypes of vertebrate retinal ganglion cells (4,5). Functional and anatomic studies have characterized these different types of ganglion cells and there is experimental evidence that some types of ganglion cells may be more susceptible to injury resulting from diseases such as glaucoma. In the human visual pathway two complementary systems are believed to exist—a color-opponency system and a "broad-band" or rapidly conducting system (6).

The **parvocellular system** appears to have evolved for detailed visual analysis with a trade-off of speed. The ganglion cells serving this visual system have small receptor fields, form part of a color discrimination system, respond well to high-contrast stimuli and conduct relatively slowly. The ganglion cells serving this system constitute a majority of the total human retinal ganglion cell population.

The **magnocellular system** appears to function as a "re-direction" system for the parvocellular system. Many of its ganglion cells are concentrated in the region of the arcuate bundles (near-periphery), the cells have large receptor fields, very little color discrimination activity, respond to minimal changes in contrast and conduct rapidly. In contrast to the parvocellular system this is a system capable of responding rapidly to changes in the visual environment but with trade-off in detail. The ganglion cells serving this system constitute a relative minority of the total human retinal ganglion cell population. Additionally, this subpopulation of ganglion cells may be more vulnerable to injury in a number of diseases including glaucoma.

Models for M-Cell (Magnocellular) Dysfunction in Glaucoma

Quigley and coworkers were able to demonstrate that in an animal model of glaucoma there is apparently selective loss of larger-diameter fibers in the earlier stages of the disease (7). Whether this is due to mechanical fragility of these larger fibers or an inherent vulnerability of the magnocellular type of ganglion cell, which is associated with this fiber is not fully clear. In subsequent work Quigley demonstrated that larger pores in the lamina cribrosa of monkeys occur near the superior and inferior poles of the optic disc and thus loss of the larger-diameter fibers that presumably are associated with the magnocellular system would correlate with patterns of vertical disc cupping which are observed clinically (8).

Psychophysical studies of changes in visual function in ocular hypertension and early glaucoma tend to support the notion of selective early damage to the magnocellular system in that depressed flicker-fusion frequency, loss of contrast sensitivity at low spatial frequencies, and loss of yellow-blue discrimination are all features attributed to the magnocellular system. While it would be overly simplistic to assume a strict paradigm of clinical progression in glaucomatous visual loss, an understanding of the function of the parvocellular and magnocellular systems helps to explain a number of observed phenomena.

Topographic Interpretation of the Human VER

The strongest component of the VER signal in humans is measured from a point just above the inion overlying the cortical representations of the retinal maculas (central fixation). The majority of visual input to the human cortex arises in the macula (Fig. 11.2). By convention, the negative electrode is situated over this area and the strong resultant negative deflection in the VER occuring at about 100 msec post-stimulus is called the P-100 and is believed to be an electrical correlate of macular function represented in the visual cortex.

Areas of the parafixational near-peripheral visual field are represented more anteriorly along the calcarine fissure in the human cortex. These areas contain some of the terminations of the rapidly conducting magnocellular fibers whose ganglion cells are located in the arcuate bundles. These areas, particularly for the inferior visual field, lie closer to the positive scalp electrode situated over the vertex and thus would be expected to contribute to a positive component in the VER. Given the rapid conduction of the magnocellular fibers, it would therefore be reasonable to associate magnocellular function from the near-peripheral visual field with the N-75 component of the VER, a positive-going deflection that precedes the P-100 (9,10).

The following two cases demonstrate the types of changes one might expect to see in the VER in the presence of two somewhat different patterns of glaucomatous optic atrophy, one in which the arcuate bundle region is predominantly affected, another in which visual field loss extends into the macular area as well.

Case 11-1. A 74-year-old white man with chronic open angle glaucoma, initially worse in the left eye, subsequently well-controlled on medications. The left eye has also undergone laser trabeculoplasty. Vision is 20/20 either eye with intraocular pressures of 15 right, 11 left. Discs are asymmetric with an enlarged cup on the left and inferotemporal thinning of the neural rim. The visual field from the right eye is full, the left eye showing a proximal arcuate (Seidel)

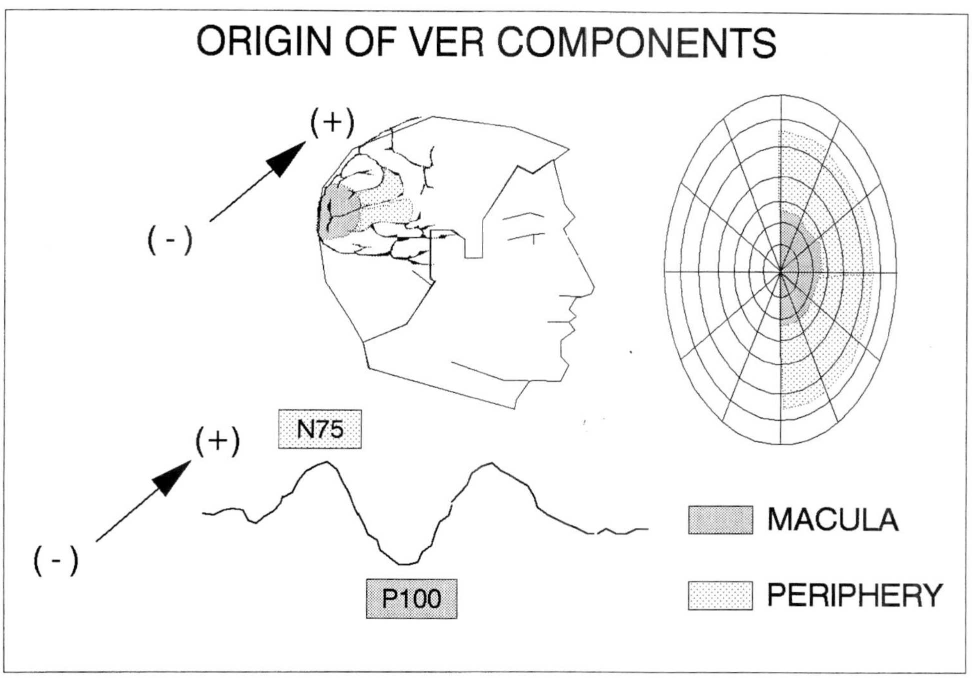

Figure 11.2. The N-75 component of the VER is believed to be associated with magnocellular function, whereas the P-100 component of the VER is thought to correlate with macular function.

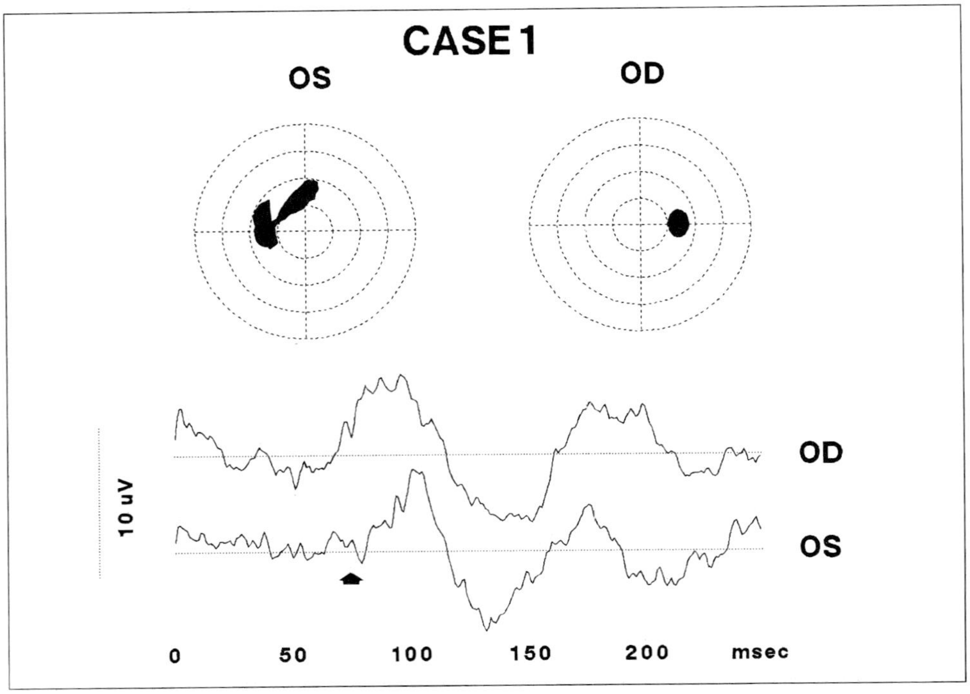

Figure 11.3. Case 11-1. Early central visual field loss OS is associated with a relative depression of the N-75 component of the flash VER OS (arrow).

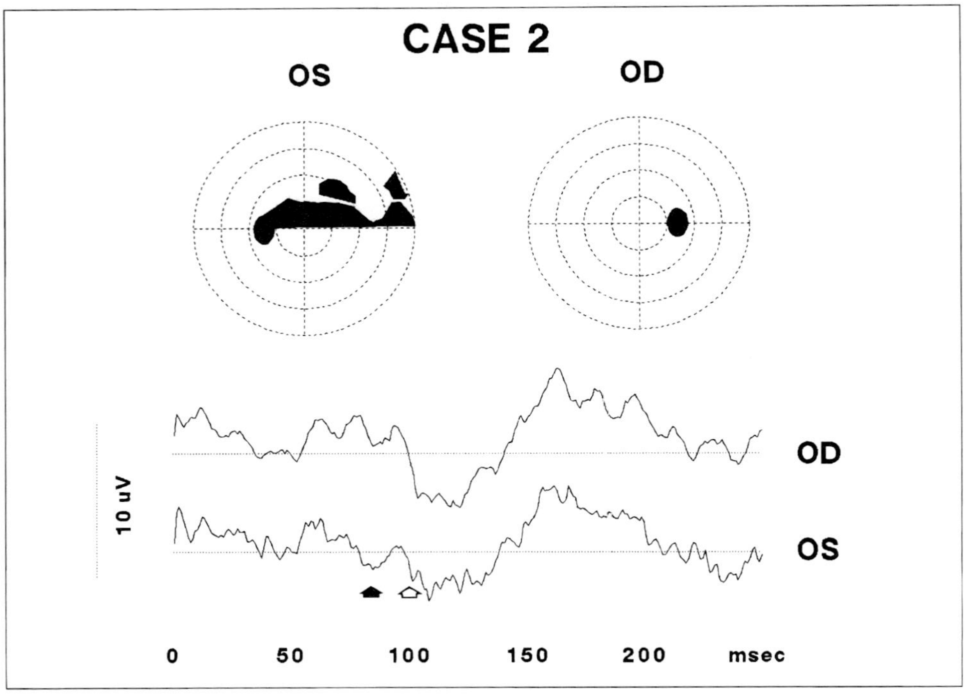

Figure 11.4. Case 11-2. A patient with more advanced visual field loss OS demonstrates reduction of both the N-75 (solid arrow) and the P-100 (open arrow) amplitude of the flash VER OS.

scotoma, indicative of damage to the proximal arcuate fibers (Fig. 11.3).

The flash VERs shown suggest a slightly smaller overall response from the left eye. Comparison of the area under the N-75 (early positive) portions shows a relative loss of energy for the left eye compared to the right—a finding we might expect if there has been loss of rapidly-conducting fibres mapping to the anterior portions of the cortex from the left eye. Though the shape of the P-100 (central troughs) differs for the two eyes the areas are roughly equal.

It is not surprising that there is only a relatively moderate difference in the VERs from the two eyes given the fact that the glaucomatous process in the left eye has been halted at a stage where there is only a limited defect in the visual field, implying focal extinction of a bundle of inferior arcuate fibers.

Case 11-2. A 61-year-old white man with chronic open angle glaucoma, worse in the left eye, subsequently well controlled. The right eye is on topical medications and has had laser trabeculoplasty, the left eye has undergone filtration. Vision is 20/20 right, 20/30 left with intraocular pressures of 21 right, 9 left. Discs are asymmetric with a significantly enlarged cup on the left and inferotemporal thinning extending around to the temporal margin. The visual field from the right eye is full; the left eye shows an arcuate scotoma which remains close to the horizontal meridian and bisects fixation (Fig. 11.4).

The flash VERs again show a relative loss of amplitude for the left eye compared with the right. In this instance both the N-75 (early positive peak) and the P-100 (central troughs) are attenuated in the left eye suggesting a pattern of nerve fiber loss in which not only fibers mapping to the anterior cortex but fibers mapping to the posterior (macular) pole of the cortex have been affected in the left eye.

This case, in comparison with the previous one, reinforces the notion that topographic mapping of visual field defects is reflected in selected components of the VER waveform.

CONCLUSION

Clinical Application of the VER in Glaucoma

The VER has been used in clinical glaucoma studies for well over a decade. Different stimulus parameters and analysis techniques have been investigated (11–15). These have been cross-sectional studies in which subjects have been characterized as 1) normal, 2) pre-glaucomatous ocular hypertensive, 3) known glaucoma. The ability of the VER to identify each of these groups has been reported. Depending on the particular method used to analyze the VER the ability to detect glaucomatous damage (sensitivity) and to exclude age-matched normals (selectivity) has approached 90%. Many studies show a range of 30 to 50% abnormal VERs in the ocular hypertensive population. The significance of this as a possible predictor of ocular hypertensives at high-risk for progression to glaucoma was reported in one study. In the group of ocular hypertensive exhibiting an abnormal VER, 30% developed field loss in 5 years, whereas individuals in the same group with normal VERs did not develop field loss in the 5-year interval (16). This suggests a possible predictive/screening role for VER testing in ocular hypertension.

Directions for Future Work

The possibility of an objective electrophysiologic test of visual function in glaucoma to characterize and follow disease progression as well as the possibility of a predictive screening test to identify high-risk ocular hypertensives motivates the continued investigation of the VER in glaucoma. A large number of case reports and limited studies exist; however, validation and acceptance of this method will depend on large-scale longitudinal studies in which the merits of this method are judged in comparison to existing diagnostic tests. As we better understand the various visual function changes in early glaucoma, a plethora of diagnostic tests emerges; however, electrophysiologic tests remain unique in that they are largely independent of subjective judgment. The complex technology initially required for electrophysiologic work has tended to relegate this diagnostic modality to laboratory investigation; however, the availability of cheaper, more-sophisticated, and accessable instrumentation for clinical electrophysiology will give this modality the popular acceptance necessary to carry out large-scale clinical studies. As confidence in the use of VERs grows, this test could potentially emerge as a valuable tool in the diagnosis of glaucoma (17).

References

1. Johnson M, Drum B, Quigley H, et al. Pattern-evoked potentials and optic nerve fibre loss in monocular laser-induced glaucoma. Invest Ophthal Vis Sci 1989;30:897.
2. Schmeisser E, Smith T. High-frequency flicker visual evoked potential losses in glaucoma. Ophthalmology 1989;96:621.
3. Fricker S, Sanders J. Clinical studies of the evoked response to rapid random flash. Electroenceph Clin Neurol 1974;36:525.
4. Hartline H. The response of single optic nerve fibres of the vertebrate eye to illumination of the retina. Am J Physiol 1938;121:400.
5. Berson E. Electrical phenomena in the retina. In: Moses R, Hart W, ed. Adler's Physiology of the Eye. C.V. Mosby Company, 1987.
6. Kaplan E. The role of P and M systems: Introductory remarks. In: Kulikowski J, Dickinson C, Murray I, eds. Seeing Contour and Colour. Pergamon Press, 1989.
7. Quigley H, Sanchez R, Dunkelberger G, et al. Chronic glaucoma selectively damages large optic nerve fibers. Invest Ophthal Vis Sci 1987; 28:913.
8. Quigley H, Addicks E. Regional differences in the structure of the lamina cribrosa and their relation to glaucomatous optic nerve damage. Arch Ophthalmol 1981;99:137.
9. Abe H, Iwata K. Checkerboard pattern reversal VER in the assessment of glaucomatous field defects. Acta Soc Ophthalmol Jpn 1976;80:127.
10. Cappin J, Nissim S. Visual evoked responses in the assessment of field defects in glaucoma. Arch Ophthalmol 1975;93:9.
11. Towle V, Moskowitz A, Sokol S, et al. The visual evoked potential in glaucoma and ocular hypertension: effects of check size, field size, and stimulation rate. Invest Ophthal Vis Sci 1983;24:175.
12. Atkin A, Bodis-Wollner I, Podos S, et al. Flicker threshold and pattern VER latency in ocular hypertension and glaucoma. Invest Ophthal Vis Sci 1983;24:1524.
13. Follman P, Kerenyi A, Vitrai J, et al. Assessment of optic nerve function by visual evoked potential recordings in the diagnosis of glaucoma. Doc Ophthal Proc Series 1984;40:265.
14. Howe J, Mitchell K. Visual evoked cortical potentials to paracentral retinal stimulation in chronic glaucoma, ocular hypertension, and an age-matched group of normals. Documenta Ophthalmologica 1986;63: 37.
15. Good P, Marsters J, Mortimer M. Flash stimulation evoked potentials in diagnosis of chronic glaucoma. Lancet 1987;1:1259.
16. Bray L, Mitchell K, Howe J. Prognostic significance of the pattern visual evoked potential in ocular hypertension. Br J Ophthalmol 1991;75:79.
17. Kass M. Foreward. Surv Ophthalmol 1989;33 Suppl:287.

Medications Used in Glaucoma Therapy II

Medications Used in Chronic Glaucoma Therapy

12

Adrenergic Agents: Blockers and Agonists

David L. Epstein

BETA BLOCKERS

Topical beta blockers decrease aqueous humor formation (1,2) and are used long term in the therapy of the chronic open angle glaucomas, and short term for various acute glaucomas. The introduction of the beta blockers about two decades ago was greeted with overwhelming enthusiasm not only because of their remarkable efficacy but because of the apparent infrequency of ocular side effects. Before the beta blockers, the only topical antiglaucoma medications available were the miotics and epinephrine-like compounds, the potential side effects from which will be discussed. In practice, the potential ocular side effects from these latter agents resulted in an appropriate hesitancy for clinicians to treat elevated IOP, even if substantial, unless there was obvious end organ damage (optic nerve), or abnormalities in (pre-automated perimetry) visual fields. The occurrence of these side effects also adversely affected patient compliance when aggressive therapy was required for advanced glaucomatous damage.

In the ensuing years, we have continued to observe that ocular side effects from the topical beta blockers are not common, and, in fact, potential long-term adverse effects of reduced aqueous humor flow on intraocular structural integrity, which some had predicted, have not occurred. However, we have become increasingly aware of the possibility of significant systemic side effects (3) from topical beta blockers, even in patients with no known systemic predisposition. In fact, systemic side effects are the major limitation to the use of topical beta blocker therapy.

Although there likely is some absorption through conjunctival blood vessels, a major site for systemic absorption of topical drugs seems to be the nasal mucosa. We therefore frequently instruct patients to perform punctal occlusion (4) for a few minutes after eye drop administration: the eye(s) are closed and the index finger(s) exert firm pressure over the (lower) punctum (punctae), conceptually thus preventing egress of excess medication in the tear film into the nasal mucosa via the occluded punctum, (Fig. 12.1). Alternatively, gentle eyelid closure for several minutes by itself without punctal occlusion (without peeping) has been reported by Zimmerman (5) to be just as effective as punctal occlusion and likely more "patient friendly".

Punctal occlusion or gentle eyelid closure is effective in some but not all patients, especially those with mild or moderate symptoms. But it is not a panacea, and one of us (DLE) has been disappointed in its efficacy in patients with advanced systemic symptoms, which most often requires discontinuation of the medication.

These **systemic symptoms from topical ocular beta blockers can be serious and even life threatening.** The most common of these symptoms are those of systemic beta blockage involving respiratory and cardiac function. The ophthalmologist needs to be alert for symptoms of bronchospasm and bradycardia. Frequently, the patient is either unaware of, or misinterprets the cause of these symptoms, attributing it to primary systemic disease. The diagnosis of a presumed systemic condition is often made by the general physician for the first time only after the patient has been placed on topical beta blockers. We have not made an effective enough effort of informing our family medicine and internal medicine colleagues about the occurrence of these systemic symptoms resulting from topical ocular medication.

It is very important to **listen to the patient breathing at the time of slit lamp examination**; patients will commonly not call symptoms of dyspnea to the attention of their ophthalmologist (because they do not associate eye drops with systemic problems), and often may not themselves be fully cognizant that "their breathing has been a little worse lately," since the topical beta blocker therapy was initiated.

Routinely check the pulse rate and blood pressure of patients receiving ocular beta blocker therapy. Patients are often unaware of bradycardia, which may not be fully symptomatic until a threshold level (that occurs subsequently) is passed.

Topical beta blockers can potentially worsen heart failure in patients by the beta-one blocking activity depressing myocardial contractility. This can also produce hypotension. Very uncommonly, patients with no apparent heart

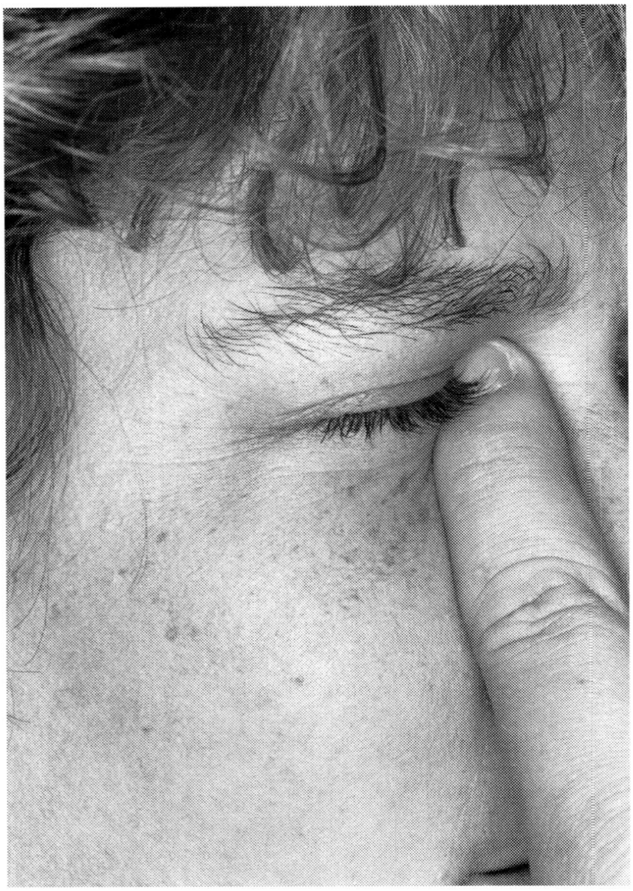

Figure 12.1. Technique of punctal occlusion. Finger is placed over the lower punctum and gentle pressure applied with eyelids closed. Pressure is removed and eyes opened after 5 minutes.

failure symptoms (but likely pre-existing maximally compensated heart function) can develop heart failure for the first time as a result of topical beta blocker therapy.

Some patients receiving topical ocular beta blockers report fatigue, which may not be due to bradycardia or heart failure, but rather might have a central (nervous system) origin. Symptoms of fatigue and depression can occur with systemic beta blocker therapy (6) and seem to represent a real potential side effect from topical beta blockers as well. Such symptoms of general fatigue and depression seem to respond better to punctal occlusion or gentle eyelid closure than those of bradycardia or bronchospasm, the latter two of which, it again needs to be stressed, can be life threatening and require discontinuation of the drug.

The true majority of glaucoma patients treated with topical beta blockers do not develop any systemic side effects, and this class of therapy has been a remarkable advance in our armentarium. But the ophthalmologist needs to be vigilant for the possible occurrence of such systemic symptoms, even in patients with no known predisposition. It is this latter group that has sensitized us all to the potential systemic hazard of this form of glaucoma therapy, because the occurrence of these serious systemic symptoms has been so unexpected but also so frequently undetected or misdiagnosed. There is no "free lunch" for either the patient with glaucoma or for us as glaucoma clinicians, and unfortunately all of our therapies have benefit/risk considerations. We have not yet developed the "magic bullet" for either the trabecular meshwork or optic nerve in glaucoma (Chapter 16), but when we do, such therapy will likely also entail benefit/risk considerations.

Other uncommon systemic side effects such as sexual dysfunction (7) and rarely Raynaud's disease-type symptoms have occasionally been attributed to topical ocular beta blocker therapy (as well as to systemic beta blocker therapy). Also, punctal occlusion or gentle eyelid closure may be effective in preventing these side effects.

Rarely reported side effects, include hypoglycemic symptoms (8) in diabetic patients, masking of symptoms of thyrotoxicosis, enhanced muscle weakness in certain myasthenic syndromes, and interactions in patients on systemic catecholamine depleting drugs such as reserpine.

Topical beta blockers, like almost all topical ocular drugs, have not been proven safe in pregnancy or in nursing mothers, and should also be used with caution in pediatric patients (Chapter 70).

Topical nonselective beta blockers may cause a small but meaningful adverse effect on blood lipoproteins presumably due to systemic absorption (9). Topical carteolol, which has in addition to its nonselective beta blocking ability, intrinsic sympathomimetic action, has been reported to have less of this effect (10). The true implications of this observation need further elucidation, and at least at the time of this book writing, this phenomenon does not, in itself, direct our choice of a beta blocker for initial therapy. On the other hand, this new observation involving systemic lipoproteins might indicate the need to have all patients taking topical beta blocker therapy perform punctal occlusion or gentle eyelid closure. It might also indicate the need to develop newer vehicle forms for low level sustained release of topical beta blockers to replace current eye drops. These systemic lipid observations in patients on topical ocular beta blockers need continued evaluation (and certainly has even more important implications for patients on systemic beta blocker therapy for various systemic diseases, where these lipid effects should be greater than after ocular administration).

Respiratory side effects with beta blockers are attributed to beta-two-type actions. Thus, one might expect that beta-one selective blockers might be free from such beta-two blocking side effects. But the key word is selective, which is a relative rather than absolute term. For example, betaxolol (Betoptic, Alcon, Ft. Worth, TX), a selective beta-one blocker, was observed in one human study to produce aqueous humor levels sufficient to produce substantial beta-two blockade (11). Thus, betaxolol can demonstrate some beta-two blockade properties, and such terminology regardless, ignores other important bio-

EVALUATING CLINICAL TRIALS

David L. Epstein

When evaluating clinical trials involving glaucoma patients, the reader should note whether the population being studied consists of patients who have never been treated with the specific medication or whether "glaucoma veterans" are studied. The latter type is what one commonly observes in pharmacological studies in the literature, and there is then an important preselection factor that the reader should understand. Not only are the latter "veteran" glaucoma patients already using the antiglaucoma therapy that is being evaluated in the study, and therefore more likely to respond with a therapeutic IOP response to the given agent (otherwise why were they being treated chronically before the study with the given agent?), but they are also preselected to not have developed untoward side effects (yet) to the given medication.

Thus the use of "glaucoma veterans" in these clinical "trials" usually underestimates the frequency of side effects and overestimates the IOP efficacy. Yet studies using such patients are the "bread and butter" of clinical pharmacological glaucoma research, in which typically patients receiving a given therapy (for a long period), have this therapy discontinued for several weeks that is termed a "washout" period, and then randomized to one of two agents, which usually includes the previous therapy. Meaningful clinical information can be obtained by such studies, which are often the only way to obtain the large numbers of patients required. However, the reader should understand that the clinical relevance to one's practice from such studies is usually more appropriately the question "if I have a patient on agent X, what is the relative benefit of switching the patient to agent Y?" There may be residual effects lasting even more than a few weeks (1,2) in washing out patients from existing therapy that can complicate the interpretation, e.g., when one is dealing with adrenergic agonists and antagonists in the same study.

It follows that for the clinical question "What antiglaucoma agent should I use in the newly diagnosed patient with glaucoma?" one would prefer a study of "ocular virgins." But as mentioned, it is harder to find patients for such a protocol. Yet this "real life" type of study is important and can offer important clinical information. Two examples may be appropriate. When we performed randomized prospective clinical trial of timolol therapy versus no treatment in "ocular virgins" with elevated IOP that demonstrated efficacy as far as end organ damage for timolol only after 2 years of therapy (3), a surprising and unanticipated substantial incidence of side effects occurred in the timolol group that resulted in cessation of therapy and complicated the statistical analysis (once randomized, always analyzed). Yet the occurrence of these side effects in patients never treated with timolol before was a clinically relevant important observation in itself. Also, although some have criticized this particular study because the sample size was too small ($n = 107$), and meaningful conclusions could only thereby be achieved in a larger multicenter study (which creates other problems of standardization and true comparison), it was often forgotten that our sample consisted only of "ocular virgins" which is an important clinical group. (In truth there are weaknesses in most clinical studies in glaucoma, if for no other reason than the likelihood that glaucoma is more than one disease, the subclassification of which we have been unable to discriminate. It is one of the challenges but also one of the charms of the field that glaucoma clinicians can thus constantly refine our understanding by performing more than a single study with the same apparent protocol. We seem to spend too much time criticizing studies, especially when they do not conform to our previous "dogma," and spend insufficient time trying to gain potentially important clinical insights within the context of the limitations of the data, which are our "constant companion").

The second example is another study in which we randomized primary open angle glaucoma "virgins" in a different proposed long-term protocol to either treatment with timolol or epinephrine. At the time, our rationale was that epinephrine was the only glaucoma agent that seemingly had been documented to alter the natural history of the disease (4,5). Hence, we wanted to compare the efficacy of timolol to this "standard." We were surprised (and it actually ruined the study) to find out that about one third of such unselected glaucoma patients did not get a clinically meaningful reduction in IOP from epinephrine (6). That is, **about one third of new glaucoma patients are nonresponders to epinephrine**. "In a newly diagnosed glaucoma patient should I utilize timolol or epinephrine as initial therapy?" is different from, "In glaucoma patients who are both 'epinephrine responders' and 'timolol responders,' which is the better therapy?" If one, as has been common in the literature, chooses patients already receiving chronic epinephrine-like antiglaucoma therapy, and thus are likely epinephrine-responders, "washes" them out, and then randomizes them to timolol or epinephrine, this potentially offers information to this second question, but not the first. (An alternative practical clinical inference from such studies might be that the clinician would have to place the patient on epinephrine first, and then determine that the patient does respond with meaningful IOP lowering (only a 67% chance). However, such a subtlety, regarding the actual clinical relevance, has not been overtly stated in many published articles).

References

1. Thomas JV, Epstein DL: Timolol and epinephrine in primary open angle glaucoma: Transient additive effect. Arch Ophthalmol 1981; 99:91–95.
2. Cyrlin MN, Thomas JV, Epstein DL: Additive effect of epinephrine to timolol therapy in primary open angle glaucoma. Arch Ophthalmol 1982;100:414–418.
3. Epstein DL, Krug Jr JH, Hertzmark E, et al: A long-term clinical trial of timolol therapy versus no treatment in the management of glaucoma suspects. Ophthalmology 1989;96:1460–1767.
4. Becker B, Morton WR: Topical epinephrine in glaucoma suspects. Am J Ophthalmol 1966;62:272–277.
5. Shin DH, et al: Longterm epinephrine therapy of ocular hypertension. Arch Ophthalmol 1976;94:2059–2060.
6. Alexander DW, Berson FG, Epstein DL: A clinical trial of timolol and epinephrine in the treatment of primary open angle glaucoma. Ophthalmology 1988;95:247–251.

SYSTEMIC BETA BLOCKERS AND PSEUDO-LOW TENSION GLAUCOMA

David L. Epstein

Systemic beta blocker therapy can explain certain patients who appear to have low tension glaucoma. The IOP was higher in the past when nerve damage apparently occurred before the patient was placed on systemic beta blocker therapy for other systemic disease.

chemical issues such as turnover time on the beta receptor and other important pharmacodynamic issues. Also, because drug systemically absorbed from ocular administration would pass first to the lung from the right side of the heart ("first pass" phenomenon), the lung tissue might experience higher drug levels than those commonly measured in the peripheral venous system. From a practical clinical point-of-view, **a beta-one selective blocker such as betaxolol is not absolutely safe for glaucoma patients with respiratory disease. In fact, in patients with respiratory disease, a beta blocker should not be the initial therapy**. In patients with respiratory disease that is not severe, a beta-one blocker can sometimes be used with great caution and close observation, but it is best to do this with the consultation of a pulmonologist. Regardless, the selective advantage of "beta-one" blockers such as betaxolol is a relative one.

Because both betaxolol, a beta-one selective blocker, and timolol, a nonselective (beta-one and beta-two) blocker, both block beta-one receptors, one would think that both drugs should produce similar degrees of bradycardia (a beta-one action). But again the selectivity of the agent should not be equated with beta blocker potency. The latter involves issues of drug turnover, bioavailability, etc. In fact, betaxolol seems to produce less bradycardia than timolol (12), and sometimes, if one has exhausted other therapeutic options, **with internal medicine consultation, one can try betaxolol in glaucoma patients in whom bradycardia has developed while receiving timolol**. One of us (DLE) has used this several times with success. However, this should never be attempted on patients with severe bradycardia or who have pre-existing bradycardia. For such patients, the risks are too great in the long run, even if it were effective in the short term.

Interactions of Topical Beta Blocker Therapy with Systemic Beta Blocker Therapy

Some have reported that topical beta blockers added to systemic beta blockers can produce apparently, for the first time, symptoms of systemic beta blocker side effects. This is very rare and unexpected in our experience considering the usual fluctuation in blood levels of drugs given systemically compared with those given topically.

A more common question is whether topical beta blockers are as effective in decreasing IOP in patients already taking systemic beta blocker therapy. Systemic beta blockers can produce IOP lowering (13,14) (this observation is what originally initiated the interest in topical beta blocker therapy for glaucoma), but the effect is usually small and somewhat variable. In practical terms, if a topical beta blocker would seem to be the logical first choice of drug, it should still be initiated in glaucoma patients who are receiving oral beta blocker therapy for systemic disease. In fact, in keeping with the above systemic blood drug level considerations, there likely is a lesser chance for systemic side effects from topical beta blockers in glaucoma patients who are already taking systemic beta blocker therapy for other medical purposes.

Why systemic beta blockers do not produce greater IOP lowering than they do has not been fully clarified, but this is most likely due to insufficient ocular levels of the drug, or possibly bioavailability factors. Beta blocker receptors in the eye are responsible for decreasing aqueous humor formation and reside on vascular or ciliary epithelial cell membrane sites. The observed weak IOP lowering effect of systemic beta blocker therapy might provide important insight into physiological mechanisms (and perhaps favor the theory of a cellular site of drug action).

TIMOLOL AND ALBINO RABBITS

David L. Epstein

Timolol produces minimal if any IOP reduction in albino rabbits (1), the usual, although questionable, model for glaucoma drug testing. This had led many to predict the unsuitability of timolol and other beta blockers for human glaucoma therapy. The differences between normal young healthy rabbits and aged humans with disease are extraordinary, yet the rabbit model for glaucoma drug screening persists. How many other potentially useful antiglaucoma therapies may have been similarly missed due to the lack of a suitable animal model for drug testing?

Reference

1. Bartels SP, Roth HO, Jumblatt MM, et al: Pharmacological effects of topical timolol in the rabbit eye. Invest Ophthalmol Vis Sci 1980; 19:1189–1197.

Ocular Side Effects

Despite great initial concern about the potential for ocular side effects when the topical beta blockers were introduced a decade and a half ago (because of the observation of an idiosyncratic reaction of a pemphigoid like syndrome with one systemic beta blocker [15,16], and also the potential of beta blockers to induce corneal anesthesia [17]), such ocular side effects have been uncommon. Topical beta blockers are probably the best tolerated topical medication for glaucoma patients. Yet occasionally symptoms of stinging, burning, redness, itching, and tearing can occur and be troublesome. Betaxolol before the recent reformulation (Betoptic S) frequently caused some symptoms of burning.

Corneal hypesthesia can definitely occur (18) and be of concern, but it is uncertain whether a small measured decrease in corneal sensitivity without any clinical symptoms or signs is clinically important. **In patients with punctate keratitis, the topical beta blocker therapy should be suspect.** Switching to another topical beta blocker (if the symptoms and signs are not severe), especially, at least theoretically, one without significant membrane stabilizing activity (which seems at least theoretically to relate to the hypesthetic potential), should perhaps be tried first and can be surprisingly effective.

Medications can produce a great variety of side effects, and this needs to be kept in mind with topical beta blocker therapy. But from a practical point of view the systemic (19) rather than the ocular side effects have been the major limitation to the use of topical beta blocker therapy for glaucoma.

"Escape" and "Drift" in IOP on Beta Blocker Therapy

The first drop of a beta blocker such as timolol applied to a glaucoma patient's eye produces a greater IOP lowering effect than the subsequent drops over the next couple days. Some have called this phenomenon beta blocker "escape" (20,21). This effect quickly plateaus in a steady state of sustained, clinically meaningful, IOP reduction for more than 90% of glaucoma patients (22). This phenomenon was extensively studied by Boger and colleagues who, along with Irving Katz, M.D., at Merck, deserve a great deal of credit for persisting and advocating continued clinical evaluation of timolol when some thought that the "escape" phenomenon was equivalent to a tachyphylaxis-type mechanism. (Zimmerman [23] and others were also important advocates and deserve our praise, but Boger and Katz deserve special credit for their elucidation of chronic dosing phenomena.)

Beyond these short-term events of "escape," which at a cellular level possibly might relate to changes in the actual receptors themselves, in glaucoma patients who were receiving long-term beta blocker therapy, there was a slow but real upward "drift" in IOP (20,21). In our studies of timolol versus no treatment in patients with elevated IOP (24), we observed this apparent "drift" in the timolol group, but we observed a similar comparable phenomenon in the no treatment group, suggesting to us that timolol, and likely other beta blockers, do not, once one is beyond the short-term "escape" phenomenon, diminish in ability to decrease the rate of aqueous humor formation in glaucoma eyes. Rather, the disease process in the trabecular meshwork in such "early glaucoma" patients continues to worsen (in both control and timolol treated patients), which results in the apparent "drift" upwards of IOP. That is, at the level of the ciliary body, timolol with chronic therapy does not progressively lose its ability to decrease aqueous humor production.

MECHANISM OF ACTION OF BETA BLOCKERS; INTERACTIONS WITH ADRENERGIC AGONISTS

Initially the fact that both beta blockers and beta agonists could each lower IOP was confusing (and in fact unanticipated from laboratory rabbit data). Combination studies

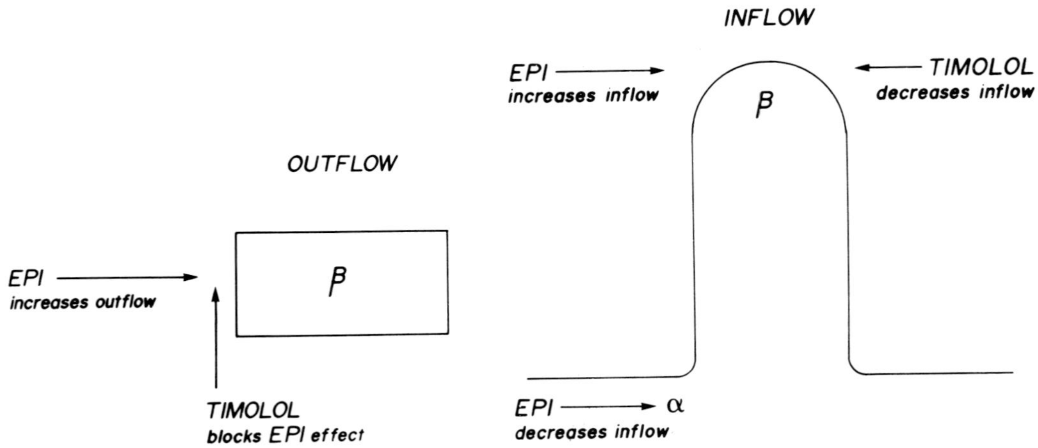

Figure 12.2. Conceptual scheme for explaining IOP effects of epinephrine, timolol, and their combination. Left, By stimulating beta receptors in the trabecular meshwork, epinephrine improves outflow facility. Timolol blocks this effect of epinephrine, but because no innervative "tone" in the primate meshwork exists, when timolol is used alone it does not impair outflow facility. Right, Epinephrine effect on inflow is mixed due to a combined beta-effect stimulating inflow and a nonbeta effect (alpha) decreasing inflow. Because there is "tone" to the ciliary body, timolol blocks beta receptors and it causes a decrease in inflow.

of agonists and antagonists have been fairly consistent in their results and led us to the following concept, which has achieved general, although perhaps not universal, acceptance.

The fact that both beta agonists and antagonists can lower IOP is explainable in part because each is believed to exert its beneficial action at a different site within the eye-the beta blocker at the ciliary body, and the beta agonist in the outflow pathways (Fig. 12.2).

Beta agonist activity is involved in the active secretion of aqueous humor (25). It is therefore likely that either sympathetic nervous system action or endogenous circulating catecholamines are involved in stimulating aqueous humor formation and somehow involved in maintaining the usual rate of production. Therefore, beta blockers block this beta-agonist driven process involved in aqueous humor formation and thus cause a decrease in aqueous humor formation (1,2) and a reduction in IOP.

It follows that beta agonistic drugs might act to increase further the rate of aqueous humor formation, unless it normally is set at a maximum rate. Epinephrine, which is used in the treatment of glaucoma, can slightly stimulate aqueous humor formation (AHF), likely through such a beta agonist mechanism (26). The reason that epinephrine does not have more of a resulting contrary effect as an antiglaucoma agent can be explained by the following: this beta effect to stimulate AHF is small (i.e., the normal "machinery" of beta "tone" is set at a near maximal level), the alpha agonistic effect of epinephrine acts in an opposite way to decrease AHF, and regardless, the primary effect of epinephrine on IOP is by an enhancement of the outflow process (Fig. 12.2) (27,28).

Beta agonists act to increase aqueous humor outflow as demonstrated tonographically in humans (27–29) and in perfusion studies in nonhuman primates (30–34). Concomitant administration of beta blockers with beta agonists blocks the latter agonist effect, presumably because as a class, adrenergic blocking agents have greater affinity for the appropriate receptor than agonists do (35). Thus simultaneous administration of timolol and epinephrine results in no improvement in outflow, whereas treatment with epinephrine alone does cause an increase in outflow. Since the epinephrine inflow action is a mix of its alpha effect to decrease inflow and its beta effect to increase inflow (which is presumably blocked by the concomitant beta blocker therapy), addition of epinephrine (or dipivefrin) to timolol therapy results in only a small further decrease in IOP due to this added (unblocked) alpha agonistic inflow effect. However, **the predominant IOP effect of epinephrine to increase outflow is blocked by the beta blocker** (Fig. 12.2).

Although timolol, for example, can block the beta effect of epinephrine on outflow, by itself, timolol does not affect outflow (27). Presumably, unlike considerations for aqueous humor production, there is no intrinsic beta driven stimulation of outflow that potentially could be blocked. The process of aqueous humor outflow through the trabecular outflow system is believed to be a passive (36), pressure driven "seepage" type process, unlike inflow which is an active, secretory process.

It has been interesting to try to discriminate between beta-one and beta-two effects in these inflow and outflow actions. Curiously, more than 90% of the beta receptors in the ciliary epithelium are of the beta-two class (37). Thus, it is surprising that beta one selective blockers such as betaxolol work well to decrease aqueous humor produc-

LABORATORY GLAUCOMA MODELS

David L. Epstein

We commonly encounter confusing data from certain laboratory glaucoma studies as far as applicability to humans, because we still do not really have adequate animal or in vitro models for what we want to study. The fact has been mentioned that albino rabbits do not show much if any reduction of IOP in response to topical beta blockers, and in truth, there are very substantial differences between rabbits and humans both in terms of ocular anatomy and tissue reactivity. It is sad, therefore, that rabbits continue to be the predominant model for glaucoma drug development.

Nonhuman primates offer more similarity to humans, but there are issues of cost, availability, and ethics. Certainly, before drugs are used on humans, it would be more appropriate to use these in nonhuman primates. But for earlier development, we are still lacking appropriate, readily available testing models. Certain in vitro models hold some promise (1,2) as do certain cell culture assays (3). In fact, assays of cell shape and attachment (4) and cell monolayer permeability (5) may be the most efficient and effective means to screen for aqueous humor outflow glaucoma drugs.

There are notable differences between nonhuman and human primates; there seems to be a substantially higher outflow through the nontrabecular unconventional outflow pathway in the nonhuman primate (Chapter 2). Further, in anterior chamber perfusion studies, the conventional trabecular outflow pathway in the nonhuman primate is believed to behave physiologically differently than humans, by demonstrating a progressive decline in outflow resistance ("washout effect") with continued perfusion (6). Further, there are, unfortunately, no animal models for human glaucoma, and diseased, aged human outflow pathway tissues (7) might respond differently from young, normal animal tissue with an anatomically and physiologically different outflow pathway. In one study, the threshold dosage for a drug outflow effect was seemingly tenfold lower in the human eye than the animal eye (8). Therefore, in vitro models will likely become even more important in the future in glaucoma drug development.

We need to keep this in mind in our research efforts in glaucoma. There likely is also much more that can be done in direct evaluation of humans with glaucoma. Tonographic studies (9) allowed the dissection of beta-one and beta-two effects directly in human glaucoma patients and helped clarify what was a confusing clinical situation at the time. Such a study was a source of much satisfaction for the clinicians involved. One thinks also of the work of Richard Brubaker and associates, who by measuring aqueous humor formation in human subjects are adding further clarity not only to antiglaucoma drug effects, but also to normal physiological influences (10).

For clinician scientists, patients with disease are a "clinical laboratory" from which it is possible to make meaningful observations from "nature's own experiments."

References

1. Erickson-Lamy K, Rohen JW, Grant WM: Outflow facility studies in the perfused human ocular anterior segment. Exp Eye Res 1991;52:723.
2. Johnson DH, Tschumper RC: Ethacrynic acid: outflow effects and toxicity in human trabecular meshwork in perfusion organ culture. Current Eye Res 1993;12:385.
3. Erickson-Lamy K, Schroeder A, Epstein DL: Ethacrynic acid induces reversible shape and cytoskeletal changes in cultured cells. Invest Ophthalmol Vis Sci 1992;33:2631.
4. Grewal A, O'Brien ET, Epstein DL: Control of cell shape in the trabecular meshwork. Invest Ophthalmol Vis Sci (Suppl) 1994;35: 2725.
5. Underwood J, Alvarado JA, Murphy CG, et al. Steroid-induced decreases in hydraulic conductivity (HC) were blocked in human trabecular meshwork (TM) cells by an antisense oligonucleotide to ZO-1. Invest Ophthalmol Vis Sci (Suppl) 1994;35:1847.
6. Erickson-Lamy K, Epstein DL, Schroeder AM, et al: Absence of time-dependent facility increase ("washout") in the perfused enucleated human eye. Invest Ophthalmol Vis Sci 1990;31: 2384–2388.
7. de Kater AW, Melamed S, Epstein DL: Patterns of aqueous humor outflow in glaucomatous and nonglaucomatous human eyes. A tracer study using cationized ferritin. Arch Ophthalmol 1989;107: 572–576.
8. Liang L-L, et al: Ethacrynic acid increases facility of outflow in the human eye in vitro. Arch Ophthalmol 1992;110:106–109.
9. Allen RC, Epstein DL: Additive effect of betaxolol and epinephrine in primary open angle glaucoma. Arch Ophthalmol 1986;104: 1178–1184.
10. Brubaker RF: Flow of aqueous humor in humans [The Friedenwald Lecture]. Invest Ophthalmol Vis Sci 1991;32:3145–66.

tion (38). We really do not know which of the ciliary body receptors are the important ones for AHF function (maybe they are mostly the beta-ones), and it also needs to be remembered that these beta-one "selective" blockers are relatively selective. Likely, we will learn more in the future about subclassification of these receptors that will provide better insight. Finally, as discussed, beta-one selective blockers such as betaxolol are not as potent as the nonselective beta blockers, e.g., timolol, in lowering IOP (12).

Tonographic studies in humans were actually the first to suggest that the beta sub-type class important for aqueous humor outflow was the beta-two (29). Timolol was observed to fully block the ability of epinephrine to increase outflow, whereas betaxolol, a beta-one blocker, did not (29). Thus, in the latter case, "unblocked" beta two receptors in the presumably trabecular outflow pathway were free to respond to epinephrine. This observation has been subsequently confirmed in perfusion studies of nonhuman primates (34). Also, predominantly beta-two receptors have been identified in human trabecular meshwork cells in culture (39–41). The clinical correlate to these findings is that although betaxolol alone is not as potent as timolol in decreasing IOP, **epinephrine-like drugs have greater additivity to betaxolol** (because of this "allowed" outflow effect) (29) than timolol. Thus, betaxolol plus epinephrine (dipivefrin) is at least equivalent to timolol plus epinephrine (dipivefrin) with regard to IOP lowering efficacy.

CHOICE OF BETA BLOCKER DRUGS (TABLE 12.1) (Figure 12.3)

Timolol (Timoptic, Merck and Co., Inc., West Point, PA) was the first topical beta blocker introduced for treating glaucoma, and there is thus perhaps the greatest experience with it. It is a nonselective (that is; both beta one and beta two) blocker and thereby is fully potent for IOP reduction. It needs to be administered twice a day, although a new once-a-day preparation has been introduced. Timolol maximally reduces the IOP because of its nonselectivity, but the latter produces the full potential for the systemic side effects mentioned. Betimol (CIBA-Vision Opthalmic, Atlanta, GA) is timolol hemihydrate, whereas Timpsotic is timolol maleate, but the two salts appear to have approximately equal efficacy.

Betaxolol (Betoptic, Alcon, Ft. Worth, TX) is a selective beta-one blocker and does not produce the same magnitude of IOP lowering as timolol (12,42). However, it has a greater systemic safety profile. Both of these phenomena are attributed to its relative beta one selectivity, which is not absolute. It should be administered twice a day and behaves in some patients as if there were a sharper 12-hour cut-off for maximal effect than with the nonselective beta blockers (43). Stinging and other external side effects have been greatly reduced by a new suspension formulation (Betoptic-S, Alcon, Ft. Worth, TX).

Table 12.1
Adrenergic Agents for the Treatment of Glaucoma

	(Trade Name)	Dosage	Frequency
Beta Blockers			
Non-Selective			
Timolol	(Timoptic, Betimol)	¼%–½%	qd–bid
Levobunolol	(Betagan)	¼%–½%	qd–bid
Carteolol	(Ocupress)	1%	bid
Metipranolol	(Optipranolol)	0.3%	bid
Selective			
Betaxolol	(Betopic)	½%	bid
	(Betoptic-S)	¼%	bid
Adrenergic Agonists			
Non-Selective			
Epinephrine		1%–2%	bid
Dipivalyl-epinephrine	(Propine)	0.1%	bid
Alpha-2 Selective			
Apraclonidine	(Iopidine)	0.5%–1%	tid
Brimonidine	(not yet commercially available)	0.2%	

Levobunolol (Betagan, Allergan Pharmaceuticals, Irvine, CA) (43) is a nonselective beta blocker that is probably equivalent to timolol in both efficacy and potential for side effects. Occasionally one observes patients who seem to respond better to timolol than levobunolol.

Metipranolol (44,45) (Optipranolol, Bausch and Lomb, Tampa, FL) is a nonselective beta blocker, whose main advantage seems to be cost. There are anecdotal accounts of greater efficacy in patients receiving timolol or levobunolol than those receiving metipranalol, which deserve further evaluation.

Carteolol (46) (Ocupress, Otsuka America Pharmaceuticals, Inc., Rockville, MD) is a new nonselective beta blocker with some intrinsic sympathomimetic activity. The implication of the latter for the ocular effects of the drug has not been defined. As mentioned, carteolol has less adverse systemic affect on lipoprotein profiles than other beta blockers (10) (Fig. 12.3).

Beta Blocker Strategy

The usual question in initiating antiglaucoma therapy with topical beta blockers (Fig. 12.3) is whether one wants maximal IOP efficacy with a nonselective agent because of the severity of the disease, or greater systemic safety at the price of slightly less IOP potency with a selective beta-one agent. **If the patient has severe disease and there is not an obvious contraindication to beta blocker therapy, we choose a nonselective agent.** If there is severe disease but a systemic concern, we choose the selective beta-one agent, as we do even without known systemic concern if maximal IOP reduction is not necessarily required. For many, but not all, patients, a selective beta-one agent such as betaxolol may produce near maximal (if not equivalent) IOP reduction, and there is always the possibility in the future of added dipivefrin therapy, which can restore full equivalency (29). Nevertheless, in patients with severe disease in which we desire maximal IOP reduction, we choose a nonselective agent if there is no systemic contraindication.

This issue of potential submaximal efficacy also relates to two other issues involving beta blockers that are often confusing to the clinician: drug concentration and dosage interval. For example, the first three topical beta blockers, timolol, levobunolol, and betaxolol, each came in two concentrations: 0.25% and 0.50%. Some have argued that for most patients, 0.25% drug concentration should be the "top of the dose response curve." This is probably true,

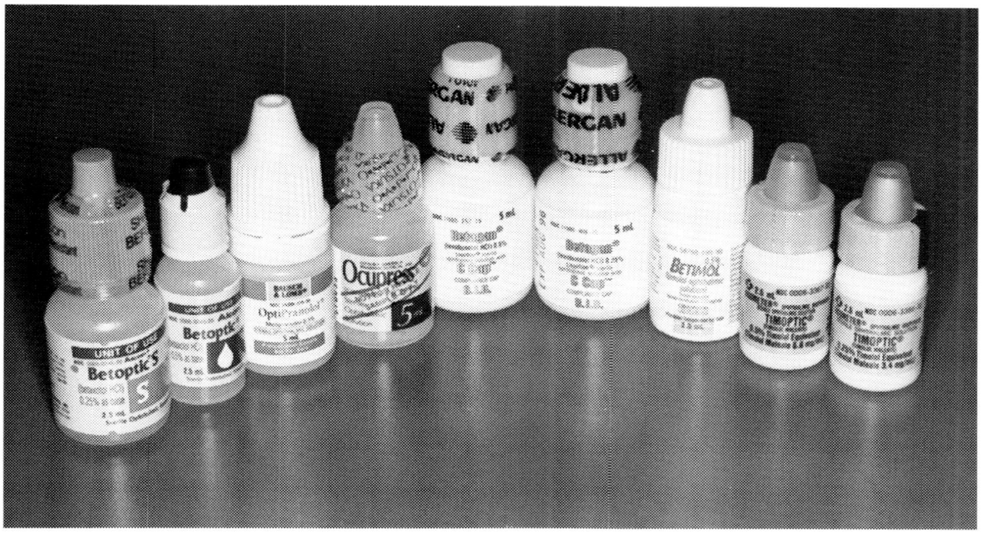

Figure 12.3. Right to left, Timoptic 1/4%, Timoptic 1/2%, Betimol 1/2%, Betagan 1/4%, Betagan 1/2%, Ocupress 1%, Optipranolol 0.3%, Betoptic 1/2%, Betoptic S 1/4%.

but in practical terms, it is difficult to be sure of this in any given patient. (Recall the discussion in Chapter 1 about how our IOP office measurements are just one "snapshot" in time, and we are in need of more extensive IOP data between visits that reflect full diurnal variation.) We suppose that one can choose to do full 24-hour diurnal IOP curves repetitively to determine equivalency between concentrations in any given patient (but remember to allow enough of a "washout" time of many weeks between the two concentrations tested), but in practical terms the decision comes down to the same basic question of the need for maximal IOP reduction or not. If maximal IOP reduction is needed, then the higher strength agent should be used. Sometimes one has no choice, as the presence of borderline side effects on the higher strength will indicate the need to try the lower strength (with punctal occlusion or gentle eyelid closure). With only anecdotal data, maximal IOP reduction is more likely to be achieved with 0.25% of a nonselective beta blocker than 0.5% of betaxolol, if the potential for systemic side effects allows the clinician this choice. (Betoptic S 0.25% due to its sustained release formulation is believed to be equivalent to 0.5% betaxolol).

There are similar considerations to the question of possible once-a-day beta-blocker therapy. Levobunolol was believed by some to be more effective for once-a-day therapy than timolol (47,48). The issue, though, has become confused. What the clinician commonly desires is a once-a-day dosage that is fully potent for the full 24 hours. It is crucial what the IOP lowering effect is during the time interval 12 to 24 hours after the once-a-day dosage. In our experience once-a-day timolol can produce IOP lowering for a full 24 hours (49), and likely once-a-day levobunolol can do somewhat better, but **if we require maximal IOP reduction for the full 24 hours, then a twice-a-day dosage for both timolol and levobunolol is commonly required**. The discussion on the next page addresses the fact that the lack of a statistically significant difference between two drugs or regimens does not necessarily mean clinical equivalency. Such issues apply not only to new formulations of once-a-day drugs, but also to new agents that are sometimes marketed with these statistical arguments to imply clinical equivalency.

EPINEPHRINE AND DIPIVEFRIN (TABLE 12.1)

As discussed, these drugs act predominantly to increase aqueous humor outflow (27–29,34) through the trabecular outflow pathway or possibly the unconventional uveal scleral outflow pathway (50). **The mechanism of enhanced outflow is believed to be by a beta-two mechanism** (29,39–41). Epinephrine-like compounds have a small but mixed effect on aqueous humor inflow (27,28) with alpha-type actions believed to decrease inflow (27,28), but beta mechanisms to actually somewhat increase inflow (25,26).

As many as one third of patients do not respond to these agents with a clinically meaningful reduction in IOP (22).

Epinephrine and dipivefrin may actually show an improved effect on IOP with time (51) (even with combination therapy with nonselective beta blockers) (28). Therefore, when therapy with these agents is initiated, efficacy should be assessed after several weeks of therapy.

The major side effect of these agents is ocular irritation, injection, and palpebral conjunctival follicle formation, that necessitates discontinuation of the agent. Patients often incorrectly attribute ocular injection to other therapeutic agents, since when these adrenergic drugs are placed in the eye, initial vasoconstriction may occur, to be followed only later (usually 1–2 hours) by rebound injection.

Dipivefrin (52) is a pro-drug of epinephrine, which was designed to decrease the ocular side effects of such therapy, by theoretically exposing the external ocular tissues to in-

STATISTICAL AND CLINICAL SIGNIFICANCE

David L. Epstein

The lack of a statistically significant difference between two drugs or regimens in clinical studies does not necessarily signify clinical equivalency. That is, one can never actually prove a negative hypothesis (i.e., that two antiglaucoma agents are not different).

A good example of this principle occurred when the selective beta one blocker betaxolol was first introduced. Some of the early studies found that the IOP reduction in betaxolol-treated patients was not statistically different from the IOP reduction in timolol-treated patients. This was true, but when one looked at the actual data, in many of these studies the mean IOP reduction was greater (albeit still not statistically significantly different) in the timolol group. Statistical significance depends on the sample size and the amount of "noise" in the study due to the design (different patients in the two groups versus crossover in the same patient, homogeneity of the patient population, number of IOP determinations, consistent time of IOP measurement, etc.). If there is too much "noise" or an insufficient sample size, mean (and clinically real) measured differences will not show statistical significance.

In our studies (1), we did observe statistically significant differences between betaxolol and timolol in IOP reduction. Our study had patients with more severe glaucoma and IOP abnormality who were more homogeneous, and perhaps our design was less "noisy" or perhaps we were fortunate, but our deduction from the study and our continuing clinical impression has been that for patients with severe glaucoma disease in whom maximal IOP reduction is desired, timolol does produce clinically meaningful, greater IOP reduction than betaxolol.

Betaxolol, also in our study, produced substantial IOP reduction, although it was not equivalent to timolol. Therefore, in a new patient when one initiates antiglaucoma therapy within the previously discussed guidelines, it may be appropriate to choose betaxolol. Our study would support this. It is a different question, however, whether patients currently well controlled on timolol can be switched to betaxolol with no change in IOP control. Our study predicted what we believe has subsequently proven to be the clinical observation (2) with such a "switch." For many patients, there is no clinically meaningful difference after the switch, but for some there is definite loss of IOP control when switched from timolol to betaxolol.

For any individual patient, there can be clinical equivalency, but it is difficult to document this with our "snapshots" of IOP, and in patients with advanced disease who need maximal IOP control continuously, our uncertainty about equivalency is an important clinical factor to consider.

The latter is also true for the questions of drug concentration equivalency or dosage interval equivalency. One can never prove a negative hypothesis. Specifically it is not sufficient (for patients with advanced disease) that for the lower concentration or less frequent dosing interval that the IOP reduction is not "statistically different" from the usual alternative.

The clinician should look closely at the actual mean differences at all the data points in these published studies, as well as critically examine the protocol and adequately assess the "noise."

References

1. Allen RC, Hertzmark E, Walker AM, et al: A double-masked comparison of betaxolol vs timolol in the treatment of open angle glaucoma. Am J Ophthalmol 1986;101:535–541.
2. Vogel R, Tipping R, Kulaga SF, et al: Changing therapy from timolol to betaxolol. Effect on intraocular pressure in selected patients with glaucoma. Timolol-Betaxolol study group. Arch Ophthalmol 1989;107:1303–7.

active compound. The drug contains two pivalyl groups that have been added to the epinephrine molecule. The pivalyl groups are cleaved when the drug passes through the cornea (53), allowing epinephrine to reach its intraocular sites of action. By means of this pro-drug approach, a lower concentration can be administered to the eye. In our experience dipivefrin is comparable to at least 1% epinephrine in IOP lowering efficacy. Some clinicians believe that 2% epinephrine, which had been used sometimes in the past (54), is more potent than dipivefrin with regard to IOP lowering efficacy (although such a concentration may be accompanied by a higher incidence of side effects). Although overall there seems to be less external irritation with dipivefrin compared with epinephrine, cases of dipivefrin sensitivity and allergy are not uncommon (55–57).

Rarely, systemic side effects relating to heart function, such as tachycardia and blood pressure elevation have been reported with the topical ocular use of these agents. Presumably these effects might be less frequent with the pro-drug, dipivefrin. Punctal occlusion or gentle eyelid closure (5) are indicated to prevent these side effects. However, the main reason these compounds need to be discontinued

MECHANISMS OF EPINEPHRINE-INDUCED CYSTOID MACULAR EDEMA

David L. Epstein

Very rarely epinephrine-like compounds can produce cystoid macular edema in phakic eyes. Ordinarily, it would seem that the presence of the crystalline lens somehow retards fluid movement from the anterior segment to the posterior segment. We do know, however, that some "aqueous humor" from the posterior chamber does make its way into the posterior segment and retinal area (Chapter 29). In experimental retinal detachment, it is believed that fluid from the vitreous moves into the subretinal space (1). However, the extreme rarity of phakic cystoid macular edema due to epinephrine-like compounds likely indicates that significant drug levels do not ordinarily develop in the retina (2). In aphakic eyes, this barrier function of the crystalline lens is obviously lost (2), but in pseudophakic eyes one would imagine there to be still some barrier function. Nevertheless, cystoid macular edema from dipivefrin has been observed in pseudophakic eyes, although the true incidence has not been determined.

There may be pathways to the posterior segment by avenues other than via the vitreous. For example, in post-surgical or inflamed eyes (or possibly eyes in the future treated with prostaglandin-like drugs), fluid potentially carrying topically applied medications may pass via the uveo-vascular-scleral outflow pathway potentially to the posterior segment uvea (Chapter 2).

References

1. Pederson JE, Toris CB: Experimental retinal detachment. IX. Aqueous, vitreous, and subretinal protein concentrations. Arch Ophthalmol 1985;103:835–6.
2. Kramer SG: Epinephrine distribution after topical administration to phakic and aphakic eyes. Trans Am Ophthalmol Soc 1980;78: 947–82.

usually relates to ocular rather than systemic side effects. The latter are, in fact, rare in our experience.

These compounds presumably need to be administered twice a day, although when discontinued, residual IOP effects can last for weeks (necessitating several weeks at least for "washout periods" in clinical pharmacological studies [28]). They can be administered 5 minutes after other ocular drugs. Theoretically it once seemed possible that by separating by many hours the time between beta agonist and beta blocker topical therapy, one might be able to lessen the ability of the blocker to interfere with the agonist on the receptor site. However, clinical studies demonstrated that such a separation did not provide better IOP lowering efficacy, thus indicating that with both the blockers and the agonists, there is a long residual effect (28,58).

Epinephrine usually comes in strengths of 1% or 2% and dipivefrin in a single strength of 0.1% (Fig. 12.4). Apparently there was a historical although anecdotal clinical impression that 2% epinephrine (54) was somewhat more potent than 1%, but there is greater potential for both ocular and systemic side effects with this higher dosage, and it was less frequently used. For most clinicians dipivefrin has replaced epinephrine for antiglaucoma therapy.

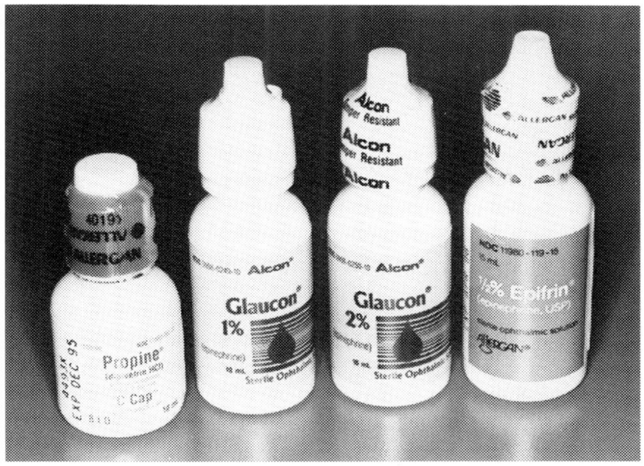

Figure 12.4. Epinephrine compounds, Propine 0.1%.

In aphakic (59,60) **and also pseudophakic eyes, epinephrine or dipivefrin can produce cystoid macular edema.** We therefore tend to avoid use of these drugs in such patients. However, not all aphakic eyes did, in fact, develop cystoid macular edema with epinephrine therapy (61), and this propensity is even less in pseudophakic compared with aphakic eyes. Therefore, as a last topical choice for antiglaucoma therapy, dipivefrin can still be considered for use in pseudophakic eyes, in which beta blockers cannot be used and miotics are ineffective. However, the macular status needs to be carefully monitored. If cystoid macular edema is detected early, it is believed to be fully reversible in almost all patients. However, chronic cystoid macular edema may produce permanent macular damage.

Because epinephrine-like compounds are only minimally additive to nonselective beta blockers (27–29), **we tend to avoid adding these agents to pseudophakic eyes already being treated with these topical beta blockers (the benefit/risk ratio does not seem appropriate).**

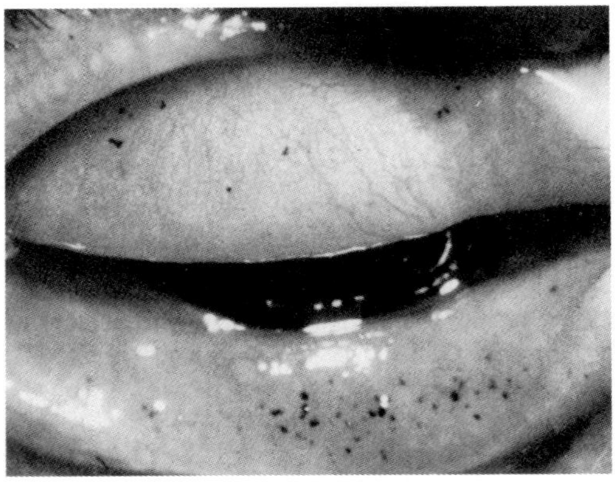

Figure 12.5. Black breakdown products from epinephrine and conjunctival injection in a patient who has topical epinephrine sensitivity.

Although epinephrine-like compounds are free from accommodative type side effects, sometimes some pupillary dilatation can be produced which can produce symptoms of visual blurring. This is especially noted when these drugs are used in combination with beta blockers (presumably because they produce now unopposed alpha adrenergic activity, although this is speculation).

Adrenachrome breakdown products can occasionally be observed on the palpebral conjunctiva (Fig. 12.5). This is more commonly seen with epinephrine use than dipivefrin.

Although approximately one third of patients do not respond to epinephrine-like compounds with a clinically meaningful reduction in IOP (22), there are patients who show a dramatic decrease in IOP, greater than from beta blockers or miotics. The explanation for this is obscure. One of us (DLE) has observed this in a few patients with pigmentary glaucoma. Although this heightened response to epinephrine-like compounds is rare, it nevertheless should be kept in mind in treating patients with glaucoma. (We have wondered whether these "super-responders" might have constitutively a lower beta receptor density and also therefore might demonstrate suboptimal IOP response to the opposite acting beta blockers, but we have not investigated this further.)

In patients who are receiving topical beta blocker therapy for glaucoma and who require a second antiglaucoma agent, we would frame the decision to possibly add epinephrine-like compounds as follows: if a selective beta-one blocker (such as betaxolol) is being used, then an epinephrine-like drug, such as dipivefrin, is a reasonable initial choice. The clinician needs to remember that approximately one third of glaucoma patients do not respond to epinephrine-like drugs with clinically meaningful IOP reduction. The potential additivity needs to be assessed after several weeks of combined therapy. Epinephrine-like drugs are potentially additive to a relatively selective beta-one blocker, because the latter does not (or minimally does) interfere with the beta-two outflow effect of epinephrine-like drugs (29).

In contrast, if a nonselective beta blocker is being used, then epinephrine-like drugs, such as dipivefrin, are minimally (27–29) if at all, additive, although there are unusual "outlier patients" who show a greater additive IOP effect than expected. The most that can be hoped for usually is a further 1–3 mm Hg IOP lowering. However, in some patients, such a slight additivity is clinically meaningful, and there may not be other therapeutic alternatives. The additive effect should be assessed after several weeks of combined therapy (28).

ALPHA-2 AGONISTS (Table 12.1)

Apraclonidine (Iopidine, Alcon Ft. Worth, TX) was originally developed to diminish iris bleeding (presumably by inducing iris vasoconstriction) during Nd:YAG laser iridectomy, but IOP was also lowered (62). Actually this is another example of how, based on detailed clinical information, a clinician-scientist, Alan Robin, contributed to an advancement in our field of glaucoma. Subsequent studies indicated that apraclonidine could also blunt the IOP spike after both Nd:YAG (63) and argon iridectomy (64), Nd:YAG posterior capsulotomy (65), and argon laser trabeculoplasty (66) and have potential efficacy for certain patients in chronic therapy (67-70).

Thus, apraclonidine has been an important addition to our glaucoma armamentarium, but there are unfortunately some misconceptions concerning its use. Apraclonidine acts to decrease aqueous humor formation (71), an effect that is partially additive in most patients to beta blockers (68), which also act to decrease aqueous humor flow. However, the mechanism for the IOP increase after laser iridectomy and trabeculoplasty involves an added obstruction to aqueous outflow possibly mechanically due to pigment and capsulotomy or lens debris or protein (Chapters 47 and 54), and not an increase in aqueous humor formation (not involved in the mechanism of any type of glaucoma). Thus there is nothing specific as to the cause of the post-laser IOP spike that apraclonidine affects. **It is a drug that effectively decreases IOP by reducing aqueous flow that thus compensates for the obstruction to outflow that actually causes the elevated IOP.** This has potential clinical consequences and is important for the glaucoma clinician to understand (especially when dealing with those "5%" of patients referred to in "Epstein's Rule of 5%," see Chapter 1).

Apraclonidine both for post-laser treatment and when used for pre-treatment is administered in either a 0.5 or 1% strength. In such short term use, side effects except for lid retraction and conjunctival blanching are uncommon.

The drug has been approved in 0.5% strength to be taken two to three times a day for the chronic treatment of the glaucomas (Fig. 12.6). In some patients, there is substantial efficacy even when added to "maximally tolerated medical therapy," but curiously in some patients there is little to no additive effect. The reason for this difference

APRACLONIDINE AND LASER INDUCED IOP ELEVATION

David L. Epstein

It is now "routine" to pre-treat patients before or after laser iridectomy trabeculoplasty, and capsulotomy procedures with apraclonidine because clinicians have observed that while the patient is in the office (1–2 hours after the laser) there is a diminished incidence of substantial IOP spikes with this regimen. This results from a nonspecific decrease in aqueous humor flow rather than a specific alleviation of the induced obstruction to aqueous outflow, which is responsible for the IOP elevation.

The patient should remain in the office for 1–2 hours after the laser and then return the next morning for an IOP check before more long-term follow up (see Chapters 52, 53, 55, 56). Although with chronic therapy, apraclonidine might have to be given every 8–12 hours some patients achieve a longer duration effect of 24 hours or a little longer from the initial instillation. Thus, there is the potential in at least a few patients ("rule of 5%") for the clinician to be lulled into a false sense of security. Even though no substantial IOP spike is observed during the observation period, it can still occur at a slightly later time when aqueous humor flow (no longer under the influence of the discontinued apraclonidine) returns to normal, thus unmasking the trabecular obstruction to outflow induced by the laser. Another consideration is that the latter may still be evolving (and getting worse in some patients) over the next few days. The key to understanding this potential is the understanding of the fact that apraclonidine acts to diminish aqueous flow and does not "treat" the underlying cause of the IOP spike.

What are potential strategies to avoid missing such a "delayed" (after 24 hours) (1) IOP spike in these probably small number of glaucoma patients at risk? One possibility would be to also perform a 2nd day (48 hour) IOP check, or at least delay the time of the next day IOP check to a time later than a true 24 hours (the next afternoon, rather than an early morning IOP check the next day after the laser). Although this sounds reasonable and probably should be implemented in patients with advanced disc cupping or susceptible optic nerves, in whom there might be even short-term adverse consequences from an untreated IOP spike, this is often not practical, especially when patients travel long distances.

Another possible strategy would be to continue the apraclonidine for a few days after the laser, and in most situations this probably is the most practical solution. However, the 1% strength apraclonidine routinely used for laser procedures was originally not approved for use in this way (although now the lower strength 0.5% (2) has been approved for short-term use), and by decreasing aqueous humor flow the drug is compensating for the induced obstruction to outflow, which has a natural history of its own.

Another strategy for trabeculoplasty, capsulotomy, and argon but not YAG iridectomy is the following: the hemostasis in the iris that is induced by apraclonidine and which, as described,was responsible for its initial development, is an important component in the YAG iridectomy procedure. Thus, there is a need to pretreat with apraclonidine before a YAG iridectomy (if a hyphema occurs post-laser this, in itself, can cause a further increase in IOP because the blood will drain through the trabecular meshwork, see Chapters 43,45). But in patients undergoing argon laser trabeculoplasty or argon laser iridectomy alone (where the argon laser actually photocoagulates the iris and this acts to prevent iris bleeding) or YAG capsulotomy, one can choose not to pretreat but to only post-treat with apraclondine after the IOP is checked 1-2 hours after the procedure. The latter IOP check, without the influence of an added aqueous humor suppressant, will identify by an IOP increase patients with trabecular obstruction to outflow (at least in the early stages). This allows one to identify those patients who need both detailed follow-up (perhaps every day for a while if their optic nerves are susceptible) and also more vigorous short-term antiglaucoma therapy. As indicated, the trabecular obstruction is evolving and may uncommonly "peak" late so this strategy might not identify all such patients at risk. Nevertheless, for the overwhelming majority of patients, the 1-2 hour IOP spike is a good predictor (3) of those patients likely to have further substantial IOP elevation in the first few days after the laser procedure. Thus by not pre-treating such patients routinely, trabecular-related IOP spikes can be more easily identified, allowing more intensive follow-up and therapy. As an added safety measure, patients (even without apparent IOP spikes) can routinely be given apraclonidine after the post-laser IOP measurement.

All these considerations must be taken in the context of the state of the patient's glaucoma in terms of severity and the potential susceptibility of the optic nerve to an IOP spike. Patients with advanced cupping or susceptible nerves need close monitoring. An undetected IOP spike into the 30s for 1-2 days likely will have little adverse consequence for patients with healthy optic nerves (as is commonly found in many patients undergoing iridectomy). However, for a patient with advanced cupping with an IOP in the teens, such an IOP spike is potentially hazardous. Therefore, care for the glaucoma patient must be individualized; this is what makes glaucoma so challenging, yet potentially rewarding for the clinician. (General "rules" apply to general patients, but as clinicians we need to treat patients individually).

References

1. Nesher R, Kolker AE: Failure of apraclonidine to prevent delayed IOP elevation after Nd:YAG laser posterior capsulotomy. Trans Am Ophthalmol Soc 1990;88:229–32.
2. Stewart WC, et al.: The efficacy of apraclonidine as an adjunct to timolol therapy. Arch Ophthalmol 1995;113:287.
3. Richter CU, et al.: Intraocular pressure elevation following Nd: YAG laser posterior capsulotomy. Ophthalmology 1985;92:636.

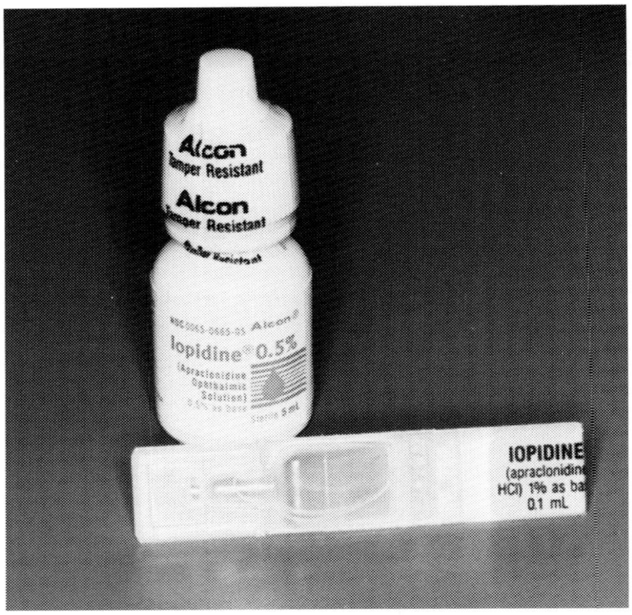

Figure 12.6. Apraclonidine 1% (front) and 1/2% (rear). The 1% solution was first approved for the treatment of post-laser IOP spikes; the 1/2% solution was later approved for short-term chronic use. The 1/2% solution is probably equally effective to apraclonidine 1%.

in clinical response is not readily apparent, but it would be interesting and potentially useful to understand this better. Like the beta blockers and the carbonic anhydrase inhibitors, apraclonidine decreases aqueous humor formation (71). Because there seems to be additivity in some patients at least, one is led to conclude tentatively that apraclonidine must be acting, at least in part, at sites in the ciliary body distinct from those where the beta blockers and carbonic anhydrase inhibitors (CAI) act. Although similar to considerations of CAIs and beta blockers themselves in combination (72) (see Chapter 14), the actions are likely not totally independent but interrelated in some manner, perhaps involving vascular or cellular targets in sequence.

By dissecting out the presence or absence of an added effect of apraclonidine with other aqueous suppressants alone or in combination, some useful insights into the aqueous humor formation process and its therapeutic modification would be possible. Since one can observe clinically a vascular response to apraclonidine in the iris and conjunctiva, one might initially hypothesize a vascular influence at the level of the ciliary body as well. On the other hand, similar to considerations for the other aqueous suppressants, alpha-two agonists might have direct cellular effects on the ciliary epithelium. Because the aged human glaucomatous eye is distinctly different from the young, healthy animal eye, final elucidation of this understanding, or even potentially the next advance in therapy, will likely require innovative clinical investigation (the dissection of the beta adrenergic agonist and antagonist efficacy conundrum really came first from clinical investigation) (27–29).

One of us (DLE) has a vague sense that perhaps patients on dipivefrin or equivalent in combination might respond less well to added apraclonidine, but this needs careful study and might be erroneous (but again, increased glaucoma understanding commonly needs to start with clinical impressions and then analysis—glaucoma is a field of study that is dependent on clinical science).

With long-term use of apraclonidine, in addition to common lid retraction and conjunctival blanching, signs of ocular allergy or sensitivity are unfortunately becoming increasingly apparent (67,73,74). Patients can develop conjunctival injection with papillary and follicular reactions. The latter may not be marked, but patients complain of ocular irritation that requires discontinuation of the medication. Although firm final numbers are not yet in, probably a third or more of patients develop such side effects.

In addition there is concern that with long-term administration (after 2–12 months), the efficacy of apraclonidine may diminish due to some form of tolerance. The data in the literature are somewhat conflicting in this regard (69,70,75) and similar to considerations of beta blocker "drift," this phenomenon possibly may reflect, at least in part, the progressive worsening of the diseases in the trabecular meshwork rather than a diminished efficacy of the drug at the level of the ciliary body. More clinical investigation, likely using fluorophotometry to directly measure flow, will be required to settle this issue.

Alpha-two agonists for the treatment of glaucoma have perhaps been late to be developed because the prototype compound, clonidine, after topical administration demonstrated dramatic systemic effects involving decreased blood pressure and other central actions. Apraclonidine was designed pharmacologically to avoid these side effects, and so far this has proven true (although constant surveillance is still advisable). Some of the newer alpha-two agonists, such as brimonidine, which has activity similar to apraclonidine, may demonstrate some clonidine-like effects (76), and the clinician needs to keep this potential in mind as these newer agents become available.

In summary, if one maintains appropriate insight into the mechanism of action to decrease aqueous inflow, apraclonidine and presumably newer alpha-two agonists currently under development have important efficacy for short-term elevations of IOP, and, more limited, but still some potential efficacy in the chronic treatment of glaucoma in responsive patients.

FUTURE DIRECTIONS

Because current topical beta blockers likely demonstrate maximal potency and even a twice-a-day dosing regimen is "patient friendly," it is unlikely that there is much potential for the future development of beta blockers with greater IOP-lowering efficacy.

Nevertheless, it is not obvious that the current beta blockers are the "best" beta blockers for glaucoma that there can be, and one wonders whether more effort should, in fact, be placed in this direction. Polansky has made the provocative suggestion that these drugs may work by affecting chloride and other cellular channels rather than the beta receptors (77–79), and this hypothesis could offer the potential for innovative new drug development.

Similarly, the adrenergic outflow effects with epinephrine-like drugs may not represent "all that there can be" with this class of drug. Better insight in the future into the exact cellular mechanism of action might open up the possibility of better therapeutic agents.

Finally, we need to consider whether there is a maximum amount of reduction in aqueous humor formation that is either possible or wise to produce. Too much reduction in aqueous flow, which carries nutrition to anterior segment structures, might potentially produce adverse consequences. It is for this reason that we have placed a major emphasis on the development of outflow rather than inflow drugs for glaucoma in the future (Chapter 16). Nevertheless, the possibility of more effective aqueous humor suppressants in the adrenergic class should continue to be explored.

References

1. Coakes RL, Brubaker RF: The mechanism of timolol in lowering intraocular pressure in the normal eye. Arch Ophthalmol 1978;96:2045–2048.
2. Yablonski ME, et al: A fluorophotometric study of the effect of topical timolol on aqueous humor dynamics. Exp Eye Res 1978;27:135–142.
3. Frishman WH, Fuksbrumer MS, Tannenbaum M: Topical ophthalmic beta-adrenergic blockade for the treatment of glaucoma and ocular hypertension. J Clin Pharmacol 1994;34:795–803.
4. Zimmerman TJ, Sharir M, Nardin GF, et al: Therapeutic index of pilocarpine, carbachol, and timolol with nasolacrimal occlusion. Am J Ophthalmol 1992;114:1–7.
5. Zimmerman TJ, Kooner KS, Kandarakis AS, et al: Improving the therapeutic index of topically applied ocular drugs. Arch Ophthalmol 1984; 102:551–553.
6. Wiklund I: Quality of life and cost-effectiveness in the treatment of hypertension. J Clin Pharm Ther 1994;19:81–87.
7. Fraunfelder FT, Meyer SM: Sexual dysfunction secondary to topical ophthalmic timolol. JAMA 1985;253:3092.
8. Silverstone BZ, Marcus T: Hypoglycemia due to ophthalmic timolol in a diabetic. Harefuah 1990;118:693–694.
9. Coleman AL, et al: Topical timolol decreases plasma high-density lipoprotein cholesterol level. Arch Ophthalmol 1990;108:1260.
10. Freedman SF, et al: Effects of ocular carteolol and timolol on plasma high-density lipoprotein cholesterol level. Am J Ophthalmol 1994;116: 600–11.
11. Vuori M, Kaila T, Jisalo E, et al: Concentrations and antagonist activity of topically applied betaxolol in aqueous humour. Acta Ophthalmol 1993;71:677–681.
12. Allen RC, Hertzmark E, Walker AM, et al: A double-masked comparison of betaxolol vs timolol in the treatment of open angle glaucoma. Am J Ophthalmol 1986;101:535–541.
13. Wettrell K, Pandolfi M: Effect of oral administration of various beta-blocking agents on the intraocular pressure in healthy volunteers. Exp Eye Res 1975;21:451.
14. Pandolfi M, Ohrstrom A: Treatment of ocular hypertension with oral beta-adrenergic blocking agents. Acta Ophthalmol 1974;52:464.
15. Rahi AHS, Chapman CM, Garner A, et al: Pathology of practolol induced ocular toxicity. Br J Ophthalmol 1976;60:312.
16. Garner A, Rahi AHS: Practolol and ocular toxicity. Antibodies in serum and tears. Br J Ophthalmol 1976;60:684.
17. Musini A, et al: Comparison of the effect of propranolol, lignocaine, and other drugs on normal and raised intraocular pressure in man. Am J Ophthalmol 1971;72:773.
18. Van Buskirk EM: Corneal anesthesia after timolol maleate therapy. Am J Ophthalmol 1979;88:739–43.
19. Van Buskirk EM: Adverse reactions from timolol administration. Ophthalmology 1980;87:447.
20. Boger WP III, Puliafito CA, Steinert RF, et al: Long-term experience with timolol ophthalmic solution in patients with open angle glaucoma. Ophthalmology 1978;85:259-267.
21. Boger WP III: Editorial: Timolol: short term "escape" and long term "drift." Ann Ophthalmol 1979;11:1239–1242.
22. Alexander DW, Berson FG, Epstein DL: A clinical trial of timolol and epinephrine in the treatment of primary open angle glaucoma. Ophthalmology 1988;95:247–251.
23. Zimmerman TJ: Timolol maleate-a new glaucoma medication? Invest Ophthal Vis Sci 1977;16:687.
24. Epstein DL, Krug Jr JH, Hertzmark E, et al: A long-term clinical trial of timolol therapy versus no treatment in the management of glaucoma suspects. Ophthalmology 1989;96:1460–1767.
25. Kacere RD, Dolan JW, Brubaker RF: Intravenous epinephrine stimulates aqueous formation in the human eye. Invest Ophthalmol Vis Sci 1992;33:2861–5.
26. Townsend DJ, Brubaker RF: Immediate effect of epinephrine on aqueous formation in the normal human eye as measured by fluorophotometry. Invest Ophthalmol Vis Sci 1980;19:256–266.
27. Thomas JV, Epstein DL: Timolol and epinephrine in primary open angle glaucoma: Transient additive effect. Arch Ophthalmol 1981;99:91–95.
28. Cyrlin MN, Thomas JV, Epstein DL: Addictive effect of epinephrine to timolol therapy in primary open angle glaucoma. Arch Ophthalmol 1982;100:414–418.
29. Allen RC, Epstein DL: Additive effect of betaxolol and epinephrine in primary open angle glaucoma. Arch Ophthalmol 1986;104:1178-1184.
30. Bill A: Early effects of epinephrine on aqueous humor dynamics in vervet monkeys (Cercopithecus ethiops). Exp Eye Res 1969;8:35–43.
31. Bill A: Effects of norepinephrine, isoproterenol and sympathetic stimulation on aqueous humor dynamics in vervet monkeys. Exp Eye Res 1970; 10:31–46.
32. Neufeld AH: Influences of cyclic nucleotides on outflow facility in the vervet monkey. Exp Eye Res 1978;27:387–397.
33. Kaufman PL: Epinephrine, norepinephrine, and isoproterenol dose-outflow facility response relationships in cynomolgus monkey eyes with and without ciliary muscle retrodisplacement. Acta Ophthalmol (Copenh) 1986;64:356–63.
34. Robinson JC, Kaufman PL: Effects and interactions of epinephrine, norepinephrine, timolol, and betaxolol on outflow facility in the cynomolgus monkey. Am J Ophthalmol 1990;109:189–94.
35. Neufeld AH: Experimental studies on the mechanism of action of timolol. Surv Ophthalmol 1979;23:363–370.
36. Van Buskirk EM, Grant WM: Influence of temperature and the question of involvement of cellular metabolism in aqueous outflow. Am J Ophthalmol 1974;77:565–572.
37. Wax MB, Molinoff PB: Distribution and properties of β-adrenergic receptors in human iris-ciliary body. Invest Ophthalmol Vis Sci 1987; 28:420–30.
38. Gaul GR, Will NJ, Brubaker RF: Comparison of a noncardioselective beta-adrenoceptor blocker and a cardioselective blocker in reducing aqueous flow in humans. Arch Ophthalmol 1989;107:1308–11.

39. Jampel HD, et al: Beta-adrenergic receptors in human trabecular meshwork. Identification and autoradiographic localization. Invest Ophthalmol Vis Sci 1987;28:772–9.
40. Wax MB, Molinoff PB, Alvarado J, et al: Characterization of beta-adrenergic receptors in cultured human trabecular cells and in human trabecular meshwork. Invest Ophthalmol Vis Sci 1989;30:51–7.
41. Polansky J, et al: Effects of betaxolol/timolol on epinephrine stimulated cyclic-AMP levels in human trabecular meshwork cells. Int Ophthalmol 1989;13:95–7.
42. Vogel R, Tipping R, Kulaga SF, et al: Changing therapy from timolol to betaxolol. Effect on intraocular pressure in selected patients with glaucoma. Timolol-Betaxolol study group. Arch Ophthalmol 1989;107:1303–7.
43. Long DA, et al: Levobunolol and betaxolol. Ophthalmology 1988;95:735.
44. Hickey-Dwyer M, Campbell SH, Harding S: Doubled-masked three-period crossover investigation of metipranolol in control of raised intraocular pressure. J Ocular Pharmacol 1991;7:277–83.
45. Serle JB, Lustgarten JS, Podos SM: A clinical trial of metipranolol, a noncardioselective beta-adrenergic antagonist, in ocular hypertension. Am J Ophthalmol 1991;112:302–7.
46. Flammer J, et al: Influence of carteolol and timolol on IOP and visual fields in glaucoma: a multi-center, double-masked, prospective study. 1992;2:169–74.
47. Wandel T, et al: Ocular hypotensive efficacy of 0.25% levobunolol instilled once daily. Ophthalmology 1988;95:252–4.
48. Derick RJ, et al: Once-daily versus twice-daily levobunolol (0.5%) therapy. A crossover study. Ophthalmology 1992;99:424–9.
49. Silverstone D, et al: Evaluation of once-daily levobunolol 0.25% and timolol 0.25% therapy for increased intraocular pressure. Am J Ophthalmol 1991;112:56–60.
50. Higgins RG, Brubaker RF: Acute effect of epinephrine on aqueous humor formation in the timolol treated normal eye as measured by fluorophotometry. Invest Ophthalmol Vis Sci 1980;19:420–423.
51. Ballintine EJ, Garner LL: Improvement of the coefficient of outflow in glaucomatous eyes. Arch Ophthalmol 1961;66:314–317.
52. Albracht DC, et al: A double-masked comparison of betaxolol and dipivefrin for the treatment of increased intraocular pressure. Am J Ophthalmol 1993;116:307.
53. Nakamura M, Shirasawa E, Hikida M: Characterization of esterases involved in the hydrolysis of dipivefrin hydrochloride. Ophthalmic Res 1993;25:46–51.
54. Garner LL, Johnston WW, Ballintine EJ, et al: Effect of 2% levo-rotary epinephrine on the intraocular pressure of the glaucomatous eye. Arch Ophthalmol 1959;62:230.
55. Theodore J, Leibowitz HM: External ocular toxicity of dipivalyl epinephrine. Am J Ophthalmol 1979;88:1013–1016.
56. Petersen PE, Evans RB, Johnstone MA, et al: Evaluation of ocular hypersensitivity to dipivalyl epinephrine by component eye-drop testing. J Allergy Clin Immunol 1990;85:954–8.
57. Boerner CF: Total punctate keratopathy due to dipivefrin. Case report. Arch Ophthalmol 1988;106:171.
58. Tsoy EA, Meekins BB, Shields MD: Comparison of two treatment schedules for combined timolol and dipivefrin therapy. Am J Ophthalmol 1986;102:320–4.
59. Kolker AE, Becker B: Epinephrine maculopathy. Arch Ophthalmol 1968;79:552.
60. Obstbaum SA, Galin MA, Poole TA: Topical epinephrine and cystoid macular edema. Ann Ophthalmol 1976;8:455.
61. Thomas JV, Gragoudas ES, Blair NP, et al: Correlation of epinephrine use and macular edema in aphakic glaucomatous eyes. Arch Ophthalmol 1978;96:625.
62. Robin AL, Pollack IP: Uses of ALO 2145 in anterior segment glaucoma laser surgery. In: Perspectives in Glaucoma: Trans 1st Sci Meet American Glaucoma Society. Shields MB, Pollack IP, Kolker AE, eds. Thorofare, NJ: Slack, 1988.
63. Kitazawa Y, Taniguchi T, Sugiyama K: Use of apraclonidine to reduce acute intraocular pressure rise following Q-switched Nd:YAG laser iridotomy. Ophthalmic Surg 1989;20:49–52.
64. Robin A, Pollack I, deFaller J: Effects of topical AL0 2145 (p-aminoclonidine hydrochloride) on the acute intraocular pressure rise after argon laser iridotomy. Arch Ophthalmol 1987;105:1208–1211.
65. Pollack I, et al: Prevention of the rise in intraocular pressure following neodymium-YAG posterior capsulotomy using topical 1% apraclonidine. Arch Ophthalmol 1988;106:754–757.
66. Robin A, Pollack I, House B, et al: Effects of AL0 2145 on intraocular pressure following argon laser trabeculoplasty. Arch Ophthalmol 1987;105:646–650.
67. Nagasubramanian S, et al: Comparison of apraclonidine and timolol in chronic open angle glaucoma. A three month study. Ophthalmology 1993;100:1318–23.
68. Morrison J, Robin A: Adjunctive glaucoma therapy: a comparison of apraclonidine to dipivefrin when added to timolol maleate. Ophthalmology 1989;96:3–7.
69. Lish A, Camras C, Podos S: Effect of apraclonidine on intraocular pressure in glaucoma patients receiving maximally tolerated medications. J Glaucoma 1992;1:19–22.
70. Stewart WC, et al: The efficacy of apraclonidine as an adjunct to timolol therapy. Arch Ophthalmol 1995;113:287.
71. Gharagozloo NZ, Relf SJ, Brubaker RF: Aqueous flow is reduced by the alpha-adrenergic agonist, apraclonidine hydrochloride (ALO 2145). Ophthalmology 1988;95:1217–1220.
72. Berson FG, Epstein DL: Separate and combined effects of timolol maleate and acetazolamide in open angle glaucoma. Am J Ophthalmol 1981;92:788–791.
73. Wilkerson M, Lewis RA, Shields MB: Follicular conjunctivitis associated with apraclonidine [letter]. Am J Ophthalmol 1991;111:105–6.
74. Butler P, et al.: Clinical experience with the long-term use of 1% apraclonidine. Arch Ophthalmol 1995;113:293.
75. Cardakli F, et al: Effect of chronic apraclonidine treatment on intraocular pressure in advanced glaucoma. J Glaucoma 1994;2:271–278.
76. Nordlund JR, Pasquale LR, Robin AL, et al: The cardiovascular, pulmonary, and ocular hypotensive effects of 0.2% brimonidine. Arch Ophthalmol 1995;113:77.
77. Cherksey BD, Fauss DJ, Alvarado JA, et al: Dose-response effectiveness for opthalmic beta blockage of ciliary epithelial anion channel: activities of metipranolol and L-bunolol metabolite compared to timolol. Invest Ophthalmol Vis Sci 1989;107:1308–1311.
78. Polansky JR: Side effects of topical ophthalmic therapy with anti-inflammatory steroids on β-blockers. Curr Op Ophthalmol 1992;3:259–272.
79. Polansky JR, Cherksey BD, Alvarado JA: Update on β-adrenergic drug therapy. In: Pharmacology of Glaucoma. SM Drance, EM Van Buskirk, AH Neufeld, eds. Baltimore, MD: Williams and Wilkins, 1992:301–321.

Medications Used in Chronic Glaucoma Therapy

13

The Miotics (Cholinergic Agonists)

David L. Epstein

Miotics, or more appropriately termed muscarinic (cholinergic-acting) agonists, have been used in the treatment of the glaucomas for more than a hundred years. It is noteworthy in our perspective that our understanding and discrimination between open angle and angle closure glaucoma has been widely recognized for only the past 50 or 60 years (Paul Chandler was an important voice in teaching this differentiation). Cholinergic-acting agonists are miotics, but this effect on the pupil is of significance only in the acute treatment of angle closure glaucoma due to pupillary block. For the chronic treatment of primary open-angle glaucoma (POAG), pupillary miosis (and accommodation) are for most patients unwanted side effects that frequently contribute to the need to discontinue the medication.

Miotics are classified as weak (e.g., pilocarpine or carbachol) or strong (e.g., echothiophate iodide). The former refers to direct-acting acetylcholine-mimicking drugs that bind directly to the receptor site, whereas the latter refer to indirect acting (acetylcholinesterase) enzyme inhibitor drugs that allow the endogenous normal transmitter, acetylcholine, to accumulate at the receptor site.

In acute angle closure glaucoma, the miotic effect of pilocarpine, the most commonly used agent, may decrease pupillary block at the level of the pupil by this miotic action on the usually semidilated pupil. But probably just as important is the drug acting to pull the iris out of the angle and to increase iris tension, that then resists more the increased pressure in the posterior chamber found in pupillary block. A more detailed description of these complicated potential vectors is found in Chapter 22, but at the level of the pupil, these cholinergic drugs may increase pupillary block if there is excessive miosis (the pupil is more closely apposed to the convex forward crystalline lens), and if the cholinergic effect on the ciliary muscle results in ciliary muscle contraction and release of zonular tension that can allow the crystalline lens to move forward to the pupil and thus actually increase pupillary block. **On occasion, patients with underlying primary open angle glaucoma thus can develop a superimposed angle closure component from the use of "miotic" therapy.** Hence, gonioscopy should be repeated in patients who have POAG and are taking miotic therapy.

In patients with POAG or with chronic forms of (noninflammatory) secondary open angle glaucoma such as exfoliation, the mechanism of IOP lowering by "miotics" has nothing to do with the pupillary effect. It is due to the contraction of the longitudinal portion of the ciliary muscle, which inserts on the scleral spur. The latter is adjacent to, and receives also the insertion of, the trabecular meshwork (see Chapter 2). **The IOP lowering effect of miotics is due almost exclusively to the outflow effect produced by mechanical traction by the longitudinal ciliary muscle on to the scleral spur and thus the trabecular meshwork.** Anatomically the spaces within the trabecular meshwork are altered and are more "open" under the influence of cholinergic therapy (1). Experimentally, when the ciliary muscle is disinserted from the scleral spur, cholinergic drugs do not improve outflow (2). (The latter observation also might have potential relevance to the clinical conditions of cyclodialysis or angle recession, although likely the overall circumferential extent of these conditions might be an important determiner of cholinergic drug efficacy.)

Some have described small effects of cholinergic-acting drugs on reducing aqueous humor formation or a potential direct effect on the trabecular meshwork. These proposed alternative actions deserve further evaluation, but the existing data strongly indicate that the effects of these muscarinic drugs on outflow are mainly mechanical from longitudinal ciliary muscle contraction. The latter action likely produces little adverse effects, except perhaps for the risk of mechanical traction on attachments to the ora serrata potentially leading to detachment of the retina. Unfortunately, it is not (yet) possible to have drugs that exert cholinergic effects on only this longitudinal portion of the ciliary muscle [although some have argued that aceclidine exerts a preferential effect on the longitudinal muscle (3)]. The necessary accompanying contraction of the circular and other portions of the ciliary muscle from cholinergic-

MIOTIC-INDUCED ANGLE CLOSURE

David L. Epstein

In discussing a miotic-induced angle closure component to an open angle glaucoma, Chandler and Grant wrote: "In cases of open-angle glaucoma in which the angle is very narrow, the strong miotics may in rare instances precipitate acute angle closure glaucoma. In eyes in which the angles were very narrow and the strong miotics are contraindicated, one tries to maintain control with weaker miotics and other medications. However, if it becomes necessary to choose between using the strong miotics or operating, one may sometimes take a chance on closure of the angle with the stronger miotics. In the eyes of one of us (PAC), the angle was extremely narrow, but when a stronger miotic was needed for control of IOP, weak echothiophate iodide was first tried. Later 0.25% was used. If the angle had closed, we were prepared for peripheral iridectomy. However, another patient might not be so understanding and so ready to accept the consequences if the angle is closed." (Of course, today we would advise performing prophylactic iridectomies in patients with potentially occludable angles.)

acting drugs produces accommodation and thus commonly unacceptable symptoms of visual blurring and myopia. In young patients, myopia-producing effects are frequently intolerable.

On the other hand, many presbyopic patients achieve a re-establishment of their near point, and if the accompanying miosis does not adversely affect their visual function (by cutting down light entering the eye, especially at night), and there are not excessive problems with the required frequency of drug administration or ocular irritation, many patients accept this therapy. **Like miosis, the effect on accommodation is not part of the IOP-lowering mechanism (and therefore not necessary for efficacy). The therapeutic efficacy is due to the contraction of the longitudinal portion of the ciliary muscle, which is mechanically connected to the trabecular meshwork via the scleral spur.**

Contraction of the ciliary muscle may obliterate some of the extracellular spaces available for uveo-scleral outflow and thus cause a decrease in outflow by this unconventional outflow pathway (4,5). Although theoretically this is both interesting and potentially important (Chapter 3), from a clinical point of view this potential phenomenon has little influence on how to treat POAG. If patients can tolerate the potential side effects of cholinergic-acting drugs and the inconvenience of the usual frequent administration (although see later for discussion of pilocarpine gel and the Ocusert), such "miotics" can be effective in lowering IOP by this mechanical outflow mechanism.

Considering the effect of miotics on anterior chamber depth and its mechanism of action, it does not come as a surprise that there are several forms of glaucoma that are not amenable to miotic therapy or are worsened by it (Table 13.1). Forms of angle closure glaucoma in which axial shallowing, such as malignant glaucoma or that following an acute central retinal vein occlusion, are worsened by miotics. Additionally, neovascular and inflammatory forms of secondary angle closure glaucoma are not amenable to miotic treatment.

Miotics have many ocular side effects that should be considered before and after initiating therapy (Table 13.2).

VISUAL SIDE EFFECTS OF MIOTICS

In patients with early cataractous lens changes, especially those close to the visual axis, miotic therapy can be visually disabling. In such patients who are well controlled on miotic therapy but have visual disability, the substitution of laser trabeculoplasty for miotics should be considered (assuming there are no other topical antiglaucomatous therapy options that could be tried first). The patient's objective and subjective vision should be assessed when miotic therapy has been stopped for a few days, if possible. Less desirable is to assess this after pupillary dilatation (which unfortunately itself, likely due to light scattering, may make cataract symptoms worse). It is useful to ask the patient about their visual function in the morning before putting their miotic drops in, for this may offer a clue as to the role of the miotics in the visual disability. In patients with early cataract formation, a substitution strategy for miotic therapy is often effective in delaying the need for cataract surgery, and thus allowing longer time for the glaucoma status to be evaluated (for example, time often can help answer the question whether cataract surgery alone or, in fact, combined cataract and filtration surgery is required).

OCULAR SIDE EFFECTS OF MIOTICS

In addition to the effects of miosis and accommodation (which by allowing the crystalline lens to move forward might have adverse effects beyond the visual, e.g., pupillary block and susceptibility to malignant glaucoma-type syndromes), cholinergic-acting drugs appear to increase vascular permeability and perhaps thereby induce some type of "pre-inflammatory" predisposition in certain eyes.

Table 13.1
Contraindications for Miotics

Contraindication	Comment
Secondary angle closure glaucomas	Worsens angle closure by shallowing anterior chamber (miotics produce forward movement of lens-iris diaphragm)
Malignant glaucoma	
Status post vitreoretinal surgery	
Status post PRP or retinal cryopexy	
Status post CRVO (acute)	
Secondary to sulfa drugs	
Associated with ciliary body swelling	
Uveitic glaucoma	Increases inflammation, may paradoxically increase IOP
Neovascular glaucoma	Increases inflammation, may produce hyphema, ineffective
Trauma (recent, with inflammation)	Increases inflammation, increases ciliary spasm and pain

These drugs should not be used in inflammatory glaucoma, and in fact may have paradoxical effects on IOP (one of the rules discussed previously is that if a patient with presumed POAG is placed on a miotic and demonstrates an increase in IOP, as always when there is an increase in IOP, gonioscopy should be repeated, with the suspicion of an induced angle closure component or an accentuated occult inflammatory trabeculitis). Furthermore, subsequent to chronic miotic therapy, at the time of surgery in addition to "small pupil" problems and suspected increased iris rigidity, the eyes are more injected, there is greater postoperative inflammation and sustained breakdown of the blood-aqueous barrier, and there is greater subconjunctival inflammation and potential scarring at the filtration site. Thus there is this clinical sense, that perhaps has been somewhat overstated, that chronic miotic therapy is not "good" for the eye.

One of us (DLE) shares this "gestalt." It also must be stated that glaucoma itself is probably not "good" for the eye, and sometimes neither is glaucoma surgery. If miotics can reasonably control the IOP in patients with various forms of open angle glaucoma, then the risk/benefit considerations indicate that this therapy should not be avoided. We are dealing again with the humbling realization that all of our treatments for glaucoma are nonspecific and have potential down-sides. Many patients appreciate the induced near point visual side effects and the pinhole effect on overall visual acuity from the miosis (except at night). Yet, there is legitimacy to the dissatisfaction that clinicians feel with the use of long-term cholinergic therapy.

Systems Side Effects

Systemic side effects from cholinergic agents (except for the use of cholinesterase inhibitors-see below) are uncommon. The most frequently seen systemic side effects are gastrointestinal, which seem to be a direct cholinergic ef-

Table 13.2
Adverse Effects of Miotics

Adverse Effect	Cause	Comment
Dimmed vision	Miosis Pre-existing cataract	Reduce concentration of miotic Trial of "slow release" miotic (Ocusert or pilocarpine gel) Strong miotics may induce cataract formation and should not be used in phakic patients
Brow ache	Ciliary muscle spasm	Symptoms usually transient if mild, reassure patient Always initiate miotic therapy with ½ to 1% pilocarpine (or carbachol equivalent) Strong miotics should only be started after pilocarpine treatment and at a low initial dose (0.03–0.06% echothiophate iodide)
Reduced visual acuity	Induced myopia Cataract	Refract patient Young patients (< 40 years) prone to induced myopia Trial low concentration miotic (½% pilocarpine), Ocusert, or pilocarpine gel Strong miotics should not be used in phakic patients (cataractogenic)
Floaters Change in visual field	Vitreous detachment Retinal detachment	Dilated exam of lens, vitreous (pigment/RBC's), and retina (rule out retinal detachment)
Increased IOP (paradoxical response to therapy)	Occult ocular inflammation Induced angle closure	Slit lamp exam for anterior segment inflammation Gonioscopy to establish angle open or closed and examine for KPS or PAS
Ocular irritation or epiphora	Drug allergy or toxicity Cicatricial pemphigoid	Examine lids, conjunctiva and cornea (punctual occlusion, follicles, corneal epithelial changes, and fornices for evidence of ocular cicatricial pemphigoid) Rule out keratitis sicca

ACETYLCHOLINESTERASE

David L. Epstein

Acetylcholine, which is commonly released at cholinergic nerve terminals in the eye, is normally inactivated by the enzyme, acetylcholinesterase. Inhibitors of the latter enzyme allow acetylcholine to accumulate at the receptor site and thus produce a cholinergic "miotic" effect of long duration. Such acetylcholinesterase enzyme inhibitors have been used as systemic nerve gases (1) or insecticides (where presumably they are lethal as a result of sustained cholinergic stimulation). It is remarkable that such agents in dilute concentrations have found use topically as antiglaucomatous agents, but, with respect for the ocular cholinergic side effects, such cholinesterase inhibitor therapy can be very effective in, for example, pseudophakic or aphakic eyes. This observation, on the one hand, makes one wonder whether all of our current glaucoma therapy is not, in fact, applied "toxicology," but on the other hand teaches us the importance of dose–response relationships and therapeutic indexes in the development of all new glaucoma medications (or for any disease). Any drug at a high enough dosage can have substantial side effects. When we screen for new drugs, we commonly use high concentrations looking for large effects (because they are easier to detect initially).

One wonders how many potentially useful drugs may have been missed because of such screening techniques. The first attempts to study topical cholinesterase inhibitor therapy to the eyes of rabbits produced a lethal result!

Reference

1. Rengstorff RH: Vision and ocular changes following accidental exposure to organophosphates. J Appl Toxicol 1994;14:115–8.

fect and likely results from drug reaching the alimentary channels directly through luminal connections from the throat. The latter derives from the topical drug reaching the nasolacrimal duct. Often this symptom responds well to punctal occlusion (or gentle eyelid closure). Theoretically, this cholinergic symptom could result also from systemic absorption (that would obviously not be responsive to punctal occlusion strategies), and despite the efficacy of punctal occlusion diminishing this symptom, such systemic absorption might be more involved than first appreciated. Rarely, cholinergic bladder symptoms have been observed from topical miotic therapy, and cerebral influences that are frequently viewed positively by the rare patients who believe they are so affected. The latter has been observed more with the use of cholinesterase inhibitors than with short-acting miotics in our (DLE) experience. Certain cholinergic therapies may positively slightly influence mental function in Alzheimer's disease (6). Regardless, the bottom line for the clinician is that one should be alert to the possibility of systemic cholinergic symptoms in patients on topical cholinergic therapy to the eye, especially the cholinesterase inhibitors, although these are decidedly uncommon.

CHOLINESTERASE INHIBITORS

The short acting "miotics" are cholinergic acting drugs that mimic and theoretically might compete at the receptor with endogenously released acetylcholine, which is the usual transmitter at cholinergic sites in the eye. Such potential competition of cholinergic drugs with acetylcholine for the receptor, while theoretically possible, does not occur from a practical clinical point of view. Cholinesterase inhibitors and cholinergic drugs are not negatively interactive on IOP (7); in fact, in some small minority of patients, there is slight additivity.

Significant systemic absorption of a topical ocular drug can occur. Therefore, it is not surprising that this happens also with cholinesterase inhibitors. The clinician should be alert to the potential for gastrointestinal, urological, or cerebral cholinergic side effects, although these are uncommon. However, what is common with the use of topical acetylcholinesterase inhibitors is the inhibition of cholinesterase activity in the blood (8). For some forms of general anesthesia, certain agents such as succinylcholine are used and require the blood enzyme for inactivation. Therefore, anesthesiologic consultation should be obtained preoperatively, and the anesthesiologist should be informed ahead of time to "flag" the chart as to the use of topical cholinesterase inhibitors. **It may require several months of cessation of such ocular therapy for blood levels of cholinesterase to return to normal.** Fortunately, many alternatives exist in the choice of general anesthesia, but the anesthesiologist needs to know ahead of time about the use of this type of medication in patients who have glaucoma.

Potential Retinal Complications

Presumably because the ciliary muscle sends extensions of its tendon to the ora serrata, there is the potential for retinal complications with use of these cholinergic agents as a result of mechanical tension from the muscle's contraction.

As part of the routine of full ophthalmological evaluation of the glaucoma patient, indirect ophthalmoscopy should be performed, with special attention to the retinal periphery looking for pre-existing retinal pathology that might be adversely affected by the mechanical actions of miotics. As part of the routine follow-up of patients with glaucoma, the pupil is periodically dilated not only to examine the optic nerve head but also to re-examine the retina.

Patients receiving miotics are told of potential symptoms of "flashes, floaters, curtains, etc." Although rare, retinal tears can occur with weak miotic therapy, e.g., pilocarpine (9). In fact, posterior vitreous detachment may occur more commonly after even weak miotic therapy than is often appreciated. It would make sense, and clinically seems to be the case, that the risk goes up with increasing concentration of miotic and therefore with use of the stronger miotics, i.e., cholinesterase inhibitors.

The potential for such rare side effects is perhaps another reason why the miotics are no longer the drug of first choice for POAG. But as discussed, even with these general cholinergic effects on the eye, these agents are still effective medications. As with all glaucoma medications, they have risk/benefit considerations that need to be appreciated by the clinician and discussed with the patient ahead of time.

Whether patients with previous retinal detachment and successful repair should be treated with strong miotics is an interesting question that requires retinal specialist consultation. Retina specialists have given their approval provided they are satisfied with the result of the retinal surgery. Thus, although these strong miotics should still be a drug of last resort, we have used them effectively in such patients. Such patients need continuing evaluation by a retina colleague.

For patients with a predisposition to retinal detachment whether due to significant myopia or identified retinal thinning, avoid these stronger miotics unless absolutely necessary. Again retinal consultation is strongly advised, and only the weakest effective solution should be used.

STRATEGIES IN CHOICE/USE OF MIOTICS

Weak Miotics

Pilocarpine is the usual first choice of miotic eye drop. Several preparations differ only in the choice of salt, buffer, preservatives, or other constituents added for comfort. Strengths of pilocarpine range from ½% to 6 %. Some glaucoma clinicians have argued that the maximally effective concentration may occur at concentrations less than 4%, whereas others have argued that 6% is probably the top of the dose response curve. There is individual variability but we believe that for most patients, except those with heavily pigmented irides, 4% is likely the clinically meaningful top of the dose response curve, and that lesser concentrations are not. Also, although 6% concentration may be slightly more effective in certain heavily pigmented non-Caucasian eyes, for practical purposes, 4% pilocarpine is still the highest concentration used except perhaps for individuals with severe glaucoma.

Even in patients in whom it is anticipated that higher strengths of pilocarpine will be required, one should still start with low strengths of ½ or 1% to allow the patient to adapt to the anticipated initial ciliary spasm. "Headaches" and "brow aches" due to miotics are common, and the clinician should spend time explaining this to the patient (e.g., "the drug makes the muscle next to the drain contract and open the spaces, and like any muscle that hasn't been used fully, some initial cramping ("Charlie horse") is to be anticipated"). These symptoms should abate after the first day or so. The patient should be told to call if they do not, or if there are any other symptoms such as flashes and floaters, etc.

It is also very useful for the clinician to assess the IOP lowering efficacy of 1% pilocarpine. Sometimes there is a surprisingly large IOP effect. In fact, many years ago a "pilocarpine drop test" for glaucoma was described in which in patients with "true glaucoma," a large decrease in IOP was anticipated. It is not certain in the era of this "pilocarpine drop test" whether all forms of chronic angle closure were well differentiated from open angle glaucoma, and there is likely great individual variability, regardless, in IOP reduction in POAG patients from miotics. The clinical point is that some patients with POAG are very responsive to lower strengths of pilocarpine. It is not possible to predict what strength of pilocarpine will be required in the individual patient. In some cases of POAG, perhaps just a slight mechanical "widening" (1) of whatever the critical space is in the outflow pathway is enough, at least initially, to substantially improve the outflow of aqueous humor from the eye.

One of the major problems with pilocarpine and short-acting cholinergic-acting agonists is the short duration of drug effect. This necessitates a need for frequent instillation, usually four times a day for pilocarpine, which represents medication every 6 hours. Patients do not have to wake up at night after 6 hours of sleep to instill the drop, but it is surprising how many patients, in fact, do this due to inadequate initial instruction! However, while the patient is awake, the drops should be spaced as far apart as possible, approximately every 6 hours. During sleep, aqueous humor formation decreases in most individuals and IOP is usually lower (Chapter 3), thus rationalizing why awakening from nighttime sleep for the potential administration of cholinergic outflow drops is not necessary. Nevertheless, there is the possibility of an IOP spike after 6 hours of sleep. Patients should administer the morning drop soon after awakening.

Clinically some patients behave as if the maximum IOP effect from pilocarpine lasts only 4 hours, and we have seen some clinicians with good documentation therefore

DRUG THERAPY COMPLIANCE

David L. Epstein

Compliance is a real issue for the frequent dosing regimen required with weak miotic therapy. Kass has documented the surprising magnitude of this problem in glaucoma therapy with the use of a special electronic monitoring eye bottle (1–3). But the clinician by simple means can also sometimes gain insight into this issue. Examination and recording of pupil size is an important part of the eye examination (Chapter 5). For example, although the degree of miosis induced by these agents may be variable among different individuals, it should be consistent within the same patient. One often finds that the pupil is somewhat larger at a subsequent visit, and it takes specific physician probing to uncover the fact that the patient (who usually wants to actually please the glaucoma clinician), failed to take the medication, at least on the day of the visit. One patient told us that she did not want to hurt her physician's feelings by telling him that she could not take her medication routinely! It goes without saying that, given the short duration of IOP effect from such therapy, failure to take the medication on the day of examination will cause an unexpectedly higher IOP. Some patients, unless counseled otherwise, routinely will omit their drops on the day of examination, this for a variety of reasons that reflect miscommunication ("the doctor puts in his own drops at the visit," "it interferes with the examination," etc.).

Patients on miotic therapy (truly, all glaucoma patients) need specific instructions (see Fig. 18.1) about these issues and about inquiry into actual medication usage. Poor compliance is a common cause of fluctuating IOP. We are aware of cases in which the clinician prescribed a miotic, but the patient, due to confusion, did not take it, and this was not picked up by the office personnel until a referral consultation was arranged, at which time, it was observed that the pupil was not miotic! Thus, the recording of the pupil size is an important part of the glaucoma examination.

References

1. Kass MA, et al: Compliance with topical pilocarpine treatment. Am J Ophthalmol 1986;101:515–23.
2. Kass MA, Gordon M, Meltzer DW: Can ophthalmologists correctly identify patients defaulting from pilocarpine therapy? Am J Ophthalmol 1986;101:524–30.
3. Kass MA, et al: Compliance with topical timolol treatment. Am J Ophthalmol 1987;103:188–93.

prescribe pilocarpine drops six times a day! We as clinicians need to appreciate how disruptive frequent drop regimens are to a patient's life style. In fact, most patients do not adhere to a QID dosage regimen (10,11). For such patients with an apparent shorter time of clinical efficacy from cholinergic therapy, one should consider a higher strength of the drug, in fact up to 6%, or perhaps, more reasonably, the use of pilocarpine ointment at night supplemented with pilocarpine drops during the day.

The need for such frequent dosing with miotics is because, pharmacodynamically, active drug is cleared from the effector site after this time interval. The other side of this issue is that very high concentrations of the drug, therefore, are applied to the eye initially because of this rapid decay. Unfortunately, this likely leads to some of the general side effects.

This rapid decay phenomenon of pilocarpine may be amenable to therapeutic innovation, and there have been several attempts. Carbachol needs to be given only every 8 hours (12). Three percent carbachol is equivalent to 4% pilocarpine. Carbachol may not penetrate the cornea (13) as well as pilocarpine in certain patients, and therefore the IOP-lowering efficacy as well as dosing frequency needs also to be established for the individual patient. However, for some patients, carbachol three times a day can be an effective and acceptable regimen. Carbachol can also be used for those who are allergic to pilocarpine.

Pilocarpine Ocusert Therapy

The Ocusert (Alza Pharmaceuticals, Palo Alto, CA) (14) (Fig. 13.1) is a continuous delivery device in which a low level of pilocarpine is constantly released into the tear film over the period of a week. Because of the low (but steady) concentration of pilocarpine in the eye at any one time, effects on miosis and accommodation are minimized (and stable), but IOP lowering effects are maintained. In most patients the pilo-40 Ocusert is equivalent to 2 to 4% pilocarpine, although in some patients the IOP lowering efficacy is less. We have had a satisfying experience with Ocusert therapy in young patients with glaucoma (who are often well motivated to use this form of therapy).

However, there are some drawbacks to Ocusert therapy; it is more expensive than pilocarpine drops, retention of the Ocusert in the eye is often a problem for most patients during the initial experience with the device, and especially some elderly patients seem to have great difficulty with placement, retention, and removal of the device long term. **For best results with the Ocusert form of therapy, it is important for the ophthalmologist or trained**

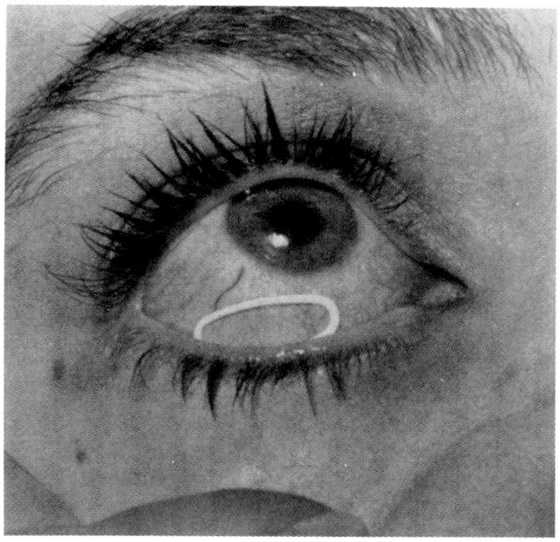

Figure 13.1. The pilocarpine Ocusert is a useful form of glaucoma therapy in young patients who cannot tolerate pilocarpine eye drops. For success, the physician or his staff should spend time personally instructing the patient in its use.

personnel to spend considerable time with the patient in teaching the placement and removal of the device.

Theoretically, the Ocusert is a wonderful solution to the previous issues because it provides sustained low levels of pilocarpine continuously over a week. For young patients with glaucoma, e.g., those with pigmentary glaucoma, it can seem almost a "miracle" if the patient previously has experienced the induced visual problems with pilocarpine drops. Young patients also have a high probability of success with the Ocusert. But because most patients with glaucoma are elderly and have problems with insertion and retention of this "one size fits all" device, they are not very successful with this regimen, unless highly motivated and possessing good hand to eye coordination.

(As an aside it is remarkable how difficult it is for most elderly glaucoma patients to put eye drops in their eyes themselves with the common inversion bottle, even if they possess fairly good hand-to-eye coordination. Many patients require the drops to be administered by spouses or relatives who may not live in the same house! The problems with self-medication with existing eye drop bottles is an underappreciated public health issue that should be addressed by industry.)

Pilocarpine Gel

Another potential solution to this problem of required frequent dosing with the shorter acting miotics has been the development of 4% pilocarpine gel (Pilopine, Alcon, Ft. Worth, TX), which was designed to be administered once a day at bedtime and provide 24-hour IOP lowering (15). In truth, this does represent an important advance, which has both efficacy and reasonable patient acceptance. Some patients do not like putting a gel (ointment) in their eye even at bedtime because of visual blurring later at night, which can persist into the morning. Clinically, there is considerable individual variability among patients in the "liquefaction " of the gel by the normal tear production. Some patients complain that no matter how little gel (16) they put in at night, there is constant blurring the next day. On the other hand, many patients tolerate the regimen without any complaint.

Of course in this ointment form, it is still 4% pilocarpine that is being placed in the eye. Some patients report less visual disturbance than with pilocarpine drops, and especially the absence of vision fluctuation. Nevertheless, unlike the pilocarpine Ocusert, the pupil does become and remain miotic on the 4% gel similar to 4% pilocarpine drops, and there is maintained accommodation in young patients.

Another issue with pilocarpine gel is that although originally designed to provide 24 hours of reduction of IOP and thus alleviate the need for pilocarpine drops during the day, there is individual variation in this effect, and many patients require supplemental pilocarpine drops at "trough" times, beginning 12 or more hours later (15). Still, the need for one or perhaps two supplemental drops of pilocarpine later the next day to maintain maximal IOP lowering is an advance over a 4 or more drop a day regimen. Also, it needs to be remembered that although potentially not providing maximal IOP lowering by itself for a full 24 hours in many patients, there is usually some submaximal IOP effect for the full 24 hours. With the known compliance problems in patients with use of pilocarpine drops (10,11), this sustained, although perhaps submaximal, effect has important therapeutic significance. In fact, in some patients with difficult glaucoma to control either perhaps because of compliance issues or the potential shortened time of pilocarpine drug efficacy to only 4 hours (possibly indicating a need for six times a day therapy at first glance), simply adding 4% pilocarpine gel at bedtime and maintaining the four times a day pilocarpine drop regimen, which is mostly but not always complied with, is a strategy that one of us (DLE) quite commonly employs.

When pilocarpine gel was first introduced a fine corneal haze was observed in several patients; that was initially a cause for concern (17). There was no effect on vision, and there have been no reported long term sequelae (18). This corneal haze seemingly has been observed less commonly more recently.

Strong Miotics

The stronger acting miotics, which for practical clinical purposes are restricted now to the acetylcholinesterase inhibitors, Phospholine Iodide (echothiophate iodide) and Humorsol (demecarium bromide), require less frequent instillation, usually only once a day (but occasionally twice

LIMITED DURATION OF ACTIVITY OF PHOSPHOLINE IODIDE

David L. Epstein

The limited duration of activity of Phospholine Iodide once prepared, and occasionally the failure of a pharmacy to mix up the solution fresh when needed, have important implications for glaucoma patient management. For example, in patients who over a prolonged period seem well controlled on Phospholine Iodide therapy, but then suddenly appear with otherwise unexplained elevation of IOP, among other issues, inactive drug should also be suspected, and prior to other maneuvers, the patient should be treated with a fresh new bottle of Phospholine Iodide, after other ocular causes for the IOP elevation have been ruled out. This strategy has quite commonly (but not always) reestablished the previous steady state. This phenomenon especially seems to occur during periods of the summer when patients carry their medication with them. Phospholine Iodide should normally be refrigerated, and with the potential for once a day dosage this should not greatly inconvenience the patient. It is useful always to ask the patient how much of the bottle has been used, and how long ago was the prescription filled.

a day). However, the potential for side effects are much greater with these agents than with the weaker miotics. In phakic eyes, these cholinesterase inhibitors are definitely cataractogenic (19,20), and therefore, these agents are avoided in phakic eyes. **However, for pseudophakic or aphakic eyes, acetylcholinesterase inhibitors can be dramatically effective and actually patient-friendly in terms of the frequency of instillation and ocular tolerance.** These agents provide greater IOP reduction than the shorter-acting miotics such as pilocarpine (21). In pseudophakic or aphakic eyes, these agents should be used (at least in a weak strength) after other topical medications are used, before consideration of filtration surgery. (It is equivocal whether laser trabeculoplasty with a more guarded prognosis for efficacy in such eyes should be tried before or after a trial of such strong miotic therapy, although most clinicians would probably proceed with laser trabeculoplasty first.)

Because these strong miotics produce greater and more sustained ciliary muscle contraction, and thereby presumably greater mechanical traction on the retina, there seems to be a greater risk of retinal detachment than with the use of the weaker miotics. The need for a detailed retinal examination on all glaucoma patients has already been mentioned. In addition, this issue of potential retinal complications needs to be specifically discussed with the patient, who is advised about warning signs and symptoms. Nevertheless, the risk/benefit considerations are such that although the risk of retinal detachment is real (although small), it certainly is appropriate to try these agents before filtration surgery, with full informed consent.

In phakic eyes, anticholinesterase agents are not used, even before filtration surgery, except with a poor surgical prognosis. Since the cataractogenic effect is dose related, the weakest strength possible of the medication should be used first in such eyes for IOP control.

Humorsol is slightly less potent than Phospholine Iodide. It probably needs to be given twice a day, but a potential advantage is that the solutions are more stable than Phospholine Iodide, which must be refrigerated, and can be carried at all times by the patient. Humorsol is prepared in 0.125 and 0.25% strengths.

Phospholine Iodide must be prepared fresh from powder, has a limited length of activity, and should be refrigerated. It is probably the most potent miotic and probably needs to be administered only once a day, at higher dosages (0.125% and 0.25%). However, this needs to be established for the individual patient by assessing IOP in the "trough" period at a time greater than 12 hours after dosage. Because it is an iodide, there is the potential for greater ocular sensitivity, and the possible rare occurrence of a pemphigoid-like ocular syndrome (22,23), which exists for all miotics but seems slightly greater for Phospholine Iodide. This has been hypothesized by Grant possibly to be due to this iodide content.

Phospholine Iodide is prepared in solution strengths from 0.03 to 0.25%. The 0.06% strength should be evaluated initially, although we have the distinct clinical impression that 0.25% represents maximum potency.

It is important to state again that even if it is extremely likely that a drug such as Phospholine Iodide will be required for miotic therapy, patients should still start with weaker and then subsequent greater strengths of pilocarpine or equivalent to allow adaptation to the ciliary muscle contraction. Placing a drug such as Phospholine Iodide on the eye that has not been previously treated with miotics causes acute ciliary spasm and severe pain that is almost always intolerable to the patient.

As mentioned, because cholinesterase inhibitors such

as Phospholine Iodide act pharmacologically to allow endogenously produced acetylcholine to accumulate and act at the receptor, one might have anticipated that a muscarinic drug such as pilocarpine would compete for the same receptor and interfere with the Phospholine Iodide IOP-lowering action. This does not in fact happen (8), and occasionally there seems to be a slight additivity that might be meaningful in a patient with severe disease. Therefore, a strategy that one of us (DLE) sometimes uses in advanced glaucoma cases is simply to add Phospholine Iodide at bedtime (once a day) to the continued pilocarpine regimen. On the one hand, this might result in some additivity, but on the other, should the Phospholine Iodide decay towards the end of the bottle, the patient still maintains a cholinergic drug effect from the pilocarpine.

Strong miotics may produce cysts at the pupillary margin which may be innocuous or produce visual symptoms. These are less common with weaker strengths of drug and perhaps with Humorsol. They can be successfully treated with weak solutions of phenylephrine if the patient needs to be maintained on the strong miotic.

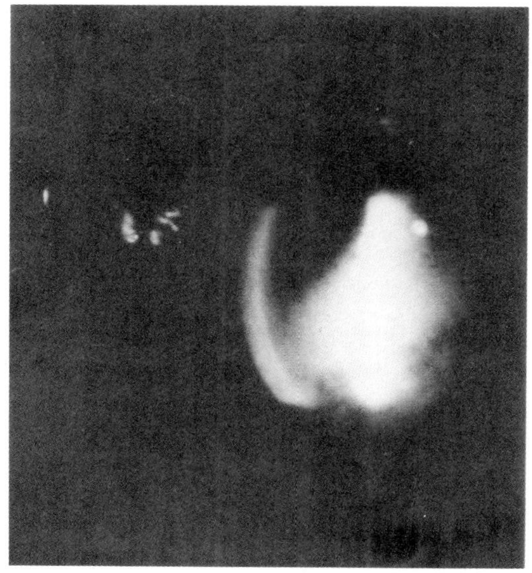

Figure 13.2. Atypical central band keratopathy believed to be due to the mercurial preservative used in certain older preparations of pilocarpine.

Ocular Irritation/Sensitivity from Miotics: Pemphigoid-Like Syndrome

All of the miotics may in certain individuals produce ocular allergy or sensitivity that is usually characterized by injection, but also papillary and follicular conjunctival reactions that may mimic and be misinterpreted as an allergy to an epinephrine-like compound, such as Propine. Corneal abnormalities including rare keratinization-type reactions have been observed. In previous times, an atypical band keratopathy (24) was observed in glaucoma patients on one particular brand of pilocarpine that was due to a phenylmercuric nitrate preservative (Fig. 13.2).

Depending on the severity, the first strategy for a presumed pilocarpine allergy might be to switch to a different brand, since commonly it is one of the other ingredients in the eye drop such as the preservative that is responsible for the sensitivity. Nevertheless, true allergies to pilocarpine itself do exist and if the miotic is efficacious for IOP (see above), carbachol should be tried and usually demonstrates little cross sensitivity (although the patient may be still intolerant of the usual miotic visual effects that are not a drug sensitivity).

The iodide in Phospholine Iodide may be sensitizing in some patients. We and others (22) have observed the occurrence of an ocular pemphigoid-like syndrome in patients on Phospholine Iodide therapy, which seems likely drug-related (e.g., unilateral cases with unilateral drug treatment). The exact incidence of this is unknown since many patients with primary ocular pemphigoid may develop POAG (23). Likely this drug-induced pemphigoid syndrome is rare, but this is another reason why such strong agents are drugs of last resort. On the other hand, this pemphigoid syndrome has also been reported after pilocarpine therapy (although our impression is much less commonly than with Phospholine Iodide), suggesting that it may represent a rare cholinergic effect. Laboratory experiments suggest that cholinergic drugs can stimulate conjunctival and corneal epithelial cell proliferation (25).

An important clinical point is that as part of one's routine ophthalmological examination, retraction of the lower lid with **examination for early symblepharon formation should be performed in all glaucoma patients** (not just those on miotics-other occurrences may thus for the first time be noted by the clinician).

In discussing glaucoma drug sensitivity, Chandler and Grant wrote:

> "Drug sensitivity not infrequently develops in patients under various forms of treatment for glaucoma. The most common manifestation of drug sensitivity is dermatitis of the lids, with drying and wrinkling of the skin of the lids, particularly the lower lid. In other cases there is no involvement of the skin of the lids but there is a beefy, fiery redness of the conjunctiva, especially in the lower fornix, usually with enlargement of conjunctival follicles. These sensitivity reactions disappear shortly after the offending drug is discontinued.
>
> A rare reaction that we have seen in only two patients developed after long-term use of pilocarpine. It consisted of a haziness of the corneal epithelium with superficial vascularization extending onto the cornea from all sides and causing marked reduction of vision. In these two cases, there were no other specific signs of drug sensitivity, except that the eyes were generally red. Improvement could be noted within 48 hours when pilocarpine was stopped. The following is a description of one of these two cases.

Case 13-1. A 77-year-old patient had been receiving treatment with pilocarpine for 8 years. IOP was right and left 17, the field in the right eye was almost full with a 10-mm test object, but there was considerable loss of field in the left eye. Fundi could not be seen. Vision was right 15/200, left, 120/200. The eyes were red with enlarged follicles in the lower fornices. The conjunctiva had a sort of opaque milky appearance. The entire cornea was hazy in both eyes due to an epithelial disturbance. With a flashlight, the surface of each cornea presented a fine ground-glass appearance. Superficial vessels came in from all sides almost to the border of a 2-mm pupil. Drops were discontinued, and within 48 hours there was considerable subjective improvement. One week later vision was right and left 6/18. A fine haze persisted in the central area of the corneas, but the blood vessels became bloodless "ghost" vessels. When the corneas cleared sufficiently, it could be seen that both discs had pathologic cupping, but most of the persisting reduction of vision was due to nuclear lens opacity rather than glaucoma. Even without further treatment, the IOP ranged only from 15 to 19 mm Hg, and the patient maintained useful vision for several remaining years of his life.

> In this case, whether the corneal and conjunctival reaction was due to the pilocarpine itself or to the chlorobutanol preservative was not determined."

ACECLIDINE

There has been periodic enthusiastic interest, especially in Europe, in this cholinergic drug, which seems in some studies to lower the IOP but not produce as many accommodative type symptoms as pilocarpine (although interestingly, miosis is reportedly similar with the two drugs) (3,26). Theoretically, if one could cause more localized contraction of the longitudinal portion of the ciliary muscle and spare the other portions, one might be able to separate the outflow effects of cholinergic drugs from their accommodative effect. There has been interest in whether there may be muscarinic receptor subtype differences in different portions of the ciliary muscle that could be exploited pharmacologically (27). However, there is the suspicion that the reported submaximal effects of this drug in certain concentrations on accommodation (again the reader needs to remember the concepts of dose-response relationships) may be accompanied by submaximal IOP effects and thus not truly represent selective cholinergic targeting of different portions of the ciliary muscle. Nevertheless, investigation toward such a selective longitudinal ciliary muscle drug should continue because it would have much merit.

MIOTICS DURING CATARACT SURGERY

Intraoperative carbachol has reduced the incidence of severity of IOP elevation occurring shortly after cataract surgery (28,29).

References

1. Grierson I, Lee WR, Abraham S: The effects of topical pilocarpine on the morphology of the outflow apparatus of the baboon (Papio cynocephalus). Invest Ophthal Vis Sci 1979;18:346.
2. Kaufman PL, Barany EH: Loss of acute pilocarpine effect on outflow facility following surgical disinsertion and retrodisplacement of the ciliary muscle from the scleral spur in the cynomolgus monkey. Invest Ophthalmol Vis Sci 1976;15:793.
3. Erickson-Lamy K, Schroeder A: Dissociation between the effect of aceclidine on outflow facility and accommodation. Exp Eye Res 1990; 50:143–147.
4. Bill A: The effects of pilocarpine on the dynamics of aqueous humor in a primate (Macaca irus). Invest Ophthalmol Vis Sci 1966;5:170–175.
5. Bill A: Effect of atropine and pilocarpine on aqueous humour dynamics in cynomolgus monkeys (Macaca irus). Exp Eye Res 1967;6:120–125.
6. Gray JA, Enz A, Spiegel R: Muscarinic agonists for senile dementia: past experience and future trends. Trends Pharmacol Sci 1989.
7. Kini MM, et al: Echothiophate, pilocarpine, and open angle glaucoma. Arch Ophthalmol 1973;89:190–2.
8. Ellis PP, Esterdahl M: Echothiophate iodide therapy in children. Effect upon blood cholinesterase levels. Arch Ophthalmol 1967;77:598.
9. Puustjarvi T: Retinal detachment during glaucoma therapy. Review. A case report of an occurrence of retinal detachment after using membranous pilocarpine delivery system [Pilokarpin lameller (Ocusert) 11 mg]. Ophthalmologica 1985;190:40–4.
10. Kass MA, et al: Compliance with topical pilocarpine treatment. Am J Ophthalmol 1986;101:515–23.
11. Kass MA, Gordon M, Meltzer DW: Can ophthalmologists correctly identify patients defaulting from pilocarpine therapy? Am J Ophthalmol 1986;101:524–30.
12. O'Brien CS, Swan KC: Carbaminoylcholine chloride in the treatment of glaucoma simplex. Arch Ophthal 1942;27:253.
13. Smolen VF, Clevenger JM, Williams EJ, et al: Biophasic availability of ophthalmic carbachol I: mechanisms of cationic polymer- and surfactant-promoted miotic activity. J Pharm Sci 1973;62:958.
14. Quigley HA, Pollack IP, Harbin RS Jr: Pilocarpine ocuserts. long-term clinical trials and selected pharmacodynamics. Arch Ophthalmol 1975; 93:771.
15. Johnson DH, et al: A one year multicenter clinical trial of pilocarpine gel. Am J Ophthalmol 1984;97:723–9.
16. Fechtner RD, Piltz JR, Starita RJ: A technique for accurate application of pilocarpine gel. Ophthalmic Surg 1988;19:823.
17. Johnson DH, Kenyon KR, Epstein DL, et al: Corneal changes during pilocarpine gel therapy. Am J Ophthalmol 1986;10:13–5.
18. Nagasubramanian S, Stewart RH, Hitchings RA: Long term effects of glaucoma therapy with 4% pilocarpine gel on corneal clarity and endothelial cell density. Int Ophthalmol 1994;18:5–8.
19. Axelsson U, Holmberg A: the frequency of cataract after miotic therapy. Acta Ophthalmol 1966;44:421.
20. Thoft RA: Incidence of lens changes in patients treated with echothiophate iodide. Arch Ophthal 1968;80:317.
21. Reichert RW, Shields MB: Intraocular pressure response to the replacement of pilocarpine or carbachol with echothiophate. Graefes Arch Clin Exp Ophthalmol 1991;229:252–3.
22. Patten JT, Cavanagh HD, Allansmith MR: Induced ocular pseudopemphigoid. Am J Ophthalmol 1976;82:272.
23. Tauber J, Melamed S, Foster CS: Glaucoma in patients with ocular cicatricial pemphigoid. Ophthalmology 1989;96:33–37.
24. Kennedy RE, Roca PD, Platt DS: Further observations on atypical band keratopathy in glaucoma patients. Trans Am Ophthalmol Soc 1974;72: 107–122.
25. Cavanagh HD, Colley AM: Cholinergic, adrenergic, and PGE1 effects on cyclic nucleotides and growth in cultured corneal epithelium. Metab Pediatr Syst Ophthalmol 1982;6:63–74.

26. Keren G, Treister G: Effect of aceclidine (+) isomer and pilocarpine on the intraocular pressure decrease and the miosis in glaucomatous eyes. Effect on accommodation in normal eyes of young subjects. Ophthalmologica 1980;180:181–7.
27. Zhang X, Hernandez MR, Yang H, et al: Expression of muscarinic receptor subtype mRNA in the human ciliary muscle. Invest Ophthalmol Vis Sci 1995;36:1645–1657.
28. Ruiz RS, Rhem MN, Prager TC: Effects of carbachol and acetylcholine on intraocular pressure after cataract extraction. Am J Ophthalmol 1989; 107:7–10.
29. Wedrich A, Menapace R: Intraocular pressure following small-incision cataract surgery and polyHEMA posterior chamber lens implantation. A comparison between acetylcholine and carbachol. J Cataract Refract Surg 1992;18:500–5.

14

Carbonic Anhydrase Inhibitors (CAIs)—Systemic Use

David L. Epstein

INTRODUCTION

By virtue of their ability to reduce aqueous secretion and thereby lower intraocular pressure (1), regardless of the nature or extent of obstruction to outflow, carbonic anhydrase inhibitors (CAIs) can be useful in the treatment of all the glaucomas.

The mechanism of their action appears to be the inhibition of bicarbonate secretion into the posterior chamber by the ciliary epithelium (2). In the past, CAIs were effective in treating glaucoma only when given systemically, but a topical agent has been developed that has the potential to broadly increase the use of this form of therapy. This will be discussed in the next chapter. As with any new agent, topical CAI agents need to be continuously evaluated by the clinician, both in terms of safety and efficacy. For example, the enzyme, carbonic anhydrase, is important for the corneal endothelium pumping function (3), and the topical application of such drugs will continuously and progressively "bathe" the corneal endothelium with this enzyme inhibitor as the drug passes into the anterior chamber (this phenomenon is true for all topical drugs). Yet so far, no adverse effects on the corneal endothelium have been reported. Nevertheless, as the use of topical CAIs increases, we need to pay special attention to patients with pre-existing corneal endothelial disease.

Another issue is whether the topical CAI drugs will produce maximal IOP lowering, equivalent to that of systemic agents. Such comparative evaluation will possibly finally answer the question of the role of metabolic acidosis, induced by systemic CAIs (4), in the reduction of IOP. (Of course, another issue is whether equivalent drug levels at the ciliary epithelium will be achieved with topical compared with systemic CAI therapy.) Finally, because the rare systemic side effects affecting the bone marrow that occur with systemic administration of CAIs can be either idiosyncratic or dose-related, the experience with topical beta blockers suggests the need for appropriate surveillance for rare idiosyncratic systemic side effects after topical use of CAIs.

Nevertheless, despite this appropriate precaution, as for any new glaucoma agent, topical CAIs represent an important new part of our antiglaucoma armamentarium that promises to have broad applicability even though CAIs are not fully additive to topical beta blocker therapy (5).

The following discussion relates to the oral use of CAI agents with which we have had broad experience and which likely will still continue to be used, although hopefully with decreased frequency, with the advent of topical CAI therapy.

Oral carbonic anhydrase inhibitors are potent antiglaucoma agents that are truly the drug of last resort because of the potential for serious, even life-threatening systemic side effects (6). Therefore, in pseudophakic eyes, strong miotics, despite all their limitations and concerns, are usually preferred to the oral CAIs. **In general, laser trabeculoplasty should be performed before use of oral CAIs.** Also, for unilateral uncontrolled glaucoma (assuming a good fellow eye) other options should be fully explored first. Yet oral CAIs are responsible for the prevention of blindness in many patients with glaucoma.

The CAIs are useful in certain secondary glaucomas to protect the eye from damage by the glaucoma until the underlying cause of the glaucoma is removed. Special considerations are involved in use of these drugs in angle-closure glaucoma. These considerations are discussed in Chapter 22. In all cases of progressive adult open-angle glaucoma we currently use oral CAI treatment in addition to standard maximal topical antiglaucoma drugs prior to considering surgery. What is written here concerns principally the use of CAI agents in the management of chronic glaucoma when various agents are to be considered. It does not include treatment of acute glaucoma, for which acetazolamide, in addition to timolol, is often utilized because of rapid action and because the course of treatment is so brief that problems of side effects are few.

Some glaucoma patients tolerate oral CAI therapy well and can be maintained on long-term therapy. However, 30 to 50% of patients are unable to take CAI medications for prolonged periods because of unpleasant and sometimes debilitating side effects. The most common side effect that results in discontinuation of long-term oral CAI therapy is **a symptom-complex of malaise, fatigue, weight loss, anorexia, depression, and often loss of libido.** Patients who have this malaise symptom complex often state that they feel "awful," "don't care whether they live or die," and that they would rather go blind than continue with this type of drug. **We have seen such patients unnecessarily hospitalized for extensive evaluation for occult**

malignancy or other disease suspected because of severe loss of weight and appetite.

The occurrence of such malaise-type symptoms is often associated with the development of systemic metabolic acidosis. All patients undergoing chronic oral CAI therapy develop systemic acidosis, but the patients with these symptoms are generally more acidotic than other patients (4). Sometimes, in stoic patients on long-term oral CAI therapy, the degree of metabolic acidosis is alarming and may lead to hospitalization on a medical ward.

Many conflicting statements have been made concerning potassium supplementation in patients on long-term oral CAI therapy. We have found that patients receiving CAI treatment tend to have only small decreases in serum potassium and the decrease in patients who have the malaise-type side effects is no different from that in patients who do not. However, patients who are concurrently taking oral CAI agents for glaucoma and a diazide diuretic for systemic hypertension often develop a large decrease in serum potassium and frequently require potassium supplementation. In such patients who have become frankly hypokalemic, potassium supplementation may alleviate some of their side effects, but in patients who are taking only CAI and no thiazide, we have found no appreciable benefit from potassium supplementation, and we do not employ it.

Some patients on chronic CAI therapy develop symptoms of abdominal distress: cramping, epigastric burning, nausea, irritation, and diarrhea. These gastrointestinal side effects, unlike the malaise symptom-complex, seem to be unrelated to the degree of metabolic acidosis. These gastrointestinal disturbances seem to be local irritative phenomena and have often responded to a simple change in regimen, such as administering the CAI with food, changing to a slow-release oral CAI preparation, or adding alkaline antacid therapy. Patients with a history of gastrointestinal disease who are on CAI therapy sometimes develop symptoms that are refractory to all attempts at relief. It is curious that CAI therapy may be expected to reduce secretion of hydrochloric acid in patients with peptic ulcer, yet such patients may not tolerate CAI therapy because of aggravation of their abdominal symptoms.

Paresthesias often occur during oral CAI therapy, but these are usually transient and only rarely are a cause for discontinuing of CAI agents. We have no explanation for their occurrence.

Patients need to be informed that CAIs do at first cause an acute diuresis, but this is short lasting.

THERAPEUTIC REGIMENS

The following are currently popular dosages of oral CAI: acetazolamide (Diamox [Lederle, Wayne, NJ]) tablets, 250 mg q.i.d.; acetazolamide slow-release capsules (Diamox Sequels [Lederle, Wayne, NJ]), 500 mg b.i.d.; and methazolamide (Neptazane [Lederle, Wayne, NJ]) tablets, 50 mg b.i.d. to t.i.d.

Methazolamide has a longer duration of action and probably needs to be administered only twice a day (7), but it is slower in onset of action than acetazolamide. Accordingly, in acute glaucoma oral acetazolamide rather than methazolamide is usually employed. Only acetazolamide is available in a form for intravenous administration.

Some ophthalmologists have the impression that methazolamide less often causes side effects than does acetazolamide, but in terms of regulating the patient's glaucoma it may be that currently employed dosages of methazolamide correspond to less than the maximum customary dosage of acetazolamide (7,8).

We have demonstrated that for maximal lowering of intraocular pressure, a dosage of methazolamide of at least 75 to 100 mg b.i.d. is required (7). This, unfortunately, produces a significant increase in side effects. It is not yet clear whether methazolamide has an advantage over acetazolamide with respect to severity of side effects when dosages that have truly equivalent influences on IOP are employed. On the other hand, **methazolamide produces less metabolic acidosis than does acetazolamide, even at therapeutically equivalent dosages.**

There are reports in the literature pointing to the effectiveness of low dosages of oral CAI agents in glaucoma therapy. Although it is true that intraocular pressure can be reduced somewhat by low dosages, such as 25 mg of methazolamide twice a day, it is incorrect to believe that such low dosages result in maximal lowering of intraocular pressure. A dosage of methazolamide of at least 75 to 100 mg b.i.d. is required for maximal lowering of intraocular pressure (Fig. 14.1). Of course, in starting treatment for chronic glaucoma with this drug it is reasonable to place the patient on only 25 to 50 mg methazolamide b.i.d. and observe the effect. If the glaucoma is not too advanced and IOP not too high, a satisfactory lowering of pressure may be obtained with such a low dosage. If greater pressure lowering is then required, the dosage should be increased unless side effects are excessive.

One acetazolamide slow-release capsule daily (which may be better tolerated in the individual patient) produces a significant lowering of intraocular pressure that lasts 24 hours (Fig. 14.2), although the magnitude of the pressure lowering during the second 12 hours is often less than with twice-a-day slow-release capsule dosage (9). Nevertheless, such a single daily slow-release capsule dosage may produce an IOP effect in the second 12 hours equivalent to that of methazolamide 50 mg b.i.d. Therefore, it is often useful to initiate therapy with once-a-day dosage of slow-release capsule and assess pressure lowering 12 to 24 hours following a dose (9,10). One acetazolamide slow-release capsule taken orally b.i.d. appears as effective as acetazolamide 250 mg. tablets taken q.i.d (9).

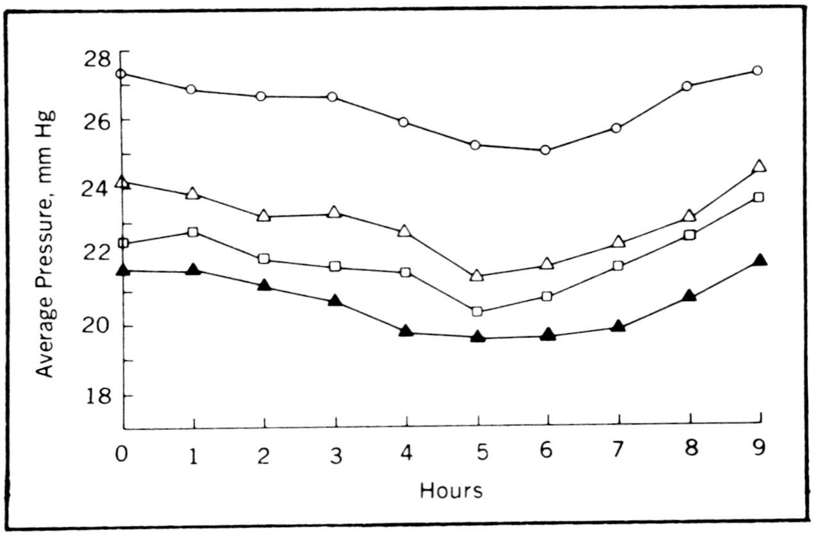

Figure 14.1. Effect of methazolamide dosage 3 times a day on IOP in patients who have glaucoma. Note an increasing effect with increasing dosage. Open circles-baseline; open triangles -25 mg; open squares-50 mg; closed triangles-100 mg. (We subsequently learned that methazolamide only needs to be given twice a day.) From Dahlen K, Epstein DL, Grant WM, et al: A repeated dose response study of methazolamide in glaucoma. Arch Ophthalmol 1978;96:2214–2218.

PRECAUTIONS; SIDE EFFECTS

CAIs should be given with caution and probably in lower dosages to patients with chronic respiratory acidosis. Such patients with chronic emphysema or bronchitis normally develop a compensatory metabolic alkalosis. As mentioned previously, CAIs produce a metabolic acidosis (4) which can interfere with these compensatory mechanisms.

Occasional patents who are receiving standard dosages of CAIs agents develop extraordinarily high serum levels of the agent (4,8,11). These patients are particularly prone to disabling malaise-type symptoms. In some such patients a decrease in dosage has resulted in a reduction of side effects, and there has been no apparent worsening of intraocular pressure (4,8).

The frequency with which serum levels higher than needed are to be found in patients with malaise-type symptoms is not yet known, but we think that excessive serum levels probably account for only a minor proportion of these symptoms. Appropriate serum levels need to be better defined. Without sufficient knowledge of the serum levels it seems reasonable in all patients with side effects to make an arbitrary trial of reducing the oral CAI dosage, but in the majority of such patients the effectiveness of regulation of the glaucoma can be expected to suffer.

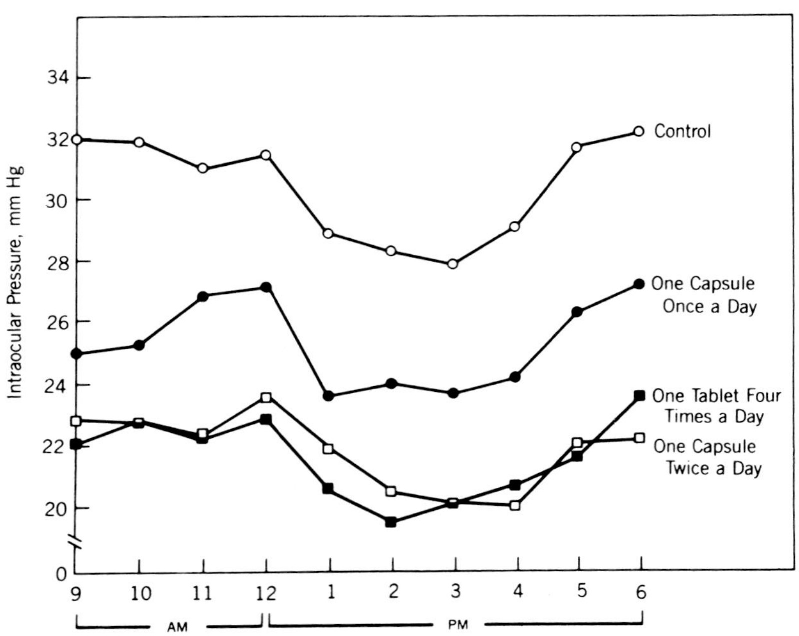

Figure 14.2. Comparison of different dosage regimens of acetazolamide in patients who have glaucoma. For one sequel a day therapy, measurements are 14 to 23 hours after that dosage. For such a once a day 500 mg sequel therapy, a 23-hour IOP lowering occurs that is submaximal during the second 12 hours. Two 500 mg sequels a day are equivalent to four 250 mg tablets. From Berson FG, Epstein DL, Grant WM, et al: Acetazolamide dosage forms in the treatment of glaucoma. Arch Ophthalmol 1980;98:1051–1054.

An extraordinarily high serum level of acetazolamide can occur occasionally in patients who are receiving standard dosage and have renal impairment, due presumably to the fact that acetazolamide is entirely excreted in the urine and is not metabolized. This is especially important in diabetic patients with retinopathy and neovascular glaucoma. These patients should be given lower than standard dosages of oral CAI agents. When methazolamide is used, renal function is of less obvious concern, because only 25% of methazolamide is known to be excreted unchanged in the urine. The fate of the remaining 75% is unknown, but presumably it is metabolized (12).

Some patients without renal impairment, as indicated by normal serum creatinine levels, also develop extraordinarily high serum levels of CAI, with no obvious cause. The elderly may be especially prone to this occurrence (11). The relationship between dosage and serum level may vary strikingly from patient to patient. Lehmann has observed that as much as a six-fold difference in acetazolamide dosage may be required to achieve a given plasma level in different patients (13).

There are a significant number of glaucoma patients for whom the benefits and risks of chronic oral CAI therapy are a preferable alternative to those of filtration surgery. Hopefully, the number of such patients will decrease with the introduction of topical CAIs. In managing patients with disabling malaise-type CAI side effects, we find the following serum chemical analyses sometimes useful: creatinine, potassium, CAI level, CO2-combining power, and chloride (4,8). Serum creatinine identifies patients with impaired renal function who should be given lower than standard dosages of oral CAI. Serum potassium helps identify those patients who are on concurrent diuretic therapy and may require potassium supplementation. The CAI level identifies those patients with apparently higher than needed serum levels of the medication, in whom a reduction in dosage is indicated. (Unfortunately, facilities for CAI serum assays are available in very few laboratories.) Serum CO2-combining power and chloride identify possible excessive acidosis as a cause of the side effects.

In excessively acidotic patients with normal serum CAI levels, preliminary studies indicate some effectiveness of additive alkali (sodium acetate) therapy in relieving symptoms (4,8,14). However, such alkali therapy potentially can lead to other symptoms such as renal stones or possibly gout, and we therefore have not pursued this strategy further, except for the very rare patient with no other therapeutic options.

Severe metabolic acidosis has been reported in some patients taking CAI and salicylates (15).

There remain significant numbers of patients who are unable to tolerate long-term oral CAI therapy. Although we have some understanding of the reason for these side effects, we still have much to learn, and newer approaches to their treatment are required.

We are intrigued by the fact that there are certain glaucoma patients who do not respond to CAI therapy with a significant lowering of intraocular pressure despite proven serum levels of the CAI agent that are therapeutically effective for other patients (7). Naturally, once it is established that a patient's IOP is not reduced, despite a serum level that should be adequate, there is no point in pursuing this form of treatment.

Kidney stones develop occasionally during oral carbonic anhydrase inhibitor therapy and are believed to be a result of calcium precipitation secondary to decrease of citrate (16) and/or magnesium excretion in the urine. The decrease of urinary citrate is thought to be a direct consequence of drug-induced metabolic acidosis. Ophthalmologists have had the impression that the incidence of kidney stones is lower with methazolamide than with acetazolamide, and, in fact, recent studies have documented less reduction of urinary citrate by methazolamide (at low dosages) than by acetazolamide (7).

Management of patients with kidney stones involves use of methazolamide in as low dosages as the severity of the glaucoma permits, restriction of dietary calcium, and use of concomitant chlorothiazide diuretics to alter the calcium/magnesium ratio in the urine. Several of our patients who have developed kidney stones on CAI therapy have been proved to have idiopathic hypercalciuria and have responded well to dietary calcium restriction. Nephrologic consultation and measurements of urinary pH, calcium, and citrate should be obtained in those patients who develop renal stones on CAIs.

A review of more uncommon side effects of CAI medications is available (6). One of the most worrisome is that of **bone marrow suppression and aplastic anemia, which can be fatal and which can occur with methazolamide** (17-19) **as well as acetazolamide.** This may result from either dose-related or idiosyncratic type of reactions. It is currently controversial whether CBC (complete blood count) profiles should routinely be performed in patients on oral CAI therapy (18). Patients need to be informed about these potential rare complications, and at a minimum, to report quickly any "sores" or lesions that do not heal, easy bruisability, etc. The issues are the cost effectiveness of routine blood profiles for this rare occurrence, and the ability to detect it by testing (18), since many cases are idiosyncratic in origin. At the current time, there is no clear answer to this question except for the clinician to do as if he/she were the patient, i.e., treat the patient as one would want one's self to be treated. Hopefully, the introduction of topical CAI therapy will reduce the frequency of occurrence of this rare but devastating side effect.

EFFICACY OF CAIs IN PATIENTS ON BETA BLOCKER THERAPY

Since both CAIs and timolol decrease aqueous humor secretion, it is reasonable to ask whether these effects are fully or only partially additive. We have observed that when

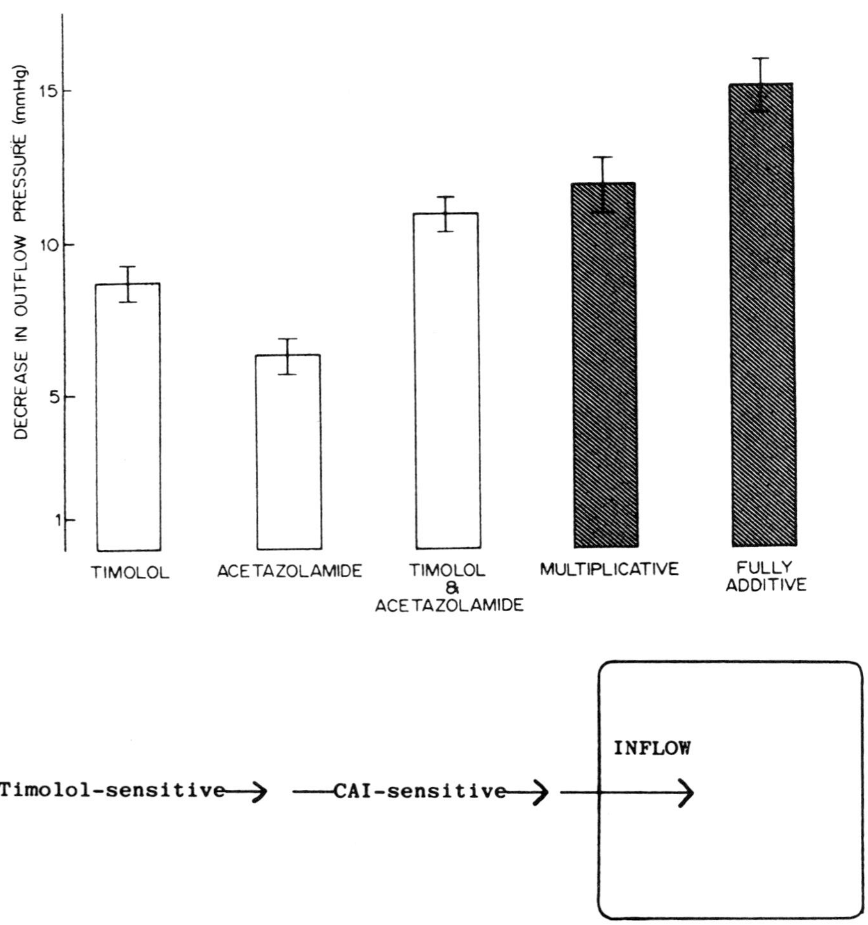

Figure 14.3. Observed (clear bars) and theoretical (slashed bars) additive effect of timolol and oral acetazolamide in glaucoma patients (top). The two drugs are not fully (independently) additive, and this suggests an inter-relationship of effects (bottom). From Berson FG, Epstein DL: Additive effect of timolol and acetazolamide in the treatment of open-angle glaucoma. Am J Ophthalmol 1981;92:788–791.

timolol and oral CAI are used together, there is greater IOP lowering than with either agent used singly, but the **apparent effects are not fully additive,** suggesting some interrelationship of carbonic anhydrase and beta adrenergic mechanisms in aqueous humor secretion (Fig. 14.3) (5,20,21).

References

1. Brubaker RF: Flow of aqueous humor in humans. Invest Ophthalmol Vis Sci 1991;32:3145–3166.
2. Maren TH: The rates of movement of Na^+, Cl-, and HCO_3^- from plasma to posterior chamber: effect of acetazolamide and relation to the treatment of glaucoma. Invest Ophthalmol 1976;15:356–364.
3. Bonanno JA: Bicarbonate transport under nominally bicarbonate-free conditions in bovine corneal endothelium. Exp Eye Res 1994;58: 415–421.
4. Epstein DL, Grant WM: Carbonic anhydrase inhibitor side effects. Serum chemical analysis. Arch Ophthalmol 1977;95:1378–1382.
5. Berson FG, Epstein DL: Additive effect of timolol and acetazolamide in the treatment of open-angle glaucoma. Arch Ophthalmol 1981;92: 788–791.
6. Grant WM: Antiglaucoma drugs: Problems with carbonic anhydrase inhibitors. In: Symposium on Ocular Therapy. Edited by I.H. Leopold. St. Louis, C.V. Mosby, 1973.
7. Dahlen K, Epstein DL, Grant WM, et al: A repeated dose response study of methazolamide in glaucoma. Arch Ophthalmol 1978;96:2214–2218.
8. Epstein DL, Grant WM: Management of carbonic anhydrase inhibitors side effects. In: Symposium on Ocular Drug Therapy. Edited by I.H. Leopold and R.P. Burns. New York, John Wiley and Sons, 1979: 51–64.
9. Berson FG, Epstein DL, Grant WM, et al: Acetazolamide dosage forms in the treatment of glaucoma. Arch Ophthalmol 1980;98:1051–1054.
10. Berson FG, Epstein DL: Carbonic anhydrase inhibitors. Perspect Ophthalmol 1980;4:91–95.
11. Charpron DJ, Gomolin IH, Sweeney KR: Acetazolamide blood concentrations are excessive in the elderly: propensity for acidosis and relationship to renal function. J Clin Pharmacol 1989;29:348–53.
12. Maren TH, Haywood JR, Chapman SK, et al: The pharmacology of methazolamide in relation to the treatment of glaucoma. Invest Ophthalmol 1977;16:730–742.
13. Lehmann B, Linner E, Wistrand PJ: The pharmacokinetics of acetazolamide in relation to its use in the treatment of glaucoma and to its effects as an inhibitor of carbonic anhydrases. In: Schering Workshop in Pharmacokinetics. Edited by G. Raspe. Oxford, Pergamon Press, 1969.
14. Arrigg CA, Giovanoni R, Epstein DL, et al: The influence of supplemental sodium acetate on carbonic anhydrase inhibitor-induced side effects. Arch Ophthalmol 1981;99:1969-1972.
15. Cowan RA, Hartnell GG, Lowdell CP, et al: Metabolic acidosis induced by carbonic anhydrase inhibitors and salicylates in patients with normal renal function. Br Med J (Clin Res Ed) 1984;289:347–348.

16. Higashihara E, Nutahara K, Takeuchi T, et al: Calcium metabolism in acidotic patients induced by carbonic anhydrase inhibitors: responses to citrate. J Urol 1991;145:942–8.
17. Werblin TP, Pollack IP, Liss RA: Blood dyscrasias in patients using methazolamide (Neptazane) for glaucoma. Ophthalmology 1980;87: 350–4.
18. Mogk LG, Cyrlin MN: Blood dyscrasias and carbonic anhydrase inhibitors. Ophthalmology 1988;95:768–71.
19. Cohen AM, Prialnik M, Ben-Nissan DS, et al: Methazolamide-associated temporary leukopenia and thrombocytopenia. DICP 1989;23:58–9.
20. Dailey RA, Brubaker RF, Bourne WM: The effects of timolol maleate and acetazolamide on the rate of aqueous formation in normal human subjects. Am J Ophthalmol 1982;93:232–7.
21. McCannel CA, Heinrich SR, Brubaker RF: Acetazolamide but not timolol lowers aqueous humor flow in sleeping humans. Graefes Arch Clin Exp Ophthalmol 1992;230:518–20.

Topical Carbonic Anhydrase Inhibitors

15

Joel S. Schuman

Carbonic anhydrase inhibitors (CAIs) have been used since 1954 in the treatment of glaucoma, following the description of their efficacy for this purpose by Becker (1) and Grant (2). Despite the fact that these agents reduce intraocular pressure (IOP), their use has been limited by side effects (3) such as malaise, fatigue, weight loss, depression, anorexia, paresthesias, loss of libido, as well as more severe side effects and toxicities, including abdominal cramping, gastric burning and irritation, nausea, diarrhea, kidney stones, teratogenicity, bone marrow depression, and even potentially fatal side effects such as aplastic anemia. To reduce the adverse effects associated with these agents, creative use has been made of alkalinizing agents, such as bicarbonate or sodium acetate, to decrease the symptom complex related to the metabolic acidosis induced by CAIs (3–5). Even with this adjunctive therapy, however, oral CAIs have found limited use in the chronic treatment of glaucoma, primarily because they are poorly tolerated by patients.

As an attempt to capture the beneficial IOP lowering action of CAIs, while minimizing their adverse effects, a topical CAI (TCAI) that could decrease IOP without producing the harmful consequences of the oral agent has long been sought. The quest for such a preparation extends back to Grant's initial publication on acetazolamide, when he found that topical or subconjunctival application of the drug was ineffective in reducing IOP (2). Over the ensuing years, several compounds were investigated for this purpose, with little success. Some of the more successful agents included dichlorphenamide, which reduced IOP in rabbits (6), ethoxzolamide analogues (7–11), ethoxzolamide gel and suspension (10–13), methazolamide and benzolamide analogues (8,9), and a compound called L-645,151, which produced corneal reactions in animals precluding its use in humans (14). Each of these agents was investigated thoroughly, but was found to be either ineffective, hazardous, or too irritating for topical use. Many of these investigations involved Thomas Maren, who also played a key role in the development of carbonic anhydrase inhibitors for systemic use.

In 1988, a breakthrough occurred, with the introduction of MK-927, a new TCAI specifically formulated for the eye produced by Merck, Sharp and Dohme Research Laboratories (15). This agent proved to be effective in humans and to be well tolerated (15–26). The first publication regarding this compound reported a 30% reduction in IOP (with a 7.2% IOP reduction in the contralateral eye) (15). Further well-designed, double-masked randomized, placebo-controlled, multicenter studies on this drug demonstrated efficacy and safety, with a peak effect approximately 2 hours after TCAI administration (16–21,23–28).

Laboratory investigation showed that this agent entered the eye not only through the cornea, but primarily via a nonaqueous, transscleral route at the limbal region (28,29). Although many of the other agents investigated for this purpose did not penetrate the eye well, after topical application, MK-927 could be found in the corneal stroma, aqueous and ciliary processes (20). Ocular penetration was most likely related to the property of the drug as an ampholyte, capable of ionizing into anionic and cationic forms. Further, the plasma concentration of the drug after a single topical ocular administration was less than 1 μM in rabbits, while at least 2 to 10 μM plasma concentration would be required for physiological effects. This indicated that systemic toxicity should be minimal or absent (20), which has been confirmed in further human studies (27,30).

Because MK-927 was a racemic mixture, its enantiomers were studied, and its s-enantiomer, MK-417 (sezolamide), was slightly more effective in IOP reduction than MK-927 itself (22, 31–33), similar in activity to timolol 0.5% (34). In a highly controlled study, sezolamide was administered over a 2-week period to healthy volunteers receiving a controlled diet; no significant changes were noted in blood or urine parameters of the subjects (27).

The most recent advance in TCAI development was the introduction of MK-507 (dorzolamide, Fig. 15.1) (26,30,35–47). Dorzolamide decreased IOP to a marginally greater degree than sezolamide (35,36,41), and was proven effective in reducing aqueous production in monkeys (45) and humans (Fig. 15.2) (46), and in reducing IOP

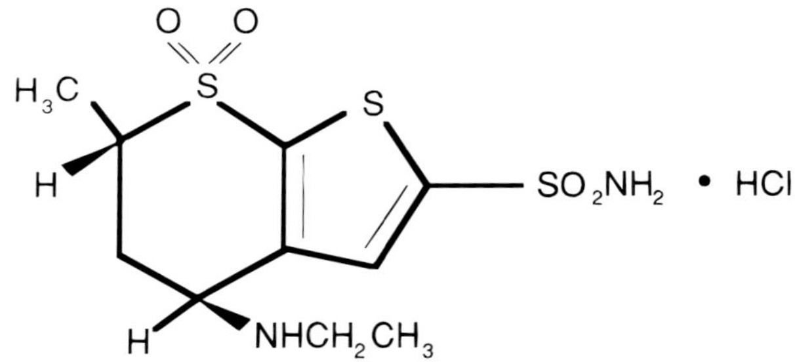

Figure 15.1. The chemical structure of dorzolamide (Trusopt).

Authors	Year	Study Duration	No. Pts*	Dosing Regimen	% IOP Reduction Trough	Peak‡	12 hours§
Bourgeois et al[5]	1990	6 Days	49	2%, bid	7.3%	17.5%	12.0%
Lippa et al[21]	1991	4 Days	82	2%, bid	19.1%†	24.4%	14.8%
				2%, tid	18.0%	26.8%	19.3%
Lippa et al[19]	1992	5 Days	73	2%, bid	18.0%†	21.8%	12.5%
				1.4%, bid	13.4%	21.7%	9.5%
				0.7%, bid	12.9%	21.4%	10.2%
		7 Days		2%, tid	21.1%	22.2%	19.2%
				1.4%, tid	16.8%	22.1%	14.2%
				0.7%, tid	17.6%	24.2%	18.9%
Kitazawa[16]	1993(A)¶	52 Weeks	98	1%, tid	15.6%†	21.2%	----
Lippa et al[20]	1993(A)¶	6 Weeks	332	0.2%, tid	9.2%†	12.5%	----
				0.7%, tid	14.1%	17.5%	----
				2.0%, tid	14.1%	17.2%	
Wilkerson et al[45]	1993	28 Days	48	2%, tid	13.3%†	18.4%	----
Strahlman et al[37]	1994(A)¶	One year	523	2%, tid	16.9%§‖	22.9%	----

* Represents the total number of patients enrolled in the study, not the total number of patients on the regimen indicated, as some patients may have been treated with placebo, other drugs, or other concentrations.
† Trough IOP is measured just before morning dosing.
‡ Peak IOP is measured 2 hours following the morning dosing.
§ IOP measured 12 hours following the morning dosing.
‖ Trough IOP is measured 8 hours after morning dosing.
¶ (A) Indicates year of publication of abstract if otherwise unpublished.

Figure 15.2. Clinical evaluations of dorzolamide (MK-507). From Serle JB, Podos SM: Topical carbonic anhydrase inhibitors in the treatment of glaucoma. Ophthalmol Clin North Am 1995;8:315–325.

in glaucomatous monkeys (26). Dorzolamide had activity comparable to 0.5% timolol in monkeys as well (44). Another study showed that the IOP reducing activity of dorzolamide was similar to betaxolol (39). The effect on IOP of dorzolamide was demonstrated to be dose dependent, with approximately a 20% reduction in IOP compared with placebo (40,42,47). When added to timolol 0.5% or to maximal medical therapy, dorzolamide provided an additional 13–21% reduction in IOP (Fig. 15.3) (43).

In toxicity studies in humans, dorzolamide had no effect on corneal thickness, corneal endothelial cell count, blood chemistry, hematology, urinalysis, or electrocardiogram after 4 weeks of drug administration (30). Tolerability was similar to timolol.

	Mean IOP (mm Hg)	±SEM	IOP Reduction (%)	No. of Patients
Day 1	19.6	1.9	-	16
Week 1	14.1*	0.9	28	16
Month 1	15.7*	1.0	24	16
Month 2	16.0	1.1	20	15
Month 8	15.3	1.4	12	8
Month 12	14.0	2.0	13	4

* IOP significantly different from study day 1, before beginning therapy with dorzolamide, by paired *t* test, $P < 0.05$.

Figure 15.3. Effect of 2% dorzolamide administered two or three times daily on IOP in glaucoma patients on maximum tolerated medical therapy not receiving systemic carbonic anhydrase inhibitors. From Serle JB, Podos SM: Topical carbonic anhydrase inhibitors in the treatment of glaucoma. Ophthalmol Clin North Am 1995;8:315–325.

Despite the findings in the toxicity studies, concern still remains, at least theoretically, regarding the effect of the TCAI on a compromised corneal endothelium. **The drug should be used with caution in patients with Fuchs' corneal dystrophy and other endotheliopathies.** Further, since aplastic anemia with oral carbonic anhydrase inhibitors is a rare idiosyncratic reaction, there is no reason to expect that it will not occur with a topical CAI, and it is not surprising that it has not been seen to date.

Dorzolamide was approved by the United States Food and Drug Administration in December 1994 for use in the treatment of glaucoma in humans, and was given the tradename, Trusopt (Merck and Co., West Point, PA). In all likelihood, dorzolamide will take its place in the glaucoma pharmacopaeia as a second-line drug, for use after beta-blockers, but before miotic agents. Because dorzolamide is a three-times-a-day drug, beta-blockers still maintain a dosing advantage, but the TCAI has the benefit of not inducing miosis, myopia or causing headache. Surely, over time, more side effects, and perhaps further toxicity, will be noted with dorzolamide, but at this point, it remains a promising and useful new agent for use in lowering IOP.

References

1. Becker B. Decrease in intraocular pressure in man by a carbonic anhydrase inhibitor, Diamox. A preliminary report. Am J Ophthalmol 1954; 37:13.

2. Grant WM, Trotter RR. Diamox (acetazolamide) in treatment of glaucoma. Arch Opthalmol 1954;51:735.
3. Epstein DL, Grant WM. Carbonic anhydrase inhibitor side effects. Serum chemical analysis. Arch Opthalmol 1977;95:1378.
4. Arrigg CA, Epstein DL, Giovannoni R, et al. The influence of supplemental sodium acetate on carbonic anhydrase inhibitor-induced side effects. Arch Ophthalmol 1981;99:1969.
5. Epstein DL, Grant WM. Management of carbonic anhydrase inhibitor side effects. Leopold & Burns, ed: Symposium on Ocular Therapy, John Wiley & Sons, Inc., 1979;II:51–64.
6. Lotti VJ, Schmitt CJ, Gatheron PD. Topical ocular hypotensive activity and ocular penetration of dichlorphenamide sodium in rabbits. Graefes Arch Clin Exp Ophthalmol 1984;222:13-19.
7. Schoenwald RD, Eller MG, Dixson JA. Topical carbonic anhydrase inhibitors. J Med Chem 1984;27:810–812.
8. Maren TH, Jankowska L. Ocular pharmacology of sulfonamides: the cornea as barrier and depot. Curr Eye Res 1985;4:399–408.
9. Maren TH, Bar-Ilan A, Caster KC, et al. Ocular pharmacology of methazolamide analogs: distribution in the eye and effects on pressure after topical application. J Pharmacol Exp Ther 1987;241:56–63.
10. Lewis RA, Schoenwald RD, Eller MG, et al. Ethoxzolamide analogue gel. A topical carbonic anhydrase inhibitor. Arch Ophthalmol 1984; 102:1821–1824.
11. Kalina PH, Shetlar DJ, Lewis RA, et al. 6-Amino-2-benzothiazole-sulfonamide. The effect of a topical carbonic anhydrase inhibitor on aqueous humor formation in the normal human eye. Ophthalmology 1988;95: 772–777.
12. Lewis RA, Schoenwald RD, Barfknecht CF, et al. Aminozolamide gel. A trial of a topical carbonic anhydrase inhibitor in ocular hypertension. Arch Ophthalmol 1986;104:842–844.
13. Lewis RA, Schoenwald RD, Barfknecht CF. Aminozolamide suspension: the role of the vehicle in a topical carbonic anhydrase inhibitor. J Ocular Pharmacol 1988;4:215–219.
14. Bar-Ilan A, Pessah N, Maren T. Ocular penetration and hypotensive activity of the topically applied carbonic anhydrase inhibitor L-645,151. J Ocular Pharmacol 1986;2:109.
15. Lippa EA, von Denffer HA, Hofmann HM, et al. Local tolerance and activity of MK-927, a novel topical carbonic anhydrase inhibitor. Arch Ophthalmol 1988;106:1694–1696.
16. Bron AM, Lippa EA, Hofmann HM, et al. MK-927: a topically effective carbonic anhydrase inhibitor in patients. Arch Ophthalmol 1989;107: 1143–1146.
17. Feicht B, Hofmann HM, Lippa E, et al. A new topical carbonic anhydrase inhibitor (MK-927). Tolerance comparison with betaxolol in healthy probands. [German]. Klinische Monatsblatter fur Augenheilkunde, 1990;197:254–257.
18. Higginbotham EJ, Kass MA, Lippa EA, et al. MK-927: A topical carbonic anhydrase inhibitor. Dose response and duration of action. Arch Ophthalmol 1990;108:65–68.
19. Lippa EA, Aasved H, Airaksinen PJ, et al. Multiple-dose, dose-response relationship for the topical carbonic anhydrase inhibitor MK-927. Arch Ophthalmol 1991;109:46–49.
20. Maren TH, Bar-Ilan A, Conroy CW, et al. Chemical and pharmacological properties of MK-927, a sulfonamide carbonic anhydrase inhibitor that lowers intraocular pressure by the topical route. Exp Eye Res 1990;50: 27–36.
21. Pfeiffer N, Hennekes R, Lippa EA, et al. A single dose of the topical carbonic anhydrase inhibitor MK-927 decreases IOP in patients. Br J Ophthalmol 1990;74:405–408.
22. Pfeiffer N, Gerling J, Lippa EA, et al. Comparative tolerability of topical carbonic anhydrase inhibitor MK-927 and its S-enantiomer MK-417. Graefes Arch Clin Exp Ophthalmol 1991;229:111–114.
23. Serle JB, Lustgarten JS, Lippa EA, et al. MK-927, a topical carbonic anhydrase inhibitor. Dose response and reproducibility. Arch Ophthalmol 1990;108:838–841.
24. Tuulonen A, Hovding G, Gustad L, et al. Multiple-dose dose-response curve of the topical carbonic anhydrase inhibitor MK-927. Invest Ophthalmol Vis Sci 1989;(suppl)30:24.
25. Wang RF, Serle JB, Podos SM, et al. The effect of MK-927, a topical carbonic anhydrase inhibitor, on IOP in glaucomatous monkeys. Current Eye Res 1990;9:163–168.
26. Wang RF, Serle JB, Podos SM, et al. The ocular hypotensive effect of the topical carbonic anhydrase inhibitor L-671,152 in glaucomatous monkeys. Arch Ophthalmol 1990;108:511–513.
27. Buclin T, Lippa EA, Biollaz J, et al. Absence of metabolic effects of the novel topically active carbonic anhydrase inhibitor MK-927 and its s-isomer during a two-week ocular administration. Eur J Clin Pharmacol 1989;36:46.
28. Michelson SR, Schwam H, Baldwin JJ, et al. Topically instilled MK-927: Lack of correlation between corneal penetration rate constant and ocular hypotensive activity in rabbits. Invest Ophthalmol Vis Sci 1989; (suppl)30:24.
29. Brechue WF, Maren TH. Correlation of drug accession with IOP reduction following local and intravenous carbonic anhydrase inhibitors (CAI). Invest Ophthalmol Vis Sci 1991;(suppl)32:1256.
30. Wilkerson M, Cyrlin M, Lippa EA, et al. Four-week safety and efficacy study of dorzolamide, a novel, active topical carbonic anhydrase inhibitor. Arch Ophthalmol 1993;111:1343–1350.
31. Bron A, Lippa EA, Gunning F, et al. Multiple-dose efficacy comparison of the two topical carbonic anhydrase inhibitors sezolamide and MK-927. Arch Ophthalmol 1991;109:50–53.
32. Gerling J, Pfeiffer N, Lippa E, et al. Local carbonic anhydrase inhibitors MK-927 and Mk-417. Effect and tolerance. [German]. Fortschritte der Ophthalmologie 1990;87:692–695.
33. George JL, Sirbat D, Lesure P. MK-417 VS. MK-927: Multiple-dose efficacy comparison of two topical carbonic anhydrase inhibitors. Invest Ophthalmol Vis Sci 1989;(suppl)30:98.
34. Lippa E, Sherwood M, Laibovitz R, et al. MK-417 vs. timolol: Comparative Activity. Invest Ophthalmol Vis Sci 1990;(suppl)31:232.
35. Bourgeois H, Bron A, Lippa E, et al. 2% L 671,152: multiple-dose activity bid. Invest Ophthalmol Vis Sci 1990;(suppl)31:233.
36. Bron A, George JL, Gunning Fea. GelriteTM solutions of MK-507 & sezolamide; comparative activity of two topical carbonic anhydrase inhibitors (CAI). Invest Ophthalmol Vis Sci 1991;(suppl)32:946.
37. Hofmann HM, Feicht B, Brunner-Ferber E, et al. MK-507 (L-671 152): local tolerance and effectiveness of a new local carbonic anhydrase inhibitor in healthy probands. [German]. Fortschritte der Ophthalmologie 1991;88:513–514.
38. Hurvitz LM, Kaufman PL, Robin AL, et al. New developments in the drug treatment of glaucoma. [Review]. Drugs 1991;41:514–532.
39. Kass MA, Laibovitz RA, Lippa EA, et al. Comparative activity of 3% MK-507, a topical CAI, with betaxolol. Invest Ophthalmol Vis Sci 1991; (suppl)1578:989.
40. Lippa EA, Carlson LE, Ehinger B, et al. Dose response and duration of action of dorzolamide, a topical carbonic anhydrase inhibitor. Arch Ophthalmol 1992;110:495–499.
41. Lippa EA, Schuman JS, Higginbotham EJ, et al. MK-507 versus sezolamide. Comparative efficacy of two topically active carbonic anhydrase inhibitors. Ophthalmology 1991;98:308–312.
42. McMahon CD, Laibovitz R. IOP Lowering Activity of the Topical CAI MK-507 at 3%. Invest Ophthalmol Vis Sci 1991;(suppl)1576:989.
43. Nardin G, Lewis R, Lippa EA. Activity of the topical CAI MK-507 bid when added to timolol bid. Invest Ophthalmol Vis Sci 1991; (suppl)1579:989.
44. Sugrue MF, Funk H, Klotzbuecher C. Comparison of the topical carbonic anhydrase inhibitor L-671,152 and timolol in glaucoma monkeys. Invest Ophthalmol Vis Sci 1990;(suppl)31:232.
45. Wang R-F, Serle JB, Podos SM, et al. L-671,152, a topically active carbonic anhydrase inhibitor reduces aqueous humor production in monkeys. Invest Ophthalmol Vis Sci 1990;(suppl)31:149.
46. Yamazaki Y, Miyamoto S, Sawa M. Effect of MK-507 on aqueous humor dynamics in normal human eyes. Jpn J Ophthalmol 1994;38:92–96.
47. Yamazaki Y, Miyamoto S, Sawa M. Effect of topical carbonic anhydrase inhibitor (MK-507) on intraocular pressure of normal human eyes. [Japanese]. Nippon Ganka Gakkai Zasshi—Acta Societatis Ophthalmologicae Japonicae, 1994;98:293–297.

Medications Used in Chronic Glaucoma Therapy

16

Potential New Drugs

David L. Epstein

The main goal of glaucoma research should continue to be the development of outflow system and optic nerve-specific therapeutic agents to correct or modify the basic abnormality in the primary open angle glaucomas (1). **None of our glaucoma medications are specific for a glaucomatous abnormality.** It will, hopefully, be possible someday to successfully answer our patients' request for a cure, rather than control of glaucoma, as has, after all, been accomplished with iridectomy for angle closure glaucoma.

A DRUG FOR THE TRABECULAR MESHWORK

The trabecular meshwork is the locus of abnormal resistance to aqueous humor outflow in POAG (2) and most other forms of open angle glaucoma (except for glaucoma secondary to increased episcleral venous pressure). (Because almost no, if any, forms of open angle glaucoma are due to hypersecretion of aqueous humor, the trabecular meshwork is thus the cause of the elevated IOP, with the exception of glaucoma secondary to increased episcleral venous pressure.) It is a fundamental tenet of medicine to develop therapies that are specifically targeted at the abnormal diseased tissue: in this case, the aqueous humor outflow pathway (3). Such a "trabecular" strategy offers the potential not only for more effective, specific glaucoma therapy by possibly reversing fundamental abnormalities present in the disease (1), but also for long duration of effects from individual therapies.

How might such long-lasting effects from specific trabecular drug therapy result? We know that in certain forms of glaucoma, e.g., exfoliation (Chapter 20), the abnormality responsible for the increased resistance to aqueous outflow is believed to be due to the mechanical effects of exfoliation material obstructing the extracellular outflow pathway (4). That is, in all but far advanced conditions in exfoliation glaucoma, the trabecular meshwork cytoarchitecture is believed to be normal. There is normally a cellular (as well as perhaps an extracellular matrix) barrier to aqueous humor outflow. If a trabecular drug could temporarily break down this barrier (1,5), the abnormal extracellular material involved in the disease process might be removable (perhaps "flushable") from the outflow pathway. Assuming a substantial time interval until this material re-accumulates, there could thus occur a long-duration effect from this therapy. In POAG, an abnormal extracellular accumulation of material is present called plaque material (6), which might be primary or secondary to some trabecular cell abnormality (Chapter 18). But even if secondary, this material probably is responsible in part for the abnormal resistance to outflow, and thus removing this material may produce a sustained beneficial effect on aqueous humor outflow. Other secondary forms of open angle glaucoma are likely where there may be primarily or secondarily extracellular obstructing material in the trabecular outflow pathway that might similarly be responsive to such a temporary elimination of the usual barrier to outflow. (One might also contemplate combination therapy of such "barrier" agents with specific "enzymes" that might dissolve and loosen extracellular deposits.)

The potential for such a "magic bullet" for the trabecular meshwork is exciting because it represents rational disease therapy. Nevertheless, whether such proposed trabecular meshwork drugs can "semi-permanently" reverse the abnormal resistance to outflow by "declogging" the extracellular obstruction to outflow, or whether they temporarily make the outflow pathway more permeable to aqueous humor ("salt water") fluid flow, i.e., function as a "trabecular diuretic" (1,3), there is the potential for improved IOP control by restoring the aqueous outflow process to "normal." Likely, different forms of open angle glaucoma will respond differently to such trabecular therapy, which hopefully will consist of more than one option.

There is much current excitement about the possibility of using **cytoskeletal drugs** for these purposes. Such drugs presumably work by changing cell shape and attachment (7-9) in the outflow pathway. They have the potential not only to improve outflow of aqueous humor by directly changing the dimensions of the outflow pathway, but also to temporarily remove the cellular barriers to outflow at the inner wall of Schlemm's canal and juxtacanalicular tis-

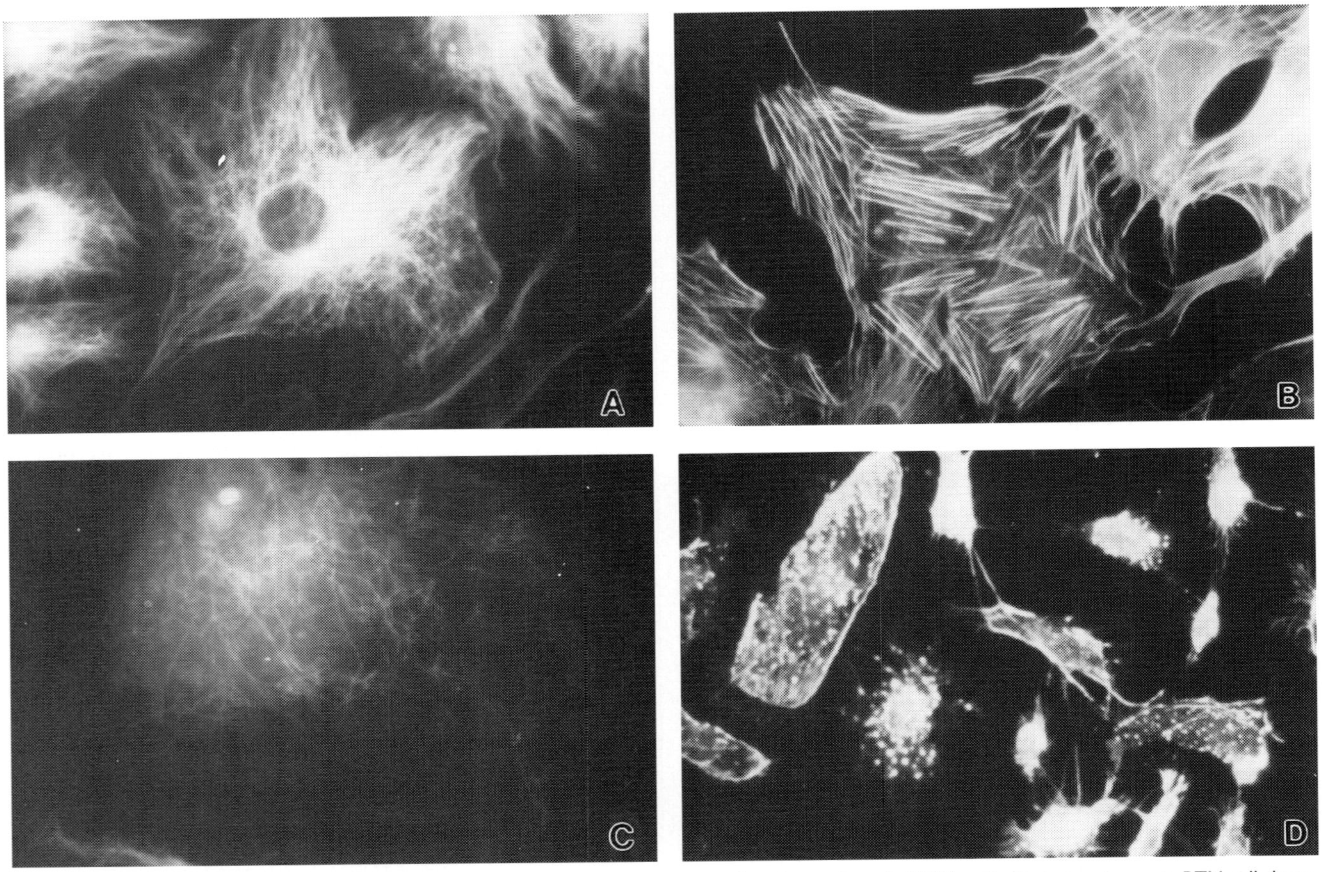

Figure 16.1. The effect of ethacrynic acid (ECA) on the cytoskeleton of bovine trabecular meshwork (BTM) cells. Note the change in BTM cell shape. BTM cells were stained for tubulin and actin before ECA treatment (A,B) and after ECA treatment (C,D), respectively. These effects on cell cytoskeleton have been correlated with increased outflow facility in animal eyes.

sue (1). In fact, a drug of this class, ethacrynic acid (10–14), (Fig. 16.1) is currently under clinical investigation for these purposes. Ethacrynic acid itself is probably not suitable for topical administration except perhaps in a pro-drug form (15). But, it is important to realize that ethacrynic acid is the first prototype of such a drug to be tried in humans, and there are many other potential agents with similar mechanisms of action. In fact, it is remarkable that the first drug that was chosen of this type, ethacrynic acid, made it into Phase III human testing. Many colleagues thought this was an impossible dream. The major importance of ethacrynic acid may prove, in the end, to have been to demonstrate that such an approach is feasible for the human eye.

The focused hypothesis remains that with such cellular therapy (1,16) targeted at the trabecular outflow pathway, more specific treatments will result in enhanced efficacy and the need for less frequent drug administration.

PROSTAGLANDIN DRUGS

In human eyes, the uveo-scleral (uveo-vascular scleral) outflow pathway through the ciliary muscle into the suprachoroidal space and then out of the eye, either through choroidal vascular or scleral absorption, accounts for less than 10% of the normal outflow of aqueous humor (Chapters 2, 3). As mentioned, in nonhuman primates, however, aqueous outflow via this pathway is much greater. Under most circumstances in human eyes, this pathway likely has little, if any, clinical significance. However, prostaglandin-type drugs break down the barrier to such unconventional outflow in human eyes (17), and this has the therapeutic potential for IOP lowering (assuming there are no adverse consequences to such enhanced fluid movement through this pathway). Thus, prostaglandin drugs theoretically could produce a form of "internal filter" directing flow of aqueous humor away from the diseased inadequate trabecular meshwork through the uveo-scleral pathway.

Breaking down this normal internal barrier might have adverse consequences. For example, in spontaneous uveitis, where the barrier to this pathway is believed to be secondarily disrupted, some feel that this pathway might cause cystoid macular edema which can follow cataract surgery and other anterior segment inflammations. In fact, the initial trials of topical ocular prostaglandin drugs produced substantial conjunctival injection and mild intraocular inflammation.

Nevertheless, despite these reservations, the early reports of new chemical modifications of certain prostaglandins at reduced dosages are promising (18–21) (there are some reports of induced change in iris color that are unexplained). This may be another example of the need for dose–response perspectives for all of our glaucoma therapy (toxicology) discussed previously (Chapter 13). The amount of IOP lowering with prostaglandin-type drugs is impressive, and if continued safety is demonstrated, these agents may represent an important new addition to the anti-glaucoma arsenal, even if the pathway for the drug action is not "usual" or "natural." In glaucoma treatment, we need all the help we can get. On the other hand, one of us (DLE) still strongly believes that an even greater advance in glaucoma therapy will eventually occur with the development of drugs that are targeted at the diseased tissue in the eye, particularly at the hydrodynamic component of glaucoma, the trabecular meshwork.

CANNABINOIDS

There has been considerable public interest in the IOP-lowering effects of cannabinoids. Unfortunately, despite the public discussion, there has been too little research and data presentation in this potentially important area. Systemic cannabinoids can acutely decrease IOP (22). The effects of chronic dosage are less clear. If the psychoactive effects can be separated from effects on IOP (23,24), then a potentially useful systemic glaucoma therapy could be developed (25,26). However, investigation into a possible topical agent (27) seemed potentially more fruitful to us. Unfortunately, cannabinoids are hydrophobic, and their poor penetration through the cornea has so far limited their topical application (28).

A GLAUCOMA DRUG FOR THE OPTIC NERVE

There are two diseased tissues in the eye in the glaucomas: the trabecular meshwork, which is responsible for the IOP component involved at least partially in almost all forms of glaucoma, and the optic nerve, which is the final end organ for damage and shows varying susceptibility to IOP effects (Chapters 18, 19). **Ultimately, ideal glaucoma treatment should involve therapy directed at the optic nerve to shift the "dose–response relationships" for IOP effects in a favorable direction, and to correct the underlying factors involved in glaucomatous cupping.** The optic nerve is a complex tissue that is part of the central nervous system, but so complex that it seems it should be easier and more immediately feasible to develop "trabecular meshwork drugs" than "optic nerve drugs," both of which are still part of the ultimate "cure" for glaucoma (1). Work in this direction should be encouraged. This latter effort will undoubtedly require intensive "bridging" type research programs between neurobiologists, basic scientists, and glaucoma clinician-scientists.

Through the use of detailed clinical examination and reflection that is part of what glaucoma clinical care practice is all about, a few therapeutic hypotheses have been developed for an optic nerve drug treatment. A few decades ago, based on retrospective clinical observations, Becker proposed that phenytoin sodium (Dilantin) might preserve visual function in patients with glaucoma (29). Subsequently there has not been unequivocal substantiation for this effect, and few, if any, glaucoma clinicians use such therapy for their glaucoma patients. (We do not.) Although it is easy to dismiss such initial observations as due to some confounding variable, we should also consider whether there is some "kernel" for future understanding and future therapeutic investigations. POAG is such a multifaceted disease, likely of multiple types, with objective assessments of visual function so imprecise, that it would be difficult to detect a moderately positive effect in a subset of the affected population. This is what makes studies of visual/optic nerve function, to say nothing about direct optic nerve therapeutic intervention, so difficult, as discussed in the introduction (Chapter 1), in which the "crudeness" of our clinical methods are described.

There has been some interest in the use of oral calcium-channel blockers to preserve visual function, at least in progressive low-tension glaucoma. The arguments for this are presented in Chapter 19. This hypothesis is unfortunately based on retrospective data with questionable small numbers of patients, which should be viewed with conservative skepticism until there is better substantiating data. But, is there a "kernel" in these data that might have implications for future investigations? One of the problems is that theoretically it is not clear at what site one wants to intervene at the level of the optic nerve, and also which effect of calcium-channel blockers, if any, might be advantageous. For example, presumably at least within the total class of calcium channel blockers, there are both direct vascular and direct axonal actions possible. **We unfortunately do not really know what it is that we want to accomplish at the level of the optic nerve** (1). We need much more information about the mechanism and events in glaucomatous cupping not only in healthy, young normal animal eyes but also the diseased, aged human eye to rationally plan therapeutic strategies for this tissue in the future. Otherwise, we will be totally dependent on a chance observation to make progress in this area, and one might anticipate several "wild goose chases" in the interval.

An optic nerve drug is the ultimate "holy grail" and we should encourage such pursuits, based on firm investigative data. The fact that we have not achieved such a similar goal with a simpler connective tissue called the trabecular meshwork should be humbling for all of us involved in this pursuit.

References

1. Epstein DL: Will there be a remedy to reverse the changes in the trabecular meshwork and the optic nerve? A personal point-of-view on glaucoma therapy. J Glaucoma 1993;2:138–140.

2. Grant WM: Experimental aqueous perfusion in enucleated human eyes. Arch Ophthalmol 1963;69:783–801.
3. Epstein DL: Open angle glaucoma: Why not a cure? (editorial). Arch Ophthalmol 1987;105:1187–1188.
4. Richardson TM, Epstein DL: Exfoliation glaucoma: a quantitative perfusion and ultrastructural study. Ophthalmology 1981;88:968–80.
5. Kaufman PL: Pharmacologic trabeculocanalotomy: facilitating aqueous outflow by assaulting the meshwork cytoskeleton, junctional complexes, and extracellular matrix [editorial]. Arch Ophthlmol 1992;110:34–6.
6. Rohen JW: Why is intraocular pressure elevated in chronic simple glaucoma? Am Acad Ophthalmol 1983;90:758–765.
7. Erickson-Lamy KA, Schroeder A, Epstein DL: Ethacrynic acid induces reversible shape and cytoskeletal changes in cultured cells. Invest Ophthalmol Vis Sci 1992;33:2631–2640.
8. Epstein DL, et al: The search for a sulfhydryl drug for glaucoma: From chemistry to the cytoskeleton. Basic aspects of glaucoma research III. Edited by Lutjen-Drecoll E. Schattauer, Stuttgart-New York, 1993; 345–353.
9. Grewal A, O'Brien ET, Epstein DL: Control of cell shape in the trabecular meshwork. Invest Ophthalmol Vis Sci 1994;35(ARVO suppl):2725.
10. Epstein DL, et al: Influence of ethacrynic acid on outflows facility in the monkey and calf eye. Invest Ophthalmol Vis Sci 1987;28:2067–2075.
11. Liang L-L, et al: Ethacrynic acid increases facility of outflow in the human eye in vitro. Arch Ophthalmol 1992;110:106–9.
12. Melamed S, Kotas-Neumann R, Barak A, et al: The effect of intracameral ethacrynic acid on intraocular pressure in glaucoma patients-a pilot study. Am J Ophthalmol 1992;113:508–12.
13. Croft MA, Hubbard WC, Kaufman PL: Effect of ethacrynic acid on aqueous outflow dynamics in monkeys. Invest Ophthalmol Vis Sci 1994; 35:1167–1175.
14. Wang RF, et al: Effects of topical ethacrynic acid ointment vs timolol on intraocular pressure in glaucomatous monkey eyes. Arch Ophthalmol 1994;112:390–4.
15. Tingey DP, Schroeder A, Epstein MPM, et al: Effects of topical ethacrynic acid adducts on intraocular pressure in rabbits and monkeys. Arch Ophthalmol 1992;110:699–702.
16. Alvarado JA, Wood I, Polansky JR: Human trabecular cells. II. Growth pattern and ultrastructural characteristics. Invest Ophthalmol 1982;23: 464–78.
17. Toris CB, Camras CB, Yablonski ME: Effects of PhXA41, a new prostaglandin F_{2a} analog, on aqueous humor dynamics in human eyes. Ophthalmology 1993;100:1297–304.
18. Nagasubramanian S, Sheth GP, Hitchings RA, et al: Intraocular pressure-reducing effect of PhXA41 in ocular hypertension. Ophthalmology 1993;100:1305–11.
19. Alm A, et al: Intraocular pressure-reducing effect of PhXA41 in patients with increased eye pressure - a one-month study. Ophthalmology 1993; 100:1314–7.
20. Rulo AH, Greve EL, Hoyng PF: Additive effect of latanoprost, a prostaglandin F_{2a} analogue, and timolol in patients with elevated intraocular pressure. Br J Ophthalmol 1994;78:899–902.
21. Alm A, et al: Latanoprost administered once daily caused a maintained reduction of intraocular pressure in glaucoma patients treated concomitantly with timolol. Br J Ophthalmol 1995;79:12–16.
22. Hepler RS, Frank IM, Petrus R: Ocular effects of marihuana smoking. In: Braude MC, Szara S. The pharmacology of marihuana. New York, Raven, 1976.
23. Weber PA, Howes JF: Lowering of intraocular pressure in normotensive human volunteers by naboctate. Invest Ophthalmol Vis Sci 1981;20: 196.
24. Tiedeman JS, et al: Effect of synthetic cannabinoids on elevated intraocular pressure. Ophthalmology 1981;88:270–277.
25. ElSohly MA, Harland EC, Benigni DA, et al: Cannabinoids in glaucoma II: the effect of different cannabinoids on intraocular pressure of the rabbit. Curr Eye Res 1984;3(6):841–850.
26. Liu JH, Dacus AC: Central nervous system and peripheral mechanisms in ocular hypotensive effect of cannabinoids. Arch Ophthalmol 1987; 105:245–8.
27. Colasanti BK: A comparison of the ocular and central effects of delta 9-tetrahydrocannabinol and cannabigerol. J Ocul Pharmacol 1990;6: 259–69.
28. Jay WM, Green K: Multiple-drop study of topically applied 1% 9-tetrahydrocannabinol in human eyes. Arch Ophthalmol 1983;101: 591–593.
29. Becker B, Stamper RL, Asseff C, et al: Effect of diphenylhydantoin on glaucomatous field loss: a preliminary report. Trans Am Acad Ophthalmol Otolaryngol 1972;76:412–22.

Management of Highly Elevated IOP 17

R. Rand Allingham

The patient with acutely elevated IOP is usually symptomatic, whereas IOP that has gradually increased, even to relatively high levels usually does not produce symptoms. Common symptoms and signs from acutely elevated IOP include dull or aching pain, blurred vision, perception of haloes, nausea or vomiting, conjunctival injection, corneal edema, and central retinal arterial or venous pulsations. Although optic nerve damage or visual field loss may not be present in cases in which IOP has increased acutely, these disorders are still referred to as glaucomas.

Most forms of glaucoma can cause extremely elevated IOP (Table 17.1). Of these, angle closure glaucoma, either primary or secondary, is a common cause of acute symptomatic IOP elevation. Acute primary angle closure glaucoma often produces the entire constellation of signs and symptoms of this group of disorders. Secondary angle closure glaucoma, particularly neovascular glaucoma, is frequently encountered in practice. Secondary open angle glaucomas, including angle recession, exfoliation, pigment dispersion, and steroid-induced glaucoma, occasionally cause a sudden, marked IOP increase. Juvenile open angle glaucoma, although rare, is the most likely primary open angle glaucoma to produce symptomatic highly elevated IOP.

DIAGNOSIS

History

A thorough ocular and general medical history frequently provides clues to the cause of highly elevated IOP. Often the cause is obvious, for example, after laser or incisional surgery. In other cases, there may be no apparent cause. An asymptomatic patient usually has had a gradual increase in IOP, which suggests chronic angle closure glaucoma or a form of open angle glaucoma. Patients who have had recent eye surgeries, those with histories of ocular inflammation, trauma, or those with chronic inflammatory medical conditions (e.g., asthma or rheumatoid arthritis) should be questioned about use of topical or systemic corticosteroids. Histories of ocular trauma are often found in those patients with angle recession glaucoma.

Episodic pain or blurred vision occurring over months or years is more commonly observed with intermittent angle closure glaucoma, whereas the sudden onset of severe unrelenting pain and blurred vision, particularly in a hyperopic patient, is most commonly seen with acute angle closure glaucoma. A history of painless loss of vision in the affected eye which occurs with a central retinal vein occlusion (CRVO), or a history of diabetes mellitus would suggest neovascular glaucoma.

In addition to information that may lead to a diagnosis, the general medical history provides essential information that is needed before initiating acute medical treatment. A history of asthma, chronic obstructive pulmonary disease, or congestive heart failure precludes use of beta blockers. In patients with metabolic acidosis (e.g., uncontrolled diabetes mellitus) or sulfa allergy, systemic carbonic anhydrase inhibitors should not be used. Hyperosmotic agents should not be administered if severe renal or heart failure is present.

Examination

Careful examination is rewarded with an accurate diagnosis in these patients. Because the mechanism of IOP elevation differs among this group of disorders, so does the initial medical management.

Obtaining the patient's refractive error is useful. Myopic patients are prone to pigment dispersion syndrome or retinal detachment (Schwartz's syndrome), whereas hyperopic patients are predisposed to angle closure glaucoma.

Visual acuity may be reduced secondary to corneal edema, media opacity, or posterior segment pathology. Good visual acuity argues against the diagnosis of CRVO in a patient with neovascular glaucoma.

The presence of an afferent pupillary defect (either consensual or reverse) suggests significant retinal or optic nerve damage which may be secondary to CRVO or long standing glaucoma.

Slit-Lamp Examination

Conjunctival injection is common in patients with acute glaucoma; however, prominent chemosis or proptosis of the globe would suggest an A-V fistula.

In cases in which the cornea is edematous, application of topical glycerin (after topical anesthetic) will often increase corneal clarity and assist in examination of the anterior segment and with gonioscopy. The cornea should be carefully examined for pigment (Kruckenberg spindles) and keratic precipitates. Patients with Posner-Schlossman syndrome may develop keratic precipitates after IOP has been elevated for a few days.

Table 17-1
Causes of Acute or Highly Elevated IOP

Primary (pupillary block) angle closure glaucoma
- Acute angle closure
- Chronic angle closure

Secondary angle closure glaucoma
- Neovascular glaucoma
- Synechial closure secondary to uveitis
- Iris bombé
- Post-operative glaucomas
  - Status post cataract surgery
  - Status post vitreoretinal surgery
  - Malignant glaucoma
- Drug (e.g. sulfa) induced
- Status post CRVO (acute)

Juvenile open angle glaucoma (rarely POAG)

Secondary open angle glaucoma
- Post-operative
  - Laser (e.g. posterior capsulotomy, laser iridectomy, laser gonioplasty or laser trabeculoplasty)
  - Cataract surgery
  - Penetrating keratoplasty
  - Closure of cyclodialysis cleft
- Exfoliation syndrome
- Pigmentary dispersion syndrome
- Angle recession
- Uveitic glaucoma
- Steroid-induced
- Carotid-cavernous fistula

The anterior chamber may contain flare or cells from ocular ischemia secondary to high IOP. However, more than a few cells would suggest uveitis or some other inflammatory disorder, whereas red cells indicate bleeding from neovascular tissue, trauma, or perhaps vitreous hemorrhage (e.g., ghost cell glaucoma). The anterior chamber depth both axially and peripherally should be noted. A peripherally shallow anterior chamber suggests angle closure glaucoma, whereas a centrally shallow anterior chamber suggests lens displacement or enlargement, posterior segment pathology, or malignant glaucoma.

The iris should be carefully examined for neovascularization. Neovascularization can be missed when IOP is extremely high because abnormal vessels may be difficult to see due both to a reduction in vessel caliber as well as corneal edema. Iridodialysis or sphincter tears indicates trauma has occurred in the past.

Although rare, a dislocated or hypermature lens can cause acute glaucoma (pupillary block or phacolytic glaucoma). The anterior lens capsule should be examined for the presence of exfoliation material.

Gonioscopy

Gonioscopy is of vital importance in these cases to determine a rational medical (and surgical) treatment strategy. As described, in cases in which there is significant corneal edema, topical glycerin will often provide an adequate view of the iris and angle structures to assess whether the angle is open or closed. Compression gonioscopy can be performed to determine which portions of the angle are appositionally versus synechially closed. If gonioscopy is not possible due to corneal opacity, ultrasound biomicroscopy can be used to establish the anatomy of the anterior segment.

Fundus

If possible, the fundus should be examined acutely for evidence of CRVO, proliferative diabetic retinopathy, retinal detachment (Schwartz's syndrome), and optic nerve damage. In those cases in which a view of the fundus is not possible due to media opacity, B-scan ultrasonography should be strongly considered. Posterior segment tumors (e.g., melanoma) and chronic retinal detachment can both present with neovascular glaucoma.

TREATMENT STRATEGY

The goal of treatment in these cases is to reduce the IOP as quickly as possible to a safe level for the optic nerve. When this has been accomplished, one can proceed with additional diagnostic tests and therapies. The approach to extremely elevated IOP can be broken down into a simple paradigm, depending on the diagnosis (Table 17.2). As stated, the treatment approach must be modified according to the patient's medical and allergic history.

IOP can be reduced by increasing outflow or reducing

Table 17-2
Medical Treatment of Dangerously Elevated IOP

Medication	Acutely Elevated IOP Marked Symptoms	Markedly Elevated IOP Mild Symptoms
Beta blockers	q 10 min × 2, then q12 hr	q 10 min × 2, then q12 hr
Alpha 2 agonists	q 10 min × 2, then q12 hr	q 10 min × 2, then q12 hr
Miotics (for pupillary block or open angle glaucoma without inflammation)	Pilocarpine 1–2% q 15 min × 2, then q 4 hr	Pilocarpine 1–2% q 15 min × 2, then q 4 hr
Carbonic anhydrase inhibitors	Acetazolamide 500 mg IV *or* topical dorzolamide 2% q 10 min × 2, then q 8 hr	Acetazolamide 500 mg (tablets) po *or* topical dorzolamide 2% q 10 min × 2, then q 8 hours
Osmotics	Mannitol 1–2 g/kg IV	Oral glycerol or isosorbide 1–1.5 g/kg PO on ice

inflow. Inflow drugs include beta blockers, alpha-2 agonists, carbonic anhydrase inhibitors, and osmotic agents. Although not strictly inflow drugs, osmotic agents reduce IOP by dehydrating ocular structures and the vitreous, and are effective in the presence of a functionally closed angle. Miotics and adrenergics primarily increase conventional outflow through action on the trabecular meshwork and can open the angle in pupillary block glaucoma.

Beta Blockers and Alpha 2 Agonists

There is considerable overlap in the mechanism in which these agents reduce aqueous inflow. The IOP lowering effect of the alpha 2 agonist apraclonidine is partially additive to timolol, which has been administered chronically (1). However, apraclonidine is not additive to timolol if both agents are given simultaneously (2). In other words, apraclonidine appears to restore the full potency of chronically administered timolol, but is no more potent than timolol when it is given acutely. This may also be true for all nonselective beta blockers. Therefore, either apraclonidine or nonselective beta blocker therapy is adequate as initial treatment for patients on no previous glaucoma therapy. Apraclonidine would be the agent of choice in cases in which there is a contraindication to using a beta blocker. However, the clinician should not be faulted for using both agents in patients with acutely elevated IOP.

Beta blockers should be given every 12 hours. Apraclonidine is given every 8 hours. There is no therapeutic benefit in treating more frequently.

Miotics

Direct-acting miotics like pilocarpine are useful in the treatment of glaucoma secondary to pupillary block, including acute and chronic angle closure, in addition to open angle glaucomas in which there is no associated anterior segment inflammation. **Indirect-acting agents (e.g., echothiophate iodide) are long lasting, difficult to reverse, more likely to increase anterior segment inflammation, and frequently cause severe pain when administered acutely. Therefore, indirect-acting miotics should not be used in treating acute glaucomas.**

Pilocarpine (1–2%) should be given every 2 hours for two doses, then once every 4 hours thereafter. More frequent administration is ineffective and can produce serious gastrointestinal and respiratory side effects (3).

Miotics are contraindicated when the angle is structurally closed by synechia (e.g., neovascularization), mechanical closure from a posterior pushing mechanism (e.g., acute angle closure after panretinal photocoagulation or malignant glaucoma), when functionally closed by inflammatory debris (uveitis), or when elevated IOP has produced anterior segment ischemia and the iris sphincter is nonfunctional. In the latter case, delaying the addition of miotics for 1 or 2 hours until the IOP has been reduced by aqueous suppressants and hyperosmotics is often as effective as starting miotic treatment initially (4).

Miotics should be used judiciously in patients with acutely elevated IOP. If there is a question as to whether miotics should be used, withhold use till the effect of aqueous suppressant and osmotic therapy can be assessed.

Cycloplegic Agents

Whereas cycloplegics such as tropicamide or cyclopentolate are not used to directly reduce IOP, they are indicated for the treatment of secondary angle closure glaucomas produced by swelling or rotation of the ciliary body and forward movement of the lens-iris diaphragm, such as malignant glaucoma or acute glaucoma after CRVO. These cases are worsened by miotic treatment.

Adrenergic Agents

Adrenergic agents, such as epinephrine and dipivefrin, are ineffective in treating high or acutely elevated IOP. Additionally, the potency of these agents is further reduced when used in conjunction with nonselective beta blockers. Adrenergic agents can be omitted from the initial treatment strategy for highly elevated IOP. If used, epinephrine compounds should be administered twice a day.

Carbonic Anhydrase Inhibitors

Carbonic anhydrase inhibitors (CAIs), such as acetazolamide and methazolamide, are sulfa derivatives that reduce aqueous inflow in a manner that is partially additive to both beta blockers and alpha-2 agonists. Methazolamide, 50–100 mg every 8 hours, or acetazolamide, 250 mg every 4–6 hours, should be given orally to adult patients. When using acetazolamide in the acute high IOP setting, two 250 mg tablets should be given, rather than 500 mg by the slow-release formulation (Diamox Sequels, Lederle Laboratories, St. Louis, MO), as the tablet formulation is more rapidly absorbed than the sustained-release preparation. Acetazolamide (500 mg) can be given intravenously for patients who have nausea.

When given systemically, CAIs produce metabolic acidosis and should be used with caution in patients with severe liver disease, renal impairment, or pulmonary insufficiency (Chapter 14).

Although likely not as potent as the oral form, the topical carbonic anhydrase inhibitor dorzolamide has been released for general use (Chapter 15) (5). This may be useful for treating acute glaucoma where nausea is present or an intravenous line cannot be placed. Because dorzolamide is also a sulfa derivative, it is contraindicated in patients who are allergic to sulfa drugs, acetazolamide, or methazolamide.

Osmotics

Osmotic agents, such as mannitol, isosorbide, and glycerol, are thought to reduce IOP by decreasing the vitreous volume (6). There may be some effect mediated through the interaction of the CNS and optic nerve, although this remains poorly understood (7).

These agents can be given orally or intravenously and are used for emergent control of dangerously elevated IOP. They should not be given chronically and can cause serious side effects (8).

Glycerol (or glycerin) is administered orally as a 50% solution. The dose is 1–1.5 g/kg lean body weight. **Glycerol is metabolized as a carbohydrate, and if given repeatedly, can cause serious metabolic disturbances in diabetic patients** (9). Peak IOP reduction after glycerol administration is reached in approximately 30 minutes and lasts for 5 hours (10).

Isosorbide is also an oral agent. The dose is 1–1.5 g/kg lean body weight. **Because it is excreted largely unmetabolized in the urine, it is safer for diabetic patients than glycerin.** The peak IOP reduction of isosorbide is reached 1 to 2 hours after administration, and lasts for 3 to 5 hours (11).

Mannitol is a potent osmotic agent that is administered intravenously. It is rapidly excreted unmetabolized in the urine. The recommended dose is 1–2 g/kg administered in a 20% solution over 20 to 30 minutes (12). The onset of action occurs within an hour and lasts for up to 6 hours. Due to the rapid infusion of a large volume of fluid, intravenous osmotic agents can precipitate renal or congestive heart failure, and consultation with an internist or family practitioner should be considered before administering mannitol to patients with clinically significant heart or renal disease (12,13).

MEDICAL MANAGEMENT

After the patient with extremely elevated IOP is examined, an initial working diagnosis is made. Patients can usually be placed into one of two groups; acutely elevated IOP with marked symptoms, or acutely elevated IOP with few or mild symptoms. Treatment can be devised accordingly (Table 17.2).

All patient groups benefit from maximal aqueous suppressant therapy. Beta blockers, apraclonidine, and carbonic anhydrase inhibitors should all be used when the patient's medical condition permits.

Miotics should only be used when the patient has pupillary block glaucoma or open angle glaucoma without associated inflammation. In all other cases, miotics should be deferred until the effect of aqueous suppressant therapy has been determined.

Osmotics should only be used when IOP is dangerously elevated and poses the threat of acutely damaging the optic nerve (e.g., acute angle closure glaucoma); they are needed to reduce IOP to clear the cornea and make a diagnostic assessment; or the patient will be going to surgery within 24 to 48 hours and the need for IOP reduction is short term. Osmotics can produce dehydration or electrolyte imbalance and should not be used for chronic therapy.

In the patient who is markedly symptomatic, especially one with acute angle closure glaucoma in which nausea and vomiting are pronounced, promptly administering acetazolamide and osmotic agents can produce a rapid reduction in IOP and avoid the problem of retention of oral medications (which can produce nausea even in the absence of acutely elevated IOP). Once IOP has been reduced to safer levels, definitive management of the underlying cause is pursued.

References

1. Gharagozloo NZ, Brubaker RF: Effect of apraclonidine in long-term timolol users. Ophthalmology 1991;98:1543–6.
2. Koskela T, Brubaker RF: Apraclonidine and timolol. Combined effects in previously untreated normal subjects. Arch Ophthalmol 1991;109: 804–6.
3. Greco JJ, Kelman CD: Systemic pilocarpine toxicity in the treatment of angle closure glaucoma. Ann Ophthalmol 1973;5:57.
4. Airaksinen PJ, Saari KM, Tiainen TJ, et al: Management of acute closed-angle glaucoma with miotics and timolol. Br J Ophthalmol 1979;63: 822.
5. Lippa EA, Carlson LE, Ehinger B, et al: Dose response and duration of action of dorzalomide, a topical carbonic anhydrase inhibitor. Arch Ophthalmol 1992:110:495–499
6. Robbins R, Galin MA: Effect of osmotic agents on the vitreous body. Arch Ophthalmol 1969;82:694.
7. Podos SM, Krupin T, Becker B: Effect of small-dose hyperosmotic injections on intraocular pressure of small animals and man when optic nerves are transected and intact. Am J Ophthal 1971;71:898.
8. Grabie MT, Gipstein RM, Adams DA, et al: Contraindications for mannitol in aphakic glaucoma. Am J Ophthalmol 1981;91:265.
9. Oakley DE, Ellis PP: Glycerol and hyperosmolar nonketotic coma. Am J Ophthalmol 1976;81:469.
10. Virno M, Cantore P, Bietti C, et al: Oral glycerol in ophthalmology. A valuable new method for the reduction of intraocular pressure. Am J Ophthalmol 1963;55:1133.
11. Mehra KS, Singh R: Lowering of intraocular pressure by isosorbide. Effects of different doses of drug. Arch Ophthalmol 1971;85:167.
12. Smith EW, Drance SM: Reduction of human intraocular pressure with intravenous mannitol. Arch Ophthalmol 1962;68:734.
13. Havener WH: Ocular Pharmacology, 4th ed. CV Mosby, St. Louis, 1978; 440.

Common Open Angle Glaucomas III

Primary Open Angle Glaucoma 18

David L. Epstein

GENERAL CONSIDERATIONS

Primary Versus Secondary

The overriding fundamental distinction is between open angle and angle closure glaucomas. These are all often called primary when there is no apparent ocular or systemic cause, and secondary when there is an initiating ocular or systemic mechanism. Because there is likely more than one mechanism of primary open angle glaucoma (POAG), the disease entity should likely be termed the primary open angle glaucomas. (Similarly, primary angle closure glaucoma is usually due to pupillary block, but plateau iris, an uncommon condition, is also often called a form of primary angle closure, Chapter 22.) In some ways, these terms are not that important except for clinical categorization because they reflect that we understand some mechanisms, but not others. For example, it is not rare for a patient with apparent "primary open angle glaucoma" to later on be discovered to have exfoliation, at which time the diagnosis is changed to that of a secondary open angle glaucoma (since we believe we now understand the mechanism of this glaucoma, Chapter 20).

Also, by analogy, secondary forms of angle closure glaucoma can involve the same mechanism for iris occlusion of the trabecular meshwork (TM) as primary causes. For example, an increase in posterior segment volume (e.g., acute central retinal vein occlusion) may move the crystalline lens forward and result in pupillary block by this means (Chapter 28). Thus, there are common final mechanisms for all the glaucomas, whether "primary" or secondary".

"Primary" open angle glaucoma is so called because it occurs spontaneously, without evident antecedent or related disease, and with no known basis other than genetic or hereditary predisposition. This is the most common variety of glaucoma in some parts of the world.

Other types of open angle glaucoma differ from the so-called primary type by the fact that they characteristically occur in conjunction with specific abnormalities or diseases of the eye that can be considered causative of the associated glaucoma. Such types of secondary open angle glaucoma include exfoliation with open angle glaucoma, amyloidosis with open angle glaucoma, pigmentary glaucoma, and in special instances, glaucoma after trauma, and glaucoma due to intraocular inflammation. These glaucomas are discussed in detail under separate headings. However, much of what is to be said concerning the treatment of primary open angle glaucoma can be applied equally well to other open angle glaucomas, except those involving active intraocular inflammation.

Primary open angle glaucoma itself is a clinically well-defined disease, having moderate variation in its characteristics. A small proportion of cases are extraordinary and fall into subcategories.

Primary Open Angle Glaucoma Is Really a Disease of Exclusion (of "Secondary" Causes)

POAG is a diagnosis of exclusion. In all cases no matter how deep the anterior chamber looks on slit-lamp examination, gonioscopy needs to be performed. One may be surprised by the observation of heretofore unsuspected angle recession, pigment dispersion or exfoliation, fine new blood vessels in the angle, partial angle closure, or inflammatory precipitates. In diabetes, neovascularization can occur in the angle before the iris is involved. **Any abnormal pigment in the angle needs to be explained** (pigmentary glaucoma, exfoliation, iris or ciliary body cysts, melanoma, etc). Chronic silent angle closure glaucoma may masquerade as "POAG."

Special mention needs to be made of the entity of **occult inflammatory precipitates in the angle.** Chandler termed this form of trabeculitis "occult KP in the angle," and stressed how it could mimic POAG. The eyes are notoriously white and quiet with no to very rare cells in the anterior chamber or precipitates on the corneal endothelium. In fact, a subtle solitary "smudge" on the corneal endothelium is often all that one sees. Thus, this diagnosis is often missed unless careful gonioscopy is performed. Patients do not have obvious uveitis. Another characteristic of this entity is the fact that patients do not respond well to standard IOP-lowering medications, especially miotics. **If patients are placed on standard anti-glaucoma therapy and do not show a therapeutic response, gonioscopy should be repeated** looking for this entity (as well as other causes such as unsuspected angle closure, neovascularization, etc.). Patients with "occult KP" in the angle commonly need to be maintained on chronic low-dose steroid therapy indefinitely to "control" the glaucoma.

Paul Chandler, MD, followed several patients with "occult KP in the angle." Commonly intervals may occur when the "trabeculitis" would slightly worsen, necessitating more intensive steroid therapy. Dr. Chandler would send the patient to the emergency room and instruct the patient not to tell the resident his or her diagnosis, but to have the resident call him. He would then ask the resident what the diagnosis was and what was seen with the "jewel" (gonioscopy lens). Thus, Dr. Chandler evaluated his residents!

The presence of "KP" on the trabecular meshwork can be subtle, mainly because in their earliest stage, they are clear, and it is easy to look right through them at the angle. One of us (DLE) recalls the first time WMG called him down to the Glaucoma Clinic to see such a patient. DLE was a pre-resident fellow at the time, eager to learn from his mentor. However, upon looking into the angle, DLE was unable to discern the KP until, after some time with the illuminator becoming hot in his hand, his hand began to slightly tremble and the light therefore caught the scleral spur adjacent to a KP and retro-illuminated it. The KP jumped out at DLE, and it was stunning that he had somehow previously missed it (he wondered what else he had missed). By using this "trick" of scleral spur retro-illumination almost a dozen KP were then identified in the entire angle circumference. This experience has been repeated (more subtly) many more times; if one suspects "occult KP" in the angle, one can view the entire 360 degrees of the angle and perhaps see one questionable area; but as one repeats the circumferential process, multiple trabecular precipitates can often be detected. One of us (DLE) always remembers that this "angle sleuthing" was how Dr. Chandler evaluated the quality of his residents.

CLINICAL CHARACTERISTICS

In POAG, the angle of the anterior chamber may be wide or narrow, but it remains open at all times, whether the disease is early or advanced, and whether IOP is normal or elevated. Even in eyes that have been blind for many years from this type of glaucoma, the angle remains open, unless neovascular glaucoma has become superimposed. **The gonioscopic appearance of the angle of the anterior chamber in most cases of POAG is no different from that in normal individuals.** Open angle glaucoma cannot be cured by presently available means, but it can often be controlled by various medical and surgical measures.

In POAG, the facility of aqueous outflow from the anterior chamber is constantly subnormal, whereas the IOP may vary in the course of a day from normal to significantly elevated pressures. This decreased facility of outflow persists throughout the rest of the patient's life and tends to worsen with the passage of time.

The clinical manifestations of POAG vary considerably. In most cases, the glaucoma develops in middle life or later, and the onset is usually gradual and asymptomatic. In the early stages, IOP may be only slightly elevated, but it is higher when the disease is more advanced.

When open angle glaucoma develops in patients under the age of 50, especially in the 20s and 30s, the onset of elevated IOP in many cases appears to be more abrupt. In this younger group, symptoms of transient blurring of vision and seeing colored holes around lights are not uncommon. At the first examination, in some younger patients one may find an IOP of 40 to 70 mm Hg, despite which the disc may be normal and the field full. These findings suggest that elevated IOP, especially to such a high level, has not been present for long. A history of transient blurred vision and seeing colored haloes is perfectly consistent in a young individual with a diagnosis of POAG. These symptoms are an indication that there is a considerable and probably rapid increase of IOP, but do not mean that an emergency has arisen and that the glaucoma cannot be controlled medically.

These symptoms occur also in angle-closure glaucoma, and the kind of glaucoma must be positively identified. In angle-closure glaucoma, the symptoms of blurring and haloes have an entirely different significance, indicating closure of a considerable portion of the angle and calling for vigorous treatment, e.g., laser iridectomy.

Not all of the younger patients have a rapid onset of open angle glaucoma. In some, the onset is gradual and asymptomatic, as it characteristically is in the older patients.

Whatever the mode of onset of open angle glaucoma, the disease tends to progress steadily with time. Whatever the cause of the impairment of outflow from the anterior chamber, **the outflow tends to become further impaired as time passes.** This may not mean in all cases that the IOP steadily rises, for in some older patients with marked obstruction to outflow, the IOP remains, or becomes in time, relatively low due to a lowered rate of aqueous formation.

DIAGNOSIS

The diagnosis of POAG is usually made by routine tonometry and by inspection of the optic nerve heads. The importance of the latter cannot be overemphasized. The IOP at a given examination may be in a normal phase, but if the disc is abnormal, suspicion is immediately aroused. If the disc is normal and routine tonometry reveals an IOP at the upper limit of normal, various tests may be used, such as tonography (Chapter 6). However, such a test is not vital in the further management of the case. Once the ophthalmologist's suspicion is aroused, he/she is bound to keep the patient under close observation. If the patient does in fact have early glaucoma, it will be apparent sooner or later in subsequent examinations.

An IOP of 22 or more mm Hg with the Goldmann applanation tonometer should arouse suspicion of glaucoma. Screening of all close relatives of a patient with glaucoma will reveal a higher incidence of glaucoma than in the general population.

Many cases of apparent POAG can be diagnosed by inspection of the optic disc. If the optic disc shows changes suggesting glaucoma, even if IOP at the time is normal, further investigation will usually lead to a definite diagnosis. One learns in time to recognize the earliest glaucomatous appearance of the optic disc (Chapter 8), so that even if the IOP is well within normal limits, one may be sufficiently suspicious to go on to additional subsequent examinations to detect the presence of POAG (or other forms of open angle glaucoma, e.g., low tension glaucoma, Chapter 19).

Asymmetry of the physiologic cup between the two eyes is a significant finding in early detection of open angle glaucoma. Even though each cup individually appears physiologic and does not reach the disc margin anywhere, if the cup in one eye is definitely different from the cup in the other eye, one's suspicions should always be aroused. Even if at first the IOP is equal in the two eyes and well within the normal limits, if the cup is definitely larger in one eye than in the other, the patient should be followed as a possible glaucoma suspect. In a large number of patients that we have seen and followed, asymmetry of the physiologic cups has been one of the most common findings in early open angle glaucoma.

As a personal illustration, when the son of Paul A. Chandler, MD, was in medical school and was practicing on his father with the ophthalmoscope, he remarked that the optic disc in one eye looked different from that in the other. Checking by a colleague, W.M. Grant, MD, confirmed the fact that the physiologic cup was a little wider in the left than in the right eye. IOP was still 18 mm Hg in both eyes. Facility of outflow was normal and equal in the two eyes on several occasions, but 5 years later, obstruction to outflow became measurable in the eye with the larger cup, and the IOP went up to a glaucomatous level.

Other early changes in the cup of the optic disc, apart from asymmetry, which suggest glaucoma, are as follows: a cup that reaches the disc margin at any point, most commonly below, a slight bending of all vessels at the margin, and an appearance, very hard to describe, in which there is little or no bending of vessels at the margin, but in which one gets the impression that the whole disc has a shallow saucer-like depression to the margins, which might be called saucerization of the disc (see Figs. 8.8 and 8.12). Many times we have suspected glaucoma from a slight bending of the vessels at the margin of the disc, or this appearance of saucerization, and the diagnosis has later been confirmed. One must practice looking at optic discs very critically and eventually one will become expert at picking out the ones that should arouse suspicion of early glaucoma. While the instrumentation described in Chapter 9 may one day make such optic nerve sleuthing obsolete, currently the clinician is obliged to identify even the most subtle disc abnormalities.

The characteristic progressive changes in the discs in glaucoma are described in greater detail, with diagrams, in Chapter 8.

An exception to be remembered is that in high myopia, it may be extremely difficult to diagnose early glaucoma by the appearance of the optic disc (see Fig. 8.20), whereas it is easier to diagnose it in the average eye. In trying to determine whether glaucoma is present in a case of considerable myopia, special care is necessary. Applanation, rather than Schiotz or other indentation tonometry, should always be performed in myopic patients because of their lower scleral rigidity. In the past decades it was common for the IOP to be in the normal range when measured with the Schiotz tonometer even though the IOP was actually in the glaucomatous range.

Another special condition of the optic nerve head that is suggestive of glaucoma is occlusion of the central retinal vein in one eye. In such a case, both eyes should be studied carefully for open angle glaucoma (especially exfoliation) because **a high percentage of patients having occlusion of the central vein in one eye turn out to have open angle glaucoma in both eyes,** either frankly present then, or diagnosed later. After occlusion of the central retinal vein, the fellow eye is usually the better eye for vision, so it should receive special attention, and early treatment for elevated IOP.

PROVOCATIVE AND CONFIRMATORY TESTS

Tonography

When suspicion of glaucoma has been aroused by a borderline IOP or a suggestive disc, tonography may reveal an impaired facility of outflow that leads to a definite diagnosis on the basis of the Po/C ratio.

Water-Drinking Test

An increase in IOP of 8 to 10 mm Hg after rapid ingestion of a quart of water strongly suggests glaucoma, but a negative test does not rule it out. Tonography plus a water-drinking test may reveal an abnormality in cases in which either test alone is inconclusive. Although theoretically useful, we have, in truth, only rarely performed a water-drinking test in recent years and do not recommend it for routine use.

Time

Once glaucoma is suspected, either on the basis of IOP or a suggestive disc, the patient should be kept under observation indefinitely. If glaucoma is developing, eventually one will find definite elevation of IOP or definite glaucomatous changes in the disc. **Stereo disc photographs are an important part of the baseline information.**

One keeps seeing the patient from one to several times a year. If the patient does have glaucoma, sooner or later unequivocally elevated IOP or optic disc change is found. Of course, during this time, close watch is kept on the optic nerve appearance to be sure no appreciable change is occurring. Such a leisurely approach is justified only in patients in whom the optic nerve heads have no more than physiologic cupping. If there is pathologic cupping, atrophy, or field loss with initial equivocal IOP measurements, one must examine the problem more intensively and not wait unduly to initiate antiglaucoma therapy. The IOP might be in a "normal phase" of diurnal fluctuation or the patient might have a form of low tension glaucoma (Chapter 19).

DIFFERENTIAL DIAGNOSIS

If IOP is definitely elevated or the disc shows definite changes characteristic of glaucoma, one must determine whether the glaucoma is primary open angle glaucoma, angle closure glaucoma, or some form of secondary glaucoma.

If gonioscopy is carried out when IOP is elevated, and the angle is seen to be open throughout, angle closure glaucoma is ruled out, no matter if the angle is narrow (Chapter 22). If the IOP is normal because the patient is already under treatment when gonioscopy is carried out, the finding of a narrow but open angle is inconclusive. Treatment must then be discontinued to allow the IOP to increase, and gonioscopy is repeated. If the angle is still open throughout, the diagnosis is open angle glaucoma. On the other hand, if one finds closure of the angle consistent with the degree of elevation of IOP (Chapters 22, 24), the diagnosis is angle closure glaucoma. Sometimes it is difficult to be sure whether a portion of the angle is closed or almost closed, and repeated examination may be necessary, especially in cases in which the IOP without treatment is only moderately elevated. If IOP without treatment increases above 35 mm Hg, in cases under investigation to determine whether one is dealing with open angle glaucoma with a narrow angle or angle closure glaucoma, it is usually not difficult to determine whether there is sufficient closure to account for the elevated IOP. If IOP without treatment increases only to 28 or 30 mm Hg, little of the angle needs be closed to account for such a moderate elevation of the IOP. It is particularly in these cases that the differential diagnosis between open angle glaucoma with a narrow angle and angle closure glaucoma is most difficult (Chapter 24).

Beta blockers, alpha-2 agonists, and carbonic-anhydrase-inhibiting drugs, due to their suppression of aqueous formation, cause some widening of the angle. One may be deceived as to the true width of the angle. In cases in which the angle appears narrow but open while the patient is using these drugs, it may appear narrower or partially closed after the drugs are discontinued (Chapter 22).

One must always rule out secondary glaucoma before deciding on a diagnosis of POAG. The possibility that the glaucoma may be secondary to some other abnormality of the eye is one of the good reasons why one should never omit gonioscopy in any case of glaucoma, no matter if it seems obvious from the appearance at slit-lamp examination that the angle must be wide and open. Findings in the angle that may not be suspected from slit-lamp examination, but that are revealed by gonioscopic examination, and that indicate that the glaucoma is secondary and not primary are peripheral anterior synechias, abnormal vessels, abnormal pigmentation, exudates (KP) on the uveal or corneoscleral meshwork, tumors in the angle, and disruption of the angle from trauma. These abnormal findings in the angle are discussed more fully in Chapter 7 and in chapters on the individual secondary glaucomas.

Finding glaucoma in only one eye while the other eye is completely normal is strongly discordant with a diagnosis of POAG and indicates that one is probably dealing with some other type of glaucoma. However, it is not unusual to have POAG advanced to a more severe stage in one eye than in the other eye, and one must have good tonographic measurements or IOP curves to be sure whether an eye in question is normal. Differential diagnosis of glaucoma restricted to one eye is discussed in Chapter 40.

NORMAL VERSUS ABNORMAL IOP

By general convention, IOPs above 22 mm Hg are considered to be either abnormal or " suspicious of being abnormal." This arose originally from population studies in which the mean IOP of "normal" individuals was determined, and thereby IOPs greater than two or three standard deviations from this "normal" mean were defined as being abnormal. However, there are several flaws in the logic of these definitions.

In population studies, patients with frank glaucomatous optic nerve changes and field loss may have a "normal" IOP, especially if only one measurement is made (1–4). As mentioned in Chapter 1, our clinical methods of detecting early optic nerve damage or unequivocal visual field loss from glaucoma are not very sensitive. To be blunt, we cannot detect early damage. Therefore, it may be difficult to categorize people as "normal." Finally the same logic if applied to systemic hypertension would result in patients at risk not receiving what is regarded as necessary therapy; with age, systemic hypertension increases in prevalence to seemingly affect as many as one third of the elderly population (with risk of future end-organ damage) (5–7). Yet, if one surveyed an elderly population and calculated the mean blood pressure and only considered abnormality as being a certain number of standard deviations from the mean, one would mislabel many patients who have systemic hypertension as being "normal." Statistical methods of identifying "normality" are useful only for establishing general guidelines rather than distinct criteria, especially when it is usual or "normal" for a disease to have a higher prevalence in a certain population.

In many ways, the glaucomas share characteristics with other diseases of aging. Although it may be "normal" to age, as physicians we want to intervene to stabilize and prevent further development of aging processes. (Death itself can be considered "normal" for a certain age group!)

We also know that progressive low-tension glaucoma (LTG) (normal pressure glaucoma) is a real entity that in the vast majority of patients has some IOP sensitive component (Chapter 19). In LTG, there is something substantially wrong with the optic nerve that we do not fully understand. Ultimately we need to develop intervention remedies that correct or treat this susceptibility of the optic nerve to glaucomatous damage. However, there is a large body of clinical evidence obtained over long periods that substantiates the clinical impression that decreasing IOP, especially to a very low level, does alter the natural history of this disease in a favorable way. Perhaps controlled clinical trials may alter this opinion, but at the present time the available clinical information strongly suggests the need to decrease IOP in LTG, which is constituted by more than one entity. The clinical implications of this are that IOP below 22 mm Hg, even if repetitive, may not be "normal," and therefore still can encompass glaucomatous disease.

Further, the original "Chandler-Grant" tenet (8) that an optic nerve damaged by glaucoma commonly requires a lower than "normal" IOP has now achieved generally wide acceptance. Therefore, for patients with known glaucoma, an IOP simply in the "normal" range is not necessarily adequate to prevent further progression of the disease (9).

What then is the clinician to do with the IOP data? What is an abnormal IOP? The diseases of glaucoma behave clinically as if individual eyes (or pairs of eyes) have an individual susceptibility to a given level of IOP that really can only be determined for that patient by long term follow up. If we only someday could understand the reasons for this individual susceptibility. We have some guidelines, but **the key to the detection of glaucoma is not simply the measurement of IOP but also the simultaneous evaluation of the optic nerve and visual field** (the methods for which have their own uncertainties in sensitivity and accuracy).

Glaucoma screenings should therefore involve not only IOP measurements but also ophthalmoscopic evaluation of the optic nerve appearance. In any suspect patient, we should obtain stereo disc photographs because in the progression of glaucoma the appearance of the "cup" of the optic nerve will change. In the long-term care of patients with glaucoma or suspicion of glaucoma, it is remarkable how often we wish we had baseline photographs from previous years to assist our clinical judgment. **It is excellent ophthalmologic care to obtain stereo disc photographs on any patient with a suspicion of glaucoma or a future risk of developing glaucoma.**

"ELEVATED" IOP ABOVE 22 MM HG

We have so far dealt with the clinical fact that a statistically "normal" IOP does not by itself indicate the absence of glaucoma. How about the opposite question: does the presence of an IOP above 22 mm Hg indicate an abnormal condition, that is, the presence of glaucoma?

For this question also, there is surprising uncertainty and varying opinions that have changed over time. Clinically a great number of patients exist whose optic nerves (and visual fields) seem to tolerate IOPs in the mid to upper 20s without apparent damage. However, the key word is "seem." Our clinical methods to detect early axonal death in the optic nerve are not very sensitive. Glaucoma for the ophthalmologist is truly the "curse" of long-term follow-up and such observations have led many to realize that elevated IOP is not as benign as once thought. Studies have indicated that there is a protective effect of lowering IOP in patients who initially had no apparent end-organ damage (10,11). Probably (although not with certainty until our methods can truly detect early damage) there are individuals with IOP elevated into the 20s who will never suffer clinically detectable optic nerve damage, but prospectively it is impossible to identify all such individuals.

One can view this in terms of relative risk. There are risk factors (12) that increase the chances for optic nerve damage, such as the degree of IOP elevation, having large cups or asymmetrical cups, or abnormal tonographic outflow (10), or the presence of myopia (13) or a strong family history, African-American race (14), or the presence of disc hemorrhages, etc. However, two recent prospective randomized studies (10,11) of "early treatment of elevated IOP" in patients not considered clinically to be at excessive risk, surprisingly showed a protective effect against end-organ damage. (In the Boston study, it was clinically sobering to realize that such a protective effect was not apparent at 2 years of follow-up, but only after longer time periods (10).)

There are strong analogies to a similar clinical question in the treatment of asymptomatic mild systemic hypertension, where controlled studies have indicated the protective effect of "early" treatment (15), and the clinical implication has been, therefore, to treat all patients with mild elevation of blood pressure, even those without additional risk factors. Yet a critical examination of the data on which this is based indicates that internists have chosen to treat perhaps a majority of such patients who seemingly will not develop end-organ damage, to protect a minority who will, because they cannot prospectively identify those individuals who will develop clinical disease.

We face the same question and dilemma in treating

(or not) asymptomatic elevation of IOP. (Glaucoma and systemic hypertension are not totally unrelated diseases from an epidemiologic point of view, Chapter 72 [16]). Although perhaps it could be argued to wait to treat elevated IOP until clinical damage is detected, we also know (from long-term clinical observations) that once a disc is damaged, it commonly requires a "progressively" lower IOP to prevent further damage. IOP elevation results in damage not only to axons, but to the supporting structures of the optic nerve itself, the cells of the lamina cribosa, and the extracellular matrix (17,18). One could hypothesize that a disc damaged by pressure is more susceptible to further damage due to the changes in the substance of the optic nerve head. The implication of this is that earlier preventative treatment could make the subsequent glaucoma less difficult to treat. (Although this latter statement has never been proven, it is the logical deduction from the clinical observation that a **disc, once damaged, requires a lower than usual IOP for stability**.)

We return again to this problem in glaucoma of individual susceptibility of the optic nerve of a given patient, in which general rules or statistical considerations are probably not as meaningful as the detailed clinical observation of the individual patient, using all the clinical means that we have available to document what is present, so that we can accurately detect future change. This individual susceptibility and variability is what makes it impossible to precisely define a "normal IOP" or an "abnormal IOP" (except for "very high" IOP levels. However, it is curious how this was defined a decade ago as IOP in the 40s, where now it is regarded as IOP in the 30s).

A further complicating factor was mentioned in Chapter 1: although the measurement of IOP is usually (but not always–see discussion of artifacts in IOP measurement in Chapter 6) an accurate data point, it is just a snapshot in time. Due to diurnal and seasonal fluctuation in IOP we are not yet able to determine the true "representative" (mean or median, time integrated, etc.) IOP of any given patient.

WHEN TO TREAT (WHEN THERE IS NO OBVIOUS END-ORGAN DAMAGE)

A decade or more ago the prevailing clinical opinion was that IOPs below a certain cut-off, usually in the 30–33 mm Hg range, did not require anti-glaucoma therapy unless there was evidence of optic nerve damage or visual field loss (for which the IOP would be vigorously treated!). There was a belief among some that elevated IOP (to even higher levels than the low 30s) could be a benign separate condition that was sometimes labeled "ocular hypertension." Regardless, probably most glaucoma clinicians did have an IOP "cut off" in the 30 mm Hg range. Today there is probably general consensus that a separate benign condition of "ocular hypertension" does not exist (or at least cannot be prospectively distinguished from "early" primary open angle glaucoma), and the "cut-off" for treating "asymptomatic" (clinical signs) elevated IOP has been lowered for most clinicians to somewhere in the 20s. There is still much discussion about where the cut-off should be (with still limited but finally some new, potentially important data).

What has been curious historically all along is that when the IOP was elevated from some secondary cause, the threshold of IOP for treatment was in many cases lower than for POAG. We practiced as if elevated IOP in POAG was somehow less damaging than in secondary causes. There is no reason to believe this is true.

The prospective randomized clinical studies of Epstein et al (10) and Kass et al (11) had different protocols but reached the same conclusion (based on surprisingly similar unexpectedly high rates of clinical failure): **lowering the IOP** (with a beta blocker) **is protective against end-organ damage**. Although neither study can be considered perfect, and in truth such randomized clinical trials can only answer one decision point-type question, and such studies need to be confirmed on larger and perhaps different populations, yet to one of us (DLE) the clinical conclusion was inescapable: the need to lower the above "cut-off" for indication of anti-glaucoma therapy from 30 mm Hg (where it had been for DLE at the start of the trial) to the mid or lower 20s.

All clinical studies should be judged by this criterion: **does it change the way one practices? A related question involves treating one's patients as one would want his or her own eyes to be treated**. The above "Boston" study (10) has, in fact changed the way the study's senior author, David L. Epstein, MD, practices, and therefore it seems appropriate to list the clinical conclusions from the study:

1. In patients with "elevated" IOP (22 to 28 mm Hg) and no obvious end-organ damage (optic nerve or abnormalities in the visual field), lowering the IOP (with a beta blocker) is protective against developing end-organ damage.
2. Although other data suggest that the risk of end-organ damage goes up fairly linearly with the degree of elevation of IOP, in this study (with two baseline IOPs), patients with baselines below 25 mm Hg were just as likely to fail as those over 25 mm Hg. Perhaps with a larger number of patients a greater risk for higher IOP would have been demonstrated for the population. However, for an individual patient, the clinician should not "relax" with **IOPs in the low 20s: such patients also require follow-up and possibly treatment.** (Our interpretation of these data relates to what has been referred to before; single measurements of IOP, although extremely accurate, are "snapshots" of only one moment in time.)

3. Patients with large optic nerve "cups" (even if deemed physiological), or slight asymmetry of their optic nerve cups, or slight asymmetry of their IOP, or with severe impairment of their tonographic outflow facility (thus indicating severe trabecular disease) are at a greater risk of failure.
4. A topical beta blocker (timolol) does not lose its ability to decrease aqueous humor formation with time in glaucoma patients. Rather POAG patients in both treated and untreated groups may show a slow upward "drift" in their IOP because the trabecular disease continues to progress. (Therefore there is no point to "withhold" use of topical beta blockers until a later stage of the disease process; this was actually advocated by some a decade ago!)

This study and the one of Kass (11) and further clinical observation (which is now entering the third decade for DLE) has convinced DLE that moderate elevation of IOP is not as benign a condition as formerly thought. Although exact cut-offs await further studies, **DLE does treat all patients (except perhaps the elderly) with IOP of 25 mm Hg or higher, and if there are large (even deemed physiological) cups, or slight asymmetry of the cups or IOP, or severely impaired outflow facility, or if the patient is myopic or has a strong family history of POAG, or is an African-American, treatment for IOPs of 23 mm Hg or higher will be initiated.** Obviously this is modified by individual factors for individual patients such as their age (since this study shows that the damage occurs over years, elevated IOP is therefore a greater risk to younger patients), side effects from medications (without obvious end-organ damage such "protective therapy" that may not truly be required for all, should not disable the patient; if medications cannot be tolerated, the balance of benefits to risks can switch to a strategy of close observation). An additional factor to be considered in myopic eyes with POAG is the possibility for the initial field loss to extend close to or actually involve central fixation.

What if the patient without apparent end-organ damage is on therapy, but the IOP exceeds these guidelines? For the patient on maximally tolerated medical therapy already, a decision for surgical intervention usually should require (in the absence of evidence of end organ damage) very high IOPs, e.g., upper 30s or greater. To perform laser trabeculoplasty, with a favorable prognosis for a clinical effect, one would probably require an IOP in the mid-20s. What is known and what is not known should be discussed with the patient who should have input with their philosophical wishes (therapeutic activism versus nihilism).

GENERAL PRINCIPLES IN TREATMENT

The goal of treatment in POAG is to prevent loss of visual function. If we prevent loss of function, our treatment is adequate. All of our treatment is designed to lower the IOP, either by increasing the facility of outflow or by suppressing formation of aqueous humor, or both. It is humbling to realize that we have no specific treatment for the outflow abnormality of POAG because the cause is still unknown.

There is no absolute level of IOP that must be obtained to ensure successful treatment in all cases. In some eyes with normal optic nerves, if treatment maintains IOP at a level in the mid or low 20s, no loss of function occurs, and the treatment may be considered successful. On the other hand, in cases of advanced glaucoma, IOP must usually be maintained at a level below 18 mm Hg to prevent continued loss of function (9). In far advanced glaucoma IOP in the low teens or lower is required (see next section). The intensity of treatment required may therefore be considerably influenced by the stage of the disease, as evidenced by the condition of the optic nerve and the visual field.

A patient with extensive cupping and considerable field loss, having an initial IOP of 20 mm Hg, should be treated just as vigorously as a patient with a normal disc and IOP in the 40s. Occasionally one sees a patient of this sort whose IOP is 20 to 22, and in whom the IOP can be reduced to less than 15 mm Hg by intensive treatment. Thus, the mere fact that an occasional patient with advanced cupping and field loss does not have a very high IOP does not mean that one should treat him with only single antiglaucoma therapy. He should be treated just as vigorously as the patient with the high IOP.

A high initial IOP, such as the 40s to the 50s, in patients with little or no field change, indicates that the patient has an extremely poor facility of outflow. In such cases we expect large fluctuations in IOP, often a considerable elevation during a particular portion of the day or night. A slight change in the rate of formation of aqueous humor in such an eye is reflected in a large change in IOP. In all patients who have a high initial IOP, before we are satisfied with the results of our medical treatment, we check the IOP at different times of the day. In the middle of the afternoon we may find that the IOP is 20 mm Hg and feel that the glaucoma is under control, but if we measure the IOP at 8 o'clock in the morning, we may find it to be 40 mm Hg!

INITIATING (AND ADVANCING) TREATMENT WITH END-ORGAN DAMAGE

Steps in medical management perhaps leading to laser trabeculoplasty and then, potentially, surgical intervention will be detailed in a subsequent chapter (and also are listed as general guidelines in Table 18.1). However in terms of general principles, **whatever the level of presenting IOP, it is obviously "too high," and therefore medical intervention is required to substantially lower the IOP**

PRIMARY OPEN ANGLE GLAUCOMA AND MYOPIA

David L. Epstein

The reader needs to be aware of an unusual, although not rare, "syndrome" that can occur with POAG and myopia (1): The earliest field loss can extend directly into fixation and involve central visual acuity. This possibility influences one's threshold IOP for treatment when POAG is associated with myopia. Careful inspection of the straight temporal margin of the disc is very important in the assessment of all glaucoma patients, but especially those who are myopic. The normal tilt of the myopic disc makes such analysis very difficult. It is particularly troublesome to be able to detect early contour changes. Thus one usually chooses a lower threshold of IOP elevation to initiate antiglaucoma therapy in such eyes.

Reference

1. Fong DS, Epstein DL, Allingham RR: Glaucoma and myopia: are they related? Int Ophthalmol Clin 1990;30:215–218.

Table 18-1
General Strategy: Steps in Medical Management

1. Beta blocker (or epinephrine compounds)
2. Add epinephrine compound (or beta blocker): expect only 1–3 mm Hg further IOP lowering with nonselective beta blocker
3. Add miotic (or apraclonidine, or topical CAI)
4. Laser trabeculoplasty (or apraclonidine, or topical CAI)
5. Add other(s) from number 4
6. (Oral CAI)
7. Filtration Surgery

Table 18-2
General Guidelines for Target IOP* Findings

	Target IOP
Suspicious appearing optic nerves; no definite field loss	21
Early glaucomatous disc damage and field loss (Fig. 18.1)	18
Moderate to advanced disc damage and field loss superiorly and inferiorly (Fig. 18.2)	15
Advanced disc damage and field loss involving areas close to fixation (Fig. 18.3)	11
Glaucoma damage with central fixation threatened	9

* Modified by IOP level at which damage occurred (see text).

by 20% to 30% below baseline. Because of the varying susceptibility of an individual's optic nerve to glaucomatous damage (cupping), there is no magical "normal" IOP that can be guaranteed to prevent further progression. As always, individual glaucoma patients require individual meticulous follow-up of the optic nerve (with photographic documentation) and visual field, even if the above target for IOP reduction is met. There are no guarantees in the glaucoma field. (Once again it needs to be mentioned that it would truly revolutionize the field if we could determine accurately what the representative IOP really was, rather than obtain "snapshot" data points.)

Once an optic nerve is damaged, clinical experience indicates that a lower than merely "normal IOP" is required. This is a clinical fact that has come from observation of many patients. Clinical appraisal influences the magnitude of the decrease in IOP that is aimed for with antiglaucoma therapy. **A damaged optic nerve requires an IOP below 18 mm Hg for stability.** However, a severely damaged optic nerve may require an IOP in the low teens or even lower (depending also on the IOP at which damage occurred) (Table 18.2) (Figs. 18.1, 18.2, 18-3,).

Central (ten degree) visual fields, probably best if automated, where actual sensitivities close to fixation are measured, are very helpful to identify how much visual field "margin" there is left to follow. That is, if one achieves significant IOP reduction to the targeted value, but follow-up proves that this target IOP was still too high and some progression does occur, if the latter involves increased density of existing scotomata or a new isolated defect away from fixation, this likely will be of little functional significance in itself, and antiglaucoma therapy can then be further escalated. But if there is total cupping, and the sensitivity close to fixation is already substantially reduced, then if one is incorrect in one's assessment of acceptable lowering of IOP, progression of loss of field here can result in substantial functional visual loss, including loss of visual acuity. In such cases with so little margin to follow, unless there is dramatic lowering of IOP to levels than can be usually achieved with glaucoma filtration surgery, e.g., below 12 mm Hg, it is often wisest to proceed rapidly to filtration surgery. (IOPs in the upper single numbers usually confer stability for such patients).

In progressive low tension glaucoma (LTG), there is an IOP sensitive component in most cases, although obviously this is not the whole answer (Chapter 19). One needs to conceptualize that the statistically "normal" level of IOP has resulted in damage to the susceptible (due to unknown causes) optic nerve, and therefore the IOP needs to be reduced at least 20%. Starting with "normal" IOPs, such a target for IOP reduction is sometimes difficult to achieve in LTG except by filtration surgery, but the usual steps

A

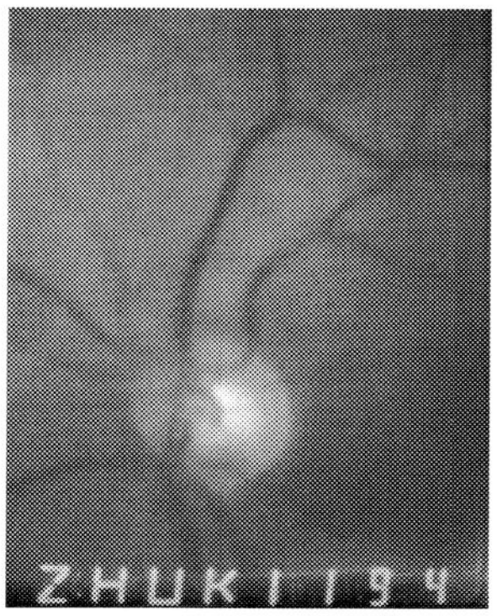

Figure 18.1. Eye with early glaucoma. This patient has early optic nerve damage but a full visual field. Target IOP is 18 (previous IOP mid twenties). A, Stereoscopic optic disc photography. B, Humphrey 24-2 visual field.

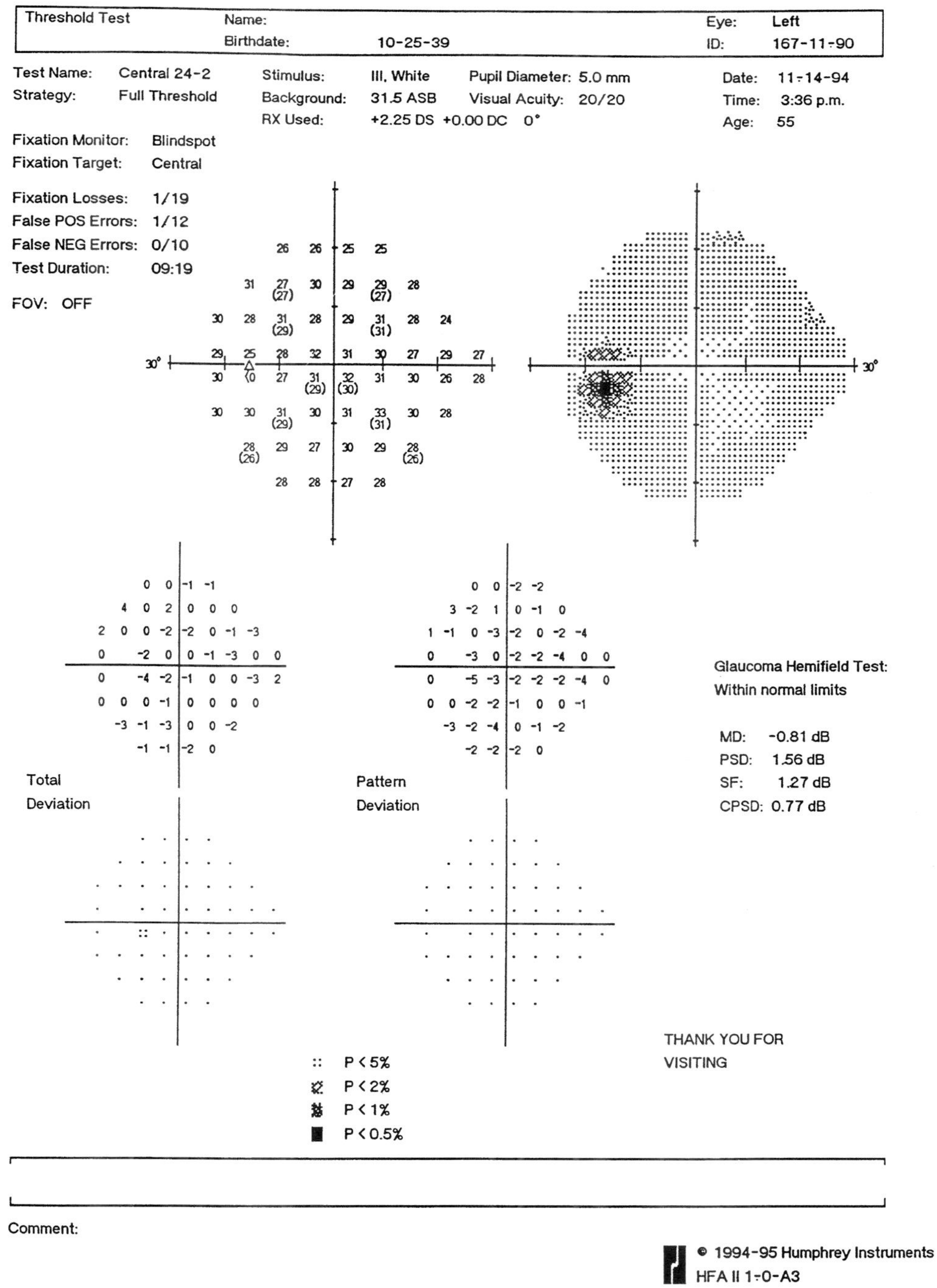

B

should be applied, unless there is no margin to follow (in which case filtration surgery should be promptly performed).

For every patient, a target for desired IOP should be set prospectively and written in the chart. This is not an exact science, and sometimes due to other considerations of age, side effects from medications, or the patient's own input after full discussion, one may modify this. (Except for advanced disease with no margin to follow, the decisions for use of oral carbonic anhydrase inhibitors or filtration surgery require documented disease progression.) However, glaucoma charts tend to get cluttered, and setting such a target pressure in writing assists clarity of thought and effective patient management.

General guidelines for "target IOP" are presented in Table 18.2. These are not "fixed in stone" and are modifiable, depending on many of the factors discussed above, including information about the level of IOP at which

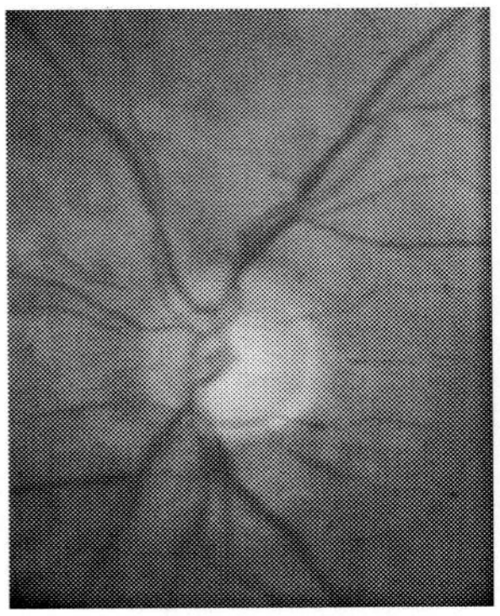

A

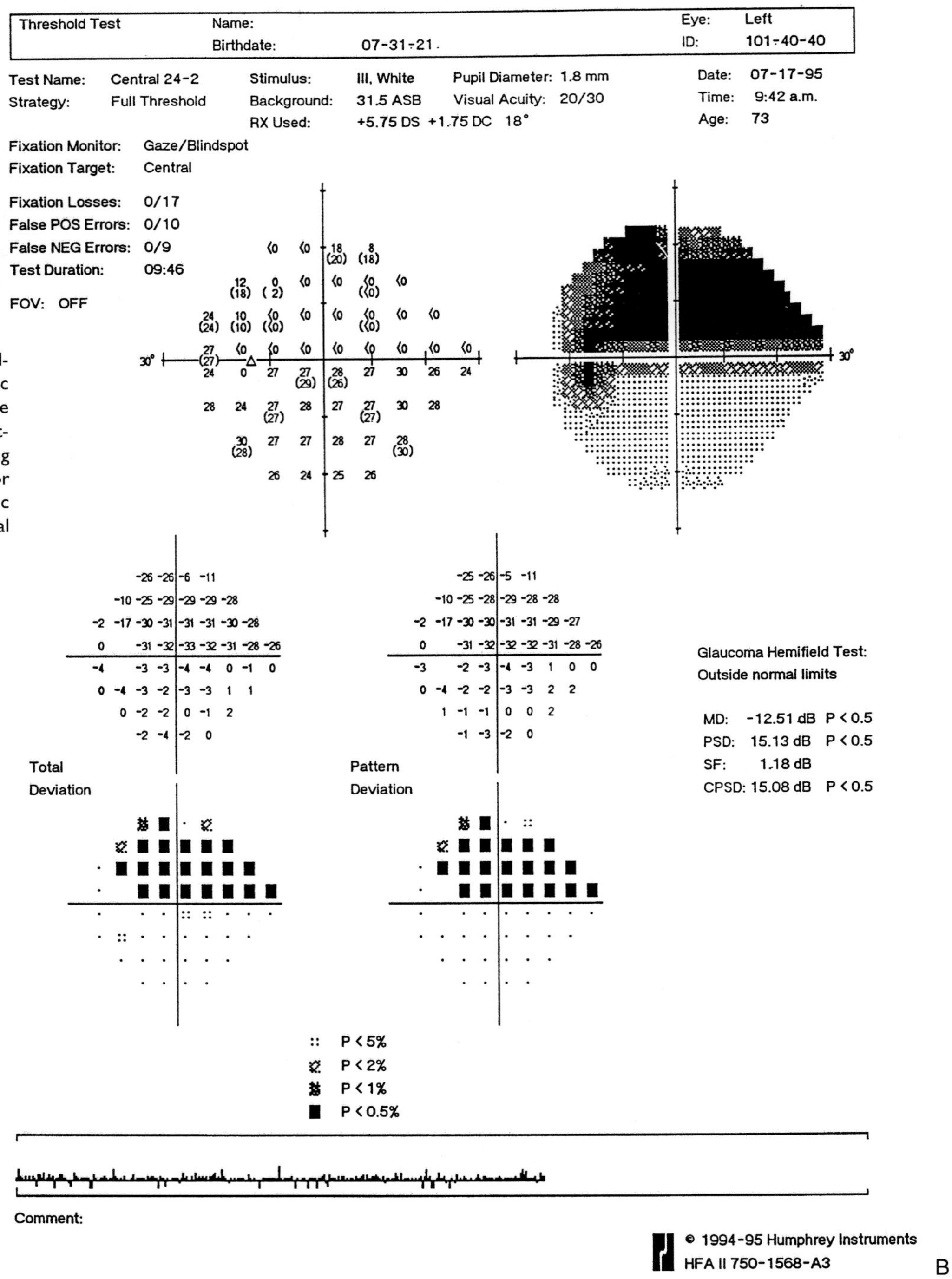

B

Figure 18.2. Eye with modest to advanced glaucoma. There is more disc damage and field loss than seen in Figure 18.1, with a dense superior scotoma splitting fixation and loss of the corresponding neuroretinal rim. Target IOP is 15 (or slightly higher). A, Stereoscopic optic disc photography. B, Humphrey 24-2 visual field.

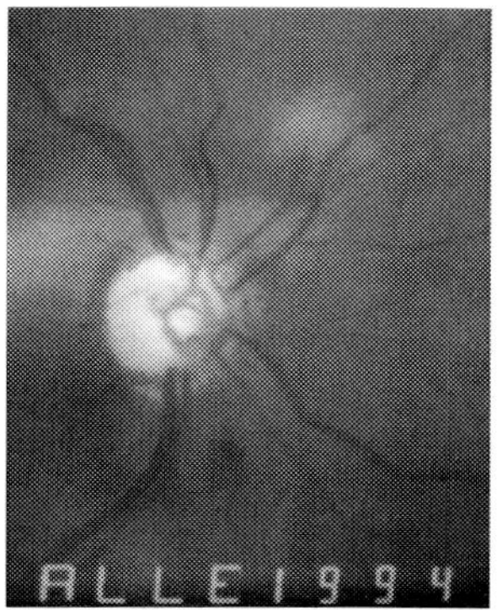

A

Figure 18.3. Eye with advanced glaucoma, and loss of visual field both above and below the horizontal meridian. Such an eye requires an IOP below 11 mm Hg. A, Stereoscopic optic disc photography. B, Humphrey 24-2 visual field.

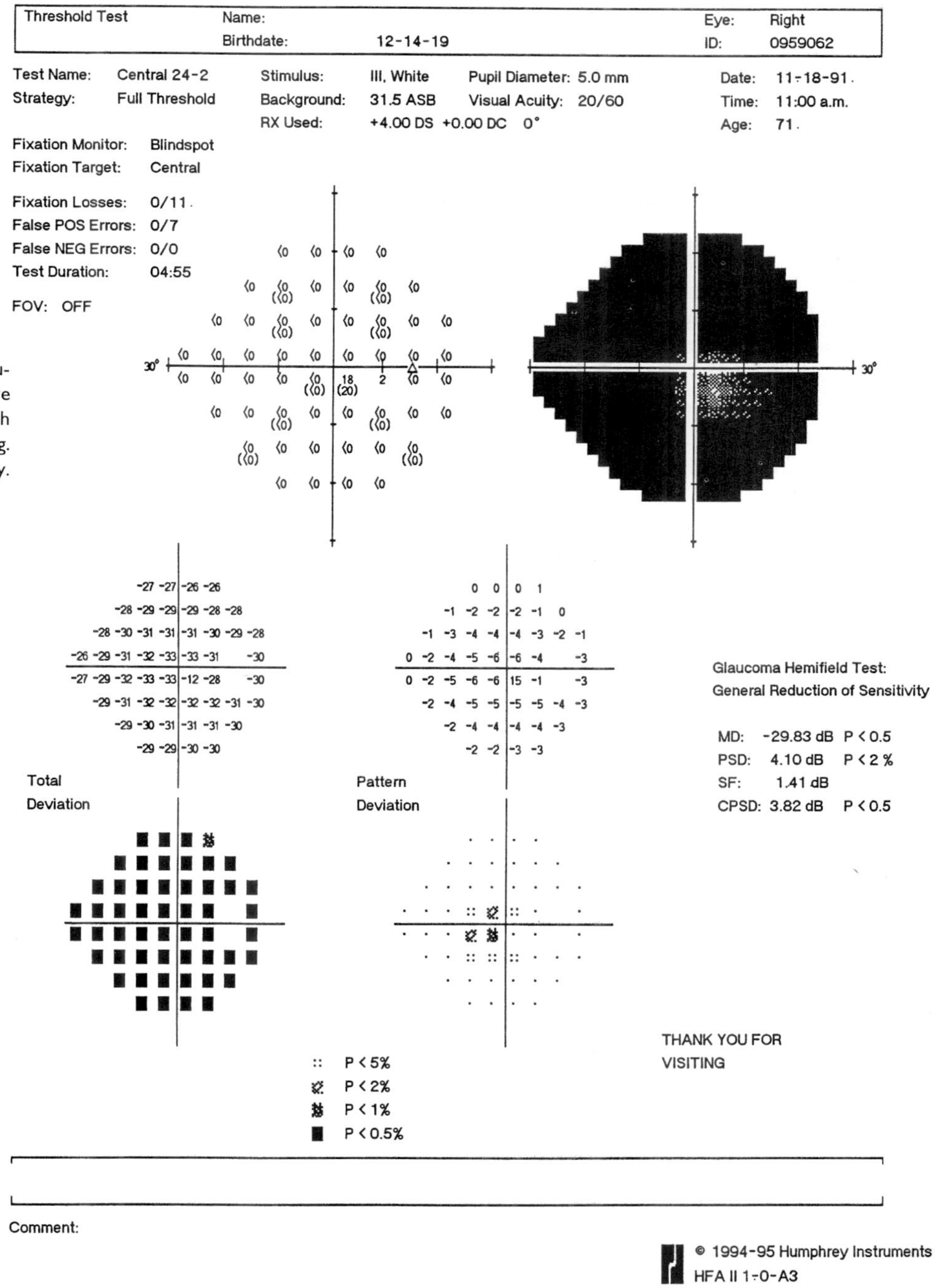

B

COMMON MISTAKES IN GLAUCOMA MANAGEMENT

David L. Epstein

1. Incorrect Diagnosis.

POAG is a diagnosis of exclusion. In addition to gonioscopy, a careful external, slit lamp (including dilated slit lamp) and fundus examination are important to rule out causes such as increased episcleral venous pressure, occult inflammation, silent angle closure, exfoliation, or retinal detachment (Schwartz's syndrome-see Chapter 43). The two most common "masqueraders" of POAG are chronic silent angle closure and occult TM inflammation (trabeculitis).

Rule: when a patient with presumed POAG returns for examination and the IOP is elevated: always perform repeat gonioscopy (look for unsuspected chronic angle closure or occult inflammation). Misinterpreting chronic angle closure as POAG is perhaps the most common diagnostic error in glaucoma.

2. Undertreating Patients with Advanced Disc Cupping and Field Loss

Such patients often require a "low normal" IOP to prevent further progression (not simply an IOP in the high teens). Depending also on the IOP level at which damage occurred, if there is severe field loss in both the superior and inferior field, a target IOP of 12 mm Hg or lower is commonly set. If field loss encroaches on fixation, a target IOP below 10 mm Hg is set. Central ten degree fields should be performed to indicate how much margin is left to follow should the target IOP be incorrect or not realized.

3. Overtreating Early POAG

Although as indicated in the text, we truly believe that elevated IOP is not as benign as once thought, it is nevertheless an error to disable patients with antiglaucoma regimens, especially without evidence of end-organ damage. For example, in such patients if a single medication decreases the IOP from the upper 20s to the lower 20s, and it would be desired to lower the IOP even further, but such medication is disabling to the patient, the risk/benefit (toxicity) ratio shifts such that it is prudent to follow the patient on the regimen with careful monitoring of the optic nerve and visual field. Obviously the presence of risk factors for optic nerve susceptibility to IOP would make one "push" more towards increased therapy, but the entire "picture" of the patient and their life needs should also be evaluated. In the absence of end organ damage, with "margin" that can be followed, and in the presence of a dedicated patient to whom the benefits, risks, and options have all been fully explained, it is permissible to closely monitor the patient on the sub-optimal regimen.

4. Talk to the Patient with Glaucoma.

Explain all the options, and have the patient participate in all decisions. Be sensitive to the potential for glaucoma medications to disable the patient. It is useful for the clinician or the office assistant to list all the medications and times of dosage on a medication card (Fig. 18.4) or equivalent. This enhances patient compliance, but also may obviously indicate the disruption in the patient's lifestyle that some therapeutic regimens are causing.

---

damage occurred. For lesser amounts of glaucomatous damage, the target IOP in the table represents to one of us (DLE) a reasonable goal for IOP, at which, if further progression were to occur due to individual susceptibility, there is sufficient "margin" to be able to assess this without the patient experiencing any (further) functional impairment. For greater amounts of glaucomatous damage indicated in the table, the target IOP chosen reflects the fact that there is progressively less "margin" available to follow the patient further without the risk of progressive functional impairment. As indicated above, in the extreme, if field loss involves central fixation, one is justified to proceed rapidly to filtration surgery to achieve the very low IOP levels required (Table 18.3).

Table 18-3
Indications for Filtration Surgery in POAG

1. Progressive field loss and/or disc cupping despite maximal medical therapy
2. Sustained high IOP, e.g., consistently in the 40s
3. Markedly advanced field loss, encroaching on central fixation, (no "margin" left to follow), with IOP at levels higher than can be achieved with filtration surgery

MECHANISM OF THE DISEASE

What are the underlying tissue abnormalities in the trabecular meshwork and optic nerve that are responsible for POAG? Possible vascular and mechanical factors involved in optic disc cupping have been alluded to in Chapter 2. We truly do not know whether the progressive cupping of the optic nerve and death of axons is a result of direct mechanical pressure on the axons at the level of the disc, or perhaps represents a vascular effect that may also involve mechanical pressure. We do know that all the features of

"TRABECULAR GLAUCOMA" VERSUS "OPTIC NERVE GLAUCOMA"

David L. Epstein

As indicated in Chapter 1, the sometimes "either/or" approach to these subjects has led to confusion, but occasionally also, suboptimal patient management. Almost all glaucomas have a hydrodynamic component involving IOP, and it is useful to frame one's thinking from the perspective of the trabecular meshwork for this component of the disease. But the "end organ" which is damaged by the "trabecular glaucoma" is the optic nerve, which has a varying susceptibility to IOP due to unknown factors that we strive to understand. Glaucoma thus is an "optic neuropathy," but by saying this, it should not connote that we should ignore the role of IOP, which is the one factor we can identify, and the only one for which we have a therapy.

It is often very useful to approach the patient with glaucoma from the perspective of both the trabecular meshwork and the optic nerve. Why is the IOP now elevated in this patient? What is the reason for this worsening of the "trabecular glaucoma"? (As suggested previously repeat gonioscopy may indicate new findings: exfoliation, occult inflammatory precipitates, partial angle closure, etc.) Why is the optic nerve showing progressive damage at this IOP? (Has the IOP been higher in the interval-what is the state of the trabecular glaucoma?) Why is this optic nerve so vulnerable? What are the systemic or ocular factors that lead to this vulnerability?

Although the last question currently has no definite answers, we are confident that by framing one's thought processes in this way, the astute clinician will eventually discover possible answers. But perhaps, even more importantly, by framing one's thoughts this way in separating "hydrodynamic disease" from varying "end organ damage," this allows more effective patient management. Patients with "melting" susceptible discs are thus clearly identified, and more vigorous "hydrodynamic" IOP lowering therapy is initiated, without specific regard for the state of the "trabecular disease." On the other hand, patients with severe trabecular disease are identified as having "real disease" (rather than some statistical variant of "normal") that is very likely, given enough time, to result in end organ damage.

We seem to be on the threshold of new specific drugs targeted at the trabecular meshwork that might "restore normal function" (Chapter 16). Obviously, these agents will treat "trabecular glaucoma" and offer nothing, except by chance, for the susceptibility factors involved in "optic nerve glaucoma." Yet if one can eliminate "trabecular glaucoma" it might greatly simplify the elucidation of these factors. Regardless, we need clear thinking about separate disease processes in the trabecular meshwork and optic nerve both for this discovery, and for optimal patient management.

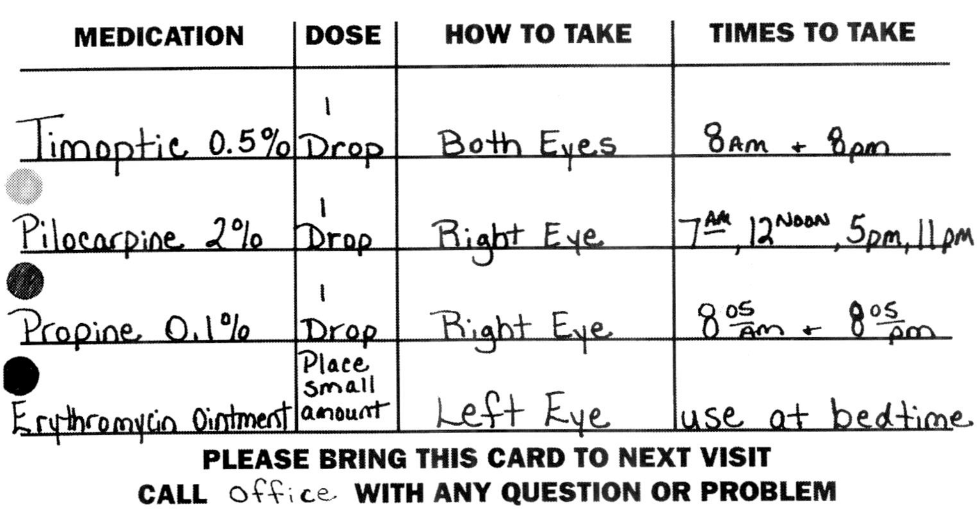

MEDICATION	DOSE	HOW TO TAKE	TIMES TO TAKE
Timoptic 0.5%	1 Drop	Both Eyes	8AM + 8pm
Pilocarpine 2%	1 Drop	Right Eye	7AM, 12NOON, 5pm, 11pm
Propine 0.1%	1 Drop	Right Eye	8:05 am + 8:05 pm
Erythromycin Ointment	Place small amount	Left Eye	use at bedtime

PLEASE BRING THIS CARD TO NEXT VISIT

CALL office **WITH ANY QUESTION OR PROBLEM**

Figure 18.4. Patients are given a medication card at their initial visit and asked to bring it with them at all subsequent examinations. One side of the card is for the right eye and the flip side for the left eye. Medications are listed with the approximate times of administration that relate to the specifics of the patient's lifestyle, bedtime, etc. For patients with impaired vision, in addition to large size letter, the eye bottles may be color coded with colored dots also placed on the medication card.

TONOGRAPHY

David L. Epstein

It is really unfortunate that tonography is so patient and physician "unfriendly." Tonography (Chapter 6) provides the only estimate of outflow function that we have. As the reader may surmise, we have had a special interest in "what's going on in the trabecular meshwork," "why," and especially "what is the severity of the trabecular disease?" In the past, we routinely obtained tonography on all new patients and found that about 1/3 of the time it did provide clinically important information. We used a qualitative approach to tonography: was outflow severely impaired, moderately abnormal, or within or close to normal? If patients had severe impairment of outflow ("almost a flat line"), these patients were believed to have "serious disease" and, all other factors being equal, were more vigorously treated hydrodynamically. For example, if outflow was severely impaired, one could logically, and with some historical validation, presume that there was the potential for more diurnal variation in IOP with small changes in aqueous humor formation. This might then indicate the need to treat rather than observe a patient with IOPs in the 20s, or to presume a significant IOP-related pathophysiological mechanism between visits for patients with progressive field loss but reasonable IOP at the "snapshot" that occurred at the time of the office visit.

But tonography is also very useful in answering the question: "is the trabecular meshwork function normal" in patients with angle recession, pigmentary dispersion syndrome, exfoliation, uveitis, puzzling apparent unilateral glaucoma, etc. Because of potential influences on aqueous humor formation in diseased eyes or the normal diurnal variation in aqueous production, a single "snapshot" IOP measurement might be misleading, especially at knowing (in an increasingly cost-effective environment) how closely to follow the patient.

Regardless, the reader is urged to always be asking the following two questions in the care of glaucoma patients: "what is going on in the trabecular meshwork?"; "what is going on in the optic nerve?."

(In the end we may discover that there are certain common pathogenetic mechanisms involved in both tissues, e.g., at the connective tissue level, but we need to include both tissues in our clinical disease framework for analysis).

typical glaucomatous cupping of the optic nerve can be produced in previously normal monkeys by induced elevation of IOP (19), and that certain features of such cupping can be correlated with certain anatomical structural aspects of the lamina cribosa (20). Yet this does not explain the varying susceptibility of the optic nerve to IOP that patients with POAG typically demonstrate, which would seem therefore to involve, in addition to IOP (but not excluding IOP), some other systemic or local optic nerve factor. An understanding, which is not yet available, of the factors truly involved in glaucomatous cupping and atrophy-whether mechanical, vascular, constitutive, or environmental, has the potential to radically re-direct and improve glaucoma therapy (21).

In the trabecular meshwork many different and sometimes conflicting histopathological correlates have been reported in POAG. Denudation of the trabecular beams with collapse of the structure and disorganization are likely only end stage phenomena. The two observations now most readily accepted by most, but not all, investigators as earlier events are 1. a decreased cellularity in the trabecular outflow pathway (22) and; 2. the presence of extracellular plaque material in the juxtacanalicular meshwork (23,24). The latter finding was discussed in Chapter 16 in terms of potential novel trabecular drug therapy that might allow this material to be removed from the outflow pathway. Some have argued that the amount of this extracellular plaque material is not sufficient, in and of itself, to mechanically obstruct the pathway for flow (25), and others have indicated that there may be other proteinaceous obstructing materials that are deposited in the outflow channels (26,27,28). Regardless, it is not known whether these extracellular accumulations are a primary or secondary process. Hypotheses concerning the former include proposed direct oxidation of extracellular proteins in the outflow pathway from oxidative species present in the aqueous humor (29,30), while those concerning the latter have involved a postulated primary trabecular cell dysfunction (31), that may also relate to the observed reduced cellularity in the trabecular meshwork (22). But, it is not clear (even in the various hypotheses!) whether the initiating pathological event for the observed increase in outflow resistance in POAG might be a direct mechanical obstruction of the spaces in the extracellular outflow pathway or a cellular defect in fluid movement (thus resulting in a secondary accumulation of extracellular proteinaceous material). Such understanding has important future therapeutic implications (21), but, regardless, it seems likely that future trabecular cellular glaucoma drug therapy will prove effective for either mechanism.

Our research has suggested an additional hypothesis concerning the possible underlying defect in the trabecular meshwork in POAG: a dynamic abnormality in cell function. Histopathological studies, that have been in some conflict, are a static "picture" "frozen in time" of the outflow pathway tissue (that is also chemically fixed for preservation). What if the trabecular cells are normally much more dynamic than these "frozen pictures" would suggest? That is, we do know that the morphology of the outflow pathway cells can change dramatically and acutely in response to different IOP conditions (32,33). We know that these cells are capable of contracting and changing their cell shape and attachment in response to pharmacological agents (34–38). Could these cells be constantly sensing their microenvironment and responding with dynamic cellular changes involving their cytoskeleton? Could such dynamic changes underlie the normal self-regulation of outflow that many have suspected to exist in the trabecular meshwork itself (since there is no innervation or feedback vascular loops in this tissue)? Could such dynamic trabecular cell events be abnormal in POAG? Could such defective dynamic cellular processes in the trabecular outflow tissue also explain the poor ability of POAG cells to grow out in tissue culture monolayers (the process of which requires normal cytoskeletal function)? These are intriguing possibilities, not only because they might point glaucoma therapy in new directions, but because it is now possible to study these dynamic cytoskeletal processes in living glaucomatous trabecular meshwork cells (without the need for a continuous monolayer) (39).

This novel, unproven, hypothesis developed as a "converse," from the trabecular drug studies (Chapter 16) that identified the cytoskeleton of the trabecular meshwork cells as the cellular target that was associated with the improved fluid outflow (34). This led to considerations that the cytoskeleton might be involved not only in such pharmacological targeting, but in normal outflow function as well (35). The corollary of this then might be that abnormalities in such dynamic cytoskeletal function might be involved in POAG, and such dynamic abnormalities would have been missed with past methods of study (hence, the lack of clarity concerning the "true" early histopathological correlate of POAG). One of us (DLE) has proposed this hypothesis, which is under active investigation, in the 16th Annual Robert N. Shaffer Lecture at the American Academy "The Glaucomas: Lessons for a Clinician-Scientist," to both honor Dr. Shaffer, who was a long-standing colleague of Drs. Chandler and Grant, but also to underscore the collective wisdom of these mentors who emphasized that future progress in glaucoma requires clinician scientists (40) to seek to creatively build upon their foundation of past (clinical and laboratory) observations.

References

1. Hollows FC, Graham PA: Intra-ocular pressure glaucoma and glaucoma suspects in a defined population. Br J Ophthalmol 1966;50:570–586.
2. Bengtsson B: The prevalence of glaucoma. Br J Ophthalmol 1981;65:46–49.
3. Sommer A, Tielsch JM, Katz J, et al: Relationship between intraocular pressure and primary open angle glaucoma among white and black Americans: the Baltimore Eye Survey. Arch Ophthalmol 1991;109:1090–1095.
4. Dielemans I, Vingerling JR, Wolfs RCW, et al: The prevalence of primary open angle glaucoma in a population-based study in the Netherlands. Ophthalmology 1994;101:1851–1855.
5. Schoenberger JA: Epidemiology of systolic and diastolic systemic blood pressure elevation in the elderly. Am J Cardiol 1986;57:45C–51C.
6. Davidson RA, Hale WE, Moore MT, et al: Incidence of hypertension in an ambulatory elderly population. J Am Geriatr Soc 1989;37:861–6.
7. Strulov A, Epstein L, Harth A, et al: Blood pressure and hypertension in an elderly population. Eur J Epidemiol 1990;6:160–5.
8. Chandler PA, Grant WM: Lectures on Glaucoma. Philadelphia, Lea & Febiger, 1965.
9. Grant WM, Burke J: Why do some people go blind from glaucoma? [Robert N. Shaffer Lecture] Ophthalmology 1982;89:991–998.
10. Epstein DL, Krug Jr JH, Hertzmark E, et al: A long-term clinical trial of timolol therapy versus no treatment in the management of glaucoma suspects. Ophthalmology 1989;96:1460–1767.
11. Kass MA, Gordon MO, Hoff MR, et al: Topical timolol administration reduces the incidence of glaucomatous damage in ocular hypertensive individuals. A randomized, double-masked, long-term clinical trial. Arch Ophthalmol 1989;107:1590–1598.
12. American Academy of Ophthalmology Quality of Care Committee Glaucoma Panel. Preferred Practice Patterns: Primary Open Angle Glaucoma. San Francisco: The Academy, 1992.
13. Fong DS, Epstein DL, Allingham RR: Glaucoma and myopia: are they related? Int Ophthalmol Clin 1990;30:215–218.
14. Tielsch JM, Sommer A, Katz J, et al: Racial variations in the prevalence of primary open-angle glaucoma. The Baltimore Eye Survey. JAMA 1991;266:369–374.
15. Gifford RW Jr: Review of the long-term controlled trials of usefulness of therapy for systemic hypertension. Am J Cardiol 1989;63:8B–16B.
16. Wilson MR, Hertzmark E, Walker AM, et al: A case control study of risk factors in open angle glaucoma. Arch Ophthalmol 1987;105:1066–1071.
17. Hernandez MR, Ye H: Glaucoma: changes in extracellular matrix in the optic nerve head. Ann Med 1993;25:309–315.
18. Yang JL, Neufeld AH, Zorn MB, et al: Collagen type I mRNA levels in cultured human lamina cribrosa cells: effects of elevated hydrostatic pressure. Exp Eye Res 1993;56:567–574.
19. Varma R, Quigley HA, Pease ME: Changes in optic disk characteristics and number of nerve fibers in experimental glaucoma. Am J Ophthalmol 1992;114:554–9.
20. Dandona L, Quigley HA, Brown AE, et al: Quantitative regional structure of the normal human lamina cribrosa. A racial comparison. Arch Ophthalmol 1990;108:393–8.
21. Epstein DL: Will there be a remedy to reverse the changes in the trabecular meshwork and the optic nerve? A personal point-of-view on glaucoma therapy. J Glaucoma 1993;2:138–140.
22. Alvarado J, Murphy C, Juster R: Trabecular meshwork cellularity in primary open-angle glaucoma and nonglaucomatous normals. Ophthalmology 1984;91:564–579.
23. Lutjen-Drecoll E, Futa R, Rohen JW: Ultrahistochemical studies on tangential sections of the trabecular meshwork in normal and glaucomatous eyes. Invest Ophthalmol Vis Sci 1981;21:563–573.
24. Rohen JW: Why is intraocular pressure elevated in chronic simple glaucoma? Ophthalmology 1983;990:758–765.
25. Alvarado JA, Yun AJ, Murphy CG: Juxtacanalicular tissue in primary open angle glaucoma and in nonglaucomatous normals. Arch Ophthalmol 1986;104:1517–1528.
26. Johnson M, Gong H, Freddo TF, et al: Serum proteins and aqueous outflow resistance in bovine eyes. Invest Ophthalmol Vis Sci 1993;34:3549–3557.
27. Epstein DL, Hashimoto J, Grant WM: Serum obstruction of aqueous

outflow in enucleated human eyes. Am J Ophthalmol 1978;86: 101–105.
28. Russell P, Koretz J, Epstein DL: Is primary open angle glaucoma caused by small proteins? Med Hypoth 1993;41:455–458.
29. Nguyen KPV, Chung ML, Anderson PJ, et al: Hydrogen peroxide removal by the calf aqueous outflow pathway. Invest Ophthalmol Vis Sci 1988;29:976–978.
30. Russell P, Garland D, Epstein DL: Analysis of the proteins of calf and cow trabecular meshwork: development of a model system to study aging effects and glaucoma. Exp Eye Res 1989;48:251–260.
31. Epstein DL: Open angle glaucoma: Why not a cure? (editorial) Arch Ophthalmol 1987;105:1187–1188.
32. Johnstone MA, Grant WG: Pressure-dependent changes in structures of the aqueous outflow system of human and monkey eyes. Am J Ophthalmol 1973;75:365–383.
33. Johnstone MA: Pressure-dependent changes in nuclei and the process origins of the endothelial cells lining Schlemm's canal. Invest Ophthalmol Vis Sci 1979;18:44–51.
34. Erickson-Lamy KA, Schroeder A, Epstein DL: Ethacrynic acid induces reversible shape and cytoskeletal changes in cultured cells. Invest Ophthalmol Vis Sci 1992;33:2631–2640.
35. Epstein DL, de Kater AW, Erickson-Lamy KA, et al: The search for a sulfhydryl drug for glaucoma: From chemistry to the cytoskeleton. Basic Aspects of Glaucoma Research III. Edited by Lütjen-Drecoll E. Schattauer, Stuttgart-New York 1993:345-353.
36. Grewal A, O'Brien ET, Epstein DL: Control of cell shape in the trabecular meshwork. Invest Ophthalmol Vis Sci 1994;35(ARVO suppl):2725.
37. Opperman AD, O'Brien ET, Roberts BC, et al: Can a rise in intracellular calcium (CA) explain the cellular effects of ethacrynic acid? Invest Ophthalmol Vis Sci 1994;35(ARVO suppl):3709.
38. Gills JP III, Roberts BC, Epstein DL: Microtubule disruption leads to active cellular contraction in human trabecular meshwork cells. Invest Ophthal Vis Sci 1996;37; (Arvo suppl):3801.
39. O'Brien, ET, Epstein DL: Observation of living glaucoma cells by video DIC microscopy. 1996;37 (ARVO suppl):4146.
40. Epstein, DL: Is the ophthalmologist as a clinician-scientist still viable? Arch Ophthalmol 1991;109:1523–1524.

Low Tension Glaucoma

19

David L. Epstein

DEFINITION

Unfortunately there is tremendous confusion about low tension glaucoma (normal pressure glaucoma) (LTG) regarding terminology, inclusion and exclusion criteria, possible different forms and pathophysiological mechanisms, and therapy. This confusion is especially nefarious because LTG is not uncommon (perhaps even increasing in prevalence as the population is aging), easily missed in its earliest stages (because the IOP is not elevated), can affect central visual function early, and is difficult to treat with less clear guidelines for the absolute level of IOP required for the IOP sensitive component (since the IOP is not elevated at baseline). **This is among the most difficult of glaucomas for the physician to manage because, unfortunately, this is a potentially blinding, most often progressive disease.** In fact, as will be discussed, we believe nonprogressive forms of this entity to be so uncommon that we use the term LTG synonymously with the older term "progressive LTG." LTG is surprisingly common in Japan (1), but we may be underappreciating its frequency in the United States.

It is useful conceptually to first take a step back and look at optic nerve cupping in response to elevated IOP in the usual forms of (high pressure) primary open angle glaucoma (POAG). As discussed previously, although elevated IOP is probably not as benign as once thought for many patients, there is an individual susceptibility of the optic nerve to cupping which exists in response to a given IOP. For example, one patient may show progressive optic nerve damage with IOP in the low 20s and another patient, with ostensibly similar IOP, may show no obvious optic nerve change. What explains the increased susceptibility of the optic nerve to IOP in the first patient? We really do not know, although there has been much discussion about various possible mechanical or vascular factors (2–5) that may lead more readily to cupping. **In high pressure glaucoma, an optic disc that has been damaged may continue to show progressive damage at "normal pressures."** We call this "LTG equivalent." This entity is further documentation of the phenomenon of individual susceptibility of the optic nerve to cupping in response to a given IOP.

Allowing that there is this varying susceptibility of the optic nerve to cupping at a given level of IOP in the POAG patient, why isn't it logical that cases of apparent LTG represent this same phenomenon, but at a more extreme point of the spectrum with respect to IOP? Just because it is logical does not make it true, but this also can be said in criticism of the school of thought that might consider LTG "logically" to be a separate disease. This book deals with the practical clinical care of the patient with glaucoma and builds on long-term clinical experience with such patients. **Our clinical experience strongly indicates that almost all patients with LTG have an IOP-sensitive component, and that adequately lowering the IOP improves the natural history of the disease.** IOP is not the whole answer and in this disease, there is an extreme susceptibility of the optic nerve to cupping (that if we could only understand, might provide important insight into mechanisms for cupping in higher IOP forms of glaucoma as well).

This "lumping" rather than "splitting" truly fits with our clinical data, and although there likely will prove to be some exceptions as we better define "the glaucomas" in the future, this concept actually simplifies and results in more effective patient management. In LTG, which in the overwhelming majority of patients is a progressive disease that can lead to blindness, there is **an IOP sensitive component combined with an extreme optic nerve susceptibility.** This concept indicates the need to substantially decrease the IOP below baseline in all patients with apparent LTG.

Nonprogressive forms (6) of LTG are rare in the authors' experience, and the burden is, therefore, on the ophthalmologist when he/she makes this rare diagnosis and chooses no therapy. Unfortunately, especially in LTG, there is the "curse of long-term follow-up," and unfortunately, as one follows such patients, it frequently becomes apparent that this is a progressive, potentially blinding, disease for most patients.

For those who might have trouble with this concept, perhaps it might be useful to consider this another way: let us suppose that the etiology of cupping in POAG (so called high pressure glaucoma) actually involves a vascular mechanism. Suppose that elevated IOP results in some type of ischemia from pressure directly on the small vessels supplying the optic nerve. The varying susceptibility of the optic nerve to cupping in high pressure glaucoma might then be due to the presence of varying small vessel disease in the optic nerve, independent of IOP. In LTG, this small vessel disease in the optic nerve might be extreme, such that "normal" levels of IOP are additive pathophysiologically. Lowering the IOP does not treat or eliminate the extreme small vessel disease, but it eliminates this additive noxious element of compromise to the vascular supply. Lowering the IOP therefore improves the natural history of the disease. This "small vessel disease" in the optic nerve might, by itself, produce damage to the optic nerve, independent of the additive noxious IOP effect.

One might argue in this construct that the patient will still ultimately go blind (from "small vessel disease"), but if one can achieve an IOP in the single numbers, our clinical experience is that stability is commonly achieved. In many cases of ("high pressure") POAG, our treatments may also only be palliative, and we are striving to delay blindness past the time of natural (whole body) death. As suggested, patients with high pressure POAG likely share this mechanism of optic nerve susceptibility (hence the varying susceptibility to a given level of IOP in different patients), and therefore lowering the IOP in POAG patients also may not be sufficient to prevent progression. Yet, because the IOP is elevated in POAG, we treat it, and if progression occurs, we treat it more vigorously and lower the IOP further. This usually, but not always, is effective, thus similar to considerations in LTG.

This discussion suggests that since there are likely some similar phenomena in these two forms of glaucoma, there likely could be similar mechanisms of pathology that, when we finally understand pathophysiological mechanisms, may more obviously be part of the same spectrum.

This discussion also implies both for POAG and LTG that, as the population ages, with the realization that our therapies are palliative for both conditions in which we seek to alter the natural history of the disease, there is the potential for blindness to increase in prevalence. Also, when the "curative drug" for the optic nerve is developed (Chapter 16), it may have effectiveness both for POAG and LTG.

Some have used the term "normal pressure" glaucoma rather than LTG. It is a matter of preference, but since it is difficult to know what "normal" IOP truly is (Chapter 18), we prefer the term "low tension."

This discussion and construct help in understanding the "spectrum" of LTG patients and moves one away from rigid inclusion and exclusion criteria. The key to all of this is the concept of "the susceptible optic nerve." There has been much effort and controversy created in patients with suspected LTG to determine whether there is ever an elevated IOP measurement "above normal," even if it occurs only once among multiple measurements. For example, some have sent "LTG" patients home with various tonometers to do diurnal curves, and if one IOP "above normal" is detected, the patient is then reclassified as POAG, but what does this observation really mean? First of all, there is the question of IOP accuracy and also the question of what is a normal IOP and how did we decide this, but regardless, this is all just begging the question.

Suppose in an accurate diurnal IOP curve of a patient with progressive LTG there is 1 elevated IOP measurement and 20 "normal " IOPs. Does this really mean that this patient with progressive field loss has POAG, when we know that there are patients who have 20 out of 20 elevated IOPs and do not have apparent optic nerve damage? We would argue that this patient has unequivocally a "susceptible optic nerve" no matter what one may choose to call it, but phenotypically it fits in our construct of LTG. If the one elevated IOP measurement would indicate to some readers that the patient has POAG and only by this diagnosis needs treatment, then how does one know in other patients with apparent LTG, that one has performed enough IOP measurements to rule out a single IOP spike?

As one carries this argument further, it is easy to see how clinical presentations may cause further confusion, unless one remembers **the unifying concept of the susceptible optic nerve combined with some IOP sensitive component**. Clearly as one part of the spectrum, there are patients with IOPs in the low teens which never go above the low teens (and by use of tonography have totally normal outflow facilities which would imply the non-occurrence of abnormally "elevated" IOPs, i.e., no IOPs in the twenties), and who nevertheless demonstrate progressive cupping and field loss. These are perhaps the most difficult of low tension glaucoma patients to treat because IOP needs to be reduced into the single numbers, but if achieved, clinical stability has, in fact, commonly been observed. But there are similar patients who present with IOPs in the mid- to upper teens (and who correspondingly have borderline abnormal tonographic outflow facilities). One can waste a lot of time looking for that "one elevated IOP measurement" or one can conceptualize that, regardless, this patient fits into the spectrum of the susceptible optic nerve" with an accompanying IOP sensitive component, and thereby **needs an IOP lowering below baseline, no matter what that absolute level of IOP is, and whether one considers it normal or "abnormal."**

Finally there is one last clinical example of the spectrum of this disease, which involves as the key unifying concept that of varying optic nerve susceptibility to IOP. Suppose a patient with a diagnosis of (former) "high pressure" glaucoma presents with documented consistent IOP in the upper teens with nevertheless continuing progressive visual field loss. **In the past, the patient was documented to have consistent IOPs in the mid twenties.** A common example of this phenomenon is a patient with exfoliation glaucoma or POAG with a good response to laser trabeculoplasty (and again here tonography can document near normal outflow facilities and implied stability of IOP) who, nevertheless, subsequently demonstrates progressive disc cupping and field loss despite these "good" IOPs. One can call such patients whatever one wishes as long as

LTG AND THE GENERAL OPHTHALMOLOGIST

David L. Epstein

The general ophthalmologist is an unsung but true hero in the detection of patients with LTG. Consider in a busy general practice a patient whose IOP is normal, where in the absence of any visual field data the general ophthalmologist is suspicious about LTG on the basis of his/her evaluation of the optic nerve. The ophthalmologist is thus a true "disc sleuth." This brings to the forefront the previously described techniques of evaluation of the optic nerve in glaucoma by assessing disc contour (Chapter 8). The goal is to detect LTG before there is much optic nerve damage and before the patient might call attention to the disease by the presence of subjective scotomata, which notoriously can involve points close to central fixation. Because this disease may be increasing in prevalence in our aging population, the "disc sleuthing" general ophthalmologist truly deserves our praise.

clinically it is clear what to do (**lower the IOP further**), but we have used the term **"low tension glaucoma equivalent"** to indicate the enhanced susceptibility of the optic nerve to these now reasonable ("normal") levels of IOP. **Regardless of terminology, these patients should be treated similarly to those with LTG**, with increased therapy to further lower the IOP. Also, consider if one did not have the history of elevated IOP in such a patient? What would one call such a patient? It doesn't really matter what one calls this patient, as long as it is clear that as for other patients with POAG, exfoliation, and low tension glaucoma, no matter what the IOP, the current level of IOP in the face of clinical progression is too high and, therefore, one needs to lower the IOP further.

For patients with both LTG and "LTG equivalent," this strategy is usually successful. There are no data that the authors are aware of that for a given level of "presenting baseline" IOP, the prognosis is any different with respect to the efficacy of further reduction of IOP in "LTG" versus "LTG equivalent" (which some would call POAG, etc). This further indicates that these conditions might share unifying features of both enhanced optic nerve susceptibility and some IOP susceptibility. Almost all clinicians would advance treatment for "LTG equivalent" with a history of previously high IOP. Yet the confusion about LTG has led some to withhold treatment for this entity. In this example, if one did not or could not know the history of elevated IOP, the patient might not be distinguishable from other cases of LTG.

Thus, there seems little merit to trying to subcategorize apparent cases of LTG. One needs to spend one's efforts vigorously lowering the IOP further and following the optic nerve appearance and the visual field closely.

There are (at least) two general rules for the practicing ophthalmologist when a suspicion of LTG is entertained:

1. **Obtain a visual field in the presence of a suspicious optic nerve.**
2. **Photograph any suspicious disc.**

The first point is obvious, but the second is often not emphasized enough. Our drawings even in the hands of "glaucoma experts" are frequently unreliable, and because the "name of the game" for all glaucomas is whether there has been disc and field progression, a baseline photograph for future comparison, even without subsequent photographs, allows one to be much more precise in one's conclusions. True stereo photographs are preferred, but if unavailable, a nonstereo baseline disc photograph can enhance good patient care in the future. In a referral glaucoma practice a common question that one constantly wishes one had the answer to is: what did the optic disc look like at a previous point in time?

"Disc sleuthing," especially in an elderly population, is challenging. In addition to other features of the aged eye such as a smaller pupil and the frequent presence of lenticular nuclear sclerosis that can give the false appearance of a disc having a "healthy" pink appearance (but remember it is contour rather than color that is the key parameter to be evaluated), there often is a "senile" sloping contour to the aged disc. Thus, one should expect to overread suspect discs in the elderly, but visual fields and disc photographs document normal limits in the former and stability in the latter.

SYMPTOMS

Most patients with LTG are asymptomatic and are detected by the ophthalmologist on a routine examination based on the optic nerve appearance. Occasionally patients present with a subjective scotoma close to fixation. Sometimes there does appear to be a credible history of sudden onset. Although one needs to rule out an acute episode of ischemic optic neuropathy, such patients typically progress as other patients with LTG with no further sudden episodes. From a pathophysiological point-of-view, this symptomatology would seem important to understand.

Patients should be asked about any neurological symptoms such as weakness in extremities, dizziness, headaches, loss of consciousness, diplopia, etc. If a patient has any such symptoms, except for typical migraine headaches, a neuro-ophthalmological evaluation is indicated. Migraine has sometimes been associated with LTG (7,8), which again raises the possibility of vascular factors involved in pathogenesis. However, it is not an indication for neurological referral unless atypical.

Raynaud's disease has been associated with LTG. Immunological disease may also be associated with LTG (9,10).

Systemic factors are probably involved in the pathogenesis of LTG that, once understood, will explain the extreme susceptibility of the optic nerve discussed. **The presence of any neurological symptom indicates the need for a neuro-ophthalmological evaluation to rule out neurological disease that might masquerade as LTG. Although the signature of glaucoma is contour changes of the optic nerve (Chapter 8), and that of neurological disease is decreased color of the optic nerve, certain nonglaucoma conditions can uncommonly cause contour changes as well.** The suggestion of other systemic disease, with the exception of migraine, in a patient with LTG would suggest the need for a medical evaluation as part of the general good care of the whole patient with eye disease that we routinely advocate. It is unlikely, however, that treatment of the systemic disease will alter the course of LTG.

DIFFERENTIAL DIAGNOSIS

Certain nonglaucoma conditions can uncommonly cause contour changes in the optic nerve that might be misinterpreted as LTG (Table 19.1).

Table 19.1
Differential Diagnosis of Low Tension Glaucoma

Disorder	Comment
Temporal arteritis	Usually acute severe unilateral vision loss, optic disc swelling, increased disc cupping occurs after acute event, systemic symptoms (myalgias, head ache), elevated ESR
Anterior ischemic optic neuropathy	Usually acute unilateral vision loss, disc swollen initially then pale, increase in disc cupping unusual, altitudinal VF loss may mimic glaucoma
Pituitary or intracranial tumors	VF usually bilateral, VF loss rarely appears glaucomatous, early loss of visual acuity and color vision, optic nerve pallor without abnormal disc cupping
Methanol intoxication	History of drinking "moonshine," acute severe bilateral vision loss, early disc swelling followed by optic nerve pallor and disc cupping
Kjer's hereditary optic neuropathy	Positive family history, usually bilateral with pallor and excavation affecting temporal disc in a young patient
Congenital optic pit or coloboma	Deeply excavated optic nerve, often unilateral, visual fields stable in absence of serous retinal detachment
Syphilitic (tertiary) optic neuropathy	Optic pallor with abnormal cupping, positive serology (FTA antibody and RPR), other evidence of tertiary syphilis
History of past elevated IOP	Resolved steroid-induced, uveitic, or trauma-induced glaucoma in the past can mimic LTG

Contour changes may occur in approximately one third or more of patients with temporal arteritis. Usually there is severe visual field and acuity loss in the cases that have these glaucoma-like contour disc changes (11), which usually are first detected a few weeks after the acute event, when the acute disc swelling has subsided. The characteristic rapid loss of vision and reduction in central visual acuity are helpful differentiating features. Other forms of ischemic optic neuropathy can rarely produce contour changes that are usually more localized on the disc.

Disc cupping rarely occurs with pituitary and other intracranial tumors. The presence of nonglaucomatous visual field loss, substantial asymmetry of the two optic nerves, or any neurological symptoms, indicate **the need for neuro-ophthalmological evaluation.** If in doubt, it is best to refer such a patient for neurological evaluation. **Not to miss an intracranial tumor is the main reason to obtain neurological evaluation and testing, but this is a rare masquerade.**

Methanol intoxication is usually obvious by history, if one remembers to ask about consumption of "moonshine" (bootleg liquor), which is probably the most common clinical situation for methanol exposure. There should be a history of acute visual loss that would be accompanied by acute disc swelling, which is later followed by atrophy of the optic nerve and occasionally contour changes as well. The rapid loss of vision and usual substantial reduction in central visual acuity that is sustained can be helpful in differentiation.

The family history (which also for many other reasons should routinely be obtained in all patients with glaucoma) should assist with the diagnosis of Kjer's and other hereditary optic neuropathies, which classically have onset at a young age (at least below the age of 20).

Lues (tertiary syphilis) has been reported to cause a pseudo-glaucomatous disc appearance, but the authors have never observed this occurrence and believe the presentation as a LTG masquerade must be rare.

Colobomas and pits can sometimes be confusing, but usually the focal, very deep excavation on careful examination helps establish the diagnosis. Field defects should be nonprogressive, unless serous macular detachment occurs.

In temporal arteritis, the disc looks glaucomatously

cupped (see Fig. 8.25). But usually the severe visual function loss and the usual unilateral condition suggests a diagnosis other than LTG. When the other conditions mentioned cause contour changes on the disc, there is usually some atypical character to the cupping, which is subjective. To us, **the most common atypical finding is the color of the rim tissue that is not involved in the contour change.** This is usually pale, i.e., demonstrating optic atrophy, in these pseudoglaucomatous conditions, unlike typical cases of glaucoma in which the unaffected disc tissue seemingly appears normal in color. However, this can be a difficult discrimination, and there do seem to be true, rare cases of intracranial tumors that appear to have glaucomatous optic nerve changes. Not to miss this rare patient with an intracranial tumor that might be confused with LTG is important, but routine CAT or MRI scans in patients with typical LTG is not prudent. On the other hand, one needs to pay attention to possible atypical (for glaucoma) visual field changes, the presence of unilaterality or substantial asymmetry between the two eyes, and the presence of any neurological symptoms, and obtain neurological evaluation in all such patients.

When discussing these conditions, some of these affected patients may develop elevated IOP and glaucoma as a separate clinical disease. One of us (DLE) has seen patients with past methanol intoxication, Kjer's hereditary optic atrophy, and a corticotrophin-secreting pituitary tumor (that caused elevated IOP that reversed after surgical resection). In addition to other considerations, these patients are a challenge to manage because of their pre-existing optic nerve changes.

In the differential diagnosis of LTG, one must include causes of past elevation of IOP, that caused optic nerve damage, but are no longer present. Examples include previous steroid usage, uveitis, or trauma-related glaucoma. Such secondary glaucoma may not have been appreciated at the time of occurrence.

WHEN TO OBTAIN NEUROLOGICAL TESTING IN A PATIENT WITH LTG

Low tension glaucoma is unfortunately not an uncommon disease. Many years ago, we stopped obtaining routine neurological evaluation. Routine scans are not performed. But if there is anything atypical, then at the slightest suggestion a full neuro-ophthalmological evaluation is obtained (Table 19.2).

One of us (DLE) would frame this as the **concept of "LTG plus."** If the patient has any neurological symptom as discussed, atypical (for glaucoma) visual field changes, or a unilateral or highly asymmetrical condition between the two eyes, or if there is something atypical about the cupping, especially the presence of atrophy in the non-contour affected portion of the disc rim, then this constitutes the "plus" and indicates the need for full neurological evaluation. **There is no such entity as unilateral LTG,** and substantial asymmetry is very uncommon. All such patients need neurological evaluation. The one diagnosis not to miss is that of an intracranial tumor, but such an apparent "masquerader" is rare and would be expected to be detected on the basis of the "plus" factors.

Table 19.2
When to Pursue Neurological Work-up in a Patient with Suspected Low Tension Glaucoma

Uniocular optic nerve involvement or marked asymmetry
Unexplained reduction in visual acuity
Color vision loss without advanced visual field loss
Visual field loss
Out of proportion to optic nerve damage
Non-glaucomatous or atypical
Optic nerve pallor instead of cupping
Neurological symptoms

THERAPY

Although there must be some systemic influence in LTG, unfortunately, there is no proven systemic therapy for this condition. There are conflicting data (12,13) about calcium-channel blockers at the time of this writing, which underscores our lack of understanding. It is not certain whether their proposed benefit might result from a vascular or direct axon effect. Different blockers have different cellular actions. Because we do not understand the mechanism for the optic nerve susceptibility in this condition (is it vascular or mechanical?), it seems quite premature to place LTG patients on such therapy. **We would not recommend calcium-channel blocker therapy until controlled prospective studies are performed.**

Since in almost all, if not all, patients with LTG we believe there to be an IOP sensitive component (14–17), therapy consists of lowering the IOP. This is all we have to offer, acknowledging that this disease involves a "sick" optic nerve involving some etiology that we do not understand. **The patient's baseline or representative IOP is very important. One aims to decrease IOP by 20—25% as a first step.** Much depends on the "margin" that is left to follow in the visual field, especially close to central fixation. **In following such patients, central 10 degree visual field programs are useful to supplement the usual 30 degree fields.** If there is little margin to follow around fixation, one must be very vigorous to obtain IOPs in the single digits. Patients with such advanced field loss should be monitored closely, e.g., three times a year.

Because in most but not all forms of LTG, outflow function through the trabecular meshwork is not substantially impaired, aqueous suppressants are usually more useful than outflow drugs. The usual first choice is the beta

OCULAR EFFECTS OF CALCIUM-CHANNEL BLOCKERS: PRESENT STATUS AND FUTURE DIRECTIONS

Peter A. Netland and Evan B. Dreyer

Calcium-channel antagonists block cell membrane-bound calcium channels and inhibit calcium influx, which can have a profound effect on cellular metabolism and function. In blood vessels, these drugs cause relaxation of smooth muscle cells in vascular walls, decrease vascular resistance, and improve blood flow. The ocular effects of calcium-channel blockers are potentially of great interest in relation to glaucoma (1).

The vascular effects of calcium-channel blockers may inhibit vasospasm or enhance ocular blood flow (2,3), which theoretically might be beneficial in glaucoma patients. In "vasospastic" patients and low-tension glaucoma patients, systemic administration of calcium-channel blockers has been associated with improvements of visual fields (4,5). We have also observed improvements or stabilization of visual fields in low-tension glaucoma patients after treatment with systemic calcium-channel blockers. We evaluated serial stereoscopic optic nerve photographs and visual fields for evidence of glaucomatous progression in low-tension glaucoma patients who were concurrently taking calcium channel blockers compared with controls (6). In this retrospective study, the use of systemic calcium-channel blockers was associated with a slowed progression of low-tension glaucoma. We have postulated that this apparent beneficial effect may be related to the inhibition of vasospasm or enhancement of optic nerve blood flow caused by these drugs.

The effect of calcium-channel blockers on intraocular pressure is also of great interest. Systemic administration of verapamil or nifedipine in rabbits sometimes caused a decrease in intraocular pressure (7,8). In humans, either no effect or sometimes a decrease in intraocular pressure after systemic administration of verapamil, nifedipine, nitrendipine, or diltiazem has been observed (9–12). However, a more pronounced effect was observed in ocular hypertensives or glaucoma patients, who demonstrated elevated intraocular pressure at baseline (9).

Topical administration of verapamil causes a significant reduction of intraocular pressure in ocular hypertensive human subjects (13). This effect was sustained after topical administration of verapamil three times daily for 2 weeks (14). Significant reduction of intraocular pressure has also been observed in normal human subjects after treatment with topical verapamil (2). Experimental studies in rabbits have shown either no effect (8) or a reduction (15) of intraocular pressure after treatment with topical calcium-channel blockers. Topical administration of higher doses of calcium-channnel blockers (1.5–5%) resulted in transient elevation of intraocular pressure (16), suggesting a dose-dependent, biphasic response at higher doses of these drugs, perhaps due to other nonspecific effects besides calcium channel blockade (1). Topical treatment with the calcium ionophores A23187 and X573A have been observed to increase intraocular pressure in rabbits (17). These agents, would be expected to demonstrate an opposite action to calcium-channel blockers.

Topical administration of the calcium-channel blocker verapamil, therefore, usually causes a reduction of intraocular pressure. The more consistent effect on intraocular pressure of topical compared with systemic treatment may be due to higher drug levels reached after topical instillation of verapamil (18). The mechanism of action may be due to enhancement of outflow facility (19,20). These studies suggest a possible future role for topical therapy in the management of glaucoma.

The clinical use of calcium-channel blockers in the management of glaucoma is currently under evaluation. We personally treat with systemic calcium-channel blockers selected low-tension glaucoma patients who continue to demonstrate disease progression despite maximal tolerated medical therapy with sustained low IOP (10–12 mm Hg). These drugs may also be the drug of first choice for patients who otherwise require calcium-channel blockers for systemic conditions. Because there is no immediately apparent clinical end-point, treatment of low-tension glaucoma patients is usually initiated with the minimal recommended systemic dose. These drugs are prescribed in consultation with an internist, and cautious use is advised in those patients taking topical ophthalmic beta blockers to avoid possible severe bradycardia (21,22).

References

1. Netland PA, Erickson KA: Calcium channel blockers in glaucoma management. Ophthalmol Clin North Am 1993;116:778–780.
2. Netland PA, Grosskreutz CL, Feke GT, et al: Color Doppler ultrasound analysis of ocular circulation after topical calcium channel blocker. Am J Ophthalmol 1995;119:694–700.
3. Harino S, Riva CE, Petrig BL: Intravenous nicardipine in cats increases optic nerve head but not retinal blood flow. Invest Ophthalmol Vis Sci 1992;33:2885.
4. Gasser P, Flammer J: Influence of vasospasm on visual function. Doc Ophthalmol 1987;66:3.
5. Kitazawa Y, Shirai H, Go FJ: The effect of Ca2+-antagonist on visual field in low-tension glaucoma. Graefes Arch Clin Exp Ophthalmol 1989;227:408.
6. Netland PA, Chaturvedi N, Dreyer EB: Calcium channel blockers in the management of low-tension and open-angle glaucoma. Am J Ophthalmol 1993;115:608.
7. Green K, Kim K: Papaverine and verapamil interaction with prostaglandin E2 and 9-tetrahydrocannabinol in the eye. Exp Eye Res 1977;24:207.

8. Payne LJ, Slagle TM, Cheeks LT, et al: Effect of calcium channel blockers on intraocular pressure. Ophthalmic Res 1990;22:337.
9. Schnell D: Response of intraocular pressure in normal subjects and glaucoma patients to single and repeated doses of the coronary drug adalat. In: Second International Adalat Symposium. Edited by Lochner W, Engel HJ, Lichtlen PR. Berlin, Springer Verlag, 1975;290.
10. Monica ML, Hesse RJ, Messerli FH: The effect of a calcium-channel blocking agent on intraocular pressure. Am J Ophthalmol 1983; 96:814.
11. Kelly SP, Walley TJ: Effect of the calcium antagonist nifedipine on intraocular pressure in normal subjects. Br J Ophthalmol 1988; 72:216.
12. Suzuki R, Hanada M, Fujii H, et al: Effects of orally administered β-adrenergic blockers and calcium-channel blockers on the intraocular pressure of patients with treated hypertension. Ann Ophthalmol 1992;24:220.
13. Abelson MB, Gilbert CM, Smith LM: Sustained reduction of intraocular pressure in humans with the calcium channel blocker verapamil. Am J Ophthalmol 1988;105:155.
14. Goyal JK, Khilnani G, Sharma DP, et al: The hypotensive effect of verapamil eye drops on ocular hypertension. Ind J Ophthalmol 1989;37:176.
15. Segarra J, Santafe J, Garrido M, et al: The topical application of verapamil and nifedipine lowers intraocular pressure in conscious rabbits. Gen Pharmacol 1993;24:1163.
16. Beatty JF, Krupin T, Nichols PF, et al: Elevation of intraocular pressure by calcium channel blockers. Arch Ophthalmol 1984; 102:1072.
17. Podos SM: The effect of cation ionophores on intraocular pressure. Invest Ophthalmol 1976;15:851.
18. Ettl A, Daxer A, Hofmann U: Calcium channel blockers in the management of low-tension and open-angle glaucoma. Am J Ophthalmol 1993;116:778.
19. Erickson KA, Schroeder A, Netland PA: Verapamil increases outflow facility in the human eye. Exp Eye Res 1995;61:565–567.
20. Schuman JS, Beaton MA, Erickson KA, Schroeder A: Effects of topical verapumil on intraocular pressure, acqueous flow, and outflow facility in humans. Invest Ophthalmol Vis Sci 1994(suppl); 35:1483.
21. Sinclair NI, Benzie JL: Timolol eye drops and verapamil- a dangerous combination. Med J Australia 1983;1:548.
22. Pringle SD, MacEwen CJ: Severe bradycardia due to interaction of timolol eye drops and verapamil. Br Med J 1987;294: 155.

blockers. There is some anecdotal data about possible adverse influences of certain nonselective beta blockers on blood flow in the posterior segment, but controlled clinical trials are needed. Because an advantage of nonselective beta blockers is the usually greater potency for IOP reduction than with the selective beta blockers (Chapter 12), and in this condition one starts with "normal" levels of IOP, the clinician usually desires full potency and chooses, if there is no systemic contraindication, a nonselective beta blocker. The condition of LTG behaves as if every millimeter mercury is important, and one is therefore striving to lower the "low IOP" as much as possible.

Therefore one begins with a beta blocker, nonselective if full potency is required, and advances therapy with epinephrine-like compounds, alpha-two agonists, miotics, topical carbonic anhydrase inhibitors, laser trabeculoplasty, and filtration surgery, as for other forms of glaucoma. These comments notwithstanding, miotics and laser trabeculoplasty can be effective in some cases of LTG. Regardless, these modalities should be tried before proceeding to filtration surgery.

As with high pressure forms of POAG it is important to establish a target pressure at the beginning. If there is margin to follow and a single beta blocker achieves 20 to 25% IOP reduction, then one can stop here but closely follow the patient. Baseline stereo disc photographs and 30 and 10 degree visual fields are important for baseline documentation and need to be re-evaluated as frequently as every 4 months.

If there is advanced field loss at presentation and little margin to follow, a greater than 25% reduction in IOP is required, and the therapy advanced. The bottom line is that many patients with LTG require an IOP in the single numbers that can only be obtained with filtration surgery (with use of antiproliferative therapy). But sometimes the medical advancement, and especially laser trabeculoplasty with concomitant medical therapy, can be surprisingly effective (18) to achieve an IOP around ten.

Many patients with progressive LTG that is not far advanced, respond to a 20% reduction in IOP with apparent stability. The key is whether there is sufficient margin in the visual field that can be accurately followed. **If there is no margin to follow around central fixation, unless IOP can be lowered to levels achievable with filtration surgery, it is justifiable in such situations to proceed rapidly to filtration surgery without the requirement of future field progression (which in such a situation, would likely affect central visual acuity).**

NONPROGRESSIVE LTG

Although much has been written about this entity wherein purported acute hemodynamic crises (19) have produced a nonprogressive form of LTG, the authors actually believe this condition to be rare. The burden is on the ophthalmologist to prove that this commonly slowly progressive disease of LTG does not in fact progress over the years. We would recommend treating all patients with apparent LTG, at least initially, unless there is good documentation for a single nonprogressive event in the past, with documented stability over many years. **Certainly in all newly diagnosed cases of LTG it should be assumed that this is a progressive disease, and therapy initiated.** Likely one might be treating some patients (uncommonly) that might prove to have a nonprogressive form, but just as likely, one treats some patients with POAG who will not progress during any given observation period (Chapter 18). Do not discriminate such patients at baseline; the consequences of not treating axonal death are greater than the risks of treating. Especially in LTG in which progression commonly involves functionally important parts of the visual field close to fixation, the benefits of treatment seem to outweigh the risks. One can never prove a negative hypothesis (and therefore prove that a patient will never progress). With increased life expectancy of the population, it likely will prove true that nonprogressive LTG is an extremely uncommon entity.

LTG "EQUIVALENT"

Chapter 18 presented the concept that an eye with POAG with glaucomatous damage and a history of elevated IOP likely required an IOP at least below 18 mm Hg to prevent further glaucomatous damage. Depending on the extent of the glaucomatous optic nerve and visual field changes, an IOP in the low teens or even single numbers might be required for stability. In this discussion, we have termed this common clinical entity "LTG equivalent" because without the known history of elevated IOP, this condition is indistinguishable from "true" LTG, and, in fact, it re-

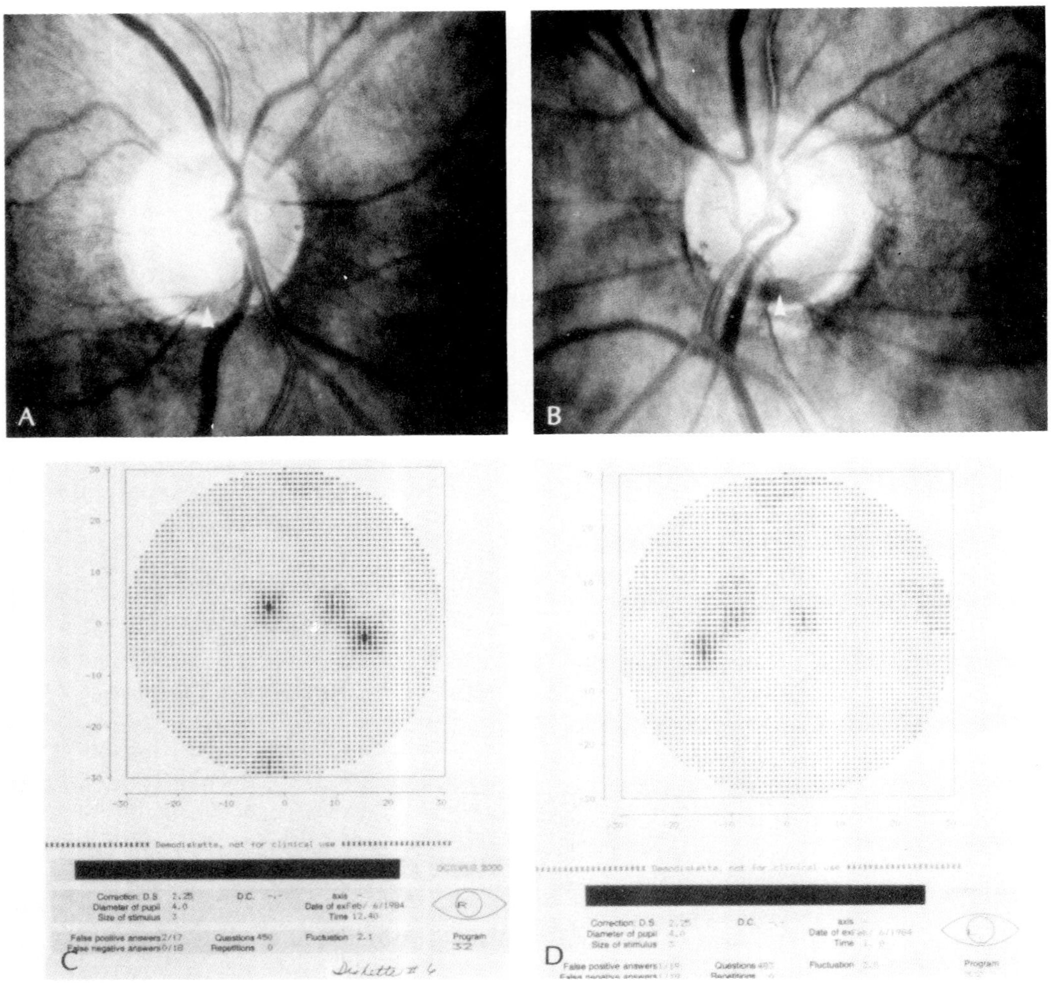

Figure 19.1. On a routine ophthalmologic examination, a 65-year-old female in good general health was observed to have abnormal disc cupping with a disc hemorrhage and an arcuate field defect OU. IOP was 15 OU and subsequently measured between 12 and 17 on multiple determinations during a 2-year period. Intermittent disc hemorrhages were documented. Outflow facility 0.33. There is inferior extension of the cups OU with disc hemorrhages (arrowheads) and superior Bjerrum scotoma OU close to fixation. During the next 3 years, medical therapy reduced IOP to consistently below 15, but there was field progression OS and recurrent disc hemorrhages OS. Laser trabeculoplasty was performed OU. Over the next 6 years, IOP was consistently in the 9 to 11 range on continued medical therapy, and the appearance of the optic discs and visual fields remained stable without further change. (Courtesy of David Hutchinson, MD).

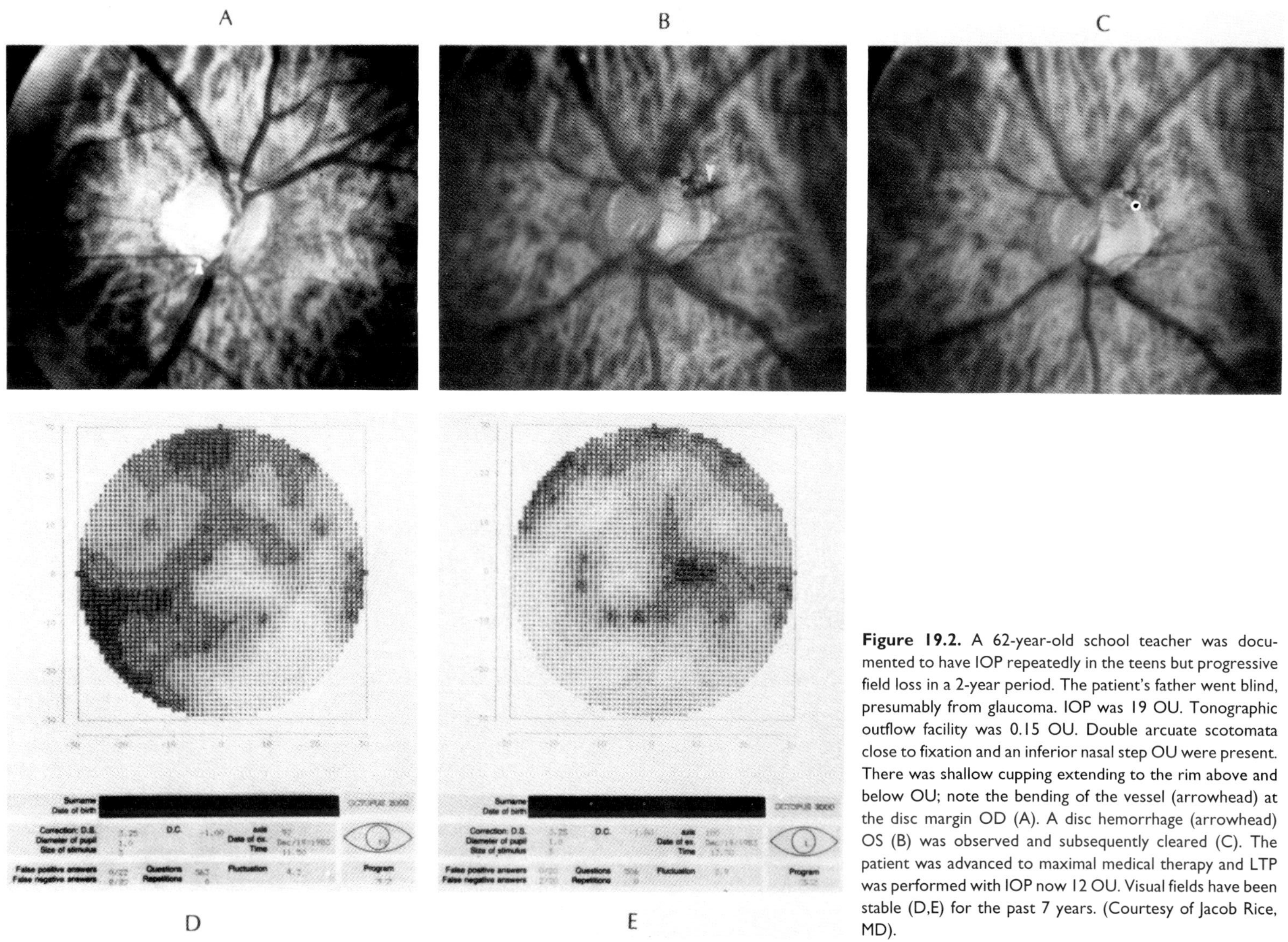

Figure 19.2. A 62-year-old school teacher was documented to have IOP repeatedly in the teens but progressive field loss in a 2-year period. The patient's father went blind, presumably from glaucoma. IOP was 19 OU. Tonographic outflow facility was 0.15 OU. Double arcuate scotomata close to fixation and an inferior nasal step OU were present. There was shallow cupping extending to the rim above and below OU; note the bending of the vessel (arrowhead) at the disc margin OD (A). A disc hemorrhage (arrowhead) OS (B) was observed and subsequently cleared (C). The patient was advanced to maximal medical therapy and LTP was performed with IOP now 12 OU. Visual fields have been stable (D,E) for the past 7 years. (Courtesy of Jacob Rice, MD).

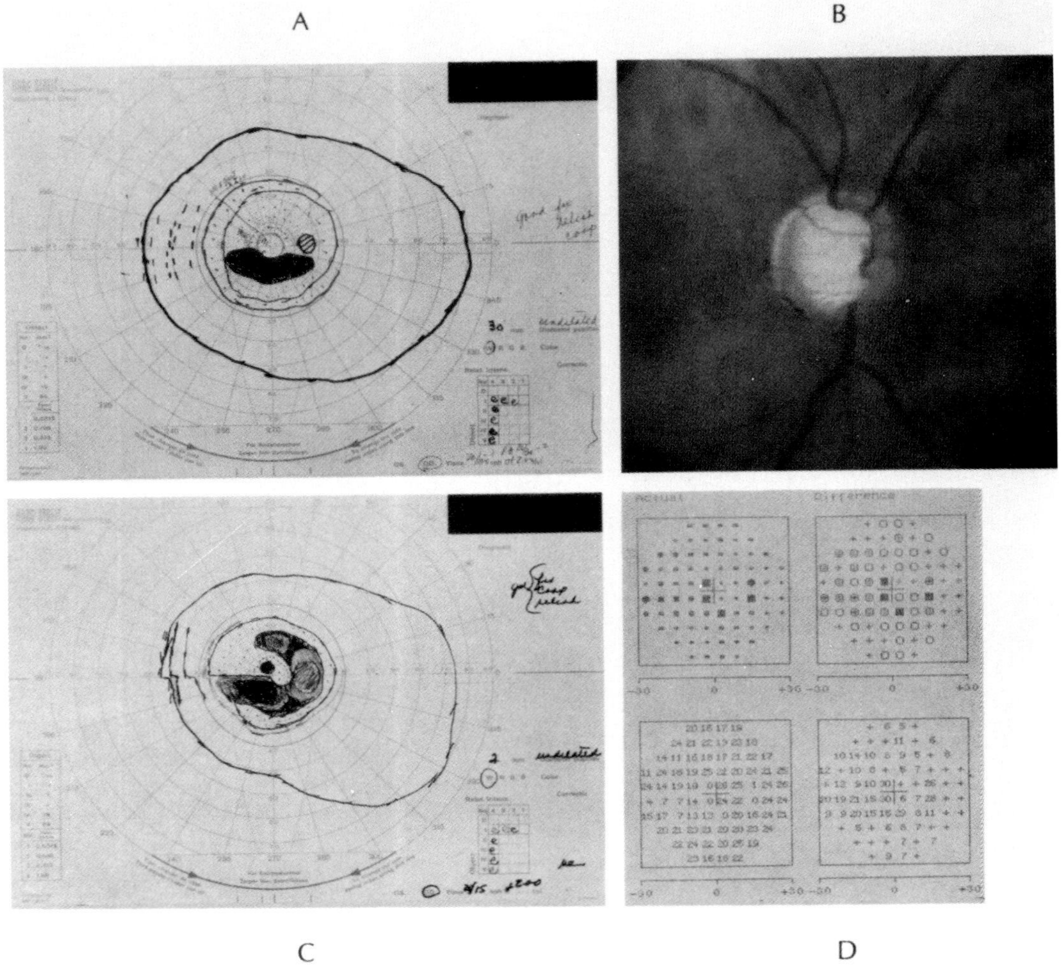

Figure 19.3. A 48-year-old male was diagnosed as having open-angle glaucoma OU with pressures in the low twenties 8 years previously. Fields revealed only a small paracentral scotoma inferiorly OD. Medical therapy was initiated with resulting IOP in the upper teens but field progression OD occurred (A, 1981). The right disc was observed to be extensively cupped both to the superior and inferior rims (B). The patient was advanced to maximal medical therapy with IOP consistently in the mid teens but further field progression was documented (C, 1982). Laser trabeculoplasty was then performed with IOP 10 OU on continued maximum medical therapy. Visual fields remained stable for the next 8 years (D) with IOP in the 10-12 range. However, 1 year later, there was a subtle increase in density of the paracentral scotoma OD, despite maintainence of 20/20 visual acuity. This patient demonstrates the condition of open angle glaucoma (with previous elevated IOP) with optic nerves that are peculiarly susceptible to "normal" levels of IOP ("LTG equivalent") (an optic nerve, once damaged from glaucoma, may require a lower than "normal" IOP).

quires the same treatment and clinical management considerations.

We will comment (Chapter 20) that **patients with exfoliation glaucoma not uncommonly develop such "LTG equivalent" features.** It is interesting to speculate whether exfoliation material in the optic nerve might be responsible for this (Chapter 1). Regardless, exfoliation glaucoma patients need to be followed with this possibility of "LTG equivalent" in mind, even if, as often occurs, at least in the short-term, there is reasonably "normal" IOP after laser trabeculoplasty.

Does sustained previously elevated IOP cause an anatomical weakening effect on the optic disc structure that results in "LTG equivalent?"

This is another way to conceptualize this entity. But from a practical point of view it still indicates the need to treat the patient the same way as "primary progressive LTG": the current IOP is too high, even if it is "normal" from a statistical population point of view, and therapy needs to be advanced to substantially lower the IOP further.

The corollary of this consideration might be that sustained elevated IOP which, in the short term, may not seem to be causing end organ damage, can, in the long

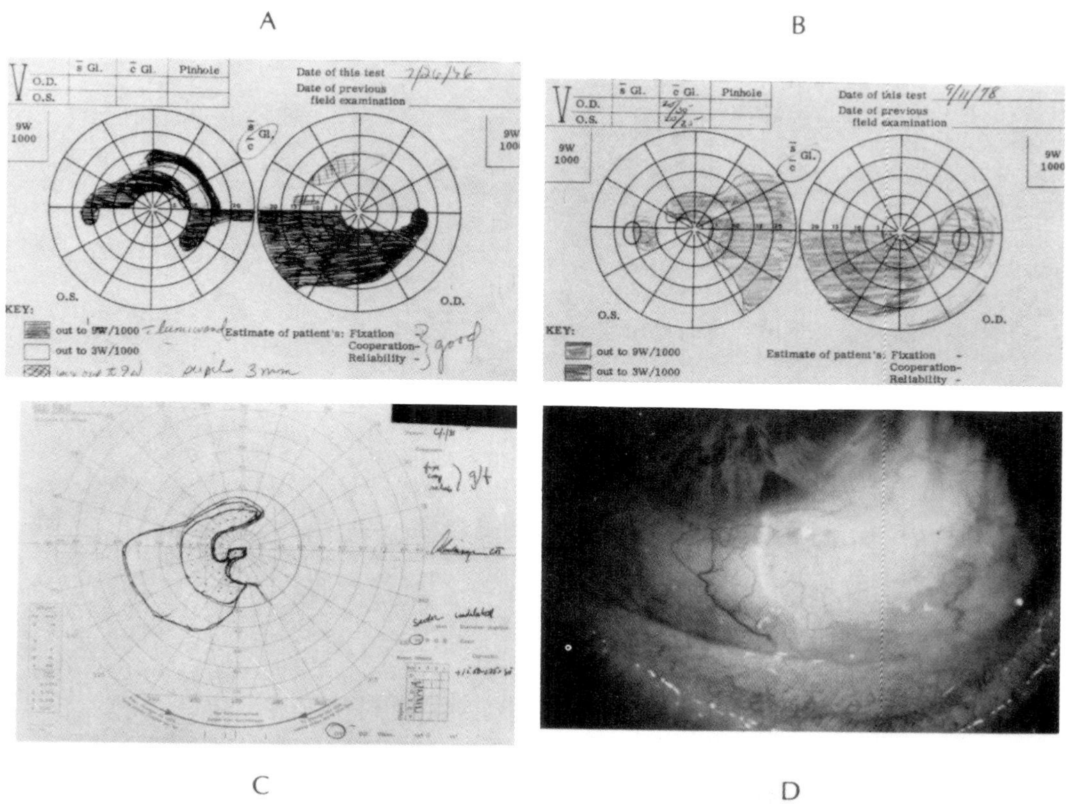

Figure 19.4. Progressive field loss OS over a 5-year period (A, 1976, B, 1978, C 1981) with IOP in the upper teens on therapy in an aphakic patient with primary open angle glaucoma and a totally cupped disc. Filtration surgery was performed from below (D) with reduction of IOP into the low to mid teens with stable vision and fields for the next 8 years.

term, produce a susceptible optic nerve, which requires a lower than statistically "normal IOP." Or, as taught by Chandler and Grant: a disc once damaged commonly requires a lower than "normal IOP" to prevent further progression.

Chandler wrote: "Progressive LTG is not a rare condition. Once the diagnosis has been established by inspection of the optic disc, repeated IOP measurement, and repeated measurement of the visual field, various medical measures are tried in an attempt to bring the IOP to lower levels. If medical treatment fails to lower the IOP significantly, and if repeated measurement of the field demonstrates progressive loss, we must come to a decision as to the future management of the case. If the patient is of advanced age, we may decide to continue with medical treatment (rather than proceeding with filtration surgery) in the hope of preserving some vision during the patient's lifetime. This is a difficult decision, for our patient might live to an advanced age and eventually become totally blind. When the situation is explained to the patient he may help us in making a decision."

For many patients with progressive LTG, medical treatment will not lower the IOP sufficiently to prevent progressive loss. Therefore for most such patients, a filtering operation has proved to be the best policy, and if it is successful in producing a low IOP, further loss of vision and field is usually prevented.

The following cases of Chandler are of interest. We consider them to be instances of progressive LTG or "equivalent" in which cupping, atrophy, and field loss progressed with IOP in the normal range, and in which progression was arrested or conspicuously slowed when IOPs were reduced surgically to low levels.

Case 19-1. A 65-year-old man, previously described by us at an earlier stage, was first seen in 1952 with IOP right 17, left 22, with cupping and field loss that during 3 years progressed seriously threatening total blindness, despite medical maintenance of IOPs in the range of 15 to 20. In 1958 at age 71, each eye was trephined. Thereafter, IOPs remained 10 or below and to at least age 89, the patient has been able to read and to carry on his profession as a lawyer.

Case 19-2. This man was always myopic and had been seen for refraction up to the age of 15 years. He was next seen at age 45

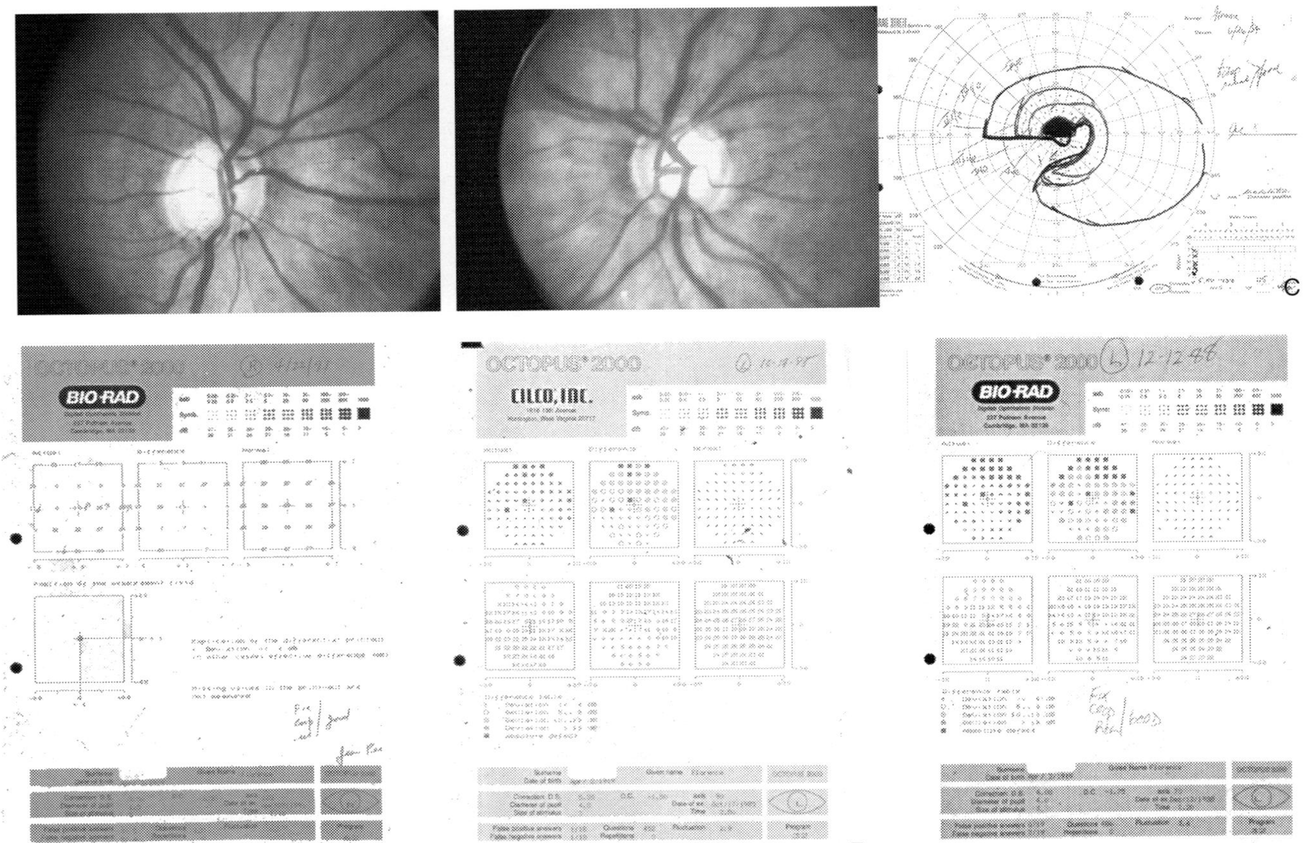

A,B C

D E F

Figure 19.5. A 72-year-old housewife with a history of migraine and a family history of glaucoma presented with IOP in the mid teens OU (outflow facility = 0.15 OU) with severe field loss and disc cupping OD (A). There was a Marcus Gunn pupillary phenomenon OD. The left eye demonstrated advanced disc cupping (B) with earlier field loss. On maximal medical therapy including laser trabeculoplasty, IOP was decreased to 12 OD but there was further field loss 18 months later (C). Filtration surgery was performed OD with resulting IOP 8-9 and stable visual fields (D) and visual acuity = 20/25 for the subsequent 6 years. In the left eye despite IOP between 11-13, there was further field progression (E,F) and disc cupping. Laser trabeculoplasty was performed OS with resulting IOP 9-11 and the fields have been stable for the subsequent 4 years.

because his ophthalmologist had found some pathologic cupping of the disc. When seen here corrected vision was 6/6 in each eye, IOP was right 20 and left 17, the angles were wide open, there appeared to be pathologic cupping of the discs, greater in the left eye. There was a double Bjerrum scotoma in the left eye with a good peripheral field, and in the right eye the field was full except for a little nasal constriction. Tonography showed a C value of 0.26 right, 0.18 left, both in the normal range. He was next seen almost 1 year later and there had been considerable loss of field and an increase in the cupping. The cup was now almost total in the left eye, came very close to the margin above and temporally in the right eye. IOP was right 20 and left 17. A trephining was done on both eyes. During the following 14 years IOP has ranged from 12 to 17. There has been an excellent bleb in the left eye, not so good in the right eye. For several years he has been pressing on the eyes four times a day to encourage the functioning of the blebs, and the IOP is temporarily reduced to a level of 10 or less after this pressure. His lenses are still clear, corrected vision 6/5, and there has been no significant change in the visual field during the last 14 years.

"This appeared to be a case of progressive low-tension glaucoma. Before operation, IOP in the upper part of the normal range was evidently too high for his eyes, and the filtering operations appear to have been of real value in slowing up the process."

The following cases (Figs. 19.1 through 19.6) illustrate several features of LTG or "LTG equivalent." Figure 19.6 provides longer term follow-up of a previously diagnosed patient with "nonprogressive LTG." Patients with progressive LTG do not form a uniform group. In some, we believe that IOP, if diurnally measured, would never exceed normal limits (as defined in population studies) (Fig. 19.1, 19.5, 19.6). We believe that the optic nerves of such patients must have an abnormal susceptibility to their given level of IOP because lowering the IOP medically or surgically can stabilize their disease process. It is not unreasonable for such a varying susceptibility to exist among different people. In other patients with progressive "LTG equivalent" as defined, the condition represents progressive damage to the optic nerve at "normal" IOP in patients with initial damage at elevated IOP. Although

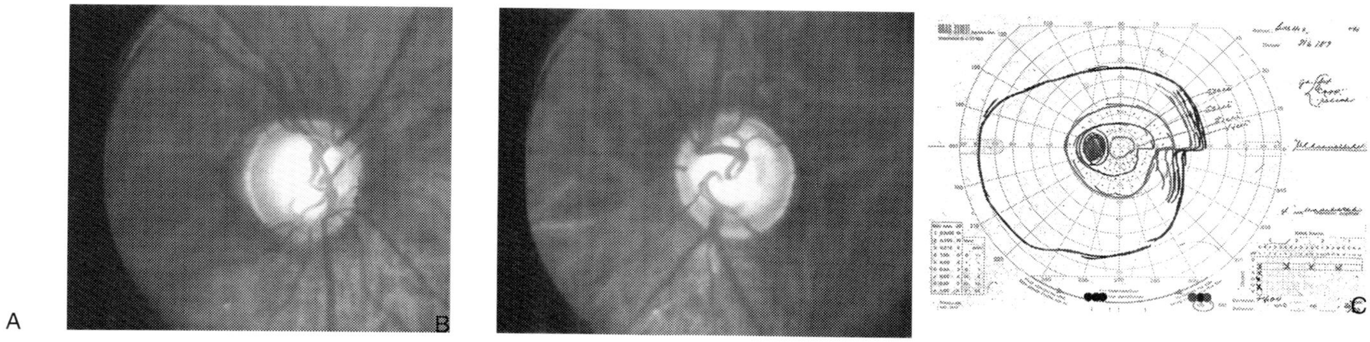

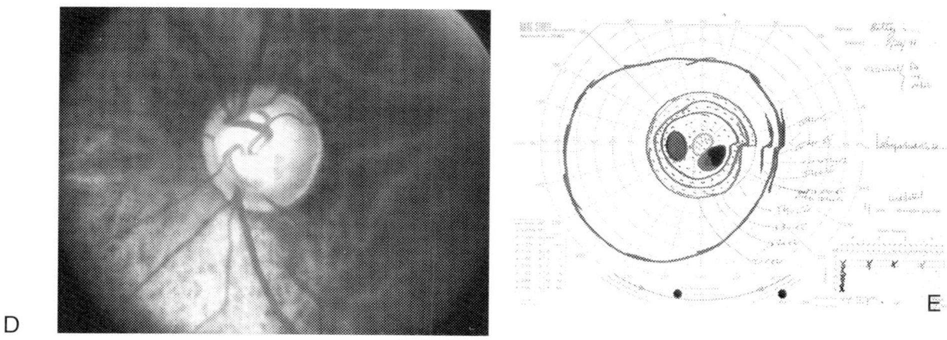

Figure 19.6. A 63-year-old businesswoman had a history of "nonprogressive LTG" after a hemodynamic crisis 5 years previously. During this interval there was reported to be a stable optic nerve (A, OD; B, OS) appearance and visual field, which was normal except for an inferior nasal step OS (C). The patient was on no antiglaucoma therapy. IOP was 16 OU (outflow values 0.20 OD: 0.17 OS). However, 4 years later there was increased cupping OU (D, OS) and field loss OS (E). Antiglaucoma therapy was initiated.

some of these may represent diurnal fluctuations in our sampling of IOP at office visits or compliance variation in patient medication, some represent the clinical fact that a damaged optic nerve will often show progressive damage with a high "normal" level of IOP. As discussed, what unites all these cases is the apparent increased vulnerability of the optic nerve to IOP.

References

1. Shiose Y, et al: Epidemiology of glaucoma in Japan—a nationwide glaucoma survey. Jpn J Ophthalmol 1991;35:133–55.
2. Usui T, Iwata K: Finger blood flow in patients with low tension glaucoma and primary open-angle glaucoma. Br J Ophthalmol 1992;76: 2–4.
3. Harris A, et al: Color doppler analysis of ocular vessel blood velocity in normal-tension glaucoma. Am J Ophthalmol 1994;118:642–9.
4. Rader J, Feuer WJ, Anderson DR: Peripapillary vasoconstriction in glaucoma and the anterior ischemic optic neuropathies. Am J Ophthalmol 1994;177:72–80.
5. Stroma GA, et al: Magnetic resonance imaging in patients with low-tension glaucoma. Arch Ophthalmol 1995;113:168–172.
6. Drance SM: Some factors in the production of low tension glaucoma. Br J Ophthalmol 1972;56:229–242.
7. Phelps CD, Corbett JJ: Migraine and low-tension glaucoma. Invest Ophthalmol Vis Sci 1985;26:1105.
8. Usui T, Iwata K, Shirakashi M, et al: Prevalence of migraine in low-tension glaucoma and primary open-angle glaucoma in Japanese. Br J Ophthalmol 1991;75:224–6.
9. Cartwright MJ, et al: Immune-related disease and normal-tension glaucoma. A case-control study. Arch Ophthalmol 1992;110:500.
10. Wax MB, Barrett DA, Pestronk A: Increased incidence of paraproteinemia and autoantibodies in patients with normal-pressure glaucoma. Am J Ophthalmol 1994;117:561–568.
11. Sebag J, Thomas JV, Epstein DL, et al: Optic disc cupping in arteritic anterior ischemic optic neuropathy resembles glaucomatous cupping. Ophthalmology 1986;93:357–361.
12. Lumme P, Tuulonen A, Airaksinen PJ, et al: Neuroretinal rim area in low tension glaucoma: effect of nifedipine and acetazolamide compared to no treatment. Acta Ophthalmol 1991;69:293–8.
13. Netland PA, Chaturvedi N, Dreyer EB: Calcium channel blockers in the management of low-tension and open angle glaucoma. Am J Ophthalmol 1993;115:608–13.
14. Chandler PA: Long-term results in glaucoma therapy. Am J Ophthalmol 1960;49:221–246.
15. Abedin S, Simmons RJ, Grant WM: Progressive low-tension glaucoma. Treatment to stop glaucomatous cupping and field loss when these progress despite normal intraocular pressure. Ophthalmology 1982;89: 1–6.
16. Cartwright MJ, Anderson DR: Correlation of asymmetric IOP in normal tension glaucoma. Arch Ophthalmol 1988;106:898–900.
17. Araie M, Sekine M, Suzuki Y, et al: Factors contributing to the progression of visual field damage in eyes with normal-tension glaucoma. Ophthalmology 1994;101:1440–1444.
18. Schulzer M: Intraocular pressure reduction in normal-tension glaucoma patients. Ophthalmology 1992;99:1468–1470.
19. Drance SM, Morgan RW, Sweeney VP: Shock-induced optic neuropathy: a cause of non-progressive glaucoma. N Engl J Med 1973; 288:392–395.
20. Chandler PA, Grant WM: Lectures on glaucoma, 1st edition. Philadelphia, Lea & Febiger, 1965;132–134.

Exfoliation and Open Angle Glaucoma 20

David L. Epstein

Once thought to be an unusual form of open angle glaucoma except in Scandinavia, we now know that exfoliation glaucoma constitutes a significant portion of most glaucoma practices in the world. We were initially surprised to learn that this disease accounted for more than 10% of glaucoma patients seen in Glaucoma Service at Mass Eye and Ear Infirmary (1). Similar findings have been observed all over the world. In many locations, initial reports indicate exfoliation to be rare, but then with more focused detection methods, a higher prevalence subsequently is observed. Several points are worth emphasizing: exfoliation open angle glaucoma mimics primary open angle in most (but not all—see below) features and therefore may be underdetected. Recognition involves meticulous observation as indicated in Chapter 5; careful attention to the crystalline lens on dilated slit lamp examination, the need to explain increased pigmentation observed on gonioscopy, the observation of white flecks in the angle, on the lens, or on the zonules or ciliary processes (when visualized), the need to explain peripupillary iris transillumination defects, etc. However, all this notwithstanding, there are seemingly valid reports of populations with a low prevalence of this disease (2–4).

Exfoliation is a disease of basement membranes of tissue lining the posterior chamber of the eye and possibly other sites (5–6). As discussed in Chapter 2, the base of the non-pigmented ciliary epithelial cell (which is head to head with the sclerad pigmented ciliary epithelial cell, Fig. 2.6) faces the posterior chamber as does the base of the posterior iris pigment epithelial cell and the base of the lens epithelial cell, which constitutes the lens capsule. The base of all three of these cells, which line the posterior chamber, "extrude" exfoliation material onto their surface where presumably the material then moves into the aqueous humor, and then with the normal flow of aqueous humor is carried into the trabecular meshwork, where it is believed to be directly responsible for the impairment in outflow (7). Exfoliation has also been reported to develop locally separate from this, possibly within the trabecular meshwork (8), and also in other intraocular sites such as corneal endothelium (9) and zonules themselves (10,11). **Exfoliation has also been reported to develop locally in the palpebral conjunctiva (12–14) and at systemic sites (6,15) and is believed to be a systemic abnormality (6,15), although it is curious that it seems to cause clinical disease only within the eye.**

The origin of exfoliation from multiple basement membrane sites within the eye is also believed to explain certain clinical features: the "weakness" of the zonules and/or lens capsule at the time of extracapsular cataract surgery (16,17); the loss of pigment from the posterior iris epithelium, either due to a "lesser integrity" of these cells or the rubbing of the iris pigment epithelium against the raised exfoliation material on the crystalline lens, especially in the pupillary area (although it is curious, given current concepts in pigmentary glaucoma (Chapter 21), that few have queried why exfoliation, that is similarly "rough," that is present on the zonules does not sometimes rub off peripheral iris pigment—presumably it is the absence of iris concavity in exfoliation) the deposition of such posterior iris pigment in the angle; and the presence of abnormal iris vascular patterns on fluorescein angiography (18–21) (presumably due likewise to a basement membrane abnormality).

DISEASE MECHANISM

A decade or more ago, considerable discussion occurred over whether exfoliation might be only an incidental finding and whether affected patients with glaucoma might actually have simply primary open angle glaucoma instead. Current thinking would not support such a tenet. Although it is true that patients can have exfoliation with no elevation of IOP (and totally normal outflow facility by tonography), there have been important studies, many from Scandinavia, that have documented the increasing risk of development of glaucoma in such patients with time (22–27). As with pigmentary dispersion syndrome, there may be patients with the distinct syndrome who do not have, and perhaps may never develop, trabecular dysfunction. These diseases may require some trabecular abnormality in addition to either the exfoliation material or pigment, but it is naive to assume that this is the same trabecular defect that is present in primary open angle glaucoma (POAG). For example, the latter may not require an "insult" such as deposited debris or pigment. However, POAG, itself, likely has more than one pathophysiological mechanism and constitutes more than one entity. Perhaps it is the presumed basement membrane abnormality within the trabecular meshwork, itself, in exfoliation that is the key to the presence or absence of abnormal outflow function.

There are also sometimes subtle but important clinical differences between exfoliation and POAG: the frequent substantial asymmetry or unilaterality (23), the potential for rapid escalation of IOP and refractoriness to antiglaucoma therapy (28), the more favorable early response to laser trabeculoplasty (29,30), and the lesser incidence of "corticosteroid responsiveness" in exfoliation (13,31,32).

Finally, important histopathological differences occur in the outflow pathway in exfoliation glaucoma compared with primary open angle glaucoma. In the latter, the specific pathological finding is not unequivocal (Chapter 18) but increased extracellular "plaque material" (33), decreased cellularity (34) and a disorganized trabecular beam structure have been observed. In contrast, in exfoliation glaucoma, the histopathology of the outflow pathway appears generally "normal" (except in far advanced stages), except for the presence of the extracellular exfoliation material (7,35). Thus we believe that **exfoliation is a secondary open angle glaucoma due to the deposited (or possibly locally produced) exfoliation material in the trabecular meshwork.**

What contributed in the past to this uncertain discrimination between exfoliation and POAG was the common occurrence of cases of apparent unilateral exfoliation but bilateral glaucoma. However, we now know from the work of Mizuno (36) that most such cases have occult exfoliation in the seemingly unaffected fellow eye. We have learned that one of the earliest sites for exfoliation to be observed is on the ciliary processes rather than the more easily viewed anterior crystalline lens surface (36). (Of course a current critical question is: are we missing detecting even earlier sites because of the limitations of our observation techniques?)

The potential for multiple ocular and systemic sites of production of exfoliation material raises another consideration that was mentioned in Chapter 19 and may oversimply be stated as follows: **there is a strong clinical sense that patients with exfoliation glaucoma who have had high IOP in the past may demonstrate optic nerves that are still "susceptible" to further damage despite normalization of the IOP that has been stabilized by laser trabeculoplasty.** Could local production of exfoliation or some related fundamental cellular abnormality within the optic nerve and especially its connective tissues explain this susceptibility? (Is there a potential unifying "thread" of a similar and possibly biochemically related phenomenon with amyloidosis? (37) (Chapters 1, 48).) We do not have an answer to this question but it deserves attention not only from the clinical management point-of-view, but also because it might lend insight into other causes for low tension glaucoma-like optic nerve susceptibility. Regardless, the clinical point is that in patients with exfoliation open angle glaucoma the clinician must pay special attention to the possibility of a "low tension glaucoma equivalent" condition (Chapter 19).

CLINICAL FINDINGS

Thus, although in many respects this type of glaucoma closely resembles primary open-angle glaucoma (POAG), there are some important differences. In addition, in open-angle glaucoma associated with exfoliation we have found in most cases an abnormal accumulation of pigment (Fig. 7.21) in the filtration portion of the corneoscleral trabecular meshwork, usually involving the whole circumference, and distinctly more than is found in normal eyes of patients of the same age or in patients who have POAG. Exfoliation is often monocular, and the associated excessive pigmentation of the trabecular meshwork and the open angle glaucoma are also commonly limited to the eye showing the exfoliation. However, sometimes in patients with bilateral exfoliation glaucoma, the severity of the glaucoma may be actually worse in the eye with lesser trabecular pigmentation (more commonly, however, the more heavily pigmented angle is associated with the more severe glaucoma).

POAG differs in that it almost always affects both eyes, although one eye may be affected more severely than the other, and in that the primary form of open angle glaucoma usually is not associated with excessive pigmentation of the trabecular meshwork. As mentioned, there is a widely held opinion, which we share, that glaucoma associated with exfoliation tends to be less responsive to medical treatment than primary open-angle glaucoma (13,28,38).

The following case illustrates some of the typical features of open angle glaucoma associated with exfoliation.

Case 20-1 An ophthalmologist, age mid-70s, had normal IOP until 1970, when routine tonometry showed IOP right 14, left 22. Exfoliation was present on the front of the lens and on the pupillary margin in the left eye. Optic discs were symmetric, normal. In 1971 IOPs were right 13, left 30. Gonioscopy showed very little pigment in the angle of the right eye at that time, but a narrow dense band of pigment in the filtration area of the trabecular meshwork in the entire circumference in the left eye. Under treatment with pilocarpine and epinephrine in the left eye, the IOP at first was reduced, then gradually rose. By 1973 the IOP left was 40 and tonography C value was 0.08 despite the use of the eye drops; the right eye remained normal. The left eye was then treated with echothiophate iodide and epinephrine, reducing the IOP to 30, but pathologic cupping of the optic disc developed, and later there was considerable loss in the lower visual field in the left eye. (The patient did not take carbonic anhydrase inhibitors because of a history of kidney stones.) By 1975 cataract had developed; combined cataract extraction and cyclodialysis was done on the left eye. Postoperatively, pilocarpine and phenylephrine were used to encourage the cyclodialysis cleft to remain open. During the next 3 years the IOP in the left eye remained 10 to 12. The right eye has continued to have normal IOP without treatment.

Exfoliation material is most commonly detected during slit lamp examination when the pupillary border and face

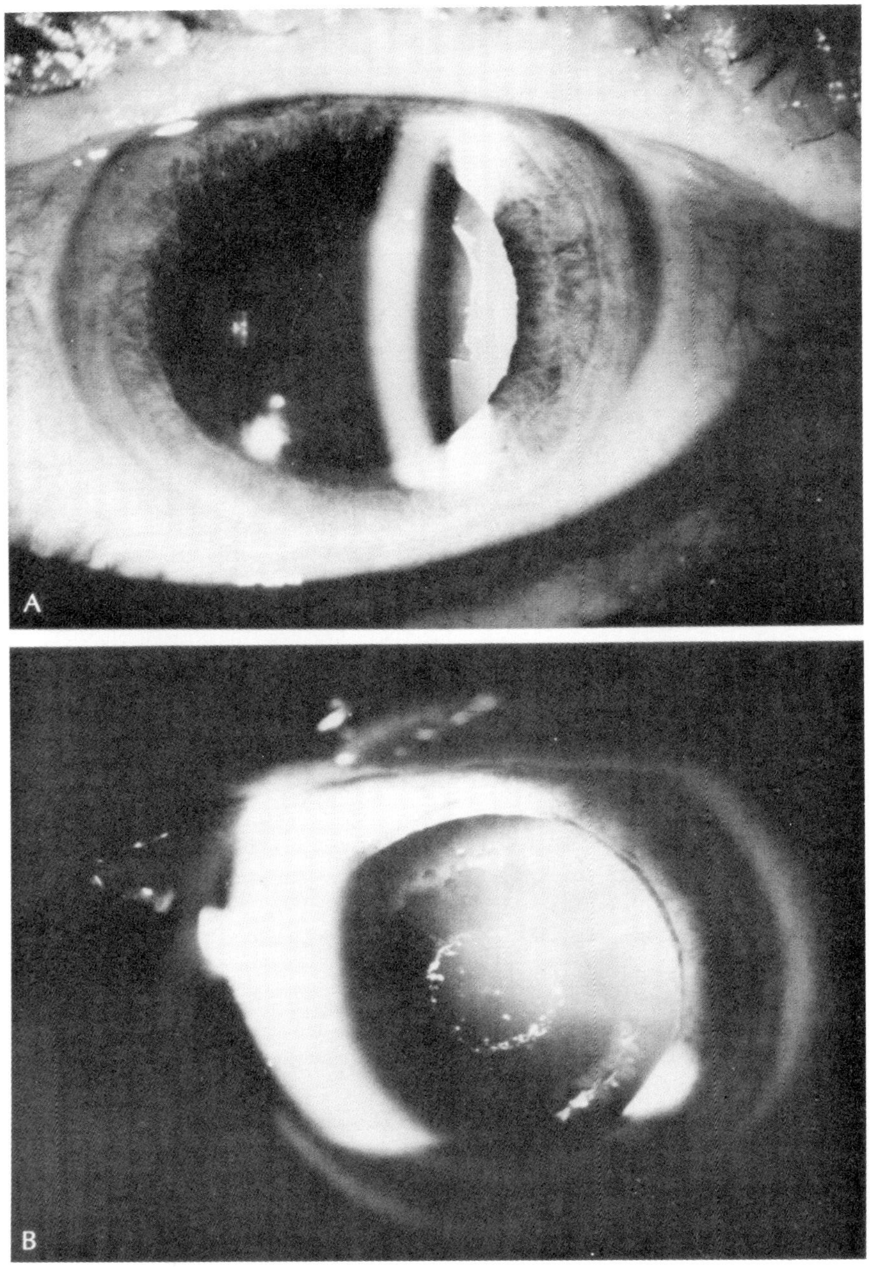

Figure. 20.1. Two examples of exfoliation of the anterior lens capsule.

of the lens are examined. **Fine light-gray amorphous flakes resembling dandruff may be noted at the pupillary margin,** or a matte gray membrane with curled edges on the anterior surface of the lens. If the pupil is small, the exfoliation material may be hidden behind the pupillary margin and may be detected only when, using gonioscopy, one looks just under the pupillary margin. If the pupil is dilated one may see on the anterior surface of the crystalline lens an area of lusterless gray that is smooth and homogeneous in the pupillary area, but ends in a series of scallops peripherally (Fig. 20.1), with the most peripheral portion of the lens capsule appearing uncoated and normally lustrous. The edges of the coating on the lens sometimes appear rolled as though a portion of the anterior capsule were being exfoliated. If there is a coloboma of the iris, one may see that the amorphous coating on the lens extends further peripherally than in the areas where the iris is intact. Examination through the gonioscope lens and examination of enucleated eyes have established that material having the same gray amorphous appearance is also present on the zonules of the lens, on the ciliary processes (Fig. 20.2), and on the posterior surface of the iris. It may also be occasionally deposited on the corneal endothelium (Fig. 20.3).

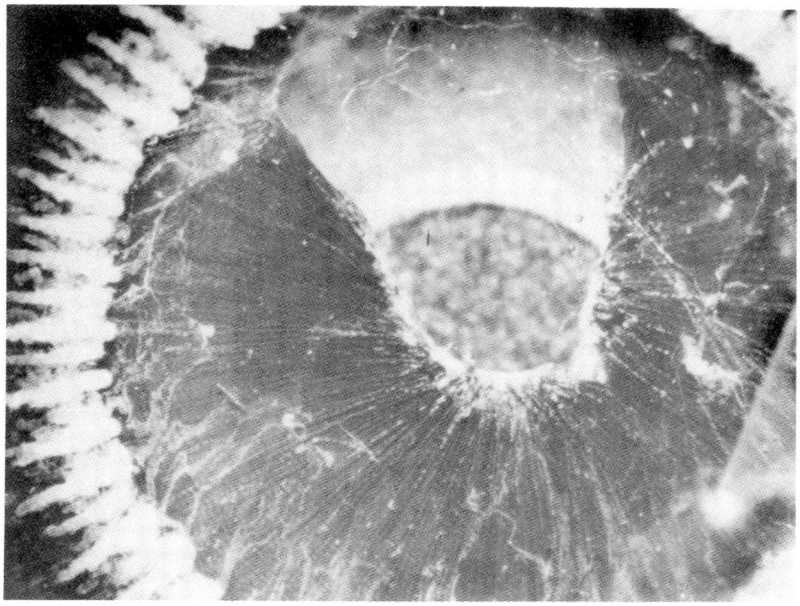

Figure. 20.2. Enucleated eye demonstrating a great amount of exfoliation material on the ciliary processes. (Courtesy of Thomas M. Richardson, M.D.)

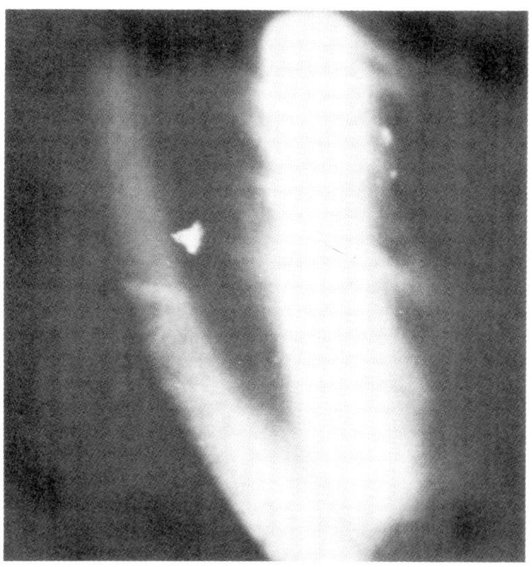

Figure. 20.3. An especially large piece of exfoliation material that was deposited on the corneal endothelium. Exfoliation flakes are occasionally seen on the corneal endothelium and in the angle.

When the material on the posterior surface of the iris is lightly brushed experimentally in an enucleated eye, particles of pigment from the pigment epithelium of the iris are released. Also, when patients with exfoliation material have their pupils dilated, a cloud of pigment particles released into the anterior chamber may be seen by slit lamp (39,40). Transillumination of the iris from behind, by light applied to the sclera near the equator, commonly demonstrates a patchy loss of pigment from the posterior pigment layer adjoining the pupil, but there is no clear indication of loss from peripheral portions of the iris. Exfoliation may be associated with cataractous lens changes (41), especially nuclear sclerosis. Presumably this relates to the basement membrane changes of the lens epithelium, which might be responsible for fluid movement changes in the crystalline lens over time.

The prevalence of exfoliation varies according to the criteria of different examiners. As mentioned, at one time exfoliation was thought to be rare outside of the Scandinavian countries, but increasing thoroughness in examination has shown it to be common worldwide, with little relation to race or geography. As a rule it is found with increasing frequency with age. Often it occurs to a much greater degree, or much earlier, in one eye than the other. A sizable minority of people who have exfoliation develop glaucoma, but many others with conspicuous amounts of exfoliaton material in their eyes apparently do not get glaucoma during observation for many years. Careful examination of patients with open-angle glaucoma in various parts of the world has disclosed that about 10 to 30% may have exfoliation material, the proportion increasing with age. From small series of tests that have been done so far, it appears that in most patients with open-angle glaucoma associated with exfoliation material, corticosteroids do not evoke an elevation of IOP of the degree or the frequency that is encountered in patients with ordinary primary open-angle glaucoma (13,31,32). This is further indication that these are fundamentally different types of glaucomas.

When open angle glaucoma is encountered with considerably elevated IOP, cupping, atrophy, and field loss in one eye, but with no evidence of glaucoma in the other eye, the most common finding is exfoliation material in the glaucomatous eye. As described, a ring of pigment is commonly found in the trabecular

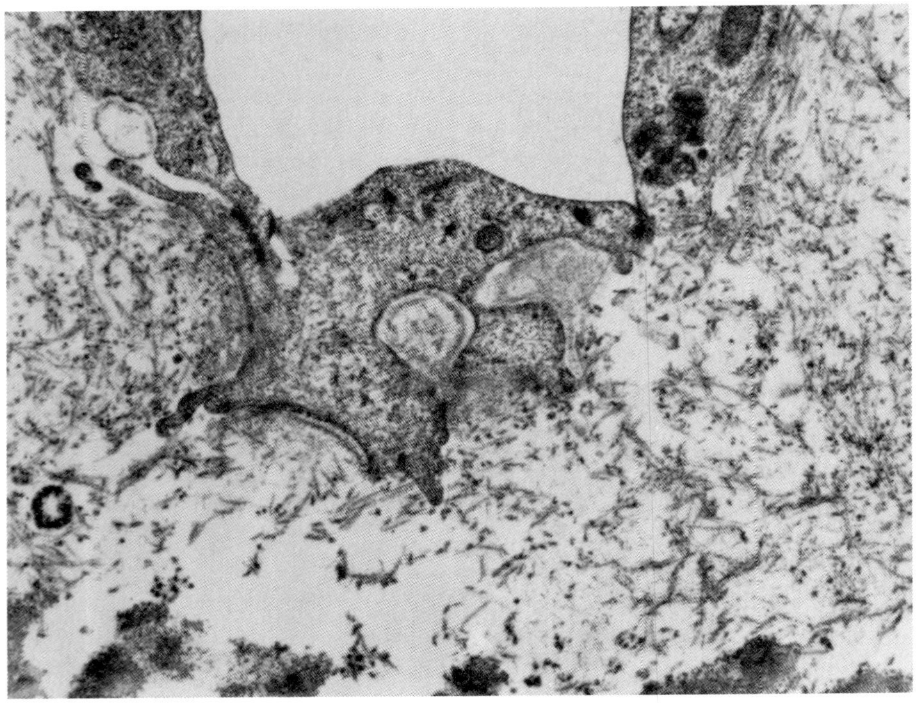

Figure. 20.4. Electron microscopy of exfoliation material in the vicinity of Schlemm's canal. The exfoliation material forms a matrix of thick and thin fibrils. (From Richardson TM, Epstein DL. Exfoliation glaucoma: A quantitative perfusion and ultrastructural study. Ophthalmology 1981; 88:968–980.)

meshwork of the glaucomatous eye, and not in the other, but this is not an essential feature. In exceptional cases there are all the features mentioned except the excess pigment, and this naturally makes it seem that pigment in the trabecular meshwork may be much less important in obstructing aqueous outflow than some other factor in glaucoma associated with exfoliation. The only other known factor is the exfoliation material itself. This is recognizable by electron microscopy as a peculiar fibrillar material, and it has been identified in the trabecular meshwork of many specimens excised during surgery on eyes with glaucoma too severe to be controlled medically (13,42,43). It is not yet proven that it is this material that obstructs the outflow, but Richardson and Epstein (7) and others (35) have demonstrated that the structure of the trabecular meshwork appears normal apart from the extracellularly deposited exfoliation material (Fig. 20.4). They hypothesize that exfoliation glaucoma may be a secondary obstruction of outflow due to this material "clogging" the aqueous humor outflow pathway (7).

Though the glaucoma associated with exfoliation material often appears monocularly as just described, when the apparently normal contralateral eye is kept under observation, usually after some years a little exfoliation material begins to make its appearance, and IOP slowly begins to rise in that eye also. As mentioned, Mizuno has demonstrated with ciliary body indentation the presence of occult exfoliation in ciliary processes in fellow eyes of patients with apparent unilateral exfoliation (36). Such occult exfoliation in the fellow eye does then likely explain the presence of bilateral glaucoma in some patients with apparent "unilateral" exfoliation (1).

ASSOCIATION WITH NARROW ANGLES

Another issue is that **it is not unusual for patients with exfoliation to have narrow angles** (44). This is important, separate from any considerations of acute angle closure, for the following reasons: patients with diagnosed exfoliation open angle glaucoma might develop a superimposed angle closure component with the passage of years. Thus this clinical worsening of the disease might be amenable to improvement with laser iridectomy. This emphasizes again the importance of the "rule": **if the IOP is elevated on a follow-up visit, always regonioscope the patient.**

In contrast, however, there may be patients presenting with narrow angles and elevated IOP (Chapter 22) who did not, in fact, have functional angle closure, but rather open angle glaucoma due to occult exfoliation. Not only might laser iridectomy not improve the IOP, but with the existing trabecular dysfunction due to exfoliation, there is the potential for a substantial acute IOP spike. The "rule" here is that **in eyes with narrow angles, the clinician,** dedicated to the rule of 5% (Chapter 5) **looks diligently and routinely for signs of occult exfoliation.**

CLINICAL COURSE

A "rule of 5%" clinical point that is not rare is as follows: in patients who have had high IOP due to exfoliation but

TONOGRAPHY IN EXFOLIATION

David L. Epstein

In cases of exfoliation one of us (DLE) has found tonography clinically useful not only to properly assess the status of the fellow eye, but also to detect the presence of severe impairment of outflow ("flat curves"). An important clinical point in dealing with exfoliation glaucoma, in contrast to most (but not all) patients with POAG, is the potential for "galloping" open angle glaucoma. That is, exfoliation glaucoma patients have the potential for dramatic further escalation of elevation of IOP between routine three- to four-month interval visits. Especially given the possible increased susceptibility of the optic nerve to glaucomatous damage in this condition, the clinician must be alert to this possibility. On the other hand, most patients with exfoliation glaucoma demonstrate the slow gradual worsening course seen in primary open angle glaucoma.

What is the strategy for not missing such "galloping" patients? The patient's past history of IOP fluctuation is a guide, but in general, exfoliation patients should be followed somewhat more closely, perhaps four times a year rather than three. In addition, one of us (DLE) has felt that if tonography demonstrated "flat outflow," that the potential, at least, for more rapid escalation was there, and, therefore, such patients should be followed even more closely.

a dramatic lowering of IOP following laser trabeculoplasty, **the clinician should be alert in his/her further follow-up to the *first* signs that the IOP, although perhaps still at an acceptable level, is "creeping up" a few millimeters of mercury.** One may find that if the next visit after this is scheduled, as is routine, four months ahead, that the patient returns then with very high IOP again and sometimes further unexpected disc and field damage. We have learned that although there are more early time period successes with laser trabeculoplasty in exfoliation glaucoma compared to POAG, there are unfortunately more longer term failures (such that the survival curves meet and may even slightly cross) (30). Regardless, the clinical point is that the trabecular abnormality present in exfoliation open angle glaucoma can dramatically worsen between routine visits, and the clinician needs to be alert to this not only following laser trabeculoplasty, but in the "routine" system follow-up of exfoliation patients in general.

A borderline IOP in an exfoliation glaucoma patient thus is a cause for concern and indicates, at a minimum, the need for closer follow-up. Another corollary of this phenomenon is that in a borderline situation it is prudent to be somewhat more aggressive with one's antiglaucomatous therapy or strategy in a patient with exfoliation glaucoma and glaucomatous end organ damage (disc cupping and field loss).

It should also be mentioned that **it is not rare to see patients with exfoliation presenting with a central (or branch) retinal vein occlusion.** Although as indicated above, there possibly might be exfoliation "processes" intrinsic to the optic nerve, we have regularly explained this clinical finding as being due to the high IOPs found in exfoliation. Thus a central retinal vein occlusion may be the first presentation of exfoliation glaucoma (and, of course, when one clinically encounters such unilateral cases, one needs to look carefully for the presumed underlying exfoliation open angle glaucoma and distinguish this unilateral exfoliation glaucoma from a secondary neovascular or angle closure disease due to the vein occlusion). Another corollary of this phenomenon is that, in known exfoliation patients the clinician needs to be alert to the occurrence of acute "vascular" events (including glaucomatous optic nerve damage) due to elevated IOP between clinical visits. The clinical point that needs to be stressed in all this is that in exfoliation glaucoma there is the definite potential for worsening of the glaucoma (both IOP and optic nerve damage) between "routine" visits.

TREATMENT

The treatment of open angle glaucoma associated with exfoliation material is the same as for POAG except that **medical treatment tends to be less effective** (13,28,38).

Exfoliation glaucoma seems to respond better in the short term than other forms of glaucoma to laser trabeculoplasty (LTP). (In view of our observations concerning the pathogenesis of exfoliation glaucoma, (7) one wonders whether the mechanism of LTP may be biologic (45–47), e.g. inducing phagocytosis of exfoliation material in the outflow channels, rather than mechanical (Chapter 54).) Despite the often dramatic IOP lowering achieved with LTP in exfoliation glaucoma eyes, late failures are unfortunately quite common (30), as indicated above. This may represent new deposition of exfoliation material in the outflow pathway. Although uncertain of the role of repeat treatment with LTP in these late failures, we currently are retreating half the angle in cases (that responded favorably to the original LTP) with initial good, but short term, results. On the other hand, as discussed in earlier chapters, it is likely true that as with all our current glaucoma therapies, none of which are "cures" (48), we are aiming mainly to slow the "rate of decay" of the disease process by usage of laser trabeculoplasty in exfoliation glaucoma. Eventually the scarring that LTP produces (49) becomes functionally significant, limiting the number of times that LTP can be repeated.

Filtration surgery is commonly required in exfoliation glaucoma. Fortunately, surgical success in exfoliation appears similar to that seen in POAG.

FURTHER QUESTIONS

The most intriguing questions about exfoliation glaucoma are: What is the exfoliation material? (50–56) Where does the material in the trabecular meshwork come from? What is its exact role in aqueous outflow obstruction? No complete answer is yet available. The chemical nature has been guessed at from results of histologic staining and electron microscopy, suggesting that it contains some noncollagenous protein and proteoglycan or glycoprotein, and that it has some resemblance to amyloid material, but no definite understanding is available.

At this time we look on open angle glaucoma associated with exfoliation as a "secondary" type of glaucoma, and we believe there is good reason to try to get at its cause or causes, hoping ultimately to retard or prevent its development. This type of glaucoma represents such a significant fraction of the glaucomas of older people, and one that is relatively refractory to medical treatment, that a means of prevention would have great overall value.

References

1. Roth M, Epstein DL: The exfoliation syndrome; a review of 74 cases. Am J Ophthalmol 1980;89:477–481.
2. Cashwell LF Jr, Shields MB: Exfoliation syndrome in southeastern United States. I. Prevalence in open-angle glaucoma and non-glaucoma populations. Acta Ophthalmol Suppl 1988;184:99–102.
3. Ball SF: Exfoliation syndrome prevalence in the glaucoma population of South Louisiana. Acta Ophthalmol Suppl 1988;184:93–98.
4. Forsius H: Exfoliation syndrome in various ethnic populations. Acta Ophthalmol Suppl 1988;184:71–85.
5. Eagle RC, Font RL, Fine BS: The basement membrane exfoliation syndrome. Arch Ophthalmol 1979;97:510–515.
6. Schlotzer-Schrehardt UM, Koca MR, Naumann GO, et al: Pseudoexfoliation syndrome. Ocular manifestation of a systemic disorder? Arch Ophthalmol 1992;110:(12):1752–1756.
7. Richardson TM, Epstein DL: Exfoliation glaucoma: a quantitative perfusion and ultrastructural study. Ophthalmology 1981;88:968–980.
8. Ringvold A, Vegge T: Electron microscopy of the trabecular meshwork in eyes with exfoliation syndrome (pseudoexfoliation of the lens capsule). Virchows Arch (Pathol Anat) 1971;353:110–127.
9. Schlötzer-Schrehardt UM, Dorfler S, Naumann GO: Corneal endothelial involvement in pseudoexfoliation syndrome. Comment in: Arch Ophthalmol 1993;111(5):666–674.
10. Schlötzer-Schrehardt U, Naumann GO: A histopathologic study of zonular instability in pseudoexfoliation syndrome. Am J Ophthalmol 1994; 118(6):730–743.
11. Assia EI, Apple DJ, Morgan RC, et al:The relationship between the stretching capability of anterior capsule and zonules. Invest Ophthalmol Vis Sci 1991;32(10):2835–2839.
12. Ringwold A: Electron microscopy of the limbal conjunctiva in eyes with pseudoexfoliation syndrome. Virchows Arch Abt A Pathol Anat 1972; 355:275–283.
13. Layden WE, Shaffer RN: Exfoliation syndrome. Am J Ophthalmol 1974; 78:835–841.
14. Streeten BW, Brookman L, Ritch R, et al: Pseudoexfoliative fibrillopathy in the conjunctiva: a relation to elastic fibers and elastosis. Ophthalmology 1987;94:1439–1449.
15. Streeten BW, Li Z–Y, Wallace RN, et al: Pseudoexfoliative fibillopathy in visceral organs of a patient with pseudoexfoliation syndrome. Arch Ophthalmol 1992;110(12):1757–1762.
16. Lumme P, Laatikainen L: Exfoliation syndrome and cataract extraction. Am J Ophthalmol 1993;116(1):51–55.
17. Lumme P, and Laatikainen LT: Risk factors for intraoperative and early postoperative complications in extracapsular cataract surgery. Eur J Ophthalmol 1994;4(3):151–158.
18. Deodati F, Labro J-B, and Poitevin B: L'angiographie fluorescéinique du segment antérieur dans la pseudo-exfoliation capsulaire. Bull Soc Ophthalmol Fr 1975;75:107–111.
19. Ghosh M, and Speakman JS: The iris in senile exfoliation of the lens. Can J Ophthalmol 1974;9:289–297.
20. Valle O, Vannas A: The cyclopentolate provocative test in suspected or untreated open angle glaucoma. Acta Ophthalmol 1976;54:783–790.
21. Konstas AG, Marshall GE, Cameron SA, and Lee WR: Morphology of iris vasculopathy in exfoliation glaucoma. Acta Ophthalmol 1993;71(6): 7511–7519.
22. Hansen E, and Sellevold OJ: Pseudoexfoliation of the lens capsule. I. Clinical evaluation with special regard to the presence of glaucoma. Acta Ophthalmol 1968;46(6):1095–1104.
23. Hansen E and Sellevold OJ: Pseudoexfoliation of the lens capsule. II. Development of the exfoliation syndrome. Acta Ophthalmol 1969;47(1): 161–173.
24. Aasved H: Intraocular pressure in eyes with and without fibrillopathia epitheliocapsularis (so-called senile exfoliation or pseudoexfoliation). Acta Ophthalmol 1971;49(4):601–610.
25. Odland M and Aasved H: Follow-up of initially nonglaucomatous patients with fibrillopathia epitheliocapsularis (so-called senile exfoliation of the anterior lens capsule). Acta Ophthalmol Suppl 1973;120:77–81.
26. Kozart DM and Yanoff M: Intraocular pressure status in 100 consecutive patients with exfoliation syndrome. Ophthalmology 1982;89(3): 214–218.
27. Henry JC, Krupin T, Schmitt M, et al: Long-term follow-up of pseudoexfoliation and the development of elevated intraocular pressure. Ophthalmology 1987;94(5):545–552.
28. Konstas AG, Jay JL, Marshall GE, et al: Prevalence, diagnostic features, and response to trabeculectomy in exfoliation glaucoma. Ophthalmology 1993;100(5):619–627.
29. Psilas K, Prevezas D, Petroutsos G, et al: Comparative study of argon laser trabeculoplasty in primary open-angle and pseudoexfoliation glaucoma. Ophthalmologica 1989;198(2):57–63.
30. Threlkeld AB, Allingham RR, Sturm R, Epstein DL: A comparative study of argon laser trabeculoplasty for exfoliation and primary open angle glaucoma. J of Glaucoma, 1996. (In Press.)
31. Gillies WE: Corticosteroid-induced ocular hypertension in pseudo-exfoliation of lens capsule. Am J Ophthalmol 1970;70:90–95.
32. Namba K, Sakuragawa M, Sakurai L: The effect of topical corticosteroid on glaucoma capsular and pseudoexfoliation of the lens capsule. Folia Ophthalmol Jpn 1977;28:1645–1649.
33. Rohen J: Why is intraocular pressure elevated in chronic simple glaucoma? Ophthalmology 1983;90:758–765.
34. Alvarado J, Murphy C, Juster R: Trabecular meshwork cellularity in primary open angle glaucoma and nonglaucomatous normals. Ophthalmology 1984;91:564–579.
35. Lutjen-Drecoll E, Shimizu T, Rohrbach M, et al: Quantitative analysis of 'plaque material' in the inner and outer wall of Schlemm's canal in normal and glaucomatous eyes. Exp Eye Res 1986;42(5):443–455.

36. Mizuno K, Muroi S: Cycloscopy of pseudoexfoliation. Am J Ophthalmol 1979;87:513.
37. Kivela T, Tarkkanen A, Frangione B, et al: Ocular amyloid deposition in familial amyloidosis, Finnish: an analysis of native and variant gelsolin in Meretoja's syndrome. Invest Ophthalmol Vis Sci 1994;35(10): 3759–3769.
38. Aasved H: The frequency of optic nerve damage and surgical treatment in chronic simple glaucoma and capsular glaucoma. Acta Ophthalmol 1971;49:589–600.
39. Krause U, Helve J, Forsius H: Pseudoexfoliation of the lens capsule and liberation of iris pigment. Acta Ophthalmol 1973;51:39–46.
40. Nagai T, Suga K, Nishi R: A clinical and histopathological study of pseudoexfoliation of the lens capsule. Folia Ophthalmol Jpn 1976;27: 185–190.
41. Puska P: Lens opacity in unilateral exfoliation syndrome with or without glaucoma. Acta Ophthalmol 1994;72(3):290–296.
42. Rodrigues MM, Spaeth GL, Sivalingam E, et al: Histopathology of 150 trabeculectomy specimens in glaucoma. Trans Ophthalmol Soc U.K. 1976;96:245–255.
43. Toriyama K, Maezawa N: Electron microscopic study on the trabecular tissues in glaucoma capsular. Acta Soc Ophthalmol Jpn 1976;80: 780–789.
44. Gross FJ, Tingey D, Epstein DL: Increased prevalence of occludable angles and angle-closure glaucoma in patients with pseudoexfoliation. Am J Ophthalmol 1993;117:333–336.
45. Van Buskirk EM, Pond V, Rosenquist RC, et al: Argon laser trabeculoplasty. Studies of mechanism of action. Ophthalmology 1984;91(9): 1005–1010.
46. Melamed S and Epstein DL: Alterations of aqueous humor outflow following argon laser trabeculoplasty in monkeys. Br J Ophthalmol 1987; 71:776–781.
47. Van Buskirk EM: Pathophysiology of laser trabeculoplasty. Surv Ophthalmol 1989;33(4):264–272.
48. Epstein DL: Will there be a remedy to reverse the changes in the trabecular meshwork and the optic nerve? A personal point-of-view on glaucoma therapy. J Glaucoma 1993;2:138–140.
49. Melamed S, Pei J, Epstein DL: Delayed response to argon laser trabeculoplasty in monkeys: Morphological study and morphometric analysis. Arch Ophthalmol 1986;104:1078–1083.
50. Streeten BW, Gibson SA, Dark AJ: Pseudoexfoliative material contains an elastic microfibrillar-associated glycoprotein. Trans Am Ophthalmol Soc 1986;84:304–320.
51. Li Z-Y, Streeten BW, Wallace RN: Association of elastin with pseudoexfoliative material: an immunoelectron microscopic study. Curr Eye Res 1988;12:1163–1172.
52. Li Z-Y, Streeten BW, Yohai N: Amyloid P protein in pseudoexfoliative fibrillopathy. Curr Eye Res 1989;8:217–227.
53. Konstas AG, Marshall GE, Lee WR: Immunogold localization of laminin in normal and exfoliative iris. Br J Ophthalmol 1990;74:450–457.
54. Schlötzer-Schrehardt U, Dörfler S, Naumann GOH: Immunohistochemical localization of basement membrane components in pseudoexfoliation material of the lens capsule. Curr Eye Res 1992;11:343–355.
55. Uusitalo M, Kivela T, Tarkkanen A: The HNK-1 epitope in the inner connective tissue layer of the human ciliary body in exfoliation syndrome and various types of glaucoma. Graefes Arch Clin Exp Ophthalmol 1994; 232(1):8–15.
56. Hietanen J, Tarkkanen A, Kivela T: Galactose-containing glycoconjugates of the ciliary body and lens in capsular glaucoma: a lectin histochemical study. Graefes Arch Clin Exp Ophthalmol 1994;232(10): 575–583.

Pigment Dispersion and Pigmentary Glaucoma

21

David L. Epstein

DIAGNOSIS

The pigment dispersion syndrome is characterized by loss of pigment from the posterior surface of the iris in the mid-periphery in both eyes, and an attendant deposition of pigment on intraocular structures such as the back of the cornea, the trabecular meshwork, the iris, and the lens. Pigment dispersion syndrome can occur with or without the pigmentary glaucoma that was first described as an entity by Sugar (1,2).

We have observed the full dispersion syndrome without glaucoma in routine eye examinations, probably as frequently as actual pigmentary glaucoma. Many pigment dispersion patients have been kept under observation for years and have not developed elevated IOP. Patients with pigmentary glaucoma whom we have seen have already had this condition or at least some abnormality in aqueous outflow when first seen by us.

Pigmentary dispersion syndrome typically occurs in people from 20 to 45 years of age, but it has been found in rare instances in teenagers and in the elderly. It is more common in men than women. Women seem to develop pigmentary glaucoma at a slightly older age than men. A family history of pigmentary glaucoma is seldom obtained, but pigmentary glaucoma has been reported in brothers (3), and we have found it in twin young women and in a father and daughter. Sometimes there is a family history of primary open angle glaucoma.

The onset of pigmentary glaucoma in some cases appears to be rapid, with elevated IOP, fine corneal edema, and symptoms of blurring of vision or seeing of haloes. These symptoms usually make the patient realize that there is a problem, though in most instances there is no pain. In a considerable proportion of cases, the diagnosis can be made before there has been much damage to the optic nerve head. However, the circumstances of onset are not always so fortunate as this. Some young men whom we have seen with this type of glaucoma had developed severe cupping and atrophy of their optic discs and loss of visual field before they became aware that something was wrong, as in the following case.

Case 21-1. A 30-year-old white man presented with a 1-year history of intermittent haloes. A diagnosis of pigmentary glaucoma had been made in Argentina. He was 6 diopters myopic in both eyes. He had fine pigment deposition on the corneal endothelium and extensive, mid-peripheral iris transillumination. Both lenses showed fine pigment dusting on the anterior capsule and pigmentation of the posterior surface peripherally. Gonioscopy revealed dense pigment bands covering the trabecular meshwork, with fine uveal meshwork ("iris processes") from iris to ciliary body band and scleral spur. IOPs were 30 right and left. There was marked glaucomatous cupping of both discs extending superiorly to the rim with extensive inferior field loss in both eyes.

Treatment was rapidly increased to maximal tolerated medical therapy. There was evidence of increasing field loss in the right eye. On this basis a filtering operation was performed on this eye. Although the bleb seemed to fail, with resumption of medical therapy, including use of pilocarpine Ocusert, and later timolol, IOPs were well controlled in the operated eye. The patient has refused operation on the left eye, but fortunately the IOP in this eye has been sufficiently controlled by topical timolol that the field has remained stable.

This case also illustrates the fact that eyes with pigmentary glaucoma, e.g., the left eye of this patient, can show spontaneous improvement in IOP control with time.

In some instances glaucoma without symptoms, but with IOP in the 40s, has been detected on routine examination in young men and occasionally in women, who have sought attention merely for refraction for myopia.

Unfortunately it is not rare for patients with pigmentary glaucoma to present with reduced vision in one eye (4), which may have been attributed to "optic neuritis" in the past. We have wondered, in such patients, whether the high IOP (that fluctuates), which can be commonly seen in this condition, may have caused a previous acute optic nerve vascular insult.

Most patients with pigmentary dispersion syndrome have deep anterior chambers and usually, but not always, are myopic. The first clue to the disease may be found during slit-lamp examination when pigment is seen on the posterior surface of the cornea, occasionally forming a Krukenberg spindle, but this is not seen in every case (Fig. 21.1). Some have little or no pigment on the back of the cornea. The reason for the variable pigment deposition on the corneal endothelium is unclear. Aqueous convection

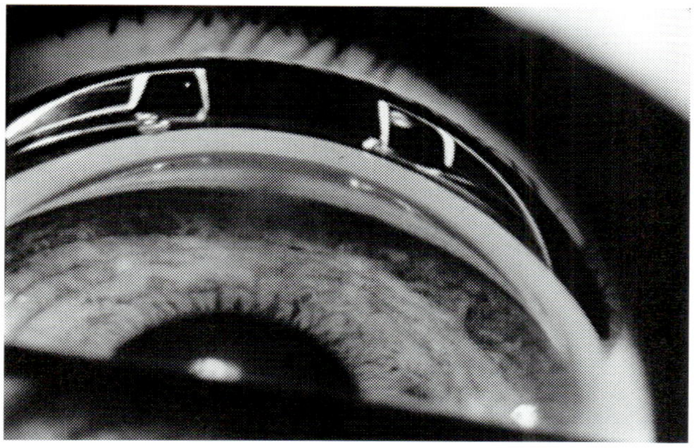

Figure 21.1. Goniophotograph of patient with pigmentary dispersion syndrome. In addition to pigment in the angle, pigment on the corneal endothelial surface is seen (Krukenburg spindle).

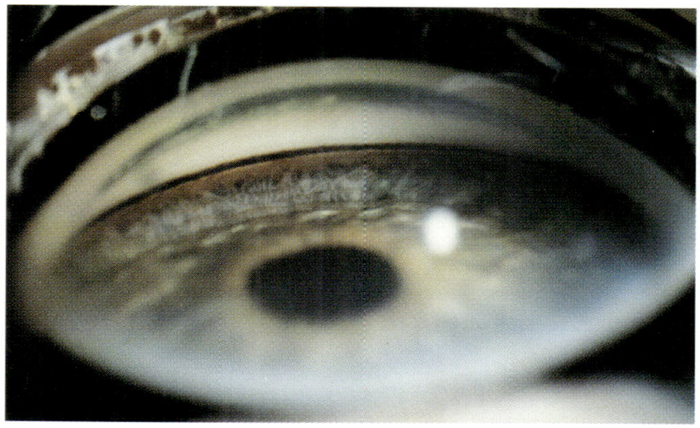

Figure 21.2. Goniophotograph demonstrating posterior iris bowing in patient with pigmentary dispersion syndrome. (Courtesy of Cynthia Mattox, MD).

currents apparently deposit the pigment on the posterior surface of the corneal endothelium, which may later engulf the pigment. Curiously, the pigment apparently does not cause corneal endothelial decompensation (5). Commonly, one can observe a sprinkling of pigment on the anterior surface of the iris stroma and on the back of the cornea.

The pigment dispersion syndrome (with or without pigmentary glaucoma) is not associated with any external or internal sign of intraocular inflammation, such as synechias or inflammatory cells in the aqueous humor or on the back of the cornea, but we have known of instances in which **pigment particles circulating in the aqueous humor have been mistaken for inflammatory cells**, and the glaucoma was erroneously attributed to uveitis, e.g., glaucomatocyclitic crisis. Attention to the brown color of the particles helps prevent this mistake. (An intriguing untested hypothesis is that there may be "something else" in addition to pigment particles (melanosomes), that may be released from the back of the iris, that might actually be producing the glaucoma in this condition (6). Perhaps in the future this might be subject to some type of novel "anti-inflammatory" therapy.)

GONIOSCOPY

Gonioscopy in pigment dispersion syndrome (with or without pigmentary glaucoma) typically shows in each eye a deep anterior chamber, with a flat and often slightly tremulous iris. A concave (posterior) iris contour is frequently observed (Fig. 21.2) (7,8). (This sometimes is more readily apparent on Koeppe gonioscopy than on mirrored slit-lamp gonioscopy.) The iris stroma appears normal, except for pigment that may be deposited on it. The angle is wide and open all around. The ciliary band is often broad, but sometimes it is not. The most essential feature in the angle is a **band of dark-brown, almost black, pigment that may strikingly delineate the filtration portion of the trabecular meshwork** in the whole circumference (Fig. 21.3). The pigment often covers not only the filtration portion, but the whole width of the trabecular meshwork in the entire circumference, including Schwalbe's line (where, similar to what can be seen in exfoliation syndrome, it can form a Sampaolesi's line). Pigment may also be deposited on the ciliary band. During gonioscopy, if one looks through the pupil toward the equator of the crystalline lens, when there is pigment dissemination one can also see an accumulation of pigment at the posterior surface of the lens (Fig. 21.4) where zonules or hyaloid face reaches the lens and form a sort of pocket. Similarly, in cases with heavy pigment dispersion there may be pigment deposition on the anterior lens surface as well (Fig. 21.5).

Although a dark, dense wide band of pigment filling the filtration portion of the trabecular meshwork is the rule in pigmentary dispersion syndrome, with or without glaucoma, in rare cases in patients examined repeatedly we have seen the density of the pigment band diminish with age, as described by Lichter and Shaffer (9). However, we are not convinced that this is accompanied necessarily by an improvement in IOP control. This same phenomenon of decreasing trabecular pigment band density was demonstrated in an experimental monkey model of pigmentary dispersion syndrome without producing chronic glaucoma (6).

In other cases, we have seen patients at a single stage with a typical transillumination pattern of the iris, but with a pigment band in the angle of only moderate density. In such cases, when the typical iris transillumination pattern has been present, we have postulated that some of the trabecular pigment may have washed out through the outflow channels or been carried away by phagocytes. The latter has also been implicated in the experimentally produced model (6).

IRIS TRANSILLUMINATION

The presence of a typical iris transillumination pattern (Fig. 21.6) is considered essential to the diagnosis of the pigmentary dispersion syndrome. **When the examiner**

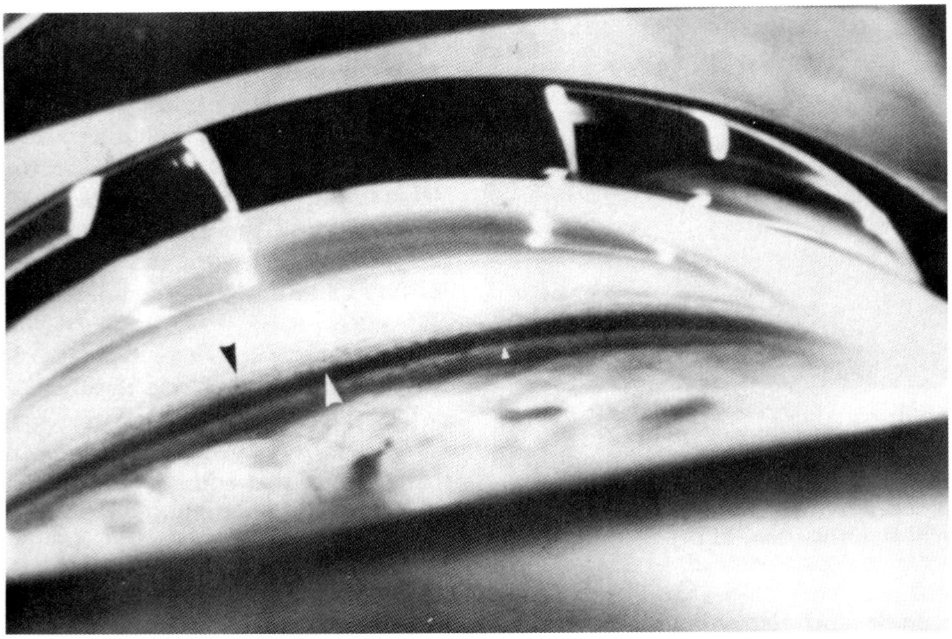

Figure 21.3. Patient with pigmentary glaucoma demonstrates angle landmarks well. The aqueous humor drains through the posterior aspect of the trabecular meshwork in which the pigment band lies (large white arrowhead). Anterior trabecular meshwork contains much less pigment. Schwalbe's line (black arrowhead) and the scleral spur (small white arrowhead) are easily defined. Reprinted with permission from Donaldson DD: Atlas of External Diseases of the Eye. Vol. IV. Anterior Chamber, Iris, and Ciliary Body. St. Louis, The C.V. Mosby Co., 1973.

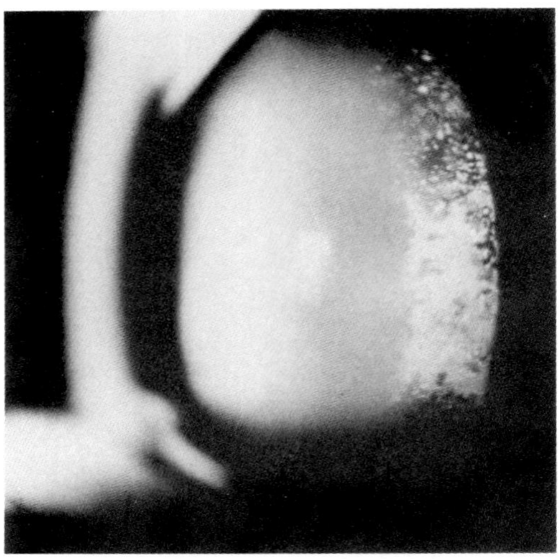

Figure 21.4. Unusually dense pigment deposition on the posterior lens surface in a patient with pigmentary dispersion syndrome.

has dark adapted for several minutes and employs a fiberoptic transilluminator in a darkened room, one sees the typical, mid-peripheral iris transillumination pattern that is initially radial and slit or wedge-like, but later may become confluent. In advanced conditions these abnormal iris transillumination defects can extend into the central third of the iris (Fig. 21.7).

To test for loss of pigment from the posterior layer of the iris, transillumination of the iris is performed by holding a shielded fiberoptic transilluminator against the lower lid temporally or against the sclera temporally, in such a way that light passing through the sclera glows bright and pink from the pupil when one looks directly at the eye. This must be done in a darkened room. In normal eyes the light does not shine through the iris in the manner characteristic of pigmentary dispersion syndrome, but in genuine cases of the syndrome, the iris transilluminates in a striking patchy ring in the mid-periphery (Fig. 21.8). This is due to loss of pigment from this particular portion of the posterior pigment layer. Elsewhere, either near the pupil (except at advanced stages) or in the periphery adjacent to the ciliary band, the pigment layer appears to remain intact. The selective loss of pigment in the mid-portion of the iris can sometimes be appreciated better if one performs the transillumination while viewing the iris through the Koeppe gonioscope lens. Alternatively, at the slit lamp, the beam may be narrowed and placed coaxial to the observer in the patient's pupil, in order to search for transillumination defects. This maneuver should be a routine part of one's slit-lamp examination.

In the absence of a characteristic iris transillumination pattern, it is difficult to make a definite diagnosis of the pigment dispersion syndrome, although there are rare patients (usually with dark irides) who demonstrate all other aspects of the syndrome but in whom the iris does not transilluminate and who have no known source for pigment dissemination other than the iris (i.e., exfoliation, iris or ciliary body cysts, or melanoma (10,11,12) were ruled out). One of us (WMG) saw one patient in whom a typical transillumination pattern disappeared, as though from new pigment formation; this patient had gradual disappearance of a pigment band from the angle several years after successful filtration surgery (in retrospect, it is possible that this may have been due to the peripheral iridectomy performed as part of the surgery).

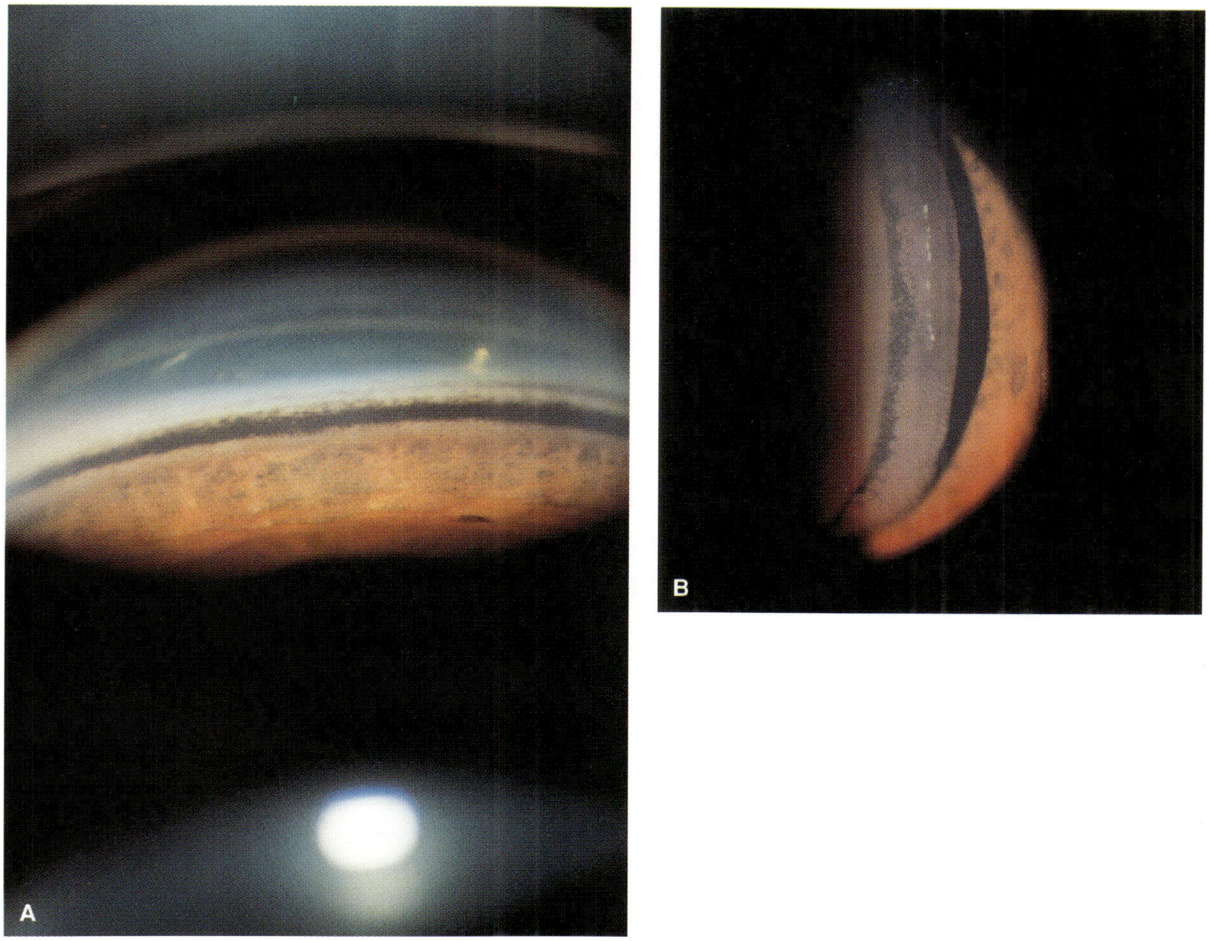

Figure 21.5. Patient with heavy accumulation of pigment in the angle (A) and on the anterior lens surface at the site of zonular attachment (B).

Case 21-2. A 29-year-old man was aware of some aching around his left eye. His ophthalmologist found IOPs of 40 mm Hg in both eyes, with pathologic cupping of both discs, worse on the left, with a Bjerrum scotoma in this eye. When seen here, without treatment, the IOP was 60 with tonographic C values of 0.05 in each eye. Both discs had deep broad cups with central vessels displaced far nasally, a thin layer of tissue preserved within the rim in most of the circumference of the right disc, but excavation to the rim lower temporally in the left. The anterior chambers were deep. By gonioscopy the irides appeared almost concave, attaching just posterior to the scleral spur in the whole circumference. A dense blackish pigment band covered the filtration portion of the trabecular meshwork in the whole circumference in both eyes. Transillumination showed a striking moth-eaten type of defect of the posterior pigment layer of each iris in a ring peripherally, characteristic of pigmentary glaucoma in both eyes. Response to treatment with pilocarpine and epinephrine was inadequate. A filtration operation was performed on the left eye, and 3 months later on the right. A better bleb was obtained on the right eye than the left. For several months the IOP was close to 7 mm Hg in the right and in the mid-20s in the left. Frequent digital pressure on the left globe was employed to try to improve the function of the bleb. A little more than a year after operation both eyes had excellent blebs and IOPs of 9 without treatment other than periodic digital pressure. The degree of cupping became notably less in each eye than when first seen, and by 8 years after the bilateral operation, the degree of cupping of both discs had decreased remarkably, though the principal vessels remained far to the nasal side of the right disc and the left was still as pale as it had been at the first observation. By that time the amount of pigment in the angles appeared to be decreasing, and the transillumination of the irides also appeared less than when the patient was first seen. At nearly 10 years after operation the blebs were not quite as good as formerly. IOPs reached the high teens, and epinephrine drops were started in each eye.

At 14 years after surgery, the IOPs were 15 in both eyes under treatment with epinephrine and digital pressure several times a day. Corrected vision was 20/25 right, 20/50 left. The Bjerrum scotoma in the left eye remained unchanged. The pigment in the angles had changed from a dense, almost black pigment band covering the filtration portion of the trabecular meshwork in the whole circumference to a thin line of a distinctly lighter brown color. The filtration blebs contained no pigment. Transillumination of the irides showed

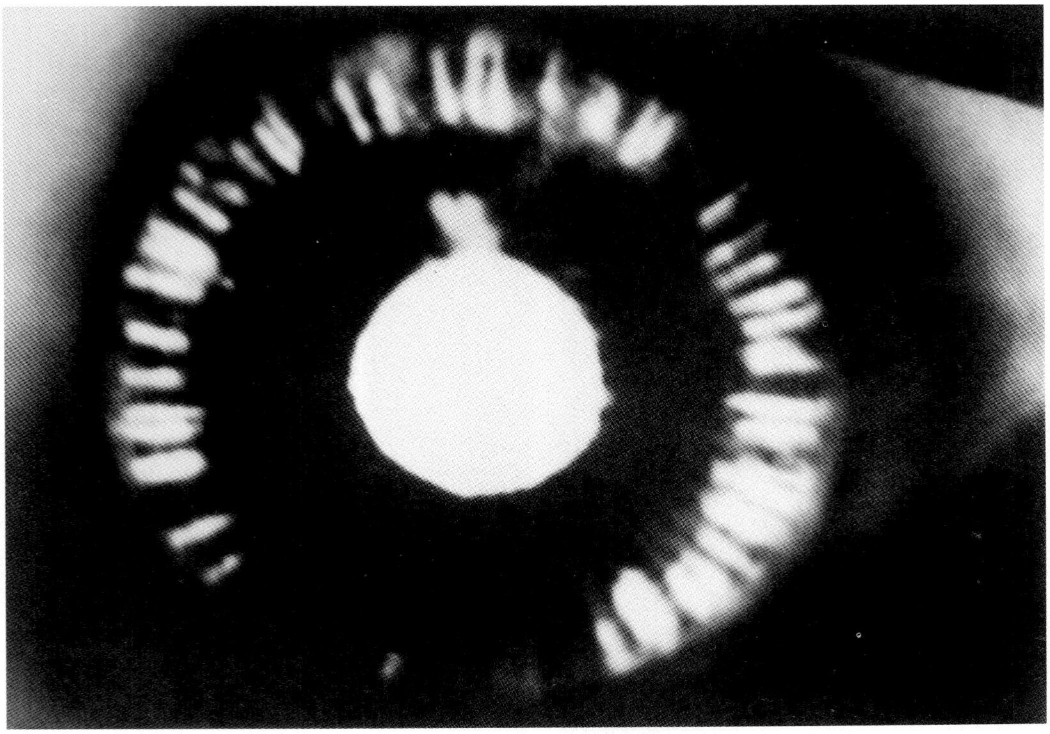

Figure 21.6. Typical transillumination pattern of the peripheral iris in a patient with pigmentary glaucoma. This patient atypically also demonstrates a small rectangular area of peripupillary transillumination. (Courtesy of David D. Donaldson, MD).

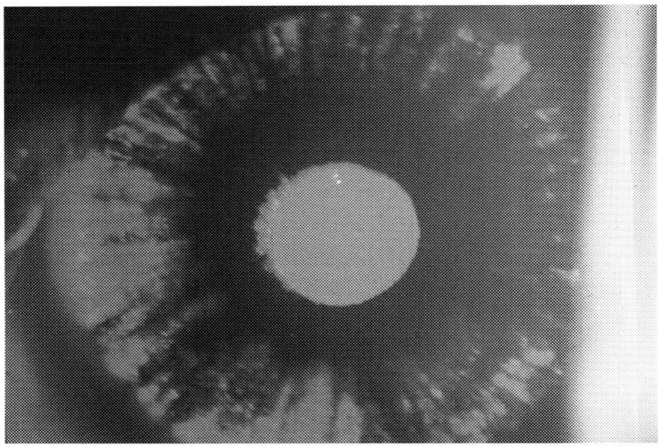

Figure 21.7. Marked loss of posterior iris pigment in a patient with pigmentary dispersion syndrome.

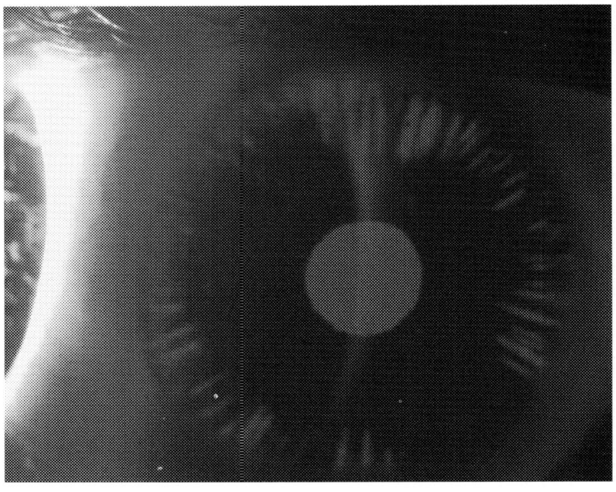

Figure 21.8. Use of fiberoptic transilluminator can be very useful in demonstrating iris transillumination in pigmentary dispersion syndrome (particularly in brown eyed patients).

no abnormal transillumination of any portion of either iris, except for the surgical colobomas, in contrast to the striking moth-eaten appearance of pigment loss from the posterior layer of the iris seen peripherally in the initial examinations performed in the same manner. There had been remarkable thinning of the pigment in the angle and disappearance of the transillumination of the irides. (On the other hand, the glaucoma was actually slowly worsening with time.)

PATHOGENESIS OF THE IRIS TRANSILLUMINATION DEFECTS AND THE PIGMENT DISPERSION

Currently, there is much clinical excitement about pigmentary glaucoma, mainly due to important new clinical observations made by observant clinicians. (Glaucoma remains a specialty where important new insights can be made by the clinician who carefully and meticulously (Chapter 5) examines patients and is an inquisitive observer). Karichoff (13,14) and Campbell (15) have observed that **the normally concave iris contour present in pigmentary glaucoma reverts to a planar configuration after laser iridectomy.** This has been confirmed by ultrasound (7). Previously Campbell had hypothesized that rubbing of the posterior iris surface against the zonules was responsible for the pigment dispersion from the posterior iris surface (16). Thus laser iridectomy, by preventing this rubbing, might have applicability in the treatment of patients with pigmentary glaucoma.

Nevertheless, it is not yet appropriate (17) to apply laser iridectomy as a potential "cure" for pigmentary glaucoma for the following reasons. The fundamental question in this disease, whether the pigment loss from the posterior iris surface represents a primary iris pigment epithelial degeneration or "abiotrophy" (a kind of presenile tissue degeneration that may be genetically predetermined) (18,19) or is, in fact, a mechanical disease due to zonular rubbing (16), has still not been totally resolved (17). The concept of zonular rubbing was ingenious and intriguing but has not, despite its ready popularity, been unequivocally established. The hypothesis was based on studies of enucleated eyes, which were fixed in a usual postmortem hypotonous state in which it might be difficult to orient zonular packets with the posterior iris defects as they might appear in a normal living eye. But further, in advanced pigmentary glaucoma the iris transillumination defects may extend well into the central third of the iris where zonules are not believed to extend. Also, the posterior surface of the iris folds on itself with pupillary dilatation (20) such that small segments should be protected from a "to and fro" rubbing, as originally proposed. The peripheral iris transillumination streaks should therefore contain small segments of less dense transillumination. (Actually a careful clinical examination does indicate that some transillumination defects in pigmentary glaucoma do show this, but this is uncommon). Of course, this "to and fro" rubbing may not be what is happening mechanically in the living eye, but rather a "ballotment" of the posterior iris surface against the zonules with eye movement as a consequence of the typical iris concavity in these usually larger myopic eyes. This then could mechanically explain the observed usually continuous iris transillumination streak.

Even more importantly, **there are patients who have the full pigmentary dispersion syndrome including iris concavity, typical transillumination defects, and angle pigmentation who do not have elevated IOP or any abnormality in outflow dynamics.** As detailed subsequently, there is a strong clinical impression with some limited data that such patients never will, in fact, develop pigmentary glaucoma. Except for the normal IOP, such pigmentary dispersion patients cannot be distinguished from those with pigmentary glaucoma. In such patients the same mechanical factors that lead to loss of iris pigment in pigmentary glaucoma must also be present, and yet there is no glaucoma. Perhaps to oversimplify this to make the point, there must then be more to pigmentary glaucoma than pigment dispersion alone. In fact, experimental studies in living monkeys have confirmed this by indicating that **one cannot in previously normal monkeys cause pigmentary glaucoma despite instilling vast quantities of pigment into the anterior chamber and producing trabecular meshwork pigment bands** (6,21). That is, experimentally one can produce pigmentary dispersion but not pigmentary glaucoma.

Most likely there is some trabecular cellular abnormality that is required in addition to the pigment dispersion for the glaucoma to occur (6). It could be argued that the pigment release is a "stress" to the trabecular meshwork in such individuals, and that by diminishing this, e.g., with laser iridectomy, it might improve the clinical condition. This needs to be evaluated by prospective randomized trials. These trials should be performed in patients with existing pigmentary glaucoma (that hopefully might be symmetrical and in which only one eye is treated), and not in patients with pigmentary dispersion syndrome without glaucoma, who as indicated have a very low probability of developing abnormal outflow function.

What also should give one caution is the observation that as patients with pigmentary glaucoma age, there is commonly a remarkable decrease in angle pigmentation (that Campbell has argued is due to the loss of iris concavity with further growth of the crystalline lens, producing an increase in relative pupillary block (16). However, we have not been impressed that the glaucoma status (except perhaps now for the absence of "attacks" of high IOP associated with "pigment storms" in the anterior chamber, that, regardless, may decrease with the passage of time) has actually concomitantly improved. One might argue in rebuttal that it is too late in the disease process for this to occur, but this still should not be used as justification to treat patients with pigmentary dispersion who have no IOP elevation with "prophylactic" laser iridectomy.

The loss of iris concavity after laser iridectomy that was originally observed by Karichoff (13,14) and Campbell (15) has been confirmed (7) but still has not had an adequate explanation. Some have proposed sudden bursts of aqueous humor flow through the pupil with reverse pupillary block temporarily ensuing (8,13,15). An alternative that needs evaluation derives from the fact that there is normally protein leakage into the anterior chamber at the base of the iris that explains the higher protein content of pre-trabecular aqueous humor compared to that in the central anterior chamber (22,23). It is conceivable that in the larger typically myopic eye involved in pigmentary dispersion, the iris may be thinner at the root (in addition to other "abiotrophic" features of such eyes), and thus there is flow of aqueous humor into the anterior chamber at this site. The latter phenomenon then could explain a slightly higher pressure occurring in the anterior chamber than the posterior chamber, and, hence, the resulting iris concavity. Alternatively, abnormalities in the iris dilator muscle have been described in pigmentary dispersion syndrome (19) and perhaps these contribute directly to the observed iris concavity. Possibly the laser-produced hole in the iris mechanically interferes with the underlying structural mechanism (e.g., interfering with circumferentially oriented iris "tone"). When the pupil is dilated with a sympathomimetic agent, the concavity of the peripheral iris of a patient with pigmentary dispersion syndrome commonly disappears, presumably due to the contraction of the iris dilator muscle. Perhaps mechanical considerations might also explain the change in iris contour with accommodation (24) that sometimes seems to occur in this condition. These are just speculations, but the effect of laser iridectomy on iris contour does not, in itself, indicate that zonular rubbing is the cause of pigment release, nor that there will be less pigment release from the posterior iris surface after the procedure. Many myopic eyes show a concave iris contour without any signs of pigment dispersion, and there may be cases of pigmentary dispersion syndrome where laser iridectomy does not alter iris concavity (25).

Despite these reservations, these new observations based on detailed clinical examination of patients with this condition (that was available to all of us but not fully appreciated in past years) offer much new information for further investigation and clarification. Certainly the time is appropriate for a randomized prospective clinical trial involving one eye, of a precisely defined population of patients with symmetrical pigmentary glaucoma. Also it would not seem wrong, as a last attempt to control pigmentary glaucoma prior to filtration surgery, to offer a laser iridectomy to one eye, after a full discussion of the benefits and risks with the affected patient. However, the clinician needs to keep the limits of our understanding firmly in mind as he/she seeks to determine whether the course of the glaucoma is truly altered, or simply the iris concavity.

PATHOGENESIS OF THE TRABECULAR GLAUCOMA

The pathogenesis of the chronic impairment in outflow function in pigmentary glaucoma is still far from clear. There is both clinical (26) and laboratory (6,27) evidence that iris pigment can acutely obstruct outflow of aqueous humor. This seems believable but leaves completely unexplained how another group of patients who appear to have the same amount of pigment in their angles have no obstruction of outflow, either by IOP measurements or tonography. Perhaps differences in the response of the trabecular endothelial cells to the pigment may be important in determining whether aqueous outflow is obstructed. Richardson reported electron micrographic evidence of trabecular sclerosis in pigmentary glaucoma, (28), but this is likely a late phenomenon. Alvarado's group has reported abnormalities in the cell lined outflow pathway in pigmentary glaucoma (29,30). Further electron microscopic examination of the pigmentary dispersion syndrome without glaucoma, as reported by Fine, Yanoff, and Scheie, (18) is needed for comparison with all these studies. Pigment alone does not appear to be obstructing the extracellular outflow pathway in chronic pigmentary glaucoma (30).

We produced a model of pigmentary dispersion syndrome in living monkeys which has provided some insight to this condition (6). Homologous uveal pigment was perfused into the anterior chamber of these monkeys. Acutely, there was a substantial lowering of outflow facility, and experimental glaucoma resulted. However, in these otherwise normal monkeys there was rapid recovery, and despite repetitive perfusions of pigment, outflow facility returned to normal. The monkeys developed trabecular pigment bands (Fig. 21.9) which often decreased in density with time. Morphologic examination indicated that the structure of the trabecular meshwork remained normal despite pigment phagocytosis and possible migration of trabecular endothelial cells. A few animals were observed for several additional years, with once again normal aqueous humor dynamics and trabecular meshwork morphology including cellularity (21). Our study also raised the issue of whether the loss observed of trabecular meshwork pigment with time was due to wandering macrophages rather than trabecular cell migration. We concluded that factors in addition to iris pigment shedding, e.g., underlying trabecular cell abnormalities, are involved in the development of chronic pigmentary glaucoma.

Some observers have interpreted pigmentary glaucoma as a congenital mesodermal angle anomaly, or simply as a variant of primary open angle glaucoma, though tests in patients with pigmentary glaucoma have indicated a different reactivity to corticosteroids than is found in primary open angle glaucoma (31). We often do observe dense or prominent uveal meshwork (so-called iris processes) in patients with pigmentary dispersion syndrome, both with and without glaucoma, but we doubt that this type of anatomy is more common in pigmentary dispersion syndrome than in similarly myopic eyes that have wide angles without excessive pigment.

DIFFERENTIAL DIAGNOSIS

In the differential diagnosis of pigmentary glaucoma, one should keep in mind open-angle glaucoma associated with exfoliation (Chapter 20), in which a smaller amount of pigment is usually seen in the trabecular meshwork, but in which transillumination shows no loss of pigment from the portion of the iris affected in "pigmentary" glaucoma,

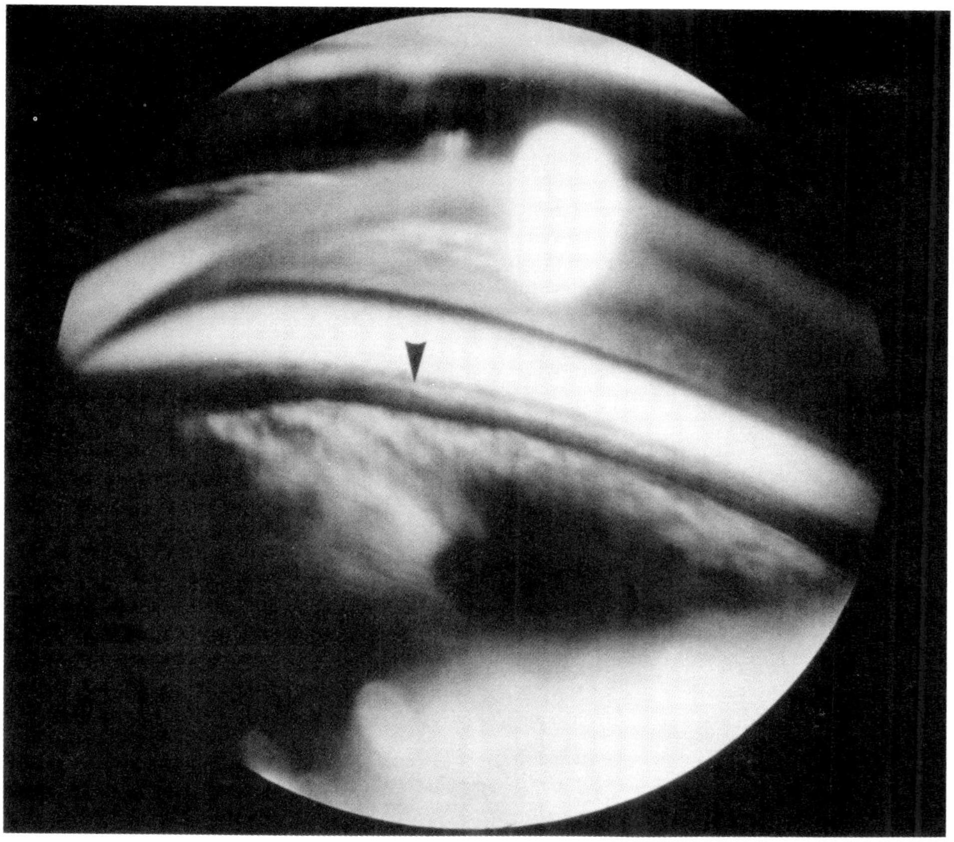

Figure 21.9. Trabecular pigment band (arrowhead) in a living monkey with experimental pigmentary dispersion syndrome. The band has decreased in density with time. The white "band" just inferior to the arrowhead is the scleral spur. Only acute glaucoma was produced. Long-term outflow facility returned to normal (see text). Reprinted with permission from Epstein DL, Freddo TF, Anderson PJ, et al. Experimental obstruction to aqueous outflow by pigment particles in living monkeys. Invest Ophthalmol Vis Sci 1986;27: 387–395.

rather only a loss near the pupil. Rarely, a pigment ring in the angle is seen in amyloidosis with glaucoma (Chapter 48). Pigment in various amounts is commonly found in the angle in elderly people either without glaucoma or with primary open-angle glaucoma, and some pigment may be found in the angle in association with uveitis (Chapter 42), with cysts of the iris and ciliary body (Chapter 34), and after operation, traumatic angle recession, or attacks of acute angle closure glaucoma. However, the pigment in most of these conditions rarely forms a uniform band in the entire circumference. In the exfoliation syndrome with glaucoma, pigment is seen in the entire circumference, but it is often narrower, coarser, and less dense than in pigmentary glaucoma. In none of these conditions does the pigment layer of the iris transilluminate abnormally in the mid-periphery as it does in pigmentary glaucoma. The clinician should always seek to explain the presence of abnormal pigmentation observed on gonioscopy.

Pigmentary dispersion syndrome nearly always affects both eyes of an individual, although it may be asymmetric. In rare instances it occurs only in one eye, but before accepting such a diagnosis one should be able to identify the iris transillumination pattern and to rule out other causes of monocular pigment dissemination, especially malignant melanoma (12) of the anterior uveal tract (Chapter 41) causing melanomalytic glaucoma (10,11).

PIGMENTARY DISPERSION WITHOUT GLAUCOMA

It is strange but true that the pigmentary dispersion syndrome can occur with or without glaucoma. Pigment dispersion with consistently normal IOPs can easily escape recognition, since transillumination is not commonly performed routinely, and a Krukenberg spindle may be overlooked or may not be present. We have discovered a number of cases of pigmentary dispersion syndrome without glaucoma by doing a screening type of transillumination during routine slit-lamp examination by narrowing the slit beam to fit into the pupil, making the beam coaxial with the microscope, and observing the iris for transillumination with low magnification. The following case is an example.

Case 21-3. A 60-year-old man presented to the emergency room with a corneal abrasion. Bilateral Krukenberg spindles were noted. The past eye history was negative except for conjunctivitis. The family history was negative for glaucoma.

Several areas of abnormal iris transillumination in the mid-periphery were noted, and gonioscopy revealed a heavy trabecular pigment band in both eyes. The discs were normal and the fields were full. Applanation IOPs were right and left 16, and tonographic C values were 0.23 right and 0.25 left. No exfoliation was seen. During 10 years of follow-up the IOPs remained in the teens.

TONOGRAPHY

David L. Epstein

We have not yet observed the onset of glaucoma, or even borderline intraocular pressure, in patients with pigmentary dispersion syndrome who initially had normal intraocular pressure and normal tonographic outflow values. We have observed late onset of glaucoma in patients with dispersion syndrome who initially had normal intraocular pressures but borderline or abnormal tonographic outflow values. Tonography may therefore be of some prognostic value in patients with pigmentary dispersion, especially since in pigmentary glaucoma the level of intraocular pressure is subject to wide fluctuations.

This man with pigmentary dispersion syndrome without glaucoma is being followed as a "pigmentary glaucoma suspect," but at his age and with his good outflow facility we do not think he will ever develop pigmentary glaucoma.

Recognizing that pigmentary dispersion syndrome without glaucoma is a real and not so rare entity raises the important question of whether these patients will eventually develop pigmentary glaucoma. Sugar has observed the onset of glaucoma 12 to 20 years after pigmentary dispersion was first detected (2). In our longest follow-up, we can say that a patient with pigmentary dispersion can go for 20 years without developing glaucoma. This occurred in the following case:

Case 21-4. A 76-year-old white man was diagnosed as having pigment dispersion without glaucoma in the Emergency Room where he sought treatment for blepharitis. According to records of his private ophthalmologist, he had been followed for the previous 20 years for heavy Krukenberg spindles in both eyes, always with normal intraocular pressures, and with no treatment. In addition to broad Krukenberg spindles, in both eyes, there were occasional pigment particles present spontaneously in the aqueous humor and moderate pigment deposition on the anterior iris surface. No exfoliation was found. The anterior chambers were deep, and marked iridodonesis was present. Striking spoke-like mid-peripheral iris transillumination was present in all quadrants in both eyes. Applanation IOP was 19 mm Hg in each eye. Gonioscopy revealed wide open angles with dense continuous pigment bands and dense but not abnormal uveal meshwork. Both optic discs had physiologic cups and the visual fields were full. Tonographic C values were 0.33 right and 0.38 left. Phenylephrine provocative testing of the right eye produced a conspicuous increase in the amount of pigment particles in the aqueous humor, but no change in intraocular pressure.

How often should one reevaluate patients who have typical pigment dispersion but apparently normal intraocular pressure? If initially several pressure determinations at different times of the day are normal, or if tonography indicates good facility of outflow, and the discs are normal, we would be content to see the patient every 6 to 12 months, depending on the "healthiness" of the optic nerve heads. We suspect that the majority of such patients with pigmentary dispersion will never develop glaucoma.

ACUTE IOP ELEVATIONS IN PATIENTS WITH PIGMENTARY GLAUCOMA ("PIGMENT STORMS")

Pigment particles in the aqueous humor are often seen in eyes with pigmentary dispersion syndrome, usually without relation to the level of intraocular pressure. **In a few cases the number of pigment particles in the aqueous humor has been observed to increase rapidly, sometimes spontaneously, or as a result of exercise** (32–34). The increase in suspended pigment has in some instances been associated with a marked rise in intraocular pressure, as exemplified in the following cases.

Case 21-5. A 30-year-old white man noticed blurring of vision and haloes on several occasions after playing basketball, greater in the right eye than in the left. IOP in each eye was found to be in the 40s on one such occasion. Pigmentary glaucoma was diagnosed. The patient was in good health, with no family history of glaucoma.

Reexamination several days later, without treatment but now asymptomatic, showed diffuse deposits of pigment on the back surface of both corneas. The anterior chambers were abnormally deep with an occasional speck of pigment circulating in the aqueous. A shadow of pigment in the angle could be demonstrated by retroillumination of the sclera at the limbus. Gonioscopy revealed an almost concave iris contour, with a dense black band of pigment in the whole circumference of the trabecular meshwork and pigment behind the equator of both lenses. The irides transilluminated in the mid-periphery. The discs had small physiologic cups. Applanation tensions were then 20 right, 19 left. Tonographic C value was 0.09 on the right, not measured on the left.

The patient agreed to go jogging to try to provoke his symptoms. After jogging, the applanation tensions were 31 right and 22 left. There were diffuse, fine clouds of pigment in the aqueous, greater on the right than the left. Tonographic C values after exercise were 0.02 right and 0.05 left. The patient stated that activity in which he "jiggled" his head, such as basketball, caused more symptoms than simple running.

Seven months later the patient returned with recurrent symptoms of haloes. IOPs were 38 right and 22 left, with a great amount of circulating pigment in the right anterior chamber, considerably less in the left.

Subsequently, when the increased IOP had spontaneously subsided, phenylephrine provocative testing was done, but it produced only an occasional pigment speck in the aqueous humor and no significant change in IOP. There was a small increase in facility of outflow.

During the next 3 years the patient had a few minor episodes of exercise-induced visual symptoms. Intraocular pressure has generally remained below 21 mm Hg in each eye without any treatment, and the discs have remained normal.

Case 21-6. In 1968 a 30-year-old white man with pigmentary glaucoma gave a history of attacks of pain, haloes, and blurred vision lasting 3 to 4 hours, sometimes in one eye and sometimes in the other. He associated these attacks with dim illumination and occasionally with emotionally upsetting circumstances, but not with exercise. When he was asymptomatic, intraocular pressures were in the low 20s in the right and low 30s in the left. The angles were open, of safe width, with dense pigment bands on the trabecular meshwork, but no pigment particles in the aqueous humor. Darkroom testing was negative. The discs had small physiologic cups. The left eye was treated with epinephrine and pilocarpine for several years.

In 1976 he had a spontaneous attack in the right eye that occurred while he was working outside in dim light at night. During the attack the intraocular pressure was 55 right and 22 left. There were many pigment particles of various sizes in the aqueous humor in the right eye, but only occasional particles in the left. Both angles were open, with dense pigment bands. The patient was treated with acetazolamide, and with pressure reduced, he was asymptomatic the following morning.

These cases and other similar cases (33,34) seem to support the concept that pigment particles under certain circumstances temporarily obstruct the aqueous outflow channels (6,27), although it is possible that the IOP elevation and pigment liberation are both secondary to some other process.

Patients with pigmentary glaucoma should be routinely queried about exercise induced or spontaneous symptoms of blurred vision and seeing "colored haloes." It is remarkable how often the patient initially denies such symptoms, but after being informed about their possible occurrence, returns at a subsequent visit now relating such symptoms in the past. These symptoms are then subsequently documented to be associated with episodic elevations of IOP.

In a few cases a pigment shower and a transitory increase of IOP have been induced by phenylephrine eye drops, and one might therefore expect this to provide the basis for a provocative test for pigmentary glaucoma. However, in systematic testing we have found the amount of pigment liberated is so varied, and the IOP increases so infrequent, that we conclude that phenylephrine testing is not useful for identifying latent glaucoma in patients with pigmentary dispersion syndrome (32). Furthermore, phenylephrine occasionally produces pigment liberation and IOP elevation in patients with primarily open angle glaucoma and in patients with exfoliation syndrome (32). It is also noteworthy that the extent of iris transillumination does not correlate with the grade of phenylephrine-induced pigment liberation.

OTHER ASSOCIATIONS

Strangely, diabetes has never to our knowledge been a cause of pigmentary glaucoma, although diabetes causes the pigment epithelium of the iris to store excessive glycogen and renders these cells so fragile that they can release great showers of pigment during intraocular surgery. Pigmentary dispersion syndrome has been rarely associated with inner ear deafness (pigment cells), congenital megalocornea, and perhaps pregnancy. The iridodonesis and possibly a higher than normal prevalence of retinal detachment are believed to result from the association of myopia with pigmentary dispersion.

TREATMENT

The IOP in pigmentary glaucoma seems to be subject to large spontaneous fluctuations, particularly in young people. In some cases, this is attributed to release of pigment particles into the anterior chamber with exercise that temporarily obstructs aqueous outflow, but in other cases the cause of this IOP fluctuation is not certain. In evaluation of the response of the IOP to medical treatment, this tendency to spontaneous fluctuation has to be kept in mind.

The principles of treatment of pigmentary glaucoma are fundamentally like those that we have described for primary open angle glaucoma (Chapter 18). Topical beta blockers or epinephrine-like compounds are the usual first choice (see Table 18.1). Because the patients are usually young and are often myopic, the use of miotic eye drops may present a considerable problem because of spasm of accommodation and blurring of vision (but see later discussion about miotics possibly preventing pigment dispersion). **However, pilocarpine Ocusert therapy (Chapter 13) is often well tolerated and effective in young patients with pigmentary glaucoma.** Several young myopic patients with pigmentary glaucoma have been described by Brachet and Chermet as having peripheral chorioretinal degeneration and retinal detachment, which they feel is another reason to be cautious about the use of miotics in these patients (35).

Sometimes epinephrine-like compounds prove remarkably effective in the control of pigmentary glaucoma, either by itself or in combination with miotics. Topical or oral carbonic anhydrase inhibitors are employed when needed. We instruct some patients who see haloes periodically to take an acetazolamide or methazolamide tablet orally or dorzolamide topically at the first symptoms. They frequently report that the episode is shortened. Apraclonidine may be used for the same purpose.

Laser trabeculoplasty (LTP) can often produce dramatic IOP lowering in pigmentary glaucoma, but the results are less uniform than with exfoliation glaucoma, and **occasional patients with pigmentary glaucoma demonstrate substantial IOP elevation, both acute and sustained, after LTP.**

CLINICAL COURSE

As mentioned, remarkable fluctuation of intraocular pressure may occur in pigmentary glaucoma. Some patients seem to have periods of "crisis" of elevated intraocular pressure and then return to more normal levels. During such crises, symptoms may be acute, with corneal edema and haloes, but usually no pain. In some patients these crises of pressure elevation seem related to excessive liberation of pigment granules into the anterior segment (Cases 21-5 and 21-6) that may be associated with exercise, but in others we have recognized no associated factor. In a few rare cases of pigmentary glaucoma we have seen the intraocular pressure return toward normal within a few years, almost as if a remission of the glaucoma is occurring, and medication can be reduced or discontinued (see Case 21-5).

Because of the tendency to transitory elevation of pressure and the possibility of some degree of remission, we are much less influenced by the height of the IOP at a given time than by the character of the optic discs and visual fields in deciding when to recommend filtration surgery in pigmentary glaucoma.

The severity of pigmentary glaucoma and the length of time it can be controlled medically vary considerably from patient to patient. We have a vague impression that the earlier the onset, the more likely the glaucoma will become too severe for medical control and will require surgery. If adequate control cannot be obtained medically, then filtration surgery should be undertaken. Fortunately, standard filtration operations are as effective for this condition as ordinary open-angle glaucoma. We have seen no tendency for filtration blebs to become obstructed by particles of pigment.

CONCLUSION

The uncertain role of laser iridectomy potentially interrupting one component in the disease mechanism in this condition by changing iris contour has been discussed at the beginning of this chapter. A major area of uncertainty is what the factors are that are responsible for the disease occurring in only certain individuals with pigmentary dispersion syndrome. This relates to trabecular meshwork events concerning which we are not fully cognizant. At a maximum, **the pigment release which is due to either intrinsic or mechanical iris factors, is only a stress to a trabecular meshwork that must be at least latently abnormal in this disease.** More information is needed on how pigment trapped in the trabecular meshwork intercellularly, and intracellularly, can slowly be disposed of by some natural mechanism. This may involve wandering macrophages rather than migration of trabecular cells. One might also speculate that clearance of the pigment particles might be favored by enlarging the spaces within the trabecular meshwork by means of newer trabecular drugs or miotics.

More information is also needed on the extent to which pigment that is lost from the posterior layer of the iris early in the disease can be regenerated later.

Campbell has hypothesized that zonular rubbing is responsible for the pigment liberation from the posterior iris surface in this syndrome (16), and this has been discussed. Most likely this involves antero-posterior iris ballotment movements against the zonules, rather than a "to and fro" friction. In the past, Campbell has queried whether chronic miotic therapy might decrease this zonular rubbing. Unfortunately, most patients with pigmentary glaucoma, due to their relatively young age, do not usually tolerate standard miotics other than Ocuserts and, therefore, it has been difficult to fully evaluate this. New alpha-blockers with pupillary effects have recently become available and might be examined. However, the recent observations about iris contour change after laser iridectomy will probably lead to a more definitive evaluation of this hypothesis, if proper prospective randomized studies of one of two symmetrical eyes with pigmentary glaucoma are performed. Although intriguing, this hypothesis still leaves unexplained the nature of the trabecular abnormality present in only certain patients with pigmentary dispersion syndrome.

The occurrence of the full pigmentary dispersion syndrome without glaucoma (or without even any abnormality in aqueous outflow function) underscores our lack of understanding about the basic mechanisms for a particular glaucoma (36). The implications of the spontaneous or exercise-induced occurrence of pigment particle floater release into the anterior chamber, the apparent "crises" of acute pressure elevation, and the frequent usefulness of adrenergic therapy in this condition are unclear. Further careful, detailed long-term serial observation of all the many parameters (37) are required to increase our understanding of this fascinating syndrome.

References

1. Sugar HS, Barbour FA: Pigmentary glaucoma: a rare clinical entity. Am J Ophthalmol 1949;32:90–92.

2. Sugar HS: Pigmentary glaucoma. A 24-year review. Am J Ophthalmol 1966;2:499–507.
3. Mauksch H: Uber idiopathischen Zerfall des retinalen Pigmentblattes der Iris bei zwei Brüdern. Z Augenheilkd 1925;57:262–268.
4. Pickett JE, Terry SA, O'Connor PS, et al: Early loss of central visual acuity in glaucoma. Ophthalmology 1985;92:891–6.
5. Lehto I, Ruusuvaara P, Setala K: Corneal endothelium in pigmentary glaucoma and pigment dispersion syndrome. Acta Ophthalmol (Copenh) 1990;68:703–9.
6. Epstein DL, Freddo TF, Anderson PJ, et al: Experimental obstruction to aqueous outflow by pigment particles in living monkeys. Invest Ophthalmol Vis Sci 1986;27:387–395.
7. Potash SD, Tello C, Liebmann JM, et al: Ultrasound biomicroscopy in pigment dispersion syndrome. Ophthalmology 1994;101:332–339.
8. Liebmann JM, Tello C, Chew SJ, et al: Prevention of blinking alters iris configuration in pigment dispersion syndrome and in normal eyes. Ophthalmology 1995;102:446–455.
9. Lichter PR, Shaffer RN: Diagnostic and prognostic signs in pigmentary glaucoma. Trans Am Acad Ophthalmol Otolaryngol 1970;74:984–998.
10. Van Buskirk EM, Leure-duPree AE: Pathophysiology and electron microscopy of melanomalytic glaucoma. Am J Ophthalmol 1978;85: 160–166.
11. Yanoff M, Scheie HG: Melanomalytic glaucoma. Arch Ophthalmol 1970;84:471–473.
12. Omulecki W, Pruszczynski M, Borowski J: Ring melanoma of the iris and ciliary body. Br J Ophthalmol 1985;9:514–8.
13. Karickhoff JR: Pigmentary dispersion syndrome and pigmentary glaucoma: a new mechanism concept, a new treatment, and a new technique. Ophthalmic Surg 1992;23:269–277.
14. Karickhoff JR: Reverse pupillary block in pigmentary glaucoma: follow up and new developments (letter). Ophthalmic Surg 1993;24:562–3.
15. Campbell DG: Iridotomy, blinking, and pigmentary glaucoma: Invest Ophthalmol Vis Sci 1993;34(ARVO Supplement):993.
16. Campbell DG: Pigmentary dispersion and glaucoma. A new theory. Arch Ophthalmol 1979;97:1667–1672.
17. Krupin T, Rosenberg LF, Weinreb RN: Pigmentary glaucoma: facts versus fiction. J Glaucoma 1994;3:273–274.
18. Fine BS, Yanoff M, Scheie HG: Pigmentary "glaucoma." A histologic study. Trans Am Acad Ophthalmol Otolaryngol 1974;78:314–325.
19. Kupfer C, Kuwabara T, Kaiser-Kupfer M: The histopathology of pigmentary dispersion syndrome with glaucoma. Am J Ophthalmol 1975; 80:857–62.
20. Kuwabara T: Unpublished observations.
21. Epstein DL, de Kater AW, Schroeder A: Long-term observation of living monkeys with experimental pigmentary dispersion. Invest Ophthalmol Vis Sci 1992;33(ARVO suppl):731.
22. Barsotti M, Bartels SP, Freddo TF, et al: The source of proteins in the aqueous humor of the normal monkey eye. Invest Ophthalmol Vis Sci 1992;33:581–595.
23. Johnson M, Gong H, Freddo TF, et al: Serum proteins and aqueous outflow resistance in bovine eyes. Invest Ophthalmol Vis Sci 1993;34: 3549–3557.
24. Pavlin CJ, Macken P, Trope G, et al: Ultrasound biomicroscopic features of pigmentary glaucoma. Can J Ophthalmol 1994;29:187–92.
25. Jampel HD: Lack of effect of peripheral laser iridotomy in pigment dispersion syndrome. Arch Ophthalmol 1993;111:1606.
26. Petersen HP: Can pigmentary deposits on the trabecular meshwork increase the resistance of the aqueous outflow? Acta Ophthalmol 1969; 47:743–749.
27. Grant WM: Experimental aqueous perfusion in enucleated human eyes. Arch Ophthalmol 1963;69:783–801.
28. Richardson TM, Hutchinson BT, Grant WM: The outflow tract in pigmentary glaucoma. A light and electron microscopic study. Arch Ophthalmol 1977;95:1015–1025.
29. Alvarado JA, Murphy CG: Outflow obstruction in pigmentary and primary open angle glaucoma. Arch Ophthalmol 1992;110:1769–1778.
30. Murphy CG, Johnson M, Alvarado JA: Juxtacanalicular tissue in pigmentary and primary open angle glaucoma. Arch Ophthalmol 1992; 110:1779–1785.
31. Zink HA, Palmberg PF, Sugar A, et al: Comparison of in vitro corticosteroid response in pigmentary glaucoma and primary open-angle glaucoma. Am J Ophthalmol 1975;80:478–484.
32. Epstein DL, Boger WP III, Grant WM: Phenylephrine provocative testing in the pigmentary dispersion syndrome. Am J Ophthalmol 1978; 85:43–50.
33. Schenker HI, Luntz MH, Kels B, et al: Exercise-induced increase of intraocular pressure in the pigmentary dispersion syndrome. Am J Ophthalmol 1980;89:598.
34. Haynes WL, Johnson AT, Alward WL: Effects of jogging exercise on patients with the pigmentary dispersion syndrome and pigmentary glaucoma. Ophthalmology 1992;99:1096–2003.
35. Brachet A, Chermet M: Association glaucome pigmentaire et décollement de rétine. Ann Oculist (Paris) 1974;207:451–457.
36. Epstein DL: Will there be a remedy to reverse the changes in the trabecular meshwork and the optic nerve? A personal point-of-view on glaucoma therapy. J Glaucoma 1993;2:138–140.
37. Richter CU, Richardson TM, Grant WM: Pigmentary dispersion syndrome and pigmentary glaucoma. A prospective study of the natural history. Arch Ophthalmol 1986;104:211–5.

Principles of Primary Angle Closure Glaucomas

22

David L. Epstein

GENERAL CONSIDERATIONS

In the various forms of angle closure glaucoma, the trabecular meshwork may have intrinsically normal function, but the position of the peripheral iris in front of the trabecular meshwork blocks access of aqueous humor to the outflow pathway. Since there is very limited circumferential flow of aqueous humor once in Schlemm's Canal (1), each portion of the trabecular meshwork circumference functions as if it were a relatively independent outflow segment. Thus the full "blockage" of a portion of the trabecular meshwork circumference by the peripheral iris, e.g., in the superior 4 hours only, results in a proportional increase in outflow resistance (the inverse of outflow facility) (Chapter 3).

Aqueous humor normally exits through the posterior half of the trabecular meshwork (TM), closest to scleral spur. This is likely related to the common observation of relatively increased pigmentation of this posterior half of the TM. Thus **when only the anterior half of the trabecular meshwork is visualized by gonioscopy, if the unseen posterior half of TM is blocked by iris apposition, there may not be aqueous outflow occurring through this segment of the angle circumference**. This observation is often misinterpreted by beginning gonioscopists who report that they "see some trabecular meshwork." Stated another way, **the full width of the trabecular meshwork needs to be visualized (without indentation) to the scleral spur to know that the angle is functionally open**. Thus the term "partial angle closure" does not mean that part of the TM is visible in one area. Rather the term refers to the fact that the angle is functionally closed (by iris apposed to at least the posterior half of the TM) in a portion of the twelve hour angle circumference (Fig. 22.1).

The peripheral iris which functionally "blocks" access to the draining (posterior half) TM in part or whole of the 12-hour (360 degree) angle circumference may be apposed without permanent adhesion or with some semi-permanent adhesion (which is called a peripheral anterior synechia). In the former situation, relief of the factors causing the movement of the peripheral iris over the TM can theoretically restore normal outflow function (although some have argued that chronic iris "touch" can cause permanent TM dysfunction without apparent synechias). In contrast, in the latter situation, i.e., with peripheral anterior synechias, relief of the factors causing movement of the peripheral iris over the TM will not by itself restore normal TM function (due to the "permanent" synechias, which can themselves potentially be broken with a technique called argon laser gonioplasty, Chapters 25, 60). The terms "chronic appositional angle closure" and "chronic synechial angle closure" are sometimes used respectively to describe these two clinical situations.

Angle-closure glaucoma differs fundamentally from open-angle glaucoma. In open-angle glaucoma, the angle of the anterior chamber is always open, at all stages of the disease, and aqueous has access to the outflow channels at all times, whether the IOP is normal or elevated. Present evidence indicates that in open-angle glaucoma there is increased resistance to outflow in the juxtacanalicular meshwork (2,3). In angle-closure glaucoma, there is no abnormal resistance to outflow in the juxtacanalicular meshwork. In this type of glaucoma, the sole cause of elevated IOP is closure of the angle. Apposition of the peripheral iris to the meshwork obstructs the access of aqueous humor to the outflow channels. Therefore, when the angle is open, the IOP is normal, the facility of outflow is normal, and there is no glaucoma. When the angle is totally closed, there is severe obstruction to outflow and the intraocular pressure (IOP) may become very high.

When the angle is closed in only a part of the circumference, IOP rises approximately in proportion to the extent of closure. However, with the angle closed in only a portion of the circumference, the level of IOP may vary in different eyes depending not only on the amount of angle closed, but also on the efficiency of the remaining open angle (Chapters 3,6). Thus in an eye that has an unusually good facility of outflow (such as 0.40 uL/min/mm Hg) when the angle is entirely open, closure of half the angle may still allow a normal or near normal IOP and a facility of outflow still within the normal range (e.g., 0.20). In another eye starting with a borderline facility of outflow (such as 0.16) when the angle is open, closure of half this angle causes a considerable elevation of IOP and a facility of outflow definitely below normal (e.g., 0.08). The following case illustrates this.

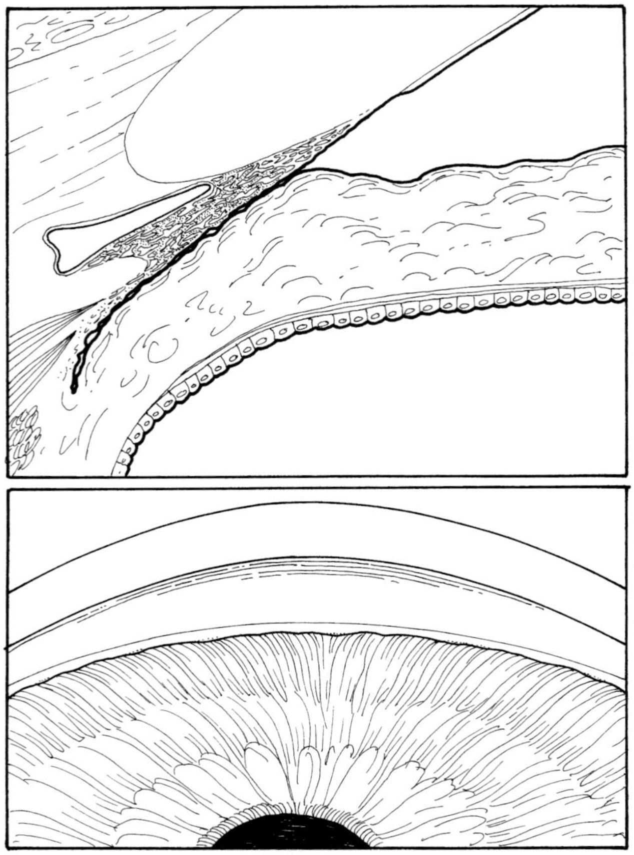

Figure 22.1. Iris apposed to posterior half of TM occludes outflow, despite anterior TM (which is non-filtering) being visible.

Case 22-1 After peripheral iridectomy exactly half the angle remained closed. The facility of outflow in the fellow eye with an open angle was 0.28. In the eye with half the angle closed facility of outflow was 0.14. It seemed probable that any residual glaucoma in the eye could be controlled medically.

Disproportion between the extent of closure and the level of IOP may in some eyes also be caused by a temporary diminution in the rate of aqueous formation. Particularly after a severe attack of acute angle-closure glaucoma, IOP may be normal or even subnormal for hours or several days, or even as long as 2 weeks, despite extensive closure of the angle. However, in such circumstances, sooner or later the IOP again rises to a level consistent with the extent of closure. In other instances, after iridectomy for angle-closure glaucoma, IOP may remain normal for weeks or even months despite synechial closure of one-quarter or more of the angle and correspondingly reduced facility of outflow. In this situation too, sooner or later IOP rises to a level proportional to the extent of closure and the residual facility of outflow.

In eyes with extensive residual peripheral anterior synechias, the variable length of time that it may take for the IOP to rise again after iridectomy is illustrated by the following two cases.

Case 22-2. A man with acute angle-closure glaucoma had a violently inflamed eye preoperatively. A chamber-deepening procedure with gonioscopy showed that the angle was closed in three-quarters of the circumference. Ordinarily this would be an indication for a filtering operation rather than iridectomy, but this eye was so inflamed that it was felt that a filtering operation would have practically no chance of working. Therefore, a peripheral iridectomy was done. The IOP stayed down for 4 or 5 weeks and then rapidly rose to a level consistent with the extent of synechial angle closure. A filtering operation was then done when the eye was less inflamed.

Case 22-3. Another patient with circumstances similar to those in the previous case had a rise of IOP to a high level within 48 hours after iridectomy.

The onset and course of angle-closure glaucoma in most cases is episodic. When the angle closes rapidly in an acute episode, the IOP rises rapidly, causing symptoms of blurred vision, pain, and sometimes an appearance of colored haloes about lights. In subacute angle-closure glaucoma, there may be a rapid rise in IOP but not to such a high level as in the acute form, since generally only a part of the angle closes. However, during an episode of closure the patient may note blurring of vision and seeing haloes about lights. In chronic angle-closure glaucoma, the closure is gradual and the patient may be asymptomatic until the glaucoma is in an advanced state. This mimics chronic open-angle glaucoma and often is misdiagnosed.

In its early stages, angle-closure glaucoma is reversible and curable. If the angle reopens throughout either spontaneously or as a result of medical treatment, the eye is again normal but predisposed to further attacks of closure. Repeated episodes of closure usually result eventually in permanent synechial closure. The tendency toward synechial closure varies greatly in different eyes. In some eyes a single severe episode of closure of the angle, especially if it is prolonged, may result in extensive synechial closure. In other eyes repeated episodes of closure over a period of a year or more may cause little or no formation of synechiae, and the angle may still be capable of opening throughout. The degree of congestion of the eye during an episode of angle-closure probably has some influence on the tendency to form peripheral anterior synechias during an episode of closure, but there must be other factors as well.

NARROW ANGLED EYES: THE "TWO POSSIBLE QUESTIONS"

In narrow angled eyes there are two common clinical situations which require a different set of questions that need to be distinguished. **If the angle is narrow but the IOP is normal, the question is whether the angle is suffi-**

ciently narrow such that there is a significant risk of spontaneous (or perhaps pharmacologically induced) angle closure. The diagnosis of occludable angles has been described (see Chapter 7) as well as the treatment with laser iridectomy (see Chapter 56). This will also be further amplified below.

The second clinical situation is when the angle is narrow but the IOP elevated. In this situation the question is different: **is there sufficient functional angle closure around the circumference to explain the IOP elevation?** That is, is the IOP elevation due to a form of chronic angle closure glaucoma, or does the patient really have primary open angle glaucoma with a narrow (potentially occludable perhaps) angle that is, however, functionally open? The need for such discrimination is not a rare clinical situation. For example, exfoliation eyes (with secondary open angle glaucoma) commonly may have narrow angles (4). Approaches to distinguish between these two different fundamental mechanisms of open angle and angle closure glaucoma will be described below and in subsequent chapters.

TERMINOLOGY

Angle closure glaucoma may be "**acute**" wherein there are symptoms of pain and blurred vision with signs of ocular injection and a fixed mid-dilated pupil, because the angle in most, if not the entire, circumference has gone suddenly from a narrow but open functional status to that of functional closure. Angle closure glaucoma may be termed "**subacute**" with milder symptoms and signs because only a portion of the twelve hour angle circumference has functionally closed. This may happen intermittently and repetitively and resolve with or without permanent peripheral anterior synechia formation. Finally angle closure may be termed "**chronic**" which usually implies an asymptomatic long term condition that mimics POAG. In fact, as indicated previously, misinterpreting and erroneously treating chronic angle closure glaucoma as POAG is perhaps the most common diagnostic error in glaucoma. In most patients with such "chronic angle closure glaucoma" there is progressive although gradual further increase in the extent of the circumference of the angle involved with the angle closure process, which usually begins in the superior angle. Because of the gradual nature of this process the IOP slowly elevates, and no acute or subacute type symptoms occur. Perhaps the term **chronic "silent" angle closure** would be more appropriate for this condition.

The terminology in the angle closure glaucomas unfortunately is not as precise as the previous paragraph indicates (or one would wish!). For example, if a patient has had repetitive episodes of acute or subacute angle closure glaucoma that perhaps were never treated, shouldn't this also be termed "chronic angle closure glaucoma"? It likely could. The main point is that one needs to organize one's thinking mechanistically, perhaps from the point of view of the TM, to understand the correct diagnosis and treatment of these various angle closure clinical situations (which will get even more complicated as we discuss unusual and secondary forms of angle closure subsequently), rather than dwell on "subacute" versus "chronic" terminology which unfortunately mixes in symptoms with concepts of what may (or may not) be happening in the angle. Such fixed terminology actually may decrease the clarity of one's understanding of what is functionally occurring in the angle.

THE CONCEPT OF PUPILLARY BLOCK

Aqueous humor is produced by the ciliary body and moves into the posterior chamber behind the iris and then moves through the pupil into the anterior chamber (Fig. 22.2). In most eyes there is some resistance to flow through the pupillary space due to the close proximity of the pupil to the crystalline lens. This phenomenon is termed relative pupillary block. Relative pupillary block is, in general, more marked in hyperopic eyes which conceptually (and oversimplified here initially for clarity) are smaller eyes with less "room" in the middle segment of the eye for structures such as the crystalline lens.

The iris functions in some ways as a valve between the posterior and anterior chambers in that the iris contour, whether convex forward towards the cornea, planar, or concave (away from the cornea) can reflect the pressure differential between the posterior and anterior chambers. For example, in most hyperopic eyes (where the hyperopia is, in fact, commonly due to the small size of the eye rather

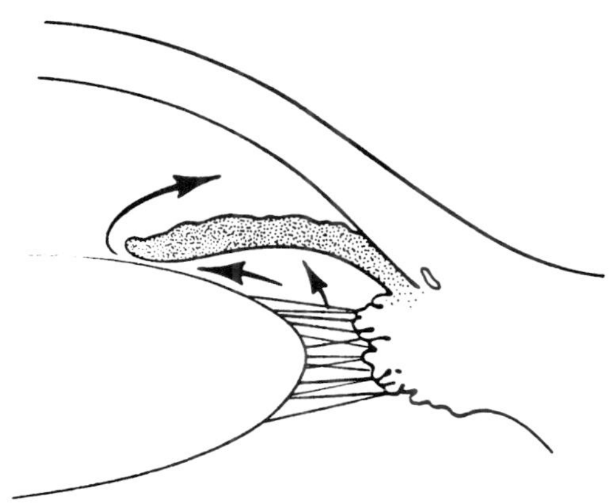

Figure 22.2. Aqueous humor is formed by the ciliary epithelium and moves across the posterior chamber between the posterior iris surface and lens, through the pupil, and into the anterior chamber. Especially in the smaller hyperopic eye, some resistance is present to flow through the pupil (relative pupillary block) that results in a slightly greater pressure in the posterior chamber than in the anterior. The result is forward iris convexity. Most emmetropic eyes demonstrate a slight iris convexity (forward) due to slight relative pupillary block. When a high degree of relative pupillary block is present, angle closure glaucoma can ensue from the resulting forward movement of the iris into the angle.

than simply abnormal corneal curvature), relative pupillary block produces by its very nature a higher pressure in the posterior chamber (since there is some resistance to forward fluid flow through the pupil). **This relatively greater pressure in the posterior chamber produces a forward convexity in iris contour.** In most clinical situations it is believed that the pressure differential that results from relative pupillary block is small in magnitude, probably less than one mm Hg. Also, as will be discussed below, forward iris convexity is a very common occurrence in aged eyes and may or may not produce a functionally narrow angle, depending on many other factors and vectors that will be described. Thus, **iris convexity by itself is not an indication for laser iridectomy.** What is the indication for laser iridectomy is the status of the angle.

In normal eyes the iris is in contact with the crystalline lens only in the immediate vicinity of the pupillary border (hence the "normal" iris convexity due to relative pupillary block), but in eyes with a shallow anterior chamber the iris may also be held forward in a convex form by the anterior surface of the lens, so that there is a greater than usual area and tightness of contact between the iris and lens.

In young eyes which are emmetropic the iris position "valve" is commonly planar indicating an absence of relative pupillary block. Interestingly, in some myopic eyes and many eyes with pigmentary dispersion syndrome (see Chapter 21) the iris contour is concave (away from the cornea), indicating possibly a relatively higher pressure in the anterior chamber than the posterior chamber. This is a fascinating, although puzzling, phenomenon since we also believe that aqueous humor flow is still forward from the posterior chamber to anterior chamber in such eyes. How then this apparent pressure differential could possibly result is a subject of much current debate. (One hypothesis that DLE favors is that in such eyes, as in certain other primates (5), in addition to the above aqueous flow directly into the posterior chamber, there is also movement of fluid into the peripheral anterior chamber through the base of the iris. This might be accentuated in myopic eyes due to anatomical features in such larger eyes, e.g., the thinness of the base of the iris, etc.). This is discussed further in Chapter 21. It is also a matter of debate whether iris concavity is fairly specific for the pigmentary dispersion syndrome or relates more to certain myopic features, themselves, of such eyes. Regardless, it must be always kept in mind that the iris contour relates very directly to the relative pressure differentials across its two surfaces. Thus, when there is posterior pole pathology, e.g. certain retinal tears where there presumably is net fluid movement posteriorly (6), the iris contour may assume a somewhat concave or retracted contour (especially when there is total pupil sequestration, i.e. true total pupillary block) (7,8).

As the eye ages, the crystalline lens increases in size and thickness producing in most eyes some iris convexity, even when there was no pre-existing hyperopia. **This iris convexity is due to relative pupillary block.** Thus some relative pupillary block is a "normal" finding in such aged eyes and does not, in and of itself (except as regards the state of the angle), require intervention. The word "relative" in relative pupillary block needs to be stressed because normally with iris convexity there continues to be fluid movement through the pupil into the anterior chamber. There is just some resistance to this flow at the level of the pupil which results in a slightly higher pressure in the posterior chamber. (The pupil in acute angle closure glaucoma may move into a position where there is presumably total or near total pupillary block, i.e., no fluid movement into the anterior chamber {although the closure of the angle and all outflow might itself result in no fluid movement into the anterior chamber]). When there are 360 degrees of posterior synechias from uveitis, total pupillary block can be said to be present from this secondary cause.

Relative pupillary block thus causes forward iris convexity which results in the movement of the peripheral iris towards the trabecular meshwork. This narrows the approach to the "angle." If the approach to the angle is sufficiently narrow (even though the angle, albeit narrow, is still functionally open, hence there is no IOP elevation), such that with slight further forward movement of the iris it could occlude the trabecular meshwork as might happen spontaneously as the pupil normally moves (that would increase relative pupillary block at one position of the pupil), or pharmacologically, then a laser iridectomy is indicated. The latter equalizes the pressures in the posterior chamber and anterior chamber by allowing free communication of fluid between the two chambers (the iris hole thus created must theoretically at least be "large enough" to allow this; 50-60 microns is probably sufficient). Obviously, correctly interpreting such a "dangerously narrow" angle is a judgment call that will be further discussed below.

When the pressure is thus equalized in the posterior and anterior chambers, the iris is no longer convex, but becomes planar. However, the key point is that **any convex iris (due to relative pupillary block) can be converted to a planar contour by creating an iridectomy opening.** It has to happen based on these "physics" principles. But the loss of iris convexity is not, in itself, an indication that the iridectomy was justified. The latter depends strictly on the assessment of the angle. Most elderly eyes have iris convexity, but only in a minority is the angle narrow enough to warrant prophylactic iridectomy.

If due to relative pupillary block and resulting iris convexity the iris comes forward enough to appose the trabecular meshwork, then as indicated, this prevents access of aqueous humor to this affected segment of the angle. Depending on the extent of nonfunctional angle thus created, the IOP will increase. The magnitude of the IOP increase (whether "subclinical," i.e., still in the "normal" range

IRIS RETRACTION SYNDROME

David L. Epstein

An appreciation of vectors affecting iris contour helps in the understanding of a peculiar condition, termed the iris retraction syndrome by Campbell (1). From a clinical point-of-view, the presence of this iris retraction syndrome (1,2) should suggest an occult rhegmatogenous retinal detachment. In this syndrome which is usually associated with pupillary seclusion, the peripheral iris demonstrates a retracted appearance. (Some have termed this the "iris suck" sign). Because of the pupillary seclusion, the patients initially might present in pupillary block associated with iris bombé, but after initiation of aqueous humor suppressant therapy, the peripheral iris surprisingly demonstrates this retracted appearance.

The explanation for this phenomenon is that aqueous humor is exiting the eye posteriorly through the retinal hole, presumably by the pumping mechanism of the retinal pigment epithelium. With reduced rates of aqueous humor formation that may be due to uveitis and, in addition, the use of aqueous humor suppressants, the amount of aqueous humor formed might become "slightly less" than the posterior pumping out rate through the retinal hole. Further, the retinal pigment epithelial pump may be stimulated by the use of carbonic anhydrase inhibitors (3). The posterior movement of fluid results in the retracted appearance of the peripheral iris. Presumably, in this unusual condition, the secluded pupil acts to keep aqueous humor in the posterior chamber from moving into the anterior chamber.

It must be remembered also that normally there is aqueous humor fluid moving posteriorly through the vitreous chamber (Chapter 29), and likely being pumped (3,4) out of the eye by the retinal pigment epithelium. In fact, interference with such pumping is one possible explanation for the sudden vitreous expansion that may occur in malignant glaucoma (Chapter 29). We obviously have much still to learn about both normal and abnormal flow of fluid from the posterior chamber to the posterior segment, but this clinical syndrome of iris retraction points out the importance of such understanding.

References

1. Campbell DG: Iris retraction associated with rhegmatogenous retinal detachment syndrome and hypotony. A new explanation. Arch Ophthalmol 1984;102:1457–63.
2. Greenfield DS, Bellows AR, Asdourian GK, et al: Iris retraction syndrome after intraocular surgery. Ophthalmology 1995;102: 98–100.
3. Kawano S, Marmor MF: Metabolic influences on the absorption of serous subretinal fluid. Invest Ophthalmol Vis Sci 1988;29(8): 1255–7.
4. Tsuboi S, Pederson JE: Volume flow across the isolated retinal pigment epithelium of cynomolgus monkey eyes. Invest Ophthalmol Vis Sci 1988;29:1652–5.

under 22 mm Hg or "abnormally" higher) depends not only on the extent of the closure but also the inherent "filterability" (outflow facility) of the unaffected part of the angle and the rate of aqueous humor formation, all of which derives from Goldmann's equation.

As indicated above, **whether there is enough functional angle closure to explain an IOP elevation is a separate question from that of whether the angle is narrow enough to develop functional angle closure in the future**. To repeat: in the presence of functional angle closure an iridectomy relieves the pressure differential factors causing the iris movement over the trabecular meshwork. The iris contour obviously becomes planar after the iridectomy, but whether there is a beneficial effect on IOP depends on whether the previous angle closure configuration was appositional or synechial. It is obvious, but sometimes confused by the early glaucoma student, that what needs to be assessed is the functional state of the angle, not just the iris contour.

FACTORS THAT MAY INCREASE RELATIVE PUPILLARY BLOCK, OR MAY OTHERWISE INFLUENCE THE OCCURRENCE OF ANGLE CLOSURE

Why do some seemingly similar narrow angles close and others do not, and why do some eyes develop chronic angle closure in only a portion of the circumference? Although there is still much that we do not know about angle closure glaucoma, there are some factors that we do know influence the process. Mapstone (9) has pointed the way towards this in the past with his discussion of the vectors (Table 22.1) that might be involved.

The Pupil

First the obvious needs to be stated concerning relative pupillary block: the size of the pupil can influence pupillary block. Classically it is taught that in mid-dilatation relative pupillary block increases, resulting in further in-

Table 22.1
Potential "Vectors" Involved in Relative Pupillary Block

1. Rate of Aqueous Humor Formation	force acting on posterior iris surface
2. Size of the Pupil	maximum dilation eliminates pupillary block mid–dilation increases pupillary block extreme miosis increases pupillary block
3. Position of the Crystalline Lens	
4. Rigidity of the Iris	
5. Potential Forward Position of the Ciliary Body	

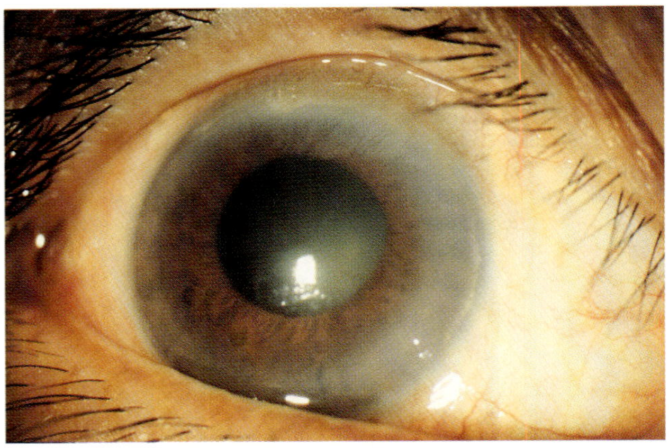

Figure 22.3. Acute angle closure. Note pupil, in classic mid-dilated position.

crease in pressure in the posterior chamber and therefore potentially sudden ballooning of the peripheral iris over the angle, and thus acute angle closure glaucoma (Fig. 22.3). Commonly in such acute angle closure eyes the pupil is observed to be fixed in this mid-dilated position, presumably from the subsequent ischemia of the iris sphincter resulting from the sudden IOP elevation. It is believed that, prior to this, the normal movement of the pupil resulted spontaneously in a mid-dilated position (e.g., classically when the patient went into a darkened movie theater), and the resulting ischemia then fixed it in this position.

In addition, dilation of the pupil to 5 or 6 mm may relax the periphery of the iris sufficiently so that the pressure in the posterior chamber can more easily push the iris forward the additional small amount needed to close the angle.

Dilation of the pupil is probably the common factor responsible in instances of angle-closure glaucoma associated with dim light or darkness, emotional disturbances, shock, physical illness, and accident. Angle-closure glaucoma may be precipitated in anatomically predisposed eyes by drugs administered as gastrointestinal or muscle relaxants, antihistaminics, or tranquilizers. Many such drugs have atropine-like, anticholinergic properties, and induce slight mydriasis. Direct sympathomimetic medications used to treat acute asthma or respiratory insufficiency have likewise been observed to precipitate acute angle-closure glaucoma (although such agents by contracting the iris dilator muscle may increase peripheral iris rigidity-see below).

Extreme dilation of the pupil is less likely to precipitate closure of the angle than is moderate dilation, because, as will be discussed later, **wide dilation may relieve pupillary block and may actually widen the angle.**

Pilocarpine therapy for acute angle closure, presumably by inducing miosis, lessens relative pupillary block by this miotic action. However, the situation is actually more complicated in that the accompanying release of zonular tension by this agent may allow the crystalline lens to move forward and increase relative pupillary block. In addition, extreme miosis, as may be achieved with stronger miotics such as 4% pilocarpine and especially cholinesterase inhibitors, may actually by the induced smaller position of the pupil, act to increase relative pupillary block. It is for such reasons that, initially at least, for acute angle closure glaucoma, the use of pilocarpine in weaker strengths, such as 1 or 2 %, is recommended. (Commonly, though due to iris sphincter ischemia, such weaker strengths do not produce miosis. As will be described in Chapter 23, the use of aqueous suppressants to lower the IOP should probably be employed first before using higher concentrations of pilocarpine, although the latter is commonly still required. Such aqueous suppressants may positively influence the vectors to be described and make it "safer" to subsequently use 4% pilocarpine.) Finally, the action of miotics to "pull" the iris out of the angle in primary acute angle closure glaucoma, may be just as important for efficacy as the accompanying change in pupil size.

The Crystalline Lens

The position of the crystalline lens influences relative pupillary block. **If the crystalline lens moves forward towards the pupil (e.g., under the influence of cholinergic drugs or secondarily from some posterior segment phenomenon) relative pupillary block is increased,** whereas if the lens moves posteriorly this lessens and can alleviate pupillary block. In fact, since cycloplegic drugs not only cause changes in lens shape but sometimes posterior movement of the crystalline lens as well, such agents have been used in certain situations to treat angle closure glaucoma. Although this might seem more obvious in certain cases of secondary angle closure glaucoma (Chapter 28) where, in addition to these factors, the resulting increase in zonular tension can act to "resist" pressure effects emanating from the posterior segment, mydriatic-cycloplegic drugs have, in fact, occasionally been used to treat primary angle closure glaucoma as well, especially when traditional therapy has failed (see Chapter 23). Obviously if the pupil can be dilated beyond the edge of the crystalline lens equator, this will, in itself, alleviate pupillary block, but the potential posterior movement of the crystalline lens is an additional potentially beneficial factor. However, for such dilation-treated eyes, even if successful in alleviating pupillary block, it is more difficult to perform a laser iridectomy, which is the definitive procedure for such eyes (and there is also the potential for placing the iridectomy in a less peripheral location with a dilated pupil). It is also possible with such therapy that the pupil will not maximally dilate beyond the lens equator, but stop at a mid-dilated position, and thereby actually increase relative pupillary block and worsen the acute angle closure glaucoma situation.

The position of the crystalline lens as one important factor in pupillary block needs to be kept in mind, and this has diagnostic as well as therapeutic implications. For example, the use of osmotics may be effective in acute angle closure glaucoma not just because of their direct IOP lowering actions, but also because they might produce some posterior movement of the crystalline lens from the dehydrating action on vitreous volume. What is not a rare clinical situation with the potential for misdiagnosis is the following: in the fellow eye under the influence of systemic osmotics, such posterior movement of the crystalline lens may result in deepening of the angle and the misinterpretation that the index eye has some form of unilateral angle closure glaucoma. Such a misdiagnosis can also result from the use of systemic aqueous suppressants such as carbonic anhydrase inhibitors, which can act to decrease the pressure vector in the posterior chamber, that will be described below.

The Rate of Aqueous Humor Formation

Aqueous humor that moves into the posterior chamber from the ciliary body epithelium (Fig. 22.2) is the "force" acting on the posterior surface of the iris to balloon the iris forward in a convex manner. **If the amount of aqueous humor formation is reduced, either by topical or systemic drugs, the "force" vectors acting on the posterior surface of the iris are reduced.** This has important therapeutic but again also diagnostic implications. For example, unless pupillary block is total, as, for example, with total seclusion of the pupil due to posterior synechias, decreasing the aqueous humor "force" in the posterior chamber not only might allow enough posterior movement of the peripheral iris to functionally open some of the angle, but it might also allow closer to an equilibrium situation between the amount of aqueous humor produced, and the amount allowed to "seep" through the pupil in the existing relative pupillary block state, this also tending to decrease the forces ballooning the peripheral iris forward. Thus, in addition to the direct IOP effect of decreasing aqueous humor flow in general, such aqueous suppressant therapy by such vector considerations might, itself, result in less iris convexity. Therefore, aqueous humor suppressants have a definite important role in the treatment of angle closure glaucoma.

But the diagnostic implications of these concepts need also to be remembered: eyes with pre-existing chronic silent angle closure, at least in part of the circumference, under the influence of topical aqueous suppressants initiated for an erroneous diagnosis of open angle glaucoma, may show deepening of the angle which results in continuation of the misdiagnosis. In patients who are initially seen on such therapy and the angle is judged to be somewhat narrow but clearly open, the clinician needs to remember the possibility of a "masquerading" chronic angle closure situation (which again may be the most common misdiagnosis in glaucoma practice). Also, as discussed above, the use of systemic aqueous suppressants for acute angle closure glaucoma may make the fellow angle, which is truly closeable, appear erroneously not closeable at the time of the initial evaluation. The clinician must remember to re-gonioscope the patient again later.

Iris Rigidity (Tension)

Another factor which influences these processes is iris rigidity, or perhaps more correctly iris tension. We don't fully understand this phenomenon, but as Mapstone (10) suggested, iris vectors do influence the process of angle closure glaucoma. The iris contains two muscles, the iris dilator and iris sphincter, whose contraction influences this tension, as seemingly does the "thickness" of the iris and other iris factors. It has been mentioned that perhaps an important action of pilocarpine in acute angle closure glaucoma is the pulling the iris out of the angle, and, also thus, increasing iris tension to resist pressure from the posterior chamber. It would seem that contraction of the iris dilator muscle, as would occur with a pure sympathomimetic drug, would act similarly to increase iris tension. In fact, when sympatholytic drugs such as the α-blocker thymoxamine or dapiprazole, have been used to produce miosis, precipitation of angle closure glaucoma has occurred rarely, presumably due to the induced "flaccidity" of the peripheral iris. Anticholinergic drugs (cycloplegics) which might exert a positive influence on these processes by actions on the crystalline lens position and zonular tension, might act at the iris level in a negative way by inducing loss of iris "tone". We previously mentioned that an additional factor leading to angle closure was the **relaxation of the peripheral iris** when the pupil might move spontaneously to a mid-dilated state. These vector considerations can certainly be complicated!

Iris rigidity considerations may also be involved in explaining the following clinical observation: full blown primary acute angle closure glaucoma is rare in African-Americans who often have thick, brown irides. In contrast, chronic or subacute forms are commonly seen (11). Al-

PSEUDOUNILATERAL ANGLE CLOSURE

David L. Epstein

As described in the text, understanding these forces or vectors has important clinical diagnostic implications. In the "old days" in the 1970s, when one of us (DLE) was an ophthalmology resident, the following scenario was common: A patient presented to the emergency room with acute angle closure glaucoma in one eye. The first year resident initiated treatment with pilocarpine (usually in too high a strength-4%, as discussed in the text), as well as systemic osmotics and systemic carbonic anhydrase inhibitors. When the supervising senior resident subsequently came to see the patient, gonioscopy of the fellow eye indicated a non-closeable angle! (due to the action of the vectors described above). Attention was then erroneously directed at causes of true unilateral angle closure glaucoma, which sometimes led to an erroneous diagnosis of acute neovascular glaucoma. Confusion increased if the affected eye with angle closure did not respond to the therapy (we know now, if not then, the possible contrary influence of stronger miotics on the factors of crystalline lens position and lack of zonular tension). Further it was not a rare occurrence in such patients, who, according to practice standards, were hospitalized for a surgical peripheral iridectomy, when the index eye was treated postoperatively with dilating drugs, for an attack of acute angle closure glaucoma to subsequently develop in the fellow eye, which had initially been judged to have a nonoccludable angle.

though not certain as an explanation, the iris texture seems thicker and/or more rigid in non-Caucasians, and it may be that the iris in African-Americans offers more resistance to forces from the posterior chamber that occur from usual relative pupillary block. On the other hand, acute angle closure glaucoma is common among Asians, such as Japanese, Chinese and those from Southeast Asia, despite thick, brown irides.

Another related observation that has been commented on in Chapter 13 is the fact that glaucoma patients on chronic miotic therapy often demonstrate increased iris rigidity at the time of intraocular (usually cataract) surgery.

The Superior Angle

In general, the superior portion of most patients' angles is the narrowest. Whether this results because the "middle segment" of the eye is just routinely smaller superiorly, or whether it results from a consideration of some of the above vector issues is not known. (Curiously, though, after iridectomy such a regional difference commonly disappears).

PUPILLARY BLOCK VERSUS OTHER FORMS OF "PRIMARY" AND SECONDARY ANGLE CLOSURE GLAUCOMA

The terms "primary" and "secondary" can be confusing when applied to angle closure glaucoma (as well as other forms of glaucoma-Chapter 18), and are not really that important. Pupillary block is the mechanism for almost, but not all cases of "primary" angle closure glaucoma (see discussion of plateau iris [Chapter 26], which can also be considered as a form of "primary" angle closure). In primary angle closure which occurs spontaneously (not presumably from secondary causes) there is usually a small "middle segment" of the eye with a relative disproportion in the size of the crystalline lens which continues to grow with advancing age. This leads to increasing relative pupillary block with resulting movement of the peripheral iris over the angle. An iridectomy (if performed at an early enough stage where there are not secondary changes in the trabecular meshwork from synechias or proposed chronic "touch") should be curative by equalizing the pressures in the posterior and anterior chambers and thus eliminating the pupillary block.

Therefore, **pupillary block should be the presumptive diagnosis in almost all forms of spontaneous angle closure glaucoma**, and, in fact, pupillary block should be treated first, and thus eliminated as a mechanism, in almost all forms of complicated angle closure glaucoma. That is, unless clearly (as will be described) not involved in the mechanism, pupillary block should always be suspected and treated first at the slightest indication in any angle closure glaucoma. For example, in Chapter 28 we will discuss secondary forms of angle closure glaucoma where pressure from the posterior segment is involved. Although such disease may involve in itself direct pressure on the peripheral iris , e.g., by the ciliary body, to close the angle (instead of fluid pressure in the posterior chamber as in "primary" angle closure glaucoma due to pupillary block), by this posterior pressure moving the crystalline lens forward to the pupil, a pupillary block condition may have been created (in an eye not otherwise predisposed to "primary" angle closure glaucoma). Many senior clinicians have learned "the hard way" to always suspect first a pupillary block mechanism to be involved even in these secondary forms of angle closure. A common example is in the secondary angle closure glaucoma which occurs directly as a result of retinal detachment surgery (see Chapter 33). It is always the debate in this condition whether the angle closure is due to direct mechanical factors of the operation, or the presence of suprachoroidal fluid, or whether pupillary block is involved, at least partially. Most of the time a pupillary block mechanism is at least partially involved, and patients do get some benefit from laser iridectomy!

PLATEAU IRIS

There is also a rare form of angle closure, which because it is spontaneous, might also be correctly described as "primary": plateau iris (12,13) (Chapter 26). In true plateau iris the mechanism for the glaucoma is the direct crowding of the peripheral iris into the angle (Fig. 22.4). The condition behaves as if the base of the iris is "hinged" too far anteriorly such that with pupillary dilatation, as the iris thickens, it obliterates access to the surface of the TM. **In plateau iris, maximal pupillary dilatation results in maximal crowding of the angle** (unlike in pupillary block where maximal dilatation of the iris relieves pupillary block if the pupil is able to clear the crystalline lens equator). Ultrasound biomicroscopic studies (Fig. 22.4) have shown in plateau iris a forward position of the ciliary processes being responsible for the forward displacement of the peripheral iris base (13).

True plateau iris (sometimes termed plateau iris syndrome) is a rare condition that can often be treated successfully with weak miotics (to prevent spontaneous pupillary dilatation), or this failing, with argon laser treatment to the iris periphery (gonioplasty) (Chapters 25 and 60) (14). However an apparent plateau iris condition (sometimes termed plateau iris configuration alone) is much more common.

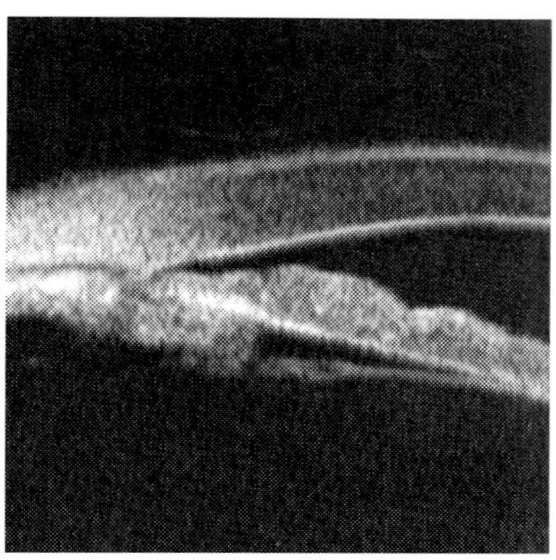

Figure 22.4. Plateau Iris. Note the flat iris plane, the narrowness of the angle, with a steep approach, and the position of the ciliary processes, which are rotated anteriorly and pushing the peripheral iris into the angle (ultrasound biomicroscopy).

Plateau iris is suspected initially based on the slit lamp examination, where unlike primary angle closure due to pupillary block, there is instead good axial depth to the anterior chamber. This is because in plateau iris there is not the relative disproportion between the size of the crystalline lens and the "middle segment" of the eye as there is in primary pupillary block. (Plateau iris is truly a "rule of 5%" condition, where meticulous ocular examination discussed in Chapter 5 is so important.) However, similar to angle closure due to pupillary block, the peripheral anterior chamber depth in plateau iris is narrow (Von Herick's Rule-see Chapter 5). **This axial/peripheral anterior chamber depth disparity is the first clue to plateau iris**, but even more definitive are the gonioscopic findings, where instead of a convex iris contour, the iris is flatter, and it is like looking "across a plateau" into a narrow angle where only anterior structures are seen (Chapter 26). There is a sense of a peripheral trough which allows there to be functional open angle just below one's view. This gonioscopic appearance, which is more easily appreciated with direct forms of gonioscopy such as the Koeppe technique, although characteristic, is subject to wide interpretation. In fact, most cases of suspected plateau iris (plateau iris configuration) angle closure glaucoma turn out to be due to pupillary block and are cured by peripheral iridectomy. In order to diagnose a true plateau iris (plateau iris syndrome) an iridectomy needs to be done first, and then the patient undergoes provocative pupillary dilatation as discussed further in Chapter 25. The important clinical point here is, once again, even with a strong suspicion of some other form of angle closure glaucoma, pupillary block should be suspected first, and eliminated by placement of an iridectomy.

HOW TO DIAGNOSE AN OCCLUDABLE ANGLE

In the era prior to laser iridectomy, where a surgical peripheral iridectomy (Chapter 67) was required, there were very rigorous protocols (that were not always successful in identifying patients at risk of subsequent angle closure), before a patient was subjected to a surgical operation, that although unequivocally successful, had a notoriously long list of possible complications. The advent of laser iridectomy has certainly changed the indications for such a procedure.

Prior to the era of the laser, provocative tests (Chapter 27) such as the "darkroom prone test" or pharmacological mydriatic tests were commonly performed to identify eyes at risk. Nowadays such provocative tests are uncommonly performed, and judgment based on the gonioscopic findings is usually the only criterion. Such an approach is justifiable if the risk/benefit considerations are such that the benefits will always far outweigh the risks, which are minimal. In truth, in equivocal situations where there is a strong suspicion of a pupillary block mechanism, the risk/benefit considerations are such that it is justifiable to perform the laser. **The glaucoma clinician needs to be able to answer this question for his/her patient: "If this were my eye, I would have this laser procedure."** This is also a good general rule for all decisions involving glaucoma care.

However, there may be certain long-term risks to laser iridectomy that are not fully appreciated at this time. We tend to think of possible short term acute complications of potentially improper laser spot placement or acute IOP elevations, but there is also a long term clinical experience from surgical peripheral iridectomy that needs to be considered. For example, there is a risk in the long term of cataract formation (15), usually nuclear sclerosis, from even a technically perfect surgical peripheral iridectomy (where the operation was truly done outside of the eye with no intraocular manipulation, Chapter 67). Thus, this potential complication likely is not a result of the surgical technique, but rather a consequence of the fact that aqueous humor is no longer flowing across the posterior chamber to the pupil and thus nourishing the anterior surface of the crystalline lens. Instead, it is now to some extent "short-circuiting" its way through the iridectomy. The occurrence after many years of follow-up of nuclear sclerosis rather than superior cortical opacity following surgical peripheral iridectomy is consistent with such a proposed mechanism. Although the laser opening in the iris is smaller, similar "short-circuiting" of the aqueous flow pathway is still possible, and in fact, there is a strong clinical suspicion that nuclear sclerotic lens changes can occur as a result of laser iridectomy after many years.

There is another long term potential complication that seems to be more common after laser iridectomy than surgical peripheral iridectomy. This is **the occurrence of "residual open angle glaucoma."** There are unequivocally more cases of "residual" open angle glaucoma in patients who have undergone laser iridectomy for "angle closure glaucoma" than there should be based on the prevalence of POAG in the same aged population. It is possible that this is partially due to incorrect diagnosis initially (the ease of doing laser iridectomy may have loosened the criteria too much). It is possible, as some have proposed, that chronic iris "touch" of the TM may cause residual open angle glaucoma (and yet the prevalence of this clinical entity is more common now than after surgical peripheral iridectomy). But more likely, the pigment and debris including inflammatory components that exit the eye through the trabecular meshwork (16) after even a technically "perfect" laser iridectomy, may take a "toll" on the ultimate function of this outflow pathway tissue in certain individuals.

Thus one wants to have certain clear guidelines as to the indications for laser iridectomy. "Above all else, do no harm" and utilize the "golden rule" in all clinical decision making.

How does one then diagnose an occludable angle? First of all, it needs to be stated again for emphasis, that one's indication for intervention depends on the appearance of the angle, not just on the presence of iris convexity. As discussed above a convex iris can always be "cured," i.e., flattened with a laser iridectomy, but the latter should be performed because of the risk based on the angle appearance.

There are no absolute rules, but one of us (DLE) will give one person's opinion based on how he would want his own eye treated. If on gonioscopy hardly any angle structure can be seen, or just the most anterior portion, or if it changes in front of one's eyes so that intermittently almost no angle structures are seen, then assuming that this is an accurate observation (and not due to improper placement of the indirect gonioscopy mirror, etc.—DLE and JSS still prefer Koeppe gonioscopy for this particular judgment), then an iridectomy is indicated without the need for further testing. If on the other extreme, despite high iris convexity, full-width trabecular meshwork to the level of scleral spur can be seen throughout most of the circumference, then this is judged to be not an occludable angle and is judged safe to dilate. (There are very, very rare exceptions to the rule that if scleral spur can be visualized, the angle is safe to dilate. DLE has seen only one or two exceptions to this and in these patients the iris convexity was extreme.)

It is when the angle is intermediate between these extremes, for example when only mid-trabecular meshwork is visualized, that judgment is less certain. In these cases there is a role for provocative tests. The "dark room-prone test" is preferred because it is deemed more physiological, and there is some clinical impression that a negative test indicates that the risk of acute angle closure is small over the subsequent six months (see Chapter 27). Pharmacological provocative dilating tests are not routinely performed, because on the one hand, they are not physiological and may pharmacologically alter the iris vectors discussed above; and on the other hand, the rapid pupillary dilatation may move the pupil rapidly past the point of greatest danger, mid-dilatation, during initial mydriasis, only to later result in angle closure (after the patient has left the office) as the pupil recovers to a smaller size. Although it is possible to keep the patient in the office all day or to use sympatholytic drugs to reintroduce miosis (which as mentioned, might however by itself lessen iris "tone" and add adversely to other vectors), it would seem that all this is cumbersome and does not relate to the fundamental question of the patient's risk of spontaneous acute angle closure under normal living conditions. However, even though the darkroom prone test is more "physiological," there is also an artificiality to the testing conditions, problems with immediate post-testing IOP measurement, and a stress to the patient.

Thus in these intermediate situations the strategy that seems best is to first consider what one would wish for one's self and consider the whole patient—if the patient is young, the problem will likely not improve with time; what is the access to care if there were to occur a spontaneous attack, etc., and, above all else, talk to the patient and fully inform them about what one's findings are, and the uncertainties in interpretation, and have the patient participate in the decision. After having done all this, if the situation is truly equivocal, to us the risk/benefit considerations are such that **with legitimate concern about the narrowness of the angle, a decision to do the laser iridectomy should be made**. But in keeping with the philosophy of the rule of 5%, accurate detailed data must be obtained first, the above points deliberated and discussed with the patient, and the patient's eye treated as if it were the physician's own.

If in the examination of the above patient, where the IOP is normal but the question is the risk of angle closure and the need for prophylactic treatment, one by compression gonioscopy identifies a definite site of peripheral anterior synechiae (PAS) formation, then this PAS, by itself (unless explained by other events such as previous inflammation or penetrating injury), is an indication for the need for laser iridectomy. There must be optimal compression whereby the area on either side of the PAS is well compressed posteriorly. Inability to compress a quadrant is not a suitable indication by itself for an iridectomy, for it may relate to technique or other factors such as the height of the IOP (Chapter 7). The presence of the PAS in a narrow angled eye "ups the ante" against a strategy of possible further observation, since it indicates that with the narrowness of the angle, there is potential for future long term possibly irreversible harm with loss of angle circumference, and hence the need for intervention. Why some patients with iris apposition to the TM readily form synechias despite the presence of a quiet eye, and others do not, is not understood. Because of the limited extent of the PAS and the presumed inherent "filterability" of the remainder of the angle, no obvious IOP elevation may be observed in this situation.

The opposite point is also worth making: in such narrow angled eyes that presumably do not have preexisting forms of latent open angle glaucoma, one would not expect more than 2 mmHg or so of IOP asymmetry between the two eyes. If this occurs, it needs to be explained, and the possibility of a few hours of functional angle closure glaucoma in one eye as a possible explanation for this small IOP asymmetry needs to be considered.

Whether the IOP is "normal," as discussed in this section, or elevated, as discussed in the next section, **the presence of definite PAS by compression gonioscopy that cannot be otherwise explained is an indication for laser iridectomy.**

HOW TO DIAGNOSE A (CHRONIC, SILENT) ANGLE CLOSURE COMPONENT WHEN THE IOP IS ELEVATED

As mentioned, chronic, silent angle closure glaucoma masquerading as "open angle glaucoma" is one of the most common misdiagnoses in clinical glaucoma practice. Further, aqueous humor suppressants by decreasing the "force" in the posterior chamber may erroneously, for a time, deepen the angle somewhat, contributing to the perpetuation of this misdiagnosis. Also, as will be discussed in Chapter 23, the use of pilocarpine due to the various "vectors" described above, can, on the one hand, convert an eye with chronic angle closure to one of seemingly open angle glaucoma, but on the other hand, convert an eye with basic open angle glaucoma into one with a superimposed angle closure component, especially with use of higher drug concentrations. All these possibilities must be kept in mind by the clinician who should perform repeat gonioscopy at various intervals, and certainly in all cases when the IOP has increased between visits.

Chronic silent angle closure thus occurs in two general clinical situations: in patients on no current antiglaucomatous therapy, and in those on such therapy. These situations require slightly different approaches.

The first consideration is the same for both situations: **what is the correlation of the angle appearance (in terms of potentially functionally closed angle) with the degree of IOP elevation?** The principles underlying this correlation have been described in Chapters 3 and 7 based on the overall concept of the segmental nature of the outflow process, and the inherent "filterability" (outflow facility) of the unaffected segments. **A key concept is that if full width of trabecular meshwork to the scleral spur can be visualized, then no matter how narrow the inlet, the angle is functionally open.** It must be stressed (although it should be obvious) that this consideration applies to the undisturbed condition of the angle. That is, one does not use one's observation on compression gonioscopy to make this correlation! Compression gonioscopy is very useful in identifying PAS which, as discussed, can constitute an indication for iridectomy. But it induces a change in the angle by moving the iris potentially away from apposition to the TM, and one has no way to correlate a true steady state IOP (at time zero) with the iris so compressed (compression actually, in all patients, by temporarily decreasing intraocular volume, increases IOP—if we could measure it simultaneously!).

For some readers this last point is obvious, but for others, there is confusion that can contribute to erroneous decision making. The overall goal is to correlate the angle appearance with the IOP, both in an unperturbed "natu-

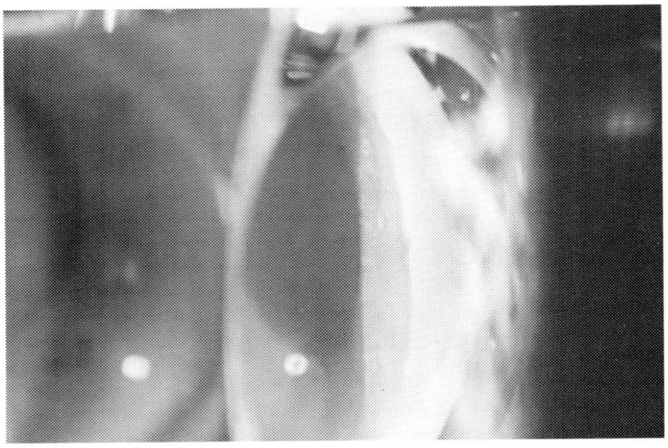

Figure 22.5. No angle structures seen on gonioscopy.

ral" state. Consider also the following: in two separate patients non-dynamic gonioscopy yields similar findings-no angle structures can be seen (e.g., Fig. 22.5) But in patient one, the IOP is 14 mm, and in patient two, it is 40 mm Hg! What explains the different IOP with two similar gonioscopic appearances? Obviously, in patient one, although the angle appears closed, it is truly functionally open (barring some other phenomenon such as hyposecretion, etc.). This means that in the undisturbed state if we could only get down there and actually view it, such as with ultrasound biomicroscopy, there must be some space for access of the aqueous humor to the TM. In patient two the angle is, in fact, functionally closed (although not to lead to confusion, it is still theoretically possible that the patient's angle access is open like patient one, but that patient two has, in addition, open angle glaucoma. This theoretical concern should be kept in mind, e.g., in eyes with exfoliation (Chapter 20), but is beside the point being made here. In both patients one and two, compression gonioscopy could indicate that with indentation the angle is "openable." This compression gonioscopy finding doesn't really help in either patient with the question: what is the correlation of the measured IOP elevation with the angle appearance? **Compression gonioscopy simply identifies the presence of PAS by its dynamic action to push the iris posteriorly, but does not help resolve whether the "undisturbed" IOP elevation can be explained by a steady state angle closure component.**

Consideration of patient one and patient two also emphasizes another point: if the angle looks open to scleral spur, it is therefore functionally open, but if TM structures cannot be seen, it could either be functionally closed or functionally open (where there must be space for access of aqueous humor to the TM).

Therefore in patients with a suspected chronic, silent angle closure component to their IOP elevation, the first question is whether there is enough of the angle circumference that appears closed (even though, as in patient one, it might truly not be functionally closed despite its appearance) to explain the IOP elevation. As indicated in Chapter 6, only a few hours of apparent (possible) functional angle closure cannot explain, by itself, a substantial elevation of IOP. For example, if the IOP is 30 mm Hg and by gonioscopy 3 hours of the angle appears possibly functionally closed (posterior TM cannot be visualized), whereas in the remainder of the circumference the inlet is narrow but scleral spur can be seen, angle closure by itself cannot explain this degree of IOP elevation (unless the functionally open portions of the angle have inherently decreased filterability—but this would indicate a coexisting open angle glaucoma process, i.e., a mixed mechanism). In such a patient the clinician performs compression gonioscopy to rule out synechias formation in the affected three hours (the presence of PAS would be an indication for iridectomy not because angle closure would explain the IOP elevation, but rather because of the risk of further angle closure in the future, discussed above; this is an important differentiation), but in the absence of this, either pharmacological testing with the equivalent of the "thymoxamine test" to be described, or clinical judgment comes into play. Reasoning that this is likely mostly, if not exclusively, open angle glaucoma accounting for the IOP of 30 mm Hg, antiglaucoma therapy for open angle glaucoma is initiated and the angle appearance continues to be monitored (as mentioned, because of the vectors involved, some antiglaucoma therapy for open angle glaucoma may actually deepen the angle—but this needs to be monitored). If over time the patient's IOP control and angle appearance remain stable and there are no PAS, one may be suspicious that the affected three hours or so that continue to appear narrow are in fact functionally open. If however, in the future, there is a slow creep upward in the IOP that can be correlated with a changing angle appearance (e.g., more than 3 hours could now be functionally closed), then the risk/benefit considerations shift in favor of an iridectomy. In fact, Paul Chandler's own combined mechanism glaucoma with exfoliation was handled in this way (surgical iridectomy was performed when later increasing IOP was accompanied by a correlating narrowed angle appearance).

Unfortunately, such a clinical situation is not rare and does not always have "crystal-clear" answers. We often must depend, instead, on clinical judgment. One might say, why not simply have performed laser iridectomy from the beginning? In addition to any long term considerations (16), in patients who have underlying open angle glaucoma with e.g., the stated IOP of 30 mm explaining this, initial iridectomy would not have produced any beneficial IOP lowering (since the basic mechanism for the elevated IOP was by an open angle mechanism). In fact, by superimposing the potential acute IOP spike seen commonly after iridectomy on an outflow system already compromised by an open angle mechanism, this might have put the patient at risk for acute adverse events. At the very least, by initiating treatment for open angle glaucoma, which would be required anyway since this is the underlying mechanism, and thus reducing the IOP it would make laser iridectomy subsequently safer from an acute IOP point-of-view. By reassessing gonioscopy on such therapy the patient might be spared a procedure which might not be necessary, and which, in the context of the "residual glaucoma" syndrome mentioned above, might actually be worsened by the procedure.

What is key is the understanding of the uncertainty of whether an angle which appears narrow or closed in a small portion of the circumference is really functionally closed. It might actually be functionally open as in patient one. If only we had better methods to accurately discriminate this, rather than relying on clinical judgment and concepts of relative risk! Regardless, there is no substitute for attempting to diagnose initially correctly the etiology of the IOP elevation (whether open angle or angle closure) and proceeding logically one step at a time. Such an approach allows one to communicate fairly and effectively with the patient, who might not respond well to the acute IOP elevation that might occur after laser iridectomy (superimposed on true underlying open angle glaucoma), when the patent had the false expectation that the laser might "cure" the glaucoma.

The principles underlying these considerations that are described in Chapter 3 and 6 need to be mastered. Suppose, in another patient, there is good correlation according to these principles of the degree of IOP elevation with the amount of the angle circumference that could be closed. **Is there any way to determine whether the seemingly closed portion of the angle to appearance is truly functionally closed?**

Several decades ago, the weak (1/4 or 1/2%) pilocarpine test was utilized with usually equivocal results to try to determine this. The rationale was that if such an agent could produce miosis that was accompanied by IOP lowering and a correlated open appearance to the angle (because of the iris movement away from the angle), then this was a positive test that indicated that the previous IOP elevation was due to a functional angle closure component. On the other hand, if the IOP was unchanged but the angle now appeared open, it was concluded that, similar to the above conundrum, although the angle previously appeared closed, it actually was functionally open all along! Thus there would be no need for iridectomy. The difficulty with this test was that pilocarpine could also lower the IOP by an open angle mechanism due to mechanical tension on the scleral spur (Chapter 13), as is commonly conceptualized to be the basis of its use in POAG. Thus the IOP lowering could result from two different mechanisms.

One of the best ideas one of us (DLE) ever saw emanating from a second year ophthalmology resident was that from Martin Wand, M.D., who reasoned that using the sympatholytic drug, thymoxamine, to produce such miosis instead of weak pilocarpine would constitute a more useful test, since thymoxamine is free from direct effects on the outflow pathway (17,18). This was documented well, and, in fact, for many years the thymoxamine test was performed in such patients at the Massachusetts Eye and Ear Infirmary Glaucoma Service, and provided much important clinical information. In addition to the positive and negative tests mentioned above (in relation to the principles of testing with weak pilocarpine), there also were equivocal cases where neither the IOP nor the angle appearance changed. In addition, there were a few cases where thymoxamine, presumably by decreasing iris tone, resulted in acute elevation of IOP due to an induced further angle closure mechanism.

In more recent times it has proven more difficult to obtain thymoxamine, but other sympatholytic drugs, such as dapiprazole, have been developed (but not tested). However, the truth is that the availability of laser iridectomy has decreased the utilization of such testing (rightfully or perhaps wrongfully).

The previous discussion in the above paragraphs should not be construed to impose a "new conservatism" away from laser iridectomy (which by alleviating pupillary block can directly answer the question at hand about a possible angle closure component). Rather it is to indicate the need to try to understand the etiology of the patient's condition ahead of time, so that the patient can be fully advised about such issues as the anticipated magnitude of the IOP spike, the chance of "residual open angle glaucoma, etc." (Most patients ask and still assume that the laser will "cure" their glaucoma, and it is very important to fully inform the patient ahead of time about the likelihood of "two causes" for their glaucoma). Also it is very important, as indicated, for the clinician to be aware when one is dealing basically with an open angle glaucoma process, and one is performing a prophylactic iridectomy for future rather than current considerations. **The rule should always be to try to accurately diagnose the patient's condition ahead of time.**

Thus, in practice one often resorts to laser iridectomy to settle this issue with full awareness of the risk/benefit considerations. And as stated previously, in an equivocal situation it is reasonable to perform the laser iridectomy.

Nevertheless, it would certainly be more satisfying if one could more accurately assess ahead of time this difficult question of a functional angle closure component. Eyes with exfoliation glaucoma on an open angle mechanism not uncommonly demonstrate narrow angles (4) that may progress with the years, and it would be ideal to not insult the diseased TM with further "debris" and pigment from laser iridectomy, unless more certain improvement in IOP control would be immediately at hand from the elimination of a true superimposed angle closure component that was functionally significant. Even ultrasound biomicroscopy, which reveals the anatomy of the angle with a resolution of 50 microns, and can determine the presence of appositional or synechial closure, or the presence of an aqueous space between the iris and trabecular meshwork, in practice seemingly cannot fully address the question of functional closure.

All patients on antiglaucoma therapy for presumed POAG (as well as patients with open angle glaucoma not under treatment) need to be periodically regonioscoped. This should always be performed in the face of an increase in IOP at the current visit. It is remarkable how rapidly the years go by and it may have been a decade since the last gonioscopy was done! In such patients the same issues, as far as the question of whether the extent of possible angle closure explains the further IOP above baseline, are involved and are handled as outlined above. In this clinical situation since the patients are commonly already on a miotic for their open angle glaucoma (and the patient was originally gonioscoped after being placed on the miotic to be sure the various vectors as a result of this therapy did not produce an unanticipated angle closure component), no "thymoxamine-type test" unfortunately could be performed (the pupil is already miotic), even if the drug were available. In this situation clinical judgment and awareness of the risk/benefit considerations will guide the clinician. Sometimes it is definitely advisable to, if possible, stop the chronic miotic therapy for a few days (depending on the status of the optic nerve), to try to assess whether the miotic itself might be involved in producing the superimposed angle closure component. (This would also apply to possibly stopping aqueous humor suppressants.) For example, if the angle is noticeably deeper and now functionally open off of the miotic therapy, one can consider substituting another antiglaucoma medication rather than performing laser iridectomy (for what is basically open angle glaucoma). On the other hand, occasionally an iridectomy might allow the continued use of miotic therapy, perhaps in even stronger concentrations, as happened to Paul Chandler himself.

Especially in patients that one sees for the first time who are on antiglaucoma therapy in whom the angle is narrow, it is worthwhile to try to assess the patient off of current antiglaucoma therapy, whether miotics or aqueous suppressants. What has to be obviously balanced is the risk to the optic nerve acutely from an untreated possible open angle glaucoma with the suspicion/likelihood that there truly is an angle closure component that needs laser iridectomy intervention. Regardless, it is essential to know the fundamental disease process that one is dealing with, for the long term benefit of the patient.

Finally, it needs to be stated here that this entire section has dealt with what was termed previously the "second" type question in narrow angled eyes: is there an angle closure component to the manifest IOP elevation? This is a separate question from the "first" which was: is this angle, which is not functionally closed now, still capable of demonstrating spontaneous angle closure in the future (and resulting in even higher IOPs)? This "first" question was discussed in the previous section in regard to patients without elevated IOP, but the main point here is this: **if the angle appearance is truly dangerously narrow, i.e., the angle is occludable, the patient should have an iridectomy even though there may be no functional angle closure involved in the current IOP elevation.** But the principle remains the same: it is very important to know exactly what type of glaucoma one is dealing with, and it is important to explain to the patient and oneself the exact reasons why some action is being initiated. (In this latest example it is to prevent further worsening of the glaucoma, not to correct the current IOP situation.)

ANGLE CLOSURE GLAUCOMA IN MYOPIA

Angle closure glaucoma is rare in myopic eyes (19) because these usually tend to be large eyes and have wide open angles. However, in rare instances in which myopia is due to an usually high index of refraction of the crystalline lens or high curvature of the cornea, the eyeball may not, in fact, be large and angle closure glaucoma due to pupillary block type mechanisms can occur; they respond, in the usual way, to iridectomy.

Eyes with previous retinopathy of prematurity, sometimes with minimal posterior pole involvement, are often myopic and can develop a progressive secondary angle closure glaucoma that may or may not respond to laser iridectomy (Chapters 68 and 71). In these cases, presumed tractional processes involving the ciliary body might cause angle closure from direct local effects on the peripheral iris (Chapter 28), or from a change in crystalline lens position causing thus "secondary" pupillary block.

NANOPHTHALMOS

Nanophthalmos (20-25) represents a special condition of high hyperopia in which there is an abnormally small (dwarfed) eyeball containing a crystalline lens of disproportionately normal size. Suspicion of this condition should be raised by hyperopia of 8 diopters or more, abnormally small corneas, and shallow anterior chambers with chronic angle-closure glaucoma. Several features make nanophthalmos special: The sclera may be more than twice as thick as normal, and there is a strong tendency to uveal effusion (20-22), which detaches the choroid and retina after operation. In suspected cases, ultrasonography is helpful in establishing the diagnosis by revealing that the globe is abnormally short and the sclera abnormally thick but that the lens is of normal size, and by detecting uveal effusion or thickening of the choroid preoperatively. Diagnosis and treatment of nanophthalmos are discussed in Chapter 30.

THE ROLE OF VASCULAR CONGESTION

In eyes with very narrow angles, engorgement of intraocular vessels such as those in the ciliary body could conceivably close the angle by pushing the iris forward. However, there is little evidence for this. In cases of shallowing of the anterior chamber or closure of the angle after central retinal vein occlusion or panretinal photocoagulation, the crystalline lens temporarily moves forward as though from an increased volume behind it, but it is unknown whether this is intravascular or extravascular. The fact that the uveal tract becomes congested after a violent attack of angle-closure glaucoma has become well established, but congestion before a spontaneous attack has not been proved.

The idea that vascular congestion is a factor in development of acute glaucoma is an old one, presumably suggested by the conspicuous shallowness of the anterior chamber and the considerable engorgement of episcleral and conjunctival blood vessels evident after a violent attack has become well established. One can demonstrate experimentally in enucleated human eyes that a rapid increase in volume of the vascular bed, by injection into the posterior ciliary arteries, can cause the lens and iris to move forward and shallow the anterior chamber, but in living patients who have threatening narrow angles, no vasodilating drug or provocative test based on vasodilation has been found effective in precipitating an attack of angle closure. Many years ago, Friedenwald succeeded in raising the pressure in dogs' eyes by injecting histamine directly into the eye, but the mechanism in those experiments appears to have been quite different from that of spontaneous acute angle-closure glaucoma in patients.

TREATMENT OF ANGLE CLOSURE GLAUCOMA WHEN ASSOCIATED WITH CATARACT

In eyes with a shallow anterior chamber and cataract, angle closure glaucoma may occur spontaneously just as in an eye without cataract, or in certain cases the angle closure may be precipitated by a change in the size of the lens associated with the development of the cataract. During the stage of intumescence or during an early stage of hypermaturity, the lens may swell sufficiently to cause closure of the angle and induce acute glaucoma. This never occurs in eyes with a normal wide angle.

Treatment in cases of hypermature cataract in which angle closure glaucoma has occurred may consist of removal of the lens after the IOP has been reduced by aqueous humor suppressants, and intravenous or oral hypertonic solutions, as needed. However, since extracapsular cataract surgery usually requires a pharmacologically dilated pupil, it may be prudent to perform laser iridectomy prior to cataract surgery.

When acute angle closure glaucoma occurs spontaneously in an eye that happens to have an immature cataract without swelling of the lens, just as it does in anatomically predisposed eyes with clear lenses, the glaucoma can be relieved by peripheral iridectomy. The mechanism for such angle closure glaucomas associated with cataract are believed to involve pupillary block. Whether the crystalline lens, itself, can force the iris into the angle, independent of any pupillary block mechanism, is discussed in Chapter 28 (but is felt to be very unlikely in usual clinical situations).

SECONDARY ANGLE CLOSURE GLAUCOMAS

We consider angle-closure glaucoma that occurs spontaneously and that can be attributed to anatomic, pharmacologic, and/or physiologic factors, such as discussed in the preceding sections, to be in one category, distinct from another category of angle closure glaucoma in which some pre-existing pathologic condition of the eye causes the angle to close secondarily.

This secondary category, in which antecedent pathologic factors are responsible for closure of the angles is encountered in the following conditions, which are discussed in separate chapters: angle-closure glaucoma 1) after scleral buckling operation for detached retina (Chapter 33); 2) from multiple cysts of the iris and ciliary body (Chapter 34); 3) secondary to occlusion of the central retinal vein (Chapter 35); 4) secondary to drug-induced acute transitory myopia (Chapter 36); 5) from contusion (with dislocation of the lens) (Chapter 43); 6) associated with spontaneous dislocation of the lens (Chapter 47); 7) due to pupillary block in aphakia (Chapter 39); 8) due to intraocular inflammation (with iris bombé) (Chapter 42); 9) associated with malignant intraocular tumors (Chapter 41); 10) after operation for congenital cataract (with pupillary block) (Chapter 71).

References

1. Van Buskirk EM, Grant WM: Lens depression and aqueous outflow in enucleated primate eyes. Am J Ophthalmol 1973;76:632–640.
2. Grant WM: Experimental aqueous perfusion in enucleated human eyes. Arch Ophthalmol 1963;69:783–801.
3. Rohen JW: Why is intraocular pressure elevated in chronic simple glaucoma? Ophthalmology 1983;90:758–765.
4. Gross FJ, Tingey D, Epstein DL: Increased prevalence of occludable angles and angle-closure glaucoma in patients with pseudoexfoliation. Am J Ophthalmol 1993;117:333–336.
5. Barsotti M, Bartels SP, Freddo TF, et al: The source of proteins in the aqueous humor of the normal monkey eye. Invest Ophthalmol Vis Sci 1992;33:581–595.
6. Pederson JE, Toris CB: Experimental retinal detachment. IX. Aqueous, vitreous, and subretinal protein concentrations. Arch Ophthalmol 1985;103:835–6.
7. Campbell DG: Iris retraction associated with rhegmatogenous retinal detachment syndrome and hypotony. A new explanation. Arch Ophthalmol 1984;102:1457–63.
8. Greenfield DS, Bellows AR, Asdourian GK, et al: Iris retraction syndrome after intraocular surgery. Ophthalmology, 1995;102:98–100.
9. Mapstone R: The syndrome of closed-angle glaucoma. Br J Ophthalmol 1976;60:120–123.

10. Mapstone R: Closed-angle glaucoma. Experimental results [Review]. Br J Ophthalmol 1974;58:41–45.
11. Salmon JF: Presenting features of primary angle-closure glaucoma in patients of mixed ethnic background. South Africa Med J 1993;83: 594–7.
12. Wand M, Grant WM, Simmons RJ, et al: Plateau iris syndrome. Trans Am Acad Ophthalmol Otolaryngol 1977;83:122–130.
13. Pavlin CJ, Ritch R, Foster FS: Ultrasound biomicroscopy in plateau iris syndrome. Am J Ophthalmol 1992;113:390–5.
14. Sassani JW, et al: Histopathology of argon laser peripheral iridoplasty. Ophthalmic Surg 1993;24:740–5.
15. Godel V, Regenbogen L: Cataractogenic factors in patients with primary angle-closure glaucoma after peripheral iridectomy. Am J Ophthalmol 1977;83:180–4.
16. Robin AL, et al: Histologic studies of angle structures after laser iridotomy in primates. Arch Ophthalmol 1982;100:1665–70.
17. Wand M, Grant WM: The thymoxamine test: A test to differentiate angle-closure glaucoma from open-angle glaucoma with narrow angles. Arch Ophthalmol 1978;96:1009–1011.
18. Wand M, Grant WM: Thymoxamine hydrochloride: Effects on the facility of outflow and intraocular pressure. Invest Ophthalmol 1976;15: 400–403.
19. Hagan JC, Lederer CM: Primary angle closure glaucoma in a myopic kinship. Arch Ophthalmol 1985;103:363–5.
20. Brockhurst RJ: Vortex vein decompression for a nanophthalmic uveal effusion. Arch Ophthalmol 1980;98:1987–90.
21. Singh OS, Simmons RJ, Brockhurst RJ, et al: Nanophthalmos: a perspective on identification and therapy. Ophthalmology 1982;89:1006–12.
22. Jin JC, Anderson DR: Laser and unsutured sclerotomy in nanophthalmos. Am J Ophthalmol 1990;109:575–80.
23. Trelstad RL, Silbermann NN, Brockhurst RJ: Nanophthalmic sclera. Ultrastructural, histochemical, and biochemical observations. Arch Ophthalmol 1982;100:1935–8.
24. Yue BY, et al: Nanophthalmic sclera. Morphologic and tissue culture studies. Ophthalmology 1986;93:534–41.
25. Stewart DH, et al: Abnormal scleral collagen in nanophthalmos. An ultrastructural study. Arch Ophthalmol 1991;109:1017–25.

Acute Angle Closure Glaucoma

23

Diagnosis and Treatment

David L. Epstein

Angle closure glaucoma that occurs spontaneously may be acute or subacute (Chapter 24). In both types, the sole cause of rise in pressure is closure of the angle, but the clinical manifestations are somewhat different in the two types. Either type may progress to a "chronic" angle closure glaucoma. This third type is a persistent, less episodic variety in which a portion of the angle is typically permanently closed by peripheral anterior synechias that are formed during attacks of acute or subacute angle closure. Chronic angle closure glaucoma often develops gradually due to synechial closure of the angle in part of the circumference, whereas open portions of the angle in the same eye are subject to episodes or attacks of reversible functional closure. On the other hand, chronic angle closure glaucoma, that may be due to potentially reversible appositional closure (as well as synechial closure) may develop silently without symptoms, and this has been referred to previously as "silent chronic angle closure glaucoma" (Chapter 22).

This chapter will discuss acute angle closure glaucoma, although many of the same considerations apply to subacute and related "chronic" angle closure glaucomas and will be presented for simplicity only in this chapter.

DIAGNOSIS

In acute angle closure glaucoma, the angle is usually extremely narrow in the whole circumference (Fig. 23.1) before closure occurs. During an attack, the entire or almost the entire angle closes, and IOP reaches high levels. Acute angle closure glaucoma represents a small fraction of all the glaucomas, but it is an important variety, because if it is not diagnosed promptly and treated properly, it can result in blindness in a matter of days. The diagnosis is usually not difficult to make, but certain points deserve emphasis.

Acute Onset

An attack of acute angle closure glaucoma has the most acute onset of any disorder involving the anterior segment. An eye may change from a normal functioning state to an acute condition of violent glaucoma in 30 to 60 minutes. No other disorder involving the anterior segment comes on with such rapidity. If an accurate history of acute onset is obtained, there can be a strong presumption, even before the patient is examined, that the diagnosis will prove to be acute angle closure glaucoma. A careful history frequently discloses that for weeks or months before the severe acute attack there were premonitory self-limited episodes of aching and blur, lasting a few hours each time and occurring with increasing frequency, until the sudden development of the latest, most severe attack.

Dilation of the Pupil

In acute angle-closure glaucoma, there is always some degree of dilation of the pupil. The diameter of the pupil ranges from 3 to 8 mm. Reaction of the pupil to light is usually minimal or absent.

Shallow Anterior Chamber

In most cases of acute angle-closure glaucoma, **the anterior chamber is very shallow axially**, but in exceptional cases the axial depth of the anterior chamber may be normal (plateau iris configuration, Chapter 26). However, the peripheral anterior chamber depth is always shallow.

Gray Atrophy of the Stroma of the Iris

After an attack of acute glaucoma, a patchy gray atrophy of the iris stroma may develop, sometimes in just one quadrant or one small sector of the iris, sometimes affecting the iris extensively (Fig. 23.2). Such atrophy is not seen during the acute phase of a first attack, becoming evident only after a few weeks. Acute glaucoma is almost the only condition that will produce this type of atrophy of the stroma of the iris. We have never seen it in any other condition except in a few cases of very high IOP after retinal detachment surgery or in cases of hyphema after contusion with high IOPs which, after all, are also forms of acute glaucoma. If there is typical gray atrophy of the stroma of the iris, one can be sure that the patient has had

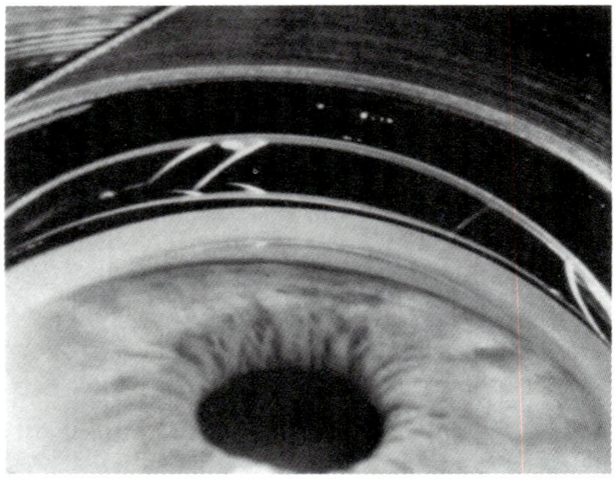

Figure 23.1. Convex iris and narrow angle in a hyperopic patient. Only midtrabecular meshwork is visible and the angle is judged to be potentially occludable. (Courtesy of David D. Donaldson, MD).

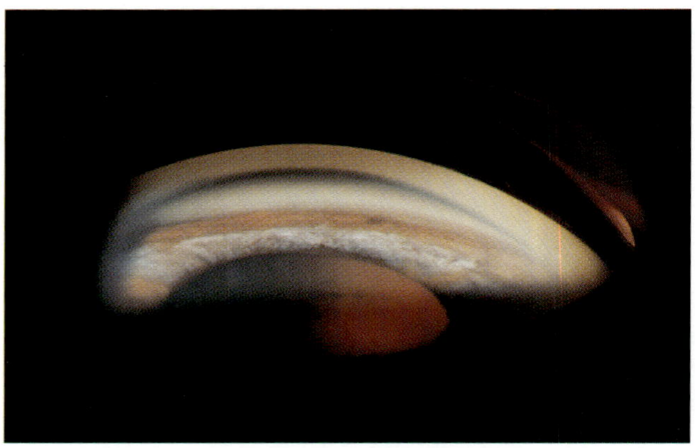

Figure 23.2. Iris stromal atrophy following acute angle closure glaucoma. Note areas of residual synechial angle closure. (Courtesy of David Campbell, MD).

an attack of acute glaucoma, especially when the characteristic atrophy is accompanied by Glaukomflecken.

Other forms of atrophy of the iris, such as may be caused by uveitis or herpes zoster, or may occur in essential atrophy of the iris, differ sufficiently in appearance from that caused by acute glaucoma that there is little chance for a diagnostic mistake.

The Glaukomflecken of Vogt

So-called Glaukomflecken (Fig. 23.3) consist of small white spots immediately in or beneath the anterior capsule of the lens in the pupillary zone, or are sometimes confluent and form sheet-like opacities. They are a positive sign of an acute attack of glaucoma. They are not seen in all cases of acute angle-closure glaucoma, but are not uncommon. Glaukomflecken may occasionally be caused by an episode of very high IOP after surgical procedure for retinal detachment or after contusion with hyphema and high IOP, but in either case they are a sign of acute glaucoma. The opacities are permanent. As time passes and new lens fibers are laid down, the opacities gradually move deeper into the anterior cortex, more rapidly in younger people. The finding of Glaukomflecken constitutes positive evidence of a previous acute episode of high IOP and in most cases means an attack of acute angle closure glaucoma. This may serve as a valuable clue, as illustrated by the following case.

Case 23-1. A 35-year-old woman had a typical attack of acute glaucoma in the left eye months previously and had a peripheral iridectomy in that eye. The referring ophthalmologist had never found an elevated IOP in the other eye. Corrected vision was right and left 6/6; IOP right 17 and left 32. There was atrophy of the stroma of the iris in both eyes and Glaukomflecken in both eyes. In the right eye most of the angle appeared to be open though excessively narrow.

The appearance of atrophy of the stroma of the iris and Glaukomflecken appeared to be positive evidence that the patient had had an attack of acute angle closure glaucoma in the right eye as well as in the left. The patient at first denied any trouble with the right eye. However, on close questioning, she admitted that for the whole day after operation on the left eye she had had severe pain in the right eye. She obviously had an attack of acute angle closure glaucoma that subsided spontaneously leaving the telltale residue of atrophy of the stroma of the iris and Glaukomflecken.

A peripheral iridectomy was advised for this eye and was subsequently done by her ophthalmologist with the result that IOP has remained normal without treatment.

Cells in the Aqueous

In acute angle closure glaucoma, cells in the aqueous are common. **Discovery of many cells in the aqueous is perfectly consistent with a diagnosis of acute angle closure glaucoma, but sometimes leads to confusion with uveitis.** If the patient is seen early, one may see only a few cells or none at all. However, if the attack has been going on for hours or days, and especially if the eye shows considerable redness from vasodilation, the aqueous may contain many cells, as well as fibrin. In neglected cases the formation of one or more posterior synechias is not uncommon. Considerable cellular debris may be seen on the back surface of the cornea, but never keratic precipitates in the form of real "mutton fat" conglomerations. The presence of typical "mutton fat" keratic precipitates is an indication of some pathologic process other than acute angle closure glaucoma.

Corneal Edema

The corneal epithelium at first develops edema of a fine ground glass sort, giving the cornea a "steamy" appearance and causing the patient to see colored haloes about lights (Fig. 23.4). Later in a severe attack, at about the stage many cells appear in the aqueous and the eye becomes

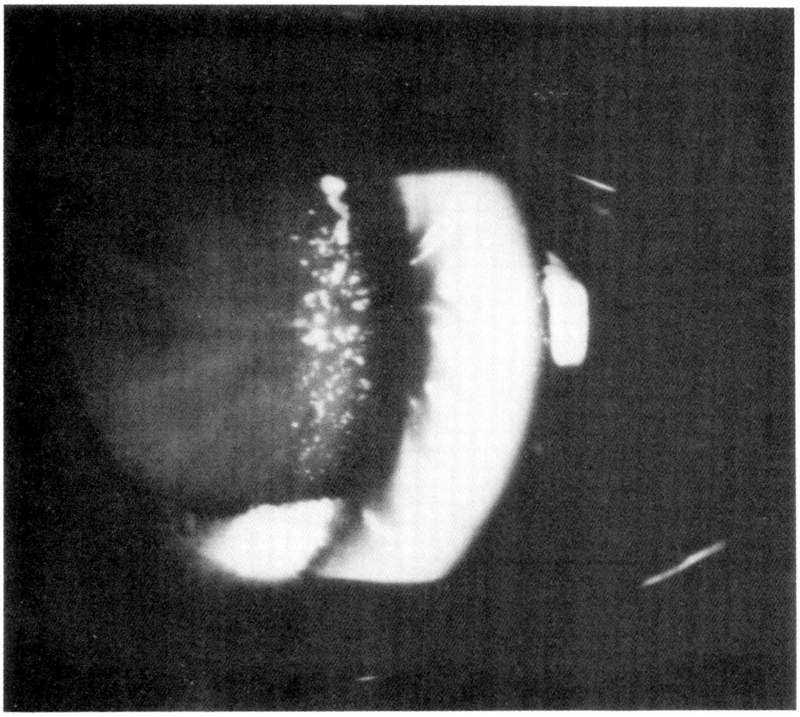

Figure 23.3. Numerous Glaukomflecken were observed subsequent to a prolonged attack of acute angle-closure glaucoma. Prominent corneal folds ultimately totally resolved.

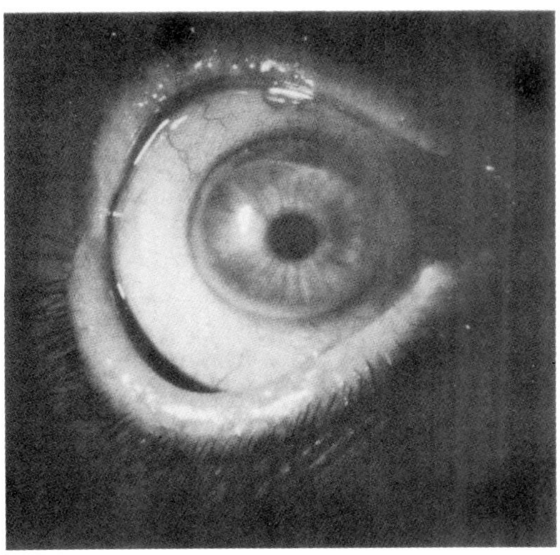

Figure 23.4. Fine corneal haze (epithelial edema) that slightly obscures iris details, caused by sudden elevation of IOP. Patient observed colored haloes around lights.

hyperemic, the whole thickness of the cornea may become swollen, with wrinkling of the posterior surface. Wrinkling of the cornea is often prominent after IOP has dropped to normal either spontaneously or as a result of treatment (Fig. 23.3). As a rule, it is not seen at the time the IOP is high.

Gonioscopy

If the cornea is sufficiently clear to permit examination of the angle, extensive closure will be found during an attack. If the cornea is too cloudy to permit accurate gonioscopy in the affected eye, **gonioscopy of the fellow eye will usually reveal a convex iris and a very narrow angle** (Fig. 23.1), which will add presumptive evidence for the diagnosis.

If in the fellow eye the anterior chamber is distinctly less shallow and the iris less convex than in the glaucomatous eye, one should look at the patient's glasses or refraction record to see if possibly the fellow eye is less hyperopic than the glaucomatous eye. If not, then one may suspect one of the secondary forms of angle closure glaucoma that are unilateral (Chapter 40). The effect of systemic aqueous suppressants and/or osmotics on the narrowness of the angle of the fellow eye needs to be evaluated (Chapter 22).

IOP

In the midst of an attack of acute angle closure glaucoma, one may find an IOP of 40 to 100 mm Hg. However, **shortly after spontaneous recovery from an attack, IOP may temporarily become subnormal or lower than the fellow eye that has not had an attack of glaucoma.**

SPONTANEOUS RECOVERY AND MISDIAGNOSIS

The following are circumstances in which the findings after spontaneous recovery from an acute attack might lead to the wrong diagnosis:

1. A patient presents a day or two after the onset of trouble in one eye. The history reveals an acute onset. Within an hour after the onset of symptoms the patient develops severe pain and blurring of vision. He takes some aspirin and goes to bed, and overnight the symptoms become less severe. The vision is much improved though still a little blurred, and there is no discomfort. Examination reveals a slightly congested eye, or it may be practically white and quiet. The pupil is somewhat dilated and reacts sluggishly. There are folds in the posterior surface of the cornea and cells in the aqueous. There may be one or more posterior synechias. Glaukomflecken may or may not be present. IOP is somewhat subnormal, lower than in the fellow eye. If the cornea is clear enough, on gonioscopy the angle can be seen to be extremely narrow or closed. The angle in the fellow eye is also found to be extremely narrow. **The findings of folds in the cornea and of cells in the aqueous and posterior synechias with a normal or subnormal IOP at first glance may point strongly toward a diagnosis of iritis.** However, the history of a typically uniocular disorder with acute onset, the dilation of the pupil, and the gonioscopic examination of the angle of the affected eye and of the fellow eye, lead to the correct diagnosis of spontaneous recovery from an attack of acute angle closure glaucoma. It is not at all uncommon in this type of case for a misdiagnosis of iritis to be made, and for atropine and corticosteroids to be prescribed. Despite this treatment, the IOP may remain normal, the eye may promptly quiet down, and the cells disappear. The patient may show up the next week or the week after with recurrence of an attack of typical acute angle closure glaucoma.

2. A patient presents with a history of an acute onset of pain and blurred vision one or more days previously, with partial recovery of vision and disappearance of pain. Examination reveals little or no congestion of the eye. There may be cells in the aqueous or folds in the cornea. IOP is normal or subnormal. Examination of the fundus reveals papilledema and many retinal hemorrhages about the posterior pole. Vision is fairly good. At first glance, one might in such a case consider a diagnosis of optic neuritis or venous occlusion, but the history of a very acute onset of trouble, with pain and blurred vision, would be inconsistent with such a diagnosis. Also the subsequent rapid return of vision to near normal would not be consistent with occlusion of the central vein or optic neuritis. **Gonioscopic examination reveals the most important clue, an extremely narrow angle that may or may not show closure.** The angle in the fellow eye is also found to be extremely narrow. Now the correct diagnosis is made. The patient has had spontaneous recovery from an attack of acute angle closure glaucoma, resulting in temporary hypotony, swelling of the disc, and hemorrhages in the posterior fundus. If the diagnosis was missed, one could expect a few weeks later a recurrence of acute angle closure glaucoma with a very high IOP and all the characteristic findings.

The following case represents an instance in which the diagnosis of acute angle closure glaucoma was not made in the beginning. Dr. Chandler wrote that, "this case illustrates the fact that 40 years ago Dr. Chandler still had a lot to learn about glaucoma."

Case 23-2 A 46-year-old woman, seen 40 years ago, gave a history of having developed "iritis" in the right eye while on a cruise and having been given atropine ointment. When she returned home her local ophthalmologist continued this treatment; finally the eye became completely quiet and she was referred for consultation. Corrected vision was 6/5 in each eye, the media were clear, discs normal, fields full. The anterior chambers were shallow. The right pupil was 4 by 5 mm and displaced slightly temporally, the left pupil was 3 mm, round and central. Atrophy of the iris was noted temporally, and on slit lamp examination there were some whitish flecks that seemed to be just beneath the anterior lens capsule. IOP was not measured. Gonioscopy was not done in those days.

There was no further trouble until 8 years later, when she developed acute glaucoma in the same eye. After miotic treatment, an iridectomy was done. Later, prophylactic iridectomy was done on the other eye at the patient's request. IOP remained normal thereafter in both eyes.

Here is a classic picture of an eye that had acute angle closure glaucoma. The so-called iritis was undoubtedly acute angle closure glaucoma and the initial treatment by mydriasis, as sometimes happens, broke the first attack.

DIFFERENTIAL DIAGNOSES

A number of disorders can produce symptoms and signs of acute angle closure glaucoma (Table 23.1). **Glaucomatocyclitic crisis, neovascular glaucoma, and glaucoma secondary to iritis or uveitis must be considered in the differential diagnosis.** In glaucomatocyclitic crisis, there may be an acute onset of blurring and haloes and occasionally some pain, but the angle is always open during an attack, and usually one or several keratic precipitates are seen. In neovascular glaucoma that is associated with occlusion of the central vein, with diabetic retinopathy, and various other conditions, pain may develop acutely with corneal edema and at first glance might be mistaken for angle-closure glaucoma. However, there is no real problem in differential diagnosis. If the slit lamp does not reveal rubeosis of the iris (Fig 23.5), the gonioscope can be depended on to show characteristic neovascularization in the angle (Fig. 23.6) if the cornea is sufficiently clear. A history of previous severe loss of vision antedating the acute attack of pain in neovascular glaucoma helps in establishing the

Table 23-1
Differential Diagnosis of Acute Angle Closure Glaucoma

Disorder	Comment
Primary open angle glaucoma with narrow angle on gonioscopy	Regardless of how narrow the angle, if posterior trabecular meshwork is visible for 360 using Goldmann or Koeppe gonioscopy in a patient with high IOP; diagnosis is usually open angle glaucoma; laser iridectomy may still be required in either case.
Neovascular glaucoma	Iris and angle neovascularization may not be apparent with high IOP or corneal edema, reexamine after IOP reduced; topical glycerin useful; angle of fellow eye usually open.
Uveitis	Anterior chamber inflammation may be present in both disorders with or without elevated IOP, KPs not seen in angle closure; angle of affected and fellow eye usually open by gonioscopy in uveitis, though focal PAS may be present; glaucomatocyclitic crisis most likely to confuse clinician.
Nanophthalmos	Patients with nanophthalmos have high hyperopia and short axial length, bilaterally.
Secondary angle closure glaucoma caused by: PRP (acute) Central retinal vein occlusion (acute) Ciliary body swelling (e.g. sulfa allergy) Malignant glaucoma Post vitreoretinal surgery Posterior segment tumors	Complete ocular history and examination will often help identify patients with secondary angle closure; fellow eye may also be narrow in patients with malignant glaucoma and those status post vitreoretinal buckling surgery; B scan to rule out posterior segment pathology is indicated in all cases where there is a poor view of the fundus and incisional surgery is being contemplated.

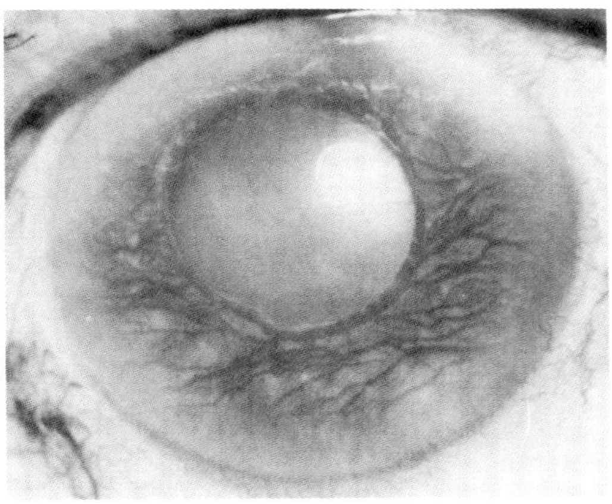

Figure 23.5. Florid neovascularization of the iris. Reprinted with permission from Donaldson DD: Atlas of external diseases of the eye. vol. iv. anterior chamber, iris, and ciliary body. St. Louis, The C.V. Mosby Co., 1973.

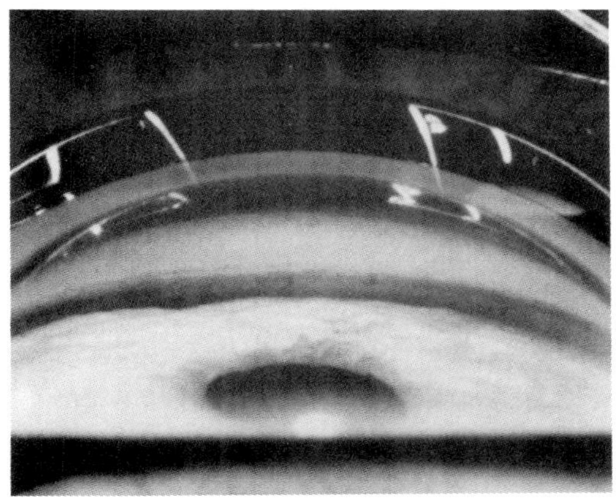

Figure 23.6. Neovascularization of the angle. Note arborization of vessels. Glaucoma can be present with the angle still open at this stage before synechial formation occurs. (Courtesy of David D. Donaldson, MD).

diagnosis in this condition. Secondary glaucoma due to iritis or uveitis should present no problem in differential diagnosis. The pupil is never dilated, generally constricted. Examination of the angle gives the answer. If it is primary angle closure glaucoma, the angle is closed.

TREATMENT

Medical therapy is used before laser iridectomy to decrease IOP and usually improve the clarity of the media for the laser procedure (Table 23.2). However, if medical therapy is not successful, laser iridectomy, or this failing, laser gonioplasty as discussed below, can be promptly performed. Sometimes pupillary block can be broken mechanically by vigorous indentation gonioscopy or placement of a muscle hook against the cornea (1).

Medical Treatment

The following sequence of medical therapy maneuvers are usually used to try to break the attack of angle closure, prior to laser iridectomy (which may not be immediately available). Nevertheless, sometimes it is more prudent to promptly perform laser iridectomy (or gonioplasty) (2–4) to break the attack, rather than to resort to substantial systemic osmotic (or even carbonic anhydrase inhibitor) therapy.

No matter how obviously hard the eye is, IOP should be accurately measured with a tonometer to provide a point of reference so that later one can tell whether IOP has changed, whether it is falling or rising. **Initial therapy consists of aqueous suppressants and weak miotics** (Table 23.3). Lower concentrations (1 to 2%) of pilocarpine

Table 23-2
Overall Treatment Strategy for Acute Angle Closure Glaucoma

Treatment	Comment
Examination of both eyes (including gonioscopy of fellow eye) prior to treatment	Aqueous suppressants and osmotics alone can dramatically deepen the anterior chamber and widen the angle of both eyes, potentially delaying definitive treatment of the occludable fellow eye.
Indentation gonioscopy with a small diameter goniolens (e.g. Zeiss lens) or by central corneal indentation with a cotton swab or muscle hook	Sometimes an attack of acute angle closure can be broken by central corneal compression which deepens the angle and can break pupillary block.
Medical treatment (see Table 23.3)	Usually it is best to reduce IOP prior to laser iridectomy; this allows corneal clearing, reduces patient discomfort, and gives time for the pupil to decrease in size making laser treatment technically easier.
Laser iridectomy	Nd:YAG is preferred for light colored irides (5–7 mJ, 1–2 bursts per pulse); for dark brown irides, a chipping technique with short pulse argon laser treatment followed by Nd:YAG is recommended (see Chapter 56).
Peripheral laser gonioplasty	To open synechially closed angle remaining after laser iridectomy or in some cases to break an attack of angle closure (see Chapter 60).
Surgical iridectomy Anterior chamber deepening Trabeculectomy	In some cases glaucoma is not controlled after laser iridectomy or it is not possible to perform laser iridectomy; in these instances multiple surgical options may be considered (see text).

Table 23-3
Medical Treatment Options for Acute Angle Closure Glaucoma

Treatment	Comment
Miotics: pilocarpine 1–2% q15 minutes times two, then q4h	Delayed miotic treatment for 2–3 hours (till after IOP has been reduced by aqueous suppressants and osmotics) is as effective as immediate treatment. 1–2% pilocarpine is as effective as higher doses and is less likely to cause additional pain and possible forward movement of the crystalline lens.
Topical aqueous suppressants: Beta blockers q12h Apraclonidine q8h Dorzolamide q8h	Prior to treatment, check medical history for asthma, pulmonary disease, history of heart failure, or bradycardia; if present use do not use beta blockers.
Systemic carbonic anhydrase inhibitors: Acetazolamide 250 mg po q6h Methazolamide 50–100 mg po q8h	Check for sulfa allergy (also for dorzolamide above). In nauseated patient one can use acetazolamide 500 mg intravenously initially.
Osmotics: Glycerine solution (1–1.5 gm/kg) Isosorbide solution (1.5 gm/kg) Mannitol solution (1–2 gm/kg) (note: dosage calculated for lean body weight)	Patients with severe heart or lung disease should have medical consult prior to using osmotics. Glycerine should not be used in diabetic patients. Glycerine and isosorbide are unpalatable. In the nauseated patient intravenous mannitol should be considered.

are chosen first, because higher concentrations can occasionally worsen pupillary block (Chapter 22), perhaps by allowing greater forward lens movement, and can cause pain.

Beta blocking agents, α-2 agonists, and topical carbonic anyhdrase inhibitors (CAIs), by decreasing aqueous humor production, decrease IOP and reduce the pressure against the iris from the posterior chamber. Systemic carbonic anhydrase inhibitors and osmotics may also be given if needed, unless there are contraindications. If the patient is not nauseated, two 250 mg acetazolamide (Diamox) tablets and glycerin 1.5 g per kg, mixed with an equal volume of cold water or fruit juice (over ice), may be given by mouth. One or two percent pilocarpine (or its equivalent in some other drug) can be given every 15 minutes for two doses then every 4 hours. If the patient is nauseated and not able to take or retain acetazolamide and glycerin, the acetazolamide can be given intravenously and at the same time mannitol 2 g per kg can be given intravenously.

In most patients treated in this way, there is a definite decrease in IOP within 2 hours. The miotic is continued every 4 hours after the first two doses, and IOP gradually decreases over the next several hours to safe or even normal or subnormal levels.

In occasional cases, despite this intensive treatment, IOP may not only fail to become lower, but may actually become higher. In this situation one should perform urgent laser iridectomy. If iridectomy cannot be performed because of the lack of clarity of the media, gonioplasty (2–4) (Chapter 60) with the argon laser to the peripheral iris can open the angle and break the attack.

The urgency of early intervention in cases in which the IOP is not falling under intensive treatment is influenced to a considerable extent by the visual acuity. Some patients at the height of an attack have vision as good as 6/12, but in other patients vision may be reduced to hand movements or counting fingers at a few feet. The fact that vision is very low is indicative of a very vulnerable eye, and it is imperative that IOP be lowered as quickly as possible. If IOP is allowed to remain very high for a further 6 or more hours, there may be irreparable damage to the eye. Therefore we feel that if there is little or no drop in IOP within 3 hours after treatment is begun, plans should be made for intervention without further delay.

In discussing intensive medical therapy for acute angle closure glaucoma, Chandler and Grant wrote:

> "Since there are occasional cases that do not respond to the customary intensive treatment, some rethinking and reevaluation of this treatment may be in order. The intensive use of miotics has been carried over, almost by habit, from times before the advent of aqueous suppressants and present hypertonic osmotic agents. Yet it is known that in some eyes the application of strong miotics can shallow the anterior chamber and precipitate or aggravate angle closure glaucoma. There is a conceptual case and some supporting evidence for starting out with less intensive miotic treatment, depending on aqueous suppressants and possibly osmotic agents to reduce the IOP sufficiently for the pupil to respond, aiming in this way to minimize contraction of the ciliary muscle that may favor unwanted forward movement of the lens. It seems to us that this less habitual but more reasoned approach to treatment of acute angle closure glaucoma merits even more extensive clinical evaluation."

For example, clinical tests in a small number of patients demonstrated that in treating acute angle closure glaucoma with intravenous acetazolamide and topical pilocarpine 2%, a single application of the miotic 3 hours after the acetazolamide was at least as good, and conceivably safer, than the more habitual immediate and frequent applications of pilocarpine (5).

Surgical (Laser) Versus Medical Management

Two decades ago there was considerable debate whether patients after acute angle closure glaucoma could be managed with chronic miotics rather than surgical peripheral iridectomy. The advent of argon laser iridectomy (see Chapter 56) has hopefully made this a moot point. The ability to cure angle closure glaucoma by an outpatient procedure truly represented a major advance in our glaucoma therapy. In our opinion, laser iridectomy should always be performed in cases of angle closure glaucoma. However, there are rare cases in which laser treatment, whether argon or YAG, is not successful and surgical iridectomy is required (Chapter 67). Before the development of laser techniques, we would have performed a surgical peripheral iridectomy for cases of angle closure glaucoma instead of using chronic medical therapy (and we still would). The reader should understand the reasoning for this. Chandler wrote:

> "In our hypothetical case in which the angle is still extremely narrow and capable of closing, one cannot predict what the subsequent course will be under miotic treatment. Since the success rate of a surgical peripheral iridectomy is very high after an attack of acute angle closure glaucoma has been brought under control with medical treatment, as in this case, we believe it is best to operate on nearly all such patients. Otherwise, without operation, the patient may suffer the second attack during a severe general illness or after injury, and then the condition may not be correctly diagnosed and treated until irreparable damage has been done. If the patient should happen to have general surgery somewhere else and be given atropine or scopolamine without appreciation of the danger, this may precipitate acute angle closure, and, in the presence of other postoperative pain and distress, the acute glaucoma may go unrecognized, even for several days. It appears that the risk of surgical peripheral iridectomy is less than the risk involved in going without operation. Far more eyes have been lost from a second or third attack of acute angle closure glaucoma than from prompt operation after medical control of the initial attack. There may, of course, be general medical contraindication to operation, such as great age or serious illness, but this is unusual."

Effect of Iris Atrophy

There is one rare circumstance in which iridectomy may be unnecessary after a violent attack of acute glaucoma. Commonly the pupil remains somewhat dilated and fixed, or dilated in one meridian after an acute attack, but this does not ordinarily prevent further attacks. **However, if the dilation is sufficiently wide overall or in one meridian to provide an easy communication from posterior to anterior chamber, and thereby relieves relative pupillary block, this can permit the angle to widen to as great an extent as after iridectomy.** Whether dilation of the pupil has been sufficient to have widened the angle can only be determined by gonioscopy. If there are permanent peripheral anterior synechias in part of the circumference but the rest of the angle has widened well, there may be residual glaucoma due to the synechias, but this patient may never again have an acute attack. In one definitive case of spontaneous cure of angle-closure glaucoma from atrophy of the iris and dilation of the pupil, the pupillary border was seen to have become retracted so far peripherally that it was actually lifted free of the lens in one quadrant and there was a space sufficient for a view of ciliary processes!

EFFECTS OF MYDRIASIS

Inclusion of weak miotic therapy has become standard in treating acute angle closure glaucoma, not only because of its potential "vector" efficacy (Chapter 22), but because it makes laser iridectomy technically easier by thinning and stretching of the iris and exposing the far peripheral iris tissue. However, a decade ago there was interest in using mydriatic rather than miotic therapy to treat acute angle closure. At the time, there were not uncommon miotic therapy failures that would sometimes respond to the opposite mydriatic therapy. The advent of potent topical aqueous suppressant therapy (combined with weak miotic therapy) has made such cases rare, but the reader should still keep the potential efficacy of such mydriatic therapy in mind in unusual circumstances dealing with refractory cases of acute angle closure glaucoma. Chandler and Grant have written:

> "Having considered spontaneous mydriasis as a possible mechanism by which angle closure may become relieved, let us consider the possibilities of mydriasis as a treatment for acute angle closure glaucoma. We have accumulated several cases in which, instead of a miotic, mydriatic treatment was used investigationally, with a prompt fall in IOP in most cases. For a case of recent onset it might be that mydriasis would be better treatment than miotic treatment. If the pupil dilates quickly and fully, this completely relieves pupillary block and the angle opens as much as it does after iridectomy. Furthermore, there may be some effect similar to that obtained in the mydriatic-cycloplegic treatment of malignant glaucoma. When mydriatic-cycloplegic treatment is used to relieve pupillary block and acute angle closure glaucoma, we are not certain how much benefit to attribute to dilation of the pupil and how much to the pulling back of the lens by tightening of the zonules. In certain instances, angle closure has been relieved by a cycloplegic, such as atropine, and in other instances by phenylephrine, which primarily affects the pupil, while in some cases better results have been obtained when both were applied.
>
> Mydriasis as a treatment for acute angle closure glaucoma is the exact opposite of the conventional treatment for this disorder and we cannot advocate it as a routine treatment. For the present it would be best to confine mydriatic treatment, if used at all, to cases known to be recent in onset. For instance, in a case of acute angle closure glaucoma in one eye, if prophylactic miotic treatment is given to the fellow eye, and this paradoxically sends the eye into an acute attack of angle closure glaucoma, then counter treatment by mydriasis may be effective and may reduce the IOP rapidly. Similarly, if a patient is in the hospital for operation for acute angle closure glaucoma in one eye, and the second eye spontaneously develops an attack, mydriatic treatment may be applicable. Mydriatic might also be justified in the treatment of acute angle closure glaucoma in the first eye, if it is known definitely that the attack is of recent origin, i.e., a matter of hours; however, in attacks of longer duration, such as several hours or a day or more, for the present it is better to employ miotic treatment.
>
> Mydriatic treatment may have a special place in angle closure glaucoma that has been provoked by miotic treatment. For instance, if in an eye with open-angle glaucoma but a very narrow angle, the use of strong miotics has provoked acute angle closure glaucoma superimposed on the open angle glaucoma, the treatment would be to use mydriatics, tropicamide or cyclopentolate, along with aqueous humor suppressants and possibly hypertonic parenteral or oral solutions to relieve the attack in preparation for iridectomy.
>
> A paradoxic and potentially hazardous aspect of mydriatic administration is that sometimes the mydriatic will precipitate an attack of angle-closure in a predisposed eye. It is likely to do this when mydriasis is incomplete. If, for instance, the pupil is semidilated, this may only slightly reduce the resistance to flow through the pupil and may relax the iris sufficiently to let the pressure in the posterior chamber push the iris forward and close the angle. The hazardous state of mydriasis probably varies with different eyes, but in general is about 4 to 7 mm. This is exemplified by the mydriatic provocative test for acute angle closure glaucoma. If the pupil dilates widely and fully the mydriasis test is usually negative, but later when the pupil is slowly becoming smaller, the patient may have acute closure.
>
> Older people in general do not get as wide dilation with mydriatics as younger people, so mydriatic treatment in acute angle-closure glaucoma would not be advisable for a patient aged 70 or 80. Also, heavily pigmented dark-brown eyes do not dilate as rapidly and fully as blue eyes and would be perhaps less good subjects for mydriatic treatment.
>
> More experience is needed to determine the most suitable cases for mydriatic treatment in angle clo-

sure glaucoma, and how best to employ it. It is intriguing and interesting, and something to think about, but for routine cases one may do well for the present to continue to treat angle closure with miotics, in the conventional way.

A possible advantage to miotic treatment is that if good miosis is achieved, there is some reason to think that this may break peripheral synechias that have recently formed, whereas mydriasis would have no such effect. Mydriasis would just allow the iris to drop back if it were not already adherent to the angle wall. Another advantage to miotic therapy is that this prepares the eye for laser iridectomy by stretching and thinning the iris. Also for the rarely performed surgical iridectomies, preoperative miotics allow easier repositing of the iris."

TIMING OF IRIDECTOMY

When should laser iridectomy be done? If the angle has opened completely under medical treatment, then there is nothing to be lost by waiting, save the risk of another attack. Too often, however, it is impossible to tell gonioscopically immediately after the attack whether or not the angle is open completely, or nearly so, and it is best to proceed at once with laser iridectomy. If some degree of closure is still present after the IOP has been brought to normal, which occurs in many cases, it may be due to adhesions that are new-formed, weak, and easily separable, but it may quickly become permanent synechial closure. Iridectomy opens all portions of the angle capable of opening and may actually release recently formed peripheral anterior synechias.

A delay of intervention "until the eye quiets down completely" or until recovery of vision can be evaluated, may allow synechial closure to become firmly established. Therefore, laser iridectomy should be performed promptly. Even when it is suspected that almost the entire angle may be closed by synechias, laser iridectomy should be performed prior to argon laser gonioplasty and consideration of filtration surgery. **With a patent iridectomy established, the patient should be regonioscoped to determine the extent of synechia formation.** Since there may be a temporary elevation of IOP from an open angle mechanism following laser iridectomy, perhaps due to liberated pigment and other debris, if the IOP is at a borderline level following laser, it is advisable to temporize for several weeks (if IOP is not too high) before deciding on the need for filtration surgery. The chances of success with a filtering operation are certainly greater if the operation is done when the eye is quiet.

CHAMBER DEEPENING

Surgical anterior chamber deepening was a technique developed to ascertain the amount of peripheral anterior synechias present following surgical peripheral iridectomy. This was developed before the use of indentation gonioscopy (6) and laser iridectomy. The technique is presented here for historical reasons, but also because of its important conceptual construct. In addition, **there are unusual situations in which argon laser gonioplasty either cannot technically be performed (shallow anterior chamber with high peripheral anterior synechias, e.g., after retinal detachment surgery) or may not be effective, when this technique might still have therapeutic use to mechanically break peripheral anterior synechias**. (Some today combine clinical mechanical chamber deepening with mechanical peripheral iris manipulation with an iris spatula through the same paracentesis site [7–9]). In addition, there may be rare occasions when a YAG or argon laser is not available, or it may be technically impossible to perform a laser iridectomy.

Basis for Choice of Operation

Before the advent of laser iridectomy, the surgeon would have to choose between surgical peripheral iridectomy or a filtration procedure. Occasionally today, one is still not able, due to corneal clouding or a "thick" inflamed iris, to achieve a patent iris opening with either the argon or YAG laser, and the surgeon is still faced with this surgical decision. What are the factors to be considered?

Chandler and Grant have written:

Since its introduction by von Graefe, peripheral iridectomy has been the most widely used operation for acute angle closure glaucoma. It is still the best operation in most cases. The principal alternative is a filtration operation. One must choose between them according to the condition of the angle. In eyes that have extensive closure after one or more acute attacks, there is no doubt that a filtration operation is necessary, but in the majority of cases, after IOP has been controlled medically and if there is no extensive synechial closure, iridectomy should be chosen.

How can one determine in an individual case whether to choose iridectomy or a filtering operation? In the first place we can say that if it is a first attack and has a known duration of 36 hours or less, iridectomy is the operation of choice, even if oral glycerol, IV mannitol, or urea is required to bring the IOP under control. Experience has shown that in a case of such short duration enough of the angle generally opens so that iridectomy will be sufficient. However, if the attack has been longer than 36 hours, even as long as several days, one should not automatically decide on a filtration operation because in certain eyes the angle may still be capable of opening sufficiently so that iridectomy will suffice.

How can one determine which operation to choose in an individual case? The level of IOP obtained with medical treatment is a poor guide and cannot be relied upon, because **even if medical measures bring the IOP to sub-**

normal levels, this does not automatically mean that the angle has opened. Carbonic anhydrase inhibitors, timolol, and hypertonic agents most obviously can cause a misleading lowering of IOP despite persistent synechias, but intensive application of miotic drops alone can also cause a remarkable drop of pressure to normal or below normal without opening the angle after an acute attack in eyes that have not previously been subjected to miotic drugs. In these special circumstances, the intensive miotic medication, added to the disturbing effects of acutely high intraocular pressure, may cause a temporary arrest of aqueous formation and lowering of pressure, with little improvement in facility of aqueous outflow. Eyes have been observed in which after an acute attack the IOP remained below 16 mm Hg for as long as 16 days due to suppression of formation of aqueous humor, even though the angle remained closed in three-quarters of the circumference, and the facility of outflow was far below normal.

The choice of whether iridectomy or a filtering operation should be performed is decided principally on the basis of preoperative gonioscopic findings, aided in some cases by gonioscopy during surgery.

If the cornea is sufficiently clear, it is usually possible to determine by preoperative gonioscopy if most of the angle has opened, to make iridectomy the obvious choice of procedure. However, in some eyes it is difficult to see definitely whether the angle has remained closed or almost closed, and it is often impossible to determine by ordinary gonioscopy whether it is simple appositional contact or synechial closure. Then, help can be obtained from gonioscopy after deepening of the anterior chamber.

Max Forbes and others have reported that using a Zeiss 4-mirror gonioscopy lens at the slit-lamp microscope (Fig. 23.7), and purposely indenting the cornea helps in demonstrating whether synechias are present (6,10). This should always be attempted preoperatively, although often corneal edema limits visualization. With indentation, areas that are not involved by synechias can be well demonstrated. However, areas that are seen as still being closed can represent either true synechias or areas of insufficient indentation. While the "indented" configuration of the iris in the suspected area can often help in interpreting the adequacy of the examination, it must be remembered that especially **when performed at a time when the IOP is elevated, insufficient distortion may be generated by this technique to reverse appositional closure.**

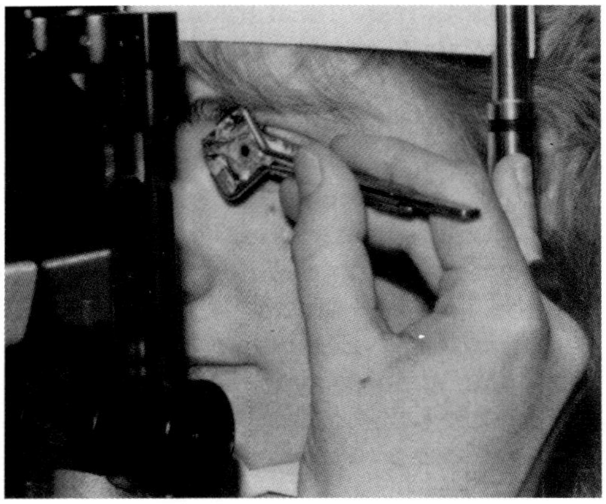

Figure 23.7. A Zeiss lens is in use at the slit lamp. This lens is useful for rapidly viewing the angle without the need for gonioscopic fluid in patients previously gonioscoped with other methods with whom differentiating angle closure from open angle glaucoma is not an issue. Indentation with this lens allows identification of peripheral anterior synechias (see text).

Definitive results can be obtained by Koeppe gonioscopy after the anterior chamber is deepened surgically. One form of gonioscopy during surgery was introduced by Shaffer in 1957 (11). Shaffer's technique consisted of performing a peripheral iridectomy, refilling the anterior chamber with saline solution, pulling up the suture, and tying one knot. He then placed a sterile Koeppe lens on the eye and examined the angle to see how much closure remained to decide whether to convert the iridectomy to a filtration procedure.

We prefer the following technique (12). After the eye is prepared and anesthetized for surgical procedure in the usual way, a slanting incision is made through the lower cornea with a Wheeler knife. The incision is enlarged upward the full width of the knife (Fig. 23.8). Then, by repeatedly depressing the posterior lip of the wound with the knife or a narrow spatula, all the aqueous possible is evacuated. It is important to persist in this maneuver long enough for aqueous to drain forward through the pupil from the posterior chamber and to drain out of the anterior chamber. This may take a full minute. Saline solution is then injected into the anterior chamber through the corneal incision until the anterior chamber has reached slightly greater than normal depth, similar to the depth observed normally in myopic eyes. (This degree of deepening of the anterior chamber would not be possible if an iridectomy had already been done, because in that case the saline solution could not be placed exclusively in the anterior chamber.)

In injecting saline solution to make the anterior chamber slightly deeper than normal, one must be careful not to make the eye too hard. If so much saline solution is injected that the eye is quite hard, it may cause epithelial edema. If this occurs, some fluid is let out of the anterior chamber so that the cornea clears.

Next, a sterile Koeppe lens is placed on the eye, and an extra drape with a 2-inch hole in the center is placed over the other drapes. The surgeon then breaks his asepsis and examines the angle with the regular hand-held microscope and the Barkan gonioscopy light, or he may use a sterile microscope and light if he prefers.

It is helpful if the assistant has a sterile muscle hook available. The tip of the muscle hook is put in the dimple of the contact glass, which can be moved in various directions to facilitate examination of the chamber angle (Fig. 23.9).

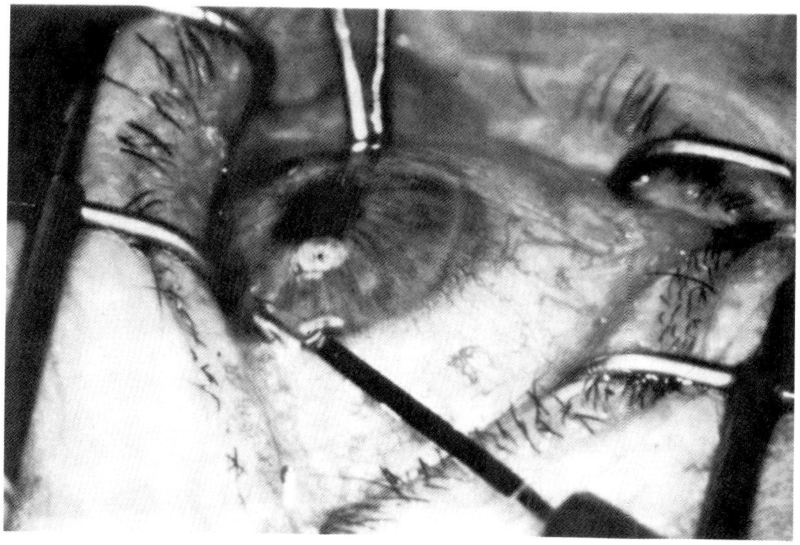

Figure 23.8. Paracentesis incision enlarged with a Wheeler knife for the chamber-deepening procedure.

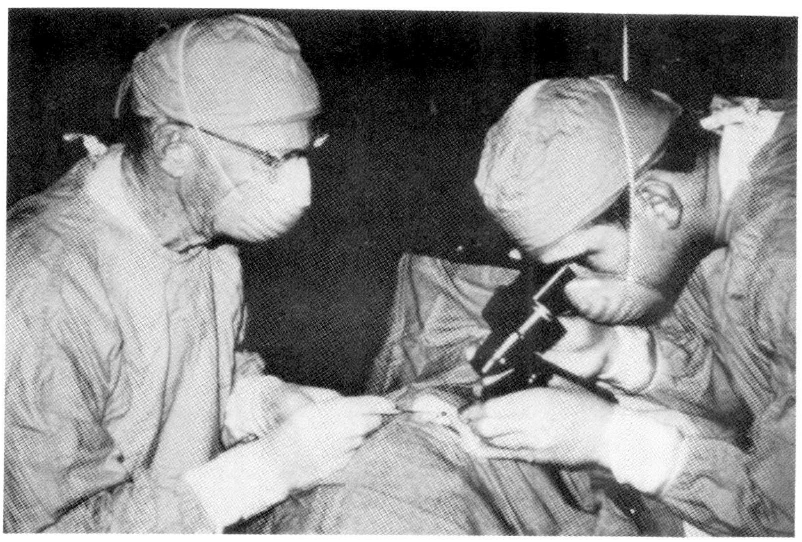

Figure 23.9. Viewing the angle after surgical deepening of the anterior chamber.

With the anterior chamber deepened at the expense of the evacuated posterior chamber in the manner described, the open portions of the angle are now seen to be wide, with scleral spur and ciliary band well exposed to view. One can readily determine just how much of the angle is closed. Any closure that is found under these conditions is synechial closure.

Peripheral anterior synechias, when present, usually extend up to or almost up to Schwalbe's line and can be seen to cover the meshwork completely. In some areas. however, the tip of the synechia may be considerably posterior to Schwalbe's line, but still covering the scleral spur. One then has to estimate to what extent the filtration area of the meshwork is covered by the synechia. One then compares such an area with an area where the angle is wide with ciliary band visible and also with an area where the synechia extends up to or almost up to Schwalbe's line. If in adjacent clearly open portions of the angle there is a line of pigment delineating the filtration area, this can be a great help. One then looks to see how much of this pigment line is hidden by synechia. One can thus make a rough but fairly accurate estimate of how much of the filtration area is covered by synechias.

After the gonioscopy is completed, the unsterile outer drape is removed, the surgeon and assistant put on sterile gloves and gown, and proceed with whatever operation has been decided upon.

The operation to be carried out is chosen according to the extent of synechial closure found. If the angle is closed in one-quarter or less of the circumference, iridectomy is always chosen. If the synechial closure involves one-third to one-half of the circumference of the angle, then information from a previous tonography may be the deciding factor. In borderline cases or when in doubt, it is generally best to try iridectomy. This should not be done at the 12 o'clock position, but at the 10:30 or 1:30 position, so that subsequently if the residual glaucoma cannot be controlled medically, an adequate portion of the superior limbus is left undisturbed to provide a place where a filtering operation can be done later.

As the basis for choice of operation, gonioscopy after surgical deepening of the anterior chamber is a simple, safe procedure, and its practical value cannot be overemphasized. **We suspect that deepening the anterior chamber in this way may actually separate recently formed, weak adhesions of iris to trabecular meshwork**, since in the opened angle one sometimes sees little tabs of tissue on the trabecular meshwork that look as though they came from the peripheral iris.

The following case illustrates this potential therapeutic benefit. In this case preoperative gonioscopy showed exactly the upper half of the angle closed, but after chamber deepening almost the entire angle was found to be open, suggesting that the procedure had broken the weak peripheral anterior synechias.

Case 23-3. A 76-year-old woman had a little nuclear sclerosis in both eyes, more in the left. Corrected vision right 6/6. Left 6/12. One month previously she had had an attack of pain and blurred vision in the left eye with nausea and vomiting. The symptoms subsided. Eighteen hours previous to her visit here the symptoms recurred—pain, nausea, vomiting, and blurring of vision. The symptoms persisted. Vision in the left eye was counting fingers at 6 feet; the cornea was edematous, pupil in mid-dilation; fundus could not be seen; IOP 76. The angle appeared to be entirely closed. Six hours after the start of intensive treatment with 4% pilocarpine, acetazolamide, and glycerin, the IOP decreased to 17. The gonioscopy revealed that exactly the lower half of the angle appeared open. Peripheral iridectomy would be the operation of choice with half the angle open. Nevertheless, a chamber deepening procedure was carried out to see if some recently formed peripheral anterior synechias could be torn off. When that was done, it was found that only about 1 hour of the angle remained closed. It appeared that the chamber deepening procedure had in fact broken nearly all the peripheral synechias in the upper half of the angle and therefore served as a therapeutic procedure. Peripheral iridectomy was done, and 2 months later IOP was 15 without treatment.

Older and stronger peripheral anterior synechias do not appear to be torn off by deepening the anterior chamber. This procedure demonstrates how much of the angle can open and can be expected to be functional. Clinical and experimental findings indicate that angles opened by this gentle procedure can be expected to be good functionally. In extreme instances, almost the entire angle may appear closed according to ordinary gonioscopy, but reexamination after deepening of an anterior chamber may establish that most or all of the angle is capable of opening.

Chandler and Simmons have reported 41 cases (53 eyes) of surgical chamber deepening and gonioscopy (12), and since that report, the procedure has been used in many more cases, with no significant complications.

The choice of operation, peripheral iridectomy or filtering operation, is greatly aided and usually easily decided by definitive gonioscopy but there are other factors also to be weighed in making the decision. These factors include the facility of outflow, the condition of the optic disc and field, and the age of the patient. Angle closure glaucoma commonly affects one eye before the other, so that the condition of the other eye with its angle still open can often provide a guide as to what to expect from synechial closure of half of the circumference. If the contralateral eye with its angle open and unmedicated has a low IOP and good facility of outflow, one can expect that synechial closure of half the circumference will not raise the IOP excessively, and peripheral iridectomy should suffice. If instead, the contralateral eye with its angle open has an IOP at the upper limit of normal, the treatment of synechial closure of half the circumference by iridectomy may not suffice, and postoperatively the additional use of antiglaucoma medications may be required, especially if there has been damage to the optic disc. The more evidence of damage to disc and field under these circumstances, the more one would favor a filtering operation, since lower IOP would be required postoperatively. Presence of lens opacities would weigh in favor of iridectomy, since an increase in opacity is more common after filtering operation. Limited life expectancy from age or disease would favor iridectomy in a borderline case.

When the circumferential extent of synechial angle closure is distinctly less than or more than half, the other factors become less important, and the choice between iridectomy and filtering operation becomes relatively easy.

PROGNOSIS FOR RECOVERY OF VISION

In acute angle-closure glaucoma the degree of recovery of vision after control of IOP varies considerably from case to case. It is, therefore, difficult to make an accurate prognosis as to recovery of vision in the individual case. In general, the better the visual acuity at the height of the attack, the better will be the vision ultimately obtained. One must take into consideration the condition of the cornea in making a prognosis. **If the cornea is clear, yet vision is low, most of the visual loss is due to damage to the optic nerve, and the prognosis for recovery of vision is more guarded.** If the cornea is cloudy with stromal and epithelial edema, the condition of the cornea itself is sufficient to cause marked reduction of vision and there may be little damage to the optic nerve. In such cases when the cornea eventually clears, there may be a remarkable recovery of vision. Many weeks must elapse after subsidence of an acute attack before one can be sure that no further recovery of vision is likely to occur.

ANTERIOR CHAMBER DEEPENING WITH MECHANICAL BREAKING OF PERIPHERAL ANTERIOR SYNECHIAS (PAS) WITH AN IRIS SPATULA

David L. Epstein

Sometimes postsurgical PAS associated with a flat anterior chamber may extend far forward anterior to Schwalbe's line and be quite firm and not amenable to argon laser gonioplasty (Chapter 60) due to the continued shallowness of the anterior chamber or other technical problems such as the lack of good corneal clarity. This clinical situation then is the one exception to the "rule" that if the PAS does not separate easily with the argon laser gonioplasty technique, further treatment of that particular PAS is not warranted. In these situations some have reported good success with surgical deepening of the anterior chamber with a viscoelastic, which itself might help break the PAS, but then subsequent entry of a fine iris spatula or equivalent into the anterior chamber to mechanically directly break the synechiae by a posterior ballotment type motion on the peripheral iris (1–3). Ideally, this should be done under gonioscopic control, as in the chamber deepening procedure, but some have described performing this without gonioscopy, especially in pseudophakic or aphakic eyes. There would be some risk of possible crystalline lens injury if gonioscopic control is not utilized.

Such a method deserves further evaluation, especially in cases in which it is not possible to perform argon laser gonioplasty. Unfortunately, in some reports this technique was combined with other antiglaucoma methods, sometimes involving ciliodestruction, so it is not always certain whether the synechialysis or the added therapy is responsible for the beneficial effects that have been reported. Also, many such anterior PAS may in fact be bridging over the trabecular meshwork, which is therefore functionally still open, but not visualized in the tunnel under the anteriorly placed synechia. The postoperative glaucoma in these complicated eyes might, despite the angle appearance, be attributable to acute open angle mechanisms involving viscoelastic, inflammation, or the use of steroids. If the latter open angle mechanisms are involved and if the IOP is not too high, "tincture of time" might also prove effective.

References

1. Forbes M: Gonioscopy with corneal indentation. Arch Ophthalmol 1966;76:488–492.
2. Shaffer RN: Operating room gonioscopy in angle-closure glaucoma surgery. Trans Am Ophthalmol Soc 1957;55:59–66.
3. Chandler PA, Simmons RJ: Anterior chamber deepening for gonioscopy at time of surgery. Arch Ophthalmol 1965;74:177–190.

MANAGEMENT OF THE FELLOW EYE

The fellow eye in cases of acute angle closure glaucoma nearly always has a narrow angle, capable of closure. In a previous era some such fellow eyes have been observed for many years with or without prophylactic miotic treatment and have remained normal. However, the incidence of involvement of the fellow eye with angle closure is extremely high. Sometimes an acute attack develops in the fellow eye while the patient is being treated for the first eye. Because it is usually not possible to predict if and when the fellow eye may suffer an attack of angle closure glaucoma, we recommend that a prophylactic laser iridectomy be performed, if the angle is at all narrow. In unusual situations such as high degrees of anisometropia we would not proceed if we felt that the fellow angle was wide open (see below). However, the burden is on the ophthalmologist to be certain that the angle of the fellow eye is not occludable. Possible factors, e.g., the use of aqueous humor suppressants, affecting vectors in the fellow eye that may falsely lead one to conclude that the angle is not closeable have been discussed in Chapter 22.

In the interval before iridectomy on the fellow eye, we prefer to leave the fellow eye without treatment. Our present custom is not to use anything in the fellow eye, because laser iridectomy will be performed within a few days and the incidence of angle closure in the interim has seemed less without miotics.

In fact, in the interval until the laser iridectomy is performed on the fellow eye, prophylactic treatment with miotics is not without hazard. **In some cases treatment with miotics, especially the stronger ones, has precipitated closure of the angle.** If miotics are to be used prophylactically for a short period before prophylactic laser surgery, it is wisest to employ no stronger miotic than ½ to 1% pilocarpine 2 or 3 times a day.

In deciding whether or not the fellow eye should have a prophylactic procedure some would employ the darkroom test or the mydriasis test. If either or both of these tests are negative, this in no way rules out the possibility of a subsequent attack of acute angle closure glaucoma, as many ophthalmologists can testify. A negative mydriasis test may be particularly misleading (Chapter 27).

Because it is impossible to predict in a given case if and when acute angle closure glaucoma may develop in the second eye and the darkroom and mydriasis provocative tests, if negative, have proved to be unreliable guides as to the possibility of later involvement in the fellow eye, use prophylactic peripheral iridectomy for all fellow eyes, unless there is some compelling reason related to the patient's physical state, or, in rare cases, because there is a great anatomical difference between the patient's two eyes.

Thus, the risk/benefit ratio of laser iridectomy is such

that we recommend it be performed for all fellow eyes of those with angle closure glaucoma, unless a rare, true unilateral angle closure condition exists. However, even before the advent of the laser procedure, we recommended that surgical peripheral iridectomy be similarly performed.

Chandler and Grant have written:

> "The risk of a properly performed surgical prophylactic peripheral iridectomy seems much less than the risk of future attacks without operation. Many instances have been observed in which prophylactic operation was not done, and the patient later had an acute attack of angle-closure glaucoma, but diagnosis and treatment were delayed, or improper treatment was carried out, and the eye was eventually lost. Prophylactic peripheral iridectomy in the fellow eye has been an important measure for the prevention of blindness in patients having proved angle closure glaucoma in one eye."

The following case illustrates the unpredictable length of time that a patient can go before developing an attack of angle closure in the fellow eye if prophylactic iridectomy is not done. The interval was 13 years and the patient would have been better off if she had had the prophylactic procedure soon after the first eye was cared for.

Case 23-4. A woman, age 67, gave a history of acute glaucoma in the left eye 4 or 5 years previously. An operation had been done, but the eye became blind. She was under treatment with 2% pilocarpine for her right eye. Corrected vision of the right eye was 6/5; the field was full: there was a little saucerization of the disc, but no pathologic excavation, IOP 15. On gonioscopy, the angle was excessively narrow, especially above and below, but the impression was that it was probably open throughout.

In view of the history of acute angle closure glaucoma in the left eye, and the excessively narrow angle in the right, peripheral iridectomy was advised for the right eye, but this was not done. The patient was next seen 13 years later with an attack of acute angle-closure in the right eye, IOP 88. She was admitted to the hospital and given intensive treatment with miotics, acetazolamide, and glycerin. IOP fell to 30. A peripheral iridectomy was done. Since that time IOP has ranged from 17 to 30, but has been mostly under 20 under treatment with 2% pilocarpine 4 times a day, epinephrine twice a day, and acetazolamide 125 mg twice a day.

If she had had prophylactic iridectomy at the time it was advised, this patient would have been spared an attack of glaucoma in her right eye and presumably would have required no medical treatment thereafter.

With limited and special exceptions, we therefore favor routinely performing laser iridectomy on all fellow eyes in patients who have had acute angle closure glaucoma in one eye.

The rare exceptions to this rule are as follows:

1. In a few patients the fellow eye may have a wide open angle. In that case we do not do the prophylactic peripheral iridectomy. However, we must be cautious about dismissing the angle as being of safe width, because we have been fooled at times, having thought that the angle of the fellow eye would not close, but it subsequently did close. **Angle width varies from time to time, and one should not conclude that the angle of a fellow eye is of safe width on the basis of a single gonioscopy.** In particular, one may get a false impression if one sees a patient who is taking a systemic carbonic anhydrase inhibitor, since this suppresses inflow of aqueous and may cause the angle to appear wider than it is when off such treatment (Chapter 22).
2. The most reliable finding of a safe wide angle in the fellow eye is made in those unusual patients who have one hypermetropic eye with a narrow angle, subject to angle closure, and the other eye myopic with the typical wide angle associated with myopia. We have occasionally seen patients in whom the glaucomatous eye had a significantly smaller cornea and shallower anterior chamber than the fellow eye, and have felt secure in judging the angle of the fellow eye to be normal and safe without iridectomy.
3. If there is little refractive error in either eye, and the fellow eye definitely has an angle of normal average width, one should consider the possibility that the shallowing of the anterior chamber and the angle closure glaucoma in the one eye may have been caused by a partial dislocation of the lens in that eye. If this is proved to be so, the entirely normal fellow eye does not need an iridectomy.

References

1. Anderson DR: Corneal indentation to relieve acute angle-closure glaucoma. Am J Ophthalmol 1979;88:1091–3.
2. Ritch R: Argon laser treatment for medically unresponsive attacks of angle-closure glaucoma. Am J Ophthalmol 1982;94:197–204.
3. Wand M: Argon laser gonioplasty for synechial angle closure. Arch Ophthalmol 1992;110:363–7.
4. Weiss HS, et al: Argon laser gonioplasty in the treatment of angle-closure glaucoma. Am J Ophthalmol 1992;114:14–18.
5. Ganias F, Mapstone R: Miotics in closed-angle glaucoma. Br J Ophthalmol 1975;59:205–206.
6. Forbes M: Indentation gonioscopy and efficacy of iridectomy in angle-closure glaucoma. Trans Am Ophthalmol Soc 1974;74:488–515.
7. Campbell DG, Vela A: Modern goniosynechialysis for the treatment of synechial angle-closure glaucoma. Ophthalmology 1984;91:1052–60.
8. Shingleton BJ, Chang MA, Bellows AR, et al: Surgical goniosynechialysis for angle-closure glaucoma. Ophthalmology 1990;97:551–6.
9. Tanihara H, Nishiwaki K, Nagata M: Surgical results and complications of goniosynechialysis. Graefes Arch Clin Exp Ophthalmol 1992;230:309–13.

Subacute (and Chronic) Angle Closure Glaucoma: Diagnosis and Treatment

24

David L. Epstein

The principles underlying the pathogenesis, diagnosis, and treatment of subacute and chronic angle closure glaucoma have been explained in the preceding two chapters. Certain important features will be highlighted in this chapter.

The incidence of subacute and chronic angle closure glaucoma is probably considerably greater than the incidence of the acute type. However, just as in acute angle closure glaucoma, the sole cause of the rise in intraocular pressure (IOP) is closure of the angle. When the angle is entirely open, the outflow is normal and there is no glaucoma. The subacute differs from the acute type in that the course may be one of small intermittent attacks usually over a long time, but symptoms are usually mild or may be absent entirely until the disease is far advanced.

As discussed in Chapter 22, the term "subacute" seems clear in that it implies "mini-attacks" of angle closure, with or without symptoms, where the whole circumference of the angle is not simultaneously involved. **The term "chronic" however is used to describe many different clinical situations: to connote the residue and continuance of these subacute episodes when peripheral anterior synechias have commonly formed; to connote residual synechial angle closure after laser iridectomy; or perhaps most commonly, to connote a totally silent progressive condition of angle closure, either appositional or synechial, that may mimic primary open angle glaucoma (POAG).** The latter entity is critically important for the clinician to diagnose and understand, and is discussed in detail in Chapter 22. The term "chronic" is thus quite imprecise. It is better to use specific descriptive terms such as silent (appositional or synechial) angle closure, residual angle closure after iridectomy, or recurrent episodes of subacute angle closure leading to formation of synechias, etc.

DIAGNOSIS

As a rule there is more variation in the width in different portions of the angle in the subacute than in the acute form. In the subacute type, some portions of the angle are excessively narrow, but other portions may be considerably wider, so that the angle does not close in the whole circumference as it usually does in the acute form. In both acute and subacute angle-closure glaucoma the anterior chamber characteristically is shallow and the iris convex, but angle closure with a relatively flat iris plane and less axial shallowing (plateau iris—Chapter 26) produces more frequently subacute than acute angle closure.

In the differential diagnosis of subacute angle closure with irregular narrowing of the angle, one should think particularly of cysts of the iris or ciliary body, which may also cause irregular closure of the angle (Fig. 24.1). This condition is discussed in Chapter 34. **Irregular synechial closure should also make one consider uveitis and, if unilateral, essential iris atrophy (Chapter 32).**

In rare cases, both open-angle and subacute or "chronic" angle closure glaucoma occur in the same eye. This is discussed in Chapter 22.

Grounds for making the diagnosis of subacute or its residue, "chronic" angle closure in typical uncomplicated cases will now be discussed. Chronic silent angle closure glaucoma has been already discussed in Chapter 22.

Intraocular Pressure (IOP) Elevations

In subacute angle closure glaucoma the rise in IOP is proportional to the extent of closure at a given time. In some cases, during an episode of partial closure there may be a considerable acute rise in IOP giving symptoms of blurred vision, discomfort, or seeing colored haloes. In other cases in which the closure is less extensive or develops more gradually (chronic silent angle closure), the patient remains asymptomatic. If episodes giving symptoms do occur they tend to recur much more frequently than do the attacks in the acute form. In subacute intermittent angle closure glaucoma, episodes of elevated IOP causing symptoms may occur every week or two, or even daily, whereas in severe acute angle closure glaucoma, episodes giving rise to symptoms usually occur at intervals of several weeks, months, or even years. Violent acute irreversible episodes do not ordinarily occur in the subacute type.

Chronic Angle Closure

As mentioned previously, cases of chronic silent angle closure glaucoma are encountered which are truly asymptomatic and which mimic chronic open angle glaucoma, for

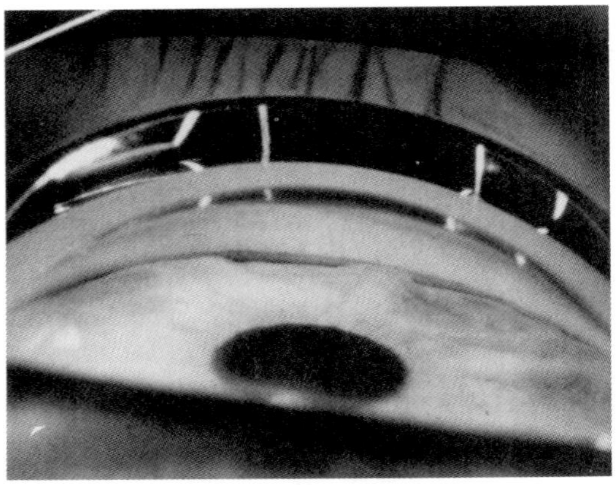

Figure 24.1. Cysts (not visible) of the posterior iris surface and ciliary body that result in an irregular bumpy contour to the peripheral iris and in focal narrowing of the angle. (Courtesy of David D. Donaldson, M.D.)

which the patients are often mistakenly treated. One of us (DLE) has been impressed that, among referral patients, cases of undetected chronic silent angle closure are the only ones in which the referral diagnoses are commonly in error. Since this condition can be cured by laser iridectomy, it is important to make this diagnosis correctly by employing the overall concepts already outlined (Chapter 22). If there is a strong suspicion of this diagnosis in a patient with elevated IOP, we usually recommend laser iridectomy be performed. In many such cases of chronic silent angle closure, the closure is appositional, rather than completely synechial, and therefore it is potentially reversible by iridectomy.

In addition to describing chronic silent angle closure glaucomas we also continue (reluctantly) to use the term "chronic" in our discussions, as indicated above, for the residuae, recurrence, and continuance of "subacute" angle closure simply because it has been used this way by others. We find the term "chronic," in general, confusing because it is defined often by past symptoms, and it sometimes obscures the understanding of the entity of chronic silent angle closure glaucoma that mimics POAG. Regardless, the treatment is the same: laser iridectomy, which is followed by a reassessment of the amount of peripheral anterior synechia formation, and further treatment and follow-up including possible gonioplasty (Chapters 25 and 60) as described for acute angle closure glaucoma (Chapter 23).

Danger of Continuing Medical Treatment

Once the diagnosis of subacute or chronic angle closure glaucoma is established, treatment should be iridectomy in nearly all cases. In the early stages of this condition when there is little or no synechial closure, the initial response to medical therapy, especially the use of miotic treatment, is normally satisfactory even without iridectomy, but this creates a dangerous long-term situation. In the short-term all portions of the angle that have not become closed by synechias may open readily with medical therapy and IOP may be brought to normal. However, in most cases in which treatment, e.g., with miotics, is continued for some time, sooner or later more synechial closure of the angle occurs, the baseline IOP gradually rises, and stronger miotics are required to bring IOP temporarily to normal levels. Aqueous humor suppressant therapy for such chronic angle closure cases also may give a false sense of security, while synechial closure of the angle relentlessly progresses. Finally, after extensive synechial closure has occurred, IOP may remain at relatively high levels and may not be lowered by medical means.

Angle Closure Glaucoma 25

Evaluation and Treatment After Iridectomy

David L. Epstein

ROUTINE FOR EVALUATION OF PATIENT AFTER LASER IRIDECTOMY

The mechanics of "handling" patients' eyes before and immediately after laser iridectomy are detailed in Chapter 56. In brief, eyes are pretreated with 1 to 2% pilocarpine to stretch and thin the iris and aid in peripheral placement of the iridectomy; and they are given apraclonidine to "blunt" a potential IOP spike post-treatment by decreasing aqueous humor formation and to lessen the chance of iris bleeding with the YAG laser by a vasoconstrictive action (Chapter 12). They are then post-treated with mild anti-inflammatory agents (e.g., weak steroids or nonsteroidal anti-inflammatory agents four times a day) for 5 days and appropriate antiglaucoma therapy. The following section deals with the conceptual steps in the subsequent post-laser management.

This begins with an evaluation before the laser as to the likely final diagnosis, i.e., the likelihood of a combined open angle and angle closure mechanism, and thus the likelihood of a laser-induced IOP spike in the short-term, and "residual open angle glaucoma" in the long term (Chapter 22). This is part of optimal patient management. This tentative understanding also aids in planning the needed frequency of patient visits after the laser procedure (Table 25.1).

The patient is seen the day after the iridectomy and every several days if the IOP is substantially elevated (in which case gonioscopy should be performed). Anti-inflammatory therapy can be extended if needed. Then the patient is routinely seen 7 to 10 days later when routine follow-up gonioscopy is performed. This visit is a convenient time to perform a prophylactic laser iridectomy on the fellow eye, assuming there are no residua in the first eye. One of us (DLE) routinely asks the patient if the first eye is "back to baseline" before performing a prophylactic iridectomy on the fellow eye (obviously this is modified if there are urgent reasons to proceed more quickly with laser iridectomy in the second eye).

Gonioscopy identifies the need for argon laser gonioplasty that might be planned a few weeks hence, and also allows correlation of the amount of synechias with the measured IOP. IOP may be elevated for a few weeks after laser (and also surgical) iridectomy by an open angle mechanism due to pigment or debris and the use of corticosteroids. Therefore, short-term antiglaucoma therapy (usually aqueous humor suppressants) is used only to protect against acute optic nerve damage, and an observed "slightly high" IOP, if safe for the optic nerve in the short-term, might be tolerated for a few weeks to evaluate, at a subsequent visit, the true "steady state." On the other hand, if more vigorous antiglaucoma therapy is initiated at this visit and the IOP later decreases into a range below the target, the need for continuation of such "strong" therapy should later be re-evaluated.

The patency of the iridectomy is assessed. At any visit during the 4 to 6 week post-laser period, late closure of the iridectomy may occur. This is much more common after argon laser iridectomy, but is still occasionally observed after YAG iridectomy. (If patent at the 6 week visit, it is rare for any laser iridectomy to close subsequently, except in patients with uveitis or neovascularization.) However, even if obviously patent, an iridectomy may be sequestered in the sense that there are adhesions between the posterior iris surface and the crystalline lens so that there is not free communication between the posterior and the anterior chamber. The iridectomy may be too central (especially if pre-laser pilocarpine was not used, or the pupil was semidilated and fixed from the acute angle closure attack) and therefore may not clear the equator of the crystalline lens. The iridectomy very rarely might be too small in size (less than 50 microns) or filled with iris stromal strands or some potentially "plugging" iris material on the posterior border. Many of these complications were more commonly encountered after argon laser iridectomy than YAG laser iridectomy, but are still sometimes observed.

Therefore, in addition to observing the apparent direct patency of the iridectomy, the functional status needs to be assessed separately by observing the contour of the iris. Has relative pupillary block been alleviated? If so, and there is resulting free communication between the posterior and anterior chambers through the

Table 25-1
Post-op Management of Laser Iridectomy

Immediate post-op (1–2 hr)	Check patency of iridectomy; IOP (at all visits); start topical steroids (qid for 5 days).
Day 1	Check patency of iridectomy.
Day 7–10	Assess location and function of iridectomy; gonioscopy to assess angle status, laser iridogonioplasty if significant portions of angle synechially closed; iridectomy for fellow eye if indicated (some clinicians prefer to do iridectomy of fellow eye at same sitting as first eye).
Week 4–6	Assess iridectomy for patency. "touch up" iridectomy if necessary, dilated exam; baseline disc photos and visual fields if indicated.
Every 3–12 months	25% of patients with acute angle closure develop an IOP rise after angle closure; (uniocular mydriatic provocative test); therefore, longterm follow-up is essential.

iridectomy, the iris contour configuration should no longer be convex forward (an effect of increased fluid pressure in the posterior chamber). Sometimes the crystalline lens convexity itself will hold the central iris forward from direct pressure, but the contour of the peripheral iris needs to be assessed by gonioscopy. (This is more easily evaluated with Koeppe gonioscopy.) Similarly, the peripheral chamber depth on slit lamp examination (Von Herick's Rule) should have also deepened, reflecting the induced loss of iris convexity. If these findings are not observed, then the clinician needs to entertain the possibility that there is not a functionally patent iridectomy, or that the patient has some other form of angle closure glaucoma such as plateau iris, or some entity with direct peripheral pressure on the peripheral posterior iris surface, e.g., ciliary body cysts or detachment.

It goes without saying, that if pupillary block has not been alleviated, then the angle may still appear closed by gonioscopy. Thus apparent synechias may not be true synechias but merely continued appositional closure. Therefore, repeat indentation gonioscopy after iridectomy with the following logic: if there is a patent iridectomy, then fluid pressure at least cannot be holding the peripheral iris in appositional closure over the TM. Therefore, with a patent iridectomy, indentation should not change the apparent amount of angle closure, which would thus have to represent peripheral anterior synechias formation. If indentation does "open the angle," then either the iridectomy is not patent, or there is some secondary cause of the closure.

This refers to opening of the angle and not a possible indentation effect on the iris. Mirrored lenses unfortunately, despite their advantages, have their greatest weakness in this post-laser iridectomy assessment of peripheral iris contour. Although there is free communication between anterior and posterior chambers, sudden indentation displacement of the anterior chamber contents with the Zeiss style indentation lenses does seemingly cause a temporary posterior indentation of the iris in many, but not all, patients (the volume displaced by the indentation from the anterior chamber cannot pass quickly enough through the iridectomy into the posterior chamber, and thus posterior iris movement is commonly produced). This induced posterior movement of the iris makes it easier to see into the angle, but should not thereby change the functional status of the angle if there is a patent iridectomy. Such persisting posterior movement of the iris after iridectomy has led to much confusion for the glaucoma student. **In an eye with a patent iridectomy and no other cause for angle closure except primary pupillary block, appositional closure of the angle can not exist by definition.** If it looked that way with this indirect approach, it was because the mirrored gonioscopy lens did not present a true view of the angle (commonly because there is a large crystalline lens holding the central half, but not the peripheral portion, of the iris forward). It is crucial to distinguish between central iris convexity, due directly to the position of the crystalline lens, and peripheral iris convexity due to increased fluid pressure in the posterior chamber, because at this post-laser visit one must be sure that relative pupillary block is no longer present (Fig. 25.1). If the examiner is uncertain, Koeppe gonioscopy should be performed as it readily allows such discrimination.

If pupillary block has been eliminated, but the angle remains either closed or very narrow and therefore occludable, and this is not due to a misinterpretation from an indirect mirrored view or a large crystalline lens, then other diagnoses should be entertained at this post-laser visit. The possibility of peripheral anterior synechias, or secondary direct mechanical closure from the ciliary body (Chapter 28) producing continuing appositional closure, or a plateau iris should be considered (Fig. 25.2, 25.3). **A mydriatic (using a sympathomimetic not a cycloplegic drug) provocative test to one eye can be performed, either at the 1-week visit, or more often at a visit several weeks later, to rule out plateau iris.**

Plateau iris (1–3) may be suspected pre-laser, or only post-laser when the access to the angle remains "narrow." Most cases of possible plateau iris (plateau iris configuration) turn out after laser iridectomy not to have the true condition. However, there are also cases in which it was not suspected ahead of time, but proven to be a true plateau iris syndrome only after laser iridectomy.

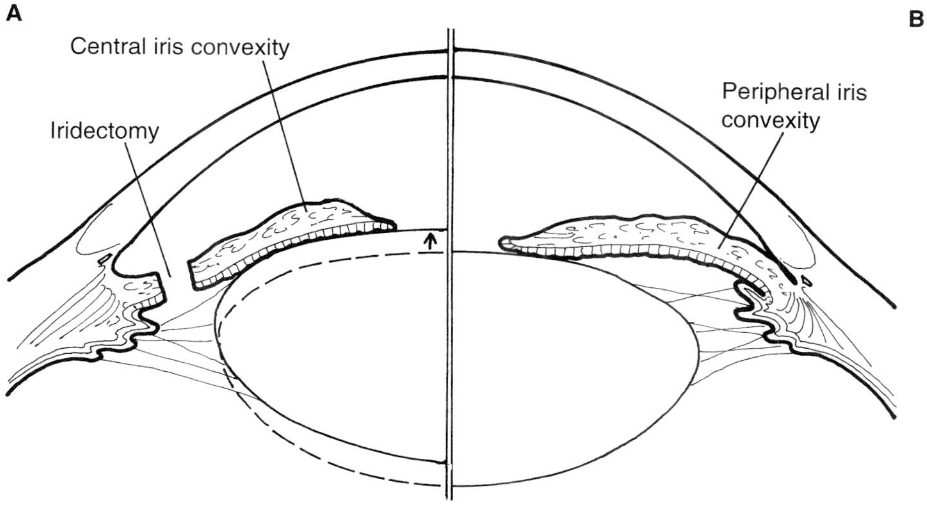

Figure 25.1. Iris convexity may be secondary to forward location of the crystalline lens (A) or due to relative pupillary block (B). Iris convexity extends more peripherally in the latter case. (Modified from Shields MB: Textbook of glaucoma. 3rd ed. Baltimore: Williams & Wilkins, 1992.)

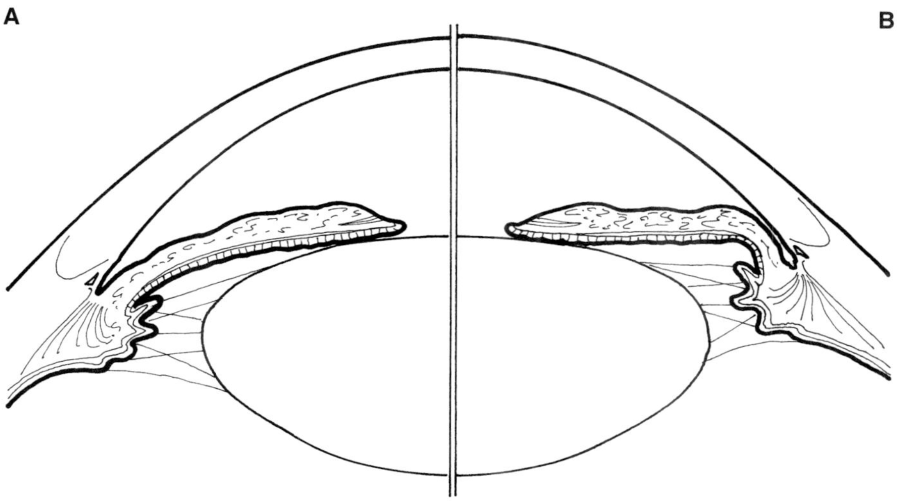

Figure 25.2. The iris configuration in pupillary block (A) demonstrates a gradual slope to the angle versus that in plateau iris syndrome (B). (Modified from Shields MB: Textbook of glaucoma. 3rd ed. Baltimore: Williams & Wilkins, 1992.)

At this post-laser visit, e.g., 1 month after the second eye has had a laser iridectomy, and all is quiet with patent iridectomies and the eyes are back to "baseline," a mydriatic provocative test should be performed in one eye only (using the fellow eye as a control and avoiding precipitating a "repeat" of bilateral angle closure in a patient who had every expectation of being "cured"). A sympathomimetic drug such as 2.5% or 5% phenylephrine is administered to one eye once or twice to try to achieve wide dilatation, after which both the IOP and gonioscopy are reassessed. This should be a routine test administered to all post-laser iridectomy patients.

Sympathomimetic drugs should not elevate IOP, but rather can cause either no change or some transitory IOP lowering from a presumed decreased inflow effect. These agents rarely can cause elevation of IOP from liberation of pigment particles (4) into the anterior chamber. This can be assessed by repeating slit-lamp examination after dilation. **An elevation of IOP of several mm Hg or more compared with the control fellow eye needs to be explained, especially since in plateau iris syndrome the amount of functional angle closure increases progressively with wider dilation and resulting iris crowding of the angle.** But regardless of the IOP change after mydriatic challenge, the patient should be regonioscoped and this documented in the chart for future reference.

Obviously, if the IOP increases during this mydriatic provocative test, gonioscopy should provide confirmation of angle closure as the responsible mechanism (otherwise, e.g., suspect pigment liberation or other open angle mech-

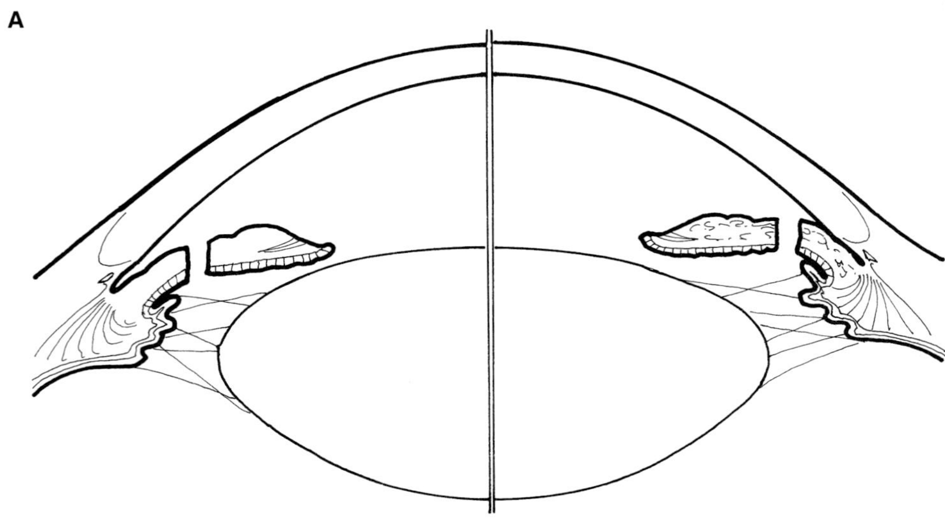

Figure 25.3. Dilation in the presence of a peripheral iridectomy does not produce angle closure when due to relative pupillary block (A). Because plateau iris configuration is not caused by relative pupillary block but rather by direct crowding of the iris into the angle, dilation does cause angle closure (B). (Modified from Shields MB: Textbook of glaucoma. 3rd ed. Baltimore: Williams & Wilkins, 1992.)

anisms). Also, the angle may look ominously closed after mydriatic treatment, even though the IOP did not increase, and this might indicate that with wider mydriasis in the future the angle might close in a plateau mechanism (not likely except when dilated in the ophthalmologist's office. There would be little risk of spontaneous closure, although long-term observations of such eyes over decades have not yet been made). Alternatively, it might indicate that the angle is functionally open beyond a peripheral iris roll, though it looks closed or "close to closed" with the mirrored gonioscopy lens. The latter appearance might be important to document in the chart for future reference when, for example, the patient might be dilated with a cycloplegic drug that could elevate the IOP on an open angle mechanism (5,6) due to interference with ciliary muscle tone—the opposite effect of pilocarpine. In such a case, the IOP increase at this subsequent visit might be misinterpreted as angle closure "due to plateau iris," and the patient would be mislabeled. Such a phenomenon is not rare, and it is surprising how many patients with prior angle closure were, at least in the previous era, both erroneously maintained on chronic pilocarpine therapy and told that their pupils should never be dilated, based on cycloplegic drug-induced IOP elevation due to a true open angle mechanism that was never correlated with gonioscopy.

Performing gonioscopy on narrow angled patients after pupillary dilation takes much experience because of the common presence of a peripheral iris roll. One learns to interpret correctly the open angle beyond this iris roll, but only if one routinely performs gonioscopy in all patients after pupillary dilatation (not just those with elevated IOP).

A cycloplegic (anticholinergic) drug, presumably by interfering with ciliary muscle tone to the outflow pathway, can cause an IOP increase with a maintained open angle in as many as one third of patients with primary open angle glaucoma (5,6). This is supposedly uncommon in "normal" patients, and thus it would be unexpected in pure forms of angle closure glaucoma. Yet this scenario of cycloplegic-induced IOP elevation on an open angle glaucoma mechanism is not rare in patients with angle closure. In some we have wondered if this is a temporary situation for the first few months after iridectomy. This phenomenon truly needs to be studied further and better explained. This might also relate to the discussion of "residual open angle glaucoma" in patients who have had iridectomy for angle closure (Chapter 22). The latter phenomenon also occurs more commonly in angle closure eyes than the expected incidence of POAG. Regardless, **the key concept is the need to correlate the gonioscopic findings with the IOP response after this mydriatic provocative test**. If the test is truly positive for plateau iris syndrome, the patient is then managed as detailed in the next chapter.

When the pupil is dilated at this postoperative visit, a dilated slit-lamp examination should be performed documenting the presence and extent of crystalline lens changes (there is a risk of lens changes long term after laser iridectomy, but also occult exfoliation should be looked for [7]), the appearance of the optic nerve including stereo disc photos (remember the risk of "residual open angle glaucoma"), and indirect ophthalmoscopy performed with examination of the retinal periphery as in any other patient with glaucoma (Chapter 5).

For practical purposes, unilateral plateau iris has not been observed, and therefore if IOP does not increase or true angle closure is not observed with this unilateral mydriatic provocative test, at subsequent visits it is safe to dilate both pupils with the physician's choice of mydriatic and/or cycloplegic.

If in the postlaser iridectomy visits it is suspected that

there is direct mechanical pressure on the posterior iris surface acting to close the angle, cycloplegic drugs can and should be used in this situation to help diagnose this. Tightening the zonules and interfering with ciliary muscle contraction could cause posterior movement of the crystalline lens and potentially also some alteration in ciliary body position. Use of cycloplegic drugs for certain forms of secondary angle closure glaucoma is described in Chapters 28 and 29.

Laser iridectomy establishes communication between the posterior and anterior chambers by creating a hole in the iris, but this does nothing to change the position of the crystalline lens. It is sometimes an illusion, especially to the beginning student of glaucoma, that the anterior chamber may have seemed to deepen centrally after laser iridectomy, but compulsive recording of the axial and peripheral chamber depth will indicate that only the peripheral chamber depth can change after iridectomy (and was responsible for this illusion). This has been confirmed by photogrammetric and biometric measurements (8–10). The recording of both peripheral and axial anterior chamber depth measured in terms of "corneal thicknesses" is important, especially in case of subsequent shallowing of the anterior chamber. In malignant glaucoma syndromes, there is axial anterior chamber (as well as peripheral) shallowing (Chapter 29). Although malignant glaucoma has not yet been unequivocally observed after laser iridectomy (although there are rare case reports [11]), it was not rare (and a very serious problem potentially progressing to blindness) after surgical peripheral iridectomy. Maybe one of the readers of this book will observe the first true postlaser iridectomy case of malignant glaucoma by meticulous attention to detail. Eyes with previous angle closure may in the ensuing years experience some new occurrence, perhaps involving the posterior segment, unrelated to the past angle closure event and it may be very important to know that the axial depth has subsequently changed.

Assuming all is well 4 to 6 weeks after the laser iridectomy in the fellow eye, the ophthalmologist should continue to follow the patient. As mentioned, "residual open angle glaucoma," possibly increasing nuclear sclerosis with the passage of time, etc., are issues in such eyes (Chapter 22). The patient should be checked 6 months later, and then at yearly intervals and subsequently, assuming all is well, every 2 years.

"RESIDUAL OPEN ANGLE GLAUCOMA AFTER LASER IRIDECTOMY"

As mentioned, there is a higher incidence of open angle glaucoma in eyes that have had laser iridectomy than what would be predicted from the prevalence of primary open angle glaucoma in the same aged population. Possible explanations include that the two diseases are linked genetically, and that certain forms of open angle glaucoma such as exfoliation commonly are associated with narrow angles (7). Chronic iris "touch" from appositional closure may perhaps cause "residual open angle glaucoma," the original diagnosis of angle closure may be in error, and laser iridectomy might cause trabecular meshwork dysfunction presumably as a result of released pigment, debris, and inflammation, which all necessarily must leave the eye via the outflow pathways (12). Possibly all of these explanations are valid.

Regardless, it behooves the clinician to establish the correct diagnosis as accurately as possible ahead of time (Chapter 22) and both inform the patient and plan one's short-term and long-term follow-up accordingly. **In a patient with exfoliation open angle glaucoma and a narrow but functionally open angle, one should anticipate a potentially large IOP spike after laser iridectomy,** which also would do nothing to improve the current IOP control (although potentially prevent future worsening). Inform the patient fully about this ahead of time. One of us (DLE) is aware of at least two cases in which this scenario was not anticipated, resulting in loss of central visual acuity from the IOP spike, leading to medicolegal discussions.

The earlier described steps in evaluating the patient and determining whether laser iridectomy is indicated needs to be followed.

Thus patients who have had laser iridectomy should be evaluated indefinitely at 1- to 2-year intervals as possible future "open angle glaucoma suspects."

LONG-TERM FOLLOW-UP AFTER IRIDECTOMY

The initial measurements of IOP after iridectomy are by no means a guide as to what the future is going to hold. Examine the angle. If much of the angle is closed by synechiae, one should not be misled if the IOP at that time happens still to be low without treatment because sooner or later IOP can be expected to increase. This may not occur for some time. If there are synechiae, gonioplasty with the argon laser should be performed. Warn the patient so that if the IOP increases to a level consistent with the extent of synechial closure, the patient is not shocked to find that medical antiglaucoma therapy, "additional" laser therapy-gonioplasty, or filtration surgery may be needed.

In addition, after laser iridectomy, IOP may be moderately elevated by an ill-defined open angle mechanism for several weeks to months after the procedure. This may relate to the increased pigmentation of the trabecular meshwork that one often sees, or perhaps to obstructing iris or inflammatory debris. Therefore, depending on the disc and field status, one would like to delay if possible a decision concerning possible filtration surgery even in a patient with residual synechias, until a month or so after the iridectomy.

TREATMENT OF RESIDUAL ("CHRONIC") SYNECHIAL ANGLE CLOSURE GLAUCOMA

Gonioscopy should always be performed at the first follow-up visit after laser iridectomy. As described, IOP can be elevated at this or subsequent visits by an open angle mechanism perhaps relating to pigment, debris or inflammation in the trabecular meshwork, or can be lowered (giving a false sense of security) by hyposecretion especially after a substantial acute attack. Regardless, **the clinician needs to ascertain the extent of residual peripheral anterior synechias in the angle, no matter what the level of IOP**.

In treating this residual synechial angle closure glaucoma, one chooses medical therapy alone if there are minimal peripheral anterior synechias, and gonioplasty with supplemental medical antiglaucoma therapy, if the synechias are extensive. If this strategy fails because of the presence of extensive residual peripheral anterior synechias, filtration surgery will be required. (The term "chronic" can also be applied to this latter angle closure entity, but it may lead to confusion and we prefer the more specific term "residual synechial" angle closure glaucoma.)

MEDICAL THERAPY

Aqueous humor suppressant therapy is most commonly used in the short and intermediate term, but long term one is free to use any and all antiglaucoma therapy, including miotics and epinephrine (in the absence of previous malignant glaucoma or plateau iris).

ARGON LASER GONIOPLASTY (IRIDOPLASTY)

If 6 or more hours of the angle have synechias, consideration should be given at a subsequent visit to performing gonioplasty (13–17) (Chapter 60) to break these synechias, if possible. The overall clinical impression is that in perhaps 50% of patients with synechias of less than 1 year's duration, this procedure can restore normal or near normal outflow function to the affected portion of the angle. Probably (although not certainly) the more recent the synechia formation the better the chances for a beneficial effect. On the other hand, the eye should be free from inflammation and "fully recovered" from the iridectomy procedure, and, therefore, the gonioplasty can usually be delayed for a few weeks after iridectomy, unless the magnitude of the IOP forces one's hand sooner. However, in the latter case the concept of correlation of the angle with the IOP needs to be remembered, for, as described, the IOP can be elevated for a few weeks after laser iridectomy on the basis of an open angle mechanism.

In doing this laser gonioplasty technique, use of the angle mirror of a gonioscopy lens is preferred to directly place the argon laser burns (e.g., 200 microns, 0.2–0.5 seconds, 300 mW) on the far peripheral iris as close to the angle as possible. Some synechias will readily separate yielding an apparent open angle to view (that still has only an approximate 50% chance of being functionally open). **Other peripheral anterior synechias do not readily separate with placement of the peripheral iris laser burn, and we recommend not persisting in treating such sites** (since even if it is anatomically possible to "open" the angle, the chance for functional recovery seems much less likely) and we recommend moving on to other sites. Because this procedure can induce inflammation in the eye and can liberate pigment debris, all of which might elevate the IOP by an open angle mechanism, this procedure should be performed in two divided sessions, perhaps weeks apart. **Pre-treating the eye with 1 or 2% pilocarpine** makes the procedure much easier to perform by stretching the peripheral iris.

Depending on other clinical factors such as the presumed "filterability" of the open angle (Chapters 3 and 7) as well as the disc and field status, gonioplasty could also be performed for lesser amounts of residual peripheral anterior synechias, e.g., 3–6 hours of the angle. Probably for 3 or fewer hours of synechias, except in unusual situations (the need for a very low IOP because of the vulnerability of the optic nerve), this procedure need not be performed. (Although an adverse effect from gonioplasty has not really been documented, theoretically, as with laser iridectomy, the induced inflammation and potential pigment liberation might have a long term adverse effect on the open portions of the angle. This is the reason we do not advocate persisting in treating synechias that do not readily separate.)

Although not all clinicians would agree that this procedure is effective (and many would argue that regardless, chronic iris "touch" to the trabecular meshwork in a narrow angled eye can cause trabecular dysfunction even if the synechias are anatomically separated), gonioplasty is gaining increased acceptance and certainly should be attempted before consideration of filtration surgery for uncontrolled residual synechial angle closure glaucoma. Some, especially after certain secondary forms of angle closure, have argued that **surgical goniosynechialysis** (18–20) should be attempted to break such peripheral anterior synechias. In certain secondary forms of angle closure, the peripheral iris adjacent to the angle may not be accessible to the argon laser through the mirrored lens, and therefore this procedure may be used (Chapter 23). However, in cases of primary angle closure glaucoma, access of the peripheral iris to the argon laser is usually technically possible, and therefore surgical chamber deepening has only rare indication. Peripheral anterior synechias that are difficult to separate with an argon laser burn probably indicate a portion of the angle with little if any chance for functional recovery.

After argon laser gonioplasty, patients are treated with topical steroids, probably a little more intensively (e.g., dexamethasone alcohol two to three times a day) than after iridectomy for 4 to 5 days.

FILTRATION SURGERY

The techniques of filtration surgery in patients with residual ("chronic") synechial angle closure glaucoma are similar to those in other patients with glaucoma, and are detailed in Chapter 62. There are, however, a few special considerations. Because the anatomy of the usual hyperopic eye is "crowded" anteriorly, special attention is made to carry the conjunctival and scleral flap incisions far enough anteriorly, to avoid entering the eye and placing the fistula too far posteriorly, over the ciliary body. **A good rule is that one is "never far enough anteriorly" and extra time is taken at the limbus to move the dissection of tissue as far anterior as possible.** Because shallowing of the anterior chamber intra- and postoperatively may be involved in the development of malignant glaucoma (Chapter 29), there is special attention to the chamber intraoperatively in such hyperopic eyes to prevent anterior chamber shallowing. The glaucoma fistula might be designed to be "tighter" rather than "looser" (with potential future use of suture lysis) to try to avoid postoperative anterior chamber shallowing. **The possibility of malignant glaucoma developing in the early postoperative period must always be on the surgeon's mind when performing filtration surgery on eyes with residual synechial angle closure.**

References

1. Tornquist R: Angle-closure glaucoma in an eye with a plateau type of iris. Acta Ophthalmol 1958;36:419–423.
2. Wand M, Grant WM, Simmons RJ, et al: Plateau iris syndrome. Trans Am Acad Ophthalmol Otolaryngol 1977;83:122–130.
3. Pavlin CJ, Ritch R, Foster FS: Ultrasound biomicroscopy in plateau iris syndrome. Am J Ophthalmol 1992;113:390–5.
4. Epstein DL, Boger WP, Grant WM: Phenylephrine provocative testing in the pigmentary dispersion syndrome. Am J Ophthalmol 1978;85: 43–50.
5. Harris LS: Cycloplegic provocative testing. Arch Ophthalmol 1969;81: 544–547.
6. Harris LS: Cycloplegic provocative testing and topical administration of steroids. Arch Ophthalmol 1971;86:12–14.
7. Gross FJ, Tingey D, Epstein DL: Increased prevalence of occludable angles and angle-closure glaucoma in patients with pseudoexfoliation. Am J Ophthalmol 1993;117:333–336.
8. Lee DA, Brubaker RF, Ilstrup DM: Anterior chamber dimensions in patients with narrow angles and angle-closure glaucoma. Arch Ophthalmol 1984;102:46–50.
9. Jin JC, Anderson DR: The effect of iridotomy on iris contour. Am J Ophthalmol 1990;110:260–3.
10. Schrems W, Hofmann G, Krieglstein GK: Zur Biometrie der Augenvorderkammer bei der Nd:YAG-Laseriridektomie. Klin Monatsbl Augenheilkd 1990;196:128–31.
11. Cashwell LF, Martin TJ: Malignant glaucoma after laser iridotomy. Ophthalmology 1992;99:651–9.
12. Robin AL, et al: Histologic studies of angle structures after laser iridotomy in primates. Arch Ophthalmol 1982;100:1665–70.
13. Ritch R: Argon laser treatment for medically unresponsive attacks of angle-closure glaucoma. Am J Ophthalmol 1982;94:197–204.
14. Wand M: Argon laser gonioplasty for synechial angle closure. Arch Ophthalmol 1992;110:363–7.
15. Weiss HS, et al: Argon laser gonioplasty in the treatment of angle-closure glaucoma. Am J Ophthalmol 1992;114:14–18.
16. Lim AS, et al: Laser iridoplasty in the treatment of severe acute angle closure glaucoma. Int Ophthalmol 1993;17:33–6.
17. Sassani JW, et al: Histopathology of argon laser peripheral iridoplasty. Ophthalmic Surg 1993;24:740–5.
18. Campbell DG, Vela A: Modern goniosynechialysis for the treatment of synechial angle-closure glaucoma. Ophthalmology 1984;91:1052–60.
19. Shingleton BJ, Chang MA, Bellows AR, et al: Surgical goniosynechialysis for angle-closure glaucoma. Ophthalmology 1990;97:551–6.
20. Tanihara H, Nishiwaki K, Nagata M: Surgical results and complications of goniosynechialysis. Graefes Arch Clin Exp Ophthalmol 1992;230: 309–13.

Plateau Iris

26

David L. Epstein

PLATEAU IRIS CONFIGURATION AND PLATEAU IRIS SYNDROME

Clinical Features

In a small proportion of eyes that develop angle closure glaucoma, the axial depth of the anterior chamber is not as shallow as we are accustomed to associate with angle closure glaucoma, and the front surface of the iris lacks the overall convex curvature that usually involves the whole iris from pupil to angle. In angle closure glaucoma associated with the so-called plateau iris or flat iris plane, the distance from cornea to lens may be equivalent to three or more corneal thicknesses, normal depth in some cases, and the surface of the iris extending from the pupil toward the angle may appear nearly flat centrally; it may be convex only in the periphery, where it conforms to the curvature of the angle wall and closes the angle. The profile of such an iris, if it could be seen in cross section, can be conceived as resembling a plateau, as pointed out by Tornquist in 1958 (1).

In most cases in which angle closure glaucoma is associated with plateau iris, the glaucoma can be eliminated as successfully by iridectomy as in the more common cases in which the whole iris is convex. Relative pupillary block and accumulation of aqueous humor in the posterior chamber must be significant factors contributing to the convexity of the iris in both the common and the plateau iris cases, though with plateau iris, the convexity is limited to the periphery, and widening of the angle is not as striking after iridectomy as in eyes in which the whole iris is convex.

Rarely, despite iridectomy and the presence of a definite surgical coloboma in the iris, the angle of an eye with plateau iris remains so narrow that the angle can be caused to close by dilating the pupil (Chapter 25), and an attack of angle closure glaucoma results. Even more rarely, angle closure glaucoma can recur spontaneously, without artificially dilating the pupil. Fortunately, as a rule, weak miotic therapy is effective in relieving this type of postiridectomy glaucoma.

We think it is desirable to distinguish the preoperative condition of the iris from the postiridectomy recurrence of angle closure glaucoma simply by calling the preoperative condition, **plateau iris configuration, and the rare postoperative recurrence of glaucoma,** the **plateau iris syndrome,** as was done in a study of these conditions reported by Wand and colleagues (2). The rarity of the plateau iris syndrome was also indicated in that report; only eight cases could be identified among a large number of glaucoma patients in the Glaucoma Service of the Massachusetts Eye and Ear Infirmary and the referral practices of two of its members. Review of the literature uncovered few reports in which this condition was clearly identified gonioscopically.

The diagnosis can only be established conclusively by gonioscopy. Other causes of IOP increase, spontaneously or from application of mydriatics, after iridectomy for angle-closure glaucoma include: 1) failure of the iridectomy to make a hole through all layers of the iris, 2) residual peripheral anterior synechias (Chapter 24), 3) presence of multiple cysts of the ciliary body (Chapter 34), or 4) presence of open-angle glaucoma (Chapter 25). Slit-lamp biomicroscopy and gonioscopy establish the diagnosis. Only if there is conspicuous axial shallowing of the anterior chamber associated with the postoperative increase of IOP and closure of the angle does one need to consider a diagnosis of malignant glaucoma (Chapter 29). However, this distinction is important because the topical treatment of plateau iris syndrome and the treatment of malignant glaucoma are totally different. Plateau iris syndrome may be precipitated by cycloplegics and relieved by pilocarpine, whereas malignant glaucoma may be precipitated or aggravated by miotics and relieved or benefited by cycloplegics.

The conspicuous axial shallowing of the anterior chamber in malignant glaucoma (Chapter 29) is the principal feature that should distinguish this condition from plateau iris syndrome. However, there is an important point in a rare case in which there is some uncertainty due to shallowness of the anterior chamber at the time of recurrent glaucoma after angle-closure glaucoma previously associated with plateau iris. The point we believe to be significant is the relationship of ciliary processes to lens equator, as viewed (when possible) through the iris coloboma (or the widely dilated pupil) with the aid of Koeppe lens gonioscopy. According to our observations so far, in malignant glaucoma the lens equator tends to extend behind and peripheral to the tips of the ciliary processes, so that the lens equator is in a position to push ciliary processes and iris forward (Chapter 28), whereas in the plateau iris syndrome, we have not seen the lens extend peripherally beyond the tips of the ciliary processes.

DIAGNOSIS

Although a true plateau iris syndrome is rare, after laser iridectomy, the pupils should be dilated in each patient whether this was one of those coincidental diurnal IOP variations of open-angle glaucoma.

To differentiate a genuinely positive (angle closure) darkroom test from a spurious coincidental increase of IOP that is not due to closure of the angle, but is due simply to the diurnal IOP variation that occurs in some patients with open angle glaucoma, apply the bright-light test immediately after the darkroom test. This is done as follows.

At the end of the darkroom test, after the IOP has been measured and the angle has been inspected in as dim illumination as possible, to see if the angle appears to have closed, the illumination is then greatly increased, to cause the pupils to constrict. This can be done by turning on bright ceiling lights while observing the angle through the goniolens. When the light is bright enough to make the angle clearly open in the entire circumference, one knows that if the IOP was elevated due to closure of the angle during the darkroom test, it should rapidly, within 5 to 15 minutes, drop back to its original level when the angle is reopened by bright light. However, if the IOP was elevated during the darkroom test due to coincidental diurnal IOP fluctuation, rather than by closure of the angle, we can expect no such rapid drop back to the original level. The time course of diurnal IOP fluctuations is much slower than the time course of the fall of IOP when a closed angle is reopened.

The bright-light test should be a routine procedure after apparently positive darkroom tests. Of course, in cases in which bright light does not open the angle, this test is of no value. Under such circumstances, one might have recourse to the bright-light and thymoxamine test.

BRIGHT-LIGHT AND THYMOXAMINE TEST

The bright-light and thymoxamine test (4,5) is the opposite of the darkroom test. The patient is placed under bright illumination to induce and maintain miosis, to favor opening of the angle. Accommodation is purposely avoided either by using diffuse illumination or by using a light source very close to the eye. (Perhaps application of plus lenses would be a worthwhile refinement.) The aim is to induce the pupillary sphincter to constrict, but to avoid constriction of the ciliary muscle, so that there will be no complicating alteration of the lens or the trabecular meshwork by the ciliary muscle.

The opening of the angle can be aided considerably by applying 0.5% thymoxamine hydrochloride eye drops in combination with exposure to bright light (4). Thymoxamine is an alpha-adrenergic blocking agent that temporarily causes the radial muscle fibers of the iris to relax and allows the pupillary sphincter muscle to act unopposed in constricting the pupil and pulling the iris away from the angle wall. **Thymoxamine does not appreciably affect the ciliary muscle, and if the angle is already open it does not influence intraocular pressure or facility of aqueous outflow** (5). (In this respect light and thymoxamine are unlike pilocarpine or cholinergic miotics, which are not well suited for use in testing for angle closure because they cause contraction of both the pupil and the ciliary muscle. By both mechanisms pilocarpine and cholinergic miotics can influence IOP and aqueous outflow so that they do not serve to distinguish clearly between angle closure and open angle glaucoma. They can normalize IOP and outflow not only in angle closure, but also in open angle glaucoma.) Thymoxamine should be administered to only one eye, and the other eye be used as a control for diurnal variation.

One precaution to observe in the use of the bright-light test with or without thymoxamine is to avoid subjecting the eye to drying under the influence of local anesthesia and its attendant reduction in blink rate. The only shortcoming of the bright-light test and thymoxamine is that in some eyes the miosis induced is not enough to open the angle and lower the IOP; however, where it is positive, this test gives clear uncomplicated evidence.

When should one perform the darkroom test and when the thymoxamine bright-light test? In patients with narrow angles but normal IOP the question is whether this narrow, but presumably still functionally open angle, is capable of spontaneous closure. Such a patient should have a darkroom test to answer this question. However, in patients with narrow angles but elevated IOP there is a separate question: is the IOP elevation that is already present due to partial angle closure? For this question the thymoxamine bright-light test should be performed first. This test, by inducing miosis, can reverse appositional (but not synechial) angle closure, and lower IOP. It is a separate question (question one above) whether in this latter condition further angle is capable of closure in a darkroom test. Because the IOP is already elevated possibly due to an open angle component, the potential for diurnal fluctuation due to open-angle glaucoma (and a spurious increase of IOP in the dark) must be kept in mind. This is further reason why a unilateral IOP lowering due to thymoxamine may be more definitive, and why the latter test should be performed initially in such patients.

MYDRIATIC PROVOCATIVE TEST

The mydriasis test, which we have never favored (Chapter 22), is performed by applying a short-acting mydriatic, such as eucatropine, homatropine, cyclopentolate, or phenylephrine, with measurement of IOP and inspection of the angle when the pupil has dilated, to determine if the angle has become closed. In many cases, the test may have been considered negative at the stage of widest mydriasis, and the patient had been dismissed to go home, with or without application of a counteracting drop of pilocarpine. After a few hours, the angle unexpectedly closed and an acute attack developed. This has had unfortunate consequences for patients who did not understand what was happening or who did not promptly obtain treatment for their condition.

The mydriasis test has many disadvantages. It is less natural and physiologic than the darkroom or bright-light test. It is often negative in eyes that are subject to actual spontaneous episodes of subacute angle closure, yet it can cause closure of narrow angles that might never close spontaneously. It is otherwise treacherous in that it may belatedly induce an angle closure attack, and for greatest safety, would require surveillance of the patient for many hours. In certain cases of open angle glaucoma (6,7), cycloplegic mydriatics can cause an increase of IOP by impairment of facility of aqueous outflow without closure of the angle, necessitating careful, critical gonioscopy to minimize the chances of misinterpretation of an IOP increase with this test. If adrenergic mydriatics are used, it must be remembered that they have potentially confusing side effects, reducing aqueous formation in some eyes, and in rare instances causing an increase of IOP in open angle glaucomatous eyes without causing the angle to close, possibly from pigment particle liberation (8) (Chapter 21).

Therefore, we rarely perform the mydriatic test to diagnose angle closure glaucoma. However, as discussed in Chapter 25, we routinely perform a phenylephrine provocative test after laser iridectomy to rule out a plateau iris syndrome and establish baseline parameters for future evaluation.

Mapstone (9) proposed that phenylephrine combined with pilocarpine might be useful as a provocative test for angle closure, but long-term observation has not substantiated this theory (10).

References

1. Hyams SW, Friedman Z, Neumann E: Elevated intraocular pressure in the prone position. A new provocative test for angle-closure glaucoma. Am J Ophthalmol 1968;66:661–72.
2. Friedman Z, Neumann E: Comparison of prone-position, dark-room, and mydriatic tests for angle-closure glaucoma before and after peripheral iridectomy. Am J Ophthalmol 1972;74:24–7.
3. Wilensky JT, Kaufman PL, Frohlichstein D, et al: Follow-up of angle-closure glaucoma suspects. Am J Ophthalmol 1993;115:338–46.
4. Wand M, Grant WM: The thymoxamine test: A test to differentiate angle-closure glaucoma from open-angle glaucoma with narrow angles. Arch Ophthalmol 1978;96:1009–1011.
5. Wand M, Grant WM: Thymoxamine hydrochloride: Effects on the facility of outflow and intraocular pressure. Invest Ophthalmol 1976;15: 400–403.
6. Harris LS, Galin MA: Cycloplegic provocative testing. Arch Ophthalmol 1969;81:544–547.
7. Harris LS, Galin MA, Mittag TW: Cycloplegic provocative testing and topical administration of steroids. Arch Ophthalmol 1971;86:12–14.
8. Epstein DL, Boger WP, Grant WM: Phenylephrine provocative testing in the pigmentary dispersion syndrome. Am J Ophthalmol 1978;85: 43–50.
9. Mapstone R: Outflow changes in positive provocative tests. Br J Ophthalmol 1977;61:634–6.
10. Wishart PK: Can the pilocarpine phenylephrine provocative test be used to detect covert angle closure? Br J Ophthalmol 1991;75:615–8.

Secondary Angle Closure Glaucomas V

Principles of Secondary Angle Closure Glaucomas

28

David L. Epstein

In Chapter 22, the mechanisms underlying the "primary" angle closure glaucomas were discussed. The fundamental concept was that of pupillary block wherein fluid pressure in the posterior chamber from the normal secretion of aqueous humor ballooned the peripheral iris forward over the trabecular meshwork and thus closed the angle (see Fig. 22.2). Peripheral iridectomy, by equalizing the pressure in the posterior and anterior chambers, eliminated this fluid pressure vector from the posterior chamber acting on the iris. The key concept in such a pupillary block mechanism is that of posterior chamber aqueous humor acting as the force, resulting in the angle closure. In contrast, in plateau iris syndrome, in addition to a relative pupillary block mechanism, direct crowding of the iris itself into the angle has been identified as another mechanism for angle closure (see Fig. 26.1). Conceptually, however, these both should be categorized as local iris or posterior chamber mechanisms.

In some secondary angle closure glaucomas such as that due the ICE syndrome (Chapter 32) or neovascular glaucoma (Chapter 31), there are other abnormal local iris and angle factors acting to close the angle directly.

In other secondary angle closure glaucomas, there is some additional force acting to close the angle. **Conceptually this additional force might: 1) act by itself to directly force the iris into the angle; or 2) by acting to move the crystalline lens forward, cause pupillary block** (wherein the resulting increased fluid pressure from aqueous humor in the posterior chamber acts to force the peripheral iris over the angle). This may be termed a **secondary pupillary block**. The possibility for either or both of these two mechanisms in the secondary angle closure glaucomas needs to be constantly kept in mind, for it is not rare for some patients in this category to respond favorably to laser iridectomy (even though primary pupillary block is not the initiating mechanism causing the disease).

Examples of the first mechanism include cysts of the ciliary body (Chapter 34) or tumors such as melanoma that mechanically may push the iris into the angle (Chapter 41); forward rotations of the ciliary body from choroidal detachment, hemorrhage, or scleral buckling that may then push the iris forward (Chapter 33); and possible cases of ciliary body "swelling," as seen in certain inflammatory syndromes and possibly after pan-retinal photocoagulation, and in cases of transient myopia due to idiosyncratic systemic drug reaction (Chapter 36). (In these cases, local accumulation of suprachoroidal fluid and forward rotation of the ciliary body may be an alternative explanation to that of ciliary body "swelling" and may also explain certain cases of so called "loose lens syndrome," Chapter 29.) In all of these conditions, **pathological processes affecting the ciliary body itself result in direct pressure of the ciliary processes on the iris to close the angle**.

In other conditions, pathology involving vitreous volume, such as malignant glaucoma (Chapter 29) and angle closure glaucoma after vitreous hemorrhage, central retinal vein occlusion (Chapter 35), and possibly panretinal photocoagulation, and certain volume-occupying massive forms of acute "macular degeneration" may result in pressure from the vitreous that shifts the entire lens-iris diaphragm forward (axial shallowing). Grant has observed that in eyes with malignant glaucoma, the crystalline lens equator tends to extend behind and peripheral to the tips of the ciliary processes so that the lens equator is in a position to push the ciliary processes and the iris forward over the angle in response to this pressure from the vitreous. Likely this relationship of the crystalline lens equator to the tips of the ciliary processes is an anatomical pre-condition in such eyes that have a narrowed "middle segment," that is accentuated by increasing lens size with increasing age. An expanded vitreous volume, as is believed to occur acutely in the various malignant glaucoma syndromes, thus results in a secondary angle closure glaucoma. However, whether angle closure in all such cases finally results from the ciliary processes themselves, in response to this posterior pressure, pushing the iris into the angle, or whether in some cases the forward shift of the lens-iris diaphragm from the increased fluid pressure in the expanded vitreous itself directly pushes the iris into the angle is not certain. Likely in such eyes with expanded vitreous volume and a forward shift in the lens-iris diaphragm, there is some distortion of the anatomy of the posterior chamber and the zonules (the posterior zonules normally merge into the anterior hyaloid [1]).

In some cases in which vitreous pressure is hypothesized to be involved, the initiating event may be an increase in retinal volume (e.g., after central retinal vein occlusion, acute exudative detachment of the macula (2), or after panretinal photocoagulation) that conceptually acts on a "noncompressible" vitreous to shift the lens-iris diaphragm forward. Alternatively these conditions may themselves result in fluid movement into the vitreous cavity, which itself is expanded in volume as presumably occurs in syndromes involving massive vitreous hemorrhage. In either case, vitre-

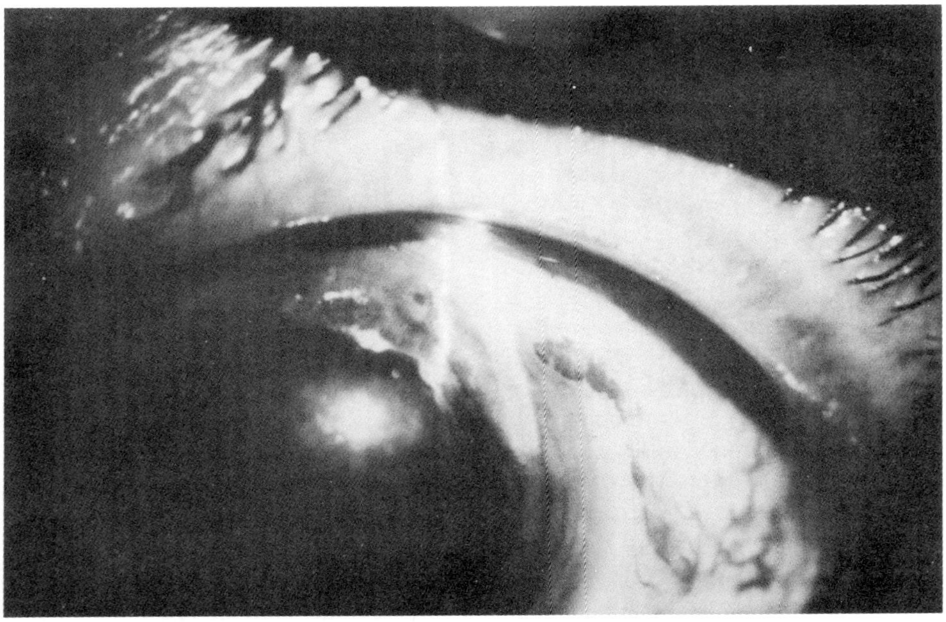

Fig. 28.1. Acute angle-closure glaucoma after a scleral buckling operation in the presence of a choroidal detachment. Although the pupil was dilated and unresponsive to miotics, laser iridectomy was nonetheless successful and lowered the IOP and opened the angle. Thus a pupillary block component to the angle closure existed, in the presence of a choroidal detachment.

ous volume acts as a "mass" to shallow the anterior chamber. The question as to why in some cases a shift in the lens-iris diaphragm occurs as a result of these diseases, and in other cases does not, will be discussed in Chapter 29, but it is believed to be a result of differences in constitutive "vitreous humor permeability" to fluid flow and transfer.

Thus these secondary angle closure glaucomas that involve "pressure from behind" the iris may result from mechanical forces from the ciliary body or the vitreous. As mentioned, the forward shift of the crystalline lens represents a separate additional mechanism–that of secondary pupillary block. A third possible mechanism, at least theoretically, is for the edge of the crystalline lens equator to itself directly push the iris into the angle. This might occur with a gross mismatch of the size of the crystalline lens to that of the middle segment of the eye, as might be conceived to occur in certain congenital conditions, nanophthalmos, or perhaps with cataract formation in certain "phacomorphic" glaucomas. We must all remember this possibility, especially as we face new entities of secondary angle closure glaucoma, but our suspicion is that such a postulated direct crystalline lens force acting on the iris itself (without an intervening effect of the crystalline lens on ciliary processes as proposed for malignant glaucoma) and independent of pupillary block, rarely if ever occurs because the equator of the crystalline lens likely does not extend far enough peripherally to close the angle. In fact, most cases of "phacomorphic glaucoma" (Chapter 47) are not due to this mechanism, but rather pupillary block (3) from the enlarged crystalline lens. Thus it is usually fluid pressure in the posterior chamber that exerts the force on the posterior iris surface to close the angle, i.e., pupillary block.

All these secondary mechanisms should be kept in mind as we now discuss the various specific entities that constitute the "secondary angle closure glaucomas" in the subsequent chapters. These mechanisms provide a unifying construct that explains how "pressure from behind" can cause the angle closure glaucoma. However, these are usually complicated cases, and we still have much to learn about the actual mechanisms involved. New syndromes or subgroups are inevitable as we increase our understanding. These concepts likely oversimplify what is occurring in individual cases, but these constructs do allow a framework in which to initially classify these conditions to eventually increase our understanding. In the short term, this will enable effective patient management. Some of these cases only behave as if the above were the mechanisms, but if these concepts result in appropriate treatment, then this is worthwhile.

It is important to remember that these conditions of "pressure from behind" can cause a **secondary pupillary block** mechanism due to the forward movement of the crystalline lens. A diagnosis of pupillary block needs to be initially entertained as at least one contributing factor, and the potential benefit of laser iridectomy contemplated (Fig. 28.1) In fact, certain conditions, such as malignant glaucoma, require the presence of a patent peripheral iridectomy for both diagnosis and therapy.

References

1. Streeten BW, Pulaski JP: Posterior zonules and lens extraction. Arch Ophthalmol 1978;96(1):132–138.
2. Wood WJ, Smith TR: Senile disciform macular degeneration complicated by massive hemorrhagic retinal detachment and angle closure glaucoma. Retina 1983;3(4):296–303.
3. Tomey KF, al-Rajhi AA: Neodymium:YAG laser iridotomy in the initial management of phacomorphic glaucoma. Ophthalmology 1992;99(5):660–665.

The Malignant Glaucoma Syndromes

29

David L. Epstein

The condition of malignant glaucoma (1,2), sometimes called "ciliary block glaucoma" (3,4) or "aqueous misdirection syndrome," either equivalently or only for certain clinical subtypes, is a dramatic form of secondary angle closure glaucoma that is sustained despite the presence of a patent peripheral iridectomy (ies). The signature of the condition is that of axial shallowing of the anterior chamber, i.e., the crystalline lens has moved forward (Table 29.1). Classically, malignant glaucoma is a postoperative condition after glaucoma filtration surgery, cataract or combined cataract/filtration surgery, or surgical peripheral iridectomy. It has not unequivocally been observed after laser iridectomy (although there have been a few reports [5-7]), in contrast to its noted occurrence after surgical iridectomy, and any explanation of possible pathogenesis must explain this difference.

Some have described forms of "malignant glaucoma" as a preoperative entity (8). Although we still have an incomplete understanding of this complicated disorder and we should not be too quick to dismiss new observations, most of these latter observations probably can be explained by other phenomena such as the normal forward movement of the crystalline lens under the influence of cholinergic drugs (9), primary choroidal detachment syndromes resulting in loosening of zonular tension and forward lens movement that accompanies the forward rotation of the ciliary body, undiagnosed crystalline lens subluxation, and certain poorly understood "loose lens" syndromes (see below). The malignant glaucoma syndromes may share certain common features, e.g., limited vitreous fluid permeability, with certain other conditions such as angle closure glaucoma secondary to central retinal vein occlusion (Chapter 35) or massive subretinal exudation (10). However, these latter conditions frequently resolve (although there may be sequelae from the angle closure episode). Malignant glaucoma is a sustained progressive process that characteristically results in blindness if not appropriately treated (11). **It is incorrect therefore to "lump" all flat chambers into a category of "malignant glaucoma."** The latter term should only be used to describe a postoperative condition of axial shallowing of the anterior chamber where other causes such as choroidal detachment and hemorrhage have been ruled out.

It is because of this characteristic progression to blindness that malignant glaucoma truly deserves to be called "malignant." (It is appropriate not to use the term "malignant" in front of patients because of the known connotation with "cancer," and therefore alternative terms may be used. However, the term "malignant glaucoma" is well established in the literature and among clinicians it seems appropriate to continue to use this and especially to avoid implications of diverse unproven mechanisms implied with use of alternative terminology.)

There is a rich heritage of thought concerning malignant (ciliary block) glaucoma. We owe a great debt to Shaffer, Chandler, Grant, and Simmons for the evolution of our concepts. The reader is referred to several classic publications (1-4,11-16).

DIFFERENTIAL DIAGNOSIS

It is important to state that not all postoperative angle closure glaucoma is "malignant glaucoma," nor are all postoperative "flat chambers" with elevated IOP (Table 29.2). **The diagnosis of malignant glaucoma requires at a minimum: 1. axial shallowing of the anterior chamber; 2. "elevated IOP"; 3. the presence of a patent iridectomy; and 4. the absence of suprachoroidal fluid or blood.**

When presented with postoperative angle closure glaucoma, even with axial shallowing, **the first diagnosis to be eliminated is pupillary block.** A patent iridectomy (that is not sequestered posteriorly) that allows free communication between posterior and anterior chambers needs to be present. The iridectomy usually placed at the time of surgery or subsequently with the laser must not be too central. If in doubt, the first step is to place another peripheral laser iridectomy. Again it must be remembered that axial shallowing of the anterior chamber, perhaps initiated by a transient wound leak, can bring the crystalline lens to the pupil and thus lead to pupillary block. (But, as discussed in Chapter 22, pupillary block by itself does not cause axial shallowing of the anterior chamber, only peripheral shallowing.)

In malignant glaucoma the IOP is "elevated." However, **in the presence of a functioning filtration bleb the IOP may not be very high**, e.g., only in the low teens. In contrast, when there is simply overfiltration and secondary choroidal detachment (Chapter 63) after filtration surgery, the shallow or flat anterior chamber is associated with a very low IOP, in the low single numbers, usually not in

Table 29.1
Features of Malignant Glaucoma

Feature	Comment
Post-operative condition	Malignant glaucoma only occurs in the post-operative setting, usually after filtering operations with or without cataract surgery, cataract surgery alone, or (historically) after surgical iridectomy.
Patient predisposition	Patients at greatest risk are those with a small, hyperopic eye, particularly those with a history of chronic angle closure glaucoma with peripheral anterior synechias.
Flat anterior chamber	Progressive axial shallowing of the anterior chamber is essential to the diagnosis.
Elevated IOP	IOP is higher than expected; with functioning filtering bleb IOP may be in the teens; however, IOP usually rises progressively.
Additional requirements	Patients should have a patent peripheral iridectomy and a dilated exam and ultrasound (B scan), if available, to rule out choroidal effusion or hemmorrhage.

Table 29.2
Differential Diagnosis of Malignant Glaucoma

Disorder	Comment
Suprachoroidal hemorrhage	Axial shallowing is often present; severe, acute pain; choroidal elevation on fundus exam or ultrasound; high IOP acutely but usually subsides within 12–24 hours.
Choroidal effusion	Usually patients are hypotonous; peripheral anterior chamber shallowing is common; axial shallowing is usually less prominent but may progress as choroidal effusions enlarge; pain is unusual; choroidal elevation is usually visible by fundus exam or ultrasound.
Secondary post-op angle closure following vitreoretinal surgery	Axial depth may be reduced in patients status post scleral buckling surgery, but usually only moderate in degree and not progressive; choroidal effusion may also be present in these patients.

the low teens. Thus, although malignant glaucoma is commonly thought of as a flat chamber with high IOP, this concept needs to be modified in the presence of a functioning filtration bleb. In fact, a good rule is that a flat or shallow anterior chamber associated with IOP in the teens after filtration surgery is malignant glaucoma (or suprachoroidal hemorrhage) until proven otherwise.

Bleeding into the suprachoroidal space, which is not rare after filtration surgery, especially when pharmacological antifibrotic therapy, e.g., with mitomycin, initially produces postoperative hypotony, actively occupies volume in the suprachoroidal space and thus acts as a "mass" that can rotate the ciliary body forward, release zonular tension, and result in forward crystalline lens movement in response to this "pressure from behind." **Delayed postoperative suprachoroidal hemorrhage can thus mimic malignant glaucoma.** This condition can be diagnosed by indirect ophthalmoscopy, ultrasound, or at the time of interventional surgery where a posterior sclerotomy is performed prior to vitreous surgery. (Such suprachoroidal bleeding occurs usually in a setting of postoperative hypotony that is accompanied by a secondary choroidal detachment with serous fluid. The latter acts to prevent clotting of the suprachoroidal blood.) Delayed suprachoroidal hemorrhage is a distinct entity and the term "malignant glaucoma " should not be used to describe it.

In contrast, the usual postoperative serous choroidal detachment associated with hypotony and overfiltration after filtration surgery is a secondary event, which may not in and of itself act as a mass to shallow the anterior chamber. One might oversimply view this as a secondary response to "fill the space" in a soft eye. However, **there are certain other conditions where a serous choroidal detachment can act as a "mass" seemingly to shallow the anterior chamber**, similar to the occurrence of suprachoroidal hemorrhage. Examples of such "primary" choroidal effusions include nanophthalmos (Chapter 30), conditions of increased orbital (and thus choroidal) venous (and accompanied episcleral venous) pressure such as dural shunt and Sturge-Weber syndrome (Chapter 46), and active uveal effusion syndromes including the one associated with HIV infection (17,18). All these conditions can cause a secondary angle closure glaucoma that is distinct from malignant glaucoma, and need to be first ruled out for a diagnosis of malignant glaucoma to be established.

At the time of this writing there seems to be a bevy of nonoperative flat chamber conditions associated with a **localized anterior choroidal detachment** that appears to be a "primary" phenomenon. These anterior uveal effusion syndromes are being defined by new ultrasound methods (19). Presumably there is some inflammatory component to these conditions as they seem to respond to corticosteroids and cycloplegics. In the past these conditions were probably described under categories of "ciliary body swelling" (20-22) or "loose lens syndromes." We have seen one similar case that appeared to be a result of an idiosyncratic systemic drug reaction (Chapter 36). We obviously have much more to learn about these conditions and other related presumed "loose lens" conditions, but these nonoperative conditions are not malignant glaucoma and do not involve a primary abnormality in the hyaloid which we believe to be the underlying and unifying mechanism involved in malignant glaucoma (23–26).

Malignant glaucoma is traditionally associated with smaller, hyperopic eyes. As will be discussed we believe that this may relate to the small "middle segment" of such eyes and the relationship to the anterior hyaloid. Certainly in such eyes which undergo cataract surgery or combined cataract/filtration surgery, the clinician should be "on guard" for postoperative malignant glaucoma. (All such eyes should have a surgical peripheral iridectomy at the time of surgery, even if simple cataract surgery alone is performed. There is a strong clinical sense that in many cases pupillary block may occur first, then is followed by malignant glaucoma, and thus this simple surgical iridectomy procedure might lessen the occurrence.) However, there are also other eyes that are not hyperopic which seem to develop a malignant glaucoma type-syndrome postoperatively. Some have used the term "aqueous misdirection" or other names to describe this occurrence, but clinically the condition behaves as malignant glaucoma and such a discrimination in terminology only can add to the confusion as to what to do clinically. As we will describe, it is proposed that a similar pathogenic mechanism is involved in "malignant glaucoma" whether the eye is hyperopic or not.

UNIFYING CONCEPTS IN PATHOGENESIS

There is much more that we need to learn about this condition that will lead to a better understanding of the events involved. One does not wish to oversimplify what is a complex process in eyes with complicated disease and the potential for multiple mechanisms of pathology. Yet there is a need for some template for our understanding, otherwise worsening confusion about what to do for the patient can result. (For example, lumping suprachoroidal hemorrhage or effusion into a malignant glaucoma category because of lack of clarity about the latter can interfere with appropriate clinical treatment.)

What do we know about malignant glaucoma clinically and also experimentally? **We know that disruption of the anterior hyaloid with the YAG laser by itself can cure phakic, aphakic, and pseudophakic forms of the disease** (25–31). We know from Chandler's observations (11,12) that puncture of the anterior hyaloid through an anterior approach can cure the condition both in phakic and aphakic eyes. We know that puncture of the hyaloid from a posterior sclerotomy approach (14,15), as will be described, can cure the condition in phakic malignant glaucoma, if one is far enough anterior. If one goes too far posterior (presumably posterior to the anterior hyaloid) in performing surgical vitrectomy, the condition of malignant glaucoma can recur (32). Also, although classically the posterior sclerotomy surgical operation was intended to aspirate a posterior pocket of aqueous humor "locked" in the vitreous, the procedure still worked even when liquid vitreous could not be aspirated (32) (presumably by the puncture itself disrupting the peripheral anterior hyaloid).

We know that mydriatic-cycloplegic therapy (13) can reverse malignant glaucoma in about 50% of affected phakic eyes, but there is risk of recurrence when the therapy is discontinued. Conversely, the use of miotics in postoperative eyes can precipitate the onset of malignant glaucoma.

We know that malignant glaucoma was not rare after surgical iridectomy, but is very rare (5–7) after laser iridectomy.

There is also a strong clinical sense that wound leak, even if transient, or overfiltration (33) may predispose an eye to malignant glaucoma, and such events seem to be a common theme in non-hyperopic eyes which develop this condition.

What do we know experimentally (23, 34)? At least in enucleated human eyes we know that if we direct the normal rate of aqueous humor flow (2-3 microliters/minute) totally into the vitreous, malignant glaucoma does not result (23,24). In fact, in such circumstances the anterior hyaloid and vitreous offer insignificant resistance to forward fluid flow. Thus, it would seem that aqueous humor secreted into the posterior chamber normally has free access into (and out of) the vitreous cavity (35). On the other hand, if one limits the amount of available hyaloid for fluid transfer (34), there is substantial resistance to forward fluid flow from the vitreous and vitreous volume continues to expand if aqueous humor continues to be directed into the vitreous cavity, and the anterior chamber then shallows. Further, when the anterior chamber is initially decompressed (then reestablished), this process is accentuated (23).

Although the above is true experimentally for the normal aged (enucleated) human eye, in certain subprimate species such as the enucleated calf eye, the hyaloid normally demonstrates much more resistance to fluid flow (23). Thus there are differences among species in hyaloid permeability and likely also among individuals. The hyperopic human vitreous may be more viscous and restrictive than that in the myopic eye.

Putting this all together we propose that **the anterior hyaloid, either because of inherent "permeability" or the amount of available hyaloid surface area for fluid transfer, is involved in the pathogenesis of the malignant glaucoma syndromes** (Fig. 29.1). **Thus, a maintained increase in total vitreous volume (rather than the presence of sequestered pockets of aqueous humor in the vitreous) is responsible for the axial flattening of the anterior chamber.** Expanded vitreous volume can obliterate available peripheral anterior hyaloid for fluid transfer by movement of the hyaloid into apposition with the posterior ciliary body. In this "silent zone" just behind the posterior chamber (and in continuity with it) there is likely great variation in the amount of space between the hyaloid and ciliary body under baseline conditions (36). In the hyperopic eye with a crowded middle segment the peripheral anterior hyaloid in its normal position is probably quite close to the posterior ciliary body.

Decompression of the anterior chamber as happens with surgical procedures (but not laser iridectomy) might pro-

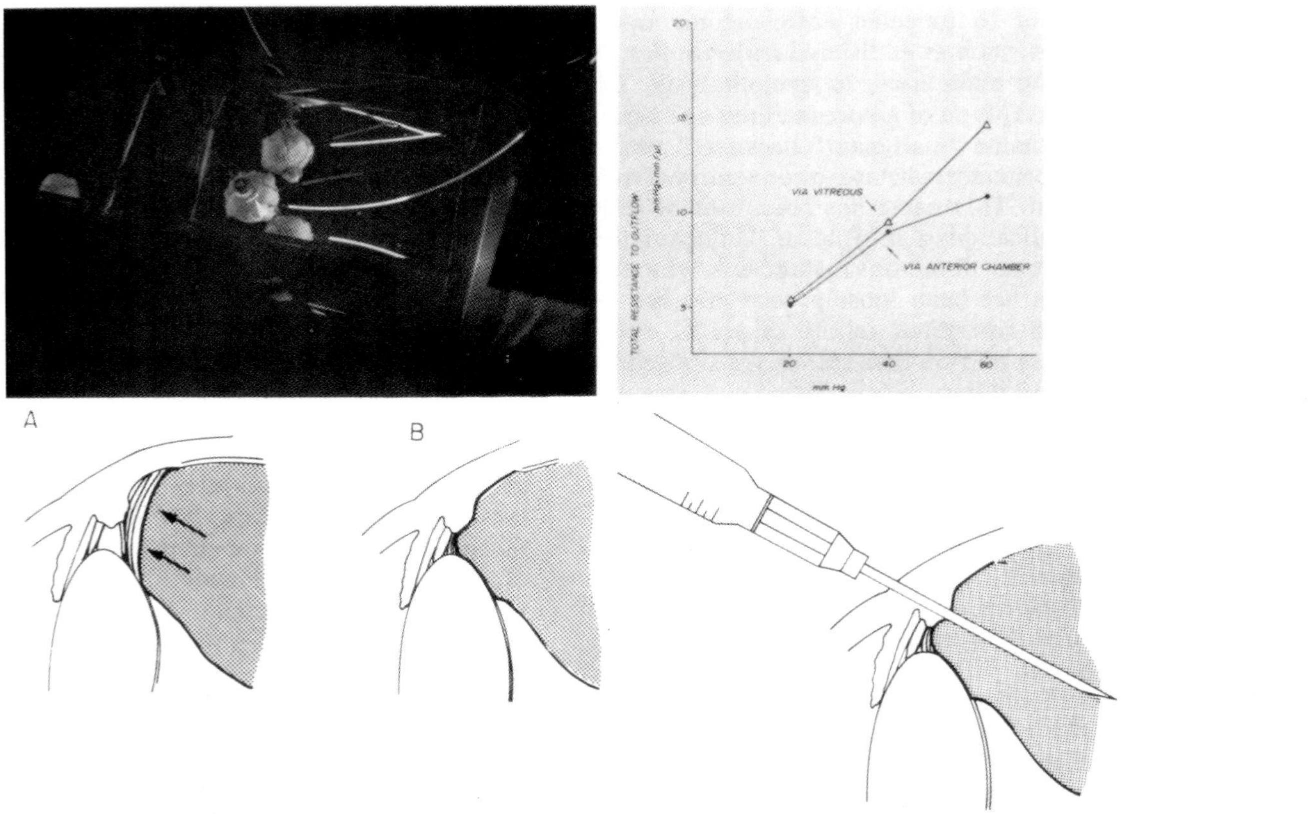

Figure 29.1. (Top left) Experimentally, if mock-aqueous humor containing fluorescein is introduced into the vitreous of an enucleated human eye, it is observed to move into the anterior chamber and to exit the eye by way of the limbus (arrowhead). (Top right) At conditions of normal IOP and flow the vitreous offers insignificant resistance to fluid flow whereas at elevated pressure and flow, substantial resistance exists to flow through the vitreous. (Bottom left) Proposed scheme to explain this observation and that of malignant glaucoma involves the expansion of vitreous volume (A) with movement of the peripheral anterior hyaloid into apposition with the posterior ciliary body (B), consequently decreasing available hyaloid surface area for fluid flow. (Bottom right) In malignant glaucoma, it is necessary to puncture this peripheral hyaloid (and perhaps also reduce vitreous volume) in order to eliminate the hyaloid as a fluid flow barrier. Reprinted with permission from Epstein DL, Hashimoto JM, Anderson PJ, et al: Experimental perfusions through the vitreous and anterior chambers; possible relationship to malignant glaucoma. Am J Ophthalmol 1979;88:1078–1086, and Epstein DL: Malignant glaucoma. In: Advanced Techniques of Ocular Surgery. Edited by F. Jakobiec and J. Sigelman. Philadelphia, W.B. Saunders Co., 1984; 158–168.

duce movement of the peripheral anterior hyaloid further forward into apposition with the ciliary body. In fact, if one accepts the concept of possible zonular distortion from anterior chamber decompression, one can hypothesize that with this forward movement the anterior hyaloid (which is continuous with the posterior zonules [37]) could be placed into direct apposition with portions of the secreting ciliary processes, even in phakic eyes. Thus aqueous humor might move directly into the vitreous cavity. This is a hypothesis (and there are other possibilities for the cause of the initial expansion of vitreous volume that is then maintained in an expanded condition from the resulting obliteration of hyaloid surface area), since this process cannot be directly visualized in the phakic eye. On the other hand, this has been directly observed to have occurred in certain aphakic eyes where the hyaloid "coated" the surface of the ciliary processes (2). Presumably this can also develop in pseudophakic eyes (26) with any type of zonular disruption.

The decompression of the anterior chamber that occurs with surgical peripheral iridectomy does not occur with laser iridectomy, and results in the movement forward (and peripheral) of the anterior hyaloid, contributing to the above events wherein the anterior hyaloid permeability/surface area is limited. **An important clinical corollary of this would seem to be to minimize this decompression—related shallowing of the anterior chamber both intra- and postoperatively.** For example, at the time of filtration surgery, especially in hyperopic eyes at greater risk, using viscoelastic in the anterior chamber to prevent shallowing intraoperatively might be useful. Using a "tighter" rather than "looser" scleral flap with judicious use of suture lysis (one suture at a time) might minimize the chance of postoperative anterior chamber shallowing due to overfiltration that could then lead to a malignant glaucoma process (33). We believe this approach is beneficial, and, in fact, is what we would recommend as a general strategy.

This concept would explain the observed efficacy (25-31) of the YAG hyaloidotomy procedure in phakic, aphakic, and pseudophakic eyes and the above clinical experience with surgical techniques that have indicated the need for anterior enough positioning (32) to disrupt the anterior hyaloid. Surgical decompression during predisposing operations could explain the initiating event that brings the hyaloid to the ciliary body, that leads to the sustaining effect of expanded vitreous volume which shallows the anterior chamber. Mydriatic-cycloplegic therapy might be effective, as originally intended, to tighten the lens-zonular diaphragm (13) to resist this "force from behind," but also because cycloplegic drugs act to dilate the ciliary body ring (38) and thus potentially could move the ciliary body outward away from the peripheral anterior hyaloid. Conversely, cholinergic miotics might narrow the ciliary body ring and move the ciliary body closer to the hyaloid.

One also could conceptualize that if it is possible to restore the normal anatomy and the small space normally present between the peripheral hyaloid and the ciliary body in the "silent zone" (36), then without other reinitiating events, such as repeat decompression of the anterior chamber, the vicious cycle could be broken. As detailed below there has been a strong clinical impression that with the surgical technique for malignant glaucoma an essential component was, in fact, to re-establish the normal anatomy and even expand the anterior chamber at the end of the operation and "push" things backward behind the iris (32).

Understanding this construct allows one to appropriately diagnose and treat affected patients clinically. For example, **an attempt should always be made, at least in the pseudophakic eye, to disrupt the hyaloid (and intervening tissue such as residual lens capsule) with the YAG laser to allow a channel for free communication between the posterior segment and anterior chamber before using surgical vitrectomy** (26). It is curious how in certain geographic locations pseudophakic eyes with malignant glaucoma are treated initially with vitrectomy. Yet the critical role of the anterior hyaloid in the pathogenesis seems clear from both clinical and experimental data.

What there is still a lingering sense of dissatisfaction with in this (and any other) construct is in understanding what, in fact, is the initiating event in this whole process; that is, how is vitreous volume initially expanded?

Decompression of the anterior chamber surgically and the resulting movement of the peripheral hyaloid to the ciliary body would explain the different incidence of malignant glaucoma between surgical and laser iridectomy (and there seem few good alternative explanations) and there is some experimental data that is consistent with this (23). With zonular distortion that might result from this anterior chamber decompression it is possible that the peripheral hyaloid might come directly into apposition with the ciliary processes, and aqueous humor could conceivably be secreted into the vitreous chamber directly across the apposed hyaloid. Yet all this doesn't seem quite "whole enough" to fully explain the true initiating event.

Perhaps with the sudden onset of pupillary block, that may precede other events, aqueous humor is suddenly forced into the vitreous. That is, some non-steady state event occurs. We do know clinically that in the surgical procedure for malignant glaucoma if one, in reforming the anterior chamber, directs too vigorously balanced salt solution over the peripheral iridectomy which is presumably close to the underlying anterior hyaloid, vitreous volume can suddenly expand and be maintained and a recurrence of malignant glaucoma produced. Alternatively, we know that there is a constant movement of fluid derived from aqueous humor posteriorly to the retina, presumably under the influence of the retinal pigment epithelium pump (39-44). It is possible that with the onset of pupillary block and high IOP this posterior pump is impaired and vitreous volume suddenly expands (45). There is a report of one human eye enucleated shortly after an attack of untreated angle closure glaucoma which purportedly did show an expanded vitreous volume (and obliteration of the space between the peripheral hyaloid and ciliary body) (46).

Understanding the initiating event is nevertheless still a "missing piece of the puzzle" which, if elucidated, might provide important new insights. Yet there still is good understanding based on both clinical experience and laboratory experimentation on which to now successfully treat most patients with this condition. In a former era malignant glaucoma syndromes were truly blinding (11). Most likely the initiating event involves some non-steady state phenomenon or anatomical distortion that results in a maintained increase in vitreous volume, which then requires disruption of the anterior hyaloid to reestablish the normal steady state. **From a clinical point of view, the (peripheral) anterior hyaloid needs to be disrupted and thus eliminated as a fluid barrier.**

(If there are sequestered spaces in the vitreous due to inflammation, etc., the hyaloid potentially needs to be disrupted in multiple locations to permit free communication between the vitreous cavity and the anterior chamber, as is normally the situation.)

CLINICAL OCCURRENCE AND THE EXAMINATION OF THE PATIENT

The usual clinical situation is that of a postoperative patient following filtration, combined cataract/filtration, or cataract surgery. Malignant glaucoma can occur any time during the usual postoperative period of day(s) to weeks to occasionally months. Commonly there is an indication of the condition on the first postoperative day.

Important times when the possibility of malignant glaucoma should be kept in mind are **following suture lysis** (33) at the filtration site (where shallowing of the anterior chamber associated with a sudden increase in outflow can subsequently lead to malignant glaucoma. Another time to keep in mind is when routine postoperative cycloplegics are stopped. In the latter situation the cycloplegics may have prevented the occurrence of the condition by their therapeutic effects of tightening the lens-zonular diaphragm and dilating the ciliary body ring.

One begins by carefully examining the filtration bleb or cataract wound. As discussed above, shallowing of the anterior chamber due either to overfiltration or a wound leak (that may have been transient) might initiate the subsequent development of a malignant glaucoma process. Further, a shallow chamber from overfiltration or a wound leak needs to be differentiated from malignant glaucoma. In the former situation the IOP is low, whereas in malignant glaucoma it is generally "high," although again it needs to be emphasized that with a functioning filtration bleb the IOP might not be very high, e.g., only in the low teens. In simple overfiltration with a shallow anterior chamber, the IOP should be in the low single numbers, not in the low teens. Or stated another way, **following filtration surgery with an IOP in the low teens the anterior chamber should not be shallow**. Special attention to possible artifacts needs to be considered when measuring the IOP in the presence of a flat chamber (47).

In a susceptible hyperopic eye a postoperative shallow anterior chamber due to overfiltration should be more vigorously treated than that in a myopic eye. Such eyes need to be followed very carefully for development of a malignant glaucoma process.

What is the axial depth of the anterior chamber (as well as peripheral depth)? Has there in fact been axial shallowing? What is the contour of the iris (is there a convex forward peripheral ballooning of the iris suggestive of pupillary block)? Is the iridectomy patent? Is it far enough peripheral beyond the lens equator? Could the iridectomy be sequestered posteriorly? Has swelling of the crystalline lens occurred (that might be simulating axial anterior chamber shallowing and malignant glaucoma)?

Gonioscopy should be performed to confirm closure of the angle, assess the contour of the iris and the patency of the iridectomy, as well as to look for retro-iridal abnormalities. In choroidal effusions the ciliary processes may be rotated forward pressing against the base of the iris. Choroidal detachments or hemorrhage, if anterior, can sometimes be seen well through the mirrored Goldmann-type examination lens. **In malignant glaucoma quite commonly the tips of the ciliary processes are observed to overlap anteriorly the edge of the crystalline lens equator.** Presumably this is a manifestation of the inherently crowded "middle segment" of the eye.

Indirect ophthalmoscopy should be performed looking for possible choroidal detachment or hemorrhage as alternative diagnoses. In addition, possible conditions of acute central retinal vein occlusion (see Chapter 35), massive submacular (10) or vitreous hemorrhage, etc., which could cause a secondary angle closure glaucoma with shallowing of the axial anterior chamber depth that may mimic malignant glaucoma (but possibly also share some common mechanisms wherein vitreous volume in only certain such patients does not decrease to accommodate the new "mass" of the lesion) should be evaluated.

Ultrasound (19,31) may aid in the determination of possible choroidal disease entities such as effusion or hemorrhage which might simulate malignant glaucoma. As might be expected from the above discussion of underlying mechanisms, ultrasound–detected abnormalities in the vitreous are not to be expected (there is an increase in total vitreous volume with perhaps the usual normal areas of less dense lacunae occasionally, but no mystical pockets of "trapped" aqueous humor). In fact, except in the case of vitreous hemorrhage producing a "pseudo-malignant" glaucoma syndrome, no vitreous pathology has been consistently observed in malignant glaucoma.

MANAGEMENT OF MALIGNANT GLAUCOMA

The approach to the management of patients with a flat anterior chamber postoperatively is methodical (Table 29.3). Any bleb or wound leak needs to be first addressed. Likely if malignant glaucoma has developed as a subsequent process, the accompanying inflammation of the eye has resulted in a stoppage of such leakage, but not always. In fact, a continued wound leak, once malignant glaucoma has occurred, may confuse the clinical picture since the IOP may not be very high. If there is any suspicion of a wound leak or overfiltration, this should be treated first while the patient is in the office. If there is no bleb, a large soft contact lens that bridges well over the surgical site can be placed on the eye, and commonly if there is a wound leak, some deepening of the anterior chamber may be observed in 30 minutes. In contrast, if there is a large bleb and if there is suspicion of overfiltration, a Simmons scleral contact lens (48-50) and/or a pressure dressing with direct pressure over the filtration site should be performed. Some anterior chamber deepening would be expected within an hour. A pressure dressing could be used also in place of a large soft contact lens for a presumed wound leak, but is less predictable (see Chapter 63).

The key to the potential success of the Simmons shell, which has a platform on the underside that can exert pressure on the filter or wound site, is the stability of the positioning. There are some eyes where the "shell" can be placed without any eye patching and good position

Table 29.3
Management of Malignant Glaucoma

	Comment
Rule out choroidal hemorrhage or effusion	Fundus exam and/or ultrasound.
Rule out overfiltration or wound leak	Seidel test; oversized contact lens, pressure patch or Simmons shell in hypotonous eyes.
Rule out pupillary block	Laser iridectomy if functional iridectomy not present.
Medical therapy	
Cycloplegics: cyclopentolate or tropicamide 1% qid	Short term cycloplegics are more potent than those that are longer acting and are therefore preferred for initial management.
Mydriatics: phenylephrine 2.5–5% qid	
Aqueous suppressants: timolol 0.5% or equivalent bid, apraclonidine 0.5% tid, acetazolamide 250 mg po q6h (or dorzolamide 2% tid)	Question patient for contraindications for phenylephrine, beta blocker, carbonic anhydrase inhibitor or osmotic therapy and monitor for systemic side effects.
Osmotics: glycerin, isosorbide, or mannitol 1–1.5 gm/kg q12h for no more than 24 hours without medical consult	Osmotics should be considered optional therapy, but there may be a rational basis for their use (see text).
Chronic medical therapy (after acute medical treatment success): atropine 1% bid or scopolamine 0.25% bid	Patients may require permanent treatment with long acting cycloplegics to prevent recurrence of malignant glaucoma; tapering medication should be done slowly and under close observation.
Hyaloidotomy with Nd:YAG laser in aphakic or pseudophakic patients	Should be performed concomitantly with medical therapy in patients who have had cataract surgery.
Surgical vitrectomy	It is essential that the retinal surgeon disrupt the hyaloid face and confirm that the normal anterior chamber depth has been restored at the end of surgery.

is maintained, at least for several hours, which will help establish the correct diagnosis. In other patients rotation and slippage (with undesired pressure on the cornea) occurs, but may respond to pressure patching over the shell tamponade site.

The use of a pressure dressing (Chapter 63), is both diagnostic and therapeutic—it seems often that once an anterior chamber deepens and presumably normal anatomy is restored, the "eye may tend to take over" and further resolution occurs (49). Obviously for this to occur the wound leak will have had to stop and/or overfiltration will have to decrease. The latter may have already begun spontaneously, but the anterior chamber is still shallow presumably because there is a "new steady state" with the choroidal detachment, although originally only a secondary occurrence, now persisting until IOP can be more dramatically elevated by the pressure dressing (which suddenly can limit the outflow from the eye).

Next the adequacy of the surgical iridectomy needs to be assessed. The iridectomy may be too central (which only became a problem when the initial overfiltration perhaps brought the crystalline lens forward), or sequestered posteriorly. Is the peripheral iris ballooned forward as if there were pupillary block? **If in doubt whether pupillary block exists, another laser iridectomy should be performed usually at a site remote from the surgical site.** (Sometimes at the surgical site zonules may be partially dehisced, allowing vitreous to come forward that will not allow free communication for aqueous humor secreted into the posterior chamber to come forward freely into the anterior chamber.) The reason a peripheral iridectomy is performed at the time of filtration surgery is to prevent pupillary block and also, perhaps even more importantly, to prevent the iris from rolling into the fistula site and thus occluding it. If there is any doubt that the original surgical iridectomy might not be accomplishing this, then a laser iridectomy at the surgical site would be indicated.

Except in this circumstance, it is usually best to place a laser iridectomy at a site remote from the fistula wound to rule out the above "complicated situation" in the posterior chamber that may have been surgically induced (broken zonules, inflammatory lacunae, etc.). The laser iridectomy should also be placed so that a YAG hyaloidotomy could be subsequently performed through it, as often there is overlying corneal edema and a hazy optical view overlying the original surgical iridectomy site. In the case of a cataract wound which may be extensive, one can still place the laser iridectomy superiorly, but perhaps away from the original iridectomy and also away from any location where there may have been an adjacent wound leak. It is technically easier in these usually "hot" eyes to perform the laser iridectomy prior to cycloplegic therapy, if this has not already been instituted, while the pupil is still somewhat small.

The next step classically (but now after laser iridectomy) would be the use of mydriatic-cycloplegic therapy (13) in phakic and pseudophakic patients with intact zonules for five days prior to surgical vitreous surgery. Nowadays with

THE HISTORY OF MYDRIATIC-CYCLOPLEGIC THERAPY

David L. Epstein

The origin in thought and history of mydriatic-cycloplegic therapy (1) for malignant glaucoma is of interest. Grant and Chandler in a dialogue about a specific patient with malignant glaucoma reasoned that if the lens-zonular diaphragm could be "tightened" by this therapy, it could resist the pressure from behind. In their first eight subsequent cases such mydriatic- cycloplegic therapy worked successfully in all eight (1). However, in their next six cases after this publication, this therapy did not work at all, and DLE and all those trained by Chandler recall with much poignancy conversations with him and Dr. Grant where they with humility and humor wondered what would have happened if the latter six cases (where the treatment was unsuccessful) had been the initial patients chosen! They wondered how many other procedures for other glaucoma conditions that ultimately would prove to be effective might have been abandoned too prematurely! In the subsequent years mydriatic-cycloplegic therapy has, in general, demonstrated a 50% success rate for the treatment of malignant glaucoma.

Reference

1. Chandler PA, Grant WM: Mydriatic-cycloplegic treatment in malignant glaucoma. Arch Ophthalmol 1962;62:353–359.

the possibility of true "cure" with a successful YAG hyaloidotomy, and considering the danger of recurrence of malignant glaucoma once cycloplegics are stopped, it is not certain in straightforward cases whether the next step should be mydriatic-cycloplegic therapy or YAG hyaloidotomy. Two points are worth making here: often these are complicated cases and it is not known what the exact diagnosis is at the beginning, and if the IOP is controlled medically (see below) and there is no cornea lens touch, it is not an emergency for YAG hyaloidotomy to be performed. In fact, there is a point to quieting the eye first with topical steroids which might make the procedure easier to perform technically (certainly after corneal edema is reversed with lowering the IOP and there is quieting of the eye). Also, there might be less chance for a recondensation of the hyaloid (25) in a quieter eye. On the other hand, the longer the angle is closed, especially in a "hot" eye, the greater the risk of permanent peripheral anterior synechias. Nevertheless, a reasonable tactic is to lower the IOP medically with aqueous suppressants (beta blockers, apraclonidine, and possibly carbonic anhydrase inhibitors) while simultaneously initiating mydriatic-cycloplegic drug therapy. Also, thought should be given to using osmotics (51) to lower the IOP but also temporarily to dehydrate and thus decrease vitreous volume. The only caution should be is that if one does too many maneuvers simultaneously, it may be difficult to define exactly what is beneficial, and also the osmotic effect on vitreous volume may be only temporary. Theoretically using the above construct of malignant glaucoma, decreasing aqueous humor formation with the aqueous suppressants might also act to decrease vitreous volume by decreasing new fluid flow into the vitreous humor cavity (35).

Mydriatic-Cycloplegic Therapy

It needs to be remembered that mydriatic-cycloplegic therapy is meant for phakic, not aphakic, eyes (where there are no zonules to tighten). In phakic eyes mydriatic-cycloplegic therapy has a 50% success rate. Also, curiously in the past there were occasional aphakic cases and patients with anterior chamber intraocular lenses after intracapsular cataract surgery where this therapy was also successful. Because cycloplegic therapy may move the ciliary body ring outward (38) away from the hyaloid, this may be explainable by this mechanism. Also, in aphakic eyes the vitreous may coat the whole posterior surface of the iris and surface of the ciliary body, thereby resulting in a limited hyaloid surface area for fluid transfer into the anterior chamber (24,26) that might respond beneficially to dilatation of the pupil (thus increasing the amount of hyaloid surface area in the pupil). Thus it may be the mydriatic effect in aphakic eyes that is beneficial rather than the cycloplegic. In previous eras there was much effort in distinguishing aphakic forms of this condition from phakic, as obviously there are gross anatomic differences between such eyes. Yet the above unifying concepts of malignant glaucoma relating to the anterior hyaloid seem applicable, and more importantly lead to effective therapeutic remedy in phakic, aphakic, and now pseudophakic forms of this condition.

The use of a sympathomimetic mydriatic in addition to a cycloplegic drug demonstrated empirical efficacy and perhaps can be explained by the above pupil effects in certain cases, perhaps also even in some phakic eyes, but more classically its effectiveness was felt to be due to the contraction of the iris dilator muscle and thus the tightening of the iris tone, which might then resist pressure from behind. In addition, the sympathomimetic drugs were believed to a minor extent to also contract the sympathetically innervated radial fibers of the ciliary muscle (52) and thus to also help tighten the zonules between the ciliary muscle and crystalline lens.

Originally very high strengths of phenylephrine (10%) and atropine (up to 4%) with frequent (four times a day) instillation were utilized, and are still advocated by some. The clinician needs to be cautious about the occurrence of systemic side effects (53-55) with this, or even with a reduced, regimen. More commonly now 1% cyclopentolate (or tropicamide) and 5% phenylephrine are instilled and the effects observed, especially on the axial anterior chamber depth. It must be remembered that the shorter acting cycloplegics such as cyclopentolate or tropicamide actually produce a greater short-term effect than the longer acting cycloplegics such as atropine or scopolamine. The latter agents are more useful in maintaining cycloplegia and mydriasis once initiated. A regimen of 1% atropine and 5% phenylephrine twice a day (with monitoring for systemic side effects) may be initiated for the first five days of therapy and if successful, the phenylephrine can be discontinued and the 1% atropine maintained once a day.

There is substantial risk of recurrence of the malignant glaucoma process once the cycloplegics are stopped. Therefore even with initial success of mydriatic-cycloplegic therapy, the performance of YAG hyaloidotomy as an elective procedure should be contemplated. In cases in which YAG hyaloidotomy is unsuccessful but cycloplegic therapy is successful, most clinicians have felt that continuance of the medical cycloplegic treatment indefinitely was indicated rather than performance of the surgical procedure. Such cases are becoming very rare as we have learned more about YAG treatments and the need to establish communication from the posterior segment to the anterior chamber by removing intervening barriers (in pseudophakic eyes) in addition to the anterior hyaloid.

YAG Hyaloidotomy

The goal of this procedure (25,26) is to disrupt the peripheral anterior hyaloid without injuring the crystalline lens (in the phakic patient), ciliary body, or zonules. **A clear view and sharp focusing is required.** Depending on circumstances this procedure may be performed without any laser contact lens or with an iridectomy or gonioscopic lens.

The usual beginning laser energy is between 4 and 6 millijoules. Obviously one needs to obtain optical breakdown at the level of the hyaloid, and with murky media or oblique angles of access, higher energy levels are sometimes required. Since with "plasma formation" (56) at the site of laser focus, energy moves anteriorly, it is common to focus posterior to the anterior hyaloid. Sometimes, in truth, one cannot visualize the hyaloid that readily, but one places the focus through the iridectomy behind the zonules but in front of the ciliary body with the plan of having forward moving energy disrupt the hyaloid.

As indicated above, with an inflamed eye with corneal edema, one may resort, after placing a new laser iridectomy, to utilize medical mydriatic-cycloplegic and antiglaucoma (aqueous suppressant) therapy for 12 hours or so. The goal of the new iridectomy is to eliminate any residual pupillary block component and permit another access site for a hyaloidotomy.

Clear media and sharp focusing are optimal requirements. Simpler aiming beam mechanisms on the YAG laser are an advantage because often there is some distortion due to the quality of the media. In choosing where to place the preliminary new iridectomy these factors affecting the potential subsequent hyaloidotomy should be considered.

One attempts to obliterate the hyaloid within the circumference of the overlying (small) iridectomy, although sometimes one "shot" is all that is required. A single burst should be used for the first "shot" until one is certain where one is in the retro-iridal space, but then a multiple burst mode can be chosen. If one uses the above retrofocusing strategy, one might then choose to come slightly forward with the second laser application. Sometimes with suboptimal media clarity one needs to proceed slowly and "feel one's way" forward in this retro-iridal space. But each shot should be precisely focused and orderly and it is important to avoid a "machine-gunner approach." That extra "wide" shot potentially could injure the crystalline lens if present, or the ciliary body and zonules.

It is usual to notice a slight deepening of the anterior chamber immediately after this YAG procedure which increases somewhat over the next hour. **Commonly dramatic deepening of the anterior chamber is not noticed until 12-24 hours after the YAG hyaloidotomy.** The explanation for this is not certain but possibly might relate to the relatively small size of the "hyaloid opening" in relation to the expanded vitreous volume. If no deepening is observed at all, then either one has not in fact obliterated the limiting anterior hyaloid membrane, or somehow, perhaps due to sequestered spaces of hyaloid due to inflammation, etc., there is still not free communication from the posterior segment into the anterior chamber (through the iridectomy). As will be discussed below, in a pseudophakic eye one needs to be certain that lens capsule, retained cortical material, inflammatory debris, or the intraocular lens is not blocking this path (26). In a phakic malignant glaucoma condition these should not be factors and one should choose to repeat this (including a new iridectomy) in another peripheral location or to do a central hyaloidotomy (27) carefully using the principle of retrofocusing (to avoid crystalline lens injury).

Many of these cases are complicated with somewhat hazy views and inexact focusing, but one of us (DLE) has had the opportunity in several, mostly pseudophakic cases to proceed step by step placing optical breakdown from the YAG in different discreet locations with the following clinical observations: in pseudophakic eyes not only the peripheral hyaloid but also all intervening tissue such as lens capsule and residual cortical lens material must be perforated to allow full access of the flow pathway from vitreous space to the anterior chamber through the iridectomy. Also, **a central hyaloidotomy may not be sufficient because the central space so created may not communicate with the anterior chamber because of the intervening lens capsule and intraocular lens.** For example, in one patient, after a central anterior hyaloidotomy that was ineffective, a subsequent posterior capsulotomy was also unsuccessful until the posterior capsule underlying a positioning hole in the intraocular lens was subsequently removed with the YAG. Then the anterior chamber suddenly deepened! In another case a peripheral and central hyaloidotomy and a central posterior capsulotomy were all unsuccessful until the posterior capsule in front of the original peripheral anterior hyaloidotomy was removed. **There must be a free path for fluid to move from the posterior segment (vitreous cavity) to the anterior chamber.** In general, this is easier to achieve through the peripheral rather than central hyaloid face.

Complicating this further has been the occurrence of inflammatory recondensations of the hyaloid. We have directly observed this in aphakic eyes (25) where the YAG procedure was initially successful, but then a recurrence of the malignant glaucoma occurred associated with an observed reformation of the anterior hyaloid (Fig. 29.2). Likely in "hot eyes" that have malignant glaucoma there is the potential for some restricted spaces in the vitreous cavity and especially in the "silent zone" of the peripheral "middle segment" of the eye, where ciliary body and hyaloid are in close proximity. We have suspected that this phenomenon may underlie some failures of the YAG procedure.

One must proceed more cautiously and deliberately in a phakic eye because of the risk and consequences of crystalline lens or zonular injury. Yet there seems to be less problems with obstructing post-surgical intervening tissue and, in fact, central hyaloidotomy has been reported to be effective by itself (27). Nevertheless, one of us (DLE) would recommend a peripheral approach through a peripheral laser iridotomy with careful retro- focusing in the retroiridal space being attentive not to be at the depth of the ciliary body, but well in front of it, and slowly moving forward but attempting to avoid the zonules (as well as the edge of the crystalline lens). The clinician must be sensitive to the sudden partial deepening of the anterior chamber (which will evolve further to full deepening without need for additional laser applications) as a sign to cease additional laser applications.

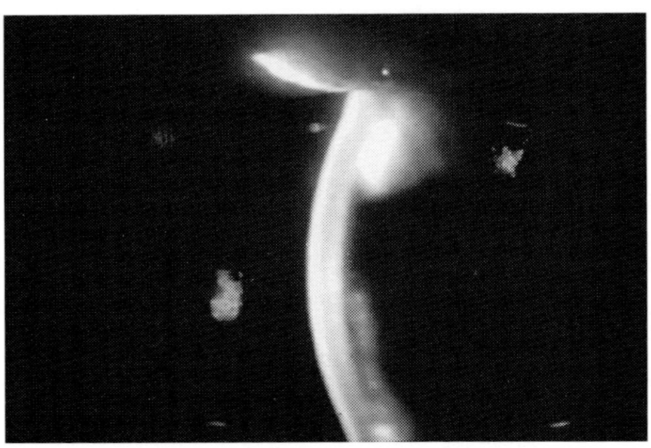

Figure 29.2. Aphakic malignant glaucoma. On two occasions YAG hyaloidotomy reversed the process, but post- treatment fibrotic recondensation of the hyaloid occurred necessitating surgical vitrectomy.

Vitreous Surgery

In patients in whom YAG hyaloidotomy and medical therapy have failed, vitreous surgery can almost always cure this condition. Pseudophakic eyes with malignant glaucoma are referred usually to the retina surgeon for vitrectomy, which can be curative if the peripheral anterior hyaloid is removed as a barrier as a result of the procedure. **The most critical portion of the operation is removal of the hyaloid barrier rather than the removal of the vitreous.** However, removal of vitreous may allow restoration of the normal anatomy more quickly by allowing anterior and mid-eye structures to move posteriorly into their more normal position. Such vitrectomy is the proper province of the retina surgeon, but it must be remembered that the original "Chandler operation" was performed by anterior segment glaucoma surgeons, and such surgery is still curative, and perhaps less involved than vitrectomy, especially if there is limited visibility.

Simmons (57) definitively described this vitreous puncture and aspiration technique for malignant glaucoma:

Corneal Paracentesis

STEP 1, CORNEAL PARACENTESIS

A beveled paracentesis incision is made peripherally in the cornea with a Wheeler knife or similar instrument to provide easy access to the anterior chamber for later injection of fluid and air. If the bevel follows a path through the cornea about 1.5 to 2 mm in length from the anterior to posterior surface of the cornea, a suture is not required at the end of the procedure to close it, because the wound will be self-sealing. This incision should be tested with a slender cannula or needle to be sure it provides easy entry.

STEP 2, EXPLORATION FOR SUPRACHOROIDAL FLUID

Radial sclerotomies are performed in both lower quadrants with a No. 15 Bard-Parker blade (or a No. 57 Beaver blade). The sclerotomies should be about 3 mm long and centered at a measured distance of 3.5 mm from the limbus

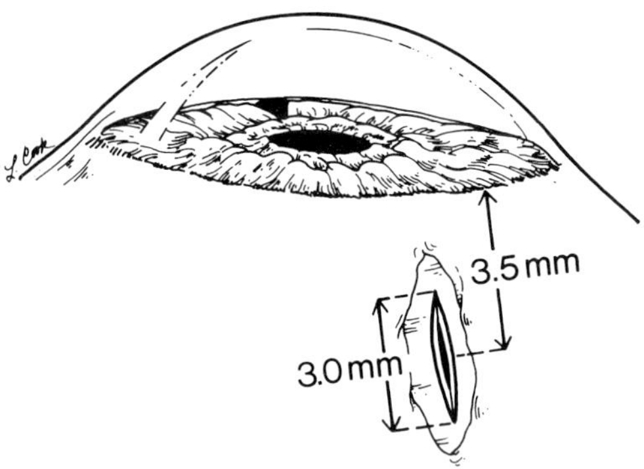

Figure 29.3. The size of the sclerotomy incision is 3.0 mm in length and it is centered 3.5 mm posterior to the limbus. Reprinted with permission from Simmons RJ, Thomas JV: Malignant glaucoma. In: The Secondary Glaucomas, Edited by R. Ritch and M.B. Shields. St. Louis, C.V. Mosby Co., 1982.

(Fig. 29.3). If a choroidal separation or suprachoroidal hemorrhage is present, suprachoroidal fluid or blood will be found, but no fluid is found in malignant glaucoma. If the fluid is found, it should be allowed to drain. Whether or not fluid or blood escapes spontaneously from the sclerotomy openings, a smooth spatula such as a standard cyclodialysis spatula should be passed circumferentially from the lips of the sclerotomy in the suprachoroidal space parallel to the limbus in both directions, since on occasion fluid or blood can be present between choroid and sclera which does not flow freely from the sclerotomy until this maneuver has been performed.

If suprachoroidal fluid is found and is drained, the anterior chamber should then be re-formed with saline solution through the preplaced corneal paracentesis wound, and the surgical procedure can be terminated, since a diagnosis of choroidal separation or suprachoroidal hemorrhage, instead of malignant glaucoma, will have been established with certainty. The sclerotomy procedure provides both diagnosis and treatment.

However, if no fluid is found and the anterior chamber remains shallow or flat, despite a patent coloboma of the iris and posterior sclerotomies, the diagnosis of malignant glaucoma is established with certainty, and it can now be treated definitively by surgery on the vitreous body.

STEP 3, VITREOUS SURGERY FOR MALIGNANT GLAUCOMA

The rationale for surgery on the vitreous body is based on the working hypothesis that aqueous humor is somehow diverted and entrapped in or behind the vitreous body, pressing lens, ciliary processes, and iris forward. The surgery is intended to establish an opening through the anterior hyaloid membrane and vitreous body for aqueous humor to escape forward to the posterior and anterior chambers.

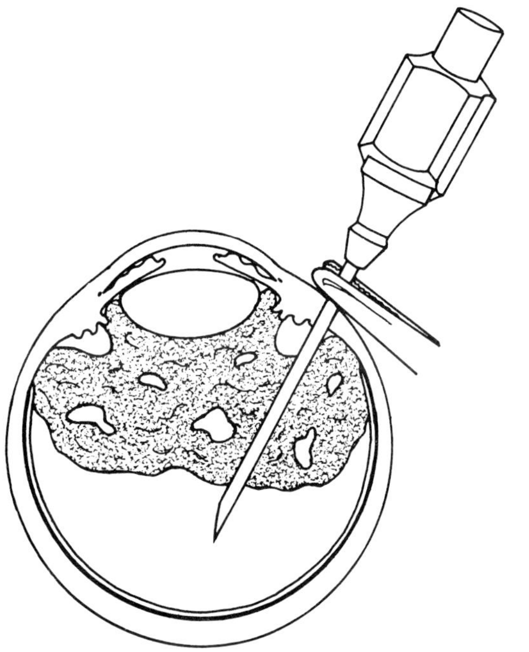

Figure 29.4. Eighteen-gauge needle is inserted 12 mm into the eye. A hemostat is used as a guard to control depth of the needle. Reprinted with permission from Simmons RJ, Thomas JV: Malignant glaucoma. In: The Secondary Glaucomas. Edited by R. Ritch and M.B. Shields. St. Louis, C.V. Mosby Co., 1982.

A ring of surface diathermy is placed around the scleral wound using a strong radio frequency diathermy current with a conical electrode and sufficient power to produce brown discoloration of the sclera, and one must be sure that the ciliary body is touched with the diathermy. This diathermy is used to prevent bleeding from the ciliary body when it is later pierced. When this has been done, bleeding has not been a problem. A Wheeler knife is plunged in a quick motion through the ciliary body 3.5 mm from the limbus into the vitreous cavity with the point of the knife aimed toward the optic nerve to avoid injuring the lens. The wound in the ciliary body is slightly enlarged anteriorly and posteriorly to a total length of about 3 mm, with its center 3.5 mm behind the external limbus.

A **sharp** 18-gauge intravenous needle is then introduced, but first a hemostat is clamped on its shaft a measured distance of 12 mm from its point in order to prevent it from penetrating excessively deep into the globe (Fig. 29.4). The needle is then passed through the scleral-uveal wound into the vitreous cavity toward the optic nerve. After it has been inserted to the measured depth of 12 mm, its tip is moved back and forth in an arc of about 4 mm, intending to cause slight separation of vitreous membranes in its path. (If the eye is extremely hyperopic, 8, 10, or more diopters, the eye is shorter axially and the needle should not be passed to a depth of more than 10 mm, because of the risk of injuring the retina in such a short eye.) Then a glass hypodermic syringe, such as a 5-

ml Luer-lock syringe, is attached to the needle. This is done by the assistant, because the surgeon must carefully observe and control the position of the needle within the eye using both hands. When the syringe is attached to the needle the surgeon continues to maintain the position of the needle with one hand, and with the other hand aspirates 1 to 1.5 ml. The fluid thus obtained may be watery or may consist of vitreous of varying consistency. Before the needle is withdrawn from the vitreous cavity, approximately 0.25 ml of what has been aspirated is injected back into the eye, in order to clear the tip of the needle of vitreous strands that may have been engaged within its lumen. The needle is then carefully drawn from the eye exactly along its path of entry. The eye at this point is expected to be markedly hypotonic, with folds in the cornea and sclera. The shape of the globe is now partially restored by injecting less than 1 ml of saline solution into the anterior chamber through the previously placed beveled corneal incision. It is important in this step that the amount of fluid injected is limited, so that the eye is not filled completely. If so much saline solution is injected that it fills the globe, it behaves in some cases as though it flows back into and behind the remaining vitreous humor and recreates the original malignant glaucoma. If this happens, a second operation must be done. Instead, after the shape of the globe is only partially restored with a limited amount of saline solution, a larger air bubble is injected into the anterior chamber to fill it completely and force the iris and lens posteriorly. The air bubble should be large enough to deepen the chamber artificially to a greater depth than is usually encountered in a normal myopic eye (Fig. 29.5). This will be a much greater depth than is naturally found in eyes predisposed to primary angle-closure glaucoma or malignant glaucoma. Even after injection of the large air bubble the eye should still be hypotonic. It is important not to fill the eye completely to normal shape or IOP. If there is measurable pressure within the eye, too much saline solution has been injected. A sterile Schiotz tonometer or palpation with a muscle hook can be used to be sure.

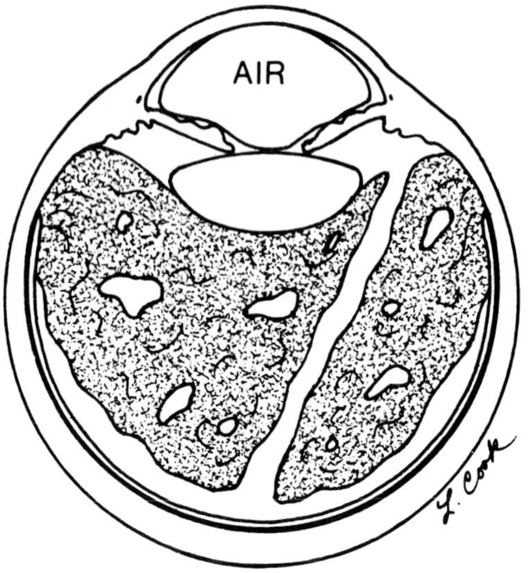

Figure 29.5. The air bubble should be large enough to deepen the chamber to a depth greater than usually encountered in a normal myopic eye. Reprinted with permission from Simmons RJ, Thomas JV: Malignant glaucoma. In: The Secondary Glaucomas. Edited by R. Ritch and M.B. Shields. St. Louis, C.V. Mosby Co., 1982.

The scleral wounds are each closed with a single interrupted suture and then the conjunctival wounds are closed.

POSTOPERATIVE CARE

Atropine is instilled at the end of the operation and is continued for several weeks or until the eye is quiet. We have had no instances of recurrence of malignant glaucoma when cycloplegics were discontinued after a successful vitreous aspiration procedure. In three additional cases, miotics were later used, without a recurrence of malignant glaucoma. If shallowing of the anterior chamber should occur in some case in the future, we would immediately resume the use of cycloplegics.

RELIABILITY AND COMPLICATIONS

This procedure for malignant glaucoma has been used extensively by us and by some of our colleagues since it was first performed by one of us (PAC) in 1965. The procedure has proved safe and effective when used precisely as described. We have learned, however, that careful attention to detail is essential. In a number of instances colleagues have discussed with us complications or failures that have occurred in their hands. In each instance, when the exact methods they used in performing the procedure were reviewed, it was found that the procedure had been altered in one way or another, departing from the recommended protocol that we have outlined. For example, a colleague reported hemorrhage into the suprachoroidal space and vitreous cavity at the time the procedure was carried out, but review of the procedure revealed that diathermy had not been applied as prescribed around the wound of entry prior to piercing the ciliary body. In another instance, colleagues reported ineffectiveness of the procedure in their hands, but when the technique that they had employed was analyzed it was found that in the last steps of the procedure they had been inserting a much smaller air bubble than recommended, too small to deepen the anterior chamber effectively. When the same surgeons instilled a large quantity of air into the anterior chamber, as recommended to force the lens, iris, and anterior vitreous body posteriorly, the procedure became effective in their hands.

Another deviation that can cause failure and that has done so in a number of cases that we have learned of, is making the incision in the sclera too far posteriorly, e.g., centered 5 or 6 mm behind the limbus instead of the 3.5 mm recommended. We think that the specified anterior placement of the wound for vitreous puncture is probably essential, since it is calculated to be anterior to the normal vitreous base, so that the anterior hyaloid membrane is punctured as the knife and the needle are introduced into the vitreous cavity. The site of this wound would be measured carefully. We think it should not be less than 3.5 mm posteriorly to the limbus for fear of injuring the lens.

Another error is not to use a sharp needle for the procedure. We are aware of surgeons who mistakenly utilized a blunt-tip vitreous aspirating needle and were unsuccessful.

Occasionally the air bubble instilled in the anterior chamber slips partially or totally behind the iris at the time of surgery or in the first day or two after surgery. The chamber then appears flat, but on careful inspection one can see that the air bubble is behind the iris. This should not be interpreted as a recurrence of malignant glaucoma. The air bubble can usually be shifted into the anterior chamber by movement of the patient's head or eye with the pupil dilated. Even if this cannot be immediately accomplished, the air bubble gradually absorbs and the anterior chamber reforms.

Small punctate retinal hemorrhages have been detected postoperatively in a few eyes when they have been examined by indirect ophthalmoscopy, but these have not caused any difficulty.

Postoperative choroidal detachment has occurred in about a third of our cases, but the choroidal separation has been transient. It is important to distinguish it from a recurrence of malignant glaucoma. With choroidal separation the anterior chamber may be shallow or flat, but the eye is soft, and choroidal elevation in the peripheral fundus is usually visible.

Despite careful adherence to the surgical protocol, we have had several cases in which malignant glaucoma was not relieved the first time the vitreous aspiration procedure was performed. In these cases we have merely resumed medical therapy for 2 to 3 days and then performed the procedure again. After the second operation, all eyes have responded with relief of the malignant glaucoma.

In three cases, all relatively young individuals, when we tried to aspirate from the vitreous cavity with the 18-gauge needle, very little fluid could be drawn into the syringe. We withdrew the needle and attempted to inject air into the anterior chamber even though it was flat, but very little air could be injected. We then resumed atropine therapy and the full medical regimen for malignant glaucoma, and to our surprise in all three cases the eye responded to the medical therapy, although it had been unresponsive prior to the surgical procedure. This suggests that the puncture of anterior hyaloid and vitreous body, even without aspiration of fluid, was enough in these cases to disrupt the malignant glaucoma mechanism. In one of these cases we found some months later that, for treatment of glaucoma due to residual peripheral anterior synechias, miotic therapy could be resumed without causing a recurrence of malignant glaucoma.

The use of a miotic after operation for angle-closure glaucoma may precipitate malignant glaucoma, but after malignant glaucoma has been relieved by vitreous puncture and aspiration, the situation is changed. The following case is an instance in which a miotic was used postoperatively without a return of the malignant glaucoma. We know of several similar cases, including one in which echothiophate iodide 0.25% was used twice daily for years without recurrence of the malignant glaucoma. Thus it appears safe to use a miotic where indicated after vitreous puncture and aspiration for malignant glaucoma.

Case 29-1. A 49-year-old woman's ophthalmologist found a closed angle in both eyes and did a peripheral iridectomy on the left eye. The anterior chamber in that eye remained shallow or flat despite atropine, acetazolamide, and mannitol. When seen here IOP was right 60 and left 30. In the right eye there was no light perception; the disc was cupped and atrophic. The left showed deep saucerization of the disc throughout; the anterior chamber, was ½ corneal thickness deep in the center, flat elsewhere.

Vitreous puncture and aspiration were done. The chamber formed but remained somewhat shallow. Two weeks later gonioscopy showed some peripheral anterior synechias, but it was thought that the residual glaucoma could probably be controlled medically. IOP was 20. One week later IOP was 27. She was given epinephrine, and 5 months later a report from her ophthalmologist stated that IOP had varied between 15 and 19, vision 6/7.5. One month later IOP was found to be 34; she was then given pilocarpine. IOP with epinephrine and pilocarpine since then has been 18 to 20, and there has been no return of the malignant glaucoma.

TREATMENT OF THE FELLOW EYE

If malignant glaucoma occurs in one eye, there is great risk of the fellow eye developing the condition postoperatively. Prophylactic laser iridectomy should almost always be performed in cases where there is evidence for chronic angle closure or an occludable angle exists. If the fellow eye is at all hyperopic, it may be wise to perform the prophylactic laser iridectomy. Chandler and Grant had a strong clinical sense that eyes with functional angle closure, especially with peripheral anterior synechias, were at greatest risk for the subsequent development of malignant glaucoma, and as mentioned, there also is a sense that pupillary block may precede the occurrence of malignant glaucoma in many cases. Thus it would seem wise to eliminate any pupillary block ahead of time in any eye that might be predisposed to malignant glaucoma.

As mentioned, at the time of intraocular surgery on such fellow eyes steps should be taken to minimize intraoperative and postoperative anterior chamber shallowing.

OTHER ENTITIES RESEMBLING MALIGNANT GLAUCOMA

Principles

There are some nonoperative conditions that may, at first blush, behave similarly to malignant glaucoma in that they are characterized by high IOP and a flat (axial) anterior chamber depth. As argued above, however, these should not be classified as malignant glaucoma because it confuses the clinical management, as well as obscures understanding. The mechanisms involved in these other entities are likely each different and probably distinct from true malignant glaucoma at least with respect to the primary mechanism (which in malignant glaucoma involves some abnormality in the anterior hyaloid). And yet secondarily these processes might share some similar mechanisms.

Prior to discussing some of these entities such as "loose lens" or "ciliary body swelling," the above principles may be easiest to understand in the context of the unusual secondary angle closure glaucoma that may occur following acute central retinal vein occlusion (Chapter 35). In this condition there is axial shallowing of the anterior chamber that is believed to be due to either an increase in retinal volume or vitreous fluid volume subsequent to the central retinal vein occlusion. Unlike true (postoperative) malignant glaucoma, this condition will spontaneously resolve.

The question for one of us (DLE) has always been not why this condition occurs, but why it occurs so uncommonly. The usual increase in retinal or vitreous volume that occurs in this condition should act as a "mass" in all patients to move the crystalline lens forward. However, it seems that in most patients this posterior volume "mass" does not transmit such a "force" through the vitreous to the crystalline lens. Rather the vitreous gives up part of its own volume to accommodate this temporary increase in posterior segment volume. Fluid must move out of the vitreous in most such patients, and as discussed, experimental data suggests that normal vitreous, in fact, offers little resistance to such fluid flow. A minority of patients develop this secondary angle closure syndrome. Perhaps it occurs in those who are hyperopic or have "restrictive" hyaloid permeability or available surface area. The vitreous does not give up volume, and therefore the increase in posterior segment volume subsequent to the central retinal vein occlusion does act as a "mass" to shallow the anterior chamber axially. If this construct is correct, YAG hyaloidotomy should act in such cases to reverse the "flat chamber," but unlike true malignant glaucoma this process will spontaneously resolve with the decrease in posterior (retinal) volume that is part of the natural history of the vein occlusion.

Thus in some cases with this "other entity" of secondary angle closure glaucoma, **some other process that occupies posterior segment volume may secondarily involve hyaloid factors in producing a shallow anterior chamber both axially and peripherally.** Similarly, in conditions where there is an increased volume in the suprachoroidal space, either from hemorrhage, tumor, or primary effusion, there may occur, depending on inherent "permeability" factors of the hyaloid and such vitreous volume considerations, flattening of the anterior chamber. Also occurring in this situation is forward rotation of the ciliary body with loss of zonular tension and the potential "loosening" of the crystalline lens position. But even if these conditions require the maintenance of normal vitreous volume to transmit the "force" from behind, this is not the same clinical condition as postoperative malignant glaucoma which arises from different causes and can only be cured through therapy directed at the hyaloid. In these other entities which involve increased posterior segment volume, the disease can be cured by, e.g., draining the suprachoroidal blood or fluid (or perhaps in the latter case treating the initiating inflammation) without the need or even indication for hyaloid therapy. Thus these conditions are not only different in regard to primary events, but also as to required therapy, and therefore the term "malignant glaucoma" is not appropriate for these other entities.

Consider also the following: there are cases of primary or secondary retinal detachment where the retina is totally detached and comes into close approximation with the posterior crystalline lens capsule, yet the observed anterior chamber depth axially is not shallow. How could this happen? Somehow the vitreous "gave up its volume" to the detached retina without itself acting as a mass to move the crystalline lens forward. In other words, the vitreous gave up fluid volume. Such eyes, that have such a voluminous retinal detachment, are commonly myopic and likely such vitreous, unlike the hyperopic vitreous seen in malignant glaucoma, is quite freely permeable to fluid. One might (with some license) simplify this and conceptualize that in such cases the vitreous had its watery fluid easily "squeezed out" in response to this force from behind, and therefore did not act as a force to move the crystalline lens forward.

There are many diseases that involve an increase in posterior segment volume as a primary process, that may or may not shallow the anterior chamber depending on the inherent vitreous hyaloid "permeability" of the individual involved, but these diseases are distinct from primary malignant glaucoma.

Purported Loose Crystalline Lens Syndromes

There are a variety of clinical cases which are characterized by a forward crystalline lens position and the absence of pupillary block. These are usually but not always nonoperative eyes, and in this way and others, distinct from malignant glaucoma. Also, in these cases there is no evidence for choroidal hemorrhage, central retinal vein occlusion, malignant melanoma, etc., that would occupy posterior segment volume. In the absence of any other apparent primary cause, they have often been called "loose lens syndrome."

These cases are typically unilateral and there is commonly no choroidal effusion visible on indirect ophthalmoscopy, otherwise they would have been classified with the known primary uveal effusion syndromes that are usually but not always felt to be inflammatory. **A recent such syndrome involves the occurrence of primary uveal effusion and secondary angle closure with HIV infection** (17,18).

New ultrasound techniques have indicated that some patients with presumed "loose lens" syndrome actually have **unsuspected small anterior choroidal detachments**. Such syndromes of far anterior choroidal detachment are probably not new and share features with what Phelps described as cases of "ciliary body swelling." (20–22). In the latter entity, which was difficult to totally define because of the uncertainty of what a "swollen" ciliary body (58) or process actually looked like when viewed gonioscopically, inflammation was felt to be involved and the eyes were commonly injected. Scleritis can cause such an inflammatory choroidal detachment syndrome (59–62). These conditions resolved (probably this was not a single homogeneous entity) with use of topical steroids and cycloplegics. However, some of these mentioned "new cases" of anterior choroidal detachment may not show obvious ocular inflammation, although they may respond to the use of cycloplegics and (often systemic) steroids.

We have observed one case of unsuspected anterior choroidal detachment, which was only visible with new ultrasound techniques, that was due to an idiosyncratic systemic drug reaction (Chapter 36). The condition resolved simply with cessation of such systemic therapy. (It failed to respond to cycloplegic therapy.) Thus, **a localized anterior choroidal (ciliary body) detachment may represent a common final mechanism from multiple causes for such an apparent syndrome.**

In these conditions the forward rotation of the ciliary body results in loosening of zonular tension and allows forward movement of the crystalline lens.

However, it is doubtful that such localized anterior choroidal detachments can explain all such cases of apparent "loose" crystalline lens. Likely there is more than one entity in this "basket," and we may learn further from some of our patients if we can understand these conditions better.

One of us (DLE) observed one such case, following blunt trauma to the eye, that demonstrated an apparent unilateral forward subluxation of the crystalline lens (without any horizontal or vertical component). The axial chamber depth shallowed further under the influence of cholinergic drugs (miotics), but did not deepen with cycloplegic therapy. No zonular dehiscence was visible with maximal pupillary dilatation, but the crystalline lens behaved as if it were "loose" in the anterior-posterior direction. Some have suggested that there are similar cases with spontaneous weak zonules due to exfoliation (63,64).

There are also some cases which may be caused by swelling of the crystalline lens and evolving (albeit slowly) cataract formation. In such cases the axial depth of the anterior chamber is somewhat shallow and asymmetrical to the fellow eye, and the normal response (in some eyes) of cholinergic therapy to cause forward crystalline lens movement (9) may then simulate a "loose lens."

In evaluating all such phenomena, it is important to contemplate and carry further the above concepts and discussion of the vitreous sometimes acting as a force to move the crystalline lens forward. We have discussed why sometimes with a new "mass" in the posterior segment, e.g., retina or choroid, the vitreous may give up volume or not, and in the latter case act as a force to move the crystalline lens forward. But here we need also to discuss the following: why in some patients with accommodation and release of zonular tension, the crystalline lens not only changes its curvature but moves anteriorly. An exact understanding of this is not available, but it seems clear that in some patients with accommodation there is anterior crystalline lens movement and in others none. It would seem that the "turgor" of the vitreous might be an important factor explaining this difference. In fact, it has been proposed that the normal mechanism of accommodation involves a narrowing of the ciliary body ring with resultant pressure on the vitreous which transmits this pressure to the crystalline lens posterior surface, with the potential, at least in some patients, for forward lens movement (38). Such a construct could also explain the clinical fact that cholinergic miotics can precipitate the onset of malignant glaucoma by moving the ciliary body inward to the hyaloid.

Regardless, it would seem plausible that with loss of zonular tension from trauma as in the above case, or from forward rotation of the ciliary body with occult anterior choroidal detachment syndromes, or with new entities that can cause an apparent loose lens syndrome that we do not yet understand, that loss of zonular tension is not enough in itself to explain forward movement of the crystalline lens. Rather the position of the crystalline lens is also determined by the support (force) from the vitreous. Obviously vitreous turgor may differ in different patients, and might be expected to be greater in hyperopic eyes (with thus the potential for more forward crystalline lens movement). However, such a mechanism is not equivalent to malignant glaucoma, although factors of vitreous "turgor" might be important in both conditions.

In these "loose lens syndromes" the mechanism of angle closure glaucoma is usually due to pupillary block which can be effectively treated with laser iridectomy. Of course the axial depth remains shallow and of concern to the clinician, especially if there is any possibility of crystalline lens-cornea touch. Very rarely (if ever) the crystalline lens might be so large (for the middle and anterior segments of the eye) that conceivably the edge of the crystalline lens might itself push the iris into the angle and cause a secondary angle closure by this mechanism (see Chapter 28). But this must be an exceptionally rare occurrence.

Of course, if there is some **dehiscence of zonules**, vitreous can come forward into the posterior chamber and cause angle closure glaucoma due to a pupillary block type mechanism (aqueous humor normally secreted into the posterior chamber does not have free circumferential access to the iridectomy because of the vitreous coming forward through the broken zonules). It is in such cases that more than one iridectomy may be required to alleviate pupillary block, and the possibility of such a condition is another reason why the general "first rule" described above for dealing with "flat chamber" cases is to place a new iridectomy. Theoretically, if there is extensive zonular dehiscence, vitreous may move forward through enough of the posterior chamber circumference so that aqueous humor is being secreted into or behind the vitreous (see Fig. 29.6), and a "malignant glaucoma"-like condition (in a non-operated eye) might be produced. One of us (DLE) has not really seen this clinical situation, although it remains a theoretical possibility. For practical purposes such cases of usually traumatic subluxed lenses usually involve mechanisms of pupillary block that respond to peripheral iridectomy (usually just one, but sometimes two in order to place one away from the area of zonular dehiscence).

This discussion should not imply that most cases of "loose crystalline lens" syndrome are in fact due to zonular dehiscence. There are likely a variety of causes that we have not fully categorized but we need to understand better. Commonly there is some cataract formation in these "unknown" cases, but even if not, all else failing, the condition seems to be "cured" by removal of the lens. It is noteworthy that the feeling among clinicians who have seen such cases is that with cataract surgery with a posterior chamber lens, such patients do well. Obviously if there were an underlying anterior choroidal detachment this might not be expected, at least in these subgroups. This clinical observation raises the possibility that the abnormality might well have been in the crystalline lens itself (and the possibility therefore, for example, of having misinterpreted the findings of an evolving cataract with a normal response to miotics in terms of crystalline lens position, or of some subclinical zonular weakness that the posterior chamber intraocular lens subsequently is not subject to). On the other hand, there might be other explanations for this observed benefit from cataract surgery.

These entities may constitute complicated clinical situations with more than one mechanism involved in individual cases. Regardless, in terms of malignant glaucoma the following differentiating points, which are generally believed to be true, should be kept in mind: **in true malignant glaucoma, cataract surgery, including the use of intracapsular surgery, was curative only when there was accompanying vitreous loss (and the hyaloid face was broken)** (11). In contrast, in loose crystalline lens syndromes that ultimately seem to come to cataract surgery, the latter is most often curative by itself without the occurrence of vitreous loss. This suggests that malignant glaucoma and certain "loose lens syndromes" share an abnormality in crystalline lens position (or size) but not in hyaloid "permeability."

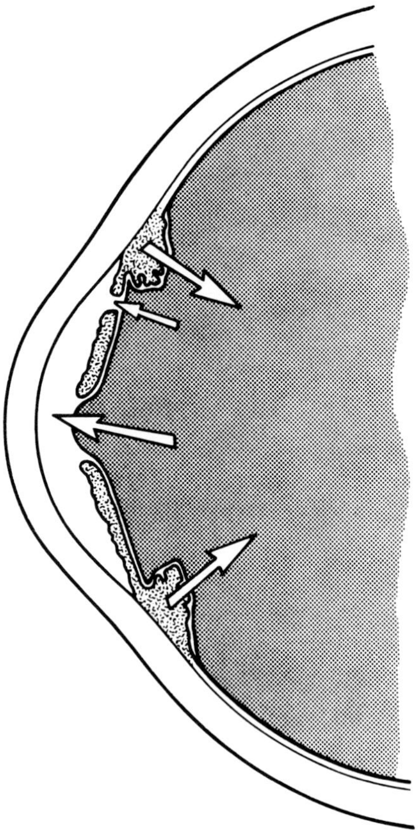

Figure 29.6. Concept of aphakic malignant glaucoma. The vitreous is apposed to the posterior iris surface and no aqueous humor-filled posterior chamber space is present. Aqueous humor moves into the vitreous (arrows) from the ciliary body and it must pass across a limited surface area of anterior hyaloid (arrows) in order to enter into the anterior chamber. The anterior hyaloid can act as a restrictive barrier to such fluid movement. Reprinted with permission from Epstein DL, Steinert RF, Puliafito CA: Nd-YAG laser therapy to the anterior hyaloid in aphakic malignant (cilio-vitreal block) glaucoma. Am J Ophthalmol 1984;98: 137–143.

MALIGNANT GLAUCOMA IN APHAKIA

With the virtual disappearance of planned intracapsular cataract surgery, cases of aphakic malignant glaucoma with or without an anterior chamber lens (Fig. 29.7) are now rarely seen.

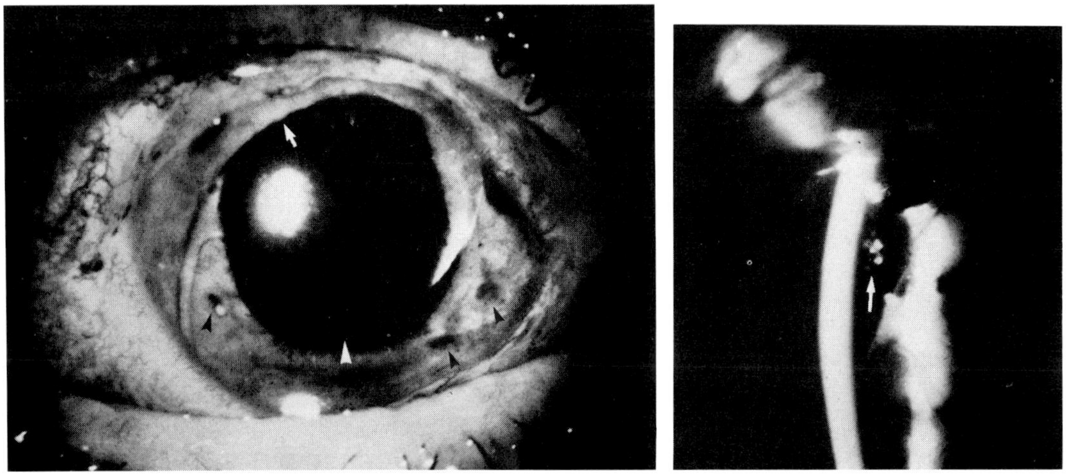

Figure 29.7. (A) On the first postoperative day after routine intracapsular cataract surgery with two peripheral iridectomies and an anterior chamber intraocular lens, the anterior chamber is shallow and IOP 53. Despite three subsequent patent argon laser iridectomies (black arrowheads), the anterior chamber remained shallow. The anterior hyaloid fills the space (white arrowhead) between the dilated iris pupillary margin and implant optic, and surrounds the optic (white arrow). (B) After Nd- YAG laser treatment to the anterior hyaloid, the anterior chamber has dramatically deepened. Loose vitreous is present in the anterior chamber (arrow). Reprinted with permission from Epstein DL, Steinert RF, Puliafito CA: Nd-YAG laser therapy to the anterior hyaloid in aphakic malignant (cilio-vitreal block) glaucoma. Am J Ophthalmol 1984;98:137–143.

The one exception is when such eyes rendered previously aphakic must now undergo filtration surgery. Therefore, the clinician should still be aware of this entity. Also the understanding and treatment of aphakic malignant glaucoma was an important milestone (25) in the development of the unifying concepts of this disease entity, which are explained above, but are now detailed further:

We explain this condition of aphakic malignant glaucoma as follows: In pure aphakic pupillary block there is an aqueous humor filled posterior chamber, at least in a portion of the circumference. Therefore a laser iridectomy, by establishing communication with this aqueous humor space behind the iris, equalizes pressure in the posterior and anterior chamber and allows free communication of aqueous humor from ciliary body to anterior chamber. However, in aphakic malignant glaucoma there is total obliteration of the posterior chamber "aqueous" space by vitreous humor and its hyaloid membrane which is apposed to the posterior iris surface (Fig. 29.6). **Aqueous humor moves directly from the ciliary body into the vitreous humor, and in order to pass into the anterior chamber must cross a limited surface area of anterior hyaloid, which may be thickened or abnormally impermeable.** When a laser iridectomy is performed, there is no free communication of aqueous humor from posterior to anterior chamber, because vitreous is present behind the iridectomy. To establish free communication and equalize pressure in the posterior and anterior segments, the limiting membrane of the vitreous, the anterior hyaloid, must be disrupted.

In the past this involved a deep surgical incision of the hyaloid or an anterior vitrectomy, but we utilized the neodymium YAG laser in several cases to disrupt the hyaloid either in the pupillary area or through the iridectomy to cure this condition (25) (Fig. 29.7). The observed dramatic cure with the YAG laser underscored the importance of the hyaloid in this condition. Often the hyaloid appears thickened in this condition, but a limited hyaloid surface area for fluid flow may also be involved as indicated by our experimental studies (23,24).

We observed this condition most commonly after anterior chamber intraocular lens implants with intracapsular surgery and wondered whether a slightly larger implant may have pushed the iris posteriorly toward the vitreous and favored the occurrence of this condition. However, it must be remembered that aphakic malignant glaucoma was a well known entity prior to the advent of intraocular lenses.

In evaluating a patient with an aphakic (or pseudophakic) flat chamber postoperatively, one wants initially to rule out wound leak and choroidal detachment. IOP is usually low in such conditions, except with suprachoroidal hemorrhage or rare forms of choroidal effusion. However, a transient wound leak can lead to pupillary block by allowing vitreous to move forward and iridectomies to become adherent to the wound. This is less of a problem with fine, permanent sutures such as 10-0 nylon which can be placed deeply, but can be quite common with sutures such as silk or various absorbable sutures that are placed too deep. Especially with silk sutures a transient shallow chamber can occur several weeks after surgery when deep sutures develop a small amount of surrounding tissue necrosis.

The wound should be inspected, a Seidel test performed, and any suspected deep suture removed (especially if it is several weeks postoperative). If a wound leak is detected, a pressure patch with local tamponade over the limbus (as with use of the glaucoma shell (48–50) or a soft contact lens or Simmon's shell should be applied. Aqueous humor suppressant therapy can be used to reduce aqueous flow through the fistula. However, obvious wound leaks should be surgically repaired, the secondary choroidal detachment drained, and the anterior chamber reformed surgically.

Most often in such cases no wound leak is apparent, and the IOP is at least moderately elevated. In these cases laser iridectomy should then be performed to rule out pupillary block. If there is already a patent surgical coloboma, it is unlikely that pupillary block is the mechanism, but it is best to perform one additional iridectomy with the laser. This is to be sure that there is not an aqueous humor filled posterior chamber space in at least one segment. If laser iridectomy fails to deepen the anterior chamber, then the YAG laser should be used to disrupt the anterior hyaloid through the iridectomy (or through the pupil if the hyaloid is easily visualized next to the pupillary margin). In several cases this proved dramatically successful in normalizing the anterior chamber depth, but in one observed case the effect was temporary, and surgical vitrectomy was required (25).

References

1. Chandler PA: Malignant glaucoma. Am J Ophthalmol 1951;34:993.
2. Shaffer RN: The role of vitreous detachment in aphakic and malignant glaucoma. Trans Am Acad Ophthalmol Otolaryngol 1954;58:217–231.
3. Weiss DI, Shaffer RN: Ciliary block (malignant) glaucoma. Trans Am Acad Ophthalmol Otolaryngol 1972;76:450–461.
4. Shaffer RN, Hoskins HD: Ciliary block (malignant) glaucoma. Trans Am Acad Ophthalmol Otolaryngol 1978;85:215.
5. Brooks AM, Harper CA, Gillies WE: Occurrence of malignant glaucoma after laser iridotomy. Br J Ophthalmol 1989;73:617–620.
6. Cashwell LF, Martin TJ: Malignant glaucoma after laser iridotomy. Ophthalmology 1992;99:651–9.
7. Aminlari A, Sassani JW: Simultaneous bilateral malignant glaucoma following laser iridotomy. Graefes Arch Clin Exp Ophthalmol 1993; 231:12–14.
8. Levene R: A new concept of malignant glaucoma. Arch Ophthalmol 1972;87:497.
9. Hitchings RA, Powell DJ: Pilocarpine and narrow-angle glaucoma. Trans Ophthalmol Soc UK 1981;101:214–17.
10. Wood WJ, Smith TR: Senile disciform macular degeneration complicated by massive hemorrhagic retinal detachment and angle closure glaucoma. Retina 1983;3:296–303.
11. Chandler PA: Progress in the treatment of glaucoma in my lifetime. Surv Ophthalmol 1977;21:412–428.
12. Chandler PA: A new operation for malignant glaucoma: a preliminary report. Trans Am Ophthalmol Soc 1964;62:408–424.
13. Chandler PA, Grant WM: Mydriatic-cycloplegic treatment in malignant glaucoma. Arch Ophthalmol 1962;62:353–359.
14. Chandler PA, Simmons RJ, Grant WM: Malignant glaucoma, medical and surgical treatment. Am J Ophthalmol 1968;66:495–502.
15. Simmons RJ: Malignant glaucoma. Br J Ophthalmol 1972;56:263.
16. Simmons RJ: In discussion of Herschler J.: Laser shrinkage of ciliary processes: a treatment for malignant (ciliary block) glaucoma. Ophthalmology 1980;87:1155.
17. Nash RW, Lindquist TD: Bilateral angle-closure glaucoma associated with uveal effusion: presenting sign of HIV infection. Surv Ophthalmol 1992;36:255–8.
18. Joshi N, et al: Bilateral angle closure glaucoma and accelerated cataract formation in a patient with AIDS. Br J Ophthalmol 1994;78:656–657.
19. Troope GE, et al: Malignant glaucoma. Clinical and ultrasound biomicroscopic features. Ophthalmology 1994;101:1030–5.
20. Phelps CD: Angle-closure glaucoma secondary to ciliary body swelling. Arch Ophthalmol 1974;92:287–90.
21. Saari KM: Acute glaucoma in hemorrhagic fever with renal syndrome (nephropathia epidemica). Am J Ophthalmol 1976;81:455–61.
22. Letocha CE: Angle-closure secondary to ciliary body swelling. Ann Ophthalmol 1977;9:597–8.
23. Epstein DL, Hashimoto JM, Anderson PJ, et al: Experimental perfusions through the vitreous and anterior chambers: possible relationship to malignant glaucoma. Am J Ophthalmol 1979;88:1078–1086.
24. Epstein DL: Malignant glaucoma. In: Advanced techniques in ocular surgery. Edited by F. Jakobiec, J. Sigelman. Philadelphia, W.B. Saunders Co., 1984:158–168.
25. Epstein DL, Steinert RF, Puliafito CA: Neodymium-YAG laser therapy to the anterior hyaloid in aphakic malignant glaucoma. Am J Ophthalmol 1984;98:137–143.
26. Epstein DL: Pseudophakic malignant glaucoma — is it really pseudomalignant? Am J Ophthalmol 1987;103:231–233.
27. Brown RH, Lynch MG, Tearse JE, et al: Neodymium-YAG vitreous surgery for phakic and pseudophakic malignant glaucoma. Arch Ophthalmol 1986;104:1464–6.
28. Luntz MH, Rosenblatt M: Malignant glaucoma. Surv Ophthalmol 1987; 32:73–93.
29. Melamed S, Ashkenazi I, Blumenthal M: Nd-YAG laser hyaloidotomy for malignant glaucoma following one-piece 7 mm intraocular lens implantation. Br J Ophthalmol 1991;75:501–3.
30. Halkias A, Magauran DM, Joyce M: Ciliary block (malignant) glaucoma after cataract extraction with lens implant treated with YAG laser capsulotomy and anterior hyaloidotomy. Br J Ophthalmol 1992;76:569–70.
31. Tello C, et al: Ultrasound biomicroscopy in pseudophakic malignant glaucoma. Ophthalmology 1993;100:1330–4.
32. Simmons RJ: Malignant glaucoma. In: Glaucoma. Edited by Chandler PA, Grant WM. Philadelphia, Lea & Febiger, 1979.
33. DiSclafani M, Liebmann JM, Ritch R: Malignant glaucoma following argon laser release of scleral flap sutures after trabeculectomy. Am J Ophthalmol 1989;108:597–8.
34. Grant WM: Experimental aqueous perfusions in enucleated human eyes. Arch Ophthalmol 1963;69:783.
35. Bleeker GM: Variation in the depth of the anterior chamber and intraocular pressure. Am J Ophthalmol 1963;55:964.
36. Jaffe NS: The vitreous in clinical ophthalmology. St. Louis, The C.V. Mosby Co., 1969.
37. Streeten BW, Pulaski JP: Posterior zonules and lens extraction. Arch Ophthalmol 1978;96:132.
38. Coleman DJ: Unified model for accommodative mechanism. Am J Ophthalmol 1970;69:1063.
39. VanHeuven WAJ, Lam KW, Ray GS: Source of subretinal fluid on the basis of ascorbate analyses. Arch Ophthalmol 1982;100:976.
40. Pederson JE, Toris CB: Experimental retinal detachment. IX. Aqueous, vitreous, and subretinal protein concentrations. Arch Ophthalmol 1985; 103:835–6.
41. Tsuboi S, Pederson JE: Permeability of the isolated dog retinal pigment epithelium to carboxyfluorescein. Invest Ophthalmol Vis Sci 1986;27: 1767–70.
42. Tsuboi S, Pederson JE: Volume flow across the isolated retinal pigment epithelium of cynomolgus monkey eyes. Invest Ophthalmol Vis Sci 1988;29:1652–5.
43. Marmor MF: Control of subretinal fluid: experimental and clinical studies. Eye 1990;4:340–4.
44. Kawano S, Marmor MF: Metabolic influences on the absorption of serous subretinal fluid. Invest Ophthalmol Vis Sci 1988;29:1255–7.
45. Robbins RM, Galin MA: Vitreous response in glaucoma. Am J Ophthalmol 1973;76:921.

46. Christensen L, Irvine AR: Pathogenesis of primary shallow chamber angle closure glaucoma. Arch Ophthalmol 1966;75:490.
47. Wright MM, Grajewski AL: Measurement of intraocular pressure with a flat anterior chamber. Ophthalmology 1991;98:1854–7.
48. Simmons RJ, Kimbrough RL: Shell tamponade in filtering surgery for glaucoma. Ophthalmic Surg 1979;10:17–34.
49. Simmons RJ: Filtering operations. In: Glaucoma, 2nd Ed. Edited by Chandler PA, Grant WM. Philadelphia, Lea & Febiger, 1979.
50. Melamed S, et al: The use of glaucoma shell tamponade in leaking filtration blebs. Ophthalmology 1986;93:839–842.
51. Weiss DI, Shaffer RN: Treatment of malignant glaucoma with intravenous mannitol infusion. Arch Ophthalmol 1963;69:154.
52. Garner LF, Brown B, Baker R, et al: The effect of phenylephrine hydrochloride on the resting point of accommodation. Invest Ophthalmol Vis Sci 1983;24:393–5.
53. Borromeo-McGrail V, Bordiuk JM, Keitel H: Systemic hypertension following ocular administration of 10 per cent phenylephrine in the neonate. Pediatrics 1973;51:1032–6.
54. Meyer SM, Fraunfelder FT: Phenylephrine hydrochloride. Ophthalmology 1980;87:1177–80.
55. Fraunfelder FT, Meyer SM: Systemic reactions to ophthalmic drug preparations. Med Toxicol Adverse Drug Exp 1987;2:287–93.
56. Steinert RF, Puliafito CA, Kittrell C: Plasma shielding by Q-switched and mode-locked Nd-YAG lasers. Ophthalmology 1983;90:1003–6.
57. Simmons RJ: Malignant glaucoma. In: Chandler and Grant's Glaucoma. 3rd Ed. Philadelphia, Lea & Febiger, 1986.
58. Frayer WC, Laties AM: Some consequences of ciliary process swelling in the rabbit and in the human. Trans Am Ophthalmol Soc 1977;74: 107–21.
59. Oksala A, Koponen J: Choroidal detachment associated with scleritis—a case report with echograms. Ultrasound Med Biol 1974;1:283–5.
60. Feldon SE, Sigelman J, Albert DM, et al: Clinical manifestations of brawny scleritis. Am J Ophthalmol 1978;85:781–7.
61. Benson WE: Posterior scleritis. Surv Ophthalmol 1988;32:297–316.
62. Mangouritsas G, Ulbig M: Secondary angle-block glaucoma in posterior scleritis. Klin Monatsbl Augenheilkd 1991;199:40–4.
63. Von Der Lippe I, Kuchle M, Naumann GO: Pseudoexfoliation syndrome as a risk factor for acute ciliary block angle closure glaucoma. Acta Ophthalmol 1993;71:277–9.
64. Schlotzer-Schrehardt U, Naumann GO: A histopathologic study of zonular instability in pseudoexfoliation syndrome. Am J Ophthalmol 1994; 118:730–43.

Nanophthalmos: Diagnosis and Treatment 30

Richard J. Simmons and Ruthanne B. Simmons

Nanophthalmos (dwarf eye) is a rare condition that we had not recognized as a unique entity until it was called to our attention by Robert Brockhurst (1). Since then, we have seen and managed more than 60 cases of nanophthalmos.

Nanophthalmos is a bilateral condition characterized by small ocular volume, usually about two-thirds of normal, typically associated with marked hypermetropia and shallow anterior chamber. Exceptionally, nanophthalmic eyes may be emmetropic or myopic. Some patients may have macular hypoplasia or retinal pigmentary degeneration (2,3). The globe has a small equatorial diameter and a small corneal diameter, but the size of the lens is normal. The disproportion between lens and ocular volume contributes to making the iris convex and the anterior chamber shallow. In nanophthalmos the lens may occupy 10 to 30 percent of the volume of the globe, compared with approximately 4 percent in normal adult eyes. The ocular pulse tends to have a greater than normal amplitude perhaps due to the abnormally thickened sclera or due to impaired drainage through the vortex veins (1,4).

The sclera in eyes with nanophthalmos is both thicker and more disorganized than normal sclera (5–8). Trelstad found that in the sclera of eyes with nanophthalmos the collagen fibrils were of normal size, but the collagen bundles were larger, less ordered, and more interwoven than normal (5). When Yue and co-workers found higher than normal levels of fibronectin, they speculated that the change in glycosaminoglycan metabolism could affect the packing of collagen fibers and lead to thickening of the sclera and occlusion of the vortex veins (6). In contrast to Trelstad, Stewart et. al. found a wide range of fibril diameters in nanophthalmic sclera as well as unusual fraying of these fibrils (7).

In some cases nanophthalmos is inherited; in other cases it is a sporadic occurrence. If inherited, transmission may be either autosomal recessive or autosomal dominant (3,4). Often the inheritance is unknown but the patients have relatives who are blind from angle closure glaucoma. Furthermore, several of our cases have a family history of consanguinity (1,9). Although the two largest case series report this observation, the number of cases reported is too small to confirm a female predominance (10,11). In fact, earlier reports described equal gender distribution (1,12). Although nanophthalmos is usually not associated with systemic abnormalities, there are cases reported with coexistent cryptorchidism (13) and Hallermann-Streiff syndrome (6).

Conventional invasive surgical operations for angle closure glaucoma can have disastrous consequences in nanophthalmos. Brockhurst pointed out that there is a strong tendency for uveal effusion and exudative retinal detachment after anterior segment surgery (Fig. 30.1). The history of disastrous results with conventional glaucoma procedures has led to the preference for medical and laser, rather than conventional surgical treatment of angle closure glaucoma in nanophthalmos.

When performing gonioscopy, we prefer to use the infant-size (12 mm) Koeppe lens, or as a second choice, a mirrored goniolens such as the Zeiss or Sussman. The advantage of the infant Koeppe lens is that it allows a clear view, simultaneous comparison of both eyes, and allows observation by multiple observers without moving the lenses. The standard adult size Koeppe lens (16, 18, or 20 mm) frequently flattens the cornea and creates folds in Descemet's membrane which blur the view and distort the configuration of the angle. The mirrored goniolenses do not distort the cornea but are less than ideal because they do not allow optimal visualization of the angle structures because of the extreme convexity of the iris in nanophthalmos.

In younger patients, the most characteristic findings are hyperopic eyes with small corneas with the lens and iris bulging forward into a shallow anterior chamber (Fig. 30.2). The central portion of the anterior chamber may appear shallower while the angle may appear wider than expected. The iris may have the peculiar appearance of conforming to the anterior surface of the lens, centrally as well as peripherally. As the lens enlarges with age, there is an increase in relative pupillary block, and the anterior chamber becomes shallow (Fig. 30.3), narrowing the angle and progressively closing the angle.

In middle aged or older patients, **spontaneous choroidal thickening and detachment** can be demonstrated by ultrasound or magnetic resonance imaging. These choroidal changes may cause a forward rotation of the ciliary body which pushes the peripheral iris forward, allows the lens to move forward, and increases relative pupillary block. The failure of iridectomy to resolve progressive angle closure demonstrates that pupillary block is not the only factor contributing to angle closure. Additional fac-

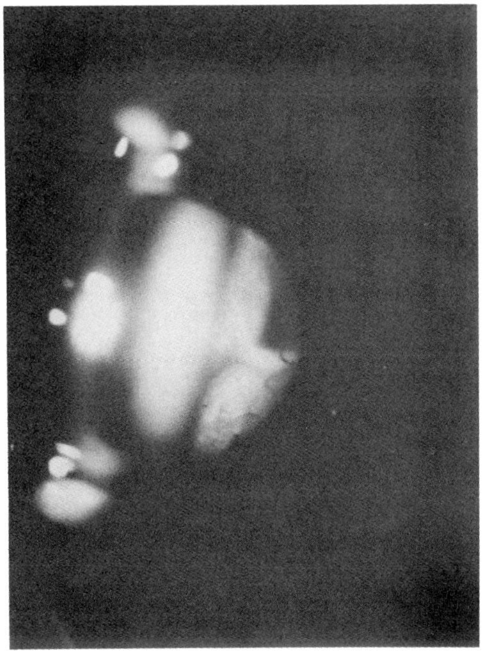

Figure 30.1. Nanophthalmos with choroidal effusion. The retina can be seen immediately behind the crystalline lens.

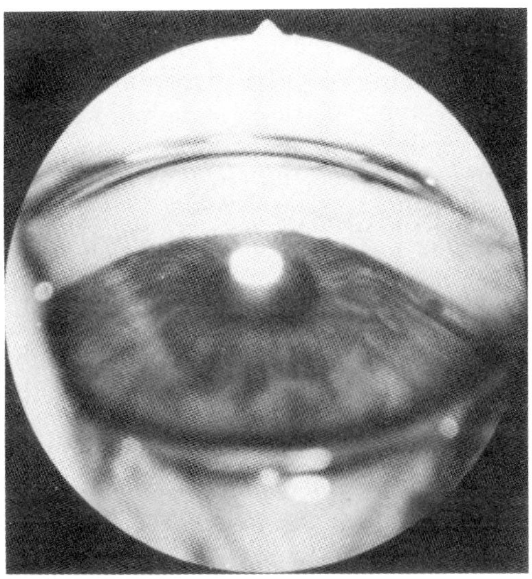

Figure 30.2. Gonioscopic view of a nanophthalmic eye showing marked iris convexity.

tors are choroidal thickening and effusions. From our surgical experience, the effusion of fluid can be intrachoroidal, suprachoroidal, or both. In some cases, we relieved the angle closure by draining an isolated pocket of fluid in the suprachoroidal space. In others, we have seen a slow exudation of fluid originating from the ciliary body and choroid. When drainage of the suprachoroidal space fails to relieve the effusion and the enlargement in the anterior choroid and ciliary body, the fluid is likely to be intrachoroidal. Shaffer has suggested that the uveal effusion in nanophthalmic eyes may be secondary to constriction of vortex veins by abnormally thickened sclera (14).

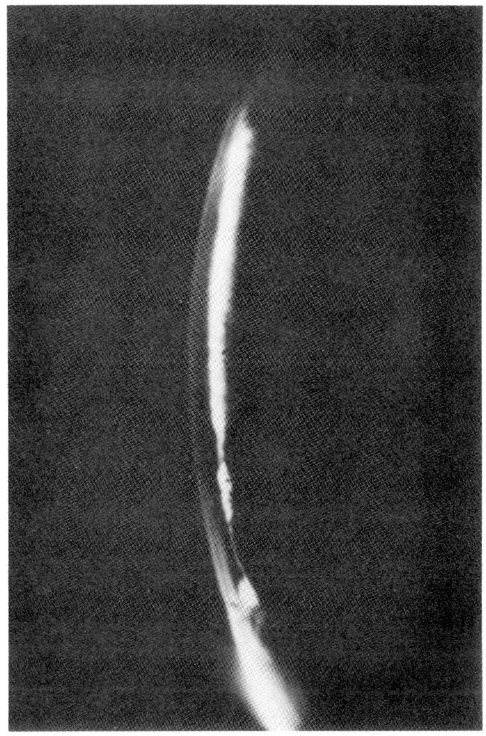

Figure 30.3. Slit-lamp demonstration of shallow anterior chamber in nanophthalmos.

Table 30.1
The Stages of Nanophthalmos

Stage 1. Narrow angle; nanophthalmos recognized; no elevation of the intraocular pressure.
Stage 2. Angle progressively more narrow; angle closure threatened but not present.
Stage 3. Angle progressively more narrow; angle partially closed.
Stage 4. Angle very narrow; extensive angle closure with increased pressure controlled with medical therapy.
Stage 5. Angle closed by synechias; intraocular pressure uncontrolled by medical therapy.

Recommendations for therapy of angle closure glaucoma in nanophthalmos are subject to change as new cases of this rare entity are treated and observed. Currently our therapeutic approach depends on the status of this condition, which may be divided into five stages (Table 30.1).

STAGE 1. NARROW ANGLE; NANOPHTHALMOS RECOGNIZED; NO ELEVATION OF THE INTRAOCULAR PRESSURE (IOP)

Early recognition of this condition is critical. Eyes with small corneal diameter and more than eight diopters of hypermetropia should be studied with ultrasonography and gonioscopy. When patients reach the fourth decade of life, one should watch carefully for choroidal separation and progressive narrowing of the angles. Our observations suggest that all untreated nanophthalmic eyes are likely to undergo gradual progressive narrowing of the angle, angle closure, formation of peripheral synechias, and elevation of intraocular pressure. We recommend examination of nanophthalmic eyes at 3-to 6-month intervals when the angle has not yet become narrow enough to require treatment. Consider early use of laser iridectomy.

STAGE 2. ANGLE PROGRESSIVELY MORE NARROW; ANGLE CLOSURE THREATENED BUT NOT PRESENT

Some patients are seen at the stage when the angles are still open but so slit-like that angle closure is threatened. In such patients, we propose prophylactic laser iridectomy. Laser iridectomy is highly preferable to surgical iridectomy because of the propensity of nanophthalmic eyes to develop intra-operative choroidal effusions at the time the anterior chamber is entered and decompressed.

We prefer to induce miosis with 2% pilocarpine, then proceed with the Nd:YAG laser for the initial attempt at iridectomy. In some cases, iris penetration cannot be achieved because the iris in nanophthalmos is thicker and more difficult to penetrate than usual. In those cases where the initial use of Nd:YAG laser is unsuccessful, the iris can be thinned with application of argon laser at the iridectomy site and then penetrated with the Nd:YAG laser. Potential damage to the crystalline lens by the Nd:YAG laser should be kept in mind, and the Nd:YAG laser should be applied to the iris as peripherally as possible to avoid this complication.

STAGE 3. ANGLE PROGRESSIVELY MORE NARROW, ANGLE PARTIALLY CLOSED

Initial therapy should consist of laser iridectomies followed by laser gonioplasty. When penetration of the iris is achieved, the peripheral iris frequently remains convex and the angle frequently remains narrow. Such narrowness can increase progressively with time in spite of a patent iridectomy. In such cases, laser gonioplasty should be applied to flatten the peripheral iris, widen the angle, and prevent angle closure (Fig. 30.4).

Gonioplasty in nanophthalmos is performed as follows. We induce miosis with 2% pilocarpine. We then set the argon laser to an initial energy level of 100 milliwatts, a 100-200 micron spot diameter, and a duration of 0.2 seconds. The central corneal portion of a goniolens is used to direct the aiming beam at the periphery of the iris. Because of the extreme convexity of the iris in nanophthalmos, it is usually necessary to aim the laser beam directly at the iris rather than attempting to reflect the laser beam off a gonio-mirror. One should aim about 1 mm on the corneal side of the limbus just far enough central to allow the laser beam to pass through clear cornea unaffected by arcus or limbal haze. Ten to 12 applications of the laser are then made to the iris in a single curved row concentric with the limbus. The iris contracts and the angle can be observed to widen. If no contracture of the iris is observed, the energy level is increased to 200 or even 300 milliwatts. Gonioplasty is applied to one or two quadrants at a sitting, enough to widen or open the most narrow portions of the angle. After treatment, a patient should have a slit-lamp examination and gonioscopy every 3 months. The widening effect of gonioplasty may gradually disappear, and either the same or another portion of peripheral iris may again bulge forward narrowing or closing the angle. If this occurs, gonioplasty is repeated.

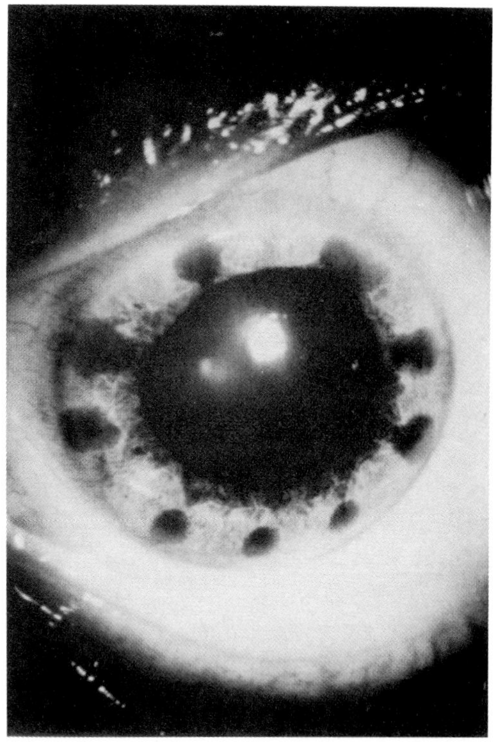

Figure 30.4. Appearance of nanophthalmic eye following successful opening of the entire angle circumference with argon laser gonioplasty.

Using this technique we have been able to keep the anterior chamber angle from closing for a period of years in several patients. The energy applied to the iris is so low that iris explosions and pigment dispersion do not occur; there is merely contracture of the surface of the iris. Peripheral synechias in early stages of formation can also be separated by this technique. The following case illustrates the use of gonioplasty.

Case 30-1. A 54-year-old man with small corneas and shallow anterior chambers was recognized by his ophthalmologist as possibly having nanophthalmos. His father and brother had nanophthalmos and had become blind from angle closure glaucoma. Ultrasound examination supported the diagnosis in this patient, establishing that the ocular volume was in the nanophthalmic range, while the volume of the lens was normal. Gonioscopy showed both angles to be narrow. In the left eye the angle appeared closed in half the circumference, and IOP was in the mid-30s under treatment with miotics and acetazolamide. Gonioplasty was applied to the closed half of the angle and succeeded in opening 4 hours. While shallowness of the anterior chamber and convexity of the iris persisted, the trabecular meshwork could be identified everywhere except for 2 hours in which synechias were still present. The patient had repeated examinations and four additional laser gonioplasty treatments at approximately 6-month intervals. IOP remained in the high-20's for 3 years, and the angle remained wider than at the initial examination. The patient was later lost to follow-up.

STAGE 4. ANGLE VERY NARROW; EXTENSIVE ANGLE CLOSURE WITH INCREASED PRESSURE CONTROLLED WITH MEDICAL THERAPY

A patent laser iridectomy should be created if one has not been done. We prefer medicines that reduce aqueous production. Although, we have tried both miotics and mydriatics, they have only helped a few eyes with nanophthalmos. If the elevated IOP due to synechial closure can not be controlled by beta blockers, alpha adrenergic agonists, and carbonic anhydrase inhibitors, laser gonioplasty is used repeatedly, attempting to open as much of the angle as possible. This is illustrated by the following case.

Case 30-2. A 17-year-old girl was referred because of elevated IOP in both eyes, right 44, left 36. Her corneas were small (horizontal diameter 10.5 mm). She was hypermetropic. Ultrasound showed bilateral nanophthalmos. Gonioscopy showed angle closure for nine clock hours in the right eye and for twelve clock hours in the left eye. In both eyes the discs were totally cupped and pale, and there were extensive Bjerrum scotomas. After treatment with carbonic anhydrase inhibitors, hyperosmotic agents, and miotics, the angle opened except for 3 clock hours. Laser iridectomies were created in both eyes. The irides remained extremely convex. Laser gonioplasty was applied to the right eye, and the angle was seen to widen. Two hours of angle closure remained. The same treatment was then applied to the left eye, with the same result. She continues on medical treatment. Her IOPs are in the teens, and she has had no further field loss. She is examined periodically and further gonioplasty will be performed as required to try to keep the angles open. Intraocular surgery is postponed unless she progresses to stage 5.

STAGE 5. ANGLE CLOSED BY SYNECHIAS; INTRAOCULAR PRESSURE UNCONTROLLED BY MEDICAL THERAPY

When there is extensive synechial closure of the angle, the problem is beyond laser iridectomy, laser gonioplasty and medical therapy. The IOP is usually high and must be lowered to preserve any vision. Two choices are currently available. One is a filtering procedure with scleral surgery, the other is a ciliary destructive procedure.

We have modified our trabeculectomy procedures to include scleral surgery performed either preoperatively or intraoperatively with the trabeculectomy. We try to avoid intraoperative and postoperative hypotony so as to minimize the chance for choroidal effusions and exudative retinal detachments. We fill the anterior chamber with a very viscous viscoelastic agent prior to performing the sclerostomy to help prevent the collapse of the globe and hypotony when entering the anterior chamber. In addition we preplace sutures in the outer trabeculectomy flap so that they may be closed immediately to prevent collapse of the globe and hypotony during surgery.

When the glaucoma is such that trabeculectomy can be deferred, we prefer that two posterior sclerectomies be done in the inferior quadrants sparing the superior conjunctiva. We prefer to do these prophylactic sclerectomies 4 to 6 weeks before the trabeculectomy to allow for full recovery. We currently recommend the technique described by Gass (15). He advocates the removal of a two-third thickness (5 mm x 7 mm) rectangle of sclera with the additional removal of a one mm full thickness piece of sclera from the scleral bed. While Gass's technique avoids the vortex veins, Brockhurst specifically recommends including vortex vein decompression with scleral thinning and posterior sclerotomies (16).

If the glaucoma is so severe that immediate surgery is necessary, we recommend that anterior sclerotomies be done at the time of the trabeculectomy. Before the eye is opened, the globe is rotated superiorly and two full thickness "V" shaped scleral flaps (4mm by 4 mm) are made in the inferior nasal and temporal quadrants. The point of the "V" should be five mm from the limbus directed toward the limbus. While Jin and Anderson (10) report uniform success leaving these flaps unsutured, we have had several unsutured flaps reseal within 7 days. If drainage of suprachoriodal fluid is observed during the procedure or if the eye is at high risk for choroidal effusion, we recommend excising the flaps at the base. This leaves four mm equilateral triangles of exposed uvea in each of the two inferior quadrants covered by conjunctiva and Tenon's capsule. While one could express concern about these large areas of uvea unprotected by sclera, one must realize that these stage 5 eyes face certain blindness unless surgery is successful. Due to this concern, however, some surgeons prefer to perform a simple linear sclerotomy centered 6 mm posterior to the limbus, similar to that made for drainage of choroidal effusions, leaving the linear incision open at the conclusion of the operation, but we have found linear sclerotomies inadequate in true nanophthalmos and have abandoned this technique.

Laser ciliary body destructive procedures can also lower

the IOP, but we reserve this until all other prior surgery has failed. We have found that nanophthalmic eyes require repeated ciliodestructive procedures for IOP control and often experience subsequent severe visual loss.

The following case of Thomas M. Richardson, MD, managed in consultation with us, illustrates the importance of prophylactic sclerotomies and the difficult course of filtering surgery in a patient with stage 5 nanophthalmos.

Case 30-3. A 27-year-old woman was seen because of gradual loss of vision, first noted approximately 4 months earlier. Her IOPs were 54 in the right eye and 58 in the left eye. She had had progressive severe loss of visual field followed by decrease of visual acuity in both eyes. The vision was hand motions inferotemporally in the right eye and 20/80 in the left eye. Both discs were totally cupped and atrophic. Both eyes were 9 diopters hyperopic and had anatomic characteristics of nanophthalmos confirmed by ultrasonography. The angles were closed in both eyes. The patient evidently had had symptomless closure of the angles without an acute attack. Because of the desperate condition of the eyes, immediate surgery was advised. A filtering procedure was performed on the left eye. It was followed by exudative retinal detachment. On the first day after operation, the retina was seen to be close behind the pupil. The lens had been forced through the sclerostomy into the filtration bleb. In the right eye the pressure persisted in the 50s and visual acuity continued to decrease. Because it appeared that no light perception would remain if intervention was postponed, a filtering procedure was performed. However, in this eye preliminary posterior sclerotomy was performed in the inferotemporal quadrant to prepare a drainage path for suprachoroidal fluid. An exudative choroidal and retinal detachment did develop postoperatively, but much less than in the first eye. Intensive corticosteroid treatment was employed, and during the next several days the choroidal and retinal detachments disappeared in both eyes. Vision improved and IOPs in the high teens prevailed in both eyes. Vision in the left eye remained hand movements, but the right eye returned to approximately preoperative levels. Ultrasonography showed return of the retinas to their normal position.

Unfortunately, several months later the filtration bleb scarred and failed in each eye and the patient was lost to follow-up.

Although angle closure glaucoma secondary to nanophthalmos can be treated with medical therapy, laser iridectomy, laser gonioplasty, and anterior or posterior sclerotomies, the prognosis remains guarded. The uveal effusion and exudative retinal detachment secondary to nanophthalmos can be treated with posterior scleral thinning, sclerotomies, and with the possible addition of vortex vein decompression.

References

1. Brockhurst RJ: Nanophthalmos with uveal effusion: A new clinical entity. Trans Am Ophthalmol Soc 1974;72:371–403, Arch Ophthalmol 1975;93:1289.
2. Ghose S, Sachdev MS, Kumar H: Bilateral nanophthalmos, pigmentary retinal dystrophy and angle closure glaucoma—a new syndrome? Br J Ophthalmol 1982;69:624–628.
3. MacKay CJ, Shek MS, Carr RE, et al: Retinal degeneration with nanophthalmos, cystic macular degeneration and angle closure glaucoma. Arch Ophthalmol 1987;105:366–371.
4. Singh OS, Simmons RJ, Brockhurst RJ: Nanophthalmos: A perspective on identification and therapy. Ophthalmology 1982;89:1006.
5. Trelstad RL, Silbermann NN, Brockhurst RJ: Nanophthalmic sclera, ultrastructural, histochemical, and biochemical observations. Arch Ophthalmol 1982;100:1935–1938.
6. Yue BY, et al: Nanophthalmic sclera. Fibronectin studies. Ophthalmology 1988;95:56–60.
7. Stewart DH, et al: Abnormal scleral collagen in nanophthalmos, an ultrastructural study. Arch Ophthalmol 1991;109:1017–1025.
8. Shrono T, Shoji A, Mutoh T, et al: Abnormal sclerocytes in nanopthalmos. Graefe's Arch Clin Exp Ophthalmol 1992;230:348–351.
9. Kimbrough RL, Trempe CS, Brockhurst RJ, et al: Angle closure in nanophthalmos. Am J Ophthalmol 1979;88:572–9.
10. Jin JC, Anderson DR: Laser and unsutured sclerotomy in nanophthalmos. Am J Ophthalmol 1990;109:575–580.
11. Singh OS, Sofinski SJ: Principles and practice of ophthalmology. D.A. Albert, F.A. Jakobiec, editors. Philadelphia, W.B. Saunders Co., 1994.
12. Calhoun FP, Jr: The management of glaucoma in nanophthalmos. Trans Am Ophthalmol Soc 1975;73:97–122.
13. Barad RF, Nelson LB, Cowchark FS, et al: Nanophthalmos associated with cryptorchidism. Ann Ophthalmol 1985;17:284–288.
14. Shaffer RN: Discussion. Trans Am Ophthalmol Soc 1975;73:119–120.
15. Gass JD: Uveal effusion syndrome, a new hypothesis concerning pathogenesis and a new technique of surgical treatment. Retina 1983;3:159–163.
16. Brockhurst RJ: Vortex vein decompression for nanophthalmic uveal effusion. Arch Ophthalmol 1980;98:1987–1990.

Neovascular Glaucoma

31

David K. Dueker

Neovascular glaucoma (NVG) is a potentially devastating secondary glaucoma that results from the growth of a fibrovascular membrane over the trabecular meshwork in the anterior chamber angle.

PREDISPOSING CONDITIONS

The changes in the anterior segment which lead to neovascular glaucoma arise in response to a predisposing condition elsewhere—most commonly to a disturbance of the retinal circulation resulting in ischemia. The two most common predisposing conditions are diabetic retinopathy and occlusion of the central retinal vein. Other forms of retinal vascular disease (e.g., Eales' disease, sickle cell retinopathy) and extraocular circulatory abnormalities affecting ocular blood flow (e.g., carotid stenosis, carotid-cavernous fistula, pulseless disease) are important though less common causes of NVG. In addition to these various types of circulatory disease, NVG may also occur in association with an intraocular neoplasm, chronic retinal detachment, and severe intraocular infection or inflammation. Thus a patient presenting with this disorder requires a rather broad-based diagnostic work-up to determine the underlying cause (1,2). Conversely, any patient with a clinical condition known to predispose an eye to NVG, deserves careful monitoring to detect the process in its earliest stages.

The conditions that predispose to NVG show large differences in their tendency to produce the disease. The incidence of NVG after central retinal vein occlusion (CRVO) is probably best known because both CRVO and NVG have clear signs and symptoms (except that a non-ischemic CRVO may be asymptomatic), and, when they occur in association, the time interval is short. Classically known as "90 day glaucoma," a high percentage of eyes which develop NVG after CRVO do so within the first 3 to 4 months after the CRVO. The risk actually extends out to 7 months, after which NVG is rare (3).

The clinical entity of central retinal vein occlusion may be subdivided into two types—ischemic and non-ischemic—with marked differences between the two both in terms of visual function and in tendency to develop NVG (4). The non-ischemic CRVO rarely develops NVG. The risk lies almost entirely with the ischemic form. About 20% of CRVOs are initially of the ischemic type (5), and approximately 50% of these will develop NVG (6).

A useful way to distinguish the two forms of occlusion is by fluorescein angiography (7–10). The ischemic form of CRVO shows large areas of retinal capillary nonperfusion, a sign of severe retinal ischemia. When the capillaries are not filled, the retina remains dark (nonfluorescent) except for the major vascular branches (Fig. 31.1). **Since the risk of subsequent neovascular glaucoma resides almost entirely with the ischemic type of central retinal vein occlusion, identifying the type of occlusion is very helpful in guiding further management.** However, a single angiogram showing well-perfused retinal capillary beds does not insure against all risk of NVG, since a percentage (approximately 15%) of non-ischemic CRVOs later convert to the ischemic form (5).

Furthermore, definitive angiograms may be unobtainable because of media opacities, widespread retinal hemorrhage, or failure to include peripheral capillary beds. Hayreh recommends a careful assessment of visual function (Table 31.1) as an aid in accurately separating ischemic from non-ischemic CRVOs (11).

The incidence of NVG in eyes with diabetic retinopathy is not as well defined as in CRVO. In unselected populations of diabetics, the incidence of neovascular glaucoma is low. However, in the presence of proliferative retinopathy, the incidence is similar to that found with central retinal vein occlusion and may actually be higher (12,13).

Among patients with one of the predisposing diseases, we do not yet know how to predict precisely which individual will develop neovascularization of the anterior segment. And if neovascularization of the iris or the angle develops, we do not yet know what factors determine which eyes will progress to neovascular glaucoma. Finally, in different patients with differing predisposing causes, the progression to full-blown NVG may take weeks, months, or years.

Against this background of multiple different causes and widely varying time course, the only sure method of detecting the earliest signs of anterior segment neovascularization is an appropriate vigilance based on knowledge of the potential causes and knowledge of the early clinical signs of anterior segment neovascularization. The reward for this vigilance is the opportunity to intervene at a relatively harmless stage of the process—slowing or even arresting it with appropriate therapy. Most often the intervention takes the form of retinal ablation, though in certain cases other forms of therapy are also useful. The rationale

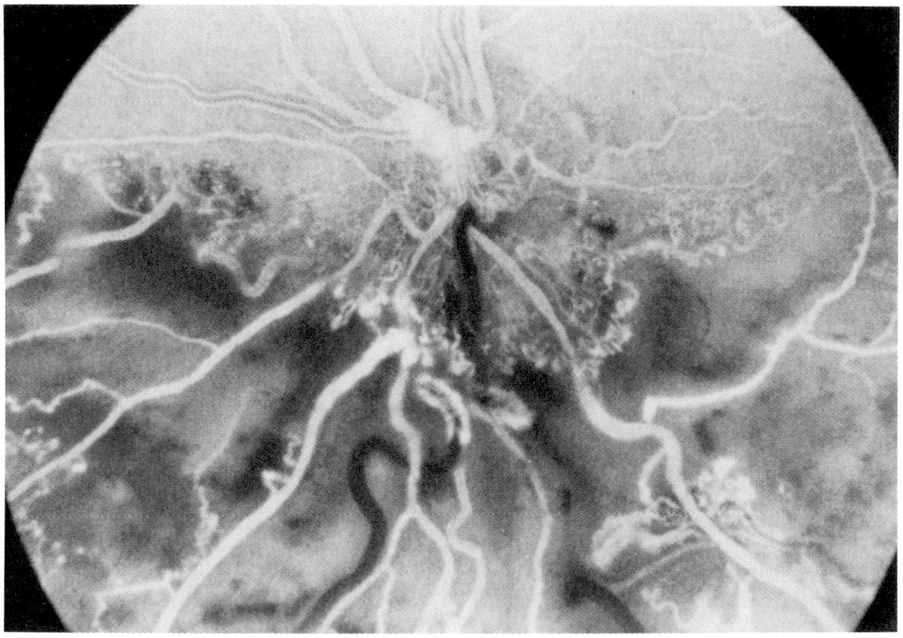

Figure 31.1. Fluorescein angiogram of a hemiretinal central vein occlusion (a variant of central retinal vein occlusion) chosen to show the appearance of capillary nonperfusion below in contrast with normal capillary filling above. An ischemic central retinal vein occlusion would show widespread capillary nonperfusion throughout the retina.

Table 31.1
Tests of Visual Function Which Help Differentiate Ischemic from Non-ischemic CRVO's (Reference 11)

Visual acuity	Visual acuity 20/200 is seen in 60% of non-ischemic and less than 2% of ischemic CRVO.
Perimetry	Goldmann VF with V4e target is normal in approx 80% of non-ischemic but less than 20% of ischemic CRVO.
Relative afferent pupillary defect (RAPD)	RAPD 0.70 log units in approximately 90% of ischemic and is normal in non-ischemic CRVO (if no other optic nerve abnormality).
ERG	Scotopic b wave is reduced in 80–90% of ischemic and is usually normal in non-ischemic CRVO.

for ablation derives from clinical observation and theoretical models of the disease (Fig. 31.2).

NATURAL CLINICAL HISTORY OF NEOVASCULAR GLAUCOMA

Although the pathologic conditions predisposing to neovascular glaucoma are numerous and varied, the sequence of anterior segment change is sufficiently uniform to suggest that the various causes of neovascular glaucoma act through a common pathway, though perhaps with variable intensities. When a patient has a disorder with a known tendency to cause neovascular glaucoma, the first sign of new vessel growth in the anterior segment is a leakage of intravenously injected fluorescein dye from vessels at the pupillary margin (Fig. 31.3). This leakage of dye may be conspicuous even when the iris appears completely normal on careful slit-lamp examination at high magnification. This abnormal permeability to fluorescein reflects an alteration of the pre-existing vasculature—an opening of the tight junctions normally found between endothelial cells in iris vessels, which is probably a necessary prelude to neovascular proliferation (Fig. 31.4). When vascular proliferation occurs, it is observable by clinical slit-lamp biomicroscopy without fluorescein, though one cannot appreciate by regular slit-lamp examination as much abnormality as is revealed by fluorescein angiography (Fig. 31.5).

Vascular proliferation is usually first evident at the pupil. Careful attention to the pupillary margin is therefore of great clinical importance for early detection of neovascularization. When an abnormality in vessels of the pupillary margin is suspected, gonioscopy should be done to search for vessels in the chamber angle. In a small proportion of patients (especially those with dark irides), there may be significant vascular proliferation in the angle before any change at the pupil is recognized by slit-lamp examination. **Therefore, any patient at risk of developing neovascular glaucoma in a useful eye should have not only a careful and repeated high-magnification slit-lamp examination of the iris (with undilated pupil), but also a periodic inspection of the anterior chamber angle by gonioscopy.**

When proliferating vessels are limited to the iris surface, they do not seem to cause clinically significant disturbance in the anterior chamber, even though they will show an abnormal permeability to fluorescein during angiography. But, when vessels proliferate in the angle, they cause a progressive decrease of outflow facility and eventu-

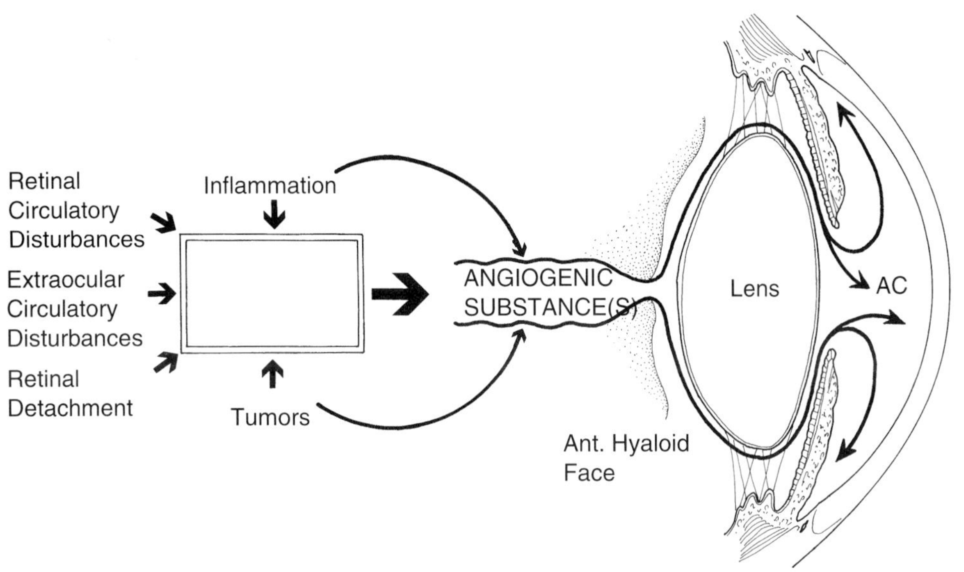

Figure 31.2. Retinal ischemia seems to be the common factor in all or most cases of anterior segment neovascularization. The pathogenic sequence leading to NVG may be modeled as depicted here. A variety of disorders may cause ischemia of the retina. The ischemic retina, in turn, produces angiogenic factor(s) which diffuse forward causing new vessel growth on the iris and angle. Forward diffusion may be impeded by the vitreous or lens, explaining why there may be a burst of angiogenic activity after vitrectomy, lensectomy, or capsulotomy. Tumors and inflammation may stimulate angiogenesis directly through elaboration of angiogenic factors or indirectly by causing retinal ischemia.

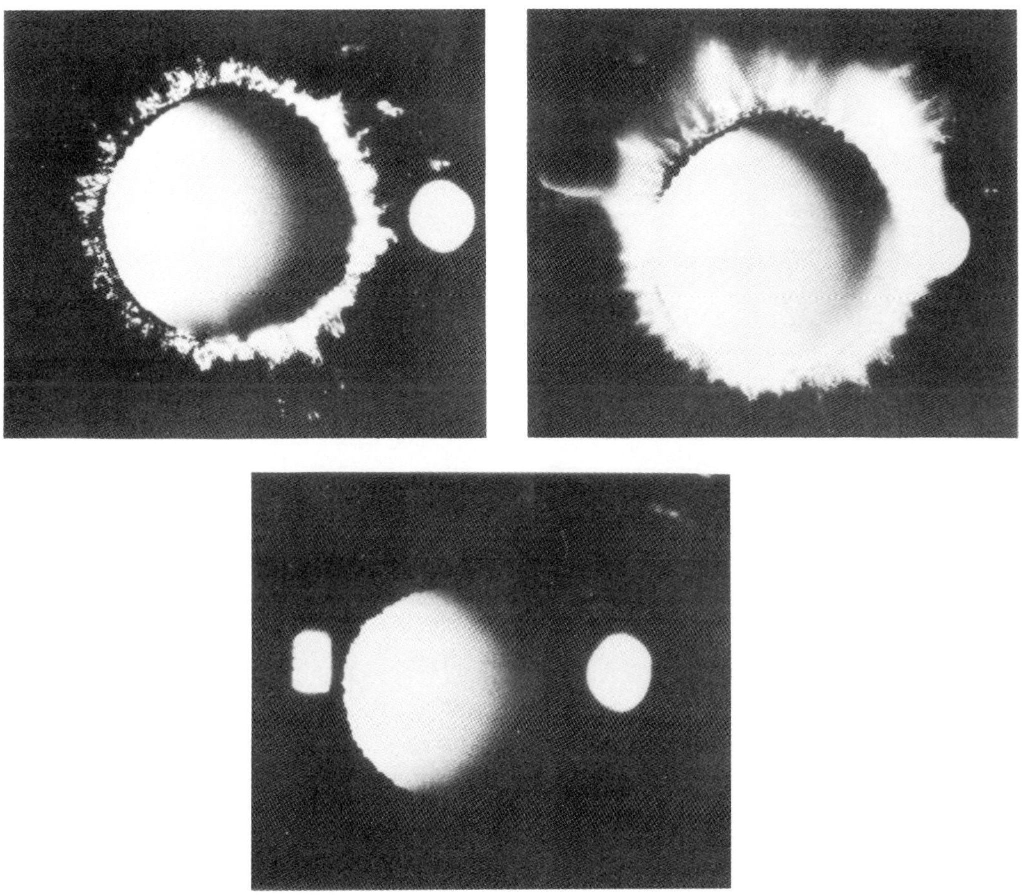

Figure 31.3. A, Fluorescein angiogram of a patient developing anterior segment neovascularization after central retinal vein occlusion. The pupillary margin had appeared normal on careful slitlamp biomicroscopy without fluorescein. B, Later stage of (A) showing dye leakage from abnormal vessels at the pupil. C, The opposite eye shows no abnormal leakage.

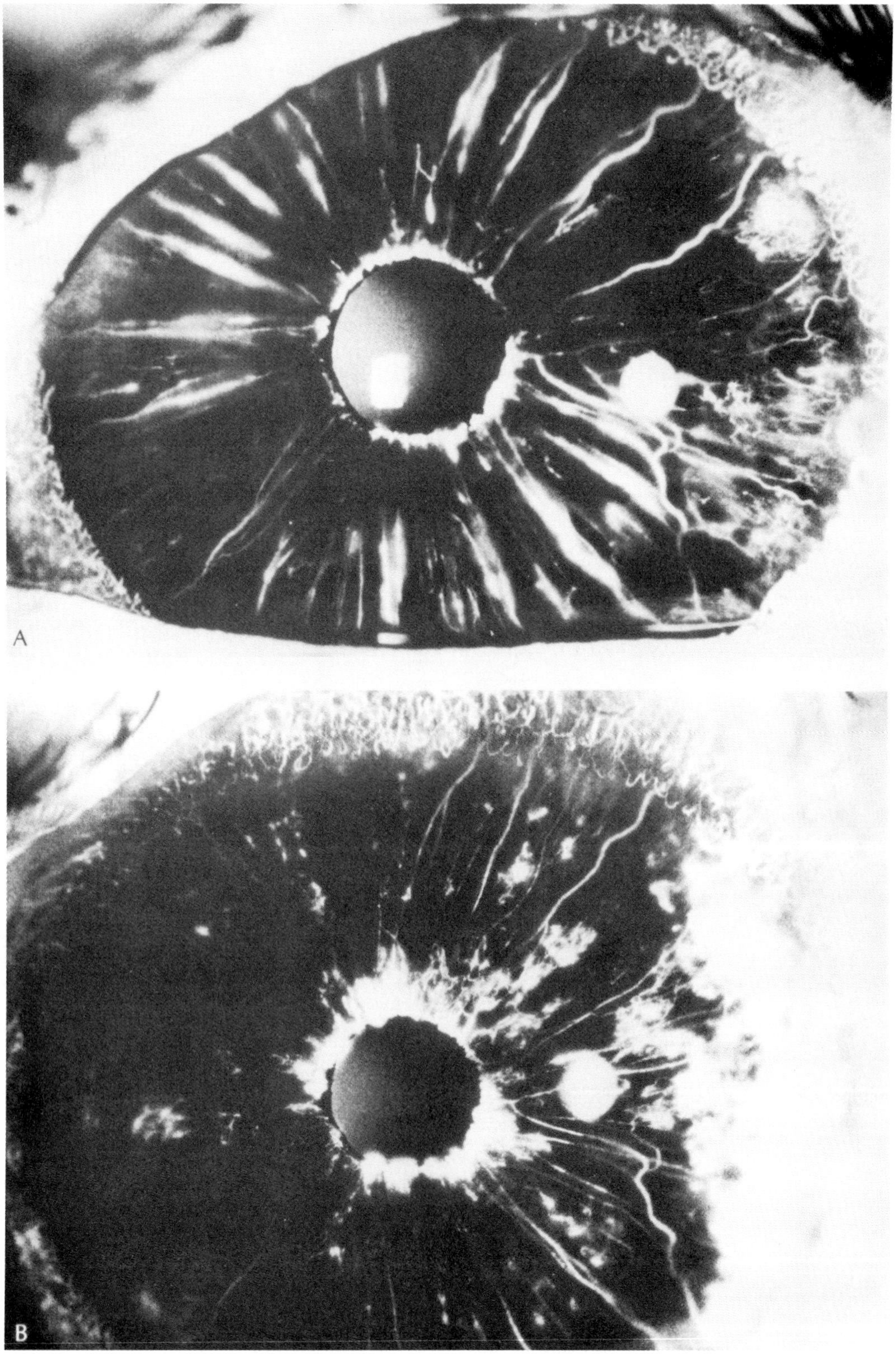

Figure 31.4. A, Fluorescein angiogram of a patient developing early iris neovascularization after central retinal vein occlusion. Prominent leakage is seen from many of the radial iris vessels. B, Repeat angiography 2 months later shows several areas of vascular proliferation, most of which developed from vessels shown to be leaking dye in the earlier angiogram.

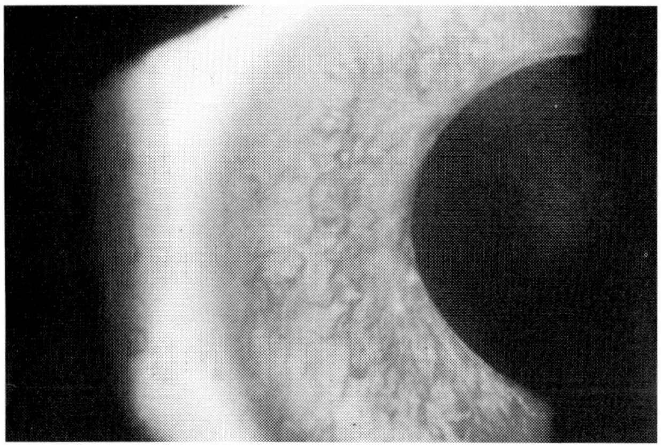

Figure 31.5. Neovascular proliferation at the pupil, though noted on slit-lamp examination, was shown by fluorescein angiography to be more extensive than otherwise would have been appreciated.

ally severe glaucoma. New vessels growing in the chamber angle develop from the base of the iris as individual trunks which cross the ciliary body and scleral spur in a direct path to the filtration area of the corneoscleral trabecular meshwork. On the meshwork the individual vessels branch into a complex pattern of fine vessels that eventually involve the entire circumference, intertwining with branches from other trunk vessels (14). **This fibrovascular tissue may severely compromise aqueous outflow, with resultant glaucoma, even while the angle remains open** (15). Next, a contractile process begins along one or more of the major vessels that run from the iris base to the trabecular meshwork, producing localized anterior synechias that tend to spread and ultimately to join, causing complete closure of the angle (Fig. 31.6).

The rate at which peripheral synechias spread to involve, eventually, the whole circumference is remarkably variable. In some eyes, once the formation of synechias is started the angle may become extensively closed within a week. In other eyes the process is much slower, for reasons unknown. The onset of high pressure is often acute and painful, whether or not the angle has been closed by neovascular tissue or synechias, and frequently the patient comes for attention as an emergency with a red eye, edematous cornea, and rubeosis of the iris.

DIAGNOSIS

A patient with acute neovascular glaucoma occasionally presents a challenge in diagnosis because the cornea may be so hazy that it obscures a view of details in the anterior chamber. Under such circumstances **the differential diagnosis includes acute angle-closure glaucoma or acute glaucoma secondary to an inflammatory disease.** A careful history is frequently helpful in diagnosing the underlying problem. For instance, most patients developing glaucoma after central retinal vein occlusion recall a painless blurring or loss of vision in the affected eye weeks or months prior to developing pain. Likewise a diabetic patient with retinal vasculopathy sufficient to cause neovascular glaucoma is almost sure to be aware that he or she has diabetes. Also a diabetic patient frequently, but not always, has a history of reduced vision before development of glaucoma. Careful examination of the patient's other eye can also provide valuable information, particularly regarding the appearance of the chamber angle, the intraocular pressure, and the condition of the retina. For example, most patients with acute primary angle closure have a predisposition to the same problem in the opposite eye (especially if the refractive error of both eyes is similar). Therefore, gonioscopy of the opposite eye will usually show a narrow angle. An elevated intraocular pressure in the opposite eye, coupled with a normal gonioscopic appearance, will suggest open angle glaucoma, a common finding in the eye opposite one with NVG after a CRVO. When diabetic retinopathy is the underlying cause for neovascular glaucoma in one eye, the opposite retina will almost always show some evidence of retinopathy as well.

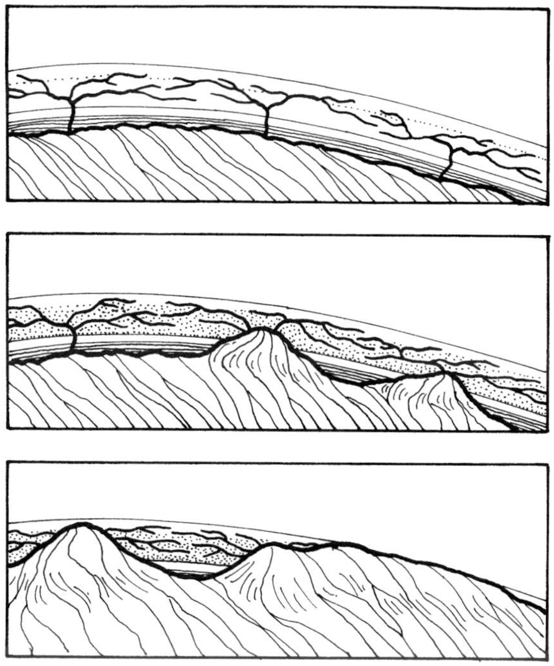

Figure 31.6. Stages of anterior segment neovascularization. New vessel proliferation begins at the pupillary margin and occurs subsequently in the anterior chamber angle. New angle vessels begin as trunks growing up from the iris base, crossing the ciliary body band and scleral spur to reach the trabecular meshwork where they branch and grow circumferentially, often connecting with branches from adjacent trunks (A). Intermediate: Contractile processes along the vessels lead to synechia formation (B). Late: The final stage is total angle closure (C).

Carotid artery disease may produce NVG (Table 31.2). These patients may demonstrate only peripheral retinal hemorrhages and a relatively low IOP despite advanced angle closure. If carotid artery disease is treated surgically, the IOP may markedly increase due to improved ocular perfusion.

Even a severely edematous cornea in the involved eye

Table 31.2
Carotid Artery Disease: Under-Appreciated Cause for NVG Unique Features

1. IOP may be normal, with poor outflow facility masked by decreased aqueous production.
2. Correction of carotid occlusion may lead to marked elevation of IOP.
3. PRP may be less effective (23).

can usually be cleared enough with topical glycerin to allow some of the superficial new vessels on the iris and angle to be seen. Occasionally, an acute iritis will cause a "rubeotic" appearance because the major vessels, and even the capillaries, may dilate markedly, becoming much more visible and imparting a red hue to the iris. But these inflamed vessels, though dilated and tortuous, are still within the iris stroma and still in a predominantly radial pattern consistent with normal iris vasculature. One must differentiate this finding from the rubeosis associated with a true vasoproliferative response that derives from the growth of irregular networks of newly formed vessels on the iris surface. Frequently a contractile element associated with these new surface vessels causes an ectropion of the posterior iris pigment epithelium: this finding can be a useful clinical clue to the diagnosis.

Having determined that the case is a true neovascular glaucoma, the clinician will then want to ensure that the underlying cause has been correctly identified. This is important because the underlying pathologic condition may require specific treatment, e.g., diabetes, systemic hypertension, carotid artery occlusion, or retinal detachment (Table 31.3). **Diagnostic ultrasound is uniquely helpful in revealing occult malignancy presenting as neovascular glaucoma and should be considered for all cases in which the cause of anterior neovascularization is unclear or the fundus cannot be seen.**

The management of neovascular glaucoma is guided by the underlying cause. Enucleation was, in the past, a common outcome for a painful and sightless eye. Enucleation may still be the proper approach for cases in which neovascular glaucoma has been caused by a posterior neoplasm or a devastating inflammation or infection. However, most cases do not fall into this category, and treatment should attempt to preserve remaining vision and maintain a comfortable eye.

PROPHYLAXIS

Before any discussion of treatment, however, **prevention of neovascular glaucoma is now possible in a large proportion of eyes that would have been destined for this disease in the past.** Preventive treatment is based on careful assessment of the setting in which anterior segment neovascularization develops and recognition of the progressive stages leading to fully manifest glaucoma. With continuing improvements in early detection and prophylaxis, the need to treat the disease in full-blown form may eventually become uncommon.

Table 31.3
Conditions Associated with Neovascular Glaucoma

Diabetic retinopathy (common)

Retinal disorders
- Vascular occlusive disorders
  - Central retinal vein occlusion (common)
  - Central retinal artery occlusion
  - Branch retinal artery or vein occlusion
- Retinal detachment (chronic)
- Retinopathy of prematurity
- Coat's disease
- Sickle cell retinopathy
- Syphilitic retinopathy
- Retinoschisis
- Radiation-induced retinopathy

Ocular tumors
- Ocular melanoma
- Retinoblastoma
- Reticulum cell sarcoma
- Metastatic tumors

Uveitis (chronic)

Vascular disorders (associated with ocular ischemia)
- Carotid artery occlusive disease (common)
- Carotid cavernous fistula
- Temporal (giant cell) arteritis
- Pulseless disease

Post surgical
- Strabismus surgery (interruption of anterior ciliary vessels)
- Vitrectomy (with associated diabetic retinopathy)
- Cataract surgery (with associated diabetic retinopathy)

The keystone for prevention of neovascular glaucoma at this time is **retinal ablation** in which, by means of photocoagulation or cryotherapy, a portion of the retinal tissue is destroyed. Reducing the mass of viable retina with photocoagulation therapy seems to inhibit and even reverse new vessel proliferation in the anterior segment. Regression of new vessels on the surface of the iris after panretinal photocoagulation has been reported by several authors (16–22), and a large retrospective study demonstrated a significantly lower incidence of neovascularization of the iris and angle in the eyes of diabetic patients treated by panretinal photocoagulation (23).

These findings are in agreement with the observation that anterior segment neovascularization characteristically occurs in close association with retinal hypoxia. This is compatible with the hypothesis put forth by Michelson (24) that ischemic retinal tissue calls forth new vessel growth by releasing a diffusible angiogenic substance. Forward diffusion of such an angiogenic factor could initiate neovascularization in the anterior segment as well (25) (Fig. 31.2). A factor with angiogenic properties has been found in solid tumors (26), and there is indication that retinal tissue also harbors an angiogenic substance (27). Vascular endothelial growth factor has been measured in the ocular fluids of eyes with ischemic retinas, suggesting it may mediate the neovascular response (28). Whatever the factors that may be active in the pathogenesis of neovascular glaucoma, large scale destruction of retinal tissue by photocoagulation plays an important role in reducing the vasoproliferative stimulus in the anterior segment. Furthermore, the retinal ablation need not be accomplished solely by photocoagulation. If media opacities preclude photocoagulation, widespread retinal cryoablation is an alternative approach which is also effective in reducing anterior segment vasoproliferation (29–30).

Although retinal ablation is the primary preventive treatment, a second means of prophylaxis using direct laser coagulation of the new vessels growing in the chamber angle, an approach developed by R.J. Simmons (31–32), may be a useful adjunct. This method, "goniophotocoagulation," requires meticulous application of small laser burns to the trunks of new vessels as they cross the ciliary band and scleral spur between the iris base and the trabecular meshwork. Successful occlusion of these vessels at the level of the ciliary band or scleral spur causes blanching of the fine vascular network which arborizes on the trabecular meshwork.

Goniophotocoagulation interrupts a critical tissue response to the angiogenic stimulus while retinal photocoagulation appears to reduce the stimulus itself. The two treatments can therefore be used in conjunction to good effect. When solid indications for panretinal photocoagulation exist (e.g., in diabetes according to Diabetic Retinopathy Study guidelines (33–34), or in ischemic retinal vein occlusion with progressive anterior segment neovascularization) (10,19,20,35,36) timely use of retinal ablation may prevent significant vasoproliferation in the chamber angle. Also, for eyes with vessels already actively growing on the chamber angle and in those with early synechia formation, rapid initiation of retinal ablation is needed to reduce the proliferative stimulus. In some cases, however, the progression to angle closure is so rapid that it occurs before the eye has time to respond to retinal treatment. In such cases goniophotocoagulation may provide a direct, though transient, interruption in the anatomic chain of events in the anterior segment, providing time for retinal treatment to achieve a reduction in the driving stimulus.

Both retinal photocoagulation and goniophotocoagulation can only prevent glaucoma if performed before permanent scarring or closure of the angle occurs. Once the meshwork is fibrosed, the glaucoma is permanently established. Early detection, before the irreversible stage, and prompt prophylactic intervention are essential. Since the time course for disease development varies greatly, a flexible schedule of examinations aimed at early detection is required. Progression to NVG, when it occurs after CRVO, tends to be rapid and dramatic. As discussed, **NVG commonly develops 3 months after a CRVO, but the period of risk actually extends from 2 weeks to about 7 months.**

Some studies support the use of pan-retinal ablation for any eye with an ischemic CRVO as soon as positive identification of the type can be made (20,35,38). Others have argued that this will result in unnecessary treatment of a high percentage of cases with a treatment method which substantially reduces the most useful remaining vision in these eyes—the peripheral field (39).

Every CRVO should be carefully evaluated when initially seen to determine if it is of the ischemic type; this subgroup must then be carefully monitored for signs of anterior segment neovascularization. The nonischemic type, once identified, cannot be dismissed, since approximately 15% of these will convert to the ischemic type and require similar close monitoring. Appropriate monitoring will include high magnification slit-lamp examination of the pupil and gonioscopy to detect angle neovascularization at closely spaced intervals (2–3 weeks) during the period of highest risk (the first 4 months) with continued less frequent (monthly) evaluation extending to 7 months.

The Central Retinal Vein Occlusion Study (CVOS) is a randomized NIH-sponsored multicenter trial of early panretinal photocoagulation for ischemic CRVO (5). In the CVOS, eyes with an ischemic CRVO are randomly assigned either to early PRP or to PRP only in the event that anterior segment neovascularization develops. After initial intervention, "panretinal photocoagulation is mandated after appropriate photographic documentation for any eye that develops 2 clock hours of INV [iris neovascularization] or any angle neovascularization (ANV) at any time during the study..." The expert panel that designed this study believed that the preferred treatment for ischemic CRVO could not be established from existing information. **The CVOS recently concluded that PRP is effective treatment for neovascularization of the anterior segment caused by ischemic CRVO (40). However, there was no benefit from PRP performed prior to the development of iris or angle neovascularization when frequent follow-up examinations were being performed (5).** It was recommended that all eyes with CRVO should be evaluated for large areas of retinal capillary nonperfusion by fluorescein angiography. Where this is not possible due to media opacity or non-availability, eyes with CRVO should be managed as if they were of the ischemic type. In cases where follow-up examinations are problematic, prophylactic PRP is recommended. The identification of early neovascularization of the pupillary border was felt to be particularly important in patients after recent CRVO to assess the need for initial or additional PRP. This study confirms the general impression that PRP is effective treatment for the prevention of NVG after CRVO, an opinion which is widely held but not universal (39,41).

In diabetes, the main risk for neovascularization of the anterior segment occurs with proliferative diabetic retinopathy. These cases should receive panretinal photocoagulation as treatment for their retinopathy (33–34), and consequently gain the additional benefits of reducing their risk for iris and angle neovascularization. However, even eyes treated with "adequate" PRP may, in fact, still have some significant retinal ischemia and a persisting risk for neovascularization of the anterior segment. Thus **patients deserve careful monitoring of the iris and angle, even after a standard course of PRP, so that further retinal ablation can be done if new vessels develop or progress in the anterior segment.**

There are other events that may initiate or aggravate new vessel growth in a previously quiet diabetic eye. One is surgical intervention. The anterior hyaloid and lens represent a barrier to forward movement of angiogenic substances from the retina (Fig. 31.2). **Removal of this barrier by vitrectomy/lensectomy or intracapsular cataract extraction may lead to rapid progression of anterior segment neovascularization in a predisposed eye (42–45).** The use of an extracapsular technique for cataract extraction seems to preserve this useful barrier, but it may be lost if posterior capsulotomy is required later (46).

Diabetics may also develop tractional retinal detachments. Since chronic retinal detachment is an important cause of neovascular glaucoma, this introduces another risk factor for NVG which requires increased monitoring of the anterior segment. Finally, diabetics may develop retinal ischemia on the basis of ocular or extraocular circulatory compromise which does not present as classic retinopathy but which can lead to neovascular glaucoma.

MEDICAL TREATMENT

Careful monitoring of at-risk eyes and vigorous use of prophylactic intervention has reduced but not eliminated the need to treat more advanced stages of neovascular glaucoma. Medical therapy of neovascular glaucoma is based on aqueous suppressants—carbonic anhydrase inhibitors, beta-adrenergic blockers, and apraclonidine. The outflow system of these eyes is usually not responsive to miotics or epinephrine, and because they may aggravate inflammation, they should be avoided. Anti-glaucoma medication is often supplemented with anti-inflammatory treatment, corticosteroids and cycloplegics. If the angle is fully closed by synechias, such combined aqueous suppressant/anti-inflammatory therapy may bring comfort and some reduction in pressure, but it will seldom provide a normal pressure. On the other hand, if the angle is wholly or partly open, and particularly if the vessels can be made to regress with retinal ablation, medical therapy may then provide adequate longterm glaucoma management.

SURGICAL TREATMENT

Surgical therapy for NVG has been considered to present the greatest challenge. Fortunately, the situation has evolved in recent years to the point that these cases can now be approached with increasing confidence, though they remain demanding and retain a higher failure rate than more routine situations. A recurring theme for NVG is the positive benefit of retinal ablation. Its earliest and most preferred use is to prevent the condition altogether. At a somewhat later stage, with new vessels on the iris and angle it remains extremely useful as a means to regress the neovascular process and salvage remaining outflow function. **Even when the angle is completely closed by irreversible fibrous contraction, retinal ablation remains extremely useful as a means to quiet the eye, reduce new vessel growth, and prepare the eye for surgery.** The full preparation of an NVG eye for surgery thus includes aqueous suppressants to reduce pressure, corticosteroids and cycloplegics to reduce inflammation, and panretinal photocoagulation to reduce the vasoproliferative stimulus (47).

If the eye has superior limbal tissue that is not heavily scarred from prior surgery, a trabeculectomy supplemented by use of an anti-metabolite is recommended (Chapter 62). Surgery along the inferior limbus should be avoided because these eyes are prone to intraoperative and postoperative bleeding, which will settle inferiorly and compromise filtration. If there is extensive scarring along the superior limbus, then a drainage implant (e.g., Baerveldt, Molteno, Krupin, Ahmed) should be considered (48–50) (Chapter 65).

The techniques do not differ for NVG except as noted—the preparation of the eye, and the avoidance of inferior placement of a sclerostomy or a drainage tube because of frequent postoperative hyphema in NVG cases. Additionally, as with all filtration surgery, control of bleeding is very important and somewhat more difficult in the face of fragile new vessels. Preoperative laser coagulation of the iris at the proposed iridectomy site is recommended by some. Others use fine bipolar cautery on the iris intraoperatively, before performing an iridectomy (51–52).

For eyes with little or no visual potential, ablation of the ciliary body has been a frequent recourse in managing neovascular glaucoma (53–57). Part of its popularity was undoubtedly related to the fairly dismal potential for success with outflow procedures. Now that success rates with filtration procedures and drainage implants are much higher, cilioablation deserves consideration principally as a final resort for eyes with little useful vision. Transscleral laser treatment of the ciliary body seems to offer some advantage over cyclocryotherapy in terms of postoperative comfort and inflammation (58).

Chronic use of steroid/cycloplegic medications can provide longterm comfort to eyes at the endstage of this disease (59). Retrobulbar alcohol injection can also be useful in relieving pain. Fortunately, the need to surgically remove eyes rendered blind and painful by NVG continues to decrease, though sometimes this is a necessary step.

CONCLUSION

Neovascular glaucoma is increasingly understood and preventable, but intervention is only maximally effective in the early stages. The clinician must be aware of the conditions that predispose to this disease, must recognize the often subtle early signs of anterior segment neovascularization, and must be ready to intervene decisively when the situation demands. Currently, the disease is more treatable in all its stages, but the most effective treatment is the earliest.

References

1. Wand M: Neovascular Glaucoma. In: Principles and Practice of Ophthalmology. Clinical Practice. Philadelphia, W.B. Saunders Co., 1994; 1485–1510.
2. Gartner S, Henkind P: Neovascularization of the iris (rubeosis iridis). Surv Ophthalmol 1978;22:291.
3. Hayreh SS, et al: Ocular neovascularization with retinal vascular occlusion - III. Incidence of Ocular Neovascularization with retinal vein occlusion. Ophthalmology 1983;90:488.
4. Hayreh SS: Classification of central retinal vein occlusion. Ophthalmology 1983;90:458.
5. Central Vein Occlusion Study Group, The Central Vein Occlusion Study, Baseline and Early Natural History Report. Arch Ophthalmol 1993;111:1087–1095.
6. Hayreh SS: Retinal Vein Occlusion. Current Ophthalmology. Indian J Ophthalmol 1994;42:3, 109–132.
7. Laatikainen L, Kohner EM: Fluorescein angiography and its prognostic significance in central retinal vein occlusion. Br J Ophthalmol 1976; 60:411.
8. Laatikainen L, Blach RK: Behaviour of the iris vasculature in central retinal vein occlusion: a fluorescein angiographic study of the vascular response of the retina and the iris. Br J Ophthalmol 1977;61:272.
9. Sinclair SH, Gragoudas ES: Prognosis for rubeosis iridis following central retinal vein occlusion. Br J Ophthalmol 1979;63:735.
10. Magargal LE, Brown GC, Augsburger JJ, et al: Neovascular glaucoma following central retinal vein obstruction. Ophthalmology 1981;88: 1095.
11. Hayreh SS, Klugman MR, Beri M, et al: Differentiation of ischemic from non-ischemic central retinal vein occlusion during the early acute phase. Graefe's Arch Clin Exp Opthalmol 1990;228:201–217.
12. Ohrt V: The frequency of rubeosis iridis in diabetic patients. Acta Ophthalmol 1971;49:301.
13. Madsen PH: Rubeosis of the iris and haemorrhagic glaucoma in patients with proliferative diabetic retinopathy. Br J Ophthalmol 1971;55:368.
14. Jocson VL: Microvascular injection studies in rubeosis iridis and neovascular glaucoma. Am J Ophthalmol 1977;483:508.
15. Grant WM: Management of neovascular glaucoma. In: Leopold IH, ed. Symposium on ocular therapy, Vol. 7. St. Louis: CV Mosby, 1974.
16. Krill AC, Archer D, Newell FW: Photocoagulation in complications secondary to branch vein occlusion. Arch Ophthalmol 1971;85:48.
17. Callahan MA, Hilton GF: Photocoagulation and rubeosis iridis. Am J Ophthalmol 1974;78:873.
18. Little HL, Rosenthal AR, Dellaports A, et al: The effect of panretinal photocoagulation on rubeosis iridis. Am J Ophthalmol 1974;78:873.
19. Laatikainen L: Preliminary report on effect of retinal panphotocoagulation on rubeosis iridis and neovascular glaucoma. Br J Ophthamol 1977; 61:278.
20. Laatikainen L, Kohner EM, Khoury D, et al: Panretinal photocoagulation in central retinal vein occlusion. A randomized controlled clinical study. Br J Ophthalmol 1977;61:741.
21. Murphy RP, Egbert PR: Regression of iris neovascularization following panretinal photocoagulation. Arch Ophthalmol 1979;97:700.
22. Tasman W, Magargal LE, Augsburger JJ: Rubeosis iridis and angle neovascularization. Ophthalmology 1980;87:400.
23. Wand M, Dueker DK, Aiello LM, et al: Effects of panretinal photocoagulation on rubeosis iridis, angle neovascularization and neovascular glaucoma. Am J Ophthalmol 1978;86:332.
24. Michaelson IC: The mode of development of the vascular system of the retina with some observations of its significance in certain retinal diseases. Trans Ophthalmol Soc UK 1948;68:137.
25. Ashton N: Retinal vascularization in health and disease. Am J Ophthalmol 1957;44:7.
26. Folkman J: The vascularization of tumors. Sci Am 1976;234–59.
27. Glaser BM, et al: The demonstration of angiogenic activity from ocular tissues. Preliminary report. Ophthalmology 1980;87:440.
28. Aiello L, Avery RL, Arrigg PG, et al: Vascular endothelial growth factor in ocular fluid of patients with diabetic retinopathy and other retinal disorders. N Engl J Med 1994;331:1480–7.
29. Hilton G: Panretinal cryotherapy of diabetic rubeosis. Arch Ophthalmol 1979;97:776.
30. May DR, Bergstrom TJ, Parmet AJ, et al: Treatment of neovascular glaucoma with transcleral panretinal cryotherapy. Ophthalmology 1980; 87:1106.
31. Simmons RJ, Dueker DK, Kimbrough RL, et al: Goniophotocoagulation for neovascul glaucoma. Trans Am Acad Ophthalmol Otolaryngol 1977; 83:80.
32. Simmons RJ, Depperman SR, Dueker DK: The role of goniophotocoagulation in neovascularization of the anterior chamber angle. Ophthalmology 1980;87:79.
33. The Diabetic Retinopathy Study Research Group: Preliminary report on effects of photocoagulation therapy. Am J. Ophthalmol 1976;81: 383.
34. Diabetic Retinopathy Study Research Group. Four risk factors for severe visual loss in diabetic retinopathy. Arch Ophthalmol 1979;97:654.
35. May DR, Klein ML, Peyman GA, et al: Xenon arc panretinal photocoagulation for central retinal vein occlusion: a randomized prospective study. Br J Ophthalmol 1979;63:725.
36. Magargal LE, Brown GC, Augsburger JJ, et al: Efficacy of panretinal photocoagulation in preventing neovascular glaucoma following ischemic central retinal vein obstruction. Ophthalmology 1982;89: 780–784.
37. May DR, Klein ML, Peyman GA, et al: Xenon are panretinal photocoagulation for central vein occlusion: a randomized prospective study. Br J Ophthalmol 1979;63:725–734.
38. Laatkainen L, Kohner EM, Khoury D, et al: Panretinal photocoagulation in central vein occlusion: a randomized controlled clinical study. Br J Ophthalmol 1977;61:741–753.
39. Hayreh SS, Klugman MR, Podhajsky P, et al: Argon laser panretinal photocoagulation in ischemic central retinal vein occlusion. Graefes Arch Ophthalmol 1990;228:281–296.
40. The Central Vein Occlusion Study Group. A randomized clinical trial of early panretinal photocoagulation for ischemic central vein occlusion. Ophthalmology 1995;102:1434–1444.
41. Hayreh SS, Klugman MR, Podhajsky P, et al: Argon laser panretinal photocoagulation in ischemic central retinal vein occlusion. Graefes Arch Clin Ophthalmol 1990;228:281–296.
42. Aiello LM, Wand M, Liang G: Neovascular glaucoma and vitreous hemorrhage following cataract surgery in patients with diabetes mellitus. Ophthalmology 1983;90:814.
43. Blankenship G: The lens influence on diabetic vitrectomy results; report of a prospective randomized study. Arch Ophthalmol 1980;98:2196.
44. Aaberg TM: Pars plana vitrectomy for diabetic traction retinal detachment. Ophthalmology 1981;88:639.
45. Rice TA, Michels RG, Maguire MG, et al: The effect of lensectomy on the incidence of iris neovascularization and neovascular glaucoma after vitrectomy for diabetic retinopathy. Am J Ophthalmol 1983;95:1.

46. Weinreb RN, Wasserstrom JP, Parker W: Neovascular glaucoma following neodymium: YAG laser posterior capsulotomy. Arch Ophthalmol 1986;104:730–731.
47. Allen RC, Bellows AR, Hutchinson BT, et al: Filtration surgery in the treatment of neovascular glaucoma. Ophthalmology 1982;89:1181.
48. Molteno ACB, Von Rooyen MMB, Bartholomew RS: Implants for draining neovascular glaucoma. Br J Ophthalmol 1977;61:120.
49. Krupin R, et al: Filtering valve implant surgery for eyes with neovascular glaucoma. Am J Ophthalmol 1980;89:338.
50. Schocket SS, Lakhanpal V, Richards RD: Anterior chamber tube shunt to an encircling band in the treatment of neovascular glaucoma. Ophthalmology 1982;89:1188.
51. Hersh SB, Kass MA: Iridectomy in rubeosis iridis. Ophthalmic Surg 1976;7:19.
52. Herschler J, Agness D: A modified filtering operation for neovascular glaucoma. Arch Ophthalmol 1979;97:2339.
53. Goldstein AL, Ide CH: Cyclocryotherapy for secondary glaucoma due to rubeosis iridis. MO Med 1972;69:736.
54. Feibel RM, Bigger JF: Rubeosis iridis and neovascular glaucoma. Evaluation of cyclocryotherapy. Am J Ophthalmol 1972;74:862.
55. Bellows AR, Grant WM: Cyclocryotherapy in advanced inadequately controlled glaucoma. Am J Ophthalmol 1973;75:659.
56. Boniuk M: Cryotherapy in neovascular glaucoma. Trans Am Acad Ophthalmol Otolaryngol 1974;78:337.
57. Krupin T, Mitchell KB, Becker B: Cyclocryotherapy in neovascular glaucoma. Am J Ophthalmol 1978;86:24.
58. Klapper R, Wandel T, Donnerfeld E, et al: Transscleral neodymium: YAG cyclophotocoagulation in refractory glaucoma: a preliminary report. Ophthalmology 1988;719:22.
59. Drews RD: Corticosteroid management of hemorrhagic glacoma. Trans Am Acad Ophthalmol Otolaryngol 1974;78:334.

Iridocorneal Endothelial Syndromes 32

M. Bruce Shields

HISTORY AND TERMINOLOGY

In the first edition of their textbook, Chandler and Grant noted that two conditions, which at that time were commonly referred to as essential iris atrophy and Chandler's syndrome, shared several common features and quite likely were variations of a spectrum of disease (1).

There were several isolated case reports in the late nineteenth century of patients with extreme iris atrophy and associated glaucoma, but it was the paper by Harms in 1903 that led to our current understanding of the condition that has been called "essential iris atrophy" or "progressive essential iris atrophy" (2). In 1956, Chandler reported cases that were similar, but differed by having less severe iris atrophy and more frequent corneal edema, which often occurred with intraocular pressures that were normal, or only slightly elevated (3). In all of his cases, Chandler noted an abnormality of the corneal endothelium, which he described as having a fine hammered silver appearance. The condition became known as "Chandler's syndrome." **In both essential iris atrophy and Chandler's syndrome, the glaucoma is associated with a characteristic, progressive closure of the anterior chamber angle.**

In 1969, Cogan and Reese described two patients with pigmented nodules of the iris (4). Malignant melanoma was suspected, and the eyes were enucleated, but the nodules were found to be benign, composed of tissue resembling that of the iris stroma. Subsequent studies revealed that these nodules may occur on the surface of the iris in association with the other changes seen with essential iris atrophy and Chandler's syndrome, and this condition became known as the "Cogan-Reese syndrome."

Continued study of these three conditions revealed the common denominator of a characteristic abnormality of the corneal endothelium, which may lead to corneal edema, progressive closure of the anterior chamber angle with associated glaucoma, and the spectrum of iris abnormalities. Scheie and Yanoff described a fourth condition with flat nevi on the surface of the iris, which they called the "iris nevus syndrome," and lumped it with the Cogan-Reese syndrome as a single entity (5). However, the iris lesions in the two conditions are distinctly different, and the iris nevus syndrome has not been shown to have the corneal endothelial abnormality, which would associate it with the other three conditions.

Eagle and associates suggested the term "iridocorneal endothelial (ICE) syndrome," and this has now become the most commonly used term for the spectrum of disease which includes essential iris atrophy, Chandler's syndrome, and the Cogan-Reese syndrome (6). Because atrophy of the iris is neither an essential nor fundamental aspect of these disorders, the term "progressive iris atrophy" may be preferable for the first of these three clinical variations. In any case, Chandler and Grant were correct in believing that **these conditions do represent a broad spectrum of ocular disease.**

CLINICAL FEATURES

The **ICE syndrome is nearly always clinically unilateral**, although subclinical abnormalities of the corneal endothelium may be seen in the fellow eye. The condition is usually recognized in early to middle adulthood, with a predilection for women. Familial cases are rare and there is no consistent association with systemic diseases.

In a study of 37 consecutive cases of the ICE syndrome, approximately half were Chandler's syndrome, while the other two clinical variations each accounted for about one fourth of all cases (7). Chandler's syndrome was characterized by more severe corneal edema, even though the glaucoma tended to be less severe than in the other two variations.

A common presenting manifestation is the recognition of an abnormal shape or position of the pupil, which the patient may describe as a localized or diffuse dark spot on the iris. Other patients may present with a chief complaint of reduced vision, which is typically worse in the morning, due to the corneal edema that develops while the lids are closed during sleep, and which improves during the day as the cornea dehydrates with exposure to air. Patients with more advanced disease may have persistent reduction in vision due to severe corneal edema or glaucomatous optic atrophy. Some patients may also present with pain, which is usually due to the corneal edema.

Clinical examination of a patient with the ICE syndrome typically reveals abnormalities of the cornea, anterior chamber angle, and iris.

The corneal abnormality, which is a common feature throughout the ICE syndrome is seen by slit-lamp examination as a **fine hammered silver appearance of the posterior cornea,** similar to that of Fuchs' dystrophy, but less coarse (Fig. 32.1). The cornea may be otherwise clear with no associated symptoms, or there may be corneal edema with variable degrees of reduced vision and pain, as noted above. In some cases, islands of the endothelial abnormality may be seen in the fellow eye, which is otherwise unaffected by the disease process.

Specular microscopy of the corneal endothelial cells reveals a characteristic, diffuse abnormality with variable degrees of pleomorphism in size and shape, dark areas within the cells, and loss of clear hexagonal margins (8). (Fig. 32.2) These cells have been called "ICE cells," and the tissue they form has been termed "ICE tissue" (9). In some cases the cells cover the entire posterior cornea while in other eyes they are scattered throughout the cornea or occur in areas that are sharply demarcated from endothelial cells that are either normal or abnormally large or small. In some cases the focal area of abnormal cells may spread over time to eventually cover the entire cornea, although one case has been reported in which the abnormal cells disappeared almost entirely over a 10-year observation period (10).

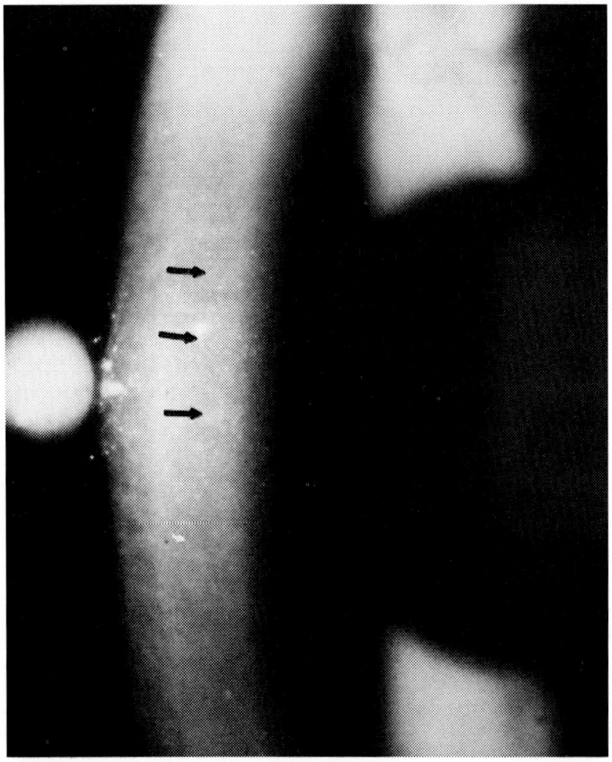

Figure 32.1. Slit-lamp view showing fine beaten metal appearance of corneal endothelial abnormality (arrows) in the ICE syndrome. Reprinted with permission from Shields MB, Campbell DG, Simmons RJ: Am J Ophthalmol 1978;85:749.

The typical anterior chamber angle abnormality, which is also common to all variations of the ICE syndrome, is seen by gonioscopy as **peripheral anterior synechiae which extend to or beyond Schwalbe's line.** The synechias are broad based and typically progress around the circumference of the angle, eventually leading to IOP elevation. Glaucoma occurs in approximately half of all patients with the ICE syndrome. It is more severe in patients with progressive iris atrophy and Cogan-Reese variations, as opposed to those with Chandler's syndrome (7). **Although glaucoma is believed to be related to the angle closure in most cases, it does not correlate precisely with the degree of synechial closure and has been observed in eyes with entirely open angles.**

The iris abnormalities constitute the primary basis for distinguishing the clinical variations within the ICE syndrome. Progressive iris atrophy is characterized by marked atrophy of the iris, associated with variable degrees of corectopia and ectropion uvea (Fig. 32.3). The latter two features are usually directed toward the quadrant with the most prominent area of peripheral anterior synechia. The hallmark of progressive iris atrophy is hole formation of the iris, which occurs in two forms: 1) stretch holes, and 2) melting holes (11). With stretch holes, the iris is markedly thinned in the quadrant away from the direction of pupil-

Figure 32.2. Specular microscopic appearance of corneal endothelial cells in the ICE syndrome showing pleomorphism in size and shape, dark areas within the cells, and loss of clear hexagonal margins. Reprinted with permission from Shields MB: Textbook of Glaucoma, 3rd ed. Baltimore: Williams and Wilkins, 1992;261.

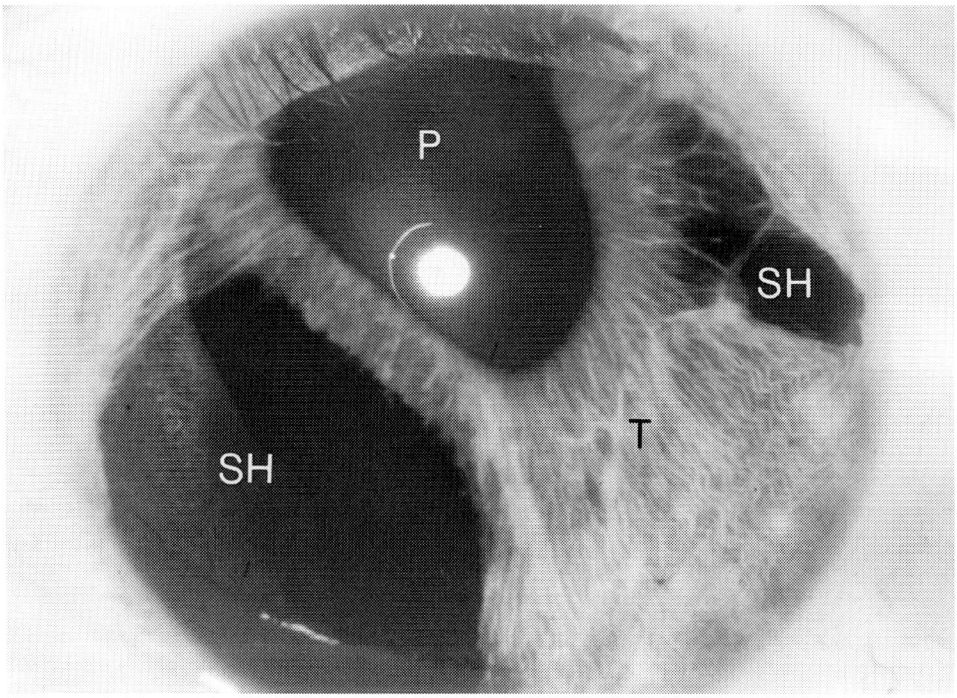

Figure 32.3. Progressive iris atrophy, a variation of the ICE syndrome, with pupillary distortion (P), thinning of the iris (T), and stretch holes (SH). Reprinted with permission from Shields MB, Campbell DG, Simmons RJ: Am J Ophthalmol 1978;85:749.

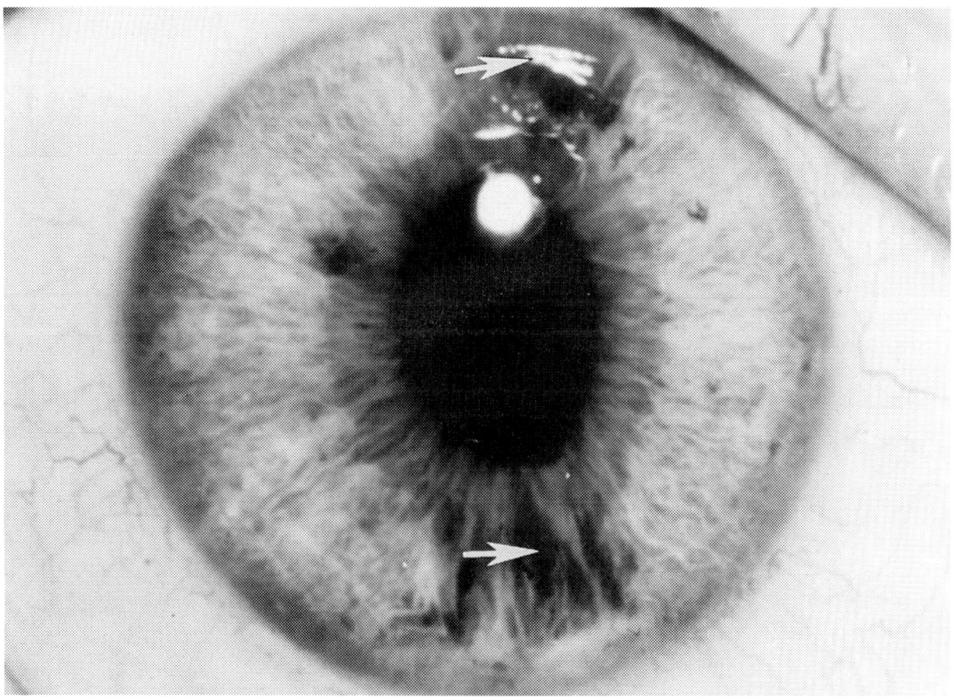

Figure 32.4. Chandler's syndrome, a variation of the ICE syndrome, with slight pupillary distortion and thinning of iris stroma at the vertical poles (arrows). Reprinted with permission from Shields MB, Campbell DG, Simmons RJ: Am J Ophthalmol 1978; 85:749.

lary distortion, and the holes develop within the stretched area. Melting holes develop without associated corectopia or iris thinning, and fluorescein angiographic studies suggest that these holes are associated with iris ischemia (11).

In Chandler's syndrome, there is typically minimal corectopia and mild atrophy of the iris stroma (Fig. 32.4). In some cases, there may be no detectable change in the iris. Intermediate variations may also occur in which the degree of corectopia and stromal iris atrophy is more extensive than that of typical Chandler's syndrome, but the characteristic hole formation of progressive iris atrophy is lacking.

Eyes with the Cogan-Reese syndrome may have any degree of iris atrophy, but are distinguished by the pres-

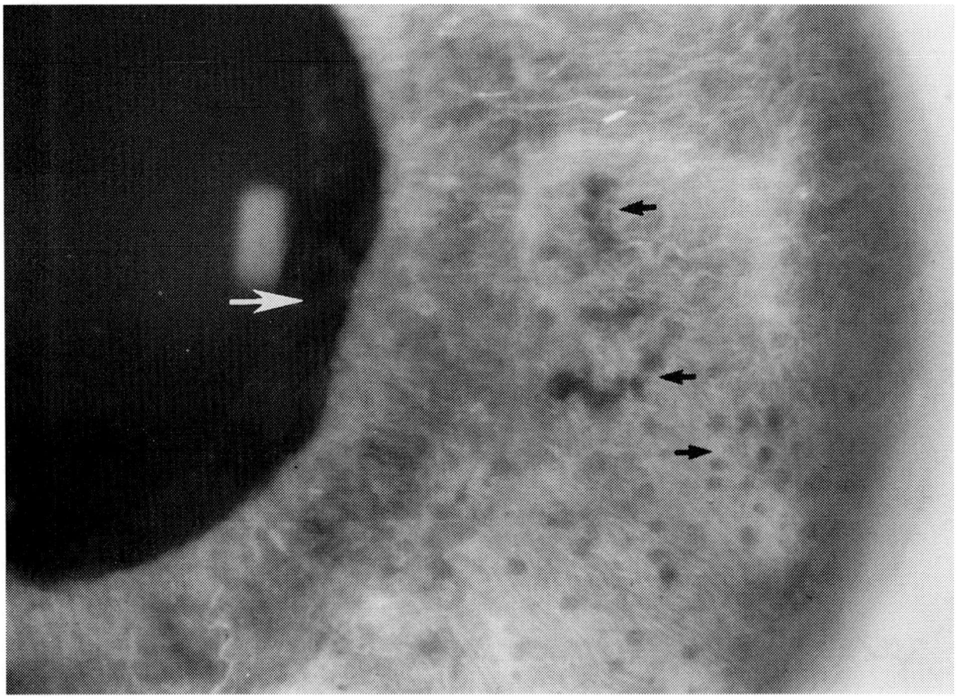

Figure 32.5. Cogan-Reese syndrome, a variation of the ICE syndrome, showing ectropion uvea (white arrow) and numerous dark nodules (black arrows) on area of flattened iris stroma. Reprinted with permission from Shields MB, Campbell DG, Simmons RJ, et al: Arch Ophthalmol 1976;96:406.

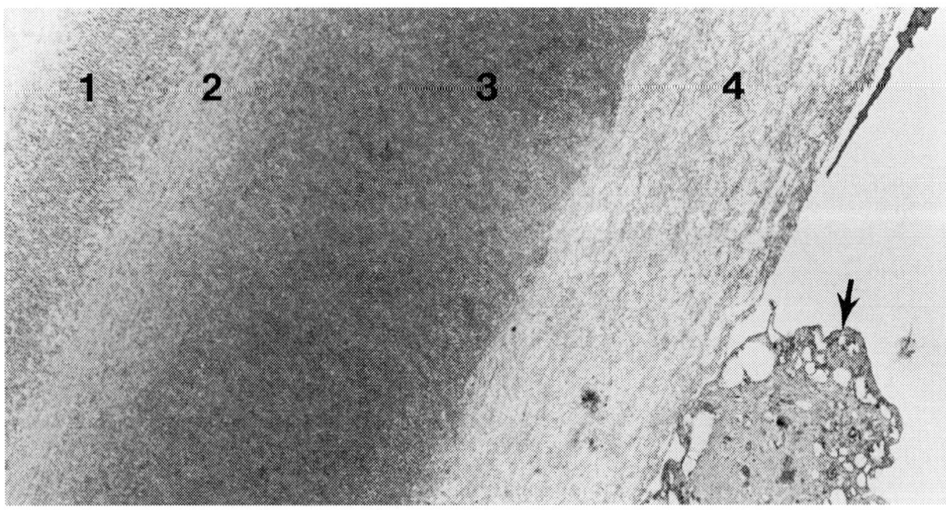

Figure 32.6. Transmission electron microscopic view of inner corneal surface in ICE syndrome showing part of an abnormal cell (arrow) on a four-layered membrane, composed of the anterior non-banded (1) and posterior banded (2) portions of Descemet's membrane with abnormal compact collagenous (3) and loose collagenous (4) layers (x6,875). Reprinted with permission from Shields MB, McCracken JS, Klintworth GK, et al: Ophthalmology 1979;86:1533.

ence of pigmented, pedunculated nodules on the surface of the iris (Fig. 32.5). The iris stroma surrounding the nodules is typically flat, with loss of the normal iris architecture. In some cases, other features of the ICE syndrome may be present for many years before the nodules appear.

HISTOPATHOLOGIC FEATURES

Electron microscopic study of the posterior cornea in advanced cases demonstrates grossly abnormal cells, lining multilayered collagenous tissue posterior to Descemet's membrane (12,13) (Fig. 32.6). In some cases, the cells are markedly attenuated or absent, exposing areas of underlying collagenous layer, whereas other specimens reveal multiple cellular layers, suggesting loss of contact inhibition. Some cells show evidence of metabolic activity, while others appear disrupted and necrotic. Cells may have filopodial cytoplasmic projections and cytoplasmic actin filaments, indicative of cellular migration (13). Some studies have revealed epithelial characteristics of the cells, including cytokeratin expression (14), although another immunohistochemical study revealed no evidence of epithelial characteristics (15). Occasional lymphocytes have been seen on or within the abnormal cellular layer (13,15). The underlying collagenous layer consists of a thin, normally-appearing Descemet's membrane bounded posteriorly by thickened layers of banded and fibrillar tissue, suggesting that the abnormal collagen was deposited by the abnormal endothelial cells in postnatal life (12,16).

Histologic studies of the anterior chamber angle reveal a cellular membrane, consisting of a single layer of endothelial cells and a Descemet's-like membrane, extending down from the peripheral cornea. The membrane may cover an open anterior chamber angle, which could explain those cases of glaucoma with open angles. Far more typically, however, the membrane is associated with synechial closure of the chamber angle.

Histopathology of the iris in all variations of the ICE syndrome includes a cellular membrane on portions of the anterior surface of the iris, which is similar to and continuous with that seen over the anterior chamber angle. The membrane is most often found in the quadrant toward which the pupil is distorted. In progressive iris atrophy, there is marked iris atrophy and hole formation in the opposite quadrant. The histopathology is the same in Chandler's syndrome with the exception of less extensive iris atrophy and no hole formation. In the Cogan-Reese syndrome, the nodular lesions have an ultrastructure similar to that of the underlying stroma of the iris and are always surrounded by the previously described cellular membrane.

THEORIES OF MECHANISM

The precise etiology of the ICE syndrome is unknown. The infrequency of familial cases and the histologic evidence that corneal alterations begin in postnatal life argues in favor of an acquired disorder, rather than an inherited or congenital condition. The observation of lymphocytes on or in the corneal endothelial layer suggests the presence of chronic inflammation and has led to the theory of a viral etiology (13). Serologic studies in 13 patients with the ICE syndrome suggested, but did not prove, a role for the Epstein-Barr virus (17). More compelling evidence from primer pair and PCR methods revealed herpes simplex viral DNA in 16 of 25 corneal specimens of ICE patients with localization within the endothelium (18). This finding was absent in normal corneas and corneas from patients with three other chronic corneal diseases.

Although the initial event in the pathogenesis of the ICE syndrome is not established, **the corneal endothelial abnormality is most likely the fundamental alteration that leads to the other clinicopathologic features.** According to the theory of Campbell and associates, the abnormality of the corneal endothelium in the ICE syndrome causes the corneal edema in some cases and leads in other cases to the proliferation of the cellular membrane across the anterior chamber angle and onto the iris surface (19). Contraction of the cellular portion of this membrane causes the formation of peripheral anterior synechias, corectopia, and ectropion uvea. Stretching of the iris in the direction away from the corectopia is believed to contribute to the atrophy and hole formation, although additional factors, such as ischemia, may also be involved. The cellular membrane is also felt to be responsible for the development of the nodular lesions of the iris in the Cogan-Reese syndrome, possibly by encircling and pinching off portions of the iris stroma (20).

The mechanism of glaucoma in the ICE syndrome, as previously noted, is also believed to be related to the cellular membrane. In some cases, the membrane may cover the trabecular meshwork, which is still visible gonioscopically, thereby obstructing aqueous outflow. In most cases, however, the IOP does not begin to rise until contraction of the membrane has led to some degree of synechial closure of the anterior chamber angle.

DIFFERENTIAL DIAGNOSIS

There are several other disorders of the cornea and iris, many of which have associated glaucoma, that could be confused with various forms of the ICE syndrome. Other conditions with corneal endothelial disorders include posterior polymorphous dystrophy and Fuchs' endothelial dystrophy. While the former condition may also have changes of the anterior chamber angle and iris that resemble the ICE syndrome, it is distinguished by a familial tendency, bilateral involvement, and a difference in the appearance of the posterior corneal abnormality by both clinical examination and specular microscopy. The corneal endothelial changes of Fuchs' endothelial dystrophy more closely resemble those of the ICE syndrome, but these patients have none of the chamber angle or iris features of the latter condition.

Other conditions with dissolution of the iris include the Axenfeld-Rieger syndrome, which has striking clinical and histopathologic similarities to the ICE syndrome, but differs by the bilateral and congenital nature of the condition and the association with systemic disorders. Aniridia and iridoschisis might be confused with the ICE syndrome, although the former is bilateral and the latter occurs in the elderly.

Nodular lesions of the iris that could be confused with the Cogan-Reese syndrome include melanomas of the iris, recalling that the first two cases were enucleated because of this confusion. Melanosis of the iris, which is characterized by verrucous-like elevations, could also be confused with the Cogan-Reese syndrome. In addition, differentiation must be made from the nodular lesions of neurofibromatosis, as well as nodular inflammatory disorders, such as sarcoidosis.

MANAGEMENT

Patients with the ICE syndrome may require treatment for corneal edema, glaucoma, or both. The glaucoma can often be controlled medically in the early stages,

IS HERPES SIMPLEX INVOLVED IN THE PATHOGENESIS OF ICE SYNDROME?

Jorge Alvarado

Iridocorneal Endothelial Syndrome: Recent Advances

The abnormalities of the corneal endothelium, trabecular meshwork, and iris tissues in the ICE syndrome have been described in extensive detail (1–4). Many clinically important diagnostic signs can now be related to ultrastructural changes affecting the corneal endothelium. Most importantly, a proposed potential viral etiology (5) raises the possibility of direct therapeutic approaches for these difficult to manage and sometimes devastating diseases.

Endothelial Involvement

Ultrastructural, immunocytochemical, and molecular biological studies have pointed out that the ICE syndrome diseases have a common underlying endothelial abnormality. This finding supports the clinical concept that Chandler's, essential iris atrophy and the Cogan-Reese iris nevus syndromes represent three different manifestations of the condition now designated the "ICE syndrome."

Normally, the endothelium remains confined to the posterior corneal surface as if held there by "contact inhibition"; in contrast, in the ICE syndrome, these cells are able to migrate peripherally. Most, if not all, of the complications associated with the ICE syndrome can be attributed to this migration. Chronic corneal edema develops when 1) cell migration results in a marked decrease in endothelial density (3), leaving tiny spaces denuded of this barrier (3); and/or when, 2) dysfunctional ICE-endothelial cells are no longer capable of maintaining a deturgesced cornea. IOP elevation and glaucomatous optic atrophy develop when migrating ICE-endothelial cells or PAS obstruct the outflow of aqueous. Iris ectropion uveae, corectopia, polycoria, transillumination defects and nevi also result from endothelial migration, with deposition and contraction of Descemet's membrane causing iris atrophy.

Nevertheless, further evidence is needed to support the hypothesis that endothelial migration is due to a loss of contact inhibition. While growth of ICE endothelial cells atop each other could reflect a loss of contact inhibition, numerous junctions bind these cells to prevent free migration (3). Moreover, there is no convincing evidence that ICE endothelial cells can migrate over an intact layer of trabecular cells.

An alternative hypothesis is that the trabecular meshwork and/or iris tissues, as well as the corneal endothelium, are primarily involved in the ICE disease process. Normally trabecular cells exert contact inhibition on the corneal endothelium so that when this barrier is broken, as in traumatic trabeculodialysis or angle recession, the corneal cells can migrate peripherally. Similarly, disease or death of trabecular cells by the ICE process could lead to abnormal endothelial migration. Regarding the iris, a primary process, such as ischemia with PAS formation, would also permit the endothelium to migrate directly onto this tissue.

In summary, the three tissues lining the anterior chamber are involved in the ICE syndrome. Although it is unclear whether all three tissues are primarily affected, the major clinical manifestations are well explained on the basis of an endothelial abnormality alone. Two appealing features of a possible viral etiology are that: it is easy to envision all three tissues being affected by such an infection; and, that loss of contact inhibition, cell transformation, and segmental iris ischemia are alterations known to be induced by viruses.

Clinical Signs

Familiarity with the salient ultrastructural features, as shown by scanning microscopy of ICE endothelial cells, makes it easier to appreciate the basis for the specular microscopy findings and to train oneself to detect these signs using slit-lamp biomicroscopy.

With the slit lamp specular reflex, one of the early signs observed in ICE patients is that the endothelial mosaic pattern is more easily recognized than that in normals. ICE cells vary widely in size and are separated by broad intercellular spaces, as if more grout has been placed between each "tile." Their extensive interdigitating intercellular processes (3) make cell borders appear wider and darker on the specular reflex. Another useful slit-lamp sign consists of white dots located near the center of each cell. These bright dots are apoptotic bodies, irregular structures which protrude into the AC (3) and disrupt the normal specular reflex. Along with the "beaten" metal appearance of the endothelium originally described by Chandler, these two signs make it possible to diagnose many ICE patients at the slit lamp without the need of special equipment.

Etiologic Considerations

To consider possible etiologies for the ICE syndrome, we compared a large series of corneal specimens from normal (1,2) and ICE patients using morphometric and advanced statistical methods to ascertain the age of onset of the endothelial derangement (3,4). Deposition of abnormal extracellular matrix on Descemet's membrane in ICE patients (4) takes place decades before disease onset but during postnatal life, in support of the hypothesis that the ICE syndrome is acquired after birth. The low-grade, chronic inflammatory response sharply confined to the corneal endothelium, in conjunction with alterations reminiscent of those present in virally-infected cells suggested that a viral antigen might also be present in the ICE endothelium.

Molecular biology methods based on the use of PCR were developed and used to demonstrate herpes simplex viral DNA in the corneal endothelium, trabecular meshwork and iris tissues of ICE patients (5). This association between the ICE syndrome and the presence of herpes simplex DNA supports the concept that there might be an underlying viral etiology for the ICE syndrome. Future investigation to demonstrate causality and to understand how the implicated virus causes the cellular derangements responsible for such devastating conditions needs to be carried out before specific treatment for the ICE syndrome may be considered.

References

1. Murphy C, Alvarado J, Juster R: Prenatal and postnatal growth of the human Descemet's membrane. Invest Ophthalmol Vis Sci 1984; 25:56–69.
2. Murphy C, Alvarado J, Juster R, et al: Prenatal and postnatal cellularity of the human corneal endothelium. Invest Ophthalmol Vis Sci 1984;25:312–322.
3. Alvarado J, Murphy C, Maglio M, et al: Pathogenesis of Chandler's Syndrome, essential iris atrophy and the Cogan-Reese Syndrome. I. Alterations of the corneal endothelium. Invest Ophthalmol Vis Sci 1986;27:853–872.
4. Alvarado J, Murphy C, Maglio M, et al: Pathogenesis of Chandler's Syndrome, essential iris atrophy and the Cogan-Reese Syndrome. II. Estimated age at disease onset. Invest Ophthalmol Vis Sci 1986; 27:873–882.
5. Alvarado J, Underwood J, Green R, et al: Detection of herpes simplex viral DNA in the iridocorneal endothelial syndrome. Arch Ophthalmol 1994;112:1601–1609.

especially with drugs that reduce aqueous production, such as beta blockers and carbonic anhydrase inhibitors. Lowering the IOP may also help to control the corneal edema, although the additional use of hypertonic saline solutions and soft contact lenses are often required.

When the IOP can no longer be controlled medically, surgical intervention is indicated. Laser trabeculoplasty is usually not effective in these cases. Filtering surgery is reasonably successful, although late failures occur, which in some cases may be due to continued growth of the endothelial membrane over the surgical fistula. It may be possible in these cases to reopen the fistula with Nd:YAG laser applications. In one report of nine eyes with the ICE syndrome, eight of which had prior unsuccessful trabeculectomies, filtration surgery with postoperative subconjunctival injections of 5-fluorouracil controlled the IOP in only four eyes, while the others required further surgery (21). The intraoperative use of mitomycin may be more effective in these cases, although there are no reports on this to date. As with other forms of glaucoma, when the IOP cannot be controlled with the more conventional therapies, cyclodestructive procedures, especially transscleral cyclophotocoagulation, may be beneficial.

In some cases, surgical reduction of the IOP may relieve the corneal edema. However, even an extremely low IOP usually will not reverse advanced corneal edema. Furthermore, corneal edema may develop as a postoperative complication of glaucoma filtering surgery in eyes with the ICE syndrome. Therefore, filtering surgery is not recommended as a specific treatment for the corneal edema. Penetrating keratoplasty is usually required for those cases that are unresponsive to saline drops or a soft contact lens, after the glaucoma has been controlled. In Chandler's syndrome, in the setting of corneal edema even at a low IOP, corneal transplantation can provide visual rehabilitation that cannot be achieved in any other way.

FUTURE CONSIDERATIONS

The ultimate treatment for all forms of glaucoma is to identify the initial events and treat these before they lead to obstruction of aqueous outflow, elevation of IOP, and glaucomatous damage. The ICE syndrome provides an example of how this concept of early glaucoma intervention may someday be invoked. For example, if the viral etiology is confirmed, this might provide a means of early diagnosis through the patient's past medical history and possibly through identification of a viral antibody or other evidence of previous viral infection. Specular microscopy, or some other screening technique, could then be used in this high risk population to detect those patients with an abnormal corneal endothelium, ideally before it leads to alterations in the anterior chamber angle. It would then be necessary to have a treatment to prevent the proliferation of the abnormal endothelium over the anterior chamber angle and iris. Fulcher and associates, for example, described an immunotoxin which inhibits the proliferation of human corneal endothelium in tissue culture (22). Alternatively, Alvardo and associates have suggested that topical and systemic anti-viral agents may one day prove to be an effective treatment (18). While there is still much work to be done before the concept of early glaucoma intervention can be applied to the treatment of the ICE syndrome, we have seen considerable advances in our understanding of this condition since it was first recognized as a spectrum of disease by Chandler and Grant more than thirty years ago.

References

1. Chandler PA, Grant WM: Lectures on Glaucoma. Philadelphia, Lea and Febiger, 1965;276.
2. Harms C: Einseitige spontane Lückenbildung der Iris durch Atrophie ohne mechanische Zerrung. Klin Monatsbl Augenheilkd 1903;41: 522–528.
3. Chandler PA: Atrophy of the stroma of the iris. Endothelial dystrophy, corneal edema, and glaucoma. Am J Ophthalmol 1956;41:607–615.
4. Cogan DG, Reese AB: A syndrome of iris nodules, ectopic Descemet's membrane, and unilateral glaucoma. Doc Ophthalmol 1969;26: 424–432.
5. Scheie HG, Yanoff M: Iris nevus (Cogan-Reese) syndrome. A cause of unilateral glaucoma. Arch Ophthalmol 1975;93:963–970.
6. Eagle RC Jr, Font RL, Yanoff M, et al: Proliferative endotheliopathy with iris abnormalities. The iridocorneal endothelial syndrome. Arch Ophthalmol 1979;97:2104–2111.
7. Wilson MC, Shields MB: A comparison of the clinical variations of the iridocorneal endothelial syndrome. Arch Ophthalmol 1989;107: 1465–1468.
8. Hirst LW, Quigley HA, Stark WJ, et al: Specular microscopy of iridocorneal endothelia syndrome. Am J Ophthalmol 1980;89:11–21.
9. Sherrard ES, Frangoulis MA, Kerr MG, et al: The posterior surface of the cornea in the iridocorneal endothelial syndrome: a specular microscopical study. Trans Ophthalmol Soc UK 1985;104:766–774.
10. Bourne WM, Brubaker RF: Progression and regression of partial corneal involvement in the iridocorneal endothelial syndrome. Am J Ophthalmol 1992;114:171–181.
11. Shields MB, Campbell DG, Simmons RJ: The essential iris atrophies. Am J Ophthalmol 1978;85:749–759.
12. Shields MB, McCracken JS, Klintworth GK, et al: Corneal edema in essential iris atrophy. Ophthalmology 1979;86:1533–1548.
13. Alvarado JA, Murphy CG, Maglio M, et al: Pathogenesis of Chandler's syndrome, essential iris atrophy and the Cogan-Reese syndrome. I. Alterations of the corneal endothelium. Invest Ophthalmol Vis Sci 1986;27: 853–872.
14. Kramer TR, Grossniklaus HE, Vigneswaran N, et al: Cytokeratin expression in corneal endothelium in the iridocorneal endothelial syndrome. Invest Ophthalmol Vis Sci 1992;33:3581–3585.
15. Rodrigues MM, Stulting RD, Waring GO III: Clinical, electron microscopic, and immunohistochemical study of the corneal endothelium and Descemet's membrane in the iridocorneal endothelial syndrome. Am J Ophthalmol 1986;101:16–27.
16. Alvarado JA, Murphy CG, Juster RP, et al: Pathogenesis of Chandler's syndrome, essential iris atrophy and the Cogan-Reese syndrome. II. Estimated age of disease onset. Invest Ophthalmol Vis Sci 1986;27: 873–882.
17. Tsai CS, Ritch R, Straus SE, et al: Antibodies to Epstein-Barr virus in iridocorneal endothelial syndrome. Arch Ophthalmol 1990;108: 1572–1576.
18. Alvarado J, Underwood J, Green R, et al: Detection of herpes simplex viral DNA in the iridocorneal endothelia syndrome. Arch Ophthalmol 1994;112:1601–1609.
19. Campbell DG, Shields MB, Smith TR: The corneal endothelium and the spectrum of essential iris atrophy. Am J Ophthalmol 1978;86:317–324.
20. Campbell DG: Formation of iris nodules in primary proliferative endothelial degeneration. Invest Ophthalmol Vis Sci 1979;(Suppl)142.
21. Wright MM, Grajewski AL, Cristal SM, et al: 5-fluorouracil after trabeculectomy and the iridocorneal endothelial syndrome. Ophthalmology 1991;98:314–316.
22. Fulcher S, Lui G, Houston LL, et al: Use of immunotoxin to inhibit proliferating human corneal endothelium. Inv Ophthalmol Vis Sci 1988; 29:755–759.

Glaucoma After Vitreo-Retinal Surgery 33

Martin Wand

Glaucoma after retinal detachment surgery is not an infrequent occurrence and requires special attention to its diagnosis, treatment, and prevention. Soon after a retina operation, the eye is often congested, painful, and with poor vision; the patient may be uncomfortable, somnolent, and at times nauseated, particularly if the surgery is performed under general anesthesia. **Thus, the signs and symptoms of a secondary glaucoma can be confused with the expected side effects of major retinal eye surgery.** An awareness of this complication and its different presentations will facilitate recognition, allow for timely treatment and, in some instances, prevention of the complication.

ANGLE CLOSURE GLAUCOMA

The reported incidence of clinically detectable angle narrowing after scleral buckle procedures ranges from 11.9% at 1 month (1) to 29% at 2 months after surgery (2); the incidence reaches 50% in eyes examined within 1 week after surgery (3). The reported incidence of actual angle closure glaucoma ranges from 1 to 4% (1,4,5,6). The etiology of the angle shallowing is probably multifactorial (Table 33.1). Experimentally, occlusion of vortex veins in monkey eyes results in uveal tract congestion, forward movement of the iris-lens diaphragm, shallowing or closure of the anterior chamber angle, and, in some eyes, elevated intraocular pressure (IOP) (7). Grant has shown that fluid injected into the choroid of human eyebank eyes results in choroidal detachment and angle closure (8). Clinically, a choroidal detachment is frequently, but not always, detectable after retinal detachment surgery (6). Ultrasound biomicroscopic studies have shown that choroidal effusion is present in eyes after scleral buckling procedures even when there are no signs of anterior chamber shallowing or clinical findings of choroidal detachment (Fig. 33.1). This confirms the impression of retinal surgeons that **virtually all eyes undergoing retinal surgery have some degree of choroidal effusion.** Angle narrowing and angle closure are just at one end of the spectrum of choroidal effusion after retinal detachment.

Other clinical situations where there is inflammation and/or swelling of the uveal tract have also been shown to result in shallowing of the anterior chamber axially, anterior rotation of the ciliary body, and shallowing or closure of the anterior chamber angle. A similar pathophysiologic process may be implicated in the following conditions, all of which have been associated with angle closure glaucoma: panretinal photocoagulation (9,10), uveal (11), and orbital pseudotumor (12), uveal effusion (13), central retinal vein occlusion (14,15), choroidal hemorrhage (16), and idiopathic ciliary body swelling (17). The ciliary body is firmly attached to the scleral spur. With uveal swelling from these diverse causes, including post-scleral buckling, there is an anterior rotation of the ciliary body with anterior movement of the lens-iris diaphragm (Fig. 33.1). In phakic or pseudophakic eyes, there may be enough forward movement to produce pupillary block with resultant angle closure glaucoma.

However, angle closure may also occur in the absence of pupillary block. In such cases, anterior rotation of the ciliary body may be limited to pushing the peripheral iris against the trabecular meshwork. The result is similar to the plateau iris syndrome, i.e., there is a relatively deep central anterior chamber depth, flat iris plane, and peripheral angle closure (18). This is attested to by the finding that angle closure glaucoma has been noted in aphakic as well as phakic eyes and in eyes with patent iridectomies (1,6). The incidence and extent of angle shallowing and closure has been related to a myriad of conditions including a pre-existing narrow angle (1,5), high myopia (5), older age of patient (5), use of an encircling band versus a scleral implant without an encircling band (3), placement of the encircling band anterior to the equator (1), episcleral implants versus intrascleral implants (6), choroidal detachment extending to the ciliary body (1), and the extent of the surgical procedure (5). In most cases, the shallowing of the angle resolves with time as the choroidal effusion is absorbed (1,2,3,5).

Prevention and Treatment

The critical point in the treatment of this problem is an awareness of the potential for angle closure after retinal detachment surgery. Frequently, there is no more discomfort or pain than from the normal sequelae of retinal surgery. Findings are minimal and a hazy cornea with a mid dilated pupil are often the only clues that glaucoma may be present (6). **Ocular rigidity is decreased to one-quarter normal after a scleral buckle (19) and Schiotz tonometry gives a falsely low IOP (2).** Thus, an applanation tension and slit-lamp examination should be done, preferably within the first 24 hours after surgery. If the cornea

Table 33.1
Risk Factors for Angle Closure Glaucoma After Scleral Buckling Surgery

Risk factors
Pre-existing narrow angles (hyperopic patient)
High myopia
Older age
Encircling band
"High scleral buckle"
Scleral buckle anterior to equator
Episcleral implants (vs. intrascleral implant)

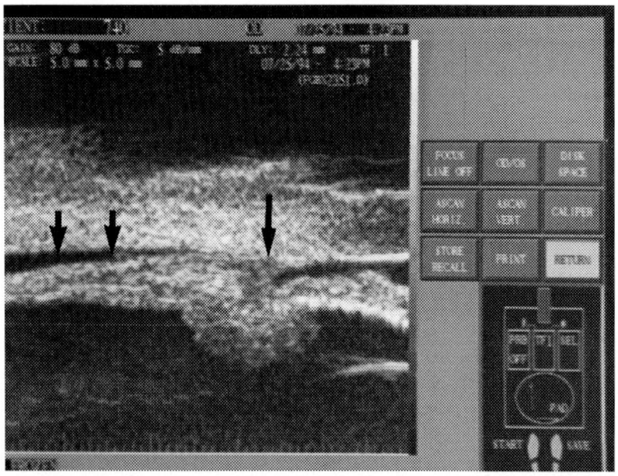

Figure 33.1. Ultrasound biomicroscopy of an eye 1 week after a 360 encircling band procedure for a rhegmatogenous retinal detachment. Postoperatively, the intraocular pressure was normal, the anterior chamber was deep, and no choroidal detachment was noted. Choroidal effusion (double arrows) was present 360 degrees with detachment of the ciliary body except for its attachment to the scleral spur (single arrow). There is anterior rotation of the ciliary processes, narrowing of the peripheral angle, anterior displacement of the lens, and relative pupillary block as shown by the anterior bowing of the iris. (Courtesy of Charles J. Pavlin, MD).

is not clear enough for gonioscopy, and the IOP is elevated, angle closure must be presumed to be present.

Treatment of angle closure glaucoma after scleral buckling surgery progresses from medical management through surgical intervention (Table 33.2). Maximal dilation and cycloplegia with atropine and phenylephrine should be aggressively continued, along with topical steroids which may decrease ocular and choroidal congestion and effusion. Miotics should be avoided; beta blockers, carbonic anhydrase inhibitors, and apraclonidine should be used as tolerated. **Regardless of the medical therapy, a laser iridectomy is indicated.** With mild cornea haziness, a Nd:YAG laser will often be successful in iris penetration where the argon laser might fail (20). If the cornea is very hazy, clarity can frequently be achieved with topical glycerin. When the cornea is too hazy to allow even Nd:YAG laser iridectomy, argon laser peripheral iridoplasty should be tried, as this has been reported to be successful in primary angle closure glaucoma under such circumstances (21). As a last resort, angle closure from pupillary block may require a surgical iridectomy, but the advent of the different lasers has virtually eliminated the need for such intervention.

When a patent laser iridectomy does not resolve the angle closure, then choroidal detachment with anterior rotation of the ciliary body is commonly the cause of the angle closure. **With the availability of argon laser gonioplasty (22), the angle can often be opened enough to lower the IOP, keeping in mind that once past the acute crisis, the choroidal effusion and secondary angle closure will resolve with time.** However, there can be so much choroidal effusion that the only solution is to drain the choroidal fluid, the traditional technique of treating this type of glaucoma (4). Surgical anterior chamber deepening and mechanical breaking of peripheral anterior synechiae can be performed at the time of this surgery, if persistent angle closure is present (Chapter 23).

Case 33-1. A 69 year-old man with a rhegmatogenous retinal detachment underwent a successful scleral buckle operation with a 200 degree scleral implant and a 360 encircling band. The course of his postoperative hospital stay was not well documented, but at his one week post-operative visit, the visual acuity was counting fingers, the IOP 40 mm Hg, and the eye was "congested." Various anti-glaucoma medications were instituted without success. At seven weeks after the retina surgery, the visual acuity was 20/100 and the IOP 57 mm Hg, the cornea clear, the anterior chamber deep, and the iris was flat with a 6 mm pupil. No pupillary block was evident, but the angle was closed 360 (Fig. 33.2). Argon laser gonioplasty was performed 360 with immediate opening of the angle and the IOP decreased to 31 mm Hg. The next day, the IOP was 21 mm Hg and the angle remained open (Fig. 33.3). Subsequently, his IOPs have remained under control on a topical beta blocker only.

This case illustrates several important points. Angle closure after retinal detachment surgery is easily overlooked if not specifically sought for and may persist long after the acute post-operative inflammatory period. It can occur in the absence of pupillary block, making the diagnosis more elusive. With the availability of laser iridectomy and laser gonioplasty, many, if not most cases of angle closure, even of several weeks duration, can now be resolved without further surgical intervention.

OPEN ANGLE GLAUCOMA

Postoperative open angle glaucoma requires special consideration because it frequently is a reflection of the preoperative status of the eye. **The prevalence of open angle glaucoma in eyes that develop retinal detachment is reported to be 4-12 times higher than that in the general population** (23). The reason is unknown, but the commonality of high myopia (24) and the use of miotics in open angle glaucoma resulting in retinal detachment (25) has been cited as a possible explanation. A higher

Table 33.2
Treatment of Angle Closure Glaucoma After Scleral Buckling Surgery

	Comments
Medical Cycloplegics Beta blockers Apraclonidine Carbonic anhydrase inhibitors Osmotics	Continue cycloplegics (pilocarpine may further shallow anterior chamber, worsen angle closure and cause pain) If more than 7–10 days since surgery, consider topical steroids as the source of elevated IOP.
Laser iridectomy	Topical glycerin may help clear cornea.
Laser gonioplasty	May help open angle enough to delay or prevent operative intervention.
Surgical intervention Choroidal tap Consider loosening excessively tight scleral buckle Trabeculectomy with anti-metabolites, seton implantation or cyclophotocoagulation in late stages	Surgical intervention is a last resort; choroidal effusions generally clear with time.

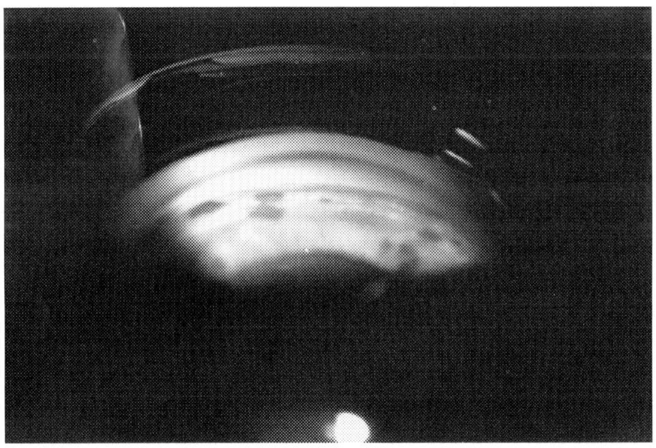

Figure 33.2. Persistent angle closure glaucoma 7 weeks after a scleral buckling procedure. Goniophotograph shows peripheral appositional angle closure without a pupillary block component.

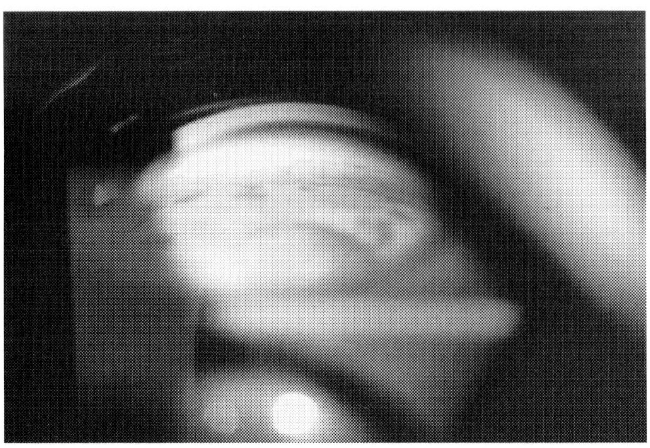

Figure 33.3. Same eye as in Figure 33.2. Goniophotograph showing open angle after argon laser gonioplasty.

incidence of both open angle glaucoma and retinal detachment in diabetics may be another factor. Since the IOP is often lower in eyes with retinal detachment due to decreased aqueous formation, successful reattachment can be expected to result in a return to at least the pre-detachment level of IOP. Additionally, debris, inflammation, blood breakdown products, and steroid response contribute to the decreased facility of outflow postoperatively (26). All things considered, re-emergence of a pre-existing open angle glaucoma should be looked for carefully after retinal detachment surgery and appropriately treated.

The obverse of postoperative open angle glaucoma is Schwartz's syndrome (27) in which the preoperative IOP elevation is caused by obstruction of the trabecular meshwork by photoreceptor outer segments from a retinal tear or dialysis (28), and is improved by retinal surgery. If the retinal break is sealed and the retina reattached, the source of trabecular meshwork obstruction (photoreceptor outer segments) is eliminated, and the secondary open angle glaucoma is resolved. In this unique situation, persistent postoperative open angle glaucoma should lead one to suspect an undetected persistent retinal detachment.

NEOVASCULAR GLAUCOMA

Chronic retinal detachment with its resultant retinal hypoxia has long been recognized as a cause of neovascular glaucoma (NVG) (29). Occasionally, the surgery for retinal detachment has been implicated in neovascularization of the iris, presumably due to anterior segment ischemia from damage to the anterior ciliary vessels (30,31). Recently, vitrectomy in diabetic eyes has been associated with a high incidence of NVG if the eye is already aphakic or has concurrent lensectomy (32). Aphakia may have resulted in the elimination of a diffusion barrier for the passage of some angiogenic substance from the posterior to the anterior segment (33). Subsequently, although the presence of the lens does seem to provide a relative protective barrier, of greater importance in the development of NVG is the presence of an angiogenic stimulus (34,35). In both diabetic and non-diabetic eyes (36) where there is posterior segment hypoxia from a persistent retinal detachment, aphakia is only of secondary importance. The highest incidence of NVG after vitrectomy for complications of diabetic retinopathy is in eyes with a persistent retinal detachment and aphakia (92%); the lowest incidence is in phakic eyes with an attached retina (0%), and intermediate incidence in phakic eyes with a detached retina (40%) (35) (Chapter 31).

In eyes already predisposed towards the development of NVG, such as eyes with diabetic retinopathy, previous central retinal vein occlusion, or carotid obstructive disease, retinal detachment surgery, with or without vitrectomy, further stimulates the inflammatory and angiogenic responses (37,38). One must be alert to the potential development of NVG post-retinal detachment surgery and one should specifically look for neovascularization of the iris on slit lamp examination. If neovascularization of the iris is detected, a dilated fundus examination with scleral depression must be performed. When a retinal detachment is found, a successful re-attachment will usually resolve the anterior segment neovascularization (39). Occasionally, neovascularization of the iris and NVG may appear after successful retinal detachment surgery. If this occurs in eyes with pre-existing diabetic retinopathy or previous central retinal vein occlusion, panretinal photocoagulation either must be performed, if not already done, and if done, it must be augmented. Indirect laser ophthalmoscopy and photocoagulation can be useful in treating the peripheral retina in this situation. With the extra inflammatory and angiogenic stimuli from the surgery, supplemental panretinal photocoagulation often needs to be performed. We and others have noted resolution of neovascularization of the iris and NVG after supplemental panretinal photocoagulation in such cases (30,34).

GLAUCOMA AFTER INTRAVITREAL GAS

The use of various intraocular gases in vitreo-retinal surgery has become increasingly popular over the past decade (40). Because of their surface tension, all gases exert a tamponading effect on the retinal breaks. However, air has the disadvantage of being absorbed (in 5 to 7 days [41]) before firm choroidal-retinal adhesions can develop. Fluorinated hydrocarbon gases have an advantage over air because they are expansile and have a longer intraocular duration, attributed to their high molecular weight, low diffusion coefficient and low water solubility. The most commonly used gases are sulfa hexafluoride (SF6) and perfluopropane (C3F8). SF6 remains in the eye twice as long as air; C3F8, with a higher molecular weight than SF6, remains in the eye even longer (40,41). When injected into the vitreous cavity, the volume of these gases expands because of diffusion of nitrogen, oxygen, and carbon dioxide from ocular tissue. Pure SF6 expands to 2 to 2½ times its original volume within 24 to 36 hours and pure C3F8 expands to 3 to 4 times its original volume within the first 3 days (40,41). With both gases, the maximum expansion occurs within the first 6 hours. When the gas gets diluted to a 40% concentration, further expansion occurs slowly and is balanced by vitreous loss (42,43).

With an expansile intravitreal gas pocket, anterior displacement of the lens can occur, despite proper positioning of the patient's head in a prone position, resulting in **pupillary block.** This can occur even after the period of maximum expansion and one must be aware of this possibility for the duration of the intravitreal gas. Because the gas bubble is compressible, high displacement tonometers, such as the Schiotz tonometer, result in significant under-evaluation of the true IOP (44). With 1 ml of intraocular gas, there is a 7 to 8 mm Hg under-evaluation when the IOP is in the 30 to 40 mm Hg range (40). Even with low displacement applanation tonometers, there can be a significant under-evaluation of the true IOP. The Tono-Pen was found to under-estimate true IOP (as measured in eyebank eyes with an intraocular manometer) by 15% and the pneumotonometer by 21% (45). **Therefore, not only is it imperative that only a low displacement tonometer, such as the Goldmann applanation tonometer, be used, but to realize that there could still be up to a 20% under-estimation in eyes with intraocular gas.**

More common than pupillary block is the glaucoma resulting directly from the expansile gas. The highest incidence and the highest IOP is during the rapid expansile phase when egress of liquid vitreous and aqueous cannot keep pace with the increasing gas volume. In an early study, 45% of 101 patients who had SF6 during surgery developed IOPs greater than 30 mm Hg within the first postoperative day; in 33 patients, the elevated IOPs persisted beyond the second postoperative day. More alarmingly, 11 of the 101 patients developed central retinal artery occlusion, 10 of whom had elevated IOPs; none of these eyes achieved functional vision (46). Eyes which developed postoperative anterior chamber fibrinous exudates appear more likely to get elevated IOPs, and diabetic eyes are more likely to develop these exudates (46). Thus, eyes likely to have retinal vascular diseases, such as with diabetes, hypertension, sickle cell trait, or chronic open angle glaucoma, may be at even greater risk for vascular occlusion associated with an elevated IOP (47).

Prevention and Treatment

Titrating the concentration and volume of these intraocular gases is the recognized approach to the safety of their use (47). Recent studies using 20% SF6 showed only 6%

INTRAOCULAR GAS AND ALTITUDE

Martin Wand

With the use of intraocular gas, another unusual complication should be considered. With any decrease in atmospheric pressure, there is a corresponding decrease in the absolute IOP which results in expansion of the intraocular gas. Because there is a delay between the decrease in the atmospheric pressure and the decrease in the absolute IOP, there is a net increase in the IOP (1). Experimental studies in monkeys show that with only .25 ml of intraocular gas, simulated decompression as experienced in commercial airline cabins (300 feet per minute to a cabin altitude of 8,000 feet above sea level) resulted in IOPs greater than 40 mm Hg (2). Transient central retinal artery occlusion was noted in these eyes. In a 79 year-old man who had undergone recent intraocular fluid-gas exchange, IOP was measured with a Tono-Pen and the intraocular gas bubble observed with an indirect ophthalmoscope during a low altitude airplane trip (3). In an unpressurized small plane, the gas fill went from 65% at sea level to 85% at 3,000 feet; the IOP went from 16 mm Hg to 49 mm Hg. Although it might be safe to fly for short periods at low altitudes, commercial air flights pose more serious potential problems. Current jets fly at up to 42,000 feet (as high as 60,000 feet for the Concorde), and cabin pressurization varies greatly from a high of 1,000 feet in a Concorde to a low of 8,000 feet in a B737; the average pressurization was 5,670 feet as measured on 204 commercial flights in different types of airplanes (4). Standard pressure differential for the commercial airline industry is 8:6:1. These pressurization levels clearly put an eye with intraocular gases at great risk. In addition, should sudden depressurization occur on a commercial airplane, the ocular consequences would be disastrous. Thus, it is essential to warn patients to avoid flying at cabin pressures less than 2,000 feet (706 mm Hg) (2) or preferably not at all until all the intraocular gas is absorbed.

In addition, rapid ascent or descent when traveling in automobiles or in high rise elevators should be avoided.

References

1. Lincoff H, Weinberger D, Reppucci V, et al: Air travel with intraocular gas: I. The mechanisms for compensation. Arch Ophthalmol 1989;107:902–906.
2. Dieckert JP, O'Connor PS, Schacklett DE, et al: Air travel and intraocular gas. Ophthalmology 1986;93:642–645.
3. Kokame GT, Ing MR: Intraocular gas and low altitude air flight. Retina 1994;14:356–358.
4. Contrell JJ: Altitude exposures during aircraft flight: flying higher. Chest 1988;92:81–84.

of eyes had an IOP greater than 30 mm Hg on one postoperative occasion (48) and only 9% had an IOP greater than 30 mm Hg when a 14% concentration of C3F8 was used (49). Regardless of the amount and concentration of gas used, close monitoring of the IOP postoperatively and attention to proper positioning of the patient's head are imperative. An unusual condition is that encountered with changes of IOP with altitude in eyes with intraocular gas (50-53) (see above). Carbonic anhydrase inhibitors, beta blockers, and alpha adrenergic agonists may be employed to control the IOP, but **if the IOP is extremely high, or in eyes susceptible to central retinal artery occlusion, aliquots of intraocular gas are sequentially removed until normotension is achieved.**

GLAUCOMA AFTER INTRAOCULAR SILICONE OIL

Silicone oil, as a vitreous substitute and for retinal tamponade, was introduced in 1962. However, serious associated complications and pending progress in modern vitreo-retinal surgery and bioengineering limited its use (54). Recently, the use of silicone oil in very complex cases has enjoyed a resurgence (55). Like air, **silicone oil is lighter than aqueous or vitreous and because of its buoyancy, it can compress the superior angle of an eye in the upright position.** In aphakic eyes it can occlude the pupil, and cause pupillary block. A 5% incidence of angle closure and a 29% incidence of angle compromise in 93 patients 3 years after intravitreal silicone use has been reported (56).

Open angle glaucoma is a more common complication after the use of silicone oil. **A definite correlation exists between the appearance of the oil in the anterior chamber and elevated IOP (57), as well as a significant decrease in the IOP with subsequent removal of the oil from the anterior chamber** (58). Silicone oil was thought to more likely to enter the anterior chamber in aphakic than phakic or pseudophakic eyes, but, with time, foamy silicone bubbles may appear in the anterior chamber of phakic eyes as well (57,60). Silicone laden microphages have been detected within the trabecular meshwork which otherwise appears normal (56), and emulsified oil in the anterior chamber may not be detectable except on gonioscopy (57). Thus, obstruction of the outflow by silicone oil appears to be at least a contributory cause of the elevated IOP. After intravitreal silicone oil, the incidence of glaucoma has been reported to be 56% (increase >10 mm Hg) in the immediate postoperative period (61). It decreases to 48% (>25 mm Hg or increase >10 mm Hg) 16 months postoperatively (62) and to 12% (>22 mm Hg) 3 years postoperatively (56). However, there are probably other contributory causes to the elevated IOP in these cases since oil in the anterior chamber is not always related to elevated IOPs and elevated IOPs have been reported in eyes with no oil in the anterior chamber (62). Peripheral anterior synechias, inflammatory cells, and debris have been implicated (61), and preoperative elevated IOP is a major risk factor (90% chance) in the development of glaucoma after intravitreal silicone oil (62).

Prevention and Treatment

To avoid angle closure from pupillary block, since silicone oil is buoyant within the eye, a prophylactic inferior peripheral iridectomy at the time of the vitrectomy, especially in aphakic eyes has been recommended (63). With an inferior peripheral iridectomy, should silicone oil get into the anterior chamber, positioning the patient in the prone position will allow the silicone oil an avenue of egress from the anterior chamber to the vitreous cavity through the pupil and ingress of aqueous through the iridectomy. In a recent study affirming the protective value of an inferior iridectomy, all 21 eyes requiring glaucoma surgery after intravitreal silicone oil either had a scleral buckle and/or lacked an intraoperative peripheral iridectomy (62). Once pupillary block is detected, an inferior peripheral iridectomy should be performed either with the laser or by surgery depending on the clarity of the cornea. Fibrinous closure of a peripheral iridectomy can occur, in which case reopening it with the Nd:YAG laser may be successful (58). In addition, as much of the silicone oil as possible should be removed, keeping in mind that there is a significant incidence of re-detachment of the retina associated with this procedure (59).

With secondary open angle glaucoma, preventive measures include avoidance of superior iridectomies or superior iris trauma at the time of vitrectomy, avoidance of overfilling the eye with silicone oil, instilling air into the anterior chamber in aphakic eyes at the time of surgery and removal of silicone oil from the anterior chamber as soon as possible when this is noted post-operatively (58). Unfortunately, even an inferior peripheral iridectomy does not always prevent the movement of silicone oil into the anterior chamber angle (57). Once glaucoma is noted, conservative measures include vigorous mydriasis-cycloplegia, topical steroids to decrease inflammation, and topical beta blockers and carbonic anhydrase inhibitors as tolerated. With concurrent removal of silicone oil from the anterior chamber, the majority (60%) (58,62), but not all, cases (64) of such a glaucoma can be controlled.

GLAUCOMA SURGERY AFTER VITREO-RETINAL DETACHMENT SURGERY

In all cases of glaucoma secondary to vitreo-retinal detachment surgery, if conservative therapy does not control the IOP, surgical intervention must be undertaken to save vision. Filtration surgery with 5-FU, (65) Molteno or other implants, Schocket procedures, and Nd:YAG laser transscleral cyclophotocoagulation have been reported to be successful (62), but the number of cases reported has been small. If filtration surgery is contemplated, because of conjunctival scarring from the vitreo-retinal surgery, antifibriotics will increase the likelihood of successful filtration. **After a retina operation, to augment the chances of successful filtration, retina surgeons should be encouraged to close the peritomy tightly with multiple sutures and eschew the tendency to use only two tack sutures at the 3:00 and 9:00 positions.** With the latter closure, the superior conjunctival flap often does not attach to the limbus, and a superior pocket is formed, sometimes extending 3 to 4 mm posterior to the limbus. Therefore, before the glaucoma surgeon starts to dissect the posterior conjunctiva for a limbus-based flap, determine the status of the conjunctiva at the limbus because it may indicate the need for a fornix-based conjunctival flap. Based on personal experience, the success rate of trabeculectomy with intraoperative mitomycin-C is not different from the success rate of other high risk glaucoma eyes, and good pressure control without anti-glaucoma medications is in the 80% success range.

References

1. Sebestyen JG, Schepens CL, Rosenthal ML: Retinal detachment and glaucoma. I. Tonometric and gonioscopic study of 160 cases. Arch Ophthalmol 1962;67:736–745.
2. Fiore JV, Newton JC: Anterior segment changes following the scleral buckling procedure. Arch Ophthalmol 1970;84:284–287.
3. Hartley RE, Marsh RJ: Anterior chamber depth changes after retinal detachment. Br J Ophthalmol 1973;57:546–550.
4. Smith TR: Acute glaucoma developing after scleral buckling procedure. Am J Ophthalmol 1967;63:1807–1808.
5. Kreiger AE, Hodgkinson BJ, Frederick AR, et al: The results of retinal detachment surgery. Arch Ophthalmol 1971;86:385–394.
6. Perez RN, Phelps CD, Burton TC: Angle closure glaucoma following scleral buckling operations. Trans Am Academy Ophthalmol Otolaryng 1976;81:247–252.
7. Hayreh SS, Baines JAB: Occlusion of the vortex veins. An experimental study. Br J Ophthalmol 1973;57:217–238.
8. Grant WM: Experimental aqueous perfusion in enucleated human eyes. Arch Ophthalmol 1963;69:783–801.
9. Mensher JH: Anterior chamber depth alteration after retinal photocoagulation. Arch Ophthalmol 1977;95:113–116.
10. Liang JC, Huamonte FU: Reduction of immediate complications after panretinal photocoagulation. Retina 1984;4:166–170.
11. Gass JD: Retinal detachment and narrow angle glaucoma. Am J Ophthalmol 1967;63:94–103.
12. Kurtz S, Moisseier J, Gutman I, et al: Orbital pseudotumor presenting as acute glaucoma with choroidal and retinal detachment. Ophthalmol 1993;2:61–62.
13. McDonald PR, de la Paz V, Sarin LK: Non-rhegmatogenous retinal

separation with choroidal detachment (uveal effusion). Am J Ophthalmol 1965;59:820–827.
14. Grant WM: Shallowing of the anterior chamber following occlusion of the central retinal vein. Am J Ophthalmol 1973;75:384–389.
15. Bloome MA: Transient angle closure glaucoma in central retinal vein occlusion. Ann Ophthalmol 1977;9:44–48.
16. Holland PM, Smith TR: Broad scleral buckle in the management of retinal detachments with giant tears. Am J Ophthalmol 1977;83: 518–525.
17. Phelps CD: Angle closure glaucoma secondary to ciliary body swelling. Arch Ophthalmol 1974;92:287–290.
18. Pavlin CJ, Ritch R, Foster FS: Ultrasound biomicroscopy in plateau iris syndrome. Am J Ophthalmol 1992;113:390–395.
19. Pemberton JW: Schiotz - applanation disparity following retinal detachment surgery. Arch Ophthalmol 1969;81:534–537.
20. Wand M: Diagnosis and management of angle closure glaucoma. Focal Points VI 1994;10:1–12.
21. Ritch R: Argon laser treatment for medically unresponsive attacks of angle closure glaucoma. Am J Ophthalmol 1982;94:197–204.
22. Wand M: Argon laser gonioplasty for synechial angle closure. Arch Ophthalmol 1992;110:363–367.
23. Phelps CD, Burton TC: Glaucoma and retinal detachment. Arch Ophthalmol 1977;95:418–422.
24. Podos SM, Becker B, Morton WR: High myopia and primary open angle glaucoma. Am J Ophthalmol 1966;62:1039–1043.
25. Ackerman AL: Retinal detachments and miotic therapy, in Pruett RL, Regan CDJ (eds): Retinal Congress New York, Appleton-Centrury-Crofts Inc, 1972;533–539.
26. Minckler D: Glaucoma after vitrectomy - role of intravitreal gas and silicone oil. J Glaucoma 1994;3:165–167.
27. Schwartz A: Chronic open angle glaucoma secondary to rhegmatogenous retinal detachment. Am J Ophthalmol 1973;75:205–211.
28. Matsuo N, Takabatake M, Ueno H, et al: Photoreceptor outer segments in the aqueous humor in rhegmatogenous retinal detachment. Am J Ophthalmol 1986;101:673–679.
29. Schulze RR: Rubeosis iridis. Am J Ophthalmol 1967;63:487–495.
30. Wand M: Neovascular glaucoma. In: Principles and practice of ophthalmology. Edited by Albert DM, Jakobiec FA. Philadelphia, W.B. Saunders Co., 1994;1485–1510.
31. Tanaka S, Ideta H, Yonemoto J, et al: Neovascularization of the iris in rhegmatogenous retinal detachment. Am J Ophthalmol 1991;112: 632–634.
32. Rice TA, Michaels RG, Maguire MG, et al: The effects of lensectomy on the incidence of iris neovascularization and neovascular glaucoma after vitrectomy in diabetic eyes. Am J Ophthalmol 1983;95:1–11.
33. Thompson JT, Glaser BM: Role of lensectomy and posterior capsule in movement of tracers from vitreous to aqueous. Arch Ophthalmol 1985; 103:420–421.
34. Kokame GT, Flynn HW, Blankenship GW: Posterior chamber intraocular lens implantation during diabetic pars plana vitrectomy. Ophthalmology 1989;96:603–610.
35. Wand M, Madigan JC, Gaudio AR, et al: Neovascular glaucoma following pars plana vitrectomy for complications of diabetic retinopathy. Ophthalmic Surg 1990;21:113–118.
36. Camaratta MR, Chang S, Sparrow J: Iris neovascularization in proliferative vitreoretinopathy. Ophthalmology 1992;99:898–905.
37. Azzolini C, Brancato R, Camesasca FI, et al: Influence of silicone oil on iris microangiopathy in diabetic vitrectomized eyes. Ophthalmology 1993;100:1152–1159.
38. Oldenoerp J, Spitznas M: Factors influencing the results of vitreous surgery in diabetic retinopathy: I. Iris rubeosis and/or active neovascularization at the fundus. Graefes Arch Clin Exp Ophthalmol 1989;227: 1–8.
39. Scuder JJ, Blumenkranz MS, Blankenship GW: Regression of diabetic rubeosis iridis following successful surgical reattachment of the retina by vitrectomy. Retina 1982;2:193–196.
40. Hilton GF, Grizzard WS: Pneumatic retinopexy. A two-step outpatient operation without conjunctival incision. Ophthalmology 1986;93: 626–641.
41. Norton EWD: Intraocular gas in the management of selected retinal detachments. Trans Am Academy Ophthalmol Otolaryng 1973;77: 85–88.
42. Peyman GA, Vygantas CM, Bennett TO, et al: Octafluorocyclobutane in vitreous and aqueous humor replacement. Arch Ophthalmol 1975; 93:514–517.
43. Killey FP, Edelhauser HF, Aaberg TM: Intraocular sulfur hexafluoride and octofluorocyclobutane. Arch Ophthalmol 1978;96:511–515.
44. Aronowitz JD, Brubaker RF: Effect of intraocular gas on intraocular pressure. Arch Ophthalmol 1976;94:1191–1196.
45. Lim JI, Blair NP, Higginbotham EJ, et al: Assessment of intraocular pressure in vitrectomized gas-containing eyes: A clinical and manometric comparison of the Tono-Pen to the pneumotonometer. Arch Ophthalmol 1990;108:684–688.
46. Abrams GW, Swanson DE, Sabates WI: The results of sulfur hexafluoride gas in vitreous surgery. Am J Ophthalmol 1982;94:165–171.
47. Sabates WI, Abrams GW, Swanson DE, et al: The use of intraocular gases. The results of sulfur hexafluoride gas in retinal detachment surgery. Ophthalmology 1981;88:447–454.
48. Silicone Study Report 1: Vitrectomy with silicone oil or sulfur hexafluoride gas in eyes with severe proliferative vitreoretinopathy: results of a randomized clinical trial. Arch Ophthalmol 1992;110:770–779.
49. Silicone Study Report 2: Vitrectomy with silicone oil or perfluoropropane gas in eyes with severe proliferative vitreopathy: results of a randomized clinical trial. Arch Ophthalmol 1992;110:780–792.
50. Lincoff H, Weinberger D, Reppucci V, et al: Air travel with intraocular gas: I. The mechanisms for compensation. Arch Ophthalmol 1989;107: 902–906.
51. Dieckert JP, O'Connor PS, Schacklett DE, et al: Air travel and intraocular gas. Ophthalmology 1986;93:642–645.
52. Kokame GT, Ing MR: Intraocular gas and low altitude air flight. Retina 1994;14:356–358.
53. Contrell JJ: Altitude exposures during aircraft flight: flying higher. Chest 1988;92:81–84.
54. Cox MS, Trese MT, Murphy PL: Silicone oil for advanced proliferative vitreoretinopathy. Ophthalmology 1986;93:646–649.
55. McCuen BW, Landers MB, Machemer R: The use of silicone oil following failed vitrectomy for retinal detachment with advanced proliferative vitreoretinopathy. Ophthalmology 1985;92:1029–1034.
56. Leaver PK, Gray RMB, Garner A: Silicone oil injection in the treatment of massive periretinal retraction. II: Late complications in 93 eyes. Br J Ophthalmol 1979;63:361–367.
57. Valone J, McCarthy M: Emulsified anterior chamber silicone oil and glaucoma. Ophthalmology 1994;101:1908–1912.
58. Gao R, Neubauer L, Tang S, et al: Silicone oil in the anterior chamber. Graefes Arch Clin Exp Ophthalmology 1989;227:106–109.
59. Pearson RV, McLeod D, Gregor ZJ: Removal of silicone oil following diabetic vitrectomy. Br J Ophthalmol 1993;77:204–207.
60. Chan C, Okun E: The question of ocular tolerance to intravitreal liquid silicone. A long-term analysis. Ophthalmology 1986;93:651–660.
61. de Corral LR, Cohen SB, Peyman GA: Effect of intravitreal silicone oil on intraocular pressure. Ophthalmol Surg 1987;8:446–449.
62. Nguyen QH, Lloyd MA, Heuer DK, et al: Incidence and management of glaucoma after intravitreal silicone oil injection for complicated retinal detachments. Ophthalmology 1992;99:1520–1526.
63. Ando F: Intraocular hypertension resulting from pupillary block by silicone oil. Am J Ophthalmol 1985;99:87–88.
64. Moisseier J, Barah A, Manaim J, et al: Removal of silicone oil in the management of glaucoma in eyes with emulsified silicone. Retina 1993; 13:290–295.
65. Ophir A, Ticho U: Trabeculectomy with 5-fluorouracil subsequent to circular buckling operation and cataract extraction. Ann Ophthalmol 1992;24:386–390.

Angle Closure Glaucoma Due to Multiple Cysts of the Iris and Ciliary Body

34

David L. Epstein

Intraepithelial cysts (1) (Figs. 34.1 and 34.2) of the iris and ciliary body, if multiple, may gradually push the peripheral iris forward so as to close the angle and cause elevated IOP. Angle closure glaucoma caused by cysts of the iris and ciliary body is rare compared with angle closure glaucoma from other causes.

The onset of the glaucoma is sometimes rapid, with the typical picture of acute angle closure glaucoma. The diagnosis may be suspected by finding on gonioscopic examination **a considerable difference in the width of the chamber angle in various parts of the circumference** (Fig. 34.2). In some areas, the angle may appear closed, but in other areas the angle may be wide, with a broad ciliary body band visible. Such marked variation in angle width is unknown in primary acute angle closure glaucoma. Also, there is often a characteristic irregularly spaced **"bumpy" contour to the peripheral iris.** Occasional patients have been observed with one or two such areas in the total angle circumference. Presumably then, occasional cysts may not be as rare as once thought. However, from a practical point-of-view, the presence of only a few such areas does not substantially affect aqueous outflow.

It is important to recognize this entity, especially from the standpoint of prognosis. In primary angle closure glaucoma, laser iridectomy, if done in time, usually effects a cure of the glaucoma. If the angle closure is caused by cysts of the iris and ciliary body, the prognosis must be more guarded.

The true state of affairs may not be recognized until after there is an iridectomy. After surgical iridectomy, e.g., in cataract or filtration surgery, one or more cysts of the ciliary processes may be seen in the coloboma. Sometimes, even through typically small laser iridectomies, cysts may occasionally be seen through the iris opening by gonioscopy. Also, either with the pupil small, or more often after dilation, an iris cyst can be seen presenting at or behind the pupillary border (Fig. 34.2). These iris cysts are dark brown and may be mistaken for a melanoma. In the area of an iris cyst, the iris is lifted off the lens sufficiently (Fig. 34.3) so that on gonioscopic examination one can look under the iris on either side of the iris cyst and one may see cysts of the ciliary processes. These cysts of the ciliary processes may be heavily pigmented like iris cysts or they may be perfectly clear.

Iris cysts can be punctured with an argon or Nd:YAG laser using a mirrored gonioscopy lens if they extend to the pupillary border or even beyond and apparently show little tendency to recur. Puncture of an iris cyst results in considerable widening of the angle in the region of the cyst if peripheral anterior synechias have not already formed. Ciliary body cysts probably would be similarly easily treated with the laser, if they could be visualized. (Occasionally, one can see 2 or 3 ciliary body cysts on either side of an iris cyst.)

In one eye that we observed after intracapsular cataract extraction, one could easily see behind the iris during gonioscopy and could view a continuous row of cysts of the ciliary processes in the entire circumference. **In some cases in which cysts of the ciliary body appear to be present in the whole circumference, the angle may remain extremely narrow after iridectomy and may close again,** causing another acute increase in IOP. In most cases, the glaucoma can be controlled medically after iridectomy, but in exceptional cases, a filtering operation may be necessary. Ciliary body cysts in particular may continue to grow and cause further closure of the angle, requiring a filtering operation.

In some cases of multiple cysts of the iris and ciliary body, a **heavy deposition of pigment is present in the corneoscleral trabecular meshwork** similar to that seen in pigmentary glaucoma and in glaucoma associated with exfoliation. This pigment can cause a permanent obstruction to outflow and a form of open angle glaucoma.

Iris and ciliary body cysts have occurred within families (2). This suggests that cysts of the iris and ciliary body may be genetically determined, and all members of the immediate family should be examined. In one member of such a family, marked fluctuations in the size of these cysts were documented (DLE) (Fig. 34.4), which may have been related to the menstrual cycle.

The following case reports are instances of angle closure glaucoma caused by cysts of the iris or ciliary body or both.

Case 34-1. A 55-year-old man had a history of an attack of acute glaucoma in the left eye. He was treated with miotics and acetazol-

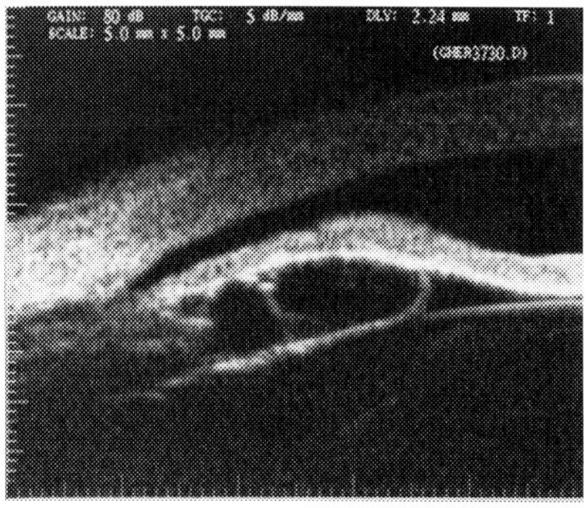

Figure 34.1. Cysts of the iris and ciliary body may be visible only as an irregular iris surface contour gonioscopically, but are visualized by ultrasound biomicroscopy.

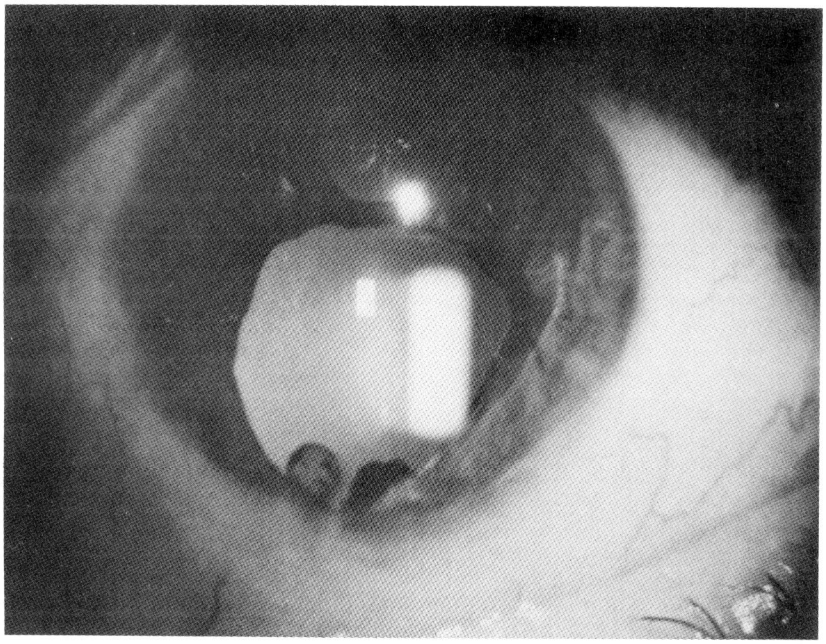

Figure 34.2. Iris and ciliary body cysts in a patient who has chronic angle closure glaucoma.

amide. When first seen 3 weeks after the attack, IOP was right 17 and left 20. The right disc was normal, the left showed no pathologic cupping but seemed a little paler than the right. Gonioscopy was as follows: in the right eye, nasally the angle was moderately wide with a fairly broad ciliary band, but below and temporally the angle was extremely narrow in 2 hours of the circumference and the iris was much more convex in this region. Above and temporally, there was another 2 hours of excessively narrow angle, very striking, and suggestive of iris and ciliary body cysts. The trabecular meshwork showed heavy pigmentation. In the left eye approximately 2/3 of the angle was open but irregularly and excessively narrow, probably closed in another 1 to 2 hours of the circumference.

A surgical peripheral iridectomy was done on the left eye (this was before the era of laser iridectomy). Two days later, the pupil was widely dilated in the right eye. One could then see a huge cyst behind the iris below and temporally. The cyst of the iris lifted the iris off the lens in this region and one could see for a short distance on either side a continuous row of cysts of the ciliary processes. An operation was done to collapse the iris cyst by inserting a Haab needle through the peripheral cornea across the anterior chamber and by incising the cyst where it was exposed behind the edge of the pupil. When the left pupil was widely dilated a large iris cyst could be seen presenting between the iris and the lens from about 3 o'clock to 5 o'clock. This cyst was similarly incised with a knife needle. During the next 8 years, the right eye required no medication, but the left required 4% pilocarpine and epinephrine to maintain IOPs under 20. Vision then was right 20/30, left 20/60. The right lens was clear, the left had a little nuclear sclerosis.

In this case, as in other similar cases, there seems to be no tendency for iris cysts to reform after they have been incised. It has been 20 years since these cysts were incised and there is still no sign of them refilling.

Case 34-2. A 35-year-old man had been told he had a "suspicion of glaucoma." He was asymptomatic. He was currently using 1%

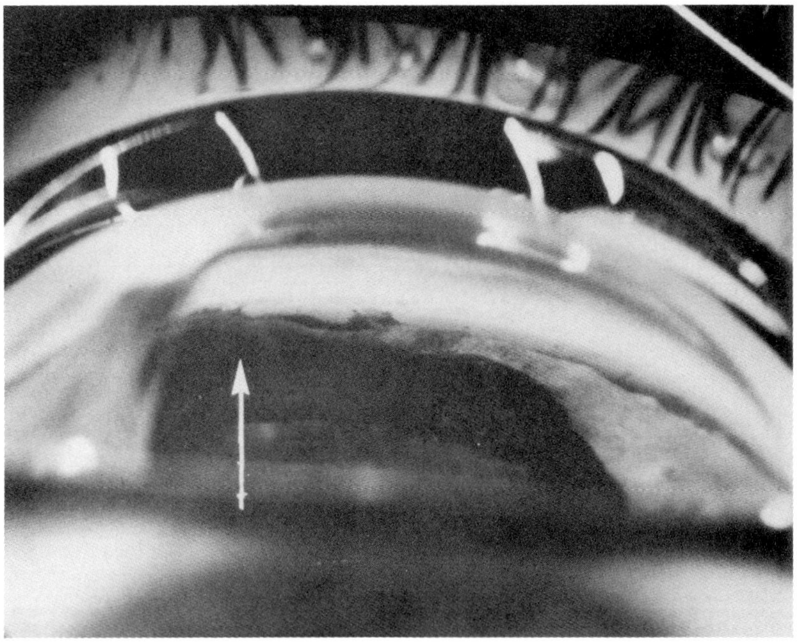

Figure 34.3. Cysts of the ciliary body (arrow) and secondary angle closure. Reprinted with permission from Donaldson DD: Atlas of external diseases of the eye. Vol. IV. Anterior chamber, iris, and ciliary body. St. Louis, The C.V. Mosby Co., 1973, courtesy of Dr. Jules H. Shaw.

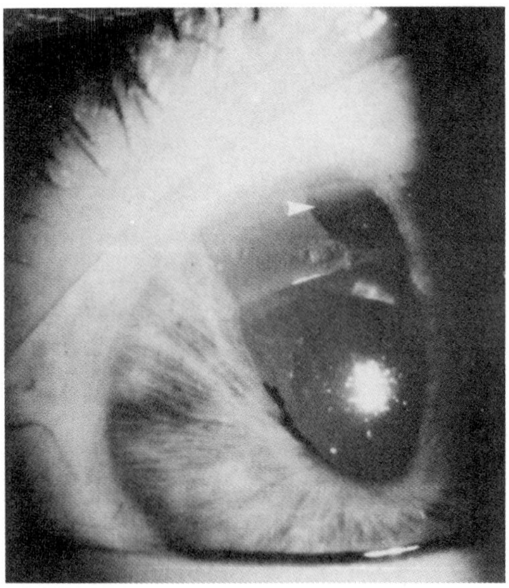

Figure 34.4. Patient with familial iris and ciliary body cysts (arrowhead) that were observed to fluctuate in size at various times. Chronic angle closure glaucoma was present.

pilocarpine tid. The discs were normal, fields full. On gonioscopy the picture was striking. In exactly the nasal half of the angle in both eyes, the iris plane was flat, the angle was wide with scleral spur visible and even a little ciliary band. In the temporal half, the iris contour was very convex, a marked contrast to the flat iris plane on the nasal side and the angle was excessively narrow, portions possibly closed. IOP in both eyes was in the mid-20s. He was seen later when off treatment. The gonioscopic picture was unchanged and the IOP was still in the mid-20s in both eyes. The pupils were then widely dilated to about 8 mm. In both eyes, there were two iris cysts temporally touching each other. In the left eye in the upper temporal quadrant the iris cyst projected a little beyond the 8-mm pupil. Elsewhere the cysts just reached the border of the 8-mm pupil. These iris cysts were treated with the argon laser. The temporal angle widened, and no iris cysts were now visible, even when the pupil was widely dilated.

This latter case reemphasizes the important point that most hyperopic narrow angled eyes are symmetrically narrow around the circumference of the angle (except for the superior angle which is narrowest in most eyes, including emmetropic eyes). If there is great disparity between the nasal and temporal halves of the angle in terms of narrowness, suspect iris or ciliary body cysts, or other ciliary body pathology, including tumors such as melanoma (Chapters 7, 41).

References

1. Shields JA: Primary cysts of the iris. Trans Am Ophthalmol Soc 1981; 79:771–809.
2. Vela A, Rieser JC, Campbell DG: The heredity and treatment of angle-closure glaucoma secondary to iris and ciliary body cysts. Ophthalmology 1984;91:332–7.

Angle Closure Glaucoma Secondary to Occlusion of the Central Retinal Vein

35

David L. Epstein

Occlusion of the central retinal vein is not ordinarily thought to affect the depth of the anterior chamber, but occasionally within a few days after vein occlusion the lens and iris move forward, producing conspicuous shallowing of the anterior chamber in the affected eye. This is especially appreciated when one compares the axial depth of the anterior chamber in the affected eye with that in the contralateral normal eye (1–4). In some cases, there has been enough shallowing to cause the angle to close. In such cases, angle closure glaucoma has usually been diagnosed within 2 or 3 weeks after vein occlusion. The shallowing is reversible, and the anterior chamber does return to its original depth within a few weeks. The problem of angle closure glaucoma then disappears if no synechias have formed, but subsequent neovascular glaucoma may develop.

In the past, before this entity was clearly distinguished from other forms of angle closure glaucoma, most cases were treated with pilocarpine and aqueous humor suppressants, which sufficed to keep the angle open until the spontaneous deepening and resolution of the glaucoma took place. We encountered one case in which treatment with pilocarpine, a carbonic anhydrase inhibitor, and oral osmotics did not relieve unilateral angle closure glaucoma secondary to occlusion of the central retinal vein. However, when the pilocarpine was discontinued and a cycloplegic (cyclopentolate) was administered, the anterior chamber deepened and the angle opened. Bloome has reported two cases in which there was a good response to a cycloplegic and acetazolamide (3). **Treatment with cycloplegic agents seems logical in this condition, and although we still have much to learn, cycloplegics should be used as initial treatment instead of miotics.**

We assume that an abnormal accumulation of blood or fluid in the posterior segment is responsible for pushing the vitreous and lens forward. This fluid is gradually reabsorbed, allowing the vitreous and lens to recede to their normal position. Angle closure appears to be caused by abnormal resistance to flow of aqueous humor through the pupil from the posterior chamber to anterior chamber due to the forward position of the lens, analogous to the mechanism in primary angle closure glaucoma in which the lens is also forward, but on a permanent rather than a transient basis; that is, the mechanism for the closure of the angle in this entity seems to involve a "secondary" pupillary block mechanism. Other possible (but unproven) secondary mechanisms for the closure of the angle are discussed in Chapter 28. Regardless, in some cases of this type, peripheral iridectomy has been done and has relieved the angle closure glaucoma, without altering the position of the crystalline lens.

Before the availability of laser iridectomy, we believed that in this particular kind of angle closure glaucoma, it was best to treat the condition medically rather than by iridectomy. We learned that in most cases the underlying condition cleared in a few weeks, even if the angle was only minimally open in this interval. With the relative ease of laser iridectomy, we now recommend that it be performed if the eye is not totally blind to prevent chronic synechial glaucoma, unless medical (cycloplegic) therapy opened the angle so well that synechia formation would be unlikely. **Gonioscopy of the fellow eye is important because it may be occludable.**

The occurrence of shallowing of the anterior chamber and angle closure glaucoma secondary to occlusion of the central retinal vein is not directly related to the risk of developing neovascular glaucoma later (5). The proportion of eyes that have developed neovascular glaucoma has not been more or less than is expected after ordinary occlusion of the central retinal vein without axial shallowing.

This condition must always be considered in the differential diagnosis of unilateral angle closure. Other causes of transient unilateral shallowing of the anterior chamber with or without angle closure glaucoma include panretinal photocoagulation (6,7), choroidal hemorrhage (8), massive retinal detachment secondary to macular degeneration (9), uveal effusion (10), and massive vitreous hemorrhage (11).

As discussed in Chapter 29, the capacity of the vitreous normally to give up fluid, and reduce its volume, to compensate for the expanded posterior segment volume from the central retinal vein occlusion, is believed to explain why this syndrome of angle closure glaucoma is uncommon. Presumably the condition occurs in patients with more "turgid" vitreous. A systematic analysis of the difference between affected and unaffected patients with central retinal vein occlusion would be of interest. However, we suspect that slight axial shallowing (without angle closure) occuring acutely after central retinal vein occlusion may be more common than realized.

References

1. Hyams SW, Neumann E: Transient angle-closure glaucoma after retinal vein occlusion. Br J Ophthalmol 1972;56:535–355.
2. Grant WM: Shallowing of the anterior chamber following occlusion of the central retinal vein. Am J Ophthalmol 1973;75:384–389.
3. Bloome MA: Transient angle-closure glaucoma in central retinal vein occlusion. Ann Ophthalmol 1977;9:44–48.
4. Mendelsohn AD, Jampol LM, Shoch D: Secondary angle-closure glaucoma after central retinal vein occlusion. Am J Ophthalmol 1985;100: 581–585.
5. Hayreh SS, Rojas P, Montague P, et al: Ocular neovascularization with retinal vascularization occlusion–III. Incidence of ocular neovascularization with retinal vein occlusion. Ophthalmology 1983;90:488–506.
6. Boulton PE: A study of the mechanisms of transient myopia following extensive xenon arc photocoagulation. Trans Ophthalmol Soc UK 1973; 93:287–300.
7. Mensher JH: Anterior chamber depth alteration after retinal photocoagulation. Arch Ophthalmol 1977;95:113–116.
8. Christensen L: Narrow angle glaucoma. Trans Am Acad Ophthalmol Otolarlyngol 1963;67:71–74.
9. Wood WJ, Smith TR: Senile disciform macular degeneration complicated by massive hemorrhagic retinal detachment and angle closure glaucoma. Retina 1983;3:296–303.
10. McDonald PR, de la Paz Jr V, Sarin LK: Nonrhegmatogenous retinal separation: With choroidal detachment (uveal effusion). Am J Ophthalmol 1965;59:820–827.
11. Doden W: Sekundarglaukom bei Periphlebitis retinae. Ophthalmologica 1961;142:506–511.

Angle Closure Glaucoma Secondary To Bilateral Transitory Myopia

36

David L. Epstein

This is a rare condition that an ophthalmologist may see once or twice in a lifetime, but it is a distinct entity that can be puzzling diagnostically. Acute transient myopia due to an idiosyncratic reaction to systemic drugs that have no cholinergic or parasympathomimetic activity is well known, but in only the rarest instances has the episode been accompanied by shallowing of the anterior chamber (1–11). More than 20 different drugs, of several different kinds, but most commonly diuretics (12–14) and sulfa-type drugs (2,4,7,10,15–17) have induced acute transitory myopia. Other drugs reported include tetracycline (3), aspirin (5), corticosteroids (18), bromocriptine (19), prochlorperazine (20), and promethazine (21).

Sometimes there is no past history of drug exposure. Typically, however, weeks or months previously the patient has taken some medication, such as a diuretic or sulfonamide antibiotic, without notable visual side effects, but after discontinuing the medication for a while and then taking it again, an acute reaction develops. Characteristically, within a few hours or a few days after resuming the medication, the patient experiences blurring of vision for distant objects, due to the development of several diopters of myopia. Visual acuity can be restored to normal with a suitable refraction, but not by anticholinergics. There is no miosis and no evidence of cyclotonia.

Good evidence, including ultrasonographic measurements (8,13), indicates that swelling of the crystalline lens is responsible, at least in part, for the myopia in most cases, and that it is reversible (4). However, others have attributed at least some of the myopia to the forward movement of the crystalline lens (7,10,11). We have seen one patient in whom accumulation of anterior choroidal fluid was implicated not only in the pathogenesis of secondary angle closure glaucoma, but also in the induced myopia (11). **The choroidal effusion** (Fig. 36.1A) **presumably caused forward rotation of the ciliary body, which led to forward movement of the entire crystalline lens due to loss of zonular tension, and angle closure** (Fig. 36.1B). The latter presumably occurred from direct mechanical pressure of the ciliary body on the iris (Chapter 28) because laser iridectomy was without effect. The forward position of the crystalline lens could explain about half of the myopic shift. A similar case of induced myopia and angle closure has been reported in which one eye had a pseudophakos, and therefore presumably lens swelling was ruled out as a cause of the myopia, which was attributed to the forward shift in the intraocular lens position (10). This condition has also been observed commonly in young women, often during the first few months of pregnancy.

When the suspect drug is discontinued, the myopia disappears spontaneously within a few days. In all cases similar changes have occurred in both eyes, except for an instance of unilateral aphakia, in which, in contrast to the aforementioned, there was no change in the refraction of the aphakic eye. **Either crystalline lens swelling or forward positioning of the crystalline lens or both may be involved in the etiology of the induced myopia.**

Only in rare cases does crystalline lens swelling and/or forward shift of the crystalline lens cause sufficient shallowing of the anterior chamber to induce bilateral angle closure glaucoma from pupillary block, and it is usually subacute rather than acute. When the process resolves in a few days, the myopia disappears, the anterior chambers return to normal depth, and the angles reopen to their former width (Fig. 36.1C). The following case is another example.

Case 36-1. A woman, aged mid-20s, accustomed to good vision without glasses, had rapid onset of blurring of vision in the course of several hours. The patient had a history of numerous allergies, but during the previous year she had taken a thiazide diuretic without adverse effect. She had stopped the diuretic 9 months before the present episode, but had resumed taking it just before the onset of the blurring of vision, having taken 5 tablets during 2 or 3 days, but none since. She had four diopters of myopia in each eye, with vision correctable to normal by lenses. The anterior chambers were shallowed to 1.5 corneal thicknesses axially, and IOP was 30 in each eye. The angles were extremely narrow and appeared closed in portions of the circumference. Pilocarpine and acetazolamide were started. The next day IOP was 14 in each eye. The media were clear and the fundi normal, but myopia had increased to 7 diopters, and the anterior chambers were still very shallow. In 2 more days, the anterior chambers regained normal depth, the angles attained normal width, vision became normal without need for glasses, and IOP was normal without further treatment.

The reversible myopia from lens swelling as an idiosyncratic reaction to drugs may be in some way allied to the changes in refraction that occasionally occur in diabetes

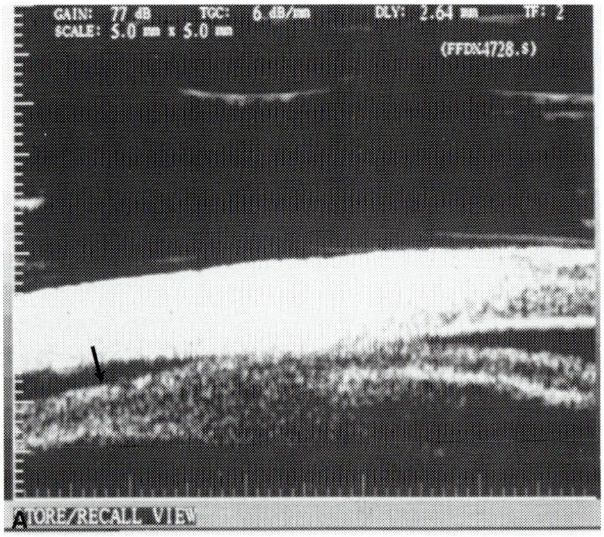

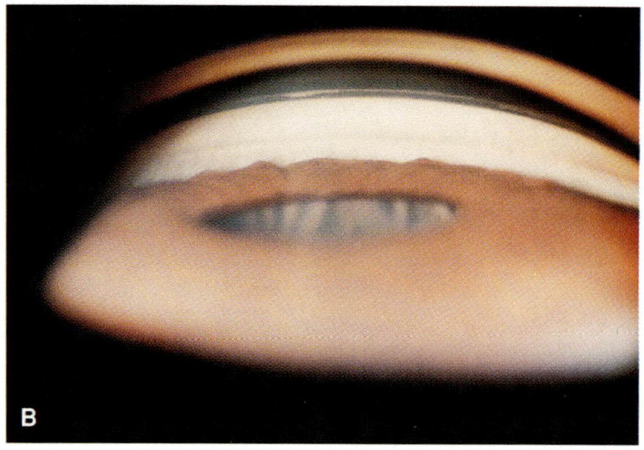

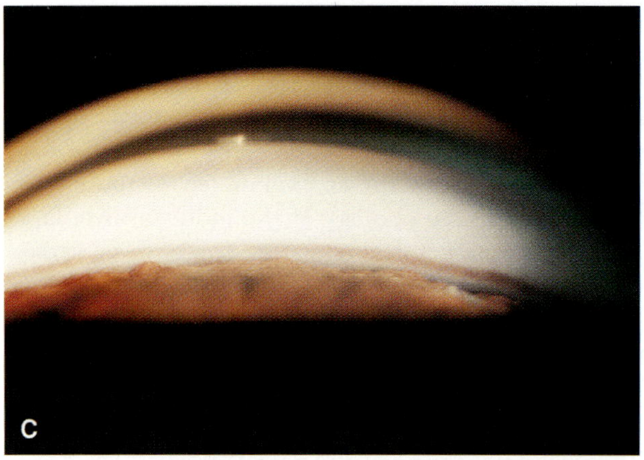

Figure 36.1. A 36-year-old white female reported progressively blurry vision beginning 1 week after bilateral lung transplantation. The anterior chamber was shallow axially and peripherally OU and there were 5-6 diopters of induced myopia OU. Ultrasound biomicroscopy revealed bilateral choroidal effusions (arrow) (A). Gonioscopy revealed no visible angle structures (B). Ciliary processes could be seen through the pupil. Laser iridectomy, performed to one eye only, was without effect, as was cycloplegic therapy. Calculations indicated that the forward position of the crystalline lenses could explain approximately half of the induced myopia. After discontinuation of oral Septra (a combination of sulfamethoxazole and trimethoprim), which she had started taking postoperatively, there was total resolution of both the angle closure glaucoma (C) and myopia OU. From Postel EA, Assalian A, Epstein DL: Drug-induced transient myopia and angle-closure glaucoma associated with supracilliary choroidal effusion. Figs. 1B and 2B. Am J Ophthalmol 1996. In press.

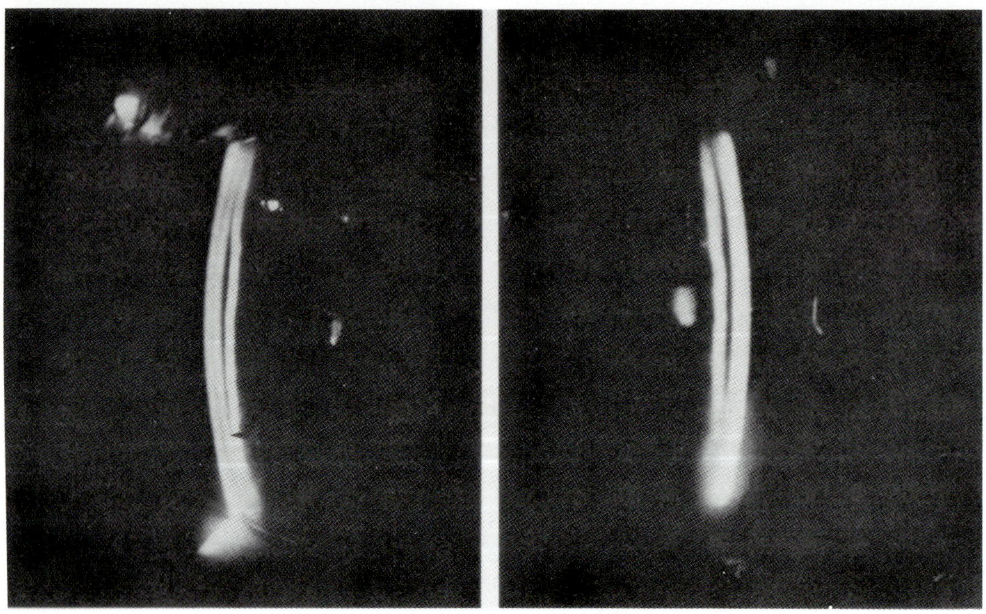

Figure 36.2. A, Shallow anterior chamber on slit-lamp examination. Note the very narrow space (black arrowhead) between peripheral iris and corneal endothelium. B, The other eye after laser iridectomy shows a deeper peripheral chamber depth.

ACUTE BILATERAL TRANSITORY MYOPIA ASSOCIATED WITH OPEN ANGLE GLAUCOMA

Joel S. Schuman

One of us (JSS) has seen a patient with bilateral transitory myopia associated with open angle, rather than angle closure, glaucoma. At the initial presentation, the patient, a 36-year-old woman, reported blurred vision after awakening. She had a low-grade fever (100 F), and a flu-like syndrome of aches, pains, and malaise. She did not recall taking any unusual medications, only loratadine (antihistamine) and nonsteroidal anti-inflammatory drugs (NSAIDs). She had no hypertension or diabetes, and a blood glucose was normal.

On examination, visual acuity was 20/200 OU, refracting to 20/25 OU with -2.00 D in each eye. Intraocular pressures (IOPs) were 23 and 24 mm Hg, and her angle was open in each eye to ciliary body band. Her examination otherwise was completely unremarkable. She was given her prescription and sent home. When she returned 3 weeks later, visual acuity was 20/20 without correction, and IOPs were 15 mm Hg in each eye. Angles were again open, and her examination was unchanged except that her axial anterior chamber depth seemed slightly greater than on the previous visit.

Two months later, the patient presented again with the same constitutional and ophthalmologic complaints. Vision was again correctable to 20/25 with -2.00 D sphere, but this time her IOPs were 36 and 38 mm Hg, although her angles were still open to scleral spur. She denied taking any new medications, but during the examination, recalled that she had taken quinine for leg cramps just before the previous episode, and again before the current episode. This was the 31st quinine tablet she had ever taken, though she had only two recognized episodes of blurred vision.

Ultrasound biomicroscopy (UBM) showed her angles to be open to ciliary body band, confirming the gonioscopy, but also revealed very anterior ciliochoroidal effusions bilaterally (Fig. 36.3). On follow-up examination 2 weeks later, the IOPs had returned to the mid-teens, the patient was again emmetropic, and the UBM demonstrated that the angles were now significantly wider than previously. The effusions were gone (Fig. 36.4). An A-scan ultrasound at the time of the myopia compared with one taken after its resolution showed deepening of the anterior chamber and thinning of the crystalline lens with the resolution of the episode.

Quinine has been associated with acute bilateral transitory myopia with angle closure glaucoma in one case (1). Our patient appears to have developed an acute sensitivity to the drug, having taken it with no known adverse effects on 29 previous occasions, but with marked systemic and ocular side effects during the last two. The mechanism for the ciliochoroidal effusion, and indeed, of the open angle glaucoma itself, remains mysterious, but the former may be related to a change in vascular permeability causing the effusion. The increased volume of the supraciliochoroidal space may have accounted for the increase in intraocular pressure, as this patient's angle was clearly open throughout each episode. Alternately, the change in the ciliary muscle (2,3) induced by the effusion may have relaxed the tone in the trabecular meshwork and Schlemm's canal, resulting in a decrease in outflow facility, thus explaning the IOP rise.

Whatever the mechanism, this rare condition of glaucoma associated with acute bilateral transitory myopia is no longer limited to angle closure alone.

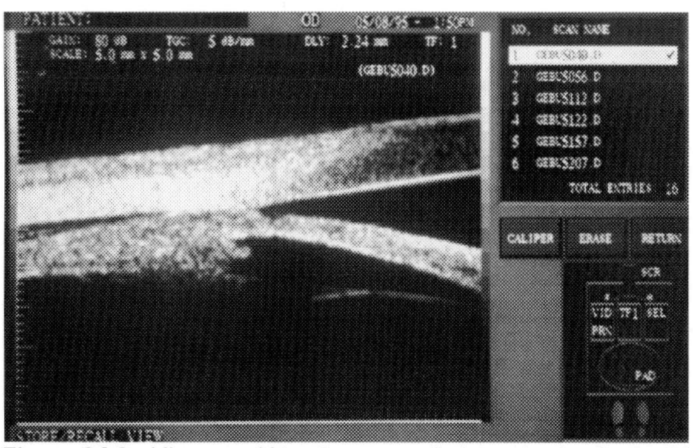

Figure 36.3. Ultrasound biomicroscopy during episode of acute bilateral transitory myopia associated with open angle glaucoma demonstrates anterior ciliochoroidal effusion with narrowing of angle inlet, but the angle is open to ciliary body band.

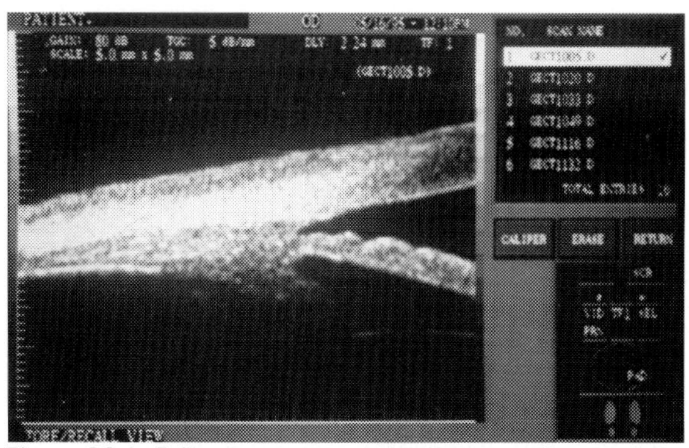

Figure 36.4. Follow-up ultrasound biomicroscopy after resolution of episode (Fig. 36.3) shows disappearance of supraciliochoroidal fluid and deepening of angle. Note change in angle configuration, although it was open both during and after the episode.

References

1. Segal A, Aisemberg A, Ducasse A: Quinine transitory myopia and angle-closure glaucoma. Bull Soc Ophthalmol France 1983;83: 247–249.
2. Grant, WM: Experimental aqueous perfusion in enucleated human eyes. Arch Ophthalmol 1963;69:783–801.
3. Rosenquist RC, Melamed S, Epstein DL: Anterior and posterior axial lens displacement and human aqueous outflow facility. Invest Ophthalmol Vis Sci 1988;29:1159–1164.

mellitus. A bilateral transitory angle-closure glaucoma has been reported in one case in an insulin-treated diabetic patient during an episode of several diopters of myopia and marked shallowing of the anterior chambers (22).

Also, acute bilateral transitory myopia with shallowing of the anterior chambers and angle-closure glaucoma has in three cases been reported in association with a febrile illness, but whether the mechanism differed from that in drug idiosyncrasy and diabetes mellitus is unproved (23).

Treatment for this particular type of angle closure glaucoma is discontinuance of any recently resumed systemic medication and temporary administration of aqueous humor suppressants. In the past miotics have been used with good success presumably due to considerations of net "vectors" discussed in Chapter 22. With lens swelling leading to pupillary block, such traditional medical therapy would make sense. However, in those cases where there may have also occurred a forward movement of the crystalline lens it is possible that miotics may actually worsen the condition. Cycloplegics theoretically might be beneficial but in a recent case (11) there was no benefit, which we attribute to the maintained forwardly rotated position of the ciliary body that resulted from the supraciliary fluid accumulation.

Supraciliary effusion resulting from idiosyncratic drug reaction may be a more common mechanism in these cases that demonstrate secondary angle closure glaucoma than is currently appreciated. **Thus there are two potential mechanisms for such secondary angle closure glaucoma: 1) pupillary block secondary to swelling of the crystalline lens or its induced forward position (as a result of loss of zonular tension accompanying suprachoroidal fluid accumulation); and 2) direct mechanical pressure (secondary to supraciliary effusion) of the forwardly rotated ciliary body on the iris forcing it into the angle** (Chapter 28). Laser iridectomy would alleviate the angle closure glaucoma only if the first mechanism were involved (Fig. 36.2). In our case (Fig. 36.1), laser iridectomy was totally without effect, thus indicating that secondary pupillary block was not involved in the mechanism for the secondary angle closure glaucoma.

We have no explanation for the mechanism of such drug-induced ciliochoroidal effusion. However, because sulfonamide drugs of the carbonic-anhydrase inhibitor type are used for glaucoma therapy and influence fluid movement at the level of the ciliary body (Chapter 3), it is theoretically possible that misdirection of flow into the suprachoroidal space might rarely occur from an idiosyncratic reaction.

References

1. Grant WM, Schuman JS: Toxicology of the eye, 4th ed. Springfield: Charles C. Thomas, 1993.
2. Muirhead JF, Scheie HG: Transient myopia after acetazolamide. Arch Ophthalmol 1960;63:315–318.
3. Edwards TS: Transient myopia due to tetracycline. J Am Med Assoc 1963;186:96–70.
4. Maddalena MA: Transient myopia associated with acute glaucoma and retinal edema following vaginal administration of sulfanilamide. Arch Ophthalmol 1968;80:186–188.
5. Sanford-Smith JH: Transient myopia after aspirin. Br J Ophthalmol 1974;58:698–700.
6. Schroeder W, Schwarzer J: Transitorische Myopie mit Winkelblockglaukom. Klin Monatsbl Augenheilkd 1978;172:762–766.
7. Bovino JA, Marcus DF: The mechanism of transient myopia induced by sulfonamide therapy. Am J Ophthalmol 1982;94:99–102.
8. Hook SR, Holladay JT, Prager TC, et al: Transient myopia induced by sulfonamides. Am J Ophthalmol 1986;101:495–496.
9. Ryan EH, Jampol LM: Drug-induced acute transient myopia with retinal folds. Retina 1986;6:220–223.
10. Fan JT, Johnson DH, Burk RR: Transient myopia, angle closure glaucoma, and choroidal detachment after oral acetazolamide. Am J Ophthalmol 1993;115:813–814.
11. Postel E, Assalian F, Epstein DL: Drug-induced transient myopia and angle closure associated with supraciliary choroidal effusion. Am J Ophthalmol, July 1996.
12. Michaelson JJ: Transient myopia due to hygroton. Am J Ophthalmol 1962;54:1146–1147.
13. Pallin O, Ericsson R: Ultrasound studies in a case of hygroton-induced myopia. ACTA Ophthalmol 1965;43:692–696.
14. Beasley FJ: Transient myopia and retinal edema during hydrochlorothiazide (hydrodiuril) therapy. Arch Ophthalmol 1961;65:212–213.
15. Granstrom KO: Transient myopia following the administration of sulphonamides. ACTA Ophthalmol 1949;27:59–68.
16. Galin MA, Baras I, Zweifach P: Diamox-induced myopia. Am J Ophthalmol 1957;35:478–484.
17. Beasley FJ: Transient myopia and retinal edema during ethoxzolamide (cardrase) therapy. Arch Ophthalmol 1962;68;490–491.
18. Stern JJ: Transient myopia in a case of dermatitis treated with corticotropin. Arch Ophthalmol 1956;54:762.
19. Manor RS, Dickerman Z, Llaron Z: Myopia during bromocriptine treatment. Lancet 1981;1(8211):102.
20. Yasuna E: Acute myopia associated with promethazine (compazine) therapy. Am J Ophthalmol 1962;54:783–796.
21. Bard L: Transient myopia associated with prochlorperazine (phenergan) therapy: report of a case. Am J Ophthalmol 1964;58:682–686.
22. Birnbaum F, Leu P: Akute Myopisierung mit intraokularer Drucksteigerung bei Entgleisung eines juvenilen Diabete mellitus. Klin Monatsbl Augenheilkd 1975;167:613–615.
23. Saari KM: Acute glaucoma in hemorrhagic fever with renal syndrome (nephropathia epidemica). Am J Ophthalmol 1976;31:455–461.

Glaucoma After Penetrating Keratoplasty 37

David L. Epstein

A common form of glaucoma that is difficult to manage is that which occurs after penetrating keratoplasty (1–3). Most often the mechanism involves peripheral anterior synechia formation and represents a form of chronic angle closure glaucoma. However, **the chronic use of topical steroids is responsible for some cases of secondary open angle glaucoma.** This latter diagnosis, which is often unrecognized because the time of onset may be late and the steroid dosage low, should always be suspected in these patients. Attempts should be made to reduce or discontinue the topical steroids. IOP may be substantially lower only a few days after steroids are totally discontinued, thus indicating an extreme sensitivity to these agents.

The mechanism of angle closure glaucoma is not well understood in these patients (Table 37.1). Pupillary block can occur, and for this reason, peripheral iridectomy should be routinely performed at the time of surgery. However, cases are encountered in which surgical iridectomy was performed, but in the postoperative period the iris and iridectomy were observed to be adherent to the cornea and the coloboma was nonfunctional (Fig. 37.1). A transient wound leak must always be suspected. However, some have questioned whether the iris may be more reactive after keratoplasty and whether iris swelling may lead to PAS formation and angle closure, especially if the iris is in contact with an intraocular lens haptic (4). Eyes with corneal disease often do demonstrate inflammatory ocular disease and the iris may thus be more "sticky." Alternatively, one of us (DLE) has questioned whether choroidal detachment may occur intraoperatively from ocular hypotension which may develop more commonly than suspected, leading to rolling forward of the ciliary body and iris into the angle. A choroidal detachment postoperatively from a transient wound leak would have the same effect. In addition, choroidal detachment may result in forward lens movement similar to that seen after retinal detachment surgery (Chapter 33), which may add a pupillary block component to the angle closure. Lens swelling, if it occurs, may also cause pupillary block.

If acute angle closure glaucoma is observed, laser iridectomy can alleviate the glaucoma. In the case of a choroidal detachment, surgical drainage may be required (Chapter 63).

More commonly, acute postoperative glaucoma is not observed in these patients, but several weeks to months after keratoplasty elevated IOP due to angle closure glaucoma is first detected. In some of these cases, earlier elevations of IOP may simply have been missed, but in others, hyposecretion, perhaps due to a choroidal detachment, may have masked the angle closure and delayed IOP elevation. It is only later after the choroidal detachment resolves, and aqueous humor production returns to normal, that elevated IOP is observed.

Unfortunately, most of these cases are complicated and the factors that have led to the chronic angle closure glaucoma are unclear. With regard to prevention, a peripheral iridectomy should be performed at the time of surgery and the period of ocular hypotony minimized. Sodium hyaluronate can be used to maintain the anterior chamber. However, this agent can cause substantial IOP elevation postoperatively (5) and should be removed from the anterior chamber at the conclusion of the operation. The anterior chamber should be well formed at the conclusion of surgery. Tightening the iris by direct suturing at the time of surgery may decrease the occurrence of angle closure (6).

Experimental tight suturing close to the limbus in enucleated eyes can cause obstruction to outflow through an "open angle" mechanism (not involving iris-trabecular apposition) (5,7,8). However if this occurs in living eyes, it most likely is a short-lived phenomenon. Slightly oversized corneal grafts may decrease the occurrence of such a secondary "open angle glaucoma" (9–11). Laser trabeculoplasty may be effective for patients with open angle glaucoma after penetrating keratoplasty (12). Secondary "pigmentary" glaucoma after anterior segment surgery can also occur (13).

However, **the major long-term clinical glaucoma problem is chronic synechial angle closure.** Medical therapy (Table 37.2) of this form of glaucoma is challenging because drugs that facilitate outflow, such as pilocarpine, are limited due to PAS formation. However, a trial of miotics is warranted because, in some cases, the PAS may be bridging over an otherwise functional trabecular meshwork to the cornea. Aqueous suppressants are useful. For surgical therapy, if PAS formation is recent, then, as discussed elsewhere, lysing of synechias should be contemplated by use of argon laser gonioplasty (Chapter 60), or surgically (14–16) (Chapter 25). In long-standing cases with good central acuity, filtration surgery should be attempted initially, but special attention to the problem of

Table 37.1
Glaucoma after Penetrating Keratoplasty

Cause	Comment
Open angle glaucoma Angle compression Postoperative inflammatory products (pigment, blood, viscoelastics) Steroids Pre-existing glaucoma	Angle compression may be reduced with meticulous wound closure and by using a donor graft which is larger than the recipient bed; viscoelastics should always be thoroughly removed at end of procedure; chronic use of topical steroids should be considered as a cause of elevated IOP.
Closed angle glaucoma Progressive angle closure Pupillary block	Iris sutures at pupillary margin to "tighten" iris plane can be used to reduce incidence of late angle closure. All patients should have a patent iridectomy.

Table 37.2
Management of Glaucoma after Penetrating Keratoplasty

Treatment	Comment
Medical management Beta blockers Adrenergic agonists Miotics (direct and indirect acting) Apraclonidine Carbonic anhydrase inhibitors	Both direct and indirect acting miotics can be very effective after the early postoperative period if the angle is open; adrenergic agents may cause or worsen cystoid macular edema.
Laser therapy Laser iridectomy Laser trabeculoplasty Laser gonioplasty	To prevent pupillary block all patients should have a patent iridectomy; laser trabeculoplasty can be effective in patients with open angles. Laser gonioplasty should be reserved for patients with PAS of recent onset (less than 1–2 months).
Surgical therapy Trabeculectomy with antimetabolites Seton implantation Cyclodestructive procedure	"Tight flap" with cautious suture lysis recommended to avoid flat chamber and graft injury, setons can be effective but may cause increased graft rejection; laser cyclodestructive procedures are useful in patients with poor potential visual acuity.

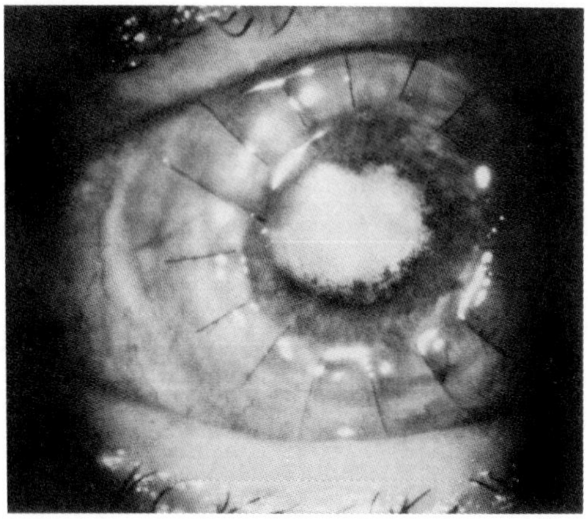

Figure 37.1. Penetrating keratoplasty was performed for a corneal perforation due to herpes simplex. A surgical iridectomy was performed. Postoperatively a flat anterior chamber with iris up to the cornea was observed with high IOP. An argon laser iridectomy was unsuccessful, but a YAG iridectomy was performed with prompt resolution of the glaucoma and deepening of the peripheral (but not central) anterior chamber. (Courtesy of Deborah Pavan-Langston, MD).

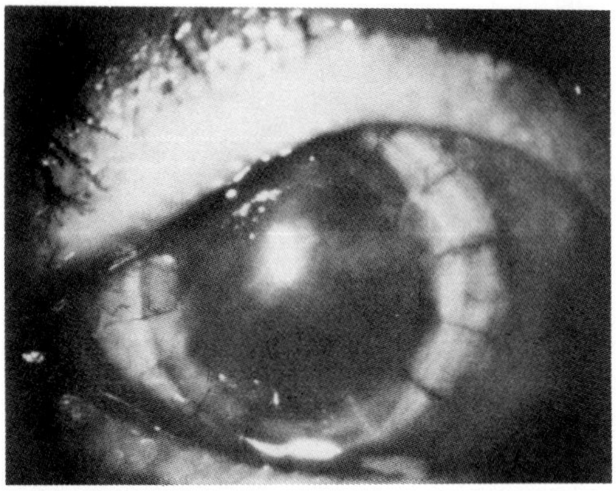

Figure 37.2. During a filtration procedure in a one-eyed aphakic patient (who had a previous penetrating keratoplasty) an expulsive hemorrhage developed. Despite three-quadrant posterior sclerotomies and an evacuation of the blood and subsequent repeat drainage of the suprachoroidal space, the eye ultimately lost light perception. The immediate postoperative appearance is shown with a dark mass, presumably pars plana, filling the anterior chamber. Although rare, this complication underscores the importance of developing more effective noninvasive methods of glaucoma therapy for these patients.

flat anterior chamber is required, due to the vulnerability of the recently transplanted cornea. **Immediate or delayed suprachoroidal hemorrhage** (Fig. 37.2) **as a complication of filtration surgery may be more common in these eyes.** Ciliodestructive procedures are an effective means of IOP control (17–21), but there is risk of macular edema in eyes with good acuity and risk of cataract formation in phakic eyes. Such treatment, however, is often the only effective means for pressure control. The use of Molteno type tubes or shunts can be effective but are accompanied by a high incidence of corneal graft rejection (22,23).

References

1. Karesh JW, Nirankari VS: Factors associated with glaucoma after penetrating keratoplasty. Am J Ophthalmol 1983;96:160–4.
2. Foulks GN: Glaucoma associated with penetrating keratoplasty. Ophthalmology 1987;94:871–874.
3. Simmons RB, Stern RA, Teekhasaenee C, et al: Elevated intraocular pressure following penetrating keratoplasty. Trans Am Ophthalmol Soc 1989;87:79–91.
4. Chu MW, Font RL, Koch DD: Visual results and complications following posterior iris-fixated posterior chamber lenses at penetrating keratoplasty. Ophthalmic Surg 1992;23:608–13.
5. Berson FG, Patterson MM, Epstein DL: Obstruction of aqueous outflow by sodium hyaluronate in enucleated human eyes. Am J Ophthalmol 1983;95:668–672.
6. Cohen EJ, Kenyon KR, Dohlman CH: Iridoplasty for prevention of post-keratoplasty angle closure and glaucoma. Ophthalmic Surg 1982;13:994–6.
7. Campbell DG, Grant WM: Unpublished data cited in Berson FG, Patterson MM, Epstein DL: Obstruction of aqueous outflow by sodium hyaluronate in enucleated human eyes. Am J Ophthalmol 1983;95:668–672.
8. Zimmerman TJ, Krupin T, Grodski W, et al: The effect of suture depth on outflow facility in penetrating keratoplasty. Arch Ophthalmol 1978;96:505–506.
9. Zimmerman T, Olson R, Waltman S, et al: Transplant size and elevated intraocular pressure postkeratoplasty. Arch Ophthalmol 1978;96:2231–2233.
10. Bourne WM, Davison JA, O'Fallon WM: The effects of oversize donor buttons on postoperative intraocular pressure and corneal curvature in aphakic penetrating keratoplasty. Ophthalmology 1982;89:242–246.
11. Heidemann DG, Sugar A, Meyer RF, et al: Oversized donor grafts in penetrating keratoplasty. A randomized trial. Arch Ophthalmol 1985;103:1807–1811.
12. Van Meter WS, Allen RC, Waring GO, et al: Laser trabeculoplasty for glaucoma in aphakic and pseudophakic eyes after penetrating keratoplasty. Arch Ophthalmol 1988;106:185–858.
13. Insler MS, Zatzkis SM: Pigment dispersion syndrome in pseudophakic corneal transplants. Am J Ophthalmol 1986;102:762–765.
14. Campbell DG, Vela A: Modern goniosynechialysis for the treatment of synechial angle-closure glaucoma. Ophthalmology 1984;91:1052–60.
15. Shingleton BJ, Chang MA, Bellows AR, et al: Surgical goniosynechialysis for angle-closure glaucoma. Ophthalmology 1990;97:551–556.
16. Tanihara H, Nishiwaki K, Nagata M: Surgical results and complications of goniosynechialysis. Graefes Arch Clin Exp Ophthalmol 1992;230:309–313.
17. West CE, Wood TO, Kaufman HE: Cyclocryotherapy for glaucoma pre- or post-penetrating keratoplasty. Am J Ophthalmol 1973;76:485–489.
18. Thoft RA, Gordon JM, Dohlman CH: Glaucoma following keratoplasty. Trans Am Acad Ophthalmol Otolaryngol 1974;78:352–364.
19. Binder PS, Abel R Jr, Kaufman HE: Cyclocryotherapy for glaucoma after penetrating keratoplasty. Am J Ophthalmol 1975;79:489–92.
20. Cohen EJ, Schwartz LW, Luskind RD, et al: Neodymium: YAG laser transscleral cyclophotocoagulation for glaucoma after penetrating keratoplasty. Ophthalmic Surg 1989;20:713–716.
21. Wheatcroft S, Singh A, Casey T, et al: Treatment of glaucoma following penetrating keratoplasty with transscleral YAG cyclophotocoagulation. Int Ophthalmol 1992;16:397–400.
22. McDonnell PJ, Robin JB, Schanzlin DJ, et al: Molteno implant for control of glaucoma in eyes after penetrating keratoplasty. Ophthalmology 1988;95:364–369.
23. Sherwood MB, Smith MF, Driebe WT Jr, et al: Drainage tube implants in the treatment of glaucoma following penetrating keratoplasty. Ophthalmic Surg 1993;24:185–189.

Combined Mechanisms VI

Combined Open Angle and Angle Closure Glaucoma

38

David L. Epstein

The obstruction to aqueous outflow in primary open angle glaucoma is due mainly to abnormalities within or just beyond the trabecular meshwork, whereas in angle closure glaucoma the cause of obstruction to aqueous outflow is a ballooning of the periphery of the iris against the corneoscleral trabecular meshwork, preventing access of aqueous humor to the normal aqueous outflow system. There is no reason why both conditions could not occur in the same eye. Because each has an independent basis, a certain number of coincidences of this sort can be expected. On the other hand, there are more cases of "residual open angle glaucoma" after laser iridectomy than would be expected by chance (Chapter 22).

There is also a hypothetical possibility that repeated episodes of angle closure could cause permanent damage to the corneoscleral trabecular meshwork even without formation of peripheral anterior synechias, and that they could in this way induce a form of permanent open angle glaucoma, which would persist between episodes of angle closure and after angle closure attacks were terminated by iridectomy. This has been mentioned previously (open angle glaucoma due to chronic iris touch in Chapter 22). As yet, however, we lack clear evidence for this mechanism.

Occasionally, patients present evidence of having both open-angle and angle closure glaucoma. In some of these patients, one may be certain that only 2, 3, or 4 hours of the angle are closed, but one may find an IOP of 40 mm Hg, and tonography may indicate an impairment of facility of outflow consistent with the IOP, but disproportionately more than the extent of angle closure. When the findings are this clear and definitive, the diagnosis is easy. One has to conclude that there is not enough angle closure to account for this amount of glaucoma.

In many other cases, it is much more difficult to establish whether one is dealing with pure angle-closure glaucoma or a combination of angle closure with open angle glaucoma. Difficulty in establishing a definite diagnosis of combined open angle and angle closure glaucoma, or of distinguishing between open angle and angle closure glaucoma, is greatest when a question of chronic appositional angle closure is involved. The other varieties of angle closure seldom present a problem in this regard. For instance, in acute angle closure glaucoma, when all the typical symptoms and signs are present, we are seldom confronted with glaucoma out of proportion to the extent of closure during an attack, or out of proportion to any residual peripheral anterior synechias after iridectomy is done. Also, in chronic synechial angle closure glaucoma in which a considerable portion of the angle has gradually become closed by synechias, it is uncommon to find glaucoma out of proportion to the extent of angle closure, or residual glaucoma after iridectomy out of proportion to the extent of synechias.

The greatest problem is encountered in eyes in which the angle is so narrow in a portion of the circumference that we think, but cannot be sure, that some of it is actually closed, while at the same time measurements of IOP and facility of outflow suggest that the glaucoma is more severe than would be expected from the conceivable extent of angle closure. When closure of only a portion of the circumference is in question, it may be very difficult to prove whether angle closure is actually taking place. If laser iridectomy is done in these cases, and the angle becomes widened so that we can rule out future episodes of angle closure, we may find that IOP and facility of outflow are not improved and that the open-angle glaucoma that is present requires continuing treatment. However, peripheral iridectomy in such cases confers the real benefit of eliminating concern about future attacks of angle closure glaucoma. The benefit/risk ratio of laser iridectomy is such that it is often used to eliminate any angle closure component. However, it is important to realize that surgical iridectomy was also previously so used. The following case illustrates this situation.

Case 38-1. A man, age 47 years with hypermetropia of 5D, a history of hypermetropia in many relatives, and acute glaucoma in his hypermetropic grandfather, was referred to us because of extremely narrow angles in both eyes. Optic nerve heads and fields were normal.

We found applanation IOPs 26 to 30 mm Hg on different occasions, and tonographic C value of 0.11, both eyes. The anterior chambers were not excessively shallow axially (equivalent to 4 or 5 corneal thicknesses) but the irides were convex peripherally, and the angles appeared to be closed in ⅓ to ½ the circumference, very narrow in the remainder. Trial of 2% and later 4% pilocarpine in one eye did not improve the facility of outflow, but under this treatment IOP was 20; the angle remained so narrow that it was impossible to say whether the angle in the superior quadrant opened; in the rest of the circumference the angle was definitely open, but extremely narrow.

The tonographic measurements indicated more obstruction to aqueous outflow than would be explained by closure of a small fraction of the angle, so we concluded that the glaucoma was mainly of the open-angle variety, but because of the extreme narrowness of the angle and probably closure of a portion, peripheral iridectomy was performed on each eye as a protective measure.

Several months after the iridectomies, when the eyes were entirely healed and quiet, examination without treatment showed applanation IOPs 25 and tonographic C values 0.12 in both eyes, all essentially the same as before the operation. The angles were only slightly less narrow than before iridectomy, but now discernibly open superiorly and definitely open in the rest of the circumference. A view obtained through the surgical colobomas suggested that the persistent narrowness of the angles might be attributable to the position of the ciliary processes, which were in contact with the back of the iris and appeared possibly to be holding the periphery of the iris forward. (Certainly the persistent narrowness of these angles could not be due to accumulation of aqueous in the posterior chamber, after iridectomy.)

We concluded that, as suspected preoperatively, the glaucoma in this patient was principally open angle glaucoma, but that the peripheral iridectomies had been worthwhile. Although the iridectomies caused only slight widening of the angles in this case, that amount appeared critical. Furthermore, by eliminating all hindrance to the flow of aqueous from posterior to anterior chamber, the iridectomies made safe and feasible the future use of all types of miotics and epinephrine-like drugs, which eventually may be needed for control of the open-angle glaucoma during the patient's expected 30 or 40 remaining years of life.

As a principle of treatment, when the angle is extremely narrow, and especially when it is certain that a portion of the angle can close when the eye is without treatment, but there is conclusive evidence of open angle glaucoma with the facility of outflow persistently subnormal when the angle is open, either spontaneously or under miotics, there is justification for performing laser iridectomy to eliminate the angle closure element and to permit use of all types of medication for the open angle glaucoma. In eyes having open angle glaucoma with a very narrow angle, which have developed acute angle closure glaucoma, the status of the previously open angle glaucoma is unchanged after iridectomy. The iridectomy is intended purely to prevent or relieve angle-closure glaucoma.

Eyes that have been under intensive treatment for open angle glaucoma, including strong miotics and epinephrine, and have angles that are only moderately narrow, with full width of trabecular meshwork visible gonioscopically and not therefore threateningly narrow, and never having closed spontaneously, merit close observation rather than either provocative testing by mydriatics or prophylactic iridectomy. Such eyes may be provocable to angle closure by mydriasis, but observation of the condition of the angle under regular treatment for the open angle glaucoma is the most meaningful guide as to whether prophylactic iridectomy is needed.

In this situation if the angles are inspected every few months, they may become more narrow. This is in part due to growth of the lens, which continues throughout life, and in part due to the action of the miotic drops. If the angle becomes so narrowed that closure appears imminent, laser peripheral iridectomy should then be done promptly, with no need for provocative testing. After laser iridectomy, widening of the angle can be expected to make subsequent use of miotics safer when they are needed.

In observing such patients, use of Zeiss indentation gonioscopy is important to be sure that PAS formation is not occurring (see Fig. 7.6). If PAS are definitely identified, then laser iridectomy should be performed.

Many of these issues have been discussed in Chapter 22, especially in terms of the indication for laser iridectomy and the categories of "residual open angle glaucoma" after iridectomy. The physiological principles of correlating the extent of angle closure with the IOP elevation have been discussed in Chapters 3 and 6. In addition to these considerations of open angle glaucoma in eyes with angle closure, the reverse category of a superimposed angle closure component to a basic open angle glaucoma process needs to be considered and has been discussed in Chapter 22. In particular, the occurrence of a subsequent additional angle closure component to an open angle glaucoma due to exfoliation (1) needs to be kept in mind: it is not rare.

Patients with presumed POAG need periodic repeated gonioscopy and should always have gonioscopy when the IOP is elevated at a follow-up visit. In addition to identifying a superimposed angle closure component, other causes such as occult inflammatory precipitates or new blood vessels, etc., need to be ruled out. When a patient with POAG seems to demonstrate some functional angle closure (usually 4 hours or more) but there is no PAS formation on indentation gonioscopy, and thus there is some uncertainty whether there is truly a functional appositional angle closure component or whether the angle is narrow but still functionally open (Chapter 22), the risk/benefit considerations are such that after fully informing the patient about these considerations as well as one's diagnostic uncertainty (and what the clinician would do if it were his/her eye) it is usually wisest to proceed with laser iridectomy. This is because in this situation the risk of not treating a possible angle closure glaucoma component is greater than the risk of the procedure.

Nevertheless, **the clinician and the patient need to be fully prepared for an IOP spike that may be substantial if, for example, the glaucoma is entirely due to an open angle exfoliation mechanism rather than**

some functional angle closure component. In this situation, pigment and other iris debris from the iridectomy and inflammation may provide further short-term and possibly long-term insult to trabecular meshwork function. Regardless, the iridectomy may be indicated for prophylactic purposes, but the patient (and clinician) need to know ahead of time that the iridectomy will not improve the IOP in the short-term and may cause a substantial acute IOP spike.

Finally, chronic silent angle closure may masquerade as "open angle glaucoma" given the absence of symptoms. The usual aqueous suppressant therapy for such presumed "open angle glaucoma," by decreasing the vectors acting on the posterior iris surface, may somewhat deepen the angle perpetuating the misdiagnosis (Chapter 22). Such an action needs to be evaluated in any patient suspected of having combined mechanism glaucoma.

References

1. Gross FJ, Tingey D, Epstein DL: Increased prevalence of occludable angles and angle-closure glaucoma in patients with pseudoexfoliation. Am J Ophthalmol 1993;117:333–336.

Glaucoma in the Pseudophakic and Aphakic Eye

39

David L. Epstein

A major revolution has occurred in the techniques of cataract surgery in the interval since the last edition of this book, with a switch from intracapsular to extracapsular surgery with smaller and smaller incisions. Many of the former seemingly "unique" aspects of glaucoma in aphakia now clearly, in hindsight, relate to the larger wounds and the removal of the mechanical support structure of the crystalline lens that occurred in intracapsular cataract surgery. Although intracapsular cataract surgery is rarely preformed today, there are still aphakic eyes from previous decades that face additional glaucoma surgery where some of the former issues still have relevance. These will be described below.

The major issue in pseudophakic and aphakic eyes is the guarded prognosis for filtration surgery because of previous cataract surgery and its attendant conjunctival manipulation. The use of antimetabolites has improved the prognosis for such eyes and is discussed in Chapter 62. **If the conjunctiva is mobile, filtration surgery with antimetabolites can and should be performed as in phakic eyes.** Sometimes if there is scarring of the conjunctiva only at the limbus, the scleral flap dissection can be used to carry the surgical site anterior to the limbus underneath this external scarring, or a fornix based conjunctival flap technique can be used. Subconjunctival fibrosis from previous cataract surgery is not simply a technical barrier to an adequate surgical procedure, but is a sign indicating the likelihood of increased post-filtration wound healing with a higher risk of bleb failure ("the conjunctiva always remembers") (Fig. 39.1). In cases in which the conjunctiva is severely scarred one may consider doing a filter inferiorly, although there is the potential for more postoperative complications with inferior blebs, including very serious ones such as endophthalmitis (1). Ciliodestructive procedures (Chapter 57) or Molteno-type shunts (Chapter 65) are other surgical options in these challenging cases (Table 39.1).

THE POSTOPERATIVE EYE WHICH IS APHAKIC

With intracapsular surgery a large wound was employed. Wound closure was frequently inadequate in these patients and there was significant potential for wound leaks to occur, which would allow the vitreous to come forward, potentially initiating pupillary block or malignant glaucoma-type conditions (Chapter 29). There were many descriptive terms used to explain a postoperative flat anterior chamber, but it often was not fully appreciated how often a wound leak, albeit transient, may have precipitated the condition. In addition, alpha-chymotrypsin was instilled into the eye to disrupt the zonules and allow intracapsular delivery of the crystalline lens, but the zonular fragments (2–4) could obstruct the trabecular meshwork and produce a temporary but substantial postoperative glaucoma (Fig. 39.2) with IOP commonly above 50 mm Hg (5). It is amazing, in retrospect, how late the understanding of this postoperative "enzyme glaucoma" was achieved, and especially the potential for acute posterior pole vascular events (Fig. 39.3) or wound leaks as a result of this severe IOP elevation. Two decades ago it was common practice to delay postoperative IOP measurement for several days because of concerns about infection! The corneal edema that was commonly observed and the usual postoperative pain that the patient experienced was likely due to the high levels of IOP.

When anterior chamber lens implant techniques were added to intracapsular surgery, the acute postoperative open angle glaucoma was further accentuated by the use of viscoelastic material that was placed into the anterior chamber. Viscoelastic was not removed because of the danger of vitreous loss in these aphakic eyes. As we now know irrigation of viscoelastic from the anterior chamber may reduce the incidence and severity of this postoperative acute IOP elevation, although in some cases the material is already present in the outflow pathway and presumably cannot be washed out (Fig. 39.4) (6).

Nowadays intracapsular cataract surgery is rarely if ever performed (except perhaps for partially dislocated crystalline lenses or in the Third World). The following is included for those rare occasions, and also for the general orientation and understanding of the reader:

Open Angle Glaucoma Due to Immediate Postoperative Reaction after Intracapsular Cataract Extraction

In the immediate postoperative period after cataract extraction, the IOP should be measured routinely.

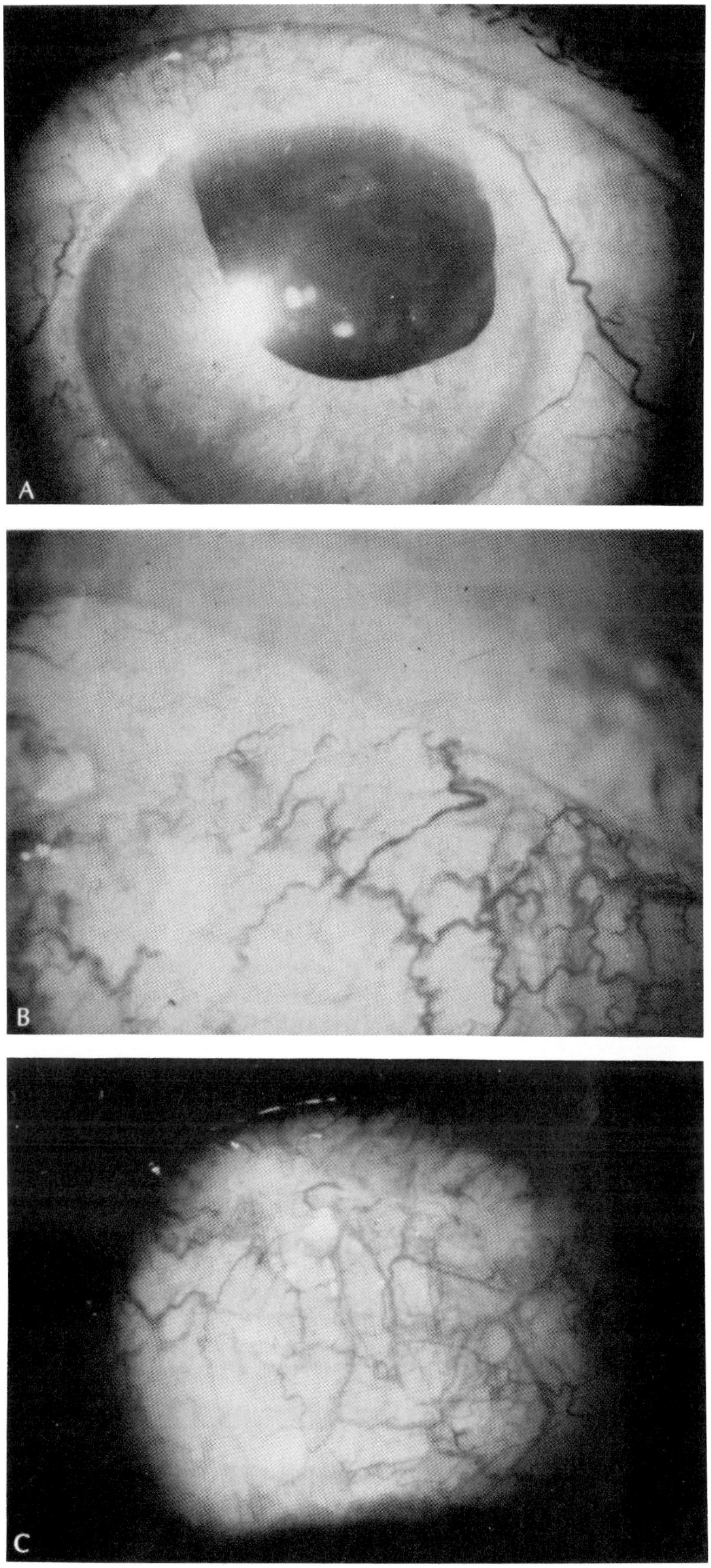

Figure 39.1. Sequence of approximate weekly photographs of the appearance of a bleb after full thickness filtration surgery superiorly in a previously aphakic eye. Conjunctival dissection superiorly was performed without difficulty and there was no substantial limbal scarring. Initially, good filtration was obtained (A) but the filtration area became progressively flatter (B) and disappeared (C). It seemed as if there must have been factors other than previous subconjunctival scarring that contributed to the lack of filtration in this aphakic eye.

GLAUCOMA SURGERY IN PSEUDOPHAKIA AND APHAKIA: WHICH PROCEDURE?

R. Rand Allingham

Glaucoma surgery is frequently required in pseudophakic, and less common today, aphakic patients. There are many options available to the surgeon and the question often arises as to how to decide which procedure to undertake. The major surgical choices include trabeculectomy with anti-metabolites, seton implantation, or laser cyclophotocoagulation. The primary determinate I use in selecting one procedure are, in order, the overall status of the patient, visual status, and ocular condition.

Status of the Patient

For patients with frail health, or who for whatever reason are unable to tolerate an incisional procedure but require IOP reduction, I use laser cyclophotocoagulation (5-7 J per pulse, 32 pulses distributed over 360 , Chapter 57).

Visual Status

In my experience, filters and seton implantation are less likely to cause postoperative vision loss than cyclodestructive procedures, which are often associated with this complication. If actual or potential visual acuity is better than 20/200 and the visual field is functional, I feel that a drainage procedure is indicated. If the visual acuity is worse than 20/200 I do laser cyclophotocoagulation. An exception is the patient with only one functional eye. In these patients, if vision is ambulatory, I favor preforming a drainage procedure before considering cyclodestruction.

Condition of the Eye

Where a drainage procedure is contemplated, the anterior chamber is deep and the conjunctiva is mobile in a superior quadrant, which is often the case in patients who have had a phacoemulsification procedure, I will do a trabeculectomy with mitomycin C (Chapter 62). If the conjunctiva is scarred and immobile, I will implant a seton (Chapter 65).

If the anterior chamber is shallow and there is insufficient room to insert a tube, I favor doing a trabeculectomy with anti-metabolites. If the patient has had a complete vitrectomy, the tube of the seton can be inserted through the pars plana, which can prevent corneal injury.

If vitreous is present in the anterior chamber, which is a particular problem in aphakic patients, a limited (but thorough) anterior vitrectomy must be performed prior to a trabeculectomy or seton implantation to prevent occlusion of the sclerotomy or tube, respectively.

For trabeculectomies in these patients, I use mitomycin C 0.3 mg/ml for 3-5 minutes. Additionally, adjunctive 5-fluorouracil (3-7 injections) can be used if there are signs of bleb failure. If an implant is required, I prefer valved setons (e.g., Ahmed or Krupin), or non-valved setons with the use of a stent or ligature, in order to prevent postoperative hypotony in these patients, who are at risk for suprachoroidal hemorrhage.

Table 39.1
Surgical Management for Glaucoma in Pseudophakia (Aphakia)

Trabeculectomy with Antimetabolites	Seton	Laser Cyclophotocoagulation
Mobile conjunctiva	Scarred conjunctiva	Scarred conjunctiva
Good visual potential (20/100 or better) or only eye	Visual potential fair to good (20/200 or better)	Fair to poor visual potential (20/200 or worse)
Little or no ocular inflammation or active neovascularization	Active ocular inflammation or neovascularization	Not a candidate for more invasive procedure

It is not uncommon for there to be substantial IOP elevation (Fig. 39.2) (5). The cornea may be deceptively clear, or show only trace edema, despite high IOP. The anterior chamber maintains normal aphakic depth throughout, and the angle remains open.

Although IOP will return to normal, usually in several days, these higher levels of pressure should be treated to prevent acute damage. Instances of optic atrophy have been observed from this temporary glaucoma. Aqueous suppressants are effective in lowering IOP in this condition (5), but osmotic therapy may also be required. The glaucoma has sometimes been blamed on postoperative iritis, but with little evidence. When alpha-chymotrypsin was introduced

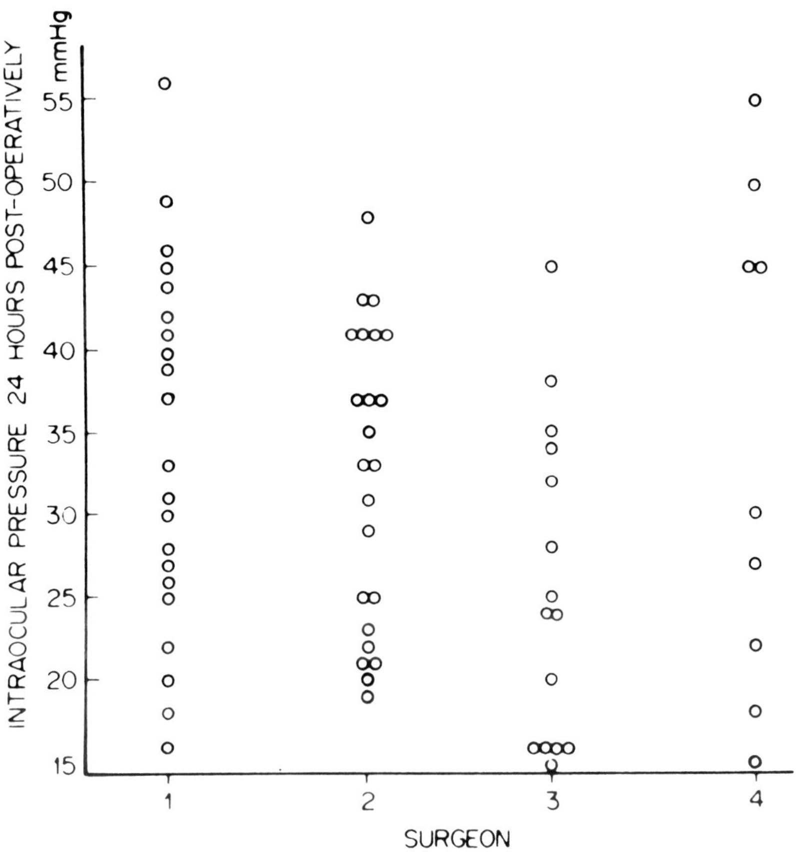

Figure 39.2. IOP measurements 24 hours following intracapsular cataract extraction with alpha-chymotrypsin in non-glaucomatous patients of four different surgeons. Reprinted with permission from Packer AJ, Fraioli AJ, Epstein DL: The effect of medical therapy on transient intraocular pressure elevation following cataract extraction using alpha-chymotrypsin. Ophthalmology 1981;86:239–243.

as an aid to intracapsular extraction, the incidence of acute, transitory, postoperative open angle glaucoma increased. In a careful study of a large series of cases, Kirsch found the incidence of transitory postoperative glaucoma to be much higher in eyes in which the enzyme was used than in a control series without the enzyme (7). This has been confirmed by other observers.

We have the clinical impression that the greater the volume of enzyme solution used, the greater the incidence of glaucoma and the higher the IOP.

The tendency for cataract surgeons to use a large number of interrupted sutures in closing the wound resulted in an increased number of cases of elevated IOP in the immediate postoperative period. In some cases the IOP reached quite high levels—50–70 mm Hg. IOP usually returned to normal within a few days. Formerly, when fewer sutures were used, these considerable elevations of IOP were less common. Perhaps a small wound-leak commonly acted as a safety valve, whereas numerous tight sutures obstructed aqueous outflow.

Clinical and experimental investigations by Campbell have shown that in patients who have had intracapsular cataract extraction with alpha-chymotrypsin and multiple sutures, the IOP is usually at its maximum on the day of the operation and gradually falls thereafter (8). Campbell found that this might be explained by a mechanism that he demonstrated in enucleated normal human eyes. In these eyes, when the facility of aqueous outflow was measured by perfusion before and after limbal sutures were inserted and were tied tightly as in cataract operations, the aqueous outflow was significantly obstructed (9). This pathologic obstruction was shown to be related to compression of limbal tissues and to gross distortion of the aqueous outflow system by the sutures. The distortion of the tissues and the obstruction to outflow were readily reversible by loosening the sutures. These effects have been confirmed by others (6,10). Kirsch has performed gonioscopy immediately after cataract surgery and has described seeing a ridge formed inside the eye (11); however, this was unrelated to sutures and appears to be different from Campbell's suture-induced effect.

In patients, the postoperative glaucoma that may be attributable to this mechanism generally subsides in a few days, presumably because the sutures spontaneously loosen and the distortion of the tissues becomes less.

Another factor that can cause impairment of out-

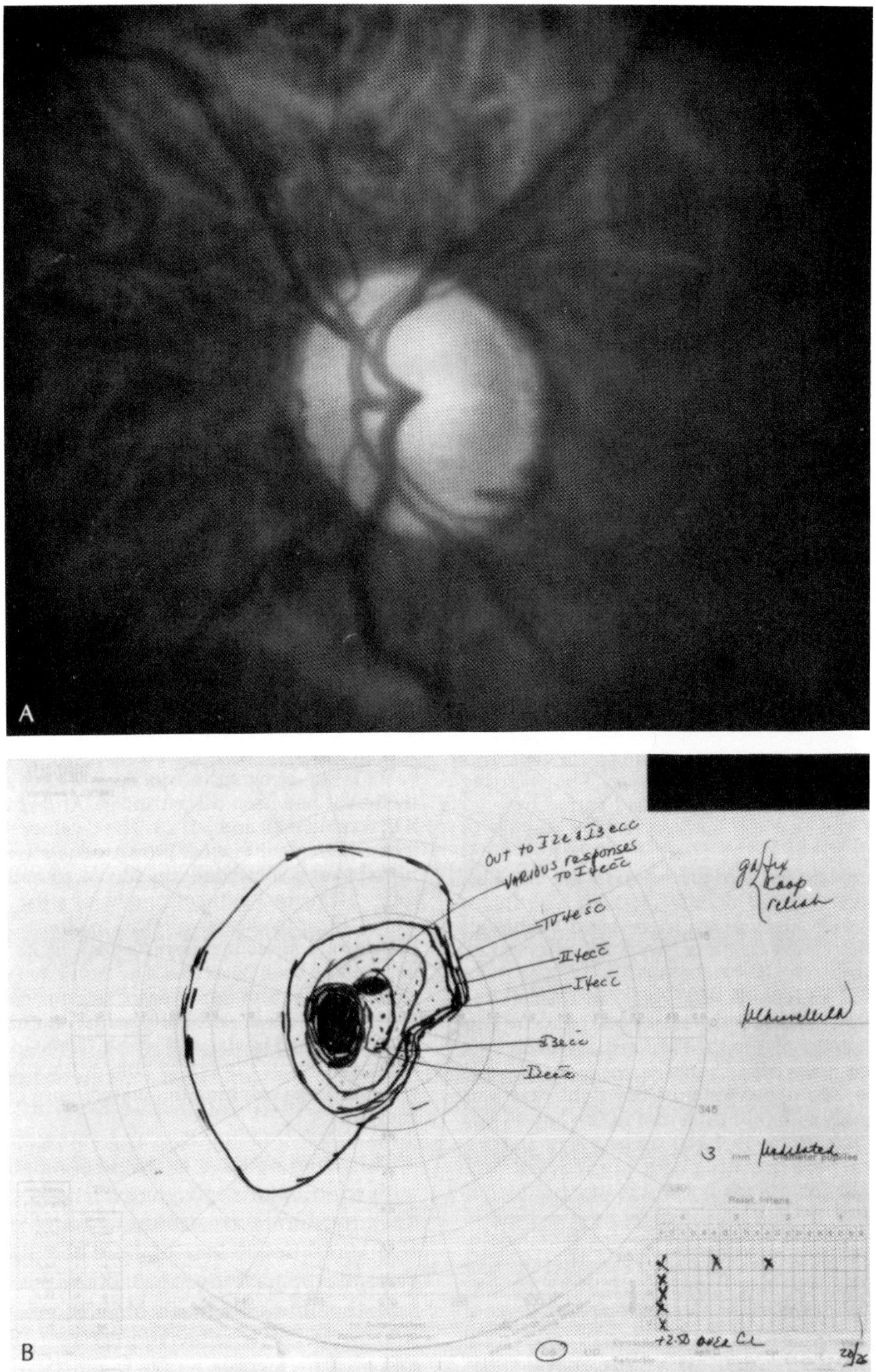

Figure 39.3. Optic atrophy (A) and dense nasal field loss (B) was believed to be due to temporary high IOP following intracapsular cataract surgery with use of alpha-chymotrypsin and fine wound closure. Note that the predominant feature of the disc is pallor (atrophy) with only slight contour changes in the shape of the cup. Findings have been stable for 3½ years. Visual acuity is 20/25.

flow facility and a postoperative elevation of IOP is the use of viscoelastics, such as sodium hyaluronate, during cataract surgery (6). Experimentally, a severe obstruction to outflow in enucleated human eyes occurs, and this is additive to the effects of limbal suture compression (Fig. 39.4) (6). Curiously, in simulated surgical maneuvers with hyaluronate it proved difficult to alleviate the impairment of outflow by irrigation of the anterior chamber. Clinically, severe postoperative glaucoma, presum-

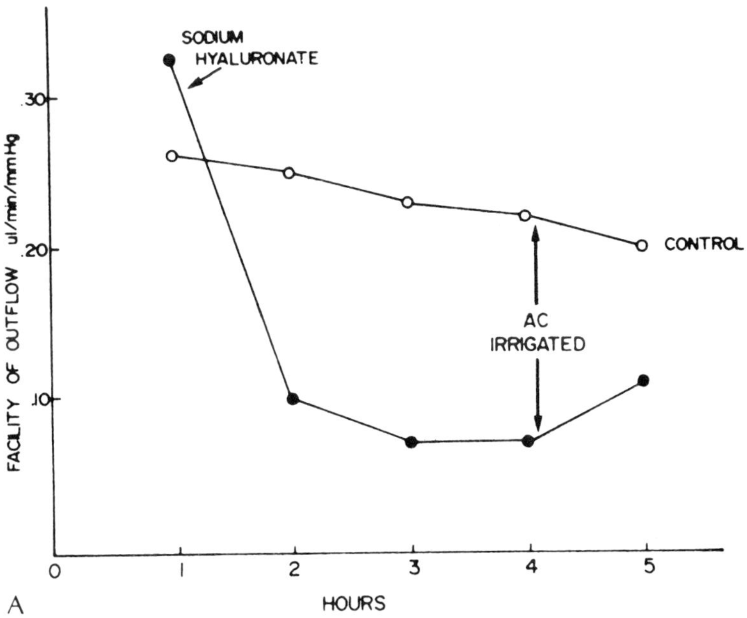

A

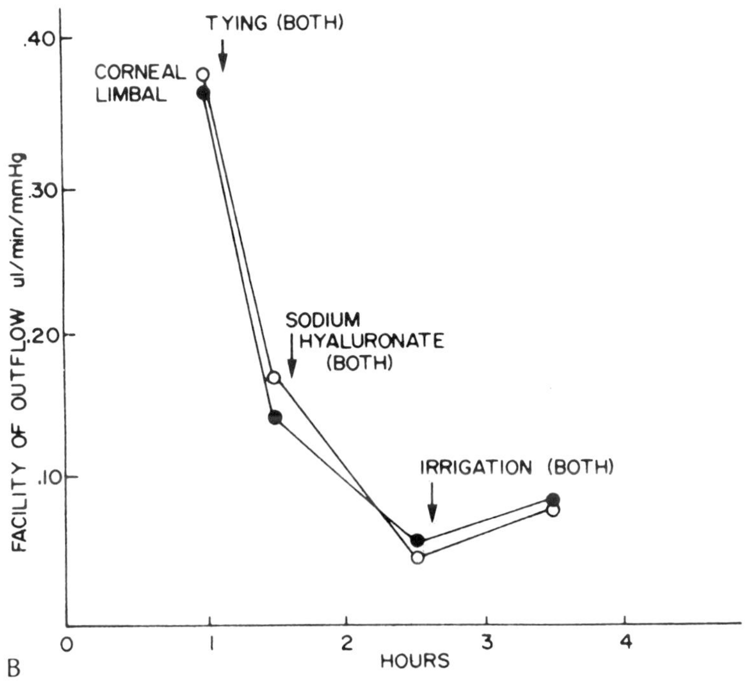

B

Figure 39.4. In experimental anterior chamber perfusion studies in excised human eyes instillation of sodium hyaluronate causes a severe obstruction of aqueous humor outflow (A). The effect is additive to that caused by limbal compression due to suture placement (B). Reprinted with permission from Berson FG, Patterson MM, Epstein DL: Obstruction of aqueous outflow by sodium hyaluronate in enucleated human eyes. Am J Ophthalmol 1983;95:668–672.

ably due to sodium hyaluronate, has been observed, sometimes persisting for several days.

Especially in patients with pre-existing glaucoma and optic nerve damage, acute IOP elevations can be dangerous and, at times, difficult to treat.

THE POSTOPERATIVE PSEUDOPHAKIC EYE

With the above historical background concerning intracapsular cataract surgery, the reader should not be surprised to learn that postoperative open angle glaucoma also occurs after modern extracapsular cataract surgery including phacoemulsification (Table 39.2). In extracapsular surgery such severe IOP elevation is much less common, owing probably to several factors: omission of alpha-chymotrypsin, the smaller size wound, and the more efficient removal of sodium hyaluronate with irrigating/aspirating devices. However, substantial residual cortical material can impair outflow facility (lens-particle glaucoma) acutely (see Chapter 47). (The IOP also needs to be carefully monitored immediately after YAG capsu-

Table 39.2
IOP Elevation Following Cataract Surgery

Cause	Comment
Early IOP elevation (first 24–48 hours) Inflammatory debris (cells, pigment, or blood) Lens products Viscoelastic Zonular fragments (ICCE with alpha chymotrypsin) Suprachoroidal hemorrhage Pupillary block	Lens products, blood, and viscoelastics should always be completely removed from the anterior chamber at the end of the procedure, especially in patients with pre-existing IOP elevation Postoperative hypotony, vitrectomized patients, and high myopia increase risk of intra- and postoperative suprachoroidal hemorrhage.
Mid term IOP elevation (2–30 days) Pupillary block (IOL or vitreous) Malignant glaucoma Steroid-induced	Pupillary block is uncommon after ECCE with posterior chamber IOL but can occur **(all eyes with an anterior chamber IOL require an iridectomy)**; axial shallowing which occurs with an elevated IOP is malignant glaucoma till proved otherwise. Topical steroids are a commonly and overlooked cause of postoperative elevate IOP.
Late onset Open angle glaucoma Synechial angle closure Pupillary block glaucoma (IOL or vitreous)	Whether late onset open angle glaucoma is secondary to surgery or is a manifestation of a preexisting process is often not known; however, treatment is the same.

lotomy which is frequently required after extracapsular surgery.)

Although postoperative glaucoma after extracapsular surgery may not be as severe or sustained as that after intracapsular surgery, it also requires the attention of the clinician, especially in patients with glaucomatous optic nerve cupping and field loss. Similar to that described above, we are learning that the IOP may be substantially elevated after extracapsular cataract extraction for the first several hours after surgery, but we have not routinely measured it at this time period.

The mechanism for an open angle glaucoma after extracapsular surgery likely involves issues of remaining viscoelastic in the eye despite intraoperative irrigation, crystalline lens fragments which may have entered the outflow pathway intraoperatively, as well as wound compression and inflammation. Postoperative hyphema can contribute to the IOP elevation since the red blood cells exit the eye through the trabecular outflow pathway (12) and can temporarily obstruct it.

Especially in patients with susceptible optic nerves, the postoperative IOP needs to be carefully monitored and preventative antiglaucoma therapy added. In patients with such susceptible nerves and especially borderline IOP control, consideration should be given to performing a combined cataract extraction/filtration procedure (Chapter 64) not just to establish better long term IOP control, but also to blunt this potentially damaging early postoperative IOP spike.

The choice of added antiglaucoma therapy depends on the patient's existing regimen. Beta blockers are commonly given at the end of surgery (if there is no contraindication), and some clinicians routinely employ a single administration of (often intravenous) carbonic anhydrase inhibitors. Except for the very small risk of blood dyscrasia (Chapter 14) in patients without a known systemic contraindication, such one time use of carbonic anhydrase therapy is usually well tolerated. Miotics should be avoided because of the usual postoperative inflammatory reaction, and epinephrine-like compounds may cause cystoid macular edema as well as unwanted vascular effects in the acute postoperative eye. The latter consideration may also be true for apraclonidine, although some clinicians have employed this agent with apparent efficacy and lack of toxicity.

It is important to measure the IOP, especially in patients at significant risk, perhaps even several hours after surgery, but certainly no later than the next day.

DIFFERENTIAL DIAGNOSIS OF ACUTE POSTOPERATIVE GLAUCOMA IN THE PSEUDOPHAKIC EYE

The key question is whether the mechanism of the postoperative glaucoma involves an open angle or an angle closure basis. This can usually be correctly inferred from the slit lamp examination evaluating the anterior chamber depth and configuration of the iris. **The clinician should not hesitate to perform gonioscopy on the eye and examine the angle. It is fundamental to know whether one is dealing with an angle closure or open angle process.** In fact one of the great lessons that was learned from the previous era of intracapsular cataract surgery and anterior chamber lenses, was how common it was for the clinician to miss a treatable form of angle closure (due to pupillary block) on the basis of the slit lamp examination alone (13). Often such **unsuspected pupillary block** had a delayed onset. Unanticipated pupillary block can also occur with use of posterior chamber intraocular lenses (14).

If one is dealing with an open angle postoperative glaucoma in the pseudophakic eye, then medical antiglaucoma therapy is utilized as above. The mechanism likely relates to retained viscoelastic material if the IOP is severely elevated and sustained. Such a viscoelastic glaucoma is usually self-limited over four to five days (although with a now discontinued viscoelastic, Orculon, it could potentially persist indefinitely [15,16]). Rarely it may be necessary to take the patient back to the operating room and irrigate the anterior chamber. This could also be employed for a postoperative hyphema which is judged to be responsible for the IOP elevation. Of course, if a combined cataract/filter was performed, suture lysis should be performed in the face of high postoperative IOP. However, in an additional four or five days the temporary added obstruction to outflow from the viscoelastic will have spontaneously cleared (by the normal vital action of trabecular meshwork cells), and therefore one does not want to have produced overfiltration by creating too loose a flap through which the now more "watery" aqueous humor is leaving the eye.

Sometimes if a paracentesis was performed at the time of surgery, the site can be gently manipulated at the slit-lamp postoperatively to temporarily lower the IOP (one should avoid substantially shallowing the anterior chamber which could produce other problems such as peripheral anterior synechia). Postoperative manipulation of the paracentesis site is commonly only effective in lowering the IOP for 1-2 hours or so, and if the glaucoma recurs, probably other choices for IOP lowering should be employed subsequently. (Experimentally such "viscoelastic open angle glaucoma" can be "cured" by placing hyaluronidase into the anterior chamber (6). Unfortunately such an "orphan drug" of very pure hyaluronidase for human use has not yet been developed).

If the angle is closed the most likely diagnosis is pupillary block. This has been discussed in Chapters 22 and 23, but the typical findings are a normal axial depth but shallow peripheral depth with a ballooning forward of the iris. Residual cortical material that has "fluffed up" behind the iris or capsular fragments may produce postoperative pupillary block. Inflammatory adhesions postoperatively may do likewise. The treatment is to either dilate the pupil or place a laser iridectomy.

It is routine now not to place a surgical peripheral iridectomy at the time of cataract surgery unless there is diabetes or a history of inflammation. However, one of us (DLE) still believes that glaucoma eyes even with POAG are "different" and are "sick eyes" and advocates the routine placement of a surgical peripheral iridectomy at the time of cataract surgery. The concept of possible "bad things" hypothesized to happen when one touches the iris during the surgery has achieved unsubstantiated popularity. When one sees these (granted occasional) postoperative eyes with pre-existing open angle glaucoma who now have developed a superimposed angle closure and then the severe complications that can ensue, one wishes that all such eyes had had routine surgical peripheral iridectomy at the time of cataract surgery. Overall, one of us (DLE) truly believes that the benefit of surgical peripheral iridectomy outweighs the risk (mainly of small postoperative hyphema) to justify its routine use in all glaucoma eyes. Especially when eyes have been on previous miotic therapy, there is both the potential for more substantial postoperative inflammation that can lead to pupillary block (most clinicians will perform an iridectomy if a patient has a history of previous uveitis), and there is also greater potential for there to be residual cortical material (due to submaximal pupillary dilatation) that also could lead to pupillary block. **All patients who have an anterior chamber IOL require an iridectomy** (Fig. 39.5).

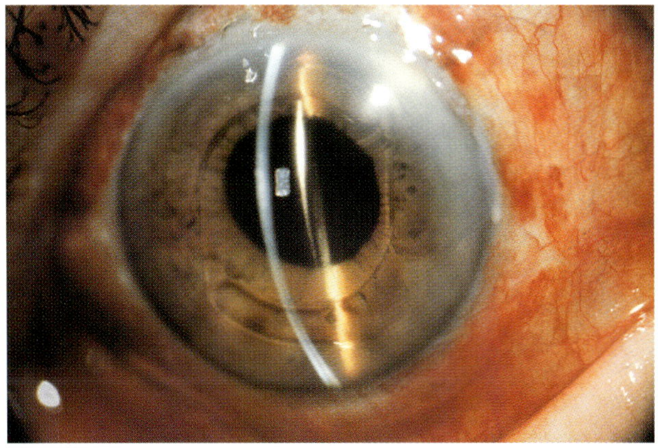

Figure 39.5. Pupillary block in a patient without a peripheral iridectomy with an anterior chamber lens.

Angle closure glaucoma postoperatively that persists despite a patent laser iridectomy is not pupillary block and is fully discussed in Chapter 29. In brief, the differential diagnosis involves choroidal hemorrhage or effusion, and this failing, the diagnosis is **malignant glaucoma** until proven otherwise.

Primary Open Angle Glaucoma and the Pseudophakic Eye

In the "old" days there was a feeling of some clinicians that (intracapsular) cataract surgery could improve long term IOP control (17,18). There was considerable controversy about this and interestingly there have been "swings of opinion."

The following is what we judge to represent current clinical information about the effect of extracapsular cataract surgery alone on the course of open angle glaucoma, but this needs to be continuously evaluated. In the immediate postoperative period (19,20) there are the problems of acute worsening of the open angle glaucoma (Table 39.2) from a few days to weeks that has been discussed above, that should have led to consideration of combined cataract/filtration surgery being performed. Beginning several months after cataract surgery (when routine corticosteroids have been stopped) there is the strong clinical impression of some beneficial effect on IOP control in some patients (21), but unfortunately not all. **Because this effect of cataract surgery on IOP is not predictable ahead of time, cataract surgery alone should not be employed as a strategy for patients with borderline IOP control,** and yet some patients do seem to benefit. Classically, it has been felt that at this intermediate time period the possible beneficial effect was due to hyposecretion of aqueous humor in the continuing "postoperative" period. However, this has not been adequately documented with respect to mechanism. One other possibility is that the usual postoperative inflammatory response may clear "debris" from the outflow pathway as has been proposed as occurring following the "inflammation" that accompanies laser trabeculoplasty (22). In fact such an occurrence might explain the generally poorer response of pseudophakic and aphakic eyes to laser trabeculoplasty—they have already participated in such a trabecular meshwork "good-type" inflammatory response.

There is the clinical sense that long term (after a year) the open angle glaucoma returns to baseline with no residual beneficial effect. (The long term beneficial effect that was reported by some in the intracapsular era was likely due to continued occult filtration that was probably initiated because of a wound that was not tightly sutured). Nevertheless, the final word may not have been spoken in this regard, especially if there were, in fact, some small beneficial effect. (For example, although it is believed by most that glaucoma status returns to "baseline" at time periods greater than a year after cataract surgery, it is possible with the natural history of open angle glaucoma to worsen over time, that the situation might naturally have been even worse; we need randomized trials to settle this issue.)

Patients with open angle glaucoma who are pseudophakic can be treated with the usual antiglaucoma medications with the exception of epinephrine-like compounds that have the potential in the pseudophakic as well as aphakic eye to produce cystoid macular edema (Chapter 12). Also miotics should be used in pseudophakic eyes with proper attention to the retina (see Chapter 13) because of the slightly increased risk of retinal detachment in pseudophakic eyes. On the other hand, miotics are usually well tolerated visually by the pseudophakic patient, and weak concentrations of strong miotics such echothiophate iodide (Phospholine Iodide) are often remarkably effective, and the once to twice a day dosage regimen is usually very "patient friendly."

Eyes with exfoliation have a tendency to cataract formation (23), and the clinician should be alert to possible previously undiagnosed exfoliation in pseudophakic eyes, especially since exfoliation eyes have some tendency for rapid worsening of glaucoma control (see Chapter 20). (Removing the cataract does not by itself improve the exfoliation glaucoma; the crystalline lens capsule is just one source for the abnormal exfoliation material). In the pseudophakic eye the light gray amorphous exfoliation material may be seen on the pupillary border, the posterior surface of the iris, the ciliary processes, the zonules, and anterior capsular remnants.

When choosing to perform cataract surgery alone on a patient with presumed well controlled POAG, it is prudent to save some of the superior conjunctiva, e.g., in the superonasal quadrant, for possible future filtration surgery, and, therefore, to perform the cataract surgery more temporally, or even better, to use a clear cornea approach.

Glaucoma due to Peripheral Anterior Synechias in Pseudophakic Eyes

Gonioscopy should be routinely performed (again) on all eyes with "open angle glaucoma" many months after cataract surgery (if not sooner in response to acute problems) to establish a new baseline. An unpleasant surprise is experienced when one views the presence of peripheral anterior synechias and thus loss of some of the angle circumference for outflow, in a situation where the outflow process was already abnormal due to POAG with a previous open angle. Such PAS formation may result from an undetected transient wound leak or pupillary block, or be a result of inflammation. Sometimes residual lens cortex will "fluff up" postoperatively in one area and mechanically focally force the iris into the angle (without pupillary block) and result in synechia formation. A forwardly positioned intraocular lens haptic may do likewise (24). After a combined cataract/filter operation where there is "overfiltration" and a transient shallow chamber, there may be resulting formation of PAS. This is much more common after (combined) cataract surgery than after filtration surgery alone, presumably because of the greater amount of usual postoperative inflammation that seals the iris to the apposed trabecular meshwork.

If extensive formation of peripheral anterior synechias is observed, then consideration should be given to laser iridogonioplasty (Chapters 25 and 60). Unfortunately, such PAS are often tightly "cemented" in the angle and not able to be broken. (We strongly recommend that such firm PAS not continue to be treated—see Chapter 25.)

Sometimes PAS formation may seem extensive, but the IOP, and especially the response to outflow drugs, such as miotics, is normal. In such cases of normal or "supernormal" response to miotics, one wants to be certain that one is not dealing with an inadvertent cyclodialysis cleft that was produced at the time of surgery (although if the IOP is controlled and not hypotonous, miotic therapy should just be continued; cyclodialysis was at one time a very useful surgical procedure for glaucoma but was unpredictable—Chapter 66). Also one wishes to be certain that the low IOP following initiation of miotic therapy is not due to a retinal detachment. However, it is also possible that the angle synechias are actually bridging the trabecular meshwork to the peripheral cornea at Schwalbe's line, and that there is functional underlying trabecular meshwork. With shallow anterior chambers due to overfiltration (and usually quiet eyes) it is not rare for such bridging synechiae to occur.

Nevertheless, it is a cause for great concern when a patient with open angle glaucoma, especially one with marginal control, now develops a superimposed chronic angle closure component. Unsuspected pupillary block (13,14) in the postoperative period may have been the cause of occult PAS. This indicates the wisdom in performing a prophylactic surgical peripheral iridectomy at the time of cataract surgery in most if not all patients with preoperative glaucoma.

APHAKIC PUPILLARY BLOCK

Aphakic pupillary block is rarely seen now except in previously aphakic eyes undergoing subsequent additional surgery. Chandler and Grant offer a "classic" description of the clinical findings, which should be treated with a laser iridectomy (perhaps following temporary "diagnostic" pupillary dilatation):

> Among the signs of pupillary block in aphakia, one occasionally observes iris bombé, but what one usually finds is overall shallowing of the anterior chamber or complete flatness, with IOP elevated. If the anterior chamber is shallow or flat in an aphakic eye and the IOP is elevated, even if only slightly, one must consider this to be positive evidence of pupillary block. If the anterior chamber is shallow or flat in association with separation of the ciliary body or choroid, IOP is almost invariably very low. (We have seen only one or two cases with choroidal separation and flat anterior chamber in which IOP was moderately elevated, among the hundreds of cases in which IOP was very low.) Less commonly, instead of uniform shallowing or absence of the anterior chamber, one finds unevenness in its depth. The anterior chamber may be normally deep in one area, shallow in another. Unevenness of depth of the anterior chamber is more common after extracapsular extraction, since there is generally more postoperative reaction than after intracapsular extraction. If there has been an unusual degree of postoperative inflammation, an unevenness in depth of the anterior chamber may sometimes be seen even after intracapsular extraction. The reason for the unevenness in depth of the anterior chamber is that there is an inflammatory membrane on the posterior surface of the iris in the area of deep anterior chamber, which prevents the iris from bowing forward. In the area where the iris bows forward, there is no inflammatory membrane behind it. The unevenness in depth of the anterior chamber is particularly common in pupillary block in children after discission or lens extraction. We know of no cause other than pupillary block for such unevenness in depth of the anterior chamber in aphakic eyes with elevated IOP.
>
> After a round-pupil intracapsular extraction with a peripheral opening or openings in the iris, these openings may become closed by adhesion to the wound, by filling with blood or fibrin, or by adhesion to the hyaloid, after which pupillary block may develop. In such cases the hyaloid membrane may herniate further and further through the round pupil until it eventually reaches the cornea (and rarely causes edema). The anterior chamber itself may remain at normal or almost normal depth for a period, but the hyaloid eventually reaches the cornea. If the block is not relieved, the anterior chamber finally becomes shallow, at least in the periphery, and the angle closes.

OPEN ANGLE GLAUCOMA DUE TO VITREOUS HUMOR FILLING THE ANTERIOR CHAMBER

In certain aphakic eyes, glaucoma is apparently due to vitreous humor completely filling the anterior chamber and blocking the corneoscleral meshwork itself (25-27). Evidence for this mechanism has been both clinical and experimental. In the laboratory, vitreous humor introduced to fill the anterior chamber of an enucleated normal human eye clearly obstructs aqueous outflow, and this obstruction is quickly eliminated by addition of hyaluronidase (28). The clinical situation may develop within a few weeks after cataract operation, but may be delayed for several months. It may be initiated, at least in some cases, by an extensive posterior vitreous detachment, so that the remaining vitreous body tends to move forward. One sees in such cases that the angle is open. On slit-lamp and gonioscopic examination the vitreous appears to fill the entire anterior chamber.

IOP is sometimes lowered by miotic treatment, but in other cases it is made higher. Mydriatic treatment is usually more effective. If the pupil is kept dilated, in most cases the IOP gradually falls, and vitreous eventually withdraws from the angle of the anterior chamber. This form of glaucoma appears to be self-limited and usually does not require surgical treatment. Aqueous humor suppressants are used during the period of elevated IOP. If this does not suffice, peripheral iridectomy and evacuation of vitreous from the anterior chamber should cure the condition.

In making a diagnosis, it is easy to be sure by gonioscopy that the angle is open. With slit-lamp examination, one must determine if the vitreous humor extends into the angle. However, clinically, it is almost impossible to be certain that it reaches the trabecular meshwork, and the diagnosis must be partially presumptive.

In 1963 one of us (WMG) collected 4 cases of this condition, but since then we have only suspected it in one or two additional cases (25). It must be an extremely rare condition.

EPITHELIZATION OF THE ANTERIOR CHAMBER

Diagnosis

After cataract extraction the eye occasionally remains injected and irritable with photophobia and discomfort. One commonly sees cells in the aqueous. **If there is little or no response to local steroid and cycloplegic treatment following cataract extraction, this should lead to a suspicion of epithelization.** (Also entities such as P. acne endophthalmitis (29–31) need to be considered.) One may see a delicate membrane on the back of the cornea advancing from the limbal area of the wound, through which it has invaded the anterior chamber. Characteristically the advancing edge appears slightly thickened. This membrane sometimes extends onto the iris (Fig. 39.6) or in aphakic eyes onto the hyaloid membrane. If it extends onto the hyaloid membrane, there are often smooth-edged holes or oval windows in the membrane. These are very suggestive that the membrane is epithelial, since one does not expect to see the same type of hole in an ordinary inflammatory membrane.

Epithelial membranes most frequently occur after cataract extraction, but have also been seen after perforating injuries in which the crystalline lens has been damaged or lost, in children as well as in adults.

In epithelization of the anterior chamber, if there is an open fistula in the wound at the site of ingrowth of epithelium, IOP may be low. When there is a fistula through the wound and the eye is soft, any evidence of a membrane on the back of the cornea or on the iris, however slight, nearly always indicates epithelization.

If there is no fistula, IOP may be normal or elevated to a varying degree. When eyes are lost as a result of epithelization of the anterior chamber, in the majority of cases it is because the eyes become blind and painful from glaucoma. In the majority of cases that we know about, the mechanism of this severe glaucoma has been pupillary block by the epithelial membrane, leading to closure of the angle and high IOP. However, in some cases of glaucoma an epithelial membrane has been described in the angle, presumably blocking the escape of aqueous humor from the angle (32). With the use of more "heroic-type" anterior segment reconstruction surgical procedures to treat this condition, this latter mechanism for secondary glaucoma is being observed more commonly.

Gonioscopically, if one can see ciliary processes through a coloboma of the iris, the processes commonly may be seen to be enveloped by a delicate gray cocoon of epithelium, which is diagnostically helpful.

When the other signs and symptoms suggestive of epithelization of the anterior chamber are present, even if no membrane is seen on cornea, iris, or hyaloid, it is appropriate to aspirate aqueous humor from the anterior chamber and examine the cellular material thus obtained. This may reveal epithelial cells and thus establish the diagnosis (33,34). Argon laser application to the involved iris produces a characteristic whitening (Fig. 39.6). A biopsy through a small limbal incision may establish the diagnosis (35,36).

After cataract extraction or penetrating injury, an implantation, serous, or pearl cyst in the anterior chamber that gradually increases in size, is almost always an epithelial cyst. **Manipulation of the cyst with laser treatment or incomplete surgical removal can produce rapidly progressive frank epithelization of the anterior chamber (37) and secondary glaucoma.**

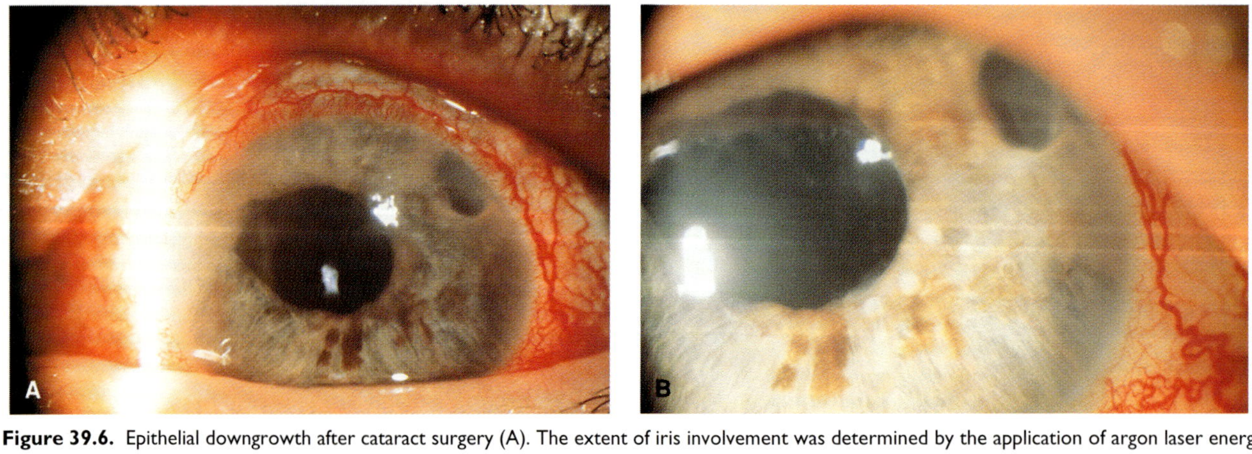

Figure 39.6. Epithelial downgrowth after cataract surgery (A). The extent of iris involvement was determined by the application of argon laser energy that produces a characteristic whitening of the involved iris (B).

Treatment

Epithelial membranes in the anterior chamber have been treated with radiation (38), beta irradiation (39), cryotherapy (40-42), curettage of the membrane from the back of the cornea and application of 70% alcohol (43-49), photocoagulation (50), and corneal transplant (51). A few eyes have been saved by one or another of these forms of treatment (52,53). Although radical procedures were once commonly favored, these are less enthusiastically embraced at the time of this writing. Instead, attention has been focused on the control of IOP to maximize the "longevity" of the affected eye. However, filtration procedures typically fail, presumably due to involvement of the epithelization process and the accompanying inflammation. In one reported case antimetabolites used for the glaucoma filtration surgery did not alter the relentless progression of epithelization (54). Sometimes ciliodestructive laser procedures are temporarily effective in controlling the secondary glaucoma. A few encouraging reports with Molteno-shunt type procedures have been made (55,56).

After an epithelial membrane has produced pupillary block, transient relief may be obtained by incising the membrane or by iridotomy or iridectomy, but no permanent relief has been obtained in this manner in any case of which we are aware, and there seems to be a strong tendency to form peripheral anterior synechias (32).

Epithelial implantation cysts have been treated by block dissection of iris, a portion of ciliary body band, and the cyst (53,57).

Prevention

If a fistula is seen in the wound shortly after cataract extraction, this calls for prompt resuturing of the wound, which is usually effective in preventing this devastating complication. A fistula found a longer time after cataract extraction is a more serious matter and may lead to epithelization. Such fistulas should be widely excised and the wound tightly closed with multiple sutures, but severe glaucoma may ensue (58).

A special point is to be made concerning eyes that have had filtration operation for glaucoma and have also had cataract extraction. A leak or rupture of a filtration bleb has different implications in an aphakic eye than in one that is phakic. In the phakic eye, on occasion a thin bleb will rupture or leak so that the anterior chamber becomes shallow or flat. This is not always a very serious matter. In most cases, one protects the eye from infection by local antibiotics, the leak gradually closes, and the anterior chamber resumes normal depth. If the leak is slow in healing, a bridging soft contact lens or glaucoma shell may be applied to promote healing, or if the anterior chamber remains flat, a "blowout patch" may be applied over the leaky bleb to reform the anterior chamber. Regardless, in the phakic eye one need not fear epithelization of the anterior chamber.

If the eye is aphakic, however, a shallow or flat anterior chamber from a leaking bleb is a far more serious matter. We have seen a few cases in which there was rapid epithelization of the anterior chamber, and the eyes were lost. We therefore feel that **if a leak develops in a bleb in an aphakic eye sufficient to produce a shallow or flat anterior chamber, surgical repair should be implemented immediately.** In a pseudophakic eye after extracapsular cataract surgery, there likely is not as great a risk as in the aphakic eye, but there is still cause for concern.

It is not yet known why epithelization of the anterior chamber only rarely develops when an intact crystalline lens is present, but as a rule it develops only when the lens has been removed or has been grossly injured.

We clearly need better understanding of the pathogenesis (59,60) of this condition. Our current treatments are vastly inadequate and most commonly ineffective. New pharmacological approaches, such as those involving immunotoxins (61), are desperately needed.

References

1. Wolner B, Liebmann JM, Sassani JW, et al: Late bleb-related endophthalmitis after trabeculectomy with adjunctive 5-fluorouracil. Ophthalmology 1991;98:1053–60.
2. Chee P, Hamasaki DI: The basis for chymotrypsin-induced glaucoma. Arch Ophthalmol 1971;85:103–6.
3. Anderson DR: Experimental alpha-chymotrypsin glaucoma studied by scanning electron microscopy. Am J Ophthalmol 1971;71:470–6.
4. Worthen DM: Scanning electron microscopy after alpha-chymotrypsin perfusion in man. Am J Ophthalmol 1972;73:637–42.
5. Packer AJ, Fraioli AJ, Epstein DL: The effects of timolol and acetazolamide on transient intraocular pressure elevation following cataract extraction with alpha-chymotrypsin. Ophthalmology 1981;88:239–243.
6. Berson FG, Patterson MM, Epstein DL: Obstruction of aqueous outflow by sodium hyaluronate in enucleated human eyes. Am J Ophthalmol 1983;95:668–672.
7. Kirsch RE: Glaucoma following cataract extraction associated with use of alpha-chymotrypsin. Arch Ophthalmol 1964;72:612–620.
8. Campbell DG: Personal communication, 1977.
9. Campbell DG, Grant WM: Unpublished data cited in Berson FG, Patterson MM, Epstein DL: Obstruction of aqueous outflow by sodium hyaluronate in enucleated human eyes. Am J Ophthalmol 1983;95: 668–672.
10. Zimmerman TJ, Krupin T, Gordski W, et al: The effect of suture depth on outflow facility in penetrating keratoplasty. Arch Ophthalmol 1978; 96:505–506.
11. Kirsch RE, Levine O, Singer JA: Further studies on the ridge at the internal edge of the cataract incision. Trans Am Acad Ophthalmol Otolaryngol 1977;83:OP-224–231.
12. Campbell DG, Simmons RJ, Grant WM: Ghost cells as a cause of glaucoma. Am J Ophthalmol 1976;81:441.
13. Van Buskirk EM: Pupillary block after intraocular lens implantation. Am J Ophthalmol 1983;95:55–59.
14. Samples JR, Bellows AR, Rosenquist RC, et al: Pupillary block with posterior chamber intraocular lenses. Arch Ophthalmol 1987;105: 335–7.
15. Siegel MJ, Spiro HJ, Miller JA, et al: Secondary glaucoma and uveitis associated with Orculon [letter]. Arch Ophthalmol 1991;109: 1496–1497.

16. Kaufman PL, Lütjen-Drecoll E, Hubbard WC, et al: Obstruction of aqueous humor outflow by cross-linked polyacrylamide microgels in bovine, monkey, and human eyes. Ophthalmology 1994;101: 1672–1679.
17. Bigger JF, Becker B: Cataracts and primary open-angle glaucoma: the effect of uncomplicated cataract extraction on glaucoma control. Trans Am Acad Ophthalmol Otolaryngol 1971;75:260.
18. Randolph ME, Maumenee AE, Iliff CE: Cataract extraction in glaucomatous eyes. Am J Ophthalmol 1971;71:328.
19. Savage JA, Thomas JV, Belcher CD III, et al: Extracapsular cataract extraction and posterior chamber intraocular lens implantation in glaucomatous eyes. Ophthalmology 1985;92:1506.
20. Krupin T, Feitl ME, Bishop KI: Postoperative intraocular pressure rise in open-angle glaucoma patients after cataract or combined cataract-filtration surgery. Ophthalmology 1989;96:579–84.
21. McGuigan LJ, et al: Extracapsular cataract extraction and posterior chamber lens implantation in eyes with preexisting glaucoma. Arch Ophthalmol 1986;104:1301–8.
22. Melamed S, Epstein DL: Alterations of aqueous humor outflow following argon laser trabeculoplasty in monkeys. Br J Ophthalmol 1987;71: 776–781.
23. Puska P: Lens opacity in unilateral exfoliation syndrome with or without glaucoma. Acta Ophthalmol 1994;72:290–6.
24. Evans RB: Peripheral anterior synechia overlying the haptics of posterior chamber lenses. Occurrence and natural history. Ophthalmology 1990; 97:415–23.
25. Grant WM: Open-angle glaucoma associated with vitreous filling the anterior chamber. Trans Am Ophthalmol Soc 1963;61:196–218.
26. Iuglio N, Tieri O: Glaucoma ad angolo aperto da vitreo in camera anteriore. Arch Ophthalmol 1964;68:481–484.
27. Schneider J: The treatment of aphakic pupillary block. Eye, Ear, Nose, Throat 1969;48:42–50.
28. Grant WM: Experimental aqueous perfusion in enucleated human eyes. Arch Ophthalmol 1963;69:783.
29. Roussel TJ, et al: Chronic postoperative endophthalmitis associated with Actinomyces species. Arch Ophthalmol 1991;109:60–2.
30. Whitcup SM, et al: Immunohistochemistry of the inflammatory response in Propionibacterium acnes endophthalmitis. Arch Ophthalmol 1991; 109:978–9.
31. Owens SL, Lam S, Tessler HH, et al: Preliminary study of a new intraocular method in the diagnosis and treatment of Propionibacterium acnes endophthalmitis following cataract extraction. Ophthalmic Surg 1993; 24:268–72.
32. Bernardino VV, Kim JC, Smith TR: Epithelization of the anterior chamber after cataract extraction. Arch Ophthalmol 1969;742–750.
33. Verrey F: Cytologie de l'humeur aqueuse et invasion epitheliale de la chambre antérieure. Ophthalmologica 1967;154:310–311.
34. Verrey F: Invasion epitheliale de la chambre antérieure: confirmation anatomique par l'examen cytologique de l'humeur aqueuse. Ophthalmoligica 1967;153:467–473.
35. Calhoun FP: An aid to the clinical diagnosis of epithelial downgrowth into the anterior chamber following cataract extraction. Am J Ophthalmol 1966;61:1055–1059.
36. Soong HK, Meyer RF, Wolter JR: Fistula excision and peripheral grafts in the treatment of persistent limbal wound leaks. Ophthalmology 1988; 95:31–6.
37. Orlin SE, et al: Epithelial downgrowth following the removal of iris inclusion cysts. Ophthalmic Surg 1991;22:330–5.
38. Gallardo E: Epithelial membrane in anterior chamber after cataract surgery: Case report and comments on X-ray treatment. Am J Ophthalmol 1955;39:868–870.
39. Zarzycka M, Kornacki B: The use of beta-rays in cases of anterior chamber epithelial ingrowth after bulbus surgery. Klin Oczna 1971;41: 401–406.
40. Maumenne AE, Paton D, Morse P, et al: Review of 40 histologically proven cases of epithelial downgrowth following cataract extraction and suggested surgical management. Am J Ophthalmol 1970;69:598–603.
41. Dixon WS, Speakman JS: Epithelial downgrowth following cataract surgery. Cryotherapy for an intraocular foreign body. Arch Ophthalmol 1970;84:303–305.
42. Brown SI: Treatment of advance epithelial downgrowth. Trans Am Acad Ophthalmol Otolaryngol 1973;77:OP-618–622.
43. Long JC: Three cases of epithelial invasion of anterior chamber treated surgically. Arch Ophthalmol 1957;58:396–400.
44. Maumenee AE: Treatment of epithelial downgrowth and intraocular fistula following cataract extraction. Trans Am Ophthalmol Soc 1964; 62:153–166.
45. Nakamura Y, Nakamura S: Two cases of epithelial downgrowth cured by a surgical technique. Folia Ophthalmol Jpn 1968;19:881–885.
46. Witmer R: Therapie der Epithelinvasion der Vorderkammer nach Staroperation. Ophthalmologica 1970;161:286–291.
47. Fock V: A case of epithelization of the anterior chamber treated operatively according to Maumenee's method. Acta Ophthalmol 1971;49: 11–15.
48. Harbin TS, Maumenee AE: Epithelial downgrowth after surgery for epithelial cyst. Am J Ophthalmol 1974;78:1–4.
49. Laflamme MY: L'invasion epitheliale de la chambre anterieure: A propos de 8 cas opérés selon la technique de Maumenee. Can J Ophthalmol 1976;11:17–20.
50. Okun E, Mandell A: Photocoagulation as a treatment of epithelial implantation cysts following cataract surgery. Trans Am Ophthalmol Soc 1974;74:170–183.
51. Sullivan GL: Epithelization of the anterior chamber following cataract extraction: a new approach to treatment. Trans Am Ophthalmol Soc 1958;56:606–654.
52. Schaeffer AR, Nalbandian RM, Brigham DW, et al: Epithelial downgrowth following wound dehiscence after extracapsular cataract extraction and posterior chamber lens implantation: surgical management. J Cataract Refract Surg 1989;15:437–41.
53. Sugar HS: Further experience with posterior lamellar resection of the cornea for epithelial implantation cysts. Am J Ophthalmol 1967;64: 291–299.
54. Loane ME, Weinreb RN: Glaucoma secondary to epithelial downgrowth and 5-fluorouracil. Ophthalmic Surg 1990;21:704–706.
55. Rubin B, et al: Histopathologic study of the Molteno glaucoma implant in three patients. Am J Ophthalmol 1990;110:371–379.
56. Costa VP, Katz LJ, Cohen EJ, et al: Glaucoma associated with epithelial downgrowth controlled with Molteno tube shunts. Ophthalmic Surg 1992;23:797–800.
57. Sugar HS: Deep lamellar resection of intra- and extraocular epithelial implantation cyst. Am J Ophthalmol 1973;76:451–454.
58. Anseth A, Dohlman CH, Albert DM: Epithelial downgrowth—fistula repair and keratoplasty. Refract Corneal Surg 1991;7:23–27.
59. Rodrigues MM, Krachmer JH, Sun TT: Clinical, electron microscopic, and monoclonal antibody studies of intraocular epithelial downgrowth. Trans Am Ophthalmol Soc 1986;84:146–169.
60. Weiner MJ, Trentacoste J, Pon DM, et al: Epithelial downgrowth: a 30-year clinicopathological review. Br J Ophthalmol 1989;73:6–11.
61. Fulcher S, et al: Suppression of human corneal epithelial proliferation with breast carcinoma immunotoxin. Cornea 1993;12:391–396.

Characteristically Unilateral Glaucomas: Differential Diagnosis

40

David L. Epstein

Certain kinds of glaucomas are typically unilateral, whereas other kinds regularly affect both eyes. This chapter is intended to provide a synopsis for differential diagnosis of certain of the unilateral glaucomas, most of which are described individually in greater detail elsewhere in this book.

In this chapter, we will provide an outline of unilateral glaucomas that belong to the following general categories: 1) unilateral angle closure glaucomas; 2) unilateral peripheral synechial glaucomas; 3) unilateral secondary open angle glaucomas.

For this synopsis, unilateral angle closure glaucomas are defined as those glaucomas in which there is axial shallowing of the anterior chamber and ballooning forward of the periphery of the iris to close the angle. Peripheral synechial glaucomas are defined for this discussion as those glaucomas in which there is no axial shallowing or pupillary block to explain the development of peripheral synechias, but peripheral anterior synechias are present. The term secondary open-angle glaucomas is self-explanatory.

UNILATERAL ANGLE CLOSURE GLAUCOMAS

In primary acute angle closure glaucoma (Chapter 23), a closed angle and elevated IOP in only one eye are very common. In the subacute and chronic forms of primary angle closure (Chapter 24), unilateral glaucoma is less common. When one finds angle closure and elevated IOP in one eye, in most cases the angle in the fellow eye is narrow and predisposed to closure. Occasionally the angle in the fellow eye appears of good width, and one might conclude that it would not close, but this is generally an erroneous conclusion, particularly if the iris is convex (Chapters 22, 23). In several cases, despite knowledge of spontaneous closure of the angle in the first eye, at our initial gonioscopic examination, we estimated that the angle in the fellow eye was of "safe" width and have been chagrined to find that it subsequently closed. **One may be misled in a single gonioscopic examination by a transient deepening of the anterior chamber and widening of the angle due to the action of agents such as aqueous humor suppressants or hypertonic agents given systemically for treatment of the contralateral glaucomatous eye** (Chapter 22).

The cases in which one can tell with some assurance that the angle in the fellow eye will not close are those in which there is considerable anatomical asymmetry, such as when one eye is hypermetropic and the other is myopic, or when the cornea is smaller in the affected eye than in the fellow uninvolved eye, and the configuration of the anterior segment is quite different in the two eyes.

True unilateral angle closure glaucoma can be produced by: 1) dislocation of the lens; 2) hypermature swollen lens; 3) intraocular tumor; 4) central retinal vein occlusion; 5) panretinal photocoagulation; 6) choroidal hemorrhage; 7) massive vitreous hemorrhage; 8) scleral buckling surgery; 9) orbital venous congestion; 10) retrobulbar tumor; 11) iris bombé from inflammation; 12) iris bombé from epithelization; 13) pupillary block or malignant glaucoma in aphakia or pseudophakia; 14) persistent primary hyperplastic vitreous in childhood.

UNILATERAL PERIPHERAL SYNECHIAL GLAUCOMAS

With the anterior chamber not significantly shallowed, unilateral glaucoma due to peripheral anterior synechias occurs in the following conditions: 1) neovascular glaucoma; 2) progressive essential iris atrophy, Chandler's syndrome, and Cogan-Reese syndrome; 3) uveitis; 4) KP on the trabecular meshwork; 5) cysts of the iris or ciliary processes; 6) malignant tumor of the ciliary body; 7) after trauma; 8) after intraocular surgery with postoperative flat chamber.

UNILATERAL SECONDARY OPEN ANGLE GLAUCOMAS

In cases in which there is unilateral glaucoma with a clearly open angle and no peripheral anterior synechias, the diagnosis is aided by special signs in the aqueous humor, on the back of the cornea, at the pupillary margin, and in the angle. These distinguish the following types: 1) exfoliation and open angle glaucoma; 2) glaucoma from contusion of the eye; 3) hemolytic or ghost-cell glaucoma; 4) lens-induced (phacolytic) glaucoma; 5) extraocular venous congestion and open angle glaucoma; 6) corticosteroid glaucoma; 7) herpes simplex keratitis, uveitis, and glaucoma; 8) herpes zoster keratitis, uveitis, and glaucoma; 9) chorioretinitis and glaucoma; 10) glaucomatocyclitic crisis; 11) heterochromic cyclitis; 12) detached retina and glaucoma (Schwartz's Syndrome); and 13) malignant melanoma.

Glaucoma Secondary to Intraocular Tumors 41

Jay S. Duker

The association between unilaterally elevated intraocular pressure (IOP) and intraocular tumors has been appreciated for many years (1). Because intraocular neoplasms are far from common, this occurrence is rarely encountered in general practice. However, when present, it is critically important to recognize. The presence of intraocular cancer represents one of the few situations in ophthalmology in which delay in diagnosis and/or inappropriate surgical intervention (i.e., filtering surgery) can not only threaten vision, but life as well.

In determining the proper treatment for elevated IOP in an eye with a tumor, the histopathologic cell type and therefore the risk of tumor growth and/or metastates may impact greatly on the treatment decisions. In these cases, definitive histologic diagnosis may be required. Contrary to widespread thought, the mere presence of elevated IOP secondary to an intraocular neoplasm does not necessarily indicate that the underlying tumor is malignant.

In a study published 100 years ago, elevated IOP was documented in more than 50% of eyes enucleated with intraocular tumors (1). Because of increased familiarity with intraocular tumors, modern improvements in diagnostic techniques including indirect ophthalmoscopy and ultrasonography, as well as earlier therapeutic interventions, at the present time only 5% of eyes harboring intraocular tumors will have elevated IOP at the time of diagnosis (2). In the setting of melanoma of the uveal tract (iris, ciliary body, and choroid), location of the tumor is key in determining the risk of IOP elevation. Elevated IOP is much more common with ciliary body melanomas (17%) than with iris melanomas (7%) or choroidal melanoma (2%). **With anterior, pigmented tumors, tumor invasion of the angle followed by pigment dispersion are the most common causes of elevated IOP. For posterior tumors, iris neovascularization with secondary angle closure is the usual cause.**

INSIGHTS INTO MECHANISMS OF ELEVATED IOP

There are nine well recognized mechanisms (Table 41.1) by which an intraocular tumor can abnormally elevate IOP (2,3):

- Direct tumor invasion and/or seeding of the angle structures
- Pigmentary dispersion mechanically obstructing the outflow apparatus.
- Melanophagic, in which macrophages with ingested melanin mechanically obstruct the outflow apparatus (melanophagic or melanomalytic)
- Hemolytic as a result of bleeding from neovascular vessels, inherent tumor vessels, tumor necrosis, or invasion of the tumor into normal vessels
- Uveitic from secondary inflammatory cells mechanically obstucting the outflow apparatus
- Iris neovascularization with secondary angle closure (neovascular glaucoma)
- Angle closure from choroidal detachment with anterior displacement of the lens/iris diaphragm
- Angle closure from massive suprachoroidal hemorrhage with anterior displacement of the lens-iris diaphragm
- Angle closure from anterior displacement of the lens-iris diaphragm due to mass effect by extremely large posterior tumors or ring melanomas

As in any case of elevated IOP, gonioscopy is the critical diagnostic procedure to determine mechanism. Whenever a diagnosis of unilateral glaucoma secondary to one of these mechanisms is made, the clinician must rule out the presence of an intraocular neoplasm with further appropriate studies. In the setting of acutely elevated IOP, clinicians must not forget to fully evaluate the mechanism of elevated IOP after the acute episode is resolved.

Ancillary testing helps greatly in determining the location, size, site of origin, and growth characteristics of intraocular masses. Depending on the clinical situation, dilated examination with indirect ophthalmoscopy, B scan ultrasonography, ultrasound biomicroscopy (UBM), transillumination, computed tomography (CT) scanning, magnetic resonance imaging (MRI) scanning, diagnostic paracentesis, fine needle aspiration biopsy, incisional biopsy and excisional biopsy may all be considered (4).

STEPS IN MANAGEMENT

The first critical step in managing patients with glaucoma secondary to an intraocular tumor is to recognize the presence of the tumor. Depending on location of the tumor, cell type, size, and growth characteristics this may be either an exercise in the obvious or an arduous undertaking punc-

Table 41.1
Mechanisms of Elevated Intraocular Pressure

Tumor invasion of the angle structures
Pigmentary dispersion
Melanophagic or melanomalytic
Hemolytic
Uveitic
Neovascular
Angle closure due to:
Choroidal detachment
Massive suprachoroidal hemorrhage
Mass effect by extremely large posterior tumors
"Ring" melanoma

tuated by multiple examinations and ancillary tests. In the setting of grossly elevated IOP, immediate medical management is usually indicated to forestall rapid optic disc damage or a retinal vascular obstruction. Further management of the glaucoma however will be intimately intertwined with the future management of the underlying tumor.

Based on patient history, clinical characteristics of the tumor and the results of ancillary testing, a systemic search for either a primary malignancy or secondary metastases from the intraocular primary lesion may be indicated. If this search yields evidence of systemic malignancy and/or metastases, then the systemic prognosis will impact further future interventions with respect to the glaucoma.

As a general rule, **treatment of the tumor should supercede treatment of the glaucoma.** When enucleation is indicated to manage the tumor, glaucoma therapy is no longer a concern. In eyes that retain useful vision, however, medical management of the elevated IOP becomes the mainstay. Alternatively, in eyes with unresponsive glaucoma, enucleation may be the only surgical option, even if therapy of the primary tumor does not require it.

Eyes that may harbor actively growing malignant tumors, especially melanomas, should not undergo filtering surgery as this may lead to orbital and eventually systemic dissemination of tumor cells. Exceptions may exist. For instance, under certain circumstances, a choroidal melanoma successfully treated with radiation therapy but complicated by secondary neovascular glaucoma could be considered for filtering surgery depending on the potential visual outcome, timing of the treatment, and location of the tumor. If indicated, ciliary body destructive procedures have been safely and effectively performed in eyes with intraocular tumors; however, ciliary body destructive procedures do lead to a breakdown in the blood-aqueous barrier. It is not currently known whether this breakdown might predispose to cellular elements (e.g., viable tumor cells) gaining access to the systemic circulation. No definite data implying an increased risk of metastases with ciliary destructive procedures exists, but common sense and caution should be used in such circumstances. Surgical intervention for glaucoma, whether laser cyclophotocoagulation or incisional, should be avoided if at all possible in the setting of an intraocular malignancy. Eyes with benign tumors such as nevi and adenomas have no contraindication to filtering surgery.

Eyes that may harbor malignant tumors should not undergo partial resection of the tumor through a full thickness scleral incision as this may presdispose to local seeding through the incision site (extrascleral extension). If biopsy is necessary several options exist:

- Complete excision for diagnosis and therapy, preferably through a "trap door" lamellar scleral incision, or, if anterior, a limbal or clear corneal incision
- Incisional biopsy with frozen section histopathologic evaluation followed by immediate enucleation if the tumor proves to be malignant
- Fine-needle aspiration biopsy through the clear cornea or trans-pars plana

In eyes with elevated IOP on the basis of pigment dispersion or melanophagic glaucoma, complete excision of the tumor can result in clearing of the pigment and/or macrophages from the trabecular meshwork with accompanying normalization of the IOP (6,7). Alternatively, radiation therapy of the underlying tumor has been noted to yield similar results in selected cases.

LOCATION: IRIS

Tumor Type: Primary

In most instances, iris tumors are easily detected at the slit–lamp. Differentiation between benign and malignant lesions may not be quite as straightforward. If definite differentiation is required by the clinical circumstances, an invasive procedure like anterior chamber paracentesis, fine-needle aspiration biospy, or excisional biopsy will be required.

Benign iris melanocytic lesions (iris nevi) rarely cause elevated IOP. When they do, pigment dispersion is the most likely mechanism. Iris nevi are usually solitary while malignant iris melanocytic lesions (Fig. 41.1) are classified as either solitary or diffuse melanomas. Diffuse iris nevus has been reported to cause elevated IOP as well (8). Iris nevi tend to be stable over time and can safely be observed.

Melanocytoma is a type of nevus that most commonly occurs in the posterior segment of the eye. Rarely they occur as solitary iris lesions that are dark brown or jet black in color. Melanocytomas have a strong tendency to undergo necrosis leading to pigment dispersion and secondarily elevated IOP (2).

An iris pigment epithelial adenoma is a rare, benign tumor arising from the posterior pigment epithelial layer. They are typically dark brown or black in color and may elevate IOP via pigment dispersion. Complete surgical ex-

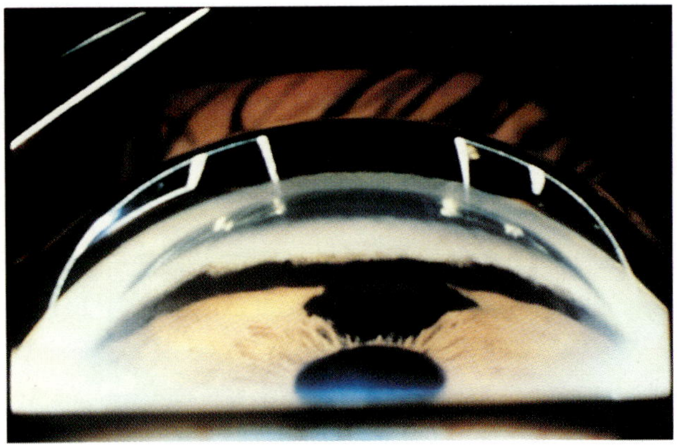

Figure 41.1. Goniophotograph of a solitary iris melanoma resulting in elevated IOP due to pigment dispersion into the angle.

cision is often possible if the tumor involves less than half the iris.

In any patient with unilateral glaucoma and acquired heterochromia, diffuse melanoma of the iris must be considered. These tumors, like their solitary counterparts, may cause elevated IOP by direct invasion of the angle structures, pigment dispersion, or, rarely, spontaneous bleeding leading to hemorrhage-associated glaucoma. **Diffuse iris melanomas are apt to be confused with congenital melanocytosis, hemosiderosis, siderosis bulbi, or one of the irido-corneal endothelial syndromes** (9).

Because iris tumors are rarely life threatening, they are typically treated by observation alone, assisted by periodic photographic documentation. Any associated increased IOP should be controlled medically. Surgery should be considered only if the glaucoma is uncontrolled medically with progressive field loss and/or unequivocal tumor growth is documented. Location of the tumor (e.g., involvement of the angle structures) alone is not an indication for surgical excision or enucleation. In a definite iris melanoma that cannot reliably be removed completely by surgical excision (i.e., greater than half the iris involved), enucleation should be considered.

Tumor Type: Metastasis

Metastases to the iris are rare. However, when they occur, elevated IOP is often a prominent finding. About 2/3 of iris metastases will show elevated IOP usually due to direct invasion of the trabecular meshwork by tumor cells (2). Lung and breast carcinoma are the most common primary sites, while cutaneous melanoma and kidney tumors may metastasize to the iris as well. Occasionally, a definite primary site is never located.

Metastatic iris carcinomas may present as either a solitary or a diffuse process. Tumor cells freely floating in the anterior chamber can mimic uveitis and layered cells may accumulate inferiorly in the angle forming a "pseudohypopyon." Uveitis, iris melanoma, intraocular lymphoma and endogenous endophthalmitis are all in the differential diagnosis.

In the presence of a known primary cancer, metastatic iris carcinoma may not be a difficult diagnosis to make. Anterior chamber paracentesis or even fine needle aspiriation biopsy can be used through the clear cornea to obtain cells for histologic diagnosis.

Beyond medical therapy, further interventions to control elevated IOP may be dependant on both the local control of the tumor as well as the systemic treatment of the primary tumor. Systemic chemotherapy can shrink intraocular metastases and local radiation therapy is highly effective for many cell types as well.

LOCATION: CILIARY BODY

Tumor Type: Primary

In contradistinction to iris masses, ciliary body masses are rarely visible with routine ophthalmologic examination techniques, including gonioscopy. Because of this fact, delay in diagnosis and/or extended treatment for a secondary manifestation of the tumor such as uveitis or elevated IOP is quite common (Case 41.1). Clinicians should be versed in the varied clinical presentations for ciliary body tumors as well as current techniques available to image such lesions like transillumination and ultrasonography.

Like their iris counterparts, benign ciliary body tumors such as nevi, melanocytomas, and pigment epithelial adenomas can lead to elevated IOP due to pigment dispersion and/or melanophagic mechanisms. Because of their location, it is virtually impossible to rule out the diagnosis of ciliary body melanoma without histopathologic examination of the lesions.

Ciliary body melanomas will result in elevated IOP in about 17% of cases (2). Along with the mechanisms mentioned above, invasion into the angle by the growing tumor can occur as well (Fig. 41.2). Diagnostic procedures that are helpful in the setting of ciliary body tumors include transillumination and ultrasound biomicroscopy (UBM). UBM is a new technique that allows very high resolution, two dimensional imaging of the angle structures, iris, ciliary body region, and pars plana. B-scan ultrasonography can be useful as well, but small, anterior tumors may not be imaged well with this technique. CT scanning and MRI scanning can also add useful information in certain cases.

Case 41.1. A 58-year-old female with a past medical history significant for chronic obstructive pulmonary disease and secondary polycythemia was referred for persistant iritis with secondary glaucoma for 7 months. At initial presentation, the visual acuity was 20/70 and a moderate non-granulomatous iritis was present with posterior synechias. Dilation of the pupil broke the synechias revealing a dense posterior subcapsular cataract with a normal fundus. The contralateral eye showed no abnormalities.

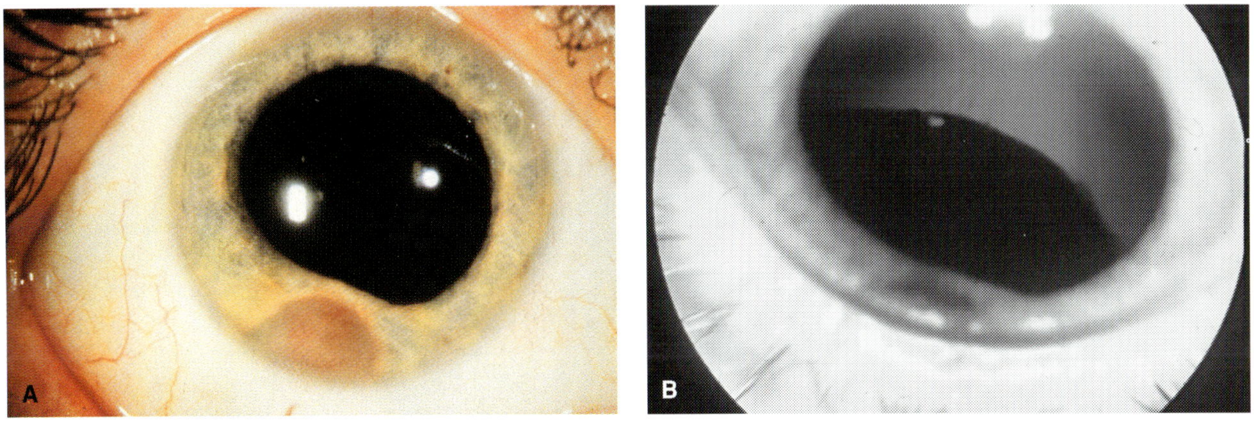

Figure 41.2. A, Slit-lamp photograph of an apparent amelanotic iris tumor. B, The same eye through the dilated pupil showing the main aspect of the tumor arising from the ciliary body.

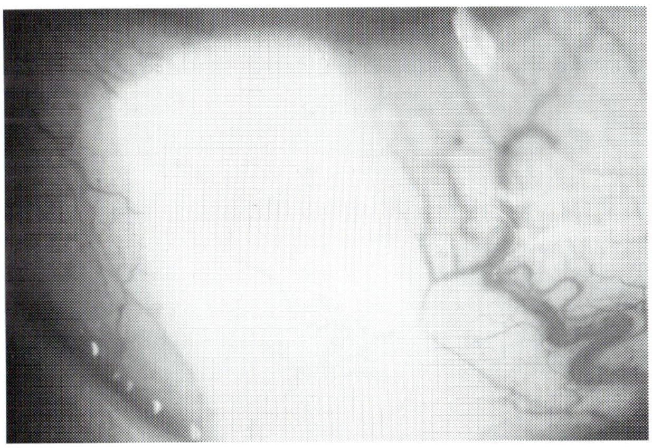

Figure 41.3. Slit-lamp photograph of the right eye of Case 1. Note sentinel vessel nasally.

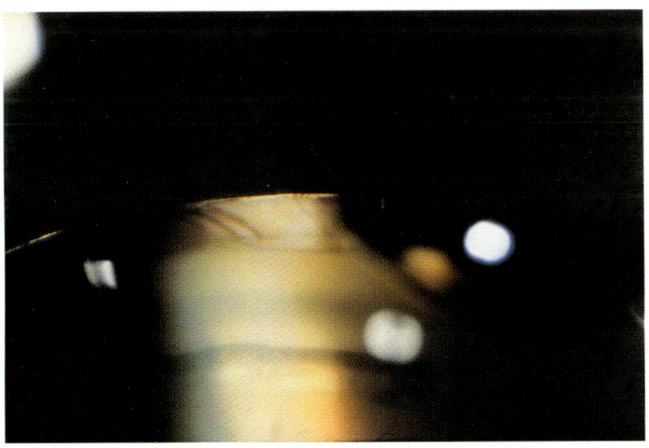

Figure 41.4. Goniophotograph of Case 41.1. There is smooth pigmentation throughout the angle.

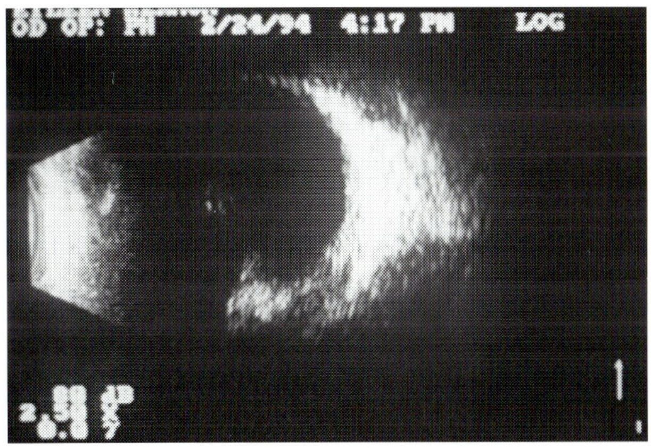

Figure 41.5. B scan ultrasonogram of Case 1 showing the anterior tumor.

Treatment with topical corticosteroids did not significantly reduce the iritis and the IOP was observed to rise to 44 mm Hg. This was believed to be a steroid response. A systemic evaluation for uveitis was unrevealing.

On initial examination by a glaucoma specialist, a visual acuity of 20/400 was noted with an IOP of 44 mm Hg. A questionable sentinal vessel was visible inferotemporally (Fig. 41.3). Gonioscopy revealed a closed angle from four to eight o'clock with dense black pigmentation in the trabecular meshwork (Fig. 41.4).

B-scan ultrasongraphy showed a ciliary body mass at approximately 5 o'clock (Fig. 41.5). This was confirmed with ultrasound biomicropscopy (UBM) (Fig. 41.6). Transillumination also revealed the ciliary body and pars plicata mass. The differential diagnosis included ciliary body melanoma, ciliary body adenoma, and ciliary body melanocytoma.

An anterior chamber paracentesis was performed which revealed pigmented cells. However, the histopathologist was unable determine the cell type.

A surgical resection of the tumor was suggested but, due to the patient's pulmonary status, it could not be safely perfomed with general anesthesia. A fine needle aspiration biopsy was then per-

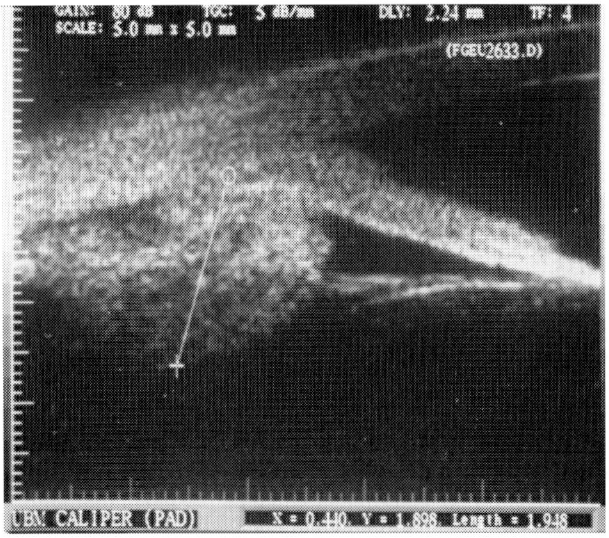

Figure 41.6. Ultrasound biomicroscopy (UBM) of the tumor in Case 41.1.

Table 41.2
Common Misdiagnoses - Anterior Tumors

Iritis
Granulomatous iris nodule (sarcoid, syphilis)
Fuchs heterochromic iridocyclitis
Iris nevus syndromes
Pigmentary dispersion syndrome
Endogenous endophthalmitis
Unilateral angle closure glaucoma without occludable contralateral angle

formed under local anesthesia followed by the placement of an episcleral radioactive iodine plaque. Evaluation of the biopsy showed positive immunoreactivity to cytokeratin, strongly suggestive of an epithelial origin (adenoma). There was negative staining for S-100, a melanoma marker.

Postoperatively, repeated UBM showed a slight reduction in the size of the mass. Because of continued elevated IOP in the 40's despite maximal medical therapy, consideration for cyclophotocoagulation versus a filtering procedure with cataract extraction or enucleation was contemplated. Based on the biopsy findings, a trabeculectomy with mitomycin C and cataract extraction was performed. One year later, the visual acuity was 20/25 and the IOP was 21 mm Hg on a topical beta blocker only. No evidence of systemic or local spread of the tumor was noted.

Medulloepithelioma (diktyoma) is an exceedingly rare, embryonal tumor that presents in infants or young children. Secondary glaucoma from a variety of mechanisms including angle closure, iris neovascularization, angle seeding, and hyphema have all been observed (10). The treatment of choice for most medulloepitheliomas is enucleation despite their frequently benign cytology. Typically, the tumors cannot be completely excised locally and end-stage glaucoma results in a blind, painful globe.

Ciliary body lesions may be amenable to surgical resection. In general, if greater than four clock hours are affected, complete surgical excision is difficult and ocular morbidity is high. Alternatively, radiation therapy can be used for growing tumors in this location.

Tumor Type: Metastasis

Isolated metastases to the ciliary body are quite rare. When they occur, however, they are notoriously difficult to diagnoses due to their protean presentation and lack of direct visibility using standard ophthalmic examination procedures. Seeding of the anterior segment may cause a uveitic syndrome and/or "pseudohypopyon" if the cells are loosely cohesive. Alternatively, a solid metastatsis may mimic a melanoma in growth characteristics.

B-scan ultrasonography and/or UBM can detect isolated ciliary body metastases reliably. Treatment will depend on cell type, location of the primary tumor, systemic prognosis, and visual prognosis.

LOCATION: CHOROID

Tumor Type: Melanocytic

While the choroid is the most common location for melanocytic tumors of the uveal tract, elevated IOP rarely results from neoplasms in this location. A recent series found the incidence of secondary glaucoma from choroidal melanomas was only 2% (2). The incidence of secondary elevated IOP from benign choroidal melanocytic lesions (choroidal nevi) is vanishingly small.

In most instances, the diagnosis of secondary glaucoma from a choroidal melanoma is not subtle. The typical mechanism is secondary angle closure from anterior segment neovascularization. Rarely, a necrotic tumor can produce a form of hemorrhagic glaucoma or inflammatory glaucoma. **The ring melanoma, a rare variant consisting of a multilobular, anterior tumor can produce secondary angle closure as well.** This variant is apt to be confused with multiple choroidal detachments. In most instances of secondary angle closure, the posterior segment tumor is large, and a secondary retinal detachment may also be present. B-scan ultrasonography, CT scanning, and MRI can be helpful when the media are opaque.

Enucleation is the treatment of choice for larger melanomas with secondary glaucoma, although rarely other modalities like radiation therapy or resection may be employed in highly selective cases. Alternatively, if advanced age, metastatic disease or poor systemic health is present, observation may be suggested.

Tumor Type: Metastases

Like their melanocytic couterparts, the choroid is the most common site in the uveal tract for a hematogenously spread metastastic tumor to develop (2). Similarly, the risk of elevated IOP in this location is quite small. Only large tumors that are accompanied by choroidal detachments, significant necrosis, or secondary retinal detachments typically produce glaucoma (11,12).

Breast and lung are by far the most common primary locations for metastases to the uveal tract. It is not uncommon for lung metastases to appear prior to detection of the primary mass. This is quite rare for breast carcinoma, however.

Management will be dependent on the systemic status of the patient, size, number and location of the choroidal metastases, cell type, and status of the fellow eye. Enucleation, radiation therapy (episcleral plaque or external beam), and observation are all possibilities. Medical management and/or ciliary body destruction procedures to manage the underlying elevated IOP may be indicated if eye-preserving therapies are to be attempted.

LOCATION: RETINA

Primary retinal tumors of adults are rare and secondary glaucoma does not usually develop. Rare cases of retinal capillary hemangioma and retinal astrocytoma in association with retinal detachment may lead to secondary iris neovascularization.

Retinoblastoma is the most common intraocular malignancy of children. **Secondary glaucoma can ensue due to a variety of mechanisms including iris neovascularization (about 20% of cases), tumor necrosis and angle closure** (13). Heterochromia may result and be a prominent presenting sign of retinoblastoma. Therapy of the secondary glaucoma is rarely an issue however, as affected eyes usually have far advanced tumors that require enucleation for treatment. In general, filtering operations should not be considered in these eyes due to the risk of extraocular spread.

LOCATION: OPTIC NERVE

Optic nerve tumors rarely result in secondarily elevated IOP. There is a single case report of a necrotic optic nerve melanocytoma resulting in a vascular obstruction and subsequent neovascular glaucoma (14).

MISDIAGNOSES

Common misdiagnoses for anterior tumors are listed in Table 41.2.

References

1. Marshall CD: On tension in cases of intra-ocular tumour. Trans Ophthalmol Soc U K 1896;16:155–170.
2. Shields CL, Shields JA, Shields MB, et al: Prevalence and mechanisms of secondary intraocular pressure elevation in eyes with intraocular tumors. Ophthalmology 1987;94:839–846.
3. Ozment R: Ocular tumors and glaucoma. In: Albert and Jakobiec, eds. Principles and Practice of Ophthalmology. vol. 3. Philadelphia: W.B. Saunders, 1994.
4. Shields JA, Shields CL: Intraocular tumors. A text and atlas. Philadelphia: W.B. Saunders Co., 1992;11–43.
5. Shields JA, Shields CL, Shields MB: Glaucomas associated with intraocular tumors. In: Ritch R, Shields MB, Krupin T, eds. The Glaucomas. St.Louis: C. V. Mosby, 1990:1111–1124.
6. Shields JA, Annesley WH, Spaeth GL: Necrotic melanocytoma of the iris with secondary glaucoma. Am J Opthalmol 1977;84:826–829.
7. Shields JA, Augsburger JJ, Sanborn GE, et al: Adenoma of the iris-pigment epithelium. Ophthalmology 1983;90:735–739.
8. Narieman AN, Ahmed H, Zimmerman LE, et al: Diffuse iris nevus manifested by unilateral open angle glaucoma. Ophthalmology 1981; 99:125–127.
9. Brown D, Boniuk M, Font RL: Diffuse malingnant melanoma of iris with metastases. Surv Ophthalmol 1990;34:357–364.
10. Broughton WL, Zimmerman LE: A clinicopathologic study of 56 cases of intraocular medulloepitheliomas. Am J Ophthalmol 1978;85:407–418.
11. Bloch RS, Gartner S: The incidence of ocular metastatic carcinoma. Arch Ophthalmol 1971;85:673–678.
12. Khawly JA, Shields NB: Metastatic carcinoma manifesting as angle-closure glaucoma. Am J Ophthamlol 1994;118:116–117.
13. Shields JA, Augsburger JJ: Current approaches to the diagnosis and management of retinoblastoma. Surv Ophthalmol 1981;25:347–367.
14. Croxatto JO, Ebner R, Crovetto L, et al: Angle closure glaucoma as initial manifestation of melanocytoma of the optic disc. Ophthalmology 1983;90:830–834.

Secondary Open Angle Glaucoma VII

Glaucoma Due to Intraocular Inflammation 42

R. Rand Allingham

Ocular inflammation may produce elevated IOP and glaucoma. The source of inflammation may be readily determined in some cases and may be obscure in others. Intraocular inflammation affects ocular structures, which may in turn alter aqueous fluid flow dynamics. These mechanisms include acute obstruction of the trabecular meshwork from inflammatory debris, angle closure from peripheral anterior synechias or pupillary block, and steroid-induced glaucoma. The clinical course may be acute, chronic, or relapsing. The symptoms can be mild or severe. Therefore, diagnosing and managing glaucoma secondary to inflammatory disease is frequently challenging to the treating ophthalmologist.

GENERAL CONSIDERATIONS

Diagnosis

A diagnosis of glaucoma because of intraocular inflammation is self-evident in cases in which glaucoma develops in conjunction with diagnosed uveitis (Fig. 42.1). However, in many instances, clinical symptoms may be mild, and the diagnosis may be made only after careful evaluation. The clinician should be alert to certain clues associated with glaucoma that might prompt one to consider intraocular inflammation as a possible cause. Especially suggestive clues are open-angle glaucoma in one eye only, and open-angle glaucoma of rapid onset. These features are atypical for primary open-angle glaucoma. Common causes of uniocular glaucoma, such as exfoliation, trauma, and pigmentary dispersion syndrome, can be eliminated by careful examination. In cases in which these causes have been excluded, one should consider inflammatory glaucoma as a possibility. **The aqueous humor may be deceptively clear with only trace flare and a rare circulating white cell.** Indications of an inflammatory process, such as collections of inflammatory cells on the trabecular meshwork, posterior synechias, or inflammatory foci in the fundus, may be present. Occasionally, the signs and symptoms of glaucoma develop rapidly over a few days, and the angle is wide and open without any evidence of inflammation. In these cases, one should carefully reexamine the eye frequently, as the first evidence of inflammation in the form of cells in the aqueous humor or keratic precipitates (KP) may make its appearance only after a few days.

The correct diagnosis must be made because in many respects, the management of glaucoma due to intraocular inflammation is different from that of other glaucomas.

OCULAR INFLAMMATION AND IOP

In association with various types of iritis or uveitis, the IOP may be normal, below normal, or raised well above normal. Inflammation can produce its effect on IOP by altering aqueous outflow resistance and aqueous humor production. **Iritis or uveitis tends to increase aqueous outflow resistance while reducing aqueous humor inflow.** Because these forces tend to act in opposite directions, IOP may be normal or low despite elevated outflow resistance. If the character or intensity of the inflammation changes and permits the formation of aqueous humor to return to a normal rate, then while the resistance to outflow remains high, the IOP will rise. The reverse is also true; if an eye has elevated IOP because of high resistance to aqueous outflow and a normal rate of aqueous formation, intraocular inflammation may reduce aqueous formation and decrease IOP.

Ocular inflammation is associated with production of prostaglandins, which have a wide variety of effects on the eye (1–5). These effects may be mediated through alteration of aqueous humor production, uveoscleral outflow, or aqueous outflow resistance through the trabecular meshwork.

The decrease in IOP associated with intraocular inflammation can be completely reversible. The IOP may return promptly to normal after the inflammation has subsided in some cases or very slowly in others. In some cases, a permanent decrease in aqueous formation appears to be induced by structural damage to the ciliary processes mediated by chronic intraocular inflammation. When this occurs, the ciliary processes, if visible, may appear atrophic. Occasionally, a distinct cyclitic membrane may be seen overlying the ciliary processes. Even in these cases, IOP may fluctuate profoundly if the resistance to aqueous outflow is high.

The character of the glaucoma associated with various types of intraocular inflammation is determined by the relative degree to which resistance to outflow and formation of aqueous humor are affected, reversibly or irreversibly, by the mechanisms just discussed. In general, the more protracted the inflammation, the more likely the changes will be permanent.

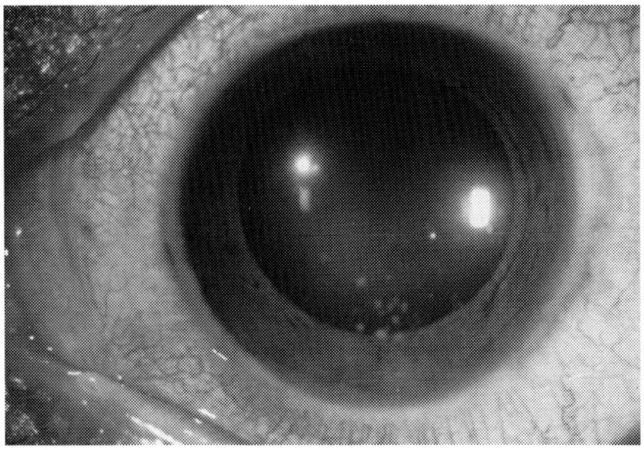

Figure 42.1. Acute anterior uveitis: Note ciliary flush and corneal precipitates in this patient with elevated IOP associated with sarcoid uveitis. (Courtesy of Glenn J. Jaffe, MD.)

Intraocular inflammation can affect aqueous outflow resistance through various mechanisms. In most cases, the cause of elevated outflow resistance cannot be detected by gonioscopy. The trabecular meshwork may be obstructed by inflammatory cells or debris (6). Experimentally, serum proteins have been shown to increase aqueous outflow resistance (7). Swelling of phagocytic cells lining the lamellae within the trabecular meshwork or adjacent to Schlemm's canal may also contribute to elevated IOP (8).

In certain types of iridocyclitis, focal accumulations of inflammatory cells resembling keratic precipitates may be visible on the inner surface of the trabecular meshwork by gonioscopy. These trabecular precipitates can completely resolve as inflammation subsides, leaving few, if any, persistent changes in the angle.

Frequently, inflammatory changes in the trabecular meshwork are not reversible. In these cases, the associated obstruction to aqueous outflow is permanent. **The most conspicuous form of irreversible obstruction to aqueous outflow is caused by peripheral anterior synechias (PAS), which form when the iris adheres to the trabecular meshwork.** PAS are produced as a result of organization of inflammatory exudates in the angle or from secondary pupillary block. Permanent obstruction can also be caused by endothelial or fibrovascular membranes that may line the inner surface of the trabecular meshwork. Within the trabecular meshwork, chronic inflammation may obliterate outflow channels.

Synechias and abnormal vessels in the angle are readily recognizable gonioscopically. Other alterations of the trabecular meshwork that may affect the permeability of the angle structures may only produce a "dirty" appearance of the trabecular meshwork gonioscopically. Occasionally, the trabecular meshwork does not have this appearance, but is blank, white, and lacking its normal finely granular surface texture.

In acute inflammation, the blood vessels of the anterior segment may be conspicuously dilated, but no demonstration has shown that this in itself has an influence on facility of aqueous outflow. Occasionally, **dilated iris vessels can be confused with those seen in neovascular glaucoma.** However, blood vessels found in association with inflammation have a normal radial pattern and do not bridge the scleral spur or arborize over the trabecular meshwork as do those seen in neovascularization of the anterior segment (Chapter 31).

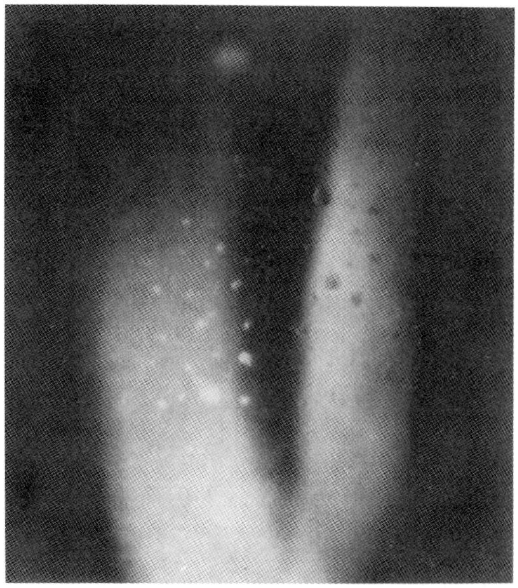

Figure 42.2. Elevated IOP in a patient who has acute anterior uveitis with corneal endothelial precipitates. Although IOP is frequently low in this situation, tonography may demonstrate impairment of outflow facility. IOP is therefore low because of relatively greater aqueous hyposecretion.

ACUTE IRITIS AND IRIDOCYCLITIS

Acute iritis is typically associated with anterior segment hyperemia, cells and flare in the anterior chamber, and miosis. Acute iridocyclitis appears clinically similar, with the addition of keratic precipitates (Fig. 42.2), and in some cases, inflammatory cells in the anterior vitreous. In most instances, IOP remains normal or low. Inflammation may not produce an increase in resistance to aqueous outflow, although commonly, the resistance to outflow is increased. However, the rate of formation of aqueous humor typically is lowered to a degree that is compensatory or even disproportionately greater. This results in a subnormal IOP.

In diagnosing acute iritis, with or without glaucoma, **a serious error that one can make is to confuse this condition with the sequelae of acute angle-closure glaucoma.** After an attack of angle-closure glaucoma, IOP is frequently normal or low, the anterior segment may be hyperemic, and the anterior chamber may contain conspicuous flare and cells as in iritis. One feature that distinguishes the two is the history. Usually, after an acute angle-closure attack, there is less photophobia and the pupil tends to be somewhat dilated. Most importantly, the anterior chamber angle is narrow by slit-lamp examination, and the angle is narrow or closed by gonioscopy. The treatment of angle-closure is, of course, entirely different from that of iritis. The clinical features of acute angle closure glaucoma are discussed more fully in Chapter 23.

In acute iritis or iridocyclitis, the angle is typically open gonioscopically. The treatment of the inflammation is the same whether glaucoma is present or not, relying principally upon topical administration of mydriatic-cycloplegic agents, such as atropine or scopolamine, and corticosteroids (except in herpetic dendritic keratopathy). If inflammation has caused an increase in outflow resistance, topical steroids may improve aqueous outflow over the short term. In a few instances, a cause for the uveitis will be discovered (e.g., syphilis) which requires specific treatment.

RECURRENT AND CHRONIC IRIDOCYCLITIS

Certain forms of recurrent or chronic iridocyclitis have distinctive characteristics and specific names, including glaucomatocyclitic crisis, heterochromic cyclitis, sarcoid uveitis, and pars planitis. Also, severe uveitis and secondary glaucoma sometimes are associated with arthritis, especially in juvenile rheumatoid arthritis, and severe glaucoma occurs in some cases of sympathetic ophthalmia. These uveitic glaucoma sub-types represent a small proportion of all cases of recurrent iridocyclitis and will be discussed individually later in this chapter.

The majority of cases of recurrent or chronic iridocyclitis lack specific or distinctive characteristics, and the causes are usually unknown. In nonspecific chronic anterior uveitis, the signs of inflammation, particularly cells, flare, and KP, come and go, or persist over a long period, responding incompletely to treatment. Glaucoma becomes a serious problem in some of these cases because of significantly elevated IOP and a chronic course.

In cases in which anterior segment inflammation has been prolonged, IOP may remain normal for a long time because of a low rate of aqueous production, but when the inflammation subsides, the rate of aqueous formation may return to normal. The IOP may then rise considerably if outflow facility remains reduced secondary to changes in the trabecular meshwork. In some instances, control of inflammation may result in an IOP that is uncontrollable by any medical means. Under these circumstances, one may be forced to choose between reducing anti-inflammatory treatment and permitting mild inflammation, or proceeding with invasive high risk glaucoma surgery. In such cases, one tries to steer a course between Scylla and Charybdis.

In certain cases of chronic uveitis, after the inflammation has subsided, one is confronted by chronic glaucoma. This may be caused by peripheral anterior synechias in some cases, but in other cases, the angle remains wide and open. Often, the angle is open but has a "dirty appearance." The details of normal angle structures may be partially obscured, as though covered with tissue. Additionally, pigment may be dispersed indiscriminately throughout the angle and extend up to or beyond Schwalbe's line.

Residual, permanent glaucoma is treated in the same manner as primary glaucoma, with beta blockers, epinephrine-like compounds, apraclonidine, and carbonic anhydrase inhibitors. Although less likely to be effective, miotics can be effective where the eye is completely quiet. Laser trabeculoplasty is not effective in these cases and may produce an acute IOP elevation. Filtering operations are performed in cases in which medical management is insufficient. If a filtering operation is required, use systemic steroids before, during, and after the operation in the hope of preventing a recurrence of active inflammation. Antimetabolites have been useful in promoting filtration success (Chapter 62).

Iris bombé is one of the complications one must guard against, particularly in active recurrent or chronic iritis or uveitis. An inflammatory membrane at the pupillary margin readily seals the iris to the lens when the pupil is small, but complete seclusion of the pupil and iris bombé can occur even with a semidilated pupil of 6 or 7 mm. When iris bombé is present, considerable elevation of IOP results. The iris is bowed forward in a characteristic fashion (Fig. 42.3) by elevated posterior chamber pressure, which closes the angle. If the angle is not held closed by formation of peripheral anterior synechias, the iris bombé and closure of the angle can be relieved immediately by making an opening in the periphery of the iris. Laser iridectomy should be performed, although in inflamed eyes, there is a tendency for closure of the iridectomy. Additional sessions may be needed, or in some cases, a surgical iridectomy (Chapter 67) may be required. If extensive synechial closure of the angle is found after iris bombé is relieved by iridectomy, a filtering operation may be necessary. If synechias are of recent onset and inflammation is well controlled, iridogonioplasty can, on occasion, restore aqueous outflow (Chapter 60).

In chronic or recurring iritis or uveitis, when there are extensive posterior synechias and a small or semidilated pupil, obstruction of the pupil may not cause the iris to assume a typical bombé appearance, but may instead lead to an uneven but progressive shallowing of the peripheral anterior chamber. This is because the iris is widely adherent to the lens, not just at the pupillary border, but well out to the periphery. These widespread adhesions prevent the iris from coming forward in typical bombé form. Once one notes progressive shallowing of the peripheral anterior chamber, one must watch the patient very closely, because sooner or later acute angle-closure glaucoma may ensue. If so, it is treated by iridec-

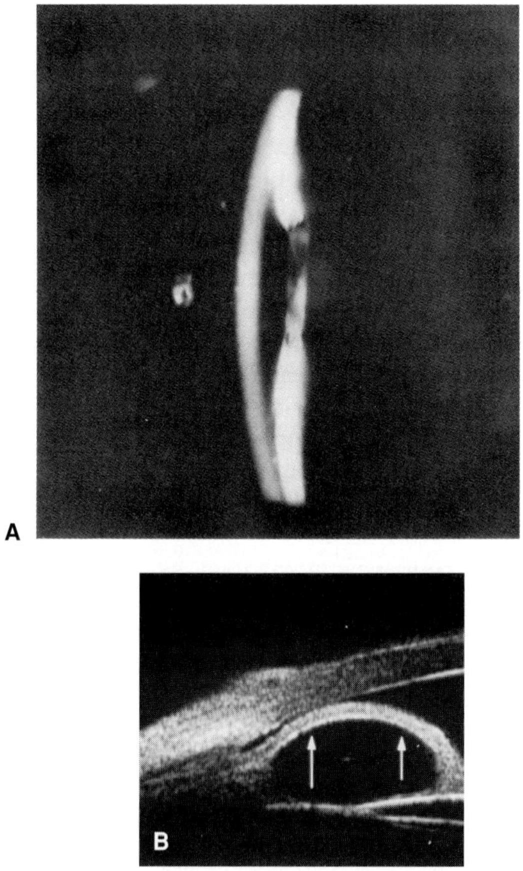

Figure 42.3. Iris bombé and angle closure glaucoma caused by posterior synechias from chronic uveitis (A). Ultrasound biomicroscopic image of patient with iris bombé and secondary angle closure (B). (Courtesy of Joel S. Schuman, MD.)

tomy or by lens extraction and iridectomy, according to the visual acuity.

In exceptional cases of iris bombé, one finds the IOP normal or even below normal. This is because of a subnormal rate of formation of aqueous humor, even though obstruction to aqueous outflow may be near complete. If the IOP is subnormal, any surgical procedure, even a surgical iridectomy, may cause the eye to become phthisical. Therefore, **in cases of iris bombé in which the IOP is normal, and especially if it is subnormal, surgical intervention is contraindicated**. In some cases, these eyes will go on to phthisis bulbi spontaneously.

TREATMENT

Medical Management

If IOP elevation secondary to iridocyclitis requires treatment, aqueous suppressants, including topical beta blockers, apraclonidine, and/or systemic or topical carbonic anhydrase inhibitors, are often effective. Topical apraclonidine is additive to beta blockers when beta blockers have been given chronically in the past. Apraclonidine is *not* additive to beta blocker therapy that is also being given acutely for IOP control (9–10).

Miotic treatment is generally contraindicated in the presence of iridocyclitis. Miotics can cause pain, intensify anterior segment inflammation, and may increase formation of posterior synechias which can produce complete block of the pupil (iris bombé).

If the optic nerve head is entirely normal, as is usual in acute iritis or iridocyclitis, treatment of moderate elevation of IOP may not be indicated. In these cases, once inflammation is controlled, the IOP will probably return to safe levels long before optic nerve damage occurs. Typically, a normal optic nerve can tolerate an IOP in the mid-thirties for many weeks without damage. Only if there are frequent recurrences, or if inflammation becomes chronic, is significant optic nerve damage likely. In eyes with corneal endothelial disease, a moderate elevation of IOP may cause corneal edema, which calls for more vigorous efforts to lower the IOP.

Use of Steroids in Ocular Inflammation

If the inflammation persists for weeks, glaucoma becomes a more pressing problem. The clinician must consider whether corticosteroids may be contributing to the elevated IOP. **Steroid induced IOP elevations typically occur after 7–10 days but may occur much sooner.** Where this is a concern, topical steroid treatment should be tapered, or less potent steroid formulations can be substituted (e.g., fluorometholone 0.12%). If possible, taper steroid therapy gradually to avoid rebound inflammation, which may occur after rapid discontinuation.

When evaluating the effect of steroids on IOP in patients with uveitis, possible separate actions on aqueous humor secretion and outflow must be considered (Fig. 42.4). Steroids may suppress inflammation in the ciliary body so that aqueous humor formation returns to a more normal rate. If outflow facility is impaired by inflammation, the improvement in aqueous humor formation may produce an increase in IOP which is not secondary to steroid-induced outflow obstruction. If there is actual inflammation in the trabecular meshwork, steroids may, in fact, improve outflow facility, but the resulting IOP represents the balance between aqueous humor inflow and outflow effects.

Immunosuppressive Therapy

Corticosteroids have a wide variety of unwanted side effects that may limit their use in the treatment of inflammatory disorders. **In selected cases, with appropriate medical consultation, immunosuppressive therapy may be considered when severe inflammation is threatening**

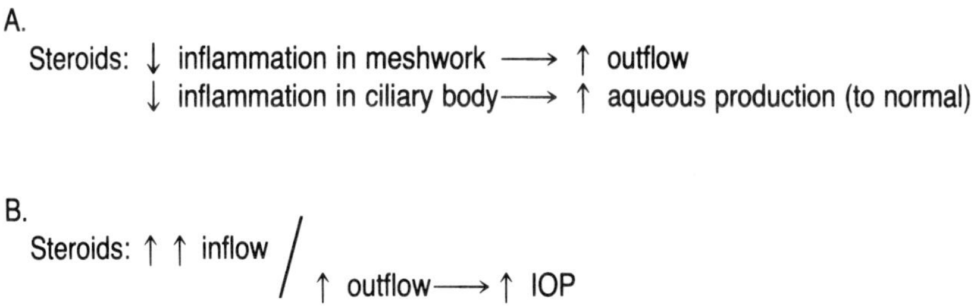

Figure 42.4. Framework in which to consider steroids' effects on IOP in uveitis. Only if steroids actually increase outflow resistance should patients be termed "steroid-responders." Most often, elevation of IOP in such patients is caused by changes in aqueous inflow.

vision or in cases in which an associated systemic disorder exists (11–13). The risks of immunosuppressive therapy should be considered carefully because potential side effects may outway benefits (14).

Novel Anti-inflammatory Agents

The pathophysiology of ocular inflammation is undergoing a continuing period of intense scrutiny. Prostaglandins, prostacyclin, thromboxane A2, cytokines, interleukins, and a variety of other agents play wide-ranging roles in mediating specific types of ocular inflammatory response and its severity (15–21). Future developments in the field of immune pathophysiology and pharmacology will greatly impact treatment for ocular inflammation and its sequelae, including glaucoma (22–25).

Surgical Management

Medical treatment may not adequately control glaucoma in cases associated with ocular inflammation. Surgical treatment must be directed at the mechanism responsible for outflow obstruction.

Laser Therapy

In cases in which pupillary block exists, (e.g., iris bombé) an iridectomy is indicated. Laser iridectomy is possible in these cases; however, in the presence of active inflammation, a strong tendency exists for these to close because fibrin and associated blood often forms a clot at the site of the iridectomy. In these cases, a surgical iridectomy may be necessary.

Laser trabeculoplasty is not only ineffective in cases in which glaucoma is secondary to an inflammatory process, but it may produce a significant increase in IOP.

Laser cyclophotocoagulation can be used in cases in which advanced optic nerve damage exists and visual potential is limited (Chapter 57) (26–29). Cycloablative procedures often increase intraocular inflammation, which can exacerbate the underlying disease in these patients.

Incisional Surgery

Filtering surgery is prone to failure in patients who have uveitis (Chapter 62). The importance of reducing ocular inflammation before surgical intervention cannot be overemphasized. This issue has been addressed in the context of cataract surgery, much of which is relevant to glaucoma surgery (30). Unfortunately, glaucoma is, at times, an immediate threat to vision and it is not possible to completely control inflammation prior to surgery. The use of adjuvant antimetabolites, such as 5-FU and mitomycin C, are becoming increasingly important in the management of these high risk patients to promote surgical success (31–34).

The role of setons in the management of patients with ocular inflammation is still undetermined, but their successful use has been documented in several recent studies (Chapter 65) (35–38).

IDIOPATHIC INFLAMMATORY GLAUCOMA

Glaucomatocyclitic Crisis (Posner-Schlossman Syndrome)

This idiopathic syndrome was first described by Posner and Schlossman in 1948 (39). **This disorder can be characterized as a trabeculitis.** The initial episode most commonly occurs between ages 20 to 50 years. Onset of symptoms is usually acute. IOP is often highly elevated. Symptoms are typically unilateral and consist of slight ocular discomfort and blurred vision. The patient may see colored halos around lights secondary to corneal edema.

Examination reveals a highly elevated IOP, usually between 40 and 70 mm Hg. The eye is generally quiet with little or no hyperemia. The cornea may have mild to moderate epithelial edema with a few fine keratic precipitates. **Keratic precipitates may not be noted for 2 or 3 days after the onset of symptoms and tend to vary in number and position from day to day.** Gonioscopy reveals a normal appearing angle, open throughout, with no abnormal pigmentation. Occasionally, one may find a few tiny inflammatory precipitates on the trabecular meshwork. Characteristically, no posterior or anterior synechias are formed. If tonography is performed, it demonstrates a highly elevated resistance to aqueous outflow in the affected eye but a normal value in the unaffected eye.

This disorder must be distinguished from an acute angle-closure glaucoma attack because treatment is radically different. The authors have seen several instances where iridectomies have been performed in an effort to treat this disorder. Iridectomies are of no use in glaucomatocyclitic glaucoma but, of course, would be indicated for angle closure glaucoma.

An attack of glaucomatocyclitic crisis generally subsides within 1 to 3 weeks, with or without treatment. Beta blockers, apraclonidine, and carbonic anhydrase inhibitors are usually given to decrease IOP and to relieve symptoms. Topical steroid therapy is used to reduce inflammation, thus improving aqueous outflow resistance. It is unclear whether mydriatic-cycloplegics are beneficial.

After the IOP is reduced and treatment is discontinued, the tonographic facility of outflow returns to normal. In many cases during an interval after the attack, the facility of outflow is even greater than in the contralateral normal eye (observation by W. Morton Grant, MD).

Glaucomatocyclitic crises are prone to recur at intervals of a few months to a year or two. Eventually, episodes appear to stop because this condition is almost never seen after age 60. Surprisingly, even repeated attacks may not damage the optic nerve. Perhaps the period of IOP elevation is insufficient to produce irreversible glaucomatous damage. However, cases exist in which the optic nerve head can be injured after repeated attacks. Therefore, **we recommend treatment of elevated IOP and inflammation for all cases.**

We have seen patients who initially experienced multiple self-limited attacks that subsided in characteristic fashion but then became chronically affected over time. These cases required continuous treatment with topical steroids to prevent recurrence of uveitis and elevated IOP.

At the outset, one cannot be sure whether one is dealing with a short case of glaucomatocyclitic crisis or with the beginning of a long-lasting iridocyclitis. In some cases, with the initial episodes of glaucomatocyclitic crisis, one finds a good response to local corticosteroid treatment; but, after this treatment is discontinued, the inflammatory precipitates recur and IOP again becomes elevated. This condition may then persist for weeks or months. In such cases, one must determine by trial and error the maintenance dose of local steroids that will prevent recurrence of the inflammation. If IOP rises when no evidence of inflammation exists, one must determine whether it is caused by the local corticosteroid therapy itself. If there is severe residual glaucoma uncontrolled by any medical means, a filtering operation may be required. In such cases, although the onset closely resembles glaucomatocyclitic crisis, the subsequent course does not support this diagnosis.

Among the seemingly typical glaucomatocyclitic crisis cases, the general belief is that no special tendency towards cataract formation exists, that heterochromia of the irides is slight and occasional rather than typical, and that repeated episodes usually occur in the same eye but rarely occur in one eye and then the other. Still, we have seen several cases in which, after repeated attacks, keratic precipitates were found continuously on the cornea unless 1 or 2 drops of topical steroid were used daily. These patients have developed a slowly progressive posterior subcapsular lens opacity; whether it is because of the disease or the topical steroid is not clear.

Repeated glaucomatocyclitic attacks have occurred during 15 to 25 years in many patients, with return of the IOP to normal levels between attacks, and without permanent damage to vision, giving the impression of a benign or harmless condition. Nevertheless, an increasing number of patients have developed glaucomatous cupping and loss of visual field, leading to the realization that a guarded prognosis and continued supervision are necessary (40). In a given case, one cannot assure the patient that it is always a benign disorder when the diagnosis of glaucomatocyclitic crisis is first made.

Iridectomy has no influence on the occurrence of attacks. Filtration surgery has been observed to prevent the rises of IOP, although cyclitic episodes continue (41). Sometimes, evidence exists of primary open-angle glaucoma in the fellow eye, but the significance of this observation is unknown (42,43).

When the patient is seen at the first attack, the differential diagnosis in suspected glaucomatocyclitic crisis includes: (1) iridocyclitis of some other type, as already mentioned; (2) chorioretinitis with associated anterior uveitis and secondary glaucoma (e.g., toxoplasmosis); and (3) retinal detachment—a rare cause of secondary glaucoma (see below). Careful examination of the fundus and visual fields is essential.

Heterochromic Iridocyclitis (Fuchs' HIC)

Fuchs' HIC is an idiopathic form of low grade iridocyclitis associated with iris stromal atrophy, cataract formation, and glaucoma (Fig. 42.5). Because of the diverse number of abnormalities that may be present, this may be one of the more difficult uveitides to diagnose. A lack of uniform diagnostic criteria exists (44,45).

Although Fuchs' HIC typically affects only one eye, it is bilateral in approximately 13% of cases (46). Onset is usually in the third or fourth decade (47). The patient is frequently either asymptomatic or complains of monocular reduced visual acuity on clinical presentation. The eye is white and quiet. Characteristically, there are fine colorless keratic precipitates; some are round, but the most typical are filamentary or star-shaped, scattered over the posterior surface of the cornea. These are best seen by retroillumina-

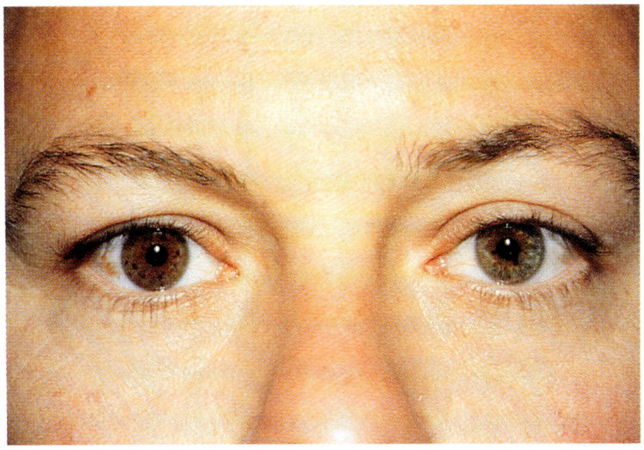

Figure 42.5. Patient with Fuchs' heterochromic iridocyclitis. Iris stromal atrophy of the left eye is responsible for the heterochromia. (Courtesy of Glenn J. Jaffe, MD.)

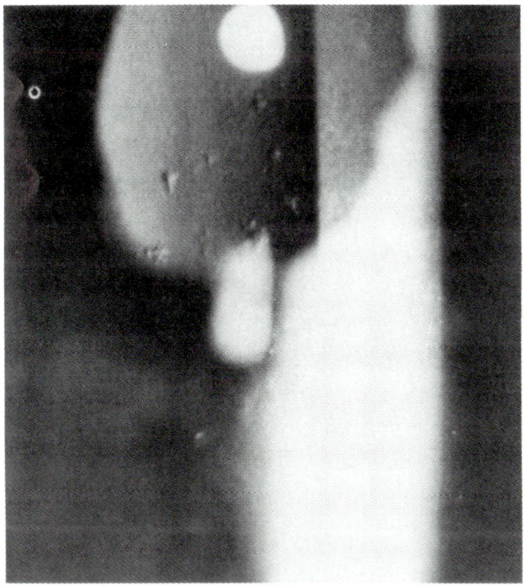

Figure 42.6. Typical filamentary star-shaped corneal endothelial precipitates seen in Fuchs' heterochromic iridocyclitis.

tion (48) (Fig. 42.6). There may be trace flare in the aqueous humor with an occasional white cell. The iris is infiltrated with plasma cells with accompanying degeneration and atrophy (49). Clinically, atrophy of the iris affects the pupil collarette (transforming it to a hyaline border) and produces hypochromia of the iris stroma with abnormal transillumination of the posterior pigment layer (50). A history of heterochromia may antedate detection of iridocyclitis. In some cases, congenital Horner's syndrome has been reported (51). Heterochromia may not be recognized in darkly pigmented irides, which can lead to diagnostic confusion (52). Fluorescein may leak from vessels at the pupil, but these are not new vessels. A cataract in the affected eye is the rule, initially presenting as a posterior subcapsular cataract. Vitreous opacities are frequent (45). Chorioretinal scars similar to those seen in toxoplasmosis have been described in Fuchs' HIC, but the association of these two diseases is unclear (53).

Glaucoma has been reported to occur in 13 to 59% of cases of Fuchs' HIC, and an overall incidence of approximately 25% seems likely (45,54–57). Typically, glaucoma is of the open angle variety, but a number of mechanisms have been observed, including secondary synechial angle closure, neovascular glaucoma, lens-induced, and glaucoma secondary to recurrent hyphemas (57–59).

Gonioscopy characteristically reveals a few fine new blood vessels wandering on the surface of the ciliary band, on the scleral spur, and on the corneoscleral meshwork. Only a few abnormal vessels may be seen in the angle. These may be overlooked easily. Abnormal vessels in the angle may also be seen in cases of heterochromia without glaucoma (60). These blood vessels appear to be different from those associated with neovascular glaucoma because they do not proliferate or produce synechial closure of the angle. If paracentesis is done, Huber has shown that filiform self-limited hemorrhage from the angle (rarely a problem at surgery) is characteristic (60). Also, hyphema can be produced by manipulation of a gonioscopy lens, without paracentesis. Blood comes either from Schlemm's canal or from the vessels, according to Huber and Francois (60–62).

Glaucoma tends to develop both gradually and late in the course of Fuchs' HIC. Glaucoma usually occurs after a cataract has formed and, in some cases, after cataract extraction. When it occurs in Fuchs' HIC, glaucoma may be well-controlled medically early in the disease course. In a large percentage of cases, it becomes increasingly difficult to control medically, eventually leading to progressive optic nerve damage and requiring surgical management (56–58).

In most cases of heterochromic iridocyclitis, once glaucoma develops, it appears to be permanent. Unfortunately, **control of the associated inflammation has little influence on the IOP.** The inflammation usually continues for many years, but even if the inflammation eventually clears, the glaucoma invariably remains. Treatment of the inflammation accomplishes little, and it is questionable whether it is even worthwhile, especially because there is little tendency to form synechias. In fact, **we do not routinely administer steroids to patients with well-defined heterochromic iridocyclitis.** We have allowed the signs of "inflammation" to persist without adverse consequences. Steroids may in fact cause elevation of IOP and accelerate cataract formation.

Medical treatment with beta blockers, apraclonidine, miotics and carbonic anhydrase inhibitors may be effective initially. As time passes, the glaucoma responds poorly to medical treatment. The angle typically remains open, with a few characteristic fine vessels. The trabecular meshwork at this stage may be covered by an inflammatory membrane that is demonstrable only histologically (63). In some cases, the canal of Schlemm appears to be collapsed (64). Once the glaucoma is well established, surgical intervention is usually necessary. Glaucoma filtration surgery is generally well tolerated and causes little or no increase in the inflammation. Argon laser trabeculoplasty in cases of Fuchs' HIC, as in other uveitides, is not effective.

In Fuchs' HIC, the lens eventually becomes opaque, but extraction of the lens has no favorable effect on the glaucoma. If cataract is present and the glaucoma is becoming difficult to control medically in this syndrome, it is best to do a filtering operation before cataract extraction. The lens may or may not be removed later, according to the visual requirements of the patient. Alternatively, a combined cataract extraction and trabeculectomy can be considered. In either case, the failure rate is substantial. Adjunctive antimetabolites appear to improve the glaucoma surgical success rate (56–58).

Keratic Precipitates on the Trabecular Meshwork

Chandler and Grant were the first to describe a relatively rare cause of idiopathic secondary glaucoma consisting of inflammatory precipitates on the trabecular meshwork (65). **Although it is uncommon, it is important to diagnose this disorder correctly because treatment with topical steroids in most cases is effective.**

Typically, the IOP is elevated in both eyes, and the eyes are white and quiet, with few (if any) inflammatory precipitates on the back of the cornea. There may be a few cells in the aqueous, but in most cases, no cells are seen.

Gonioscopy is crucial to differentiate this condition from primary open-angle glaucoma. When gonioscopy is done, one finds inflammatory precipitates projecting from the surface of the corneoscleral meshwork. These are generally colorless or tapioca colored and tend to be broader and flatter than KP seen on the back of the cornea, and they may be confluent.

In rare instances, the KP in the angle are large and striking in appearance (Fig. 42.7). We have seen large KP in only two patients. In all other cases, the KP have been small and inconspicuous and therefore easily overlooked. It is not unusual that after careful examination of the entire angle only a few KP may be identified; however, if one immediately repeats the examination a second or third time, more KP may be observed. One should also look for irregularity in the level of the attachment of the iris root. KP in the angle tend to organize and thus cause irregularities in the width of the angle. In primary open-angle glaucoma, although the angle may be narrower above or below, there are never any abrupt changes in the width of the angle. Such abrupt changes are almost certainly the result of organization of KP in the angle or trauma. The only other conditions in which such abrupt changes in the width of the angle are seen include old interstitial keratitis and multiple cysts of the iris and ciliary body, essential atrophy of the iris, and Chandler's syndrome. All of these conditions are identified and readily differentiated from trabeculitis.

The level of IOP elevation may not be proportional to the number of inflammatory precipitates observed in the angle. In some cases, one may find many KP in the angle, but the IOP is normal or only slightly elevated. Or, one may identify only a few KP in the angle, yet the IOP may

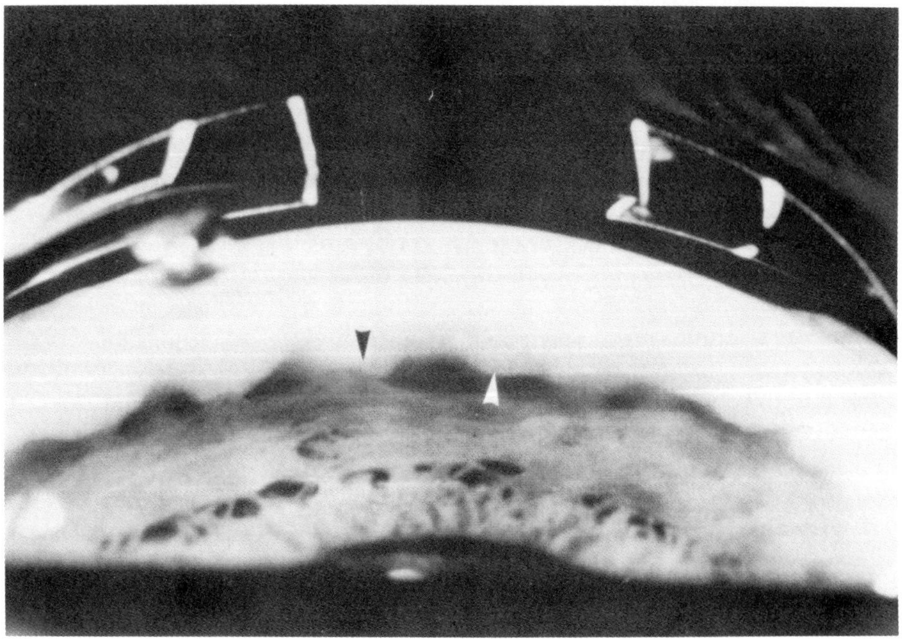

Figure 42.7. "Giant" KP's in the angle (arrowheads) with early organization involving the iris surface and synechia formation in a patient with sarcoidosis. Such KP can be very subtle and are difficult to photograph, especially in the condition of "occult" KP in the angle associated with little or no anterior chamber reaction. (Courtesy of David D. Donaldson, MD.)

be considerably elevated. In one notable case during the follow-up period, careful search revealed only one KP in the angle, yet IOP was 40, and IOP returned to normal in a few days with topical steroid treatment. This suggests that inflammatory debris must be present within the trabecular meshwork which is blocking the outflow pathways but cannot be seen gonioscopically.

In early cases of glaucoma associated with inflammatory precipitates on the trabecular meshwork, the disc is normal and the field is full, but in longstanding cases, one may find cupping of the disc with field loss. If the true condition is not recognized and the patient is treated mistakenly as primary open-angle glaucoma, there is usually a poor response. **This is especially true for pilocarpine therapy, in which marked IOP elevation may be observed.** If the condition is unrecognized and the eye is treated for primary open-angle glaucoma, the exudates in the angle may gradually organize to bring about synechial closure of the angle and permanent glaucoma.

In early cases with no synechial closure of the angle, medical treatment consists of topical corticosteroids, beta blockers, apraclonidine, and carbonic anhydrase inhibitors as required. Topical corticosteroids are at first given every hour during the day, then every 2 hours, and then gradually tapered. Trabecular precipitates typically clear over a 1 to 2 week period and, in the absence of advanced peripheral synechial closure, the IOP returns to normal levels.

In some cases, there is no recurrence after the initial treatment, but **in the majority of cases when the topical corticosteroids are reduced below a certain level or discontinued, the precipitates in the angle tend to recur and IOP again becomes elevated.** In such cases, the maintenance dose of topical steroids in preventing recurrence is determined by trial and error.

Once the KP have cleared after treatment, one expects the IOP to return to normal, but if there are many recurrences, eventually the patient may have a permanent open-angle glaucoma. When one is sure there is no activity in the angle, one can treat this residual open-angle glaucoma with miotics. Individuals with this condition should be monitored indefinitely because of a significant risk of recurrence. The recurrence is not likely to be noted by the patient because the patient is usually asymptomatic.

If there is extensive synechial closure of the angle when the diagnosis is first established, one may improve the condition and eliminate the precipitates in the open portions of the angle, but there may be severe residual glaucoma because of the secondary angle closure. In such cases, a glaucoma filtering operation may be necessary.

The cause of this disorder is unknown. Some patients who initially present with this disorder will develop other inflammatory conditions such as sarcoidosis, ankylosing spondylitis, rheumatoid arthritis, or chronic uveitis (6).

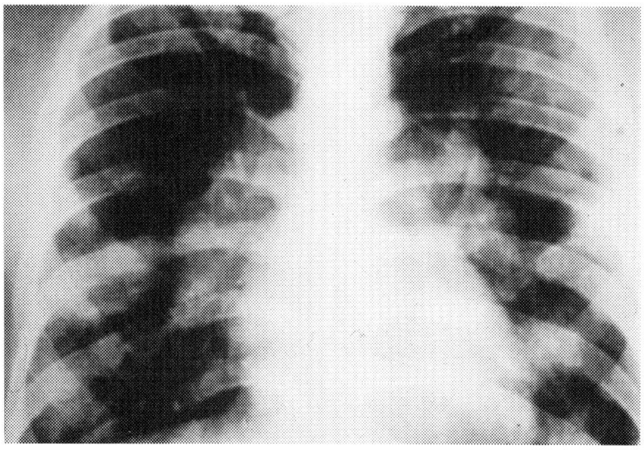

Figure 42.8. Sarcoidosis: Chest radiograph demonstrating hilar adenopathy from pulmonary involvement. (Courtesy of Glenn J. Jaffe, MD.)

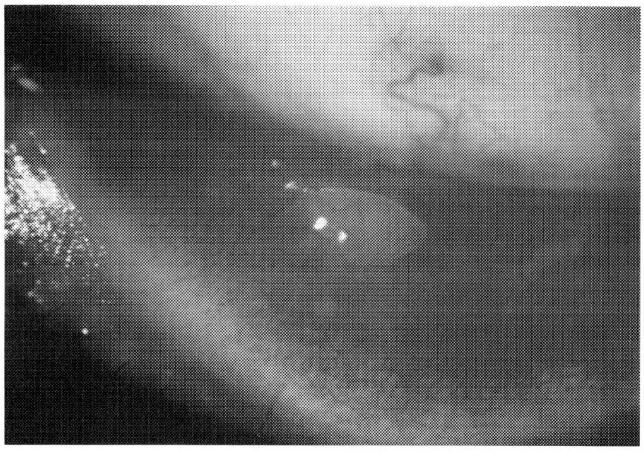

Figure 42.9. Sarcoidosis: Conjunctival nodule. Histological evaluation demonstrated non-caseating granulomas. (Courtesy of Glenn J. Jaffe, MD.)

SARCOID UVEITIS

Sarcoidosis is a multisystem disease of unknown etiology which is characterized by the formation of noncaseating granulomas and a pattern of remissions and exacerbations. Sarcoidosis is commonly manifested by pulmonary, cutaneous, and ocular involvement (Fig. 42.8, 42.9) (66–68). As discussed in the foregoing section, **sarcoidosis has been associated with inflammatory precipitates on the trabecular meshwork**.

Sarcoidosis is more common in young adults and in black patients compared to white patients. Ocular manifestations of sarcoidosis include iridocyclitis, retinal phlebitis, optic disc inflammation, and vitritis (Fig. 42.10). One or more of these findings occurs in a large number of patients, perhaps as many as 20–70% or more of patients with systemic disease (69–71). Glaucoma occurs in a variable number of those afflicted by ocular sarcoidosis. In one study, glaucoma was diagnosed in approximately 10% of those patients with iridocyclitis (68).

The appearance of the iris seen at an early stage of irido-

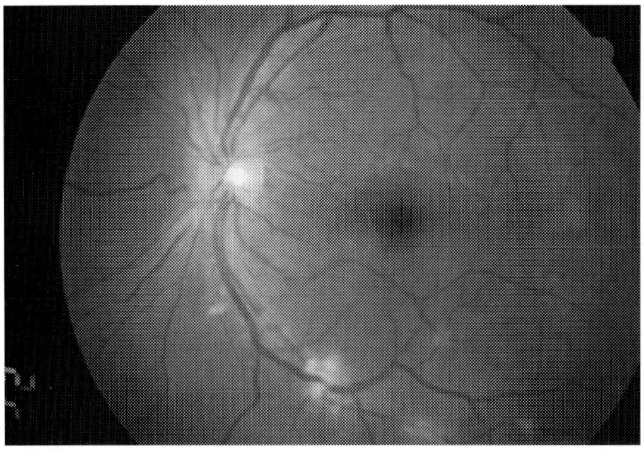

Figure 42.10. Sarcoidosis: Retinal phlebitis with typical "candlewax drippings" appearance. (Courtesy of Glenn J. Jaffe, MD.)

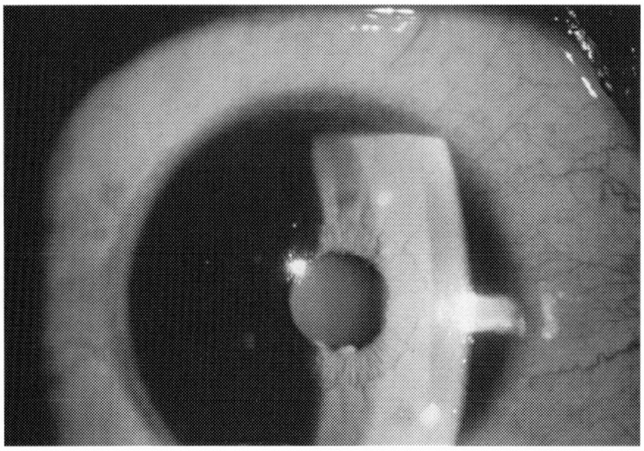

Figure 42.11. Sarcoidosis: Anterior uveitis with mutton fat keratic precipitates. Note Koeppe nodules on pupillary border. (Courtesy of Glenn J. Jaffe, MD.)

cyclitis may have a grossly and irregularly elevated stromal surface due to sarcoid nodules (Fig. 42.11). There is a strong tendency for large peripheral anterior synechias to form between the KP on the trabecular meshwork and the iris, especially in an area of iris elevated by nodules. Additionally, there is a tendency for posterior synechias to form. Small grayish white balls ("snowballs") of inflammatory cells may be seen in the vitreous. The inflammation is chronic and long standing. In its later stages, thickened areas of the iris may clear and the anterior chamber may become conspicuously deep. The iris may change from an irregularly rounded convex shape to a strikingly concave form, held forward only in the angle by thick columns of synechias to the full width of trabecular meshwork.

The glaucoma associated with sarcoid uveitis is subject to the same principles and variables as that due to intraocular inflammation from other causes and from inflammatory deposits on the trabecular meshwork in general. Glaucoma may respond well to topical corticosteroids early in the disease course. Later, it may become increasingly difficult to control, especially when peripheral anterior synechias are extensive. Oddly, in some cases, despite extensive peripheral anterior synechias, IOP may remain well controlled on few if any medications for years. Topical steroid treatment employed in this last situation may serve only to create a greater problem with the glaucoma. This can occur because of increased aqueous humor formation with decreased aqueous outflow secondary to anterior synechias (Fig. 42.4), or in conjunction with a true steroid response. As stated before, it may be difficult to distinguish between the two.

Pars Planitis

Pars planitis is a chronic inflammatory disorder primarily involving the peripheral retina and pars plana and vitreous base. It is frequently associated with cystoid macular edema. Secondary glaucoma probably occurs in less than 10% of cases (72–74). When it has occurred, the anterior chamber angle has mainly been open, but scattered peripheral anterior synechias also have been observed, with inflammatory precipitates on the trabecular meshwork. If medical treatment, including topical steroids, topical beta blockers, apraclonidine and carbonic anhydrase inhibitor, proves inadequate, peripheral cryotherapy has been used with some success to treat the inflammation (74). Chronic steroid use is frequently required with this disorder. Whether given systemically, topically, or by retrobulbar injection, the IOP can become markedly elevated. In these cases, non-steroidal antiinflammatory agents or anti-metabolites (the latter used in consultation with an internist) may be required to control the inflammation and reduce corticosteroid therapy.

Scleritis and Episcleritis

Scleritis is a disorder characterized by severe pain in association with variable anterior or posterior segment inflammation. A number of diseases are associated with the development of scleritis, and the most common associated condition is rheumatoid arthritis. Other disorders associated with scleritis include herpes zoster ophthalmicus, IgA nephropathy, acanthamoeba keratitis, toxoplasmosis, systemic lupus erythematosis, and other systemic immune-mediated conditions (75–80).

Anterior scleritis can be divided into diffuse, nodular, or necrotizing types. Diffuse and nodular scleritis are characterized by pain with variable degrees of erythema (Fig. 42.12). Clinically, these forms are more benign. Necrotizing scleritis is associated with rheumatoid arthritis. It presents with severe inflammation and, if untreated, may result in irreversible destruction of ocular tissues. This form of scleritis accounts for approximately 10% of scleritis cases and has a higher risk of glaucoma than with other forms of anterior scleritis.

Secondary glaucoma may occur in either anterior or pos-

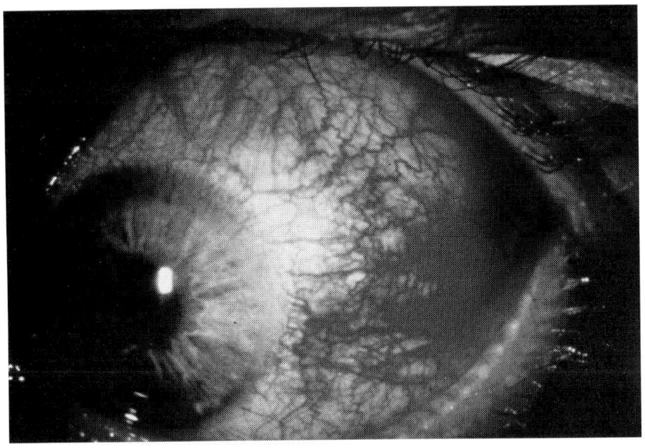

Figure 42.12. Anterior nodular scleritis: Although painful, glaucoma is unusual in this form of scleritis in contrast to necrotizing scleritis. (Courtesy of Glenn J. Jaffe, MD.)

terior forms of scleritis but is more common in the former. It has been reported to develop in 11% or more of cases of anterior scleritis but to be rare in association with posterior scleritis or with episcleritis (81). The mechanism of glaucoma varies but is usually secondary to damage to the trabecular meshwork by iridocyclitis or peripheral anterior synechias (75). **Glaucoma in posterior scleritis is usually caused by secondary angle closure produced by ciliochoroidal effusion** and subsequent detachment (Fig. 42.13) (78,80,82,83).

Episcleritis is typically a benign, self-limited syndrome consisting of mild to moderate pain and episcleral injection and edema; it is often recurrent. Permanent damage to ocular structures is rare. Steroids and nonsteroidal antiinflammatory agents do not appear to shorten the clinical course of episcleritis and may cause IOP elevation, glaucoma, or cataracts (81,84–86).

Treatment for glaucoma in scleritis is directed at the specific mechanism of IOP elevation. Topical or systemic steroids and nonsteroidal antiinflammatory agents are frequently required to treat these disorders. Steroids, of course, may induce a secondary IOP elevation. Aqueous suppressants, including topical beta blockers, apraclonidine, and carbonic anhydrase inhibitors, are useful. Miotics are generally not effective. Treatment for secondary angle closure due to ciliochoroidal effusion is with cycloplegics and aqueous suppressants; miotics are contraindicated in these cases as they may further shallow the anterior chamber, making angle closure worse (76,80,82,83). Surgical intervention should only be used when intact conjunctiva and sclera are present and inflammation is controlled.

GLAUCOMA ASSOCIATED WITH ARTHRITIS AND UVEITIS

Juvenile Rheumatoid Arthritis

Juvenile rheumatoid arthritis (JRA) is the most common disorder associated with uveitis in children. This disorder

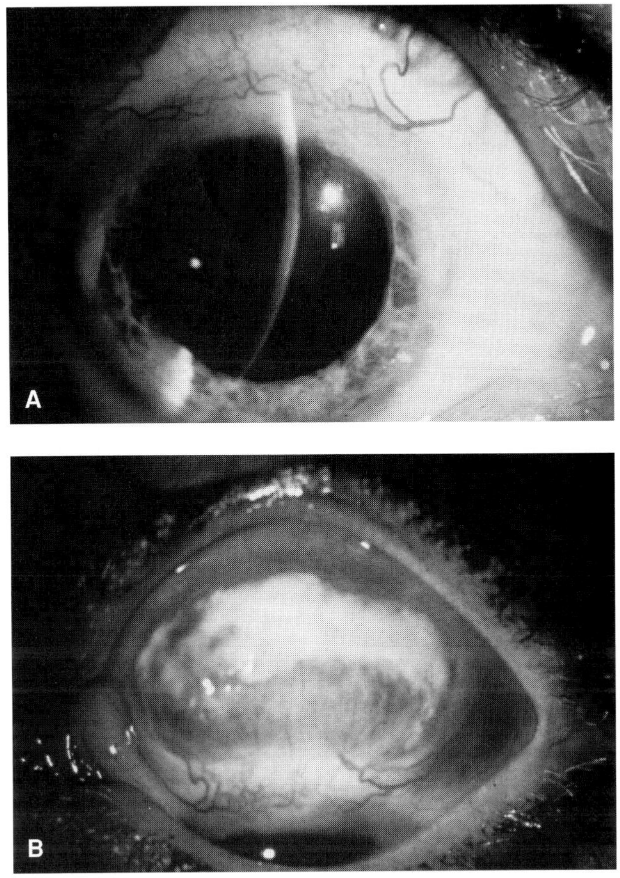

Figure 42.13. Posterior scleritis: Primary gaze (A) and down gaze (B). Glaucoma is usually caused by secondary angle closure from ciliochoroidal effusions. (Courtesy of Glenn J. Jaffe, MD.)

accounts for approximately 70% of all cases of juvenile arthritis. There are three major forms. Systemic onset JRA is associated with fever, generalized lymphadenopathy, hepatosplenomegaly, pericarditis or rash and accounts for 20% of cases. Polyarticular onset JRA affects five or more joints within the first three months. The type of JRA most commonly associated with uveitis is pauciarticular, which affects four or fewer joints that are affected within the first three months. Uveitis occurs rarely in systemic onset JRA, in about 10–15% of those children with polyarticular onset JRA, but in over 75% of those with pauciarticular onset JRA (87,88). For this reason, the patients in this latter group require regular (monthly) follow-up to monitor uveitis control (89,90).

Although JRA is more common in boys, girls appear to have a higher risk of developing uveitis (88). Uveitis is bilateral in over two-thirds of the cases (88,91). Patients with uveitis are usually asymptomatic even when inflammation is marked (Fig. 42.14). The uveitis is typically non-granulomatous in nature. Keratic precipitates are small and frequently confined to the inferior cornea. When inflammation is marked, there may be cells in the anterior vitreous.

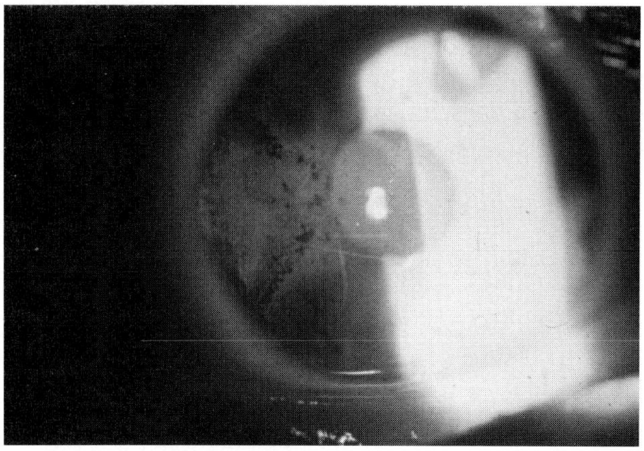

Figure 42.14. Juvenile rheumatoid arthritis: Patient with a long history of anterior uveitis. Note band keratopathy. Patient has had a cataract extraction. Glaucoma in these patients is frequently difficult to control. (Courtesy of Glenn J. Jaffe, MD.)

Secondary glaucoma is a major cause of visual loss in JRA and carries a poor prognosis. In one study, 35% of patients with JRA and secondary glaucoma progressed to no light perception (88). Aqueous suppressants, including carbonic anhydrase inhibitors, are useful in managing glaucoma. Systemic carbonic anhydrase inhibitors should be used with caution in these patients. Carbonic anhydrase inhibitors can produce metabolic acidosis, which is particularly hazardous in patients receiving aspirin (salicylates) for arthritis (92) (see Chapter 70 regarding management of glaucoma in children). Unfortunately, medical management successfully controls no more than 30–50% of these patients. The remainder require surgical intervention.

Because of chronic inflammation and the "vitality" of ocular tissues in young children, the success rate for filtration surgery is poor. Additionally, these patients frequently require cataract surgery, which may affect glaucoma control (93). The adjunctive use of antimetabolites with filtration surgery or setons may prove useful in this population. **Trabeculodialysis,** a modification of goniotomy, has been more successful than traditional filtration surgery in a number of studies (Chapter 70) (94–96). Additionally, **Nd:YAG goniotomy** has been effective in some cases (Chapter 50). Cyclocryotherapy typically reduces IOP only transiently. The role of laser cyclophotocoagulation in this disorder is unclear at this time.

HLA-B27 ASSOCIATED UVEITIS

Individuals with human leukocyte antigen (HLA) B27 are at an increased risk of developing acute anterior uveitis, ankylosing spondylitis, Reiter's syndrome, and juvenile rheumatoid arthritis (97–100). The incidence of acute anterior uveitis in patients with HLA-B27 is between 33 and 88%, depending on the population studied (97,101,102).

Clinically, the uveitis is typically unilateral and self limited. Recurrence is common and is usually in the same eye. Glaucoma may occur secondary to synechia formation or because of steroid treatment.

INFLAMMATORY GLAUCOMA SECONDARY TO VIRAL DISEASES

Herpes Simplex Keratitis and Uveitis

Ocular involvement secondary to herpes simplex virus (HSV) infection includes conjunctivitis, keratitis, and uveitis. **HSV keratouveitis is often accompanied by IOP elevation and secondary glaucoma.** In one study, 28% of patients with ocular HSV developed secondary glaucoma, over 90% of whom had corneal stromal disease (103). Increased IOP is usually related to obstruction of the trabecular meshwork by trabeculitis or inflammatory debris (104,105). Secondary angle closure may occur in cases in which penetrating keratoplasty has been performed. A devastating condition consisting of anterior segment ischemia secondary to chronic keratouveitis has been reported (106). In these cases, glaucoma was secondary to extensive corneoscleral and intraocular inflammation and secondary angle closure. Glaucoma was unresponsive to maximal medical therapy.

Medical therapy for glaucoma when HSV keratouveitis exists consists of aqueous suppressants in conjunction with antiinflammatory and antiviral treatment. Miotics can be tried in cases in which intraocular inflammation is not present, but these agents are frequently ineffective. When medical treatment has failed, glaucoma filtering surgery or seton placement may be successful. In eyes with poor visual potential, laser cyclophotocoagulation may be used.

Herpes Zoster Keratitis and Uveitis

Herpes zoster ophthalmicus involves the ophthalmic division of the fifth cranial nerve. A small proportion (approximately 10%) of cases of general herpes zoster develop ophthalmic manifestations of the disease, including keratitis, iridocyclitis, and secondary glaucoma (107). Of those with keratouveitis, approximately one-third develop elevated IOP (107,108). Ocular involvement typically occurs 1 to 2 weeks after the appearance of the skin lesions. In these cases, the ipsilateral eye demonstrates anterior chamber cells and flare, often with associated keratic precipitates. The precipitates tend to become dark with pigment. The IOP may rise to 30 to 50 mm Hg, with the angle remaining open. Obstruction to aqueous outflow causes glaucoma and it is generally reversible, but the pathogenesis of the obstruction is unknown. Although posterior synechias may develop, formation of peripheral anterior synechias is uncommon. **The stroma of the iris in the affected eye may develop one or more gray atrophic patches which**

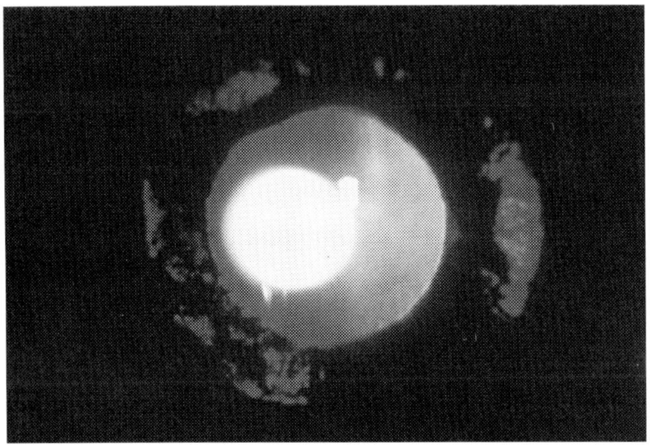

Figure 42.15. Herpes zoster keratouveitis: Note large areas of iris transillumination from iridocyclitis. (Courtesy of Glenn J. Jaffe, MD.)

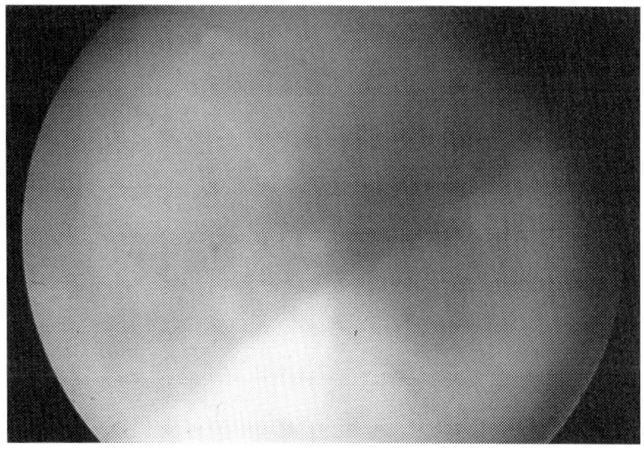

Figure 42.16. Acute retinal necrosis: Note the sharply demarcated gray area of retinal necrosis. The hazy view is caused by associated vitritis. This disorder can produce both open angle and secondary angle closure glaucoma. (Courtesy of Glenn J. Jaffe, MD.)

transilluminate (Fig. 42.15). This presumably results from virus-induced arteritis that causes ischemic necrosis of the iris stroma and posterior pigmented epithelium. Fluorescein iris angiography demonstrates areas of abnormal leakage of iris blood vessels.

Usually there is inconspicuous localized irregularity of the corneal epithelium at the onset of ocular involvement, but later, deep keratitis may develop, and the zoster virus can cause dendritic ulcers resembling those of herpes simplex.

Because of the varied pathology associated with ocular involvement with herpes zoster, treatment can be complex (109). Treatment for uveitis and secondary glaucoma is usually necessary for several months, but it may be required indefinitely. Clinical experience shows that in glaucoma secondary to herpes zoster, miotics should generally be avoided. Corticosteroid eye drops should be used for the inflammation and aqueous suppressants for reduction of IOP. Cycloplegic medications may be useful to relieve ciliary pain and, if significant inflammation exists, to prevent formation of posterior synechia. If, despite maximal medical treatment, the IOP remains high and damaging to the eye, a filtering operation may be required.

Acute Retinal Necrosis

Acute retinal necrosis (ARN) is a clinical syndrome characterized by confluent peripheral necrotizing retinitis in association with retinal arteritis and phlebitis, an optic neuropathy, and vitritis (Fig. 42.16) (110,111). Herpes zoster and herpes simplex types I and II are identified most frequently as the etiologic agent (112,113). Patients may be immunocompromized; however, in many cases no predisposing conditions can be identified (114–116).

Glaucoma has not been reported frequently (117). **Glaucoma, seen by the author, in association with ARN includes both open angle glaucoma in association with mild anterior chamber inflammation and iris bombé with secondary angle closure.** In several cases, despite iris bombé and secondary angle closure, the IOP was normal or low. Presumably, damage to the ciliary body reduced aqueous production in these cases.

The association of glaucoma with herpetic diseases involving primarily the anterior segment is well known; glaucoma in association with posterior segment herpetic disease may be more common than previously thought.

Acquired Immune Deficiency Syndrome (AIDS)

Acquired immune deficiency syndrome is a disorder secondary to HIV infection which is characterized by severe immunocompromise. Patients are subject to opportunistic infections, many of which involve the eye. These include cytomegalovirus, herpes simplex and zoster, syphilis, Toxoplasma gondii, HIV, mycobacterial disease, Pneumocystis carinii, Histoplasma capsulatum, Candida, and others (118,119). Secondary glaucoma can occur in many of these disorders, some of which have been described elsewhere. The most commonly described glaucoma affecting AIDS patients has been **acute bilateral angle closure secondary to choroidal effusion** (120–122). These cases have been treated successfully with cycloplegics, corticosteroids, and aqueous humor suppressants. Miotics exacerbate this form of angle closure and are, therefore, contraindicated. Drainage of suprachoroidal fluid may be required to reverse the angle closure.

Congenital Rubella

Congenital rubella infection within the first trimester of pregnancy is associated with a high incidence of ophthalmic, auditory, cardiac, and a wide variety of other anomalies (123,124). Ocular abnormalities include microphthalmia, cataract, iris stromal atrophy, corneal clouding, and glaucoma. Glaucoma may occur early in life and is frequently associated with cataract and microphthalmia (125,126). Typically, glaucoma occurs within the first few decades of life. In some cases, there are keratic precipitates signaling an inflammatory component to the glaucoma (125). Usually, the anterior chamber shows little evidence of active inflammation and the angle is open to gonioscopy. **In our experience, glaucoma may present with acute elevations of IOP which are controlled initially with intensive medical treatment with aqueous humor suppressants and topical steroids.** These acute exacerbations may be followed by long periods of good IOP control, not unlike that seen in patients with glaucomatocyclitic glaucoma. In most of these patients, control of glaucoma proves increasingly difficult and ultimately requires surgical intervention. **The glaucoma seen in congenital rubella patients is frequently severe and difficult to manage.** In one study, 8 of 15 children were blinded by glaucoma (127).

INFLAMMATORY GLAUCOMA SECONDARY TO BACTERIAL DISEASES

Syphilis and Secondary Glaucoma

Glaucoma is associated most commonly with congenital syphilis in the form of interstitial keratitis and in the adult acquired form of the disease. In rare instances, glaucoma may present in conjunction with acute uveitis in patients with acquired syphilis (Fig. 42.17).

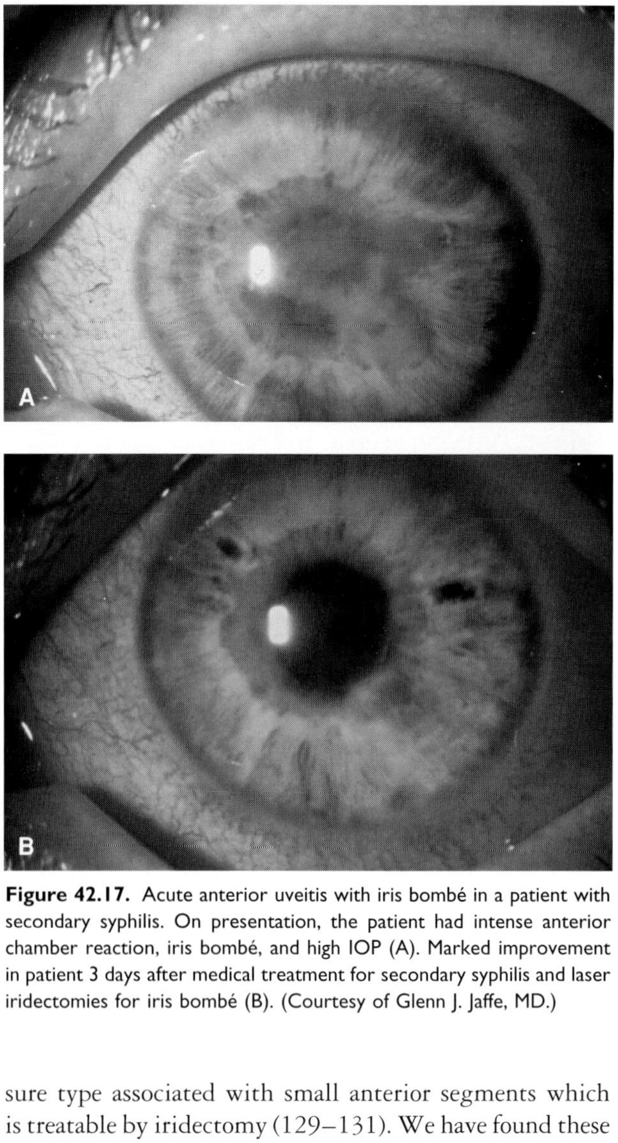

Figure 42.17. Acute anterior uveitis with iris bombé in a patient with secondary syphilis. On presentation, the patient had intense anterior chamber reaction, iris bombé, and high IOP (A). Marked improvement in patient 3 days after medical treatment for secondary syphilis and laser iridectomies for iris bombé (B). (Courtesy of Glenn J. Jaffe, MD.)

EARLY ACUTE SECONDARY GLAUCOMA

Interstitial keratitis occurs in about 15% of cases of congenital syphilis. The onset of symptoms is usually in the first two decades of life and consists of lacrimation and photophobia and is usually bilateral. Vascularization of the deep layers of the cornea, corneal infiltrates, and iridocyclitis are typically present. Glaucoma can develop in congenital syphilis during attacks of acute interstitial keratitis or soon after the inflammation has subsided. With the advent of early diagnosis and treatment of syphilis, patients with acute interstitial keratitis and secondary glaucoma are rare today.

The common sequelae of interstitial keratitis include ghost vessels in the deeper layers of the cornea, peripheral anterior synechias, irregular pigmentation of the open portions of the filtering angle, and chorioretinal atrophy (128). Patients who have had interstitial keratitis in youth commonly have peripheral anterior synechias, usually with no history of glaucoma at the time of the acute disease. The extent of synechial angle closure varies greatly from patient to patient.

Two predominant types of glaucoma occur in patients with old interstitial keratitis: a deep-chamber type superimposed on old inflammatory changes, and an angle-closure type associated with small anterior segments which is treatable by iridectomy (129–131). We have found these two types of glaucoma to be about equal in frequency in a series of patients with a history of interstitial keratitis (128).

DEEP-CHAMBER TYPE OF LATE GLAUCOMA

In patients with the "deep-chamber" type of glaucoma, the axial depth of the anterior chamber tends to be normal, and the iris is flat centrally. There are no signs of active inflammation. In the angle, there are varying amounts of synechias, which appear to be postinflammatory and old. Portions of the angle that are open have a "dirty" appearance. The IOP in most cases is higher, and the facility of aqueous outflow worse, than one would anticipate from the extent of visible synechias. Glaucoma may be present in one or both eyes. Commonly, the optic discs and visual fields are already severely damaged when IOP is discovered to be elevated, but in some eyes the discs and fields show little damage although the IOP is 30 to 40. This suggests that the IOP probably had not been elevated to that degree since childhood and that glaucoma developed, or became exacerbated, in recent years.

In several cases we have documented worsening of the glaucoma without an increase in the extent of peripheral anterior synechias during that time. In most cases of the deep-chamber type of glaucoma there is a poor response to medical treatment, and a filtering operation is required. With modern techniques, the results of filtering operations appear to be as good as in primary open-angle glaucoma.

There is little information on the pathology of this condition, but enough exists to permit us to **postulate that the late-appearing, deep-chamber type of glaucoma that is refractory to medical treatment may be caused by endothelization of open portions of the angle** and by formation of an impermeable membrane (128). Additionally, there have been recent reports of iridoschisis and glaucoma in patients with luetic interstitial keratitis (133,134).

ANGLE-CLOSURE TYPE OF LATE GLAUCOMA

Approximately equally common are patients with a shallow-chamber, angle-closure type of glaucoma that occurs many years after interstitial keratitis. The eyes of these patients characteristically have small anterior segments, possibly as a consequence of the childhood disease. The portions of the angle that are open are subject to reversible closure by forward ballooning of the iris, as in primary angle-closure glaucoma. The onset of angle-closure glaucoma is occasionally acute, but more often is subacute. When the closure is mostly appositional and reversible, peripheral iridectomy is curative. With extensive synechial closure, a filtering operation is indicated.

ACUTE ANTERIOR UVEITIS, LATE SECONDARY GLAUCOMA

We have seen four adult cases of active anterior uveitis with secondary glaucoma in patients who had had interstitial keratitis in youth, with the typical interstitial vessels and peripheral anterior synechias. However, the number of cases is small. There were no other distinguishing features.

Leprosy (Hansen's Disease)

Leprosy remains a significant cause of preventable blindness in developing nations of the world (135). Uveitis is a common finding and a major cause of blindness in those patients with ocular disease (136–138). In one study of treated patients who were institutionalized with leprosy and in whom glaucoma was seen in approximately 10% of those examined, over half of these patients had active uveitis. Uveitis may occur acutely (plastic iridocyclitis) or may be chronic. The iris may have miliary or nodular lepromata (nodules) (139). Treatment with appropriate antimicrobials and antiinflammatory medications may reduce ocular complications (140). Low grade iridocyclitis is common and requires periodic examinations for early detection and treatment (138).

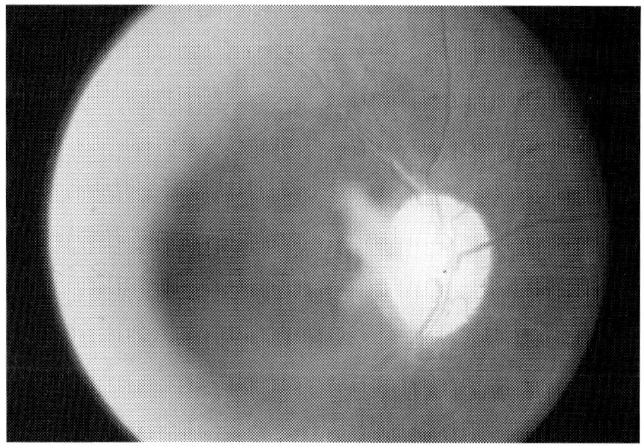

Figure 42.18. Behcet's disease: Optic nerve is pale but not cupped in this patient. Optic atrophy is secondary to vasculitis. (Courtesy of Glenn J. Jaffe, MD.)

MISCELLANEOUS TYPES OF UVEITIS

Behcet's Disease

Behcet's is a multisystem disease characterized by the triad of recurrent iritis and oral and genital ulcerative lesions. It is an immune complex disease which produces an occlusive vasculitis. It is rare in the United States but occurs more commonly in the Middle and Far East. In one report, loss of useful vision occurred in nearly three-fourths of those studied over a period of 10 years (13) (Fig. 42.18). Glaucoma secondary to uveitis, including formation of anterior and posterior synechias, has been reported in approximately 10% of cases (141). If ocular surgery is required, complete preoperative control of inflammation is essential (142).

Coccidioidomycosis

In very rare instances, this infection has resulted in secondary glaucoma in association with anterior segment inflammation and exudate, leading to enucleation (143,144).

Mumps

This infection has been rarely complicated by transient secondary glaucoma in one or both eyes, is associated with redness of the eyes, but shows little or no other sign of iritis (145).

Onchocerciasis

This disease occurs in individuals infected by *Onchocerca volvulus*. Larvae of the nematode are transmitted to humans by the bite of the black fly genus *Simulium*. Onchocerciasis is prevalent throughout much of the Third World. It is complicated by a high incidence of uveitis with frequent chorioretinal disease (146). Severe secondary open-angle glaucoma may also occur in young adults (ages 10 to 40); it is a significant cause of blindness in countries where it is widespread, especially in Africa. Microfilariae may be seen by slitlamp in the anterior chamber, in the aqueous humor, or on the iris (147–149). Community based treatment with ivermectin (microfilaricide) reduces the incidence of ocular manifestations of the disease, including anterior uveitis (150).

Retinal Detachment, Uveitis, and Glaucoma (Schwartz's Syndrome)

In the majority of cases of retinal detachment, IOP is normal or subnormal. (Special forms of glaucoma that sometimes occur after operation for retinal detachment are discussed in Chapter 33.) **In a small percentage of patients with retinal detachment or dialysis, the IOP may become elevated to a moderate or high level in association with a mild anterior chamber reaction.** Local treatment with steroids, cycloplegics, and aqueous suppressants may be of some benefit temporarily, but typically these interventions fail to control the anterior chamber reaction or glaucoma. Interestingly, glaucoma is frequently controlled after successful scleral buckling surgery.

Clinically, this entity may present with a fairly rapid onset of uveitis and glaucoma in one eye. Visual field loss that is not typical for glaucoma, or is observed in the presence of a normal appearing optic nerve, may raise the index of suspicion for this disorder. Even in the absence of a visual field defect, a thorough dilated examination of the peripheral retina may reveal a retinal detachment or retinal dialysis. (A dilated retinal exam is strongly recommended as part of any initial evaluation of a glaucoma patient if only to rule out asymptomatic retinal breaks that need treatment, and which might contraindicate miotic therapy.) In our experience, it is not uncommon for glaucoma to be diagnosed months or years before making the correct diagnosis of retinal detachment with associated glaucoma. This is unfortunate because surgical reattachment of the retina has resulted in prompt and permanent IOP control.

The first mention of this form of anterior segment inflammation and glaucoma was by Shaffer in 1963 (151). In a short paragraph he stated, "Retinal detachment produces flare, cells, and usually a soft eye. Occasionally an extremely resistant form of secondary glaucoma ensues. Typically this condition is caused by a small retinal break with a limited peripheral retinal separation which is easily missed if peripheral fields are not determined. The condition can easily masquerade as chronic iritis with glaucoma. Cure of the detachment often cures the glaucoma." Ariah Schwartz (152) presented 11 cases of severe anterior inflammation with glaucoma in which he found retinal detachment. Approximately half of the cases were secondary to ocular trauma with resultant peripheral retinal dialysis. In each case, when the retina was reattached, the anterior chamber reaction and glaucoma resolved.

It is currently believed that the anterior chamber reaction and the glaucoma in this condition are **secondary to the release of photoreceptor outer segments through the retinal break into the aqueous humor, which then obstruct aqueous outflow pathways** (153–155). Recently, Matsuo has written a review of this unusual disorder (156).

Sympathetic Ophthalmia

This fortunately rare but potentially devastating inflammatory disorder occurs most commonly after penetrating injury to the fellow eye (157). Recently, there have been a number of reports of sympathetic ophthalmia following cyclodestructive treatment (158–160). The pathology is similar to that seen in Vogt-Koyanagi-Harada syndrome, although chorioretinal scarring may be more severe in the latter (161). **Secondary glaucoma occurred in over 40% of cases in one study** (157). Modern immunosuppressive therapy may help reduce the necessity for systemic corticosteroids (162).

Toxocariasis

This disorder commonly presents as a uniocular painless white retinal mass in a child's eye and can be confused with retinoblastoma (Fig. 42.19). Although posterior segment pathology is most common, anterior uveitis may occur (163). In these cases, posterior synechias may cause iris bombé (164).

Toxoplasmosis

Toxoplasmosis is a common cause of vitritis and necrotizing retinitis (Fig. 42.20) (165). Although posterior seg-

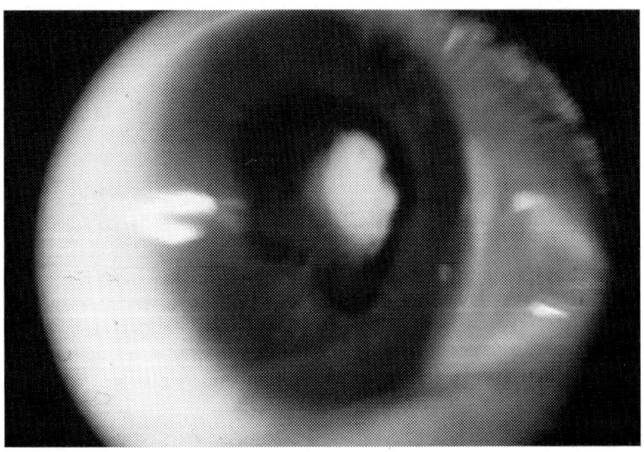

Figure 42.19. Toxocara: This child presented with a posterior segment mass, visible through the pupil. Glaucoma associated with anterior segment inflammation is common in these patients. The angle is usually open. (Courtesy of Glenn J. Jaffe, MD.)

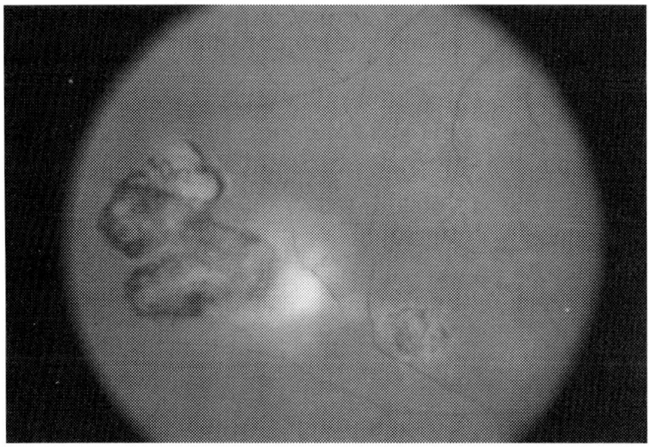

Figure 42.20. Toxoplasmosis: An active retinal lesion adjacent to an old chorioretinal scar. "Spillover" of posterior segment inflammation into the anterior segment frequently causes acute glaucoma. The condition may masquerade as glaucomatocyclitic crisis. Glaucoma usually resolves with successful treatment of the retinitis. (Courtesy of Glenn J. Jaffe, MD.)

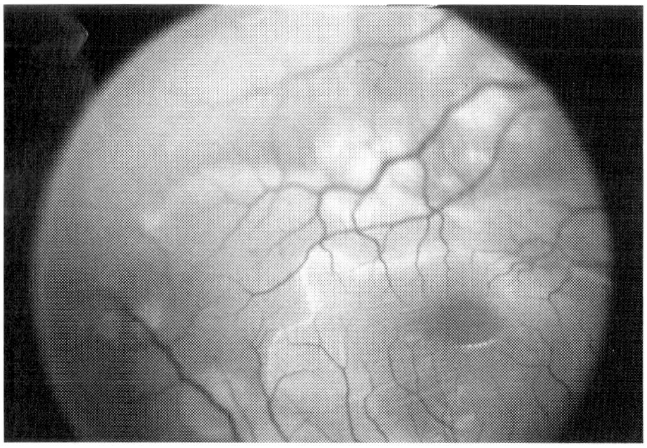

Figure 42.21. Vogt-Koyanagi-Harada syndrome: Exudative retinal detachment, seen here, can produce glaucoma from secondary angle closure. (Courtesy of Glenn J. Jaffe, MD.)

ment involvement is most common, anterior uveitis may occur. Secondary glaucoma is commonly attributed to this disorder, yet few reports exist in the literature (166).

Vogt-Koyanagi-Harada Syndrome

This disease is characterized by alopecia, vitiligo, poliosis, dysacousia, and meningeal irritation. Bilateral posterior uveitis with exudative retinal detachment occurs, and it may be complicated by secondary glaucoma (Fig. 42.21) (167). In one study, glaucoma requiring medical or surgical management was found in 38% of cases (16 of 42) (168). Of those with glaucoma, open angle glaucoma occurred in over half of eyes and angle closure glaucoma was seen in 43%. Surgical management consisting of laser iridectomy, surgical iridectomy, trabeculectomy or seton implantation was required in over two-thirds of cases. Glaucoma is often secondary to forward displacement of the lens-iris diaphragm, causing angle-closure glaucoma, which may be acute and cause extensive peripheral anterior synechias to form (169–171). Treatment with systemic corticosteroids is frequently effective (172). Cycloplegics and aqueous suppressants may be useful adjuncts.

References

1. Chiang YD, Thomas RP: Ocular hypertension following intravenous infusion of prostaglandin E_1. Arch Ophthalmol 1972;88:418.
2. Chiang TS, Thomas RP: Consensual ocular hypertensive response to prostaglandin E_2. Invest Ophthalmol Vis Sci 1972;11:845.
3. Kass MA, Podos SM, Moses RA, et al: Prostaglandin E_1 and aqueous humor dynamics. Invest Ophthalmol Vis Sci 1972;11:1022.
4. Podos SM, Becker B, Kass MA: Prostaglandin synthesis, inhibition, and intraocular pressure. Invest Ophthalmol Vis Sci 1973;12:426.
5. Bengtsson E: The effect of theophylline on the breakdown of the blood-aqueous barrier in the rabbit eye. Invest Ophthalmol Vis Sci 16:636, 1977.
6. Roth M, Simmons RJ: Glaucoma associated with precipitates on the trabecular meshwork. Ophthalmology 1979;86:1613.
7. Epstein DL, Hashimoto J, Grant WM: Serum obstruction of aqueous outflow in enucleated human eyes. Am J Ophthalmol 1978;86: 101–105.
8. Freddo TF, Patterson MM, Scott DR, et al: Influence of mercurial sulfhydryl agents on aqueous humor outflow pathways in enucleated eyes. Invest Ophthalmol Vis Sci 1984;25:278–285.
9. Koskela T, Brubaker RF: Apraclonidine and timolol. Combined effects in previously untreated normal subjects. Arch Ophthalmol Vis Sci 1991;109(6):804–806.
10. Gharagozloo NZ, Brubaker RF: Effect of apraclonidine in long-term timolol users. Ophthalmology 1991;98(10):1543–1546.
11. Wong VG, Hersch EM: Methotrexate in the therapy of cyclitis. Trans Am Acad Ophthalmol Otolaryngol 1965;69:279.
12. Andrasch RH, Pirofsky B, Burns RP: Immunosuppressive therapy for severe chronic uveitis. Arch Ophthalmol Vis Sci 1978;96:247.
13. Benezra D, Cohen E: Treatment and visual prognosis in Behcet's disease. Br J Ophthalmol 1986;70:589.
14. Svenson K, Bohman SO, Hallgren R: Renal interstitial fibrosis and vascular changes. Occurrence in patients with autoimmune diseases treated with cyclosporine. Arch Intern Med 1986;146:(10): 2007–2010.
15. Bhattacherjee P, Paterson CA: Studies on prostanoid receptors in ocular tissues. J Ocul Pharmacol 1994;10(1):167–175.
16. de Vos AF, Hoekzema R, Kijlstra A: Cytokines and uveitis. Curr Eye Res 1992;11:581–597.
17. de Vos AF, Klaren VNA, Kijlstra A: Expression of multiple cytokines and interleukin-1 receptor antagonist in the uvea and retina during endotoxin-induced uveitis in the rat. Invest Ophthalmol Vis Sci 1994; 35:3873–3883.
18. Malecaze F, Chollet P, Cavrois E, et al: Role of interleukin 6 in the inflammatory response after cataract surgery. An experimental and clinical study. Arch Ophthalmol Vis Sci 1991;109:1681–1683.
19. Srinivasan BD, Kulkarni PS: The role of arachidonic acid metabolites in the mediation of the polymorphonuclear leukocyte response following corneal injury. Invest Ophthalmol Vis Sci 1980;19:1087–1093.
20. Li Q, Fujino Y, Caspi RR, et al: Association between mast cells and the development of experimental autoimmune uveitis in different rat strains. Clin Immunol Immunopathol 1992;65:294–299.
21. Wakefield D, Lloyd A: The role of cytokines in the pathogenesis of inflammatory eye disease. Cytokine 1992;4(1):1–5.
22. Weiner HL, Friedman A, Miller A, et al: Oral tolerance: immunologic mechanisms and treatment of animal and human organ-specific autoimmune diseases by oral administration of autoantigens. Annu Rev Immunol 1994;12:809–837.

23. Li Q, Lopez JS, Caspi RR, et al: Suppression of S-antigen-induced experimental autoimmune uveoretinitis in Lewis rats by oral administration with CGS-13080, a thromboxane synthetase inhibitor. Exp Eye Res 1993;57:601–608.
24. Woodward DF, Lawrence RA, Fairbairn CE, et al: Intraocular pressure effects of selective prostanoid receptor agonists involve different receptor subtypes according to radioligand binding studies. J Lipid Mediat 1993;6(1-3):545–553.
25. Bito LZ, Stjernschantz J, Resul B, et al: The ocular effects of prostaglandins and the therapeutic potential of a new PGF2 alpha analog, PhXA41 (latanoprost), for glaucoma management. J Lipid Mediat 1993;6(1-3):535–543.
26. Schuman JS, Bellows AR, Shingleton BJ, et al: Contact transscleral continuous wave neodymium:YAG laser cyclophotocoagulation. Midterm results. Ophthalmology 1992;99:1089–1094.
27. Hampton C, Shields MB, Miller KN, Blasini M: Evaluation of a protocol for transscleral neodymium: YAG cyclophotocoagulation in one hundred patients. Ophthalmology 1990;97(7):910–917.
28. Hennis HL, Stewart WC: Semiconductor diode laser transscleral cyclophotocoagulation in patients with glaucoma. Am J Ophthalmol 1992; 113(1):81–85.
29. Hawkins TA, Stewart WC: One-year results of semiconductor transscleral cyclophotocoagulation in patients with glaucoma. Arch Ophthalmol 1993;111(4):488–491.
30. Akova YA, Foster CS: Cataract surgery in patients with sarcoidosis-associated uveitis. Ophthalmology 1994;101(3):473–479.
31. Jampel HD, Jabs DA, Quigley HA: Trabeculectomy with 5-fluorouracil for adult inflammatory glaucoma. Am J Ophthalmol 1990;109: 168.
32. Smith MF, Sherwood MB, Doyle JW, et al: Results of intraoperative 5-fluorouracil supplementation on trabeculectomy for open-angle glaucoma. Am J Ophthalmol 1992;114(6):737–741.
33. Jones NP. Glaucoma in Fuchs' heterochromic uveitis: aetiology, management and outcome. Eye 1991;6:662–667.
34. Ophir A, Ticho U: Treatment of anterior uveitis with 5-fluorouracil. Harefuah 1992;122(1):21–23.
35. Smith MF, Sherwood MB, McGorray SP. Comparison of the double-plate Molteno drainage implant with the Schocket procedure. Arch Ophthalmol 1992;110(9):1246–1250.
36. Freedman J, Rubin B: Molteno implants as a treatment for refractory glaucoma in black patients. Arch Ophthalmol 1991;109 (10): 1417–1420.
37. Lloyd MA, Baerveldt G, Fellenbaum PS, et al: Intermediate-term results of a randomized clinical trial of the 350-versus the 500mm2 Baerveldt implant. Ophthalmology 1994;101(8):1456–1463.
38. Hill RA, Nguyen QH, Baerveldt G, et al: Trabeculectomy and Molteno implantation for glaucomas associated with uveitis. Ophthalmology 1993;100(6):903–908.
39. Posner A, Schlossman A: Syndrome of unilateral recurrent attacks of glaucoma with cyclitic symptoms. Arch Ophthalmol 1953;39: 517–535.
40. Mattson R. Ueber glaukomatozylklitische Krissen. Acta Ophthalmol Vis Sci 1954;32:523–533.
41. Hung PT, Chang JM: Treatment of glaucomatocyclitic crises. Am J Ophthalmol 1974;77:169–172.
42. Kass MA, Becker B, Kolker AE: Glaucomatocyclitic crisis and primary open-angle glaucoma. Am J Ophthalmol 1973;75:668–673.
43. Raitta C, Vannas A: Glaucomatocyclitic crisis. Arch Ophthalmol 1977; 95:608–612.
44. Bloch-Michael E. Fuchs' heterochromic cyclitis: current concepts. J Fr Ophtalmol 1983;6(10):853–858.
45. La Hey E, Baarsma GS, De Vries J, et al: Clinical analysis of Fuchs' heterochromic cyclitis. Doc Ophthalmol 1991;78(3-4):225–235.
46. Franceschetti A. Heterochromic cyclitis (Fuchs' syndrome). Am J Ophthalmol 1995;39:50.
47. Kimura SJ, Hogan MJ, Thygeson P: Fuchs' syndrome of heterochromic cyclitis. Arch Ophthalmol 1955;54:179.
48. Franceschetti A. Heterochromic cyclitis (Fuchs' syndrome). Am J Ophthalmol 1955;39:50–58.
49. Wobmann P. Die Heterochromiecyclitis Fuchs. Graefes Arch Ophthalmol 1976;199:167–178.
50. Saari M, Vuorre I, Nieminen H: Infra-red transillumination stereophotography of the iris in Fuchs's heterochromic cyclitis. Br J Ophthalmol 1978;62:110.
51. Regenbogen LS, Naveh-Floman N: Glaucoma in Fuchs' heterochromic cyclitis associated with congenital Horner's syndrome. Br J Ophthalmol 1987;71:844.
52. Tabbut BR, Tessler HH, Williams D: Fuchs' heterochromic iridocyclitis in blacks. Arch Ophthalmol 1988;106:1688.
53. Arffa RC, Schlaegel TF, Jr. Chorioretinal scars in Fuchs' heterochromic iridocyclitis. Arch Ophthalmol 1984;102(8):1153–1155.
54. Liesegang TJ. Clinical features and prognosis in Fuchs' uveitis syndrome. Arch Ophthalmol 1982;100:1622.
55. Daus W, Kraus-Mackiw E. Fuchs' heterochromic cyclitis. Case reports of patients treated at Heidelberg University Eye Hospital since 1978. Klin Monatsbl Augenheilkd 1984;185:410.
56. La Hey E, DeVries J, Langerhorst CT, et al: Treatment and prognosis of secondary glaucoma in Fuchs' heterochromic iridocyclitis. Am J Ophthalmol 1993;116(3):327–340.
57. Jones NP. Glaucoma in Fuchs' heterochromic uveitis: aetiology, management and outcome. Eye 1991;5(6):662–667.
58. Jones NP. Fuchs' heterochromic uveitis: an update. Surv Ophthalmol 1993;37(4):253–272.
59. Liesegang TJ. Clinical features and prognosis in Fuchs' uveitis syndrome. Arch Ophthalmol 1982;100(10):1622–1626.
60. Huber A. Das Glaukom bei komplizierter heterochromie Fuchs. Ophthalmologica 1961;141:122–135.
61. François J. Nouvelle contribution à l'hétérochromie de Fuchs. Bull Soc Belge Ophtalmol 1952;102:607–624.
62. François J, Beheyt J. Hétérochromie de Fuchs bilatérale. Ann Ocul (Paris) 1955;188:55–63.
63. Perry HD, Yanoff M, Scheie HG: Rubeosis in Fuchs heterochromic iridocyclitis. Arch Ophthalmol 1975;93:337.
64. Benedikt O, Roll P, Zirm M: The glaucoma in heterochromic cyclitis Fuchs. Gonioscopic studies and electron microscopic investigations of the trabecular meshwork. Klin Monatsbl Augenheilkd 1978;173(4): 523–533.
65. Chandler PA, Grant WM: Lectures on glaucoma. Philadelphia: Lea & Febiger, 1954:257.
66. Callen JP, Mahl CF: Oculocutaneous manifestations observed in multisystem disorders. Dermatol Clin 1992;10(4):709–716.
67. Muthiah MM, Macfarlane JT: Current concepts in the management of sarcoidosis. Drugs 1990;40(2):231–237.
68. Obenauf CD, Shaw HE, Sydnor CF, Klintworth GK: Sarcoidosis and its ophthalmic manifestations. Am J Ophthalmol 1978;86:648.
69. Karma A: Diagnostic aspects of ocular sarcoidosis. Sarcoidosis 1994; 11(1):58:60.
70. Ohara K, Okubo A, Sasaki H, Kamata K: Intraocular manifestations of systemic sarcoidosis. Jpn J Ophthalmol 1992;36(4):452–457.
71. Ohara K: Clinical manifestations of ocular sarcoidosis in Japanese patients. Nippon Rinsho 1994;52(6):1577–1581.
72. Kenyon KR, Pederson JE, Green WR, et al: Fibroglial proliferation in pars planitis. Trans Ophthalmol Soc UK 1975;95:391–397.
73. Smith RE, Godfrey WA, Kimura SJ: Complications of chronic cyclitis. Am J Ophthalmol 1976;82:277–282.
74. Henderly DE, Genstler AJ, Rao NA, et al: Pars planitis. Trans Ophthal Soc UK 1986;105:227.
75. Wilhelmus KR, Grierson I, Watson PG: Histopathologic and clinical associations of scleritis and glaucoma. Am J Ophthalmol 1981;91(6): 697–705.
76. Pavlin CJ, Easterbrook M, Harasiewicz K, et al: An ultrasound biomi-

croscopic analysis of angle-closure glaucoma secondary to ciliochoroidal effusion in IgA nephropathy. Am J Ophthalmol 1993;116(3): 341–345.

77. Bacon AS, Frazer DG, Dart JK, et al: A review of 72 consecutive cases of Acanthamoeba keratitis. Eye 1993;7(6):719–725.
78. Wagemans MA, Bos PJ: Angle-closure glaucoma in a patient with systemic lupus erythematosus. Doc Ophthalmol 1989;72(3-4): 201–207.
79. Sainz de la Maza M, Foster CS, Jabbur NS: Scleritis associated with rheumatoid arthritis and with other systemic immune-mediated diseases. Ophthalmology 1994;101(7):1281–1286, discussion 1287–1288.
80. Benson WE: Posterior scleritis. Surv Ophthalmol 1988;32 (5): 297–316.
81. Watson PG, Hayreh SS: Scleritis and episcleritis. Br J Ophthalmol 1976;60:163–191.
82. Quinlan MP, Hitchings RA. Angle-closure glaucoma secondary to posterior scleritis. Br J Ophthalmol 1978;62(5):330–335.
83. Fourman S. Angle-closure glaucoma complicating ciliochoroidal detachment. Ophthalmology 1989;96(5):646–653.
84. Lloyd-Jones D, Tokarewicz A, Watson PG: Clinical evaluation of clobetasone butyrate eye drops in episcleritis. Br J Ophthalmol 1981;65: 641.
85. Watson PG, McKay DA, Clemett RS, et al: Treatment of episcleritis: a double blind trial comparing beta-methasone 0.1%, oxyphenbutazone 10% and placebo eye ointments. Br J Ophthalmol 1973;57:866.
86. McGavin DDM, Williamson J, Forrester JV, et al: Episcleritis and scleritis. A study of their clinical manifestations and association with rheumatoid arthritis. Br J Ophthalmol 1976;60:192.
87. Chylack LT Jr, Bienfang DC, Bellows R, et al: Ocular manifestations of juvenile rheumatoid arthritis. Am J Ophthalmol 1975;79:1026–1033.
88. Kanski JJ, Shun-Shin GA: Systemic uveitis syndromes in childhood: An analysis of 340 cases. Ophthalmology 1984;91:1147–1151.
89. Chung YM, Yeh TS, Liu JH: Clinical manifestations of HLA-B27-positive acute anterior uveitis in Chinese. Chung Hua I Hsueh Tsa Chih (Taipei) 1989;43(2):97–104.
90. Petty RE: Ocular complications of rheumatic diseases of childhood. Clin Orthop 1990:(259):51–59.
91. Kanski JJ: Uveitis in juvenile chronic arthritis: incidence, clinical features and prognosis. Eye 1988;2:641–645.
92. Cowan RA, Hartnell GG, Lowdell CP, et al: Metabolic acidosis induced by carbonic anhydrase inhibitors in patients with normal renal function. Br Med J 1984;289:347–348.
93. Fox GM, Flynn HW Jr, Davis JL, et al: Causes of reduced visual acuity on long-term follow-up after cataract extraction in patients with uveitis and juvenile rheumatoid arthritis. Am J Ophthalmol 1992;114(6): 708–714.
94. Hass J: Goniotomy in aphakia. In: Welsh RC, ed. The Second Report on Cataract Surgery, Proceedings of the Second-Biennial Cataract Surgery Congress. Miami, Miami Educational Press, 1971:551–554.
95. Kanski JJ, Crick MDP: Trabeculodialysis for inflammatory glaucoma in children and young adults. Ophthalmology 1985;92:927–929.
96. Hoskins HD Jr, Hetherington J Jr, and Shaffer RN: Surgical management of inflammatory glaucoma. Perspect Ophthalmol 1977;1: 173–181.
97. Brewerton DA, Caffrey M, Nicholls A, et al: Acute anterior uveitis and HLA 27. Lancet 1973;i:994–996.
98. Brewerton DA: The histocompatibility antigen (HLA-27) and acute anterior uveitis. Trans Ophthalmol Soc UK 1974;94:735–741.
99. Nicholls A: Reiter's disease and HLA-B27. Ann Rheum Dis 34 1975; (suppl):27–28.
100. Ansell BM: Chronic arthritis in childhood. Ann Rheum Dis 1978;37: 107–120.
101. Derhaag PJRM, Linssen A, Broekema N, et al: A familial study of the inheritance of HLA-B27 anterior uveitis. Am J Ophthalmol 1988;105: 603–606.
102. Toivanen A, Granstors K, Lahesmaa-Rantala R, et al: Pathogenesis of Yersinia-triggered reactive arthritis: immunological microbiological and clinical aspects. Immunol Rev 1985;86:47–70.
103. Falcon MG, Williams HP: Herpes simplex kerato-uveitis and glaucoma. Trans Ophthal Soc UK 1978;98:101.
104. Hogan MJ, Kimura SJ, Thygeson P: Pathology of herpes simplex keratitis. Trans Am Ophthalmol 1963;Soc 61:75.
105. Townsend WM, Kaufman HE: Pathogenesis of glaucoma and endothelial changes in herpetic kerato-uveitis in rabbits. Am J Ophthalmol 1971;71:904.
106. Johns KJ, O'Day DM, Webb RA, et al: Anterior segment ischemia in chronic herpes simplex keratouveitis. Curr Eye Res (Suppl) 1991;10: 117–124.
107. Nigam P, Kumar A, Kapoor KK, et al: Clinical profile of herpes zoster ophthalmicus. J Indian Med Assoc 1991;89(5):117–119.
108. Jampel HD, Jabs DA, Quigley HA: Trabeculectomy with 5-fluorouracil for adult inflammatory glaucoma. Am J Ophthalmol 1990;109: 168.
109. Harding SP: Management of ophthalmic zoster. J Med Virol (Suppl) 1993;1:97–101.
110. Uryama A, et al: Unilateral acute uveitis with retinal periarteritis and detachment. Jpn J Clin Ophthalmol 1971;25:607–619.
111. Wilkerson D, Aaberg TM, Reeser FH: Necrotizing vaso-occlusive retinitis. Am J Ophthalmol 1977;84:209–219.
112. Culbertson WW, Blumenkranz, Pepose JS, et al: Varicella zoster virus is a cause of the acute retinal necrosis syndrome. Ophthalmology 1986; 93(5):559–569.
113. Schulman JA, Peyman GA: Management of viral retinitis. Ophthalmic Surg 1988;19(12):876–884.
114. Fisher JP, Lewis ML, Blumenkranz M, et al: The ARN syndrome. Part 1: Clinical manifestations. Ophthalmology 1982;89:1309–1316.
115. Gorman BD, Nadel AJ, Coles RS: Acute retinal necrosis. Ophthalmology 1982;89:809–814.
116. Duker JS, Blumenkranz MS: Diagnosis and management of the acute retinal necrosis (ARN) syndrome. Surv Ophthalmol 1991;35(5): 327–343.
117. Kalman A, Vogt M, Bernasconi E, et al: Bilateral acute retinal artery necrosis—healing of the second affected eye. Klin Monatsbl Augenheilkd 1994;204(4):235–240.
118. Blumenkranz MS, Penneys NS: Acquired immunodeficiency syndrome and the eye. Dermatol Clin 1992;10(4):777–783.
119. Rao NA: Acquired immunodeficiency syndrome and its ocular complications. Indian J Ophthalmol 1994;42(2):51–63.
120. Ullman S, Wilson RP, Schwartz L: Bilateral angle-closure glaucoma in association with the acquired immune deficiency syndrome. Am J Ophthalmol 1986;101(4):419–424.
121. Meige P, Cohen H, Morin B, et al: Acute bilateral glaucoma in an LAV-positive subject. Bull Soc Ophtalmol Fr 1989;89(3):449–454.
122. Nash RW, Lindquist TD: Bilateral angle-closure glaucoma associated with uveal effusion: presenting sign of HIV infection. Surv Ophthalmol 36 1992;(4):255–258.
123. Freij BJ, South MA, Sever JL: Maternal rubella and the congenital rubella syndrome. Clin Perinatol 1988;15(2):247–257.
124. Sever JL, South MA, Shaver KA: Delayed manifestations of congenital rubella. Rev Infect Dis (Suppl) 1985;7(1):S164–S169.
125. Boger WP: Late ocular complications in congenital rubella syndrome. Ophthalmology 1980;87(12):1244–1252.
126. Givens KT, Lee DA, Jones T, et al: Congenital rubella syndrome: ophthalmic manifestations and associated systemic disorders. Br J Ophthalmol 1993;77(6):358–363.
127. Sundmacher R, Neumann-Haefelin D: Herpes simplex virus isolations from the aqueous of patients suffering from focal iritis, endotheliitis, and prolonged disciform keratitis with glaucoma. Klin Monatsbl Augenheilkd 1979;175:488.
128. Grant WM: Late glaucoma after interstitial keratitis. Am J Ophthalmol 1975;79:87.

129. Knox DL: Glaucoma following syphilitic interstitial keratitis. Arch Ophthalmol 1961;64:44.
130. Sugar HS: Late glaucoma associated with inactive syphilitic interstitial keratitis. Am J Ophthalmol 1962;53:602.
131. Tsukahara S: Secondary glaucoma due to inactive congenital syphilitic interstitial keratitis. Ophthalmologica 1977;174:188.
132. Lichter PR, Shaffer RN: Interstitial keratitis and glaucoma. Amer J Ophthalmol 1969;68:241–248.
133. Salvador F, Linares F, Merita I, et al: Unilateral iridoschisis associated with syphilitic interstitial keratitis and glaucoma. Ann Ophthalmol 1993;25(9):328–329.
134. Foss AJ, Hykin PG, Benjamin L: Intersitial keratitis and iridoschisis in congenital syphilis. J Clin Neuroophthalmol 1992;12 (3):167–170.
135. Stilma JS, Franken S, Hogeweg M, Hardus P: Points of action in the campaign against blindness in developing countries. Doc Ophthalmol 1991;78(3-4):285–305.
136. Reddy SC, Raju BD, Achary NR: Survey of eye complications in leprosy in Prakasam District (Andhra Pradesh). Lepr India 1981;53(2): 231–237.
137. Kagame GK: Ocular leprosy in Africa. Soc Sci Med 1983;17(22): 1737–1742.
138. Espiritu CG, Gelber R, Ostler HB; Chronic anterior uveitis in leprosy: an insidious cause of blindness. Br J Ophthalmol 1991;75(5):273–275.
139. Michelson JB, Roth AM, Waring GO III: Lepromatous iridocyclitis diagnosed by anterior chamber paracentesis. Am J Ophthalmol 1979; 88:674.
140. Spaide R, Nattis R, Lipka A, et al: Ocular findings in leprosy in the United States. Am J Ophthalmol 1985;100:411
141. Mishima S, Masuda K, Izawa Y, et al: Behçet's disease in Japan. Ophthalmologic aspects. Trans Am Ophthalmol Soc 1979;77:225.
142. Foster CS, Fong LP, Singh G: Cataract surgery and intraocular lens implantation in patients with uveitis. Ophthalmology 1988;96:281.
143. Pettit TH, Learn RN, Foos RY: Intraocular coccidioidomycosis. Arch Ophthalmol 1967;77:655–661.
144. Bell R, Font RL: Granulomatous anterior uveitis caused by coccidioides immitis. Am J Ophthalmol 1972;74:93–98.
145. Polland W, Thorburn W: Transient glaucoma as a manifestation of mumps. Acta Ophthalmol 1976;54:779–782.
146. Newland HS, White AT, Greene BM, et al: Ocular manifestations of onchocerciasis in a rain forest area of West Africa. Br J Ophthalmol 1991;75 (3):163–169.
147. Ben-Sira I, Yassur Y: Ocular onchocerciasis in Malawi. Br J Ophthalmol 1972;56:617–620.
148. Berghout E: Onchocerciasis and glaucoma in the forest area of Ghana. Trop Geogr Med 1973;25:233–237.
149. Langham ME, Frentzel-Beyme RR, Traub ZD: Intraocular pressure and onchocerciasis infection in Liberia. Ophthalmic Res 1975;7:368–380.
150. Somo RM, Ngosso A, Dinga JS, et al: A community-based trial of ivermectin for onchocerciasis control in the forest of southwestern Cameroon: clinical and parasitologic findings after three treatments. Am J Trop Med Hyg 1993;48(1):9–13.
151. Shaffer RN: Glaucoma in uveitis. In Ocular Pharmacology and Therapeutics and the Problems of Medical Management. Philadelphia, FA Davis Co., 1963.
152. Schwartz A: Chronic open-angle glaucoma secondary to rhegmatogenous retinal detachment. Trans Am Ophthalmol Soc 70:178-189, 1972. Am J Ophthalmol 1973;75:205–211.
153. Matsuo N, Takabatake M, Ueno H, et al: Photoreceptor outer segments in the aqueous humor in rhegmatogenous retinal detachment. Am J Ophthalmol 1986;101(6):673–679.
154. Lambrou FH, Vela MA, Woods W: Obstruction of the trabecular meshwork by retinal rod outer segments. Arch Ophthalmol 1989;107(5): 742–745.
155. Netland PA, Mukai S, Covington HI: Elevated intraocular pressure secondary to rhegmatogenous retinal detachment. Clinical Pathological Review 1994;39(3):234–240.
156. Matsuo T: Photoreceptor outer segments in aqueous humor: key to understanding a new syndrome. Surv Ophthalmol 1994;39(3): 211–233.
157. Lubin JR, Albert DM, Weinstein M: Sixty-five years of sympathetic ophthalmia. A clinicopathologic review of 105 cases (1913-1978). Ophthalmology 1980;87:109.
158. Edward DP, Brown SV, Higginbotham E, et al: Sympathetic ophthalmia following neodymium:YAG cyclotherapy. Ophthalmic Surg 1989; 20(8):544–546.
159. Lam S, Tessler HH, Lam BL, et al: High incidence of sympathetic ophthalmia after contact and noncontact neodymium:YAG cyclotherapy. Ophthalmology 1992;99(12):1818–1822.
160. Sabates R: Choroiditis compatible with the histopathologic diagnosis of sympathetic ophthalmia following cyclocryotherapy of neovascular glaucoma. Ophthalmic Surg 1988;19(3):176–182.
161. Marak GE Jr: Recent advances in sympathetic ophthalmia. Surv Ophthalmol 1979;24:141.
162. Hakin KN, Pearson RV, Lightman SL: Sympathetic ophthalmia: visual results with modern immunosuppressive therapy. Eye 1992;6(5): 453–455.
163. Smith PH, Greer CH: Unusual presentation of ocular toxocara infestation. Br J Ophthalmol 1971;55:317–320.
164. Shields JA: Ocular toxocariasis. A review. Surv Ophthalmol 1984;28: 361.
165. Perkins ES: Ocular toxoplasmosis. Br J Ophthalmol 1973;57:1.
166. O'Connor GR: Manifestations and management of ocular toxoplasmosis. Bull NY Acad Med 1974;50(2):192.
167. Ohno S, Char DH, Kimura SJ, et al: Vogt-Koyanagi-Harada syndrome. Am J Ophthalmol 1977;83:735–740.
168. Forster DJ, Rao NA, Hill RA, et al: Incidence and management of glaucoma in Vogt-Koyanagi-Harada syndrome. Ophthalmology 1993; 100(5):613–618.
169. Kimura R, Suzuki A, Maekawa N: Four cases of secondary angle closure glaucoma caused by Harada's disease. Jpn J Clin Ophthalmol 1972; 26:827–830.
170. Lugossy G: Le syndrome de Vogt-Koyanagi-Harada et la cortisone. Bull Soc Fr Ophtalmol 1975;87:44–46.
171. Perry HD, Font RL: Clinical and histopathologic observations in severe Vogt-Koyanagi-Harada syndrome. Am J Ophthalmol 1977;83: 242–254.
172. Shirato S, Hayashi K, Masuda K: Acute angle closure glaucoma as an initial sign of Harada's disease: report of two cases. Jap J Ophthalmol 1980;24:260.

Glaucoma Due to Trauma

43

Bradford J. Shingleton

INTRODUCTION

Glaucoma due to trauma is a multi-factorial disease. Intraocular pressure (IOP) may increase after blunt trauma, lacerating trauma, chemical exposure, electromagnetic radiation, or surgery. Elevated IOP may develop immediately after the injury or years later. The angle may be open or closed. The injured eye may demonstrate obvious signs of damage or clinical signs of trauma may be largely inapparent. Eyes that are predisposed to glaucoma after ocular injury may actually have a low IOP initially, rather than a high IOP. Low IOP may result from aqueous hyposecretion due to ciliary contusion and inflammation, increased uveoscleral/vortex outflow due to a cyclodialysis cleft, tears through trabecular meshwork into Schlemm's canal, or loss of integrity of the globe due to scleral or corneal perforation (Table 43.1). Low IOP can often convert to high IOP as a result of treatment, normal healing processes and the long-lasting effect of the injury itself on trabecular meshwork outflow. Elevated IOP has multiple causes, but they all tend to reflect a reduced facility of outflow of aqueous humor through the trabecular meshwork drainage channels (1) (Table 43.2).

Injuries to the anterior segment, which cause glaucoma, most commonly follow blunt injury. The impact from the blunt injury results in a sudden compressive deformation of the eye. The cornea and anterior sclera are displaced posteriorly and there is a compensatory expansion of the globe in the equatorial direction (2). Campbell (3) has graphically described seven rings, or circles of tissue, anterior to the equator of the globe that suddenly expand with blunt impact. Because the internal fluids of the eye cannot compress, the forces are transmitted to the seven rings of tissue. This often results in splitting or tearing of tissues which may manifest as radial sphincter tears, iridodialysis, angle recession, cyclodialysis, trabecular meshwork tears, zonule separation, or peripheral retinal dialysis. Damage in many of these areas may result in both early onset or delayed onset glaucoma.

EARLY ONSET GLAUCOMA AFTER EYE INJURY

Contusion with Intraocular Inflammation

Blunt trauma commonly results in inflammation of the anterior segment visualized as flare and cells at the slit lamp. Red blood cells and gross angle disruption are often not identified, but IOP may still be elevated. The elevation of IOP in this setting is presumably due to reduced aqueous outflow, as a result of inflammatory cells and debris obstructing trabecular meshwork outflow channels. Edema and direct damage to trabecular meshwork beams may not be identified on gonioscopy, but may still contribute to a temporary rise in IOP. This situation tends to be self-limited and clears spontaneously or with the use of topical steroids.

Trabecular Meshwork Damage

Herschler has shown that gonioscopy early after blunt injury may demonstrate trauma-related changes in the trabecular zone (4). A full-thickness tear in trabecular meshwork may occur and a trabecular flap may be created at the point of rupture. This tends to arise just below the insertion of the trabecular sheets at Schwalbe's line. Inflammation is invariably associated with this type of injury. IOP may or may not be elevated, depending on the amount of aqueous production. Indeed, **IOP may actually be subnormal in the early peritraumatic period, due to direct access of aqueous to Schlemm's canal, bypassing the trabecular meshwork.** A small clot may be noted in the area of trabecular meshwork tears due to bleeding from Schlemm's canal. Healed trabecular meshwork tears are difficult to see, as gonioscopy is more commonly performed at a time remote from the injury. If IOP elevation develops at a later time, it is probably associated with more extensive angle recession.

Traumatic Hyphema

Significant bleeding in the anterior chamber associated with blunt ocular trauma increases the chance for elevation of IOP. The IOP may be elevated due to all the factors noted under contusion injury and trabecular meshwork damage as well as red blood cell obstruction of the outflow pathway.

Moderate IOP elevation up to 10 mm Hg above baseline may occur in as many as 30% of patients with traumatic hyphema (5). Because the vast majority of these patients have healthy optic nerves, they can tolerate an elevation of IOP for a moderate period of time. The elevation tends to be self-limited and clears as the blood cells are normally processed through the aqueous drainage channels. A given

Table 43.1
Low Intraocular Pressure After Trauma

IOP after trauma may be *low*
Aqueous hyposecretion due to ciliary body contusion
Increased uveoscleral/vortex outflow due to cyclodialysis cleft
Full thickness corneal or scleral laceration

Table 43.2
Differential Diagnosis

High IOP after trauma
Early onset
Contusion with inflammation
Trabecular meshwork tears
Hyphema
Chemical trauma
Late onset
Angle recession
Ghost cell
Lens-induced
Peripheral anterior synechias
Cyclodialysis cleft closure
Epithelial downgrowth
Retinal detachment

Table 43.3
Common Misdiagnosis

Sickle cell disease and hyphema
You must not overlook the possibility of sickle cell disease or trait in hyphema patients. IOP may rise dramatically in these patients and only mild IOP elevation can compromise optic nerve function.

patient's susceptibility to IOP elevation in the setting of trauma is highly variable. Read and Goldberg (5) found that IOP levels to 35 mm Hg or more that persist beyond 5 to 7 days may be associated with an increased risk of glaucomatous optic atrophy, particularly in the presence of sickle cell disease, but not restricted to that group. Higher pressures for a shorter period may be even more poorly tolerated.

One of the groups at highest risk for optic nerve damage in the setting of traumatic hyphema are those patients with sickle cell hemoglobinopathy (6). These patients are susceptible to even marginal IOP elevation and are also predisposed to profound IOP spikes (Table 43.3). The sensitivity of the optic nerve to marginal IOP elevation is presumably related to restricted blood flow to the optic nerve in the setting of the sickle cell disease. A high increase of IOP that may occur in these patients seems to be related to the restricted egress of rigid, sickled red blood cells through the trabecular meshwork outflow pathway. A vicious circle develops in that the sickle cells cannot clear from the anterior chamber and there is a stagnation of cells. A relatively acidotic pH develops in the anterior chamber, leading to further sickling. The accumulating sickled red cells have no greater chance of clearing through the trabecular outflow pathway and the cycle feeds on itself. Our traditional means for treating glaucoma in this setting may actually contribute to an exacerbation of the sickling process. These are theoretical concerns without confirmation clinically, but these factors must be considered by any physician treating patients with sickle disease or sickle trait. Use of a carbonic anhydrase inhibitor and the associated metabolic acidosis that results may increase sickling. Methazolamide theoretically causes less systemic acidosis than acetalzolamide. If a systemic carbonic anhydrase inhibitor is required in this situation, methazolamide may be the preferred choice. Epinephrine derivatives may exacerbate sickling due to their vasoconstrictive effect and subsequent hypoxia that develops in the anterior chamber. Miotics may increase inflammation. Topical aqueous suppressants are the treatment of choice and the role of topical apraclonidine remains to be determined.

In patients with normal hemoglobin, the greatest concern for serious elevation of IOP is in those hyphema patients who suffer rebleeding. The incidence of rebleeding is highly variable depending on type of injury and patient population. If rebleeding occurs, it tends to occur in the first 2 to 5 days after the injury. Although the majority of patients who lose vision in the setting of traumatic hyphema do so secondary to macular problems rather than secondary to glaucoma, every effort should be made to minimize the risk for sudden elevation of IOP. Treatment is directed toward minimizing the rate of rebleeding.

Several prospective studies (7,8) prove the efficacy of aminocaproic acid in reducing the rate of rebleeding; however, there is variability in the reports dealing with its side effects (nausea, vomiting, postural hypotension). **Some patients have a dramatic elevation of IOP on cessation of aminocaproic acid** (9), and for this reason we rarely use this drug. **In low-risk groups, the side effects of aminocaproic acid therapy may actually outweigh the risks of no treatment at all. Groups that appear to be at higher risk of hyphema from rebleeding are African-Americans, patients who present more than 24 hours after injury (10), and patients taking anticoagulants.** Aminocaproic acid is not the only oral medicine used to decrease rate of rebleeding. A study in 1992 by Farber et al (11) claimed efficacy for systemic prednisone at a dosage of 40 mg per day to reduce rebleeding. This dosage was equivalent in effect to the reduction in rebleeding obtained at the same institution several years earlier with aminocaproic acid.

Medical treatment for glaucoma in the setting of traumatic hyphema involves aqueous suppressants as the first line of defense (Table 43.4). Cycloplegic agents and topical steroids are often used to reduce the associated iritis and minimize outflow pathway edema.

Surgical treatment is indicated for those patients who do not respond satisfactorily to medical therapy (Table

Table 43.4
Management of Hyphema Associated with Glaucoma

First line of therapy: medical management
- Aqueous suppressants
- Topical steroids
- Cycloplegic agents

If medical management is ineffective, with concern for glaucomatous optic nerve damage and/or corneal blood staining, then surgical therapy is indicated.
- Anterior chamber washout
- Expression of blood clot
- Delivery of clot with cryoprobe
- Ultrasonic emulsification of clot
- Peripheral iridectomy
- Trabeculectomy

Generally, washing out of the circulating red cells from the anterior chamber is all that is required. The entire clot does not need to be removed because only the circulating red blood cells obstruct the outflow pathways. If that does not lower IOP to an acceptable level, the washout can be repeated or additional techniques employed as noted.

43.4). A host of surgical procedures have been described, including anterior chamber washout (12), clot expression (13), delivery of the clot with a cryoprobe (14), automated hyphemectomy (15), ultrasonic emulsification (16), and peripheral iridectomy and/or trabeculectomy (17,18). Washing out of the circulating red cells from the anterior chamber may be all that is required. If that does not lower IOP to an acceptable level, the washout can be repeated or additional techniques employed as noted above. **Paracentesis and anterior chamber washout seems to be the simplest procedure** (12), and this may be coupled with a coaxial manual irrigation system. The entire clot does not need to be removed, as only the circulating red blood cells obstruct the outflow pathways.

Chemical Trauma

Alkaline agents have the capability of penetrating ocular tissues and may lead to glaucoma. This is uncommon with acid burns. A number of researchers have studied the nature of the intraocular pressure rise following alkali exposure (19). A "dicrotic" pressure rise has been noted with an immediate IOP rise up to the level of 40 to 50 mm Hg within the first 10 minutes of the injury. The pressure tends to return to normal after a short time and then gradually rises to high levels at the end of the first hour or two. It is believed that shrinkage of the outer collagen coats of the eye may cause the initial IOP spike. Prostaglandin release has been implicated as the major factor in the second hypertensive phase. Weeks to months later, the IOP may be elevated due to angle closure as a result of peripheral anterior synechia formation.

Because of the impressive corneal changes that may arise from a chemical injury, IOP elevation may be overlooked. Treatment for the IOP elevation, if necessary, is focused on aqueous suppressant therapy, both topically and systemically. Miotics are generally avoided because of the intense inflammation that is associated with chemical burns. Topical steroids, if not contraindicated from a corneal basis, may reduce inflammation, and cycloplegic agents may maximize comfort and help to stabilize the blood-aqueous barrier. Anterior chamber paracentesis had been favored by some in the past, but this is less commonly used at this time.

LATE ONSET GLAUCOMA AFTER EYE INJURY

Angle Recession

A tear in the ciliary body results in angle recession. The typical tear occurs between the circular and longitudinal muscles in the ciliary body. There is a resulting posterior displacement of the iris root, which results in the clinical appearance of a broadening of the ciliary body band. Collins was the first to give a pathologic description of angle recession in 1892 (20). Wolff and Zimmerman presented a classic correlation between traumatic glaucoma and angle recession in 1962 (21).

Angle recession is remarkably common after blunt injury. The incidence of angle recession in the setting of traumatic hyphema has been reported from 50 to 100% (10,22,23). The incidence of glaucoma with angle recession appears to be directly related to the extent of angle involvement. **The risk of glaucoma appears to be greatest if 240 degrees or more of the angle are involved. The elevation in IOP after blunt trauma with angle recession may occur months or years after the initial injury.** Blanton observed a bimodal pattern with glaucoma occurring within the first year or after 10 years of injury (23).

The diagnosis of angle recession is made by careful gonioscopic examination (Fig. 43.1). The ciliary body band tends to be broader in certain zones and there may be baring of ciliary processes. The scleral spur may appear abnormally white. Differences between the eyes may be remarkably subtle. The most useful technique for documenting angle recession is to compare quadrants between the injured eye and the noninvolved eye of a given patient. Bilateral, simultaneous Koeppe gonioscopy (24) with two lenses is an excellent way to detect these differences.

The treatment of angle recession glaucoma follows the pattern used for primary open angle glaucoma. Inadequate control with topical and oral therapy may lead one to consider laser trabeculoplasty. Argon laser trabeculoplasty (LTP) is rarely effective and may also be associated with a higher incidence of acute IOP elevation. Filtration surgery is often required.

The mechanism for glaucoma in angle recession depends on the timing of the IOP elevation after injury. Early IOP increase is due to trabecular inflammation and the presence of circulating blood and inflammatory products.

HYPHEMA AND SECONDARY GLAUCOMA IN BLACK PATIENTS

Morton F. Goldberg

Approximately 9% of North American black individuals carry the gene for sickle cell hemogloblin. When this mutation is inherited from only one parent, creating the heterozygous condition called sickle cell trait, this unique cell trait is considered nonpathologic, because sickling of erythrocytes is uncommon. This valid principle does not apply to the anterior chamber, where all sickle cell hemoglobinopathies can induce a specific type of secondary glaucoma.

Sickled erythrocytes are elongated and rigid (like miniaturized pencils), and, unlike normal, pliable red blood cells, are not easily pushed through the interstices of the trabecular meshwork into Schlemm's canal. The logjam of sickled and non-sickled erythrocytes produces mechanical blockade of these outflow channels, creating mild to severe elevation of the intraocular pressure (IOP). This sequence of events can occur even when the total amount of blood in the aqueous humor is small (e.g., a 1 or 2 mm layered hyphema and, occasionally, even a dispersed "microhyphema" showing no gravitational settling). The elevation in IOP can occur when only a relatively small percentage of erythrocytes (e.g., 5–15%) becomes sickled. These events also occur regardless of the etiology of the hemorrhage, e.g., blunt trauma, perforating trauma, or postoperatively (for example, with passage of red cells from the vitreous to the aqueous humor after vitrectomy in an aphakic eye, or after cataract surgery, etc.).

The physico-chemical environment of the aqueous humor is uniquely constituted, i.e., in comparison with circulating whole blood. The aqueous has a low $p0_2$, low pH, high pCO_2, and a particularly high concentration of ascorbate (a reducing agent). These parameters, individually and in the aggregate, are capable of initiating and maintaining the sickled, rigid conformation of affected erythrocytes. Moreover, the presence of nonaerobically metabolizing erythrocytes and aerobically metabolizing leukocytes in the stagnant, sequestered aqueous humor contributes to further acidosis, hypoxia, and hypercarbia, thereby making a bad situation worse, by contributing to a vicious cycle, as follows:

> trabecular blockade, then sequestered blood in the anterior chamber, then sickling, then trabecular blockage (which, of course, can lead to elevated IOP).

Secondary glaucoma appears to be substantially more dangerous for the optic nerve in patients with a sickle cell hemoglobinopathy than in individuals with normal hemoglobin. Permanent, visually disabling infarctions of the optic nerve have occurred in several sickle cell hemoglobinopathy patients with only small amounts of intracameral blood and only mildly or transiently elevated IOPs (e.g., low 30s mm Hg). The mechanism is somewhat unclear, but may involve insufficient perfusion pressure within the small vessels of the optic nerve that are subjected to modest, but sudden, elevation of the IOP. Sluggish flow can lead to excessive oxygen extraction from the blood (inducing intravascular sickling), increased viscosity of the blood, and in some cases, total cessation of flow, with infarction of dependent tissue.

Conventional treatment regimens for hyphema-induced secondary glaucoma are inherently conservative and are often ineffective in the sickle cell patient. Some components of the usual treatment program, such as frequently repeated doses of osmotic agents or acetazolamide, may be deleterious, because they can exacerbate the sickling process in the anterior chamber and elsewhere. Therefore, serious consideration should be given to the following clinical guidelines: all black patients (and possibly individuals with Mediterranean or Hispanic ancestry) should have a routine, quick solubility screening test for the presence of sickle cell hemoglobin (a formal hemoglobin electrophoresis is not necessary for initial clinical decision-making); patients who are known or discovered to be positive should have regular measurements of IOP every 6 hours around the clock; whenever the measurements during any consecutive 24-hour period of time exceed 24 mm Hg (mnemonic: "24 for 24") or demonstrate spikes >30 mmHg, some of the blood should be removed from the anterior chamber to lower the burden of cells within the outflow pathways. If the hyphema is small, a simple paracentesis (which can be repeated if necessary) is usually sufficient; if the hyphema is large and blocks the pupil, a more extensive surgical wash-out is often indicated. Concomitant usage of the following regimen is sometimes effective: topical beta-blockers, atropine, and corticosteroids, plus oral epsilon-aminocaproic acid and/or corticosteroids.

These suggestions are based on clinical success in a limited number of patients. Optic nerve function cannot easily be assessed during the period of time when blood is in the anterior chamber. Because the optic nerve may be undergoing occult infarction during this time, a high index of suspicion accompanied by aggressive attempts to lower the IOP, as suggested above, may well be in the best interests of this physiologically vulnerable group of patients.

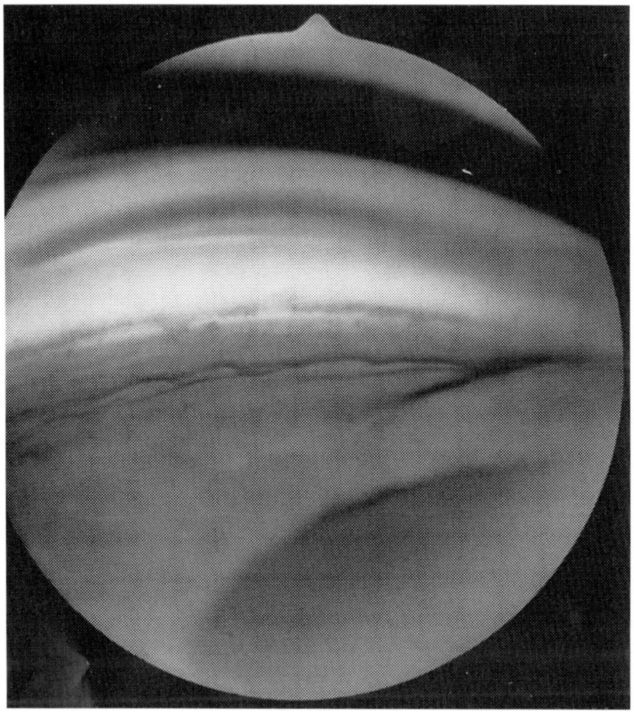

Figure 43.1. Angle recession must always be considered in the setting of asymmetrical IOP or unilateral glaucoma. Careful gonioscopy is critical. This figure demonstrates classic findings of a broadened ciliary body band with iris retrodisplacement, reduced ciliary processes and an abnormally white scleral spur. IOP did not rise to treatable levels in this patient until 10 years after injury.

This often resolves within weeks to months, and the patient may enter a "honeymoon period," with normalization of IOP. The ophthalmologist must be aware that this period of normal IOP can be short lived; such eyes deserve close follow-up, at least every 6 months.

Late angle recession glaucoma is secondary to the formation of a "glass membrane" over the trabecular meshwork, thought to be an extension of Descemet's membrane. This explains the poor response to conventional medical and laser treatment in angle recesssion glaucoma. Indeed, in such eyes treated with LTP, the surgeon may see a spreading whitening of "cracked glass" appearance at the site of laser impact. In contrast, if instead of LTP the surgeon performs Nd:YAG laser goniopuncture (Chapters 50 and 60), a transient reduction in IOP is seen, supporting the suggestion that obstruction to outflow in angle recession glaucoma is due to the presence of a "glass membrane" covering the trabecular meshwork. Unfortunately, such IOP reductions tend to be short lived, as Melamed has shown in monkeys that the openings made by goniopuncture tend to be covered by Descemet's membrane over time (25,26).

Ghost Cell Glaucoma

Ghost cell glaucoma can occur when injury to the globe causes disruption of the anterior hyaloid face and is associated with blood accumulation in the vitreous (Fig. 43.2); however, disruption of the hyaloid face is not a prerequisite for the development of ghost cell glaucoma (Chapter 45). Campbell and others (27) have shown that 1 to 3 weeks after the injury, or rarely even sooner, a secondary elevation of IOP can occur. This occurs when red blood cells, usually in the vitreous, but occasionally in longstanding hyphema, convert to less pliable, rigid, khaki-colored ghost cells that do not pass easily through the trabecular meshwork. The cells obstruct aqueous outflow with a resulting rise in IOP. The khaki ghost cells can often be identified at the slit lamp and may occasionally layer in the inferior angle recess as a **"tan hypopyon."** Anterior chamber aspirates demonstrate cells with a characteristic shrunken appearance by phase contrast microscopy. Heinz bodies represent denatured hemoglobin present in the cytoplasm of some ghost cells (28).

The treatment of ghost cell glaucoma includes conventional medical therapy, with surgery as necessary (Table 43.5). Anterior chamber washout may temporarily control IOP. If the reservoir of khaki ghost cells is large enough, there may be recurrent elevation of IOP despite anterior chamber washout. A pars plana vitrectomy may be necessary to insure complete removal of all blood components trapped in the vitreous. Filtration surgery is sometimes coupled with anterior chamber washout and pars plana vitrectomy.

Lens-induced Glaucoma

Lens-induced glaucoma is a varied group of secondary glaucomas that has the lens as a factor in the cause of IOP elevation (Chapter 47). The four major categories include lens dislocation, lens swelling, phacolytic glaucoma and

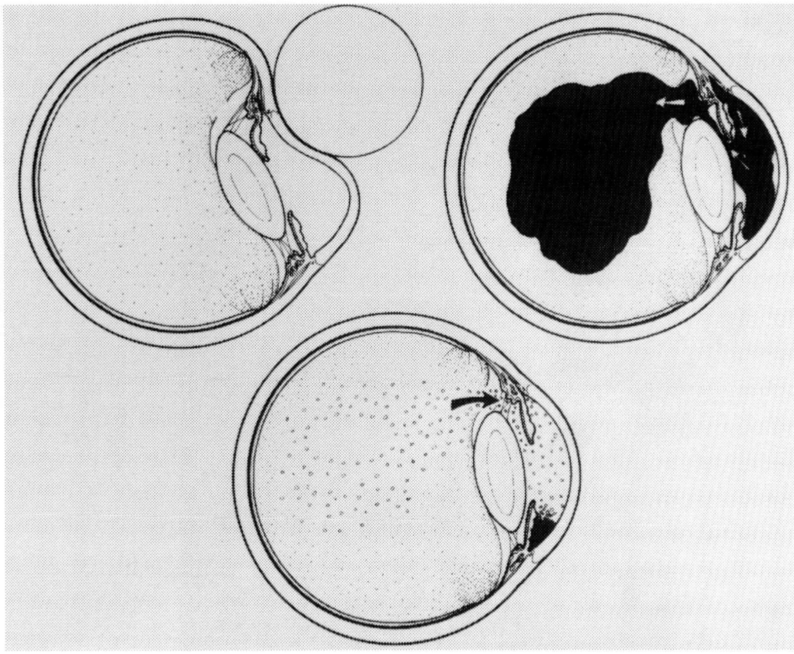

Figure 43.2. The mechanism involved in the development of ghost cell glaucoma is critical to diagnosis and management. This schematic demonstrates the effects of blunt injury, equatorial globe expansion, hyphema and vitreous hemorrhage, disruption of the anterior hyaloid face, passage of rigid khaki-colored ghost cells into the anterior chamber and blockage of trabecular meshwork. If medical therapy of glaucoma fails, treatment must involve removal of the ghost cells via anterior chamber washout, usually combined with a pars plana vitrectomy. Reprinted with permission from Campbell DG: Traumatic glaucoma. In: Eye Trauma. Edited by Shingleton BJ, Hersh PS, Kenyon KR. St. Louis, Mosby Yearbook, Inc., 1991.

Table 43.5
Management of Ghost Cell Glaucoma

Initial management
Aqueous suppressants
Miotics
Carbonic anhydrase inhibitors
Surgical management, if intraocular pressure rise is prolonged, or optic nerve is at risk, a stepwise surgical approach is taken, with each procedure following upon the other as needed:
Anterior chamber washout
Pars plana vitrectomy
Filtration surgery

Table 43.6
Insights into Mechanisms of Lens Induced Glaucomas

Lens-induced glaucoma
Lens dislocation/subluxation—pupillary block with secondary angle closure, direct mechanical angle closure or vitreous block glaucoma
Lens swelling—mass effect leading to direct mechanical angle closure or pupillary block glaucoma
Phacolytic—high molecular weight proteins obstructing trabecular meshwork with an open angle
Lens particle—lens and inflammatory material obstructing trabecular meshwork with an open angle

lens particle glaucoma. Each type may arise with trauma to the globe (29) (Table 43.6).

LENS DISLOCATION OR SUBLUXATION

Dislocation or subluxation of the crystalline lens most commonly occurs with blunt trauma. Disruption of the zonules allows the lens to move anteriorly or posteriorly. Depending on the position of the lens and vitreous status, pupillary block may occur. Pupillary block may lead to angle closure with a precipitous increase in IOP. Creeping angle closure may develop in a more sub-acute or chronic form, leading to late onset development of glaucoma. Rarely, complete dislocation of the lens may allow vitreous to come forward to fill the anterior chamber and lead to vitreous block glaucoma.

Treatment of lens-induced glaucoma depends on the type of glaucoma presenting. Careful examination is critical to determine the presence or absence of pupillary block. If pupillary block is present, a laser iridectomy or surgical iridectomy is indicated. Lensectomy may be required for visual reasons and for recurrent episodes of pupillary block. The technique of lensectomy will depend on the degree of subluxation. Surgical removal may involve a planned extracapsular or phacoemulsification approach, intracapsular extraction or pars plana lensectomy with vitrectomy.

LENS SWELLING

Blunt or penetrating trauma may alter lens fibers or capsule sufficiently to result in lens swelling. The lens may hydrate and become a mature cataract with development of phacomorphic glaucoma. Pupillary block may occur or the lens may swell enough to directly close angle structures. Cataract surgery is required for visual rehabilitation and correction of the glaucoma. Gonioscopy at the time of surgery is helpful because residual peripheral anterior synechias may best be treated directly at that time with surgical goniosynechialysis.

PHACOLYTIC GLAUCOMA

Phacolytic glaucoma is seen in the setting of a mature cataract. Open angle glaucoma occurs as a result of leakage of high molecular weight proteins through an intact lens capsule (30). Macrophages also are present in the anterior chamber. This entity is described in detail in Chapter 47.

LENS PARTICLE GLAUCOMA

Frank disruption of the lens due to penetrating trauma, and rarely blunt trauma, may lead to fragments of lens material in the anterior chamber. This will be obvious at the time of initial injury and will require surgical decision-making based on other associated findings. Most of these cases are associated with corneo-scleral lacerations that require primary repair. A primary lensectomy may be required at the time of operative corneoscleral repair.

Peripheral Anterior Synechias

Ocular injury often results in inflammation and blood in the anterior chamber. If these persist and there is pupillary block, then apposition may be possible in the angle. Peripheral anterior synechias may form. Hyphemas that persist for an extended period of time in the setting of significant inflammation are the most common cause of peripheral anterior synechia formation in the setting of blunt trauma. Stagnant clots may be an indication for AC washout (31). Penetrating trauma commonly results in peripheral anterior synechia formation, particularly if the laceration crosses the limbus. Careful attention to an intraoperative sweep of the angle and avoiding iris apposition to the wound will minimize peripheral anterior synechia formation when corneoscleral lacerations are repaired. If peripheral anterior synechias have not been firmly established, argon laser gonioplasty (Chapter 60) may be one means of reducing synechias, or surgical goniosynechialysis may be performed (32,33). If synechial closure is restricted to one quadrant, no treatment may be required.

Late Closure of a Cyclodialysis Cleft

A separation of ciliary body from the scleral spur results in a cyclodialysis cleft (Chapter 66). This may occur following blunt trauma or after surgical intervention. This can result in temporary or permanent hypotony. Goldmann (34) has postulated that a reduction in the normal flow of aqueous across the trabecular meshwork results in a reduced permeability of the meshwork to aqueous outflow. This may account for the marked, acute IOP elevation that can occur following closure of cyclodialysis clefts. The IOP increase tends to be severe and is associated with significant pain. Treatment involves use of aqueous suppressants, oral or intravenous hyperosmotics as well as alpha-agonists. Most cases can be managed medically through the short period of time that the IOP is elevated. Miotics are avoided because they can lead to recurrence of the cleft.

Epithelial Downgrowth

Lacerating trauma to the eye may lead to a fistula that develops from the external surface of the eye to the anterior chamber. This provides a conduit for epithelium to enter the anterior segment. This is an uncommon problem in the setting of microsurgical repair, but must be searched

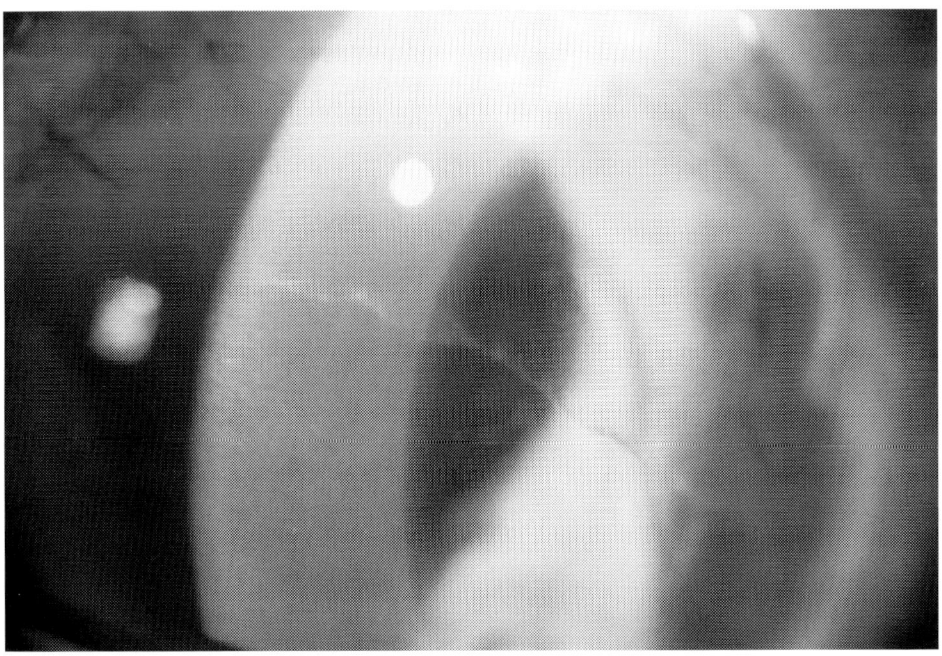

Figure 43.3. This figure demonstrates the classic, scalloped advancing border of epithelial cells on the endothelium of a patient with epithelial downgrowth. At this stage, IOP is usually elevated and patients are troubled by photophobia and eye pain. Argon laser applications (100 microns, 0.1 seconds, 300 milliwatts) to areas of iris involved with epithelium will blanch white to aid diagnosis, but occasionally, incisional biopsy is required.

IRIS RETRACTION SYNDROME

Joel S. Schuman

An interesting phenomenon can occur in some cases of Schwartz's syndrome. Exceptional patients with the syndrome and posterior synechias will develop an excessively deep anterior chamber, with dramatic iris concavity, when placed on aqueous suppressants, especially carbonic anhydrase inhibitors. The chamber will return to normal depth when the medications are discontinued and can be made extremely deep again with their reinstatement. Dramatic presentations can even have an initially elevated intraocular pressure with iris bombé, alternating with hypotony and an exceedingly deep anterior chamber once aqueous suppressants are started. The presumed mechanism for this occurrence, called "iris retraction syndrome," by David Campbell, who described the entity (1) requires the presence of both a retinal hole and 360 degrees posterior synechias and depends on a decrease in aqueous production and an increase in aqueous outflow by an unconventional route—through the retinal pigment epithelium. Aqueous humor moves freely through the vitreous cavity, (2) and the subretinal fluid of some eyes with retinal detachment has contained a high ascorbic acid level, suggesting the presence of aqueous humor in this space (3). Carbonic anhydrase inhibitors can stimulate the retinal pigment epithelial pump, and so are particularly likely to result in this uncommon circumstance, given the proper underlying conditions. This is essentially a situation of reverse pupillary block, with a lower pressure occuring in the posterior segment than the anterior, due to the 360 degree posterior synechias, the decreased aqueous production and the aqueous outflow via the retinal pigment epithelium through the retinal hole. Although a peripheral iridectomy will eliminate the anterior chamber deepening and is required given the pupillary block, a more definitive cure is repair of the retinal break.

References

1. Campbell DG: Iris retraction associated with rhegmatogenous retinal detachment syndrome and hypotony: a new explanation. Arch Ophthalmol 1984;102:1457.
2. Epstein DL, Hashimoto JM, Anderson PJ, et al: Experimental perfusions through the vitreous and anterior chambers; possible relationship to malignant glaucoma. Am J Ophthalmol 1979;88:1078–1086.
3. Van Heuven WAJ, Lam KW, Ray GS: Source of subretinal fluid on the basis of ascorbate analyses. Arch Ophthalmol 1982;100:976.

for in eyes that develop glaucoma at a time remote from the initial lacerating injury. The characteristic slit lamp appearance of a scalloped endothelial membrane is diagnostic for epithelial downgrowth (Fig. 43.3). Argon laser applications to involved iris make a white spot. These two findings confirm the diagnosis, although histopathologic confirmation via iris biopsy may be required in certain cases. Treatment involves excision of all involved iris and explantation of the intraocular lens, if present. Cryotherapy is applied to the involved ciliary body and cornea. Visual prognosis is guarded in these cases. Tube-shunt procedures may also be effective.

Retained Intraocular Foreign Body

A rare and late manifestation of iron-containing foreign bodies is siderotic glaucoma. The classic slit-lamp findings include iris heterochromia, mydriasis and rust-like discoloration of the anterior subcapsular lens surface. If these findings are present, foreign bodies should be searched for carefully with a complete ophthalmoscopic examination. Further studies may include plain radiographs, CT scanning, and ultrasound. Electroretinography may be helpful in advanced cases of siderosis.

RHEGMATOGENOUS RETINAL DETACHMENT

Rhegmatogenous retinal detachment is most commonly associated with ocular hypotension due to a decrease in aqueous production (35). However, 5 to 10% of the patients may develop elevated IOP (Schwartz's Syndrome). The mechanism for increased IOP is most likely due to direct photoreceptor obstruction of aqueous outflow in the anterior segment (36). Schwartz's syndrome can be difficult to diagnose, and commonly occurs in the setting of a shallow, peripheral retinal detachment with the appearance of an anterior chamber inflammatory reaction. In fact, the "cells" in the anterior chamber may be photoreceptor outer segments. It is not unusual for Schwartz's syndrome to be misdiagnosed as inflammatory glaucoma, and it is the ophthalmologist who is alert to the possibility of rhegmatogenous retinal detachment as a cause of elevated IOP who will make the correct diagnosis. For this reason, consider this diagnosis in any case of uveitic glaucoma and dilate all such patients, with a full examination of the peripheral retina to rule out the possibility of Schwartz's syndrome.

It is of particular importance to establish the correct

diagnosis of Schwartz's syndrome, as it is a curable entity, with a treatment different from that for inflammatory glaucoma. Repair of the retinal detachment most commonly results in a prompt and permanent return of IOP to normal, assuming there are no associated problems in the anterior segment that might exacerbate a tendency toward glaucoma.

References

1. Tingey DP, Shingleton BJ: Glaucoma associated with ocular trauma. In: Principles and Practice of Ophthalmology: The Harvard System. Edited by Albert DM, Jakobiec FA. Philadelphia, W. B. Saunders Co., 1993;1436–1444.
2. Thompson JT: Traumatic retinal tears and detachments. In: Eye Trauma. Edited by Shingleton BJ, Hersh PS, Kenyon KR. St. Louis, Mosby Year Book, Inc., 1991;196.
3. Campbell DG: Traumatic Glaucoma. In: Eye Trauma. Edited by Shingleton BJ, Hersh PS, Kenyon KR. St. Louis, Mosby Year Book, Inc., 1991;117–125.
4. Herschler J: Trabecular damage due to blunt anterior segment injury and its relationship to traumatic glaucoma. Trans Am Acad Ophthalmol Otolaryngol 1972;83:229.
5. Read J, Goldberg MF: Comparison of medical treatment for traumatic hyphema. Trans Am Acad Ophthalmol Otolaryngol 1974;78:799.
6. Goldberg MF: The diagnosis and treatment of sickled erythrocytes in human hyphemas. Trans Am Ophthalmol Soc 1978;76:481.
7. McGetrick JJ, Jampol LM, Goldberg MF, et al: Aminocaproic acid decreases secondary hemorrhage after traumatic hyphema. Arch Ophthalmol 1983;101:1031.
8. Palmer DJ et al: A comparison of two dose regimens for epsilon-aminocaproic acid in the prevention and management of secondary traumatic hyphemas. Ophthalmology 1986;93:102–108.
9. Dieste MC, Hersh PS, Kylstra JA, et al: Intraocular pressure increase associated with epsilon-aminocaproic acid therapy for traumatic hyphema. Am J Ophthalmol 1988;106:383–390.
10. Volpe NJ, Larrison WI, Hersh PS, et al: Secondary hemorrhage in traumatic hyphema. Am J Ophthalmol 1991;112:507–513.
11. Farber MD, Fiscella R, Goldberg MF: Aminocaproic acid versus prednisone for the treatment of traumatic hyphema. Ophthalmology 1991;98: 279–286.
12. Belcher CD, Brown SVL, Simmons RJ: Anterior chamber washout for traumatic hyphema. Ophthalmic Surg 1985;16:475.
13. Sears ML: Surgical management of black ball hyphema. Trans Acad Ophthalmol Otolaryngol 1970;74:820.
14. Hill K. Cryoextraction of total hyphema. Arch Ophthalmol 1968;80: 368.
15. McCuen BW, Fang WE: The role of vitrectomy instrumentation in the treatment of severe traumatic hyphema. Am J Ophthalmol 1979;71: 930.
16. Kelman CD, Brooks DL: Ultrasonic emulsification and aspiration of traumatic hyphema: A preliminary report. Am J Ophthalmol 1971;71: 1289.
17. Parrish RK, Bernardino V: Iridectomy in the surgical management of eight ball hyphema. Arch Ophthalmol 1982;100:435.
18. Weiss JS, Parrish RK, Anderson DR: Surgical therapy of traumatic hyphema. Ophthalmic Surg 1983;14:343.
19. Paterson CA, Pfister RR: Intraocular pressure changes after alkali burns. Arch Ophthalmol 1974;91:211.
20. Collins ET: On the pathologic examination of three eyes lost from concussion. Trans Ophthalmol Soc UK 1992;12:180.
21. Wolff SM, Zimmerman LE: Chronic secondary glaucoma associated with retrodisplacement of iris root and deepening of the anterior chamber angle secondary to contusion. Am J Ophthalmol 1962;84:547.
22. Canavan YM, Archer DB: Anterior segment consequences of blunt ocular injury. Br J Ophthalmol 1982;66:549.
23. Blanton FM. Anterior chamber angle recession and secondary glaucoma. A study of the after effects of traumatic hyphema. Arch Ophthalmol 1964;72:39.
24. Alper MG: Contusion angle deformity and glaucoma: Gonioscopic observation and clinical course. Arch Ophthalmol 1963;69:455.
25. Melamed S, Pei J, Puliafito CA, et al: Q-switched neodymium-YAG laser trabeculopuncture in monkeys. Arch Ophthalmol 1985;103: 129–133.
26. Epstein DL, Melamed S, Puliafito CA, et al: Neodymium-YAG laser trabeculopuncture in open-angle glaucoma. Ophthalmology 1985;92: 931–937.
27. Campbell DG, Simmons RJ, Grant WM: Ghost cells as a cause of glaucoma. Am J Ophthalmol 1973;97:2141.
28. Campbell DG: Ghost cell glaucoma following trauma. Ophthalmology 1981;88:1151.
29. Irvine JA, Smith RF: Lens injuries. In: Eye Trauma. Edited by Shingleton BJ, Hersh PS, Kenyon KR. St. Louis, Mosby Year Book, Inc., 1991;126.
30. Epstein DL: Diagnosis and management of lens-induced glaucoma. Ophthalmology 1982;89:227.
31. Deutsch TA, Feller DB: Paton and Goldberg's management of ocular injuries, ed 2. Philadelphia, W.B. Saunders, 1985.
32. Weiss HS, Shingleton BJ, Bellows AR, et al: Argon laser gonioplasty for the treatment of angle-closure glaucoma. Am J Ophthalmol 1992; 114:14–18.
33. Shingleton BJ, Chang MA, Bellows AR, et al: Surgical goniosynechialysis for angle-closure glaucoma. Ophthalmology 1990;97:551–556.
34. Goldmann H: Klinische Studien zum Glaucomproblem. Ophthalmologica 1953;125:16.
35. Cinner E: Intraocular pressure in retinal detachment. Arch Ophthalmol 1966;84:101.
36. Matsuo N, Takabatake M, Ueno H, et al: Photoreceptor outer segment in the aqueous humor in rhegmatogenous retinal detachment. Am J Ophthalmol 1986;101:673.

Corticosteroid Glaucoma

44

Douglas H. Johnson

Corticosteroid-induced elevation of intraocular pressure (IOP) may accompany the use of both topical and systemic corticosteroids. The widespread use of corticosteroids after intraocular surgery and in treating inflammatory conditions of the eye makes the possibility of a steroid-induced IOP increase part of the differential diagnosis of elevated IOP in these situations. In addition, the potential for steroids to increase IOP mandates the regular monitoring of IOP in patients on steroids.

Use of corticosteroids in ophthalmic conditions started within 2 years of the preparation and clinical use of cortisol by Kendall and Hench at the Mayo Clinic in 1949 (1,2). Although systemic ACTH was associated with elevated IOP as early as 1950, the ability of corticosteroids to elevate IOP was not widely appreciated until the early 1960s (3–6). Landmark studies by Armaly and Becker in 1963 lead to a profusion of studies on the effect of corticosteroids on intraocular pressure in the years to follow (7–13).

The clinical resemblance of corticosteroid-induced glaucoma to primary open angle glaucoma led to the initial hope that corticosteroids could be used to create a model of primary open angle glaucoma, allowing insights into its development and possible genetic nature (7–14). In addition, the finding of "high responder" patients, with a marked elevation of intraocular pressure after steroid provocative tests, was hoped to identify patients at risk for the later development of primary open angle glaucoma. The similarities between corticosteroid-induced glaucoma and primary open angle glaucoma are indeed striking: asymptomatic, quiet eyes with open angles and no distinguishing or specific findings on clinical examination. Unfortunately, the relationship between the two conditions may not be as close as was originally thought, as these initial hopes were not realized in later studies (15–17).

KEY CLINICAL POINTS

1. **How common is corticosteroid glaucoma?** Although all patients may respond with some change in pressure after prolonged corticosteroid use, studies by Armaly and Becker indicate 30 to 40% of the normal population may be "intermediate responders," with a pressure increase of at least 6 mm Hg or attain pressure levels of 20 mm Hg or higher (7–13). A small group of "high" responders had elevations of 16+ mm Hg or achieved levels of 32+ mm Hg (Table 44.1)
2. **How soon after starting steroids can intraocular pressure increase?** Although most prospective studies used topical corticosteroids for 3 to 6 weeks to assess pressure response, some elevation of pressure can be found in most patients as early as the first or second week (7–11). Armaly noted a hypertensive effect at the end of the first week in normal patients, with a mean increase in pressure of 19%. "High responders" had more rapid and higher increases in pressure, with a few patients developing an increase of 60% at the end of the first week of therapy (7,8). Patients with primary open angle glaucoma, most of whom were considered "high responders," also show a faster rate of pressure increase than normal patients. One study found more than 50% of patients with primary open angle glaucoma developed elevations of pressure 15 mm Hg higher than baseline by the end of the second week. (In some cases elevation in IOP from the use of frequent, potent topical steroid preparations such as hourly prednisolone acetate 1% may occur within 3–5 days. Additionally, patients on chronic lower dose steroids may not develop IOP elevation for months which may make this diagnosis more problematic.)

   It is unknown whether patients with little elevation of pressure after a 6-week steroid provocative test would develop higher pressures with prolonged use.
3. **How long will the elevated pressure remain once corticosteroids are stopped?** The IOP increase is usually short-lived. Both Armaly and Becker reported pressures to return to baseline values in a matter of days to weeks after stopping steroids in the majority of subjects; Armaly found this to occur by 2 weeks in all subjects (7,11). The duration of corticosteroid use, or the height of the pressure, may not necessarily predict the time course for the decrease of pressure. Case reports include that of increased pressure discovered in a patient after 1 year of topical corticosteroid use in which the pressure returned to normal 19 days after discontinuing the medication, whereas a second patient with a pressure increase that occurred after 8 weeks of corticosteroid use required 5 weeks to decrease (18). Pressure elevation accompanying several years of steroid use may not decrease, however, once steroids are discontinued

Table 44.1
Corticosteroid Testing and Intraocular Pressure

	Response		
Patient Group	*Low* Armaly <6 mm Hg Becker: IOP <20	*Intermediate* Armaly: 6–15 mm Hg Becker: IOP 20–31	*High* Armaly: 16+ mm Hg Becker: IOP 32+
Normals			
Armaly	66%	29%	5%
Becker	58%	36%	6%
Primary open angle glaucoma			
Armaly	6%	48%	46%
Becker	0%	8%	92%

From Armaly (9) and Becker (13).

(19). In other situations pressure may attain such a high level, or enough damage may have occurred, that laser trabeculoplasty or filtering surgery is required before the IOP would have a chance to diminish.

4. **Are certain patients more likely to develop the problem?** Patients with primary open angle glaucoma are particularly susceptible to the pressure elevating effect of corticosteroids. Steroid provocative tests in this population indicate that 94 to 100% of these patients will develop IOP increases of at least 6 mm Hg, or IOPs between 20 and 31 mm Hg (8,9,11,13). At least one half of these were actually considered "high responders," with pressures elevating at least 16 mm Hg, or to levels above 31 mm Hg. **Studies in patients with secondary open angle glaucoma generally do not find such high response rates** (20).

   Reports of other risk factors are mixed. Infants and children under 10 years of age may have a marked IOP response, although not all studies agree (21–22). This potential should be kept in mind when prescribing steroids after strabismus or other surgery in children, especially as lack of cooperation may make it difficult to measure the intraocular pressure in these patients. First-degree relatives of patients with primary open angle glaucoma, diabetics, high myopes, and patients with rheumatoid arthritis or other connective tissue diseases have also been reported to be likely steroid responders (10,12,15,23–25).

5. **Can systemic or other forms of corticosteroids elevate IOP?** All methods of corticosteroids use have the potential to elevate intraocular pressure. Systemic steroids were reported to elevate pressures as early as 1962; the initial link between steroids and intraocular pressure was reported in a patient who received systemic ACTH (2,6). Systemic steroid use is less likely to cause elevations of IOP than topical application; one study found a 10% incidence of ocular hypertension in renal transplant patients receiving systemic steroids after transplant, although pretreatment pressures were not obtained (26).

   Endogenous corticosteroids may cause elevation of IOP in patients with Cushing's syndrome and other forms of hypersecretion.

   Periocular injections of corticosteroids may elevate intraocular pressure. Long-acting preparations such as triamcinolone acetonide (Kenalog) may be especially likely to cause increases, as reports indicate active steroid may be released for months (27). In one group of 12 patients, the average time from injection of repository steroid to discovery of pressure elevation was 10 weeks, although the range of times varied from 1 to 26 weeks (27). Most of these patients did not previously show elevated IOP while taking topical steroid therapy. **Some patients may require the surgical removal of a repository steroid injection for IOP control.** In consideration of this such injections should be given in an easily retrievable spot, such as the inferior fornix (Fig. 44.1). **Dermal applications of corticosteroids have caused elevation of IOP,** whether administered to the periocular region or at distant sites (28). **Inhaled corticosteroids** may also cause an increase in pressure (29).

6. **Steps in management of corticosteroid-induced glaucoma.** Recognition of the condition is the most important step in its management. **Measurement of IOP on a regular basis in any patient placed on long term topical corticosteroids is essential.** Prevention is also key: use of nonsteroidal antiinflammatory agents rather than steroids, use of steroid preparations less likely to elevate intraocular pressure when possible (30–32) (rimexolone: Vexol, fluorometholone: FML, medrysone: HMS), and avoidance of using extremely long acting steroid preparations for subconjunctival injections. Prevention of unmonitored use of steroids by patients should be considered by writing nonrefillable prescriptions, for only small quantities of corticosteroids, when possible.

Once the possibility of steroid glaucoma is seriously considered, stopping steroid treatment, and observation of

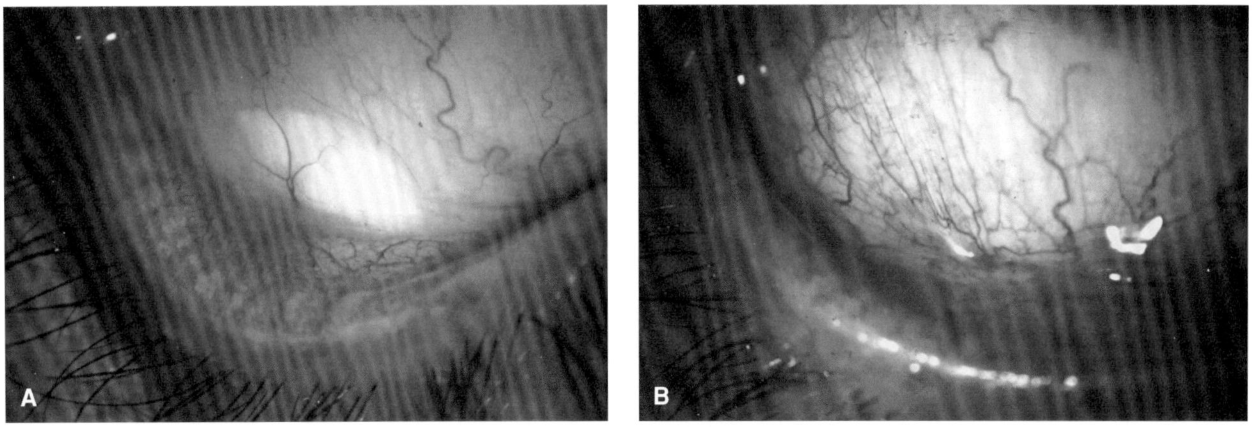

Figure 44.1. A 38-year-old patient with subconjunctival triamcinolone acetonide injection (A) after pterygium resection. IOP became elevated 3 weeks after injection to the mid 40s on maximally tolerated medications. IOP elevation persisted until the steroid was removed surgically (B) 4 months later. IOP returned to normal without medications within 1 week after surgical removal. (Courtesy of R. Rand Allingham, MD).

the eye for several weeks will usually result in spontaneous lowering of the IOP. If the IOP has reached a dangerous or worrisome level, the temporary use of IOP lowering agents may be required. No specific treatment, such as an antisteroid eyedrop, is available.

More perplexing is the situation of elevation of IOP in an eye that has been on steroid therapy for chronic iritis or uveitis (Chapter 42). It is difficult to know if the inflammatory condition has worsened and caused elevation of the pressure, or whether the patient has now become a steroid responder. It is usually advisable to increase the steroid therapy for several days to attempt to suppress any increase in inflammation. **If the IOP decreases with the increased steroid, inflammation, not a steroid "response," was the explanation for the increased IOP. If, however, the IOP remains unchanged or elevates, then a steroid response in IOP, whether due to obstruction of aqueous outflow or increased aqueous inflow, is likely, and the amount of steroid use must be decreased.** This may entail use of drops less often, decreasing the strength of the drops, or switching to a preparation less likely to affect IOP. Addition of an IOP lowering agent may also be considered if steroid use cannot be decreased.

CORTICOSTEROID PREPARATIONS

Corticosteroids are a family of compounds related in structure to the cholesterol molecule from which they are derived. They share structural similarities with the two other major classes of steroids, mineralocorticoids and sex steroids (Fig. 44.2). Addition of an extra double bond in the ring structures or small modifications of side groups of the steroid base molecule may cause significant changes in both effect and potency; prednisolone, which has a second double bond in the A ring, has significantly greater antiinflammatory activity and less fluid retaining effects than cortisol (Table 44.2) (33,34). The creation of derivative compounds (i.e., the addition of an acetate group) can also change the clinical effect of the base molecule by affecting its penetration into the eye, release characteristics, and degradation rate. Although these factors determine bioavailability, other factors, such as affinity of binding to the steroid receptor, are also involved in determining antiinflammatory activity (33). In topical therapy, experimental studies of inflammatory keratitis indicate that the acetate derivative is the most effective, followed by the alcohol and finally the steroid-phosphate compounds (35).

Table 44.2
Relative Potency of Corticosteroids

Steroid Base	Relative Anti-inflammatory Activity
Short acting (8–12 hr)	
Cortisone	0.8
Cortisol	1.0
Intermediate acting (12–36 hr)	
Prednisone	4.0
Prednisolone	4.0
Triamcinolone	5.0
Long acting (36–72 hr)	
Dexamethasone	25
Betamethasone	25

Modified from Haynes and Murad (34).

Attempts to separate the IOP elevating effect from the anti-inflammatory effect have met with mixed results. While studies indicate that rimexolone (Vexol), fluormetholone (FML) and medrysone (HMS) are less likely to cause elevation of IOP (30–32), they also appear less efficacious for intraocular inflammation than prednisolone or dexamethasone (Table 44.3) (33,35). The decreased tendency of fluorometholone to elevate IOP may be due to an increased degradation rate in the ocular tissues, resulting in a shorter duration of action or a smaller amount reaching the target tissue (33).

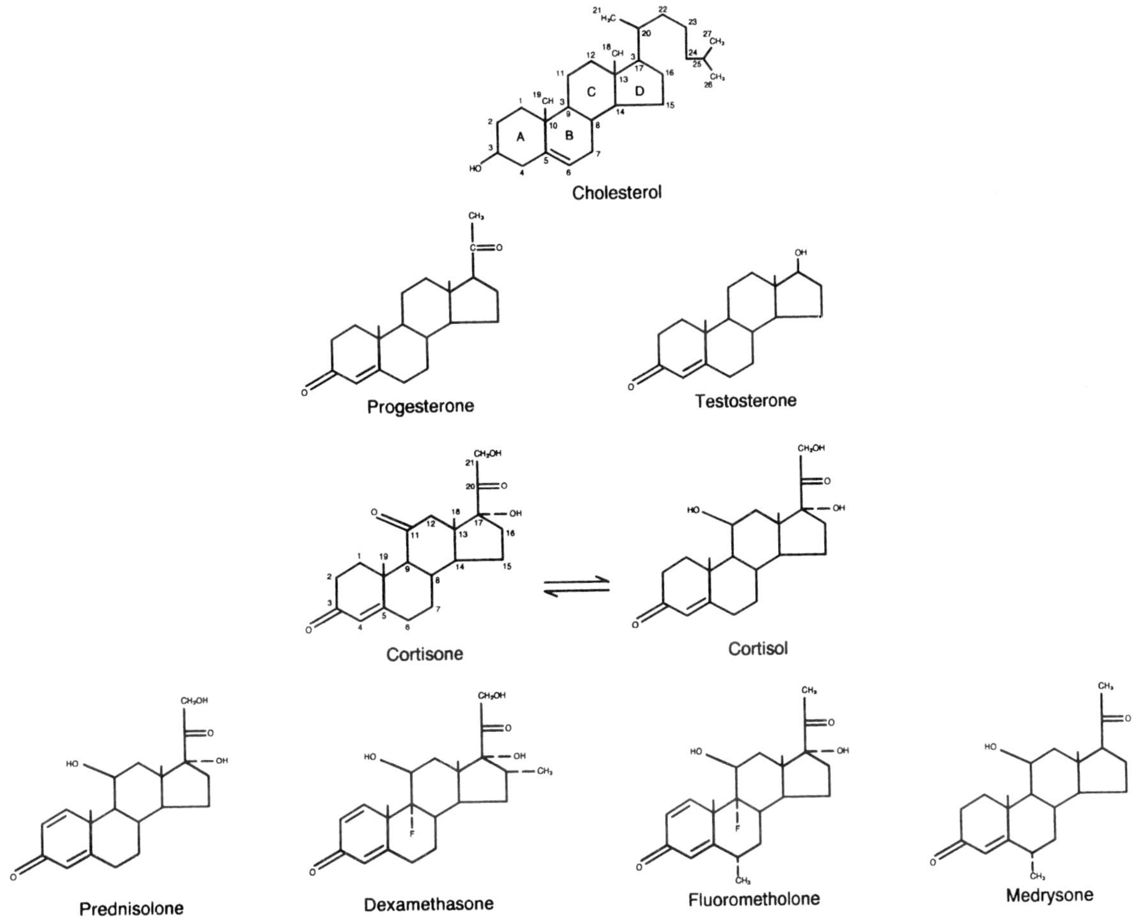

Figure 44.2. Structures of commonly used steroids. The parent molecule, cholesterol has 4 rings and 27 carbon atoms. Progesterone and the corticosteroids keep the basic four ring structure and have 21 carbon atoms, testosterone has 19. Cortisone, initially termed "compound E," has a keto group at position 11, while cortisol, "compound F," has an hydroxyl group in this position.

Table 44.3
Anti-inflammatory Activity of Topical Corticosteroids in Experimental Keratitis

Steroid compound	Anti-inflammatory Activity (%)
Dexamethasone acetate 0.1%	55
Prednisolone acetate 1% (Pred Forte; Enconopred Plus)	51
Dexamethasone alcohol 0.1% (Maxidex)	40
Fluorometholone alcohol	
0.25% (FML Forte)	35
0.1% (FML)	31
Prednisolone phosphate 1% (Inflamase Forte)	28
Dexamethasone phosphate 0.1% (Decadron Phosphate)	19
Medrysone (HMS)	not tested

Modified from Leibowitz (34).

Table 44.4
Injectable Corticosteroids

Short acting
- Dexamethasone sodium phosphate (Decadron)
- Hydrocortisone sodium succinate (Solu-Cortef)
- Methylprednisolone sodium succinate (Solu-Medrol)

Intermediate acting
- Triamcinolone diacetate (Aristocort)
- Methylprednisolone acetate (Depo-Medrol)

Long acting
- Triamcinolone acetonide (Kenalog)
- Triamcinolone hexacetonide (Aristospan)

From Herschler (27).

The efficacy and duration of action of periocular injections of corticosteroids is dependent on both the steroid base and the derivative formulation. The solubility of the compound appears to play a major role in its duration of action. Poorly soluble compounds are considered long acting while water soluble compounds are considered short acting (Table 44.4) (27,33).

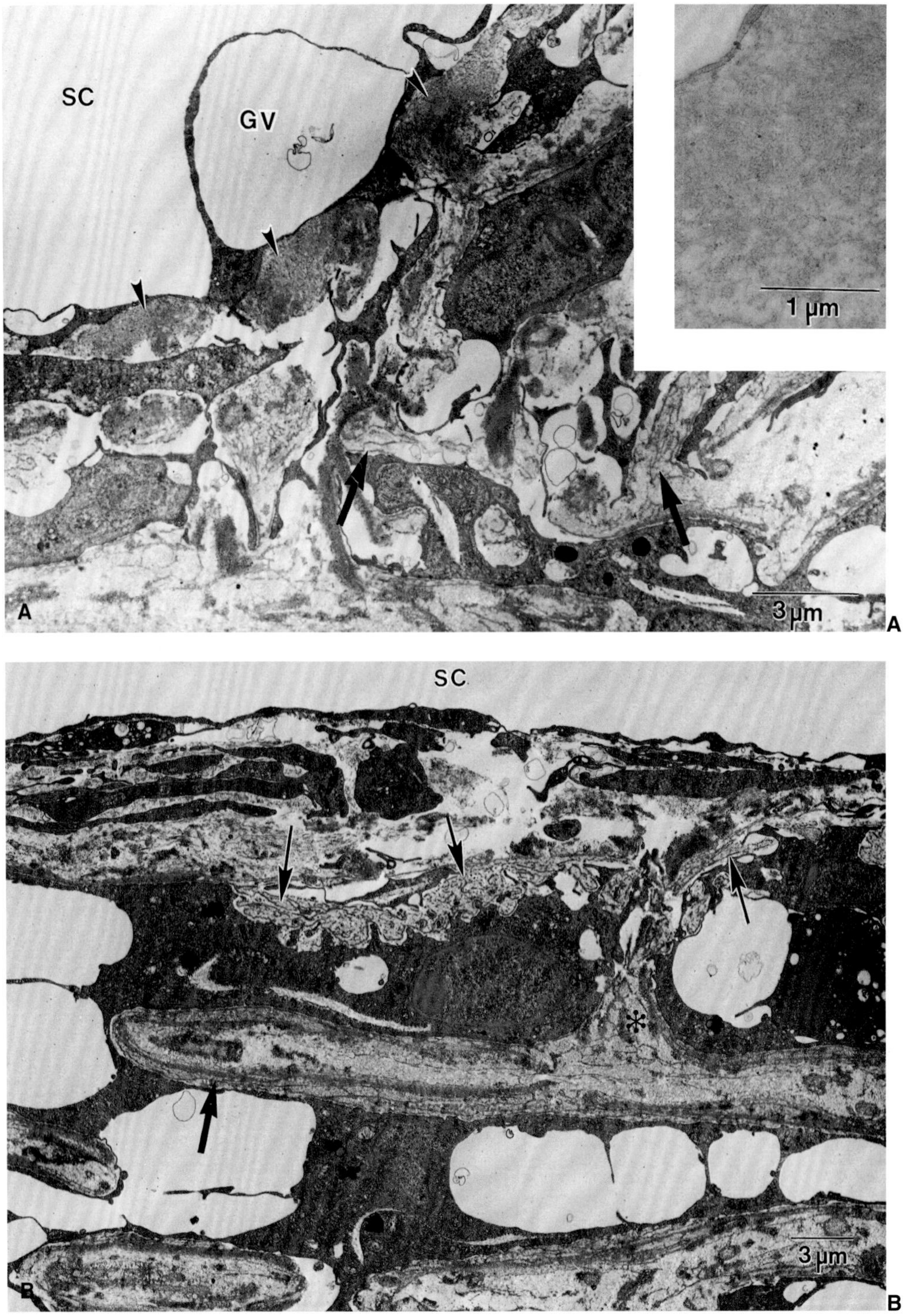

Figure 44.3. Ultrastructural findings in steroid glaucoma. The patient was a 60-year-old female who had been treated with systemic prednisone for more than 5 years. IOPs were 16 mm Hg at the start of therapy and had risen to 28 OD, 27 OS 5 years later. Eyes were obtained at autopsy. A, Dense plaques of fibrillar collagen (arrowheads) beneath the inner wall of Schlemm's canal (SC). This material is characteristic of steroid glaucoma. Fibrous band-like basement membrane appears adjacent to cells (arrow). GV: giant vacuole. Inset: Fibrillar plaque consists of closely-packed, fine fibrillar collagen. B, Fibrous band-like ("fingerprint") collagen (arrows) in juxtacanalicular region. Early reports considered this to be pathognomonic of steroid treatment. This collagen follows outline and convolutions of cell, suggestive of a basement membrane. Outer corneoscleral lamella has duplication of cortical basement membrane (thick arrow), similar in appearance to the fingerprint collagen. Branching area of lamella has exposed areas of this basement membrane collagen (asterisk). SC: Schlemm's canal.

PATHOPHYSIOLOGY

A decrease in outflow facility occurs in conjunction with the elevation of IOP (7,11). Reports of histologic findings in the trabecular meshwork of eyes with corticosteroid glaucoma are variable. Some reports find no pathological change, whereas others have described the accumulation of excess basement membrane-like material (26,36–41; Fig. 44.3). The variable time course for both the development and resolution of the IOP increase makes it likely that several mechanisms may be involved. A short-term biochemical change such as alteration of the proteoglycans of the extracellular matrix may occur initially, followed in some eyes by the structural changes pictured in Figure 44.3. Biochemical changes would be expected to be reversible within days to weeks, while structural changes would be much slower to resolve or could become permanent.

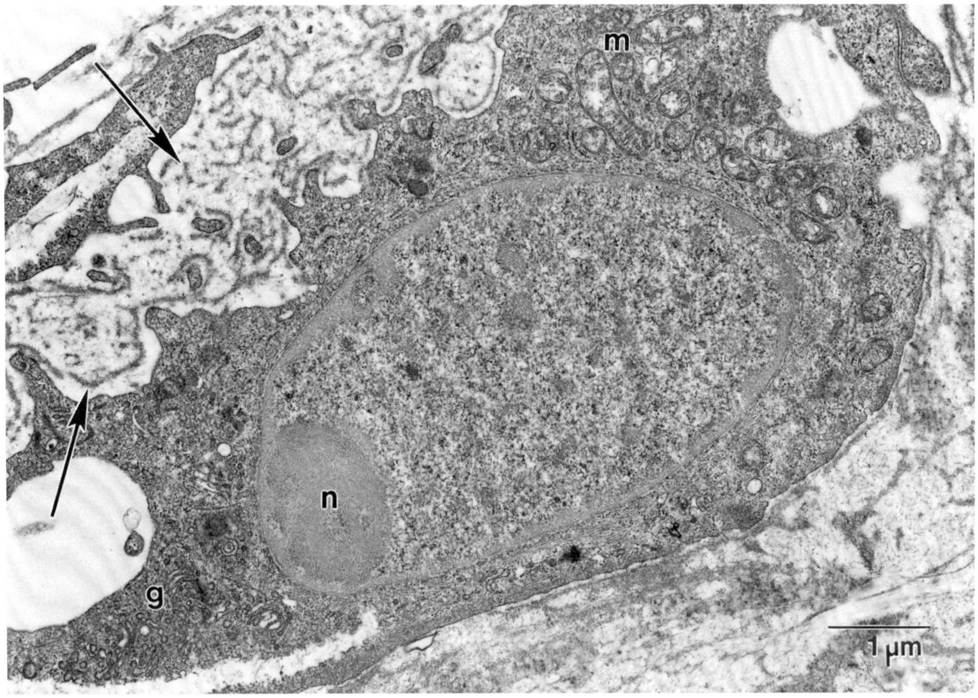

C

Figure 44.3. *(continued)* C, Enlargement of cell in Figure 44.3B. Fingerprint collagen (arrows) has a component of a finer, fibrillar collagen. Cell appears metabolically active, with prominent nucleolus (n), numerous mitochondria (m), and golgi apparatus (g).

Armaly (7) and Francois (42) postulated that changes in the mucopolysaccharides (glycosaminoglycans and proteoglycans) of the trabecular meshwork may cause the increased outflow resistance in this condition. Experimental work in human eyes and cell cultures confirms that corticosteroids can change the synthetic profile of these and other elements of the extracellular matrix through which the aqueous must flow (43–45). An inhibition of phagocytosis by the trabecular cells has also been suggested (46). This could result in the accumulation of debris in the meshwork and could ultimately increase outflow resistance. More recently, investigators have suggested that dexamethasone may alter fluid hydraulic conductivity by increasing the expression of cellular tight junction protein Z0-1 (47). This has been demonstrated in a sophisticated trabecular meshwork cell culture model.

RELATIONSHIP TO PRIMARY OPEN ANGLE GLAUCOMA

The marked sensitivity to corticosteroids of "high responder" normal eyes and eyes with primary open angle glaucoma led to initial thought that such patients had a similar genetic inheritance of a recessive gene for glaucoma (10,12). **High responders were thought to be at risk for the later development of primary open angle glaucoma. Subsequent work did not support this hypothesis; high responders did not develop primary open angle glaucoma with the frequency predicted from such a model** (15,17). An explanation for the large number of "high responders" among primary open angle glaucoma patients may be the pre-existing condition of the meshwork (7). Eyes with primary open angle glaucoma have compromised outflow channels, and small changes in glycosaminoglycans or other components may have a greater effect in these already obstructed eyes than in normal eyes. In normal eyes a small amount of "plugging" of the meshwork caused by corticosteroids would result in only a small change in outflow facility.

THE FUTURE

Diurnal Variations

Numerous studies have examined the relationship between the diurnal variation in IOP, aqueous humor flow, and the diurnal pattern of endogenous cortisone secretion, yet the exact relationship remains unclear (48–51). Several studies have found a 3- to 4-hour lag time between the administration of systemic corticosteroids and an elevation in IOP (52–54). Interestingly, this elevation of IOP lasts only a few hours. Understanding the mechanism of corticosteroids in elevating IOP, and understanding their presumed role in the diurnal variations in aqueous humor flow, will provide fundamental insights into the mechanisms controlling aqueous dynamics. Such an understanding may help with the design of new and more effective therapy for glaucoma.

Antisteroids

Outflow facility increases during pregnancy, and several studies have considered the elevated progesterone levels during this time to be responsible (55,56). The effect of other steroids and their metabolites have been examined, with the recent finding that a metabolite of cortisol, 3α, 5β-tetrahydrocortisol, may lower IOP in patients with primary open angle glaucoma (57). An anabolic androgenic steroid, 17α-methyltestosterone, reversed the steroid-induced elevation of IOP in a series of monkeys (58). This compound also possesses angiostatic activity and may represent a new class of therapeutic agents (59). RU486 is a progesterone blocker and a corticosteroid blocker which has been shown to decrease IOP when administered topically or subconjunctivally in a rabbit model (60,61). This agent has not been investigated in humans for this purpose to date. None of these studies have looked at the potential inflammatory effect that such blocking of normal steroid metabolism may cause, however.

Although steroids may play a key role in understanding fundamental aspects of aqueous inflow and outflow, and antisteroid compounds hold promise for the future at the present time, corticosteroids must still be used with discretion and the awareness of their potential to elevate IOP.

References

1. Hench PS, Kendall EC, Slocumb CH, et al: The effect of a hormone of the adrenal cortex (17-hydroxy-11-dehydrocorticosterone: compound E) and of pituitary adrenocorticotropic hormone on rheumatoid arthritis. Proc Staff Meetings Mayo Clinic 1949;24:181.
2. Woods AC: Clinical and experimental observation on the use of ACTH and cortisone in ocular inflammatory disease. Am J Ophthalmol 1950; 33:1325.
3. McLean JM: In discussion of Woods AC. Clinical and experimental observation on the use of ACTH and cortisone in ocular inflammatory disease. Trans Am Ophthalmol Soc 1950;48:259.
4. Francois J: Cortisone et tension oculaire. Ann Oculist 1954;187:805.
5. Goldmann H: Cortisone glaucoma. Arch Ophthalmol 1962;68:621.
6. Berstein HN, Schwartz B: Effects of long-term systemic steroids on ocular pressure and tonographic values. Arch Ophthalmol 1962;68:742.
7. Armaly MF: Effect of corticosteroids on intraocular pressure and fluid dynamics. I. The effect of dexamethasone in the normal eye. Arch Ophthalmol 1963;70:482.
8. Armaly MF: Effect of corticosteroids on intraocular pressure and fluid dynamics. II. The effect of dexamethasone in the glaucomatous eye. Arch Ophthalmol 1963;70:492–499.
9. Armaly MF: Statistical attributes of the steroid hypertensive response in the clinically normal eye. Invest Ophthalmol Vis Sci 1965;4:187.
10. Armaly MF: The heritable nature of dexamethasone-induced ocular hypertension. Arch Ophthalmol 1966;75:32.
11. Becker B, Mills DW: Corticosteroids and intraocular pressure. Arch Ophthalmol 1963;70:500.
12. Becker B, Hahn KA: Topical corticosteroids and heredity in primary open-angle glaucoma. Am J Ophthalmol 1964;57:543.
13. Becker B: Intraocular pressure response to topical corticosteroids. Invest Ophthalmol Vis Sci 1965;4:198.
14. Grant WM: Glaucoma from topical corticosteroids. Arch Ophthalmol 1963;70:445.
15. Armaly MF: Inheritance of dexamethasone hypertension and glaucoma. Arch Ophthalmol 1967;77:747.
16. Kitazawa Y, Horie T: The prognosis of corticosteroid-responsive individuals. Arch Ophthalmol 1981;99:819.
17. Lewis JM, et al: Intraocular pressure response to topical dexamethasone as a predictor for the development of primary open-angle glaucoma. Am J Ophthalmol 1988;106:607.
18. Epstein DL (ed): Chandler and Grant's Glaucoma, 3rd ed. Philadelphia, Lea & Febiger, 1986.
19. Espildora J, Vicuna P, Diaz E: Cortisone-induced glaucoma: a report on 44 affected eyes. J Fr Ophthalmol 1981;4:503.
20. Becker B: The effect of topical corticosteroids in secondary glaucomas. Arch Ophthalmol 1964;72:769.
21. Kass MA, Kolker AE, Becker B: Chronic topical corticosteroid use simulating congenital glaucoma. J Pediatr 1972;81:1175.
22. Ohji M, Kinoshita S, Ohmi E, et al: Marked intraocular pressure response to instillation of corticosteroids in children. Am J Ophthalmol 1991; 112:450.
23. Podos SM, Becker B, Morton WR: High myopia and primary open-angle glaucoma. Am J Ophthalmol 1966;62:1039.
24. Becker B: Diabetes mellitus and primary open-angle glaucoma. The XXVII Edward Jackson Memorial Lecture. Am J Ophthalmol 1971;71: 1.
25. Gaston H, Absolon MJ, Thurtle OA, et al: Steroid responsiveness in connective tissue diseases. Br J Ophthalmol 1983;67:487.
26. Adhikary HP, Sells RA, Basu PK: Ocular complications of systemic steroids after renal transplantation and their association with HLA. Br J Ophthalmol 1982;66:290.
27. Herschler J: Increased intraocular pressure induced by repository corticosteroids. Am J Ophthalmol 1976;82:90.
28. Spaeth GL, Rodrigues MM, Weinreb S: Steroid-induced glaucoma: A. Persistent elevation of intraocular pressure. B. Histopathological aspects. Tr Am Ophthalmol Soc 1977;75:353.
29. Dreyer EB: Inhaled steroid use and glaucoma. N Engl J Med 1993;329: 1822.
30. Cantrill HL, Palmberg PF, Zink HA, et al: Comparison of in vitro potency of corticosteroids with ability to raise intraocular pressure. Am J Ophthalmol 1975;79:1012.
31. Stewart RH, Kimbrough RL: Intraocular pressure response to topically administered fluorometholone. Arch Ophthalmol 1979;97:2139.
32. Kass M, Cheetham J, Duzman E, et al: The ocular hypertensive effect of 0.25% fluorometholone in corticosteroid responders. Am J Ophthalmol 1986;102:159.
33. Polansky JR, Weinreb RN: Anti-inflammatory agents. Steroids as anti-inflammatory agents. In: Handbook of Experimental Pharmacology, Vol. 69. Edited by Sears ML. Berlin Heidelberg, Springer-Verlag, 1984.
34. Haynes RC, Murad F: Adrenocorticotropic hormone; adrenocortical steroids and their synthetic analogs; inhibitors of adrenocortical steroid biosynthesis. In: The Pharmacological Basis of Therapeutics, 7th edition. Edited by AG Gilman, LS Goodman, TW Rall, F Murad. New York, MacMillan Publishing Co., 1985.
35. Leibowitz HM: Management of inflammation in the cornea and conjunctiva. Ophthalmology 1980;87:753.
36. Rohen JW, Linnér E, Witmer R: Electron microscopic studies on the trabecular meshwork in two cases of corticosteroid-glaucoma. Exp Eye Res 1973;17:19.
37. Toriyama K: An electron microscopic study on the trabecular meshwork in corticosteroid-glaucoma. Bull Jpn Ophthalmol 1979;30:1583.
38. Roll P, Benedikt O: Elektronenoptische Untersuchung des Trabekelwerkes bei einem Kortikosteroidglaukom. Klin Mbl Augenheilk 1979; 174:421.
39. Kayes J: Pore structure of the inner wall of Schlemm's canal. Invest Ophthalmol 1967;6:381.
40. Kayes J, Becker B: The human trabecular meshwork in corticosteroid-induced glaucoma. Tr Am Ophthalmol Soc 1969;67:339.
41. Sano T, Miyata Y: Autopsy findings in a case with steroid glaucoma. Jpn J Clin Ophthalmol 1971;25:17.
42. Francois J: The importance of the mucopolysaccharides in intraocular regulation. Invest Ophthalmol 1975;14:173.
43. Johnson DH, Bradley JMB, Acott TS: The effect of dexamethasone on glycosaminoglycans of human trabecular meshwork in perfusion organ culture. Invest Ophthalmol Vis Sci 1990;31:2568.
44. Hernandez MR, et al: The effect of dexamethasone on the synthesis of

collagen in normal human trabecular meshwork explants. Invest Ophthalmol Vis Sci 1985;26:1784.
45. Partridge CA, Weinstein BI, Southren AL, et al: Dexamethasone induces specific proteins in human trabecular meshwork cells. Invest Ophthalmol Vis Sci 1989;30:1843.
46. Bill A: The drainage of aqueous humor. Invest Ophthalmol Vis Sci 1975;14:1.
47. Underwood JL, Alvarado JA, Murphy CG, et al: Steroid-induced decreases in hydraulic conductivity were blocked in human trabecular meshwork cells by an antisense oligonucleotide to 70-1. Invest Ophthalmol Vis Sci 1994;35(ARVO Suppl):2737.
48. Linnér E: Adrenocortical hormones and glaucoma. Acta Ophthalmologica 1966;44:299.
49. Smith JL, et al: Diurnal variation of plasma 17-hydroxycorticoids and intraocular pressure in glaucoma. Am J Ophthalmol 1962;54:411.
50. Maus TL, Young Jr WF, Brubaker RF: Aqueous flow in humans after adrenalectomy. Invest Ophthalmol Vis Sci 1994;35:3325.
51. Sheridan PT, et al: The effect of oral dexamethasone on the circadian rhythm of aqueous humor flow in humans. Invest Ophthalmol Vis Sci 1994;35:1150.
52. Weitzman ED, Henkind P, Leitman M, et al: Correlative 24-hour relationships between intraocular pressure and plasma cortisol in normal subjects and patients with glaucoma. Br J Ophthalmol 1975;59:566.
53. Boyd TAS, McLeod LE, Hassard DTR, et al: Relation of diurnal variation of plasma corticoid levels and intraocular pressure in glaucoma. Can Med Ass J 1962;86:772.
54. Weinreb RN, Polansky JR, Kramer SG, et al: Acute effects of dexamethasone on intraocular pressure in glaucoma. Invest Ophthalmol Vis Sci 1985;26:170.
55. Becker B, Friedenwald JS: Clinical aqueous outflow. Arch Ophthalmol 1953;50:557.
56. Ziai N, Ory SJ, Khan AR, et al: β-human chorionic gonadotropin, progesterone, and aqueous dynamics during pregnancy. Arch Ophthalmol 1994;112:801.
57. Southren AL, Wandel T, Gordon GG, et al: Treatment of glaucoma with 3 alpha, 5 beta-tetrahydrocortisol: a new therapeutic modality. J Ocular Pharmacol 1994;10:385.
58. Knepper PA, et al: Effect of 17-alpha-methyl-testosterone on IOP and GAG profile of dexamethasone-induced ocular hypertension in primates. Invest Ophthalmol Vis Sci 1991;32:871.
59. Clark AF, McNatt L, Knepper PA: Angiostatic steroids as a new class of IOP lowering compounds. Invest Ophthalmol Vis Sci 1994;35(ARVO Suppl):1483.
60. Tsukahara S, Sasaki T, Phillips CI, et al: Subconjunctival injection of RU486 lowers intraocular pressure in normal rabbits. Br J Ophthalmol 1986;70:451–455.
61. Green K, Phillips CI, Gore SM, et al: Ocular fluid dynamics response to topical RU486, a steroid blocker. Curr Eye Res 1985;4:605–612.

Hemolytic or Ghost-Cell Glaucoma 45

David L. Epstein

CLINICAL FINDINGS

The term "hemolytic glaucoma" was introduced by Fenton and Zimmerman to describe the clinical and histologic findings in a patient who had spontaneous hemorrhage into the vitreous humor and several weeks later had high IOP and pain, leading to enucleation (1). Hemorrhagic debris and pigment-laden macrophages were found in sections of the anterior chamber angle. Fenton and Zimmerman postulated that the glaucoma was caused by a mechanical blockage of aqueous outflow by broken-down red blood cells and macrophages, analogous to phacolytic glaucoma, which was conceived of as being due to obstruction by lens material and macrophages. Clinical and experimental investigations by our colleague David Campbell (2–5) have led us to believe that ghost cells, resulting from degeneration of red blood cells, are a particularly important factor in obstructing aqueous outflow and causing glaucoma as an occasional consequence of hemorrhage in the vitreous humor, and also in some cases of glaucoma associated with hemorrhage into the anterior chamber from blunt injury to the globe.

Retinal vascular disease or injury often produces hemorrhage into the vitreous humor, but the blood seldom passes the barrier of the anterior hyaloid membrane to reach the anterior chamber. However, a few such cases have been reported in phakic eyes (6,7). Most commonly the anterior hyaloid is not intact, often from accidental injury or surgery, particularly after cataract extraction or vitrectomy, and thereby the products of hemorrhage can enter the anterior chamber and produce severe open angle glaucoma. Fresh hemorrhage into the vitreous humor appears red when viewed with the slit-lamp biomicroscope, but within 2 to 4 weeks the color of the material in the vitreous changes to a light tan or khaki color, due to loss of the red-colored hemoglobin and degeneration of the red cells to ghosts (Fig. 45.1). The red blood cells change from biconcave discs to spherical forms with Heinz bodies. Ghost cell glaucoma tends to develop within 3 to 4 weeks after the occurrence of a hemorrhage into the vitreous humor in an eye with a defective anterior hyaloid membrane. Myriads of small cells appear in the aqueous humor, and the IOP rises into the range of 30 to 70 mm Hg, with the angle remaining open.

In many instances, the appearance of a myriad of cells in the aqueous humor associated with a severe open angle glaucoma has been misinterpreted as an iritis or uveitis, in the belief that the cells were inflammatory cells. In such cases, topical or systemic treatment with corticosteroids has often been used, generally to no avail. In fact, corticosteroids may delay the "reabsorption" of the blood cells from the eye. (It is interesting to contemplate how corticosteroids might interfere with this blood reabsorption within the trabecular meshwork by interfering with normal trabecular cell actions. Similar cellular actions may be involved in steroid-induced open angle glaucoma (Chapter 44) or even POAG).

Ghost cell glaucoma with such tan-colored cells in the anterior chamber may be misinterpreted as post-surgical endophthalmitis. In these cases, there are no inflammatory keratic precipitates. If, with the slit-lamp biomicroscope, the color of the light tan old blood in the vitreous is compared with that of the fine cells circulating in the anterior chamber, they have the same hue, characteristic of ghost cells.

Aspiration of material from the anterior chamber in a series of cases of this sort, and immediate examination of the fluid by phase-contrast microscopy, without drying, staining, or filtering, has shown great numbers of ghost cells with characteristic Heinz bodies (Fig. 45.2). These cells have occasionally been called "erythroclasts." Their identity has been confirmed by transmission and scanning electron microscopy both in the aqueous and vitreous humors. Variable amounts of amorphous debris accompany the ghost cells, but in at least 15 samples of aqueous humor from eyes with "hemolytic" glaucoma examined by Campbell, macrophages were remarkably scarce, and there was no cellular evidence of inflammatory reaction (2).

By gonioscopy, the angle may appear normal, but if there are many ghost cells in the anterior chamber they may form a khaki-colored layer on the filtration portion of the trabecular meshwork, occasionally resembling a layer of butter. In more extreme cases the ghost cells may fill the dependent angle. The tan or yellowish color distinguishes this accumulation from an exudate or hypopyon of inflammatory cells.

The main causes of ghost-cell glaucoma in our experience have been 1) cataract extraction complicated by hemorrhage into the anterior chamber or vitreous cavity; 2) blunt or penetrating trauma with hemorrhage into the anterior chamber or vitreous cavity; 3) closed vitrectomy

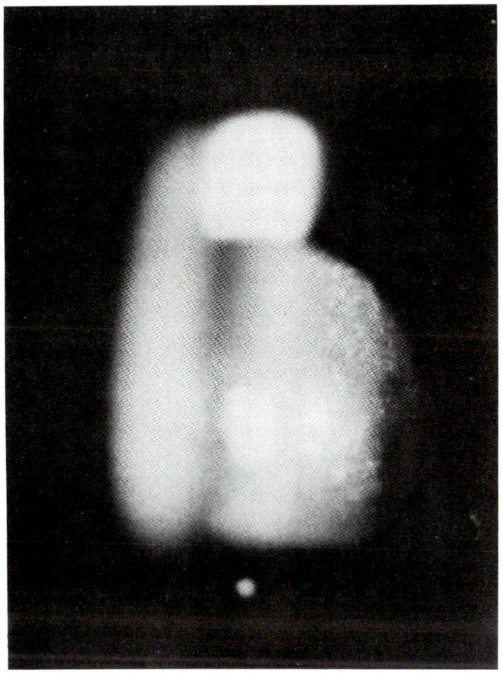

Fig. 45.1. Ghost cells in the vitreous subsequent to a contusion injury.

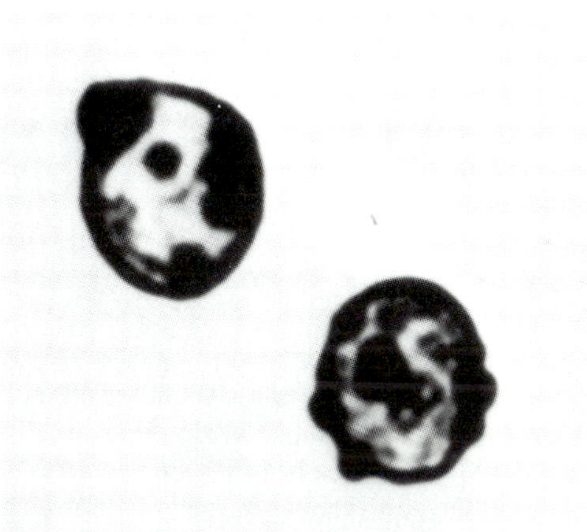

Fig. 45.2. Erythrocyte ghost cells with Heinz bodies as seen by phase-contrast microscopy in aqueous humor aspirated from the eye of a patient with hemolytic or ghost-cell glaucoma. These were found after a hemorrhage into the vitreous body and elevation of IOP associated with the appearance of myriads of ghost cells in the anterior chamber. (Courtesy of David G. Campbell).

for removal of vitreous hemorrhage for the purpose of improving vision. **Ghost cell glaucoma can also result from extensive hyphema formation alone, but is is most commonly associated with vitreous hemorrhage that acts as a reservoir for these cells to come into the anterior chamber after a subsequent interval of time.**

DIAGNOSIS

The diagnosis of hemolytic or ghost-cell glaucoma should be suspected whenever hemorrhage into the vitreous cavity has occurred and has been followed within 3 or 4 weeks by elevated IOP in the range of 30 to 70 mm Hg, associated with myriads of very small cells circulating in the anterior chamber, with no conglomerate KP on the corneal endothelium. There may be a **tan hyphema**, sometimes mixed with red blood (Fig. 45.3). When there has been trauma, gonioscopy may also show contusion-disruption of angle structures, but this should not distract attention from the importance of the fine cells in the aqueous humor. The diagnosis can be most securely established by aspirating the aqueous humor from the anterior chamber and examining it immediately by phase-contrast microscopy, without centrifuging, filtering, drying, or staining. Characteristically no inflammatory cells are seen, but a rare macrophage may be found, with innumerable erythrocyte ghost cells.

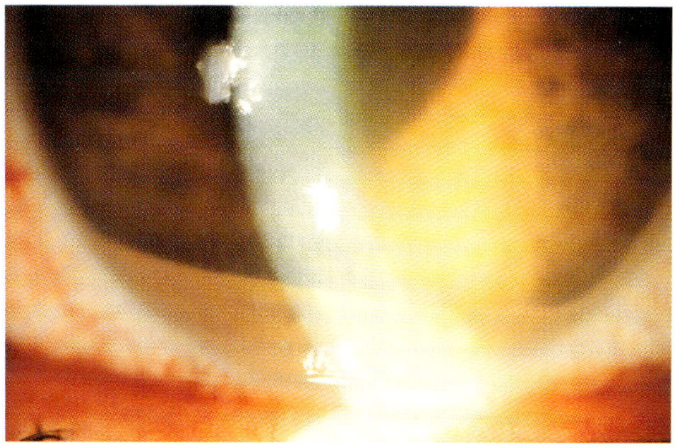

Fig. 45.3. Tan hyphema, which may at times be mixed with red blood cells, associated with glaucoma. Tan layer is comprised of ghost cells, red blood cells which have lost their hemoglobin and elasticity. These cells are responsible for the obstruction of outflow that results in ghost cell glaucoma.

MECHANISM

Campbell's experiments have provided evidence that permits one to explain the development of high IOP in this condition (2,3,5). **Normal red blood cells are so pliable that they pass readily through spaces smaller than the ordinary diameter of these cells (that are presumably present in the outflow pathway), but when they degenerate to ghost cells they lose this pliability and are unable to pass through the same small spaces.** This has been well demonstrated in vitro with standard microporous filters. Campbell has confirmed that fresh human red blood cells pass readily from the anterior chamber through the outflow system to the aqueous veins in enucleated normal human eyes, producing only a modest decrease in facility of aqueous outflow, and he has demonstrated that human erythrocyte ghosts differ from the fresh cells in being rigid and unable to pass from the anterior chamber through the aqueous outflow system (2). Instead, they obstruct and cause a marked reduction in facility of aqueous outflow, leading to the elevation of IOP.

TREATMENT

Treatment may be medical or surgical, depending on the seriousness of the situation. If IOP is not high, it may respond to medical therapy (aqueous suppressant therapy). Although miotics have been used with occasional success in the past by presumably mechanically widening the outflow channels to allow egress, this also may be counterproductive as in any eye with inflammation. If the IOP can be kept down to the 30 to 40 mm Hg range with this treatment, and the cornea is not edematous, and the patient is not in pain, the ghost cells may gradually clear in the course of some weeks (but remember the above potential contrary effect of corticosteroids), and the IOP may fall. However, if the amount of old hemorrhagic material in the vitreous is large, it may take too long to clear by slow diffusion forward into the anterior chamber and out the drainage system. When the IOP is in the 60 to 70 mm Hg range it is rare for medical treatment to reduce the IOP sufficiently, and surgical treatment is required. Systemic hyperosmotic agents usually help only temporarily. Surgical treatment is indicated also in those cases in which IOP in the 40 to 50 mm Hg range persists for weeks despite medical treatment. **In eyes prone to retinal or optic nerve vascular occlusion such as those with sickle cell anemia or trait, there is a much lower IOP threshold for surgical intervention (24–30 mm Hg)** (Chapter 43).

The surgical treatment consists of making a small paracentesis in the cornea, draining the contents of the anterior chamber, and irrigating the anterior chamber with a physiologic saline solution to wash out as many of the ghost cells as possible. If the ghost cells have come from a hemorrhage in the anterior chamber with little or no hemorrhage into the vitreous cavity, this treatment can be very effective, but if the ghost cells come from a large reservoir of old hemorrhagic material in the vitreous cavity, usually a single evacuation and irrigation of the anterior chamber is insufficient for lasting control. After a few days, the anterior chamber commonly again contains myriads of cells that have come from the vitreous chamber, the IOP is again high, and repeat evacuation and aspiration are required. In such cases, proceed to surgical vitrectomy rather than repeat anterior chamber irrigation. (Anterior chamber irrigation probably does not remove ghost cells from the interstices of the outflow pathway. Rather it eliminates a future load of such cells from going into the trabecular meshwork, and allows endogenous processes within this latter tissue to act to break down and remove the blood elements. It is this process that corticosteroids may interfere with, within the outflow pathway tissue.)

Vitrectomy has been effective in a number of cases in removing the reservoir of old blood from the vitreous cavity, allowing the anterior chamber to clear, and IOP to come down. Experience with vitrectomy suggests that to be effective in relieving the glaucoma, it must include thorough irrigation of the vitreous cavity, to leave behind as little of the old blood as possible.

This inference is drawn from a study in which patients who had old hemorrhage in the vitreous cavity, but no glaucoma, were subjected to closed vitrectomy to improve vision (8). In some of these cases, glaucoma developed within 2 to 10 days after the procedure. This was associated with a flooding of the anterior chamber with ghost cells, presumably entering through some breach in the anterior hyaloid membrane. This complication occurred less frequently when thorough irrigation was performed to remove as much old blood as possible from the vitreous cavity. In cases of ghost-cell glaucoma precipitated by closed vitrectomies with less thorough irrigation, the IOP characteristically was greater than 40 mm Hg, sometimes higher than 60 mm Hg. Some of these cases were controlled medically, and others required repeated irrigation of the anterior chamber. When only a small amount of the old blood remained in the vitreous cavity, there was less tendency for recurrence of glaucoma than when a larger reservoir of ghost cells was left in the vitreous cavity.

After vitrectomy, an increase of IOP can be produced in other ways. One must also consider the possibilities of corticosteroid glaucoma, lens-induced glaucoma, neovascular glaucoma, and obstruction of the outflow system by sickle cells in a patient with this disease (9). However, persistent ghost-cell glaucoma has been the most commonly observed cause of an increase of IOP after vitrectomy.

If despite these measures, there is reaccumulation of many cells in the anterior chamber and high IOP, other procedures must be considered. Cyclocryotherapy or newer ciliary destructive techniques have been effective in reducing the IOP in some cases, presumably by reducing the rate of aqueous formation.

The following case illustrates a typical course of ghost-cell glaucoma from contusion of the eye.

Case 45-1. A middle-aged man was struck in one eye by a block of wood, causing a small conjunctival laceration, moderate hyphema, and IOP below normal. Surgical exploration of the outer surface of the globe showed no rupture. In a few days, the hyphema spontaneously cleared from the anterior chamber. Gonioscopy showed contusion-disruption of angle structures superiorly, and the anterior chamber was abnormally deep superiorly, with a slight posterior subluxation of the upper portion of the lens. The pupil was not appreciably distorted and the lens was clear, but there was no fundus reflex due to extensive hemorrhage into the vitreous cavity. In about 2 weeks the IOP became normal. In 3 weeks, the IOP was in the 60s with diffuse corneal edema, pain, and myriads of fine cells in the anterior chamber, but no KP. Although the eye did not appear inflamed, the cells were misinterpreted as a sign of "iritis," and anti-inflammatory treatment was started with atropine and frequent application of corticosteroid. Oral glycerin produced only transient reduction of IOP. After 2 or 3 days with fundamentally no change, the patient was seen by one of us. A presumptive diagnose of ghost-cell glaucoma was made and diagnostic aspiration of aqueous humor and therapeutic washing out of the anterior chamber were done. Phase-contrast microscopy of the aqueous humor immediately after removal from the anterior chamber showed innumerable ghost cells, but no inflammatory cells or macrophages. For a day or two, IOP was normal, but soon more ghost cells leaked from the reservoir in the vitreous cavity to the anterior chamber, presumably through a defect in the anterior hyaloid membrane produced when the lens was subluxated, and the IOP increased again.

In contemplating the pathogenesis of various types of glaucoma and the mechanism by which they respond to various treatments and in thinking about how to evolve better treatments, it is interesting to consider that both in ghost-cell glaucoma and in lens-induced glaucoma, there is a good clinical response to washing out the anterior chamber, provided that there is no reservoir of ghost cells or lens material to replenish what was washed out (10). Usually in the following days, the IOP is normal, suggesting that the aqueous outflow system has become cleared of the obstructing material. Yet, when the conditions are reproduced experimentally in an excised human eye by introducing ghost cells or lens proteins (11) into the anterior chamber, clearly obstructing outflow of aqueous fluid from the anterior chamber, we find no immediate relief of the obstruction when we wash out the anterior chamber. Therefore, in vivo there must be some vital aid to clearing the outflow channels after the bulk of the material has been removed from the anterior chamber. Corticosteroids may interfere with these trabecular cellular processes. We wonder if macrophages are helping to clear the outflow system, and whether there could be some advantage in stimulating their activity. Other therapeutic approaches might conceivably include use of enzymes to break down ghost cells or lens proteins to fragments that might more easily pass through the aqueous outflow system and obstruct it less.

HEMOSIDEROTIC GLAUCOMA

The discussion in this chapter has been limited to the acute problems posed by erythrocyte ghost cells; we have not considered the late consequence of leaving blood degenerating in the eye for a long time, which may lead to a different condition, called hemosiderotic glaucoma, which usually is diagnosed histologically after enucleation of a blind eye. That condition is characterized by degeneration of the trabecular meshwork, with positive staining for iron (12,13).

References

1. Fenton RH, Zimmerman LE: Hemolytic glaucoma. Arch Ophthalmol 1963;70:236–239.
2. Campbell DG, Simmons RJ, Grant WM: Ghost cells as a cause of glaucoma. Am J Ophthalmol 1976;81:441–450.
3. Campbell DG, Essigmann EM: Hemolytic ghost cell glaucoma. Further studies. Arch Ophthalmol 1979;97:2141–6.
4. Campbell DG: Ghost cell glaucoma following trauma. Ophthalmology 1981;88:1151–8.
5. Lambrou FH Jr, Aiken DG, Woods WD, et al: The production and mechanism of ghost cell glaucoma in the cat and primate. Invest Ophthalmol Vis Sci 1985;26:893–7.
6. Mansour AM, Chess J, Starita R: Nontraumatic ghost cell glaucoma—a case report. Ophthalmic Surg 1986;17:34–6.
7. Frazer DG, Kidd MN, Johnston PB: Ghost cell glaucoma in phakic eyes. Int Ophthalmol 1987;11:51–4.
8. Campbell DG, Simmons RJ, Tolentino FI, et al: Glaucoma occurring after closed vitrectomy. Am J Ophthalmol 1977;83:63–69.
9. Wilensky JT, Goldberg MF, Alward P: Glaucoma after pars plana vitrectomy. Trans Am Acad Ophthalmol Otolaryngol 1977;83:OP-114–121.
10. Phelps CD, Watzke RC: Hemolytic glaucoma. Am J Ophthalmol 1975; 80:690–695.
11. Epstein DL, Jedziniak JA, Grant WM: Obstruction of aqueous outflow by lens particles and by heavy molecular weight soluble lens protein. Invest Ophthalmol Vis Sci 1978;17:272–277.
12. Benson WE, Spalter HF: Vitreous hemorrhage. Surv Ophthalmol 1975; 15:297–311.
13. Wollensak J: Phakolytisches und Hämolytisches Glaukom. Klin Monnatsbl Augenheilkd 1976;168:447–452.

Glaucoma Associated With Extraocular Venous Congestion (Increased Episcleral Venous Pressure)

46

David L. Epstein

INTRODUCTION

Increased episcleral venous pressure may be seen in the following clinical situations: (1) carotid-cavernous sinus fistulas and dural shunts; (2) Sturge-Weber syndrome; and (3) an idiopathic type (1–5).

Glaucoma due to increased episcleral venous pressure is not rare. It is common for clinicians to focus in on the slit-lamp examination of the cornea, anterior chamber, or posterior segment and perhaps overlook the presence of abnormally prominent episcleral veins. Routinely evaluating eyes with a penlight (Chapter 5) can greatly assist in making the diagnosis in these "red eye" glaucomas. **Both the "idiopathic" type and that due to a subclinical dural shunt are underdiagnosed.**

When an antiglaucoma therapy does not decrease the intraocular pressure (IOP), in addition to repeating gonioscopy, it is important to carefully re-examine the episcleral vessels. (Because the IOP cannot be lowered below the draining "downstream pressure" in this condition, the IOP remains elevated after initiation of medical therapy).

Whenever blood in Schlemm's canal is observed spontaneously in an eye with elevated IOP, this diagnosis should also be entertained.

Many such cases, especially the idiopathic and Sturge-Weber types, come to filtration surgery because of the persistent elevation of IOP despite medical therapy. **The increased episcleral venous pressure causing the elevated IOP via the anterior segment is an indicator of an increase in orbital venous pressure.** Thus, when such eyes are decompressed through the usual limbal incision for the filtration fistula, the transmitted elevation in choroidal venous pressure may result in transudation of fluid into the suprachoroidal space (2), which then forces intraocular contents forward through the fistula. Prophylactic posterior sclerotomies performed before entry into the anterior chamber can diminish the severity of this occurrence and also the postoperative sequelae (2). Smaller incision/excision trabeculectomy techniques with use of anterior chamber viscoelastics or maintainers should also be used.

INCREASED ORBITAL VENOUS PRESSURE

Increasing the venous pressure in the head and orbit causes the IOP to increase. Some of the pathophysiology of this relationship has been studied experimentally by Comberg and Pilz (6). Clinically, the causes of elevation of venous pressure that are of particular significance to the eye include carotid-cavernous sinus fistula, thrombosis of orbital veins or cavernous sinus, dural arteriovenous shunts, endocrine exophthalmos (7), pulmonary venous obstruction by tumors or cardiopulmonary disease, and obstruction of the superior vena cava. Congestive heart failure causes only a slight increase in IOP (8).

The venous abnormalities of the head and orbit are often unilateral and affect only one eye, whereas compression of veins in the neck or chest usually affects both eyes. There are other conditions in which both the extraocular venous pressure and the IOP are elevated, but their exact mechanism for this elevation of venous pressure is as yet unclear. This includes certain cases of hemangioma with glaucoma (Sturge-Weber syndrome) and the above mentioned particular combination of conspicuously dilated episcleral vessels with open angle glaucoma, but without other demonstrated extraocular vasculopathy (that we have termed "idiopathic") (Fig. 46.1).

Signs and Symptoms

The signs and symptoms of thrombosis of orbital veins or arteriovenous fistula may have rapid onset, sometimes with pain on the same side of the head (9). The episcleral veins appear dilated on the affected side. Chemosis and exophthalmos may develop within hours or days. The exophthalmos may be pulsating if an arteriovenous fistula is present. The retinal veins may appear dilated on the same side. The IOP becomes elevated, most commonly to the mid-20s to mid-30s, and the ocular pulse is increased. These changes are most pronounced in cases of arteriovenous communication. **If pressure is measured in the episcleral or orbital veins, the increase of IOP is about the same as the increase of venous pressure above its ordinary baseline of approximately 8 to 10 mm Hg.**

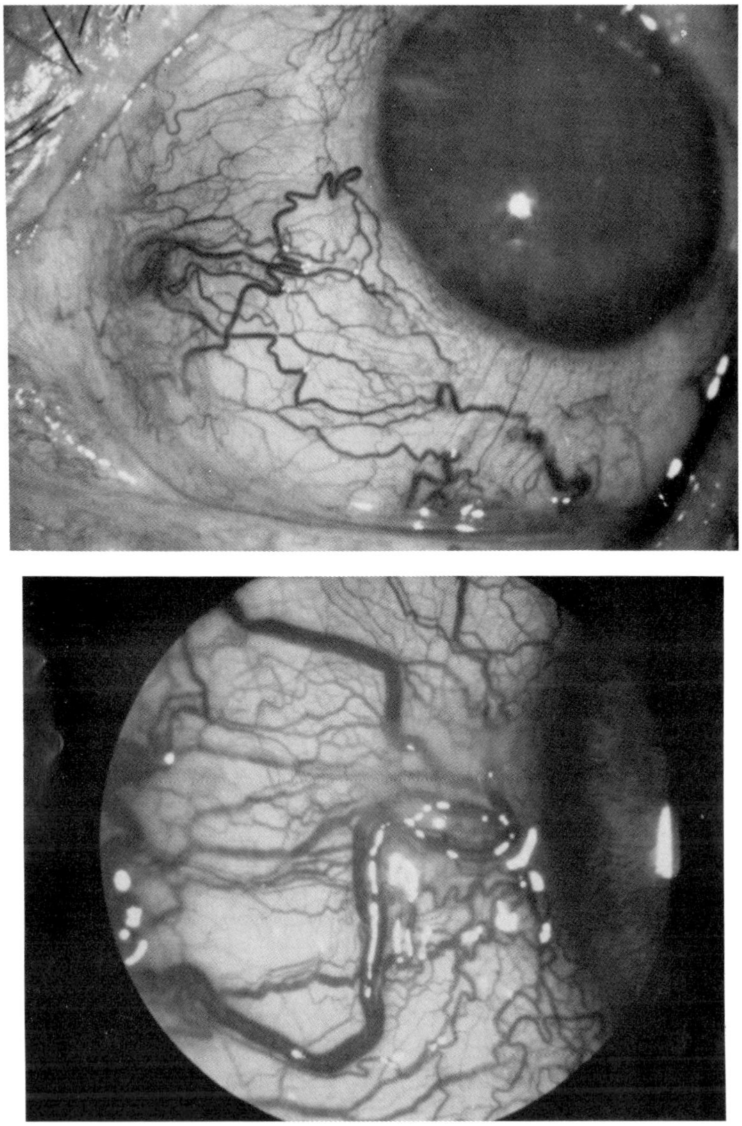

A

B

Figure 46.1. Prominent episcleral veins, increased episcleral venous pressure and glaucoma due to dural shunt (A), Sturge-Weber disease (B), and in an idiopathic condition (C). Compare the episcleral vessels in these conditions to those in a normal patient (D).

A rare complication of elevated orbital venous pressure is shallowing of the anterior chamber on the affected side (10–12); angle closure glaucoma may result. The shallowing is attributable to increased venous volume or edema fluid in the posterior segment, in some cases visible as choroidal detachment (10,11).

In rare cases of carotid-cavernous sinus fistula not only may there be elevated orbital venous pressure, but the arterial blood supply to the eye may be partially obstructed, and the rate of aqueous formation may be reduced. Then the IOP may remain low despite elevated venous pressure. In rare instances anterior segment necrosis has occurred under these circumstances (13,14). The danger appears to be greatest when the arteriovenous fistula has been treated by occluding the feeding artery.

A further complication in cases of long-standing elevated venous pressure and reduced arterial supply is growth of new blood vessels on the iris and in the angle, leading potentially to neovascular glaucoma (12,15).

In dural shunts (Fig. 46.1A) (16), which are lower pressure arteriovenous shunts than the above, the signs and symptoms may be much more subtle. Patients may actually be unaware of their "red eye." This is also true in the idiopathic variety of increased episcleral venous pressure. Also, many patients with Sturge-Weber syndrome, although fully aware of their facial hemangioma, do not appreciate well the episcleral involvement, which as will be discussed, may not become prominent until teenage years.

In most cases of elevated orbital venous pressure with secondary modest elevation of IOP, the angle remains open, and in most cases the tonographic facility of outflow remains normal. In these cases, if the orbital venous pressure subsequently becomes normal, either spontaneously or as a result of treatment, the IOP

Figure 46.1. *(continued)*

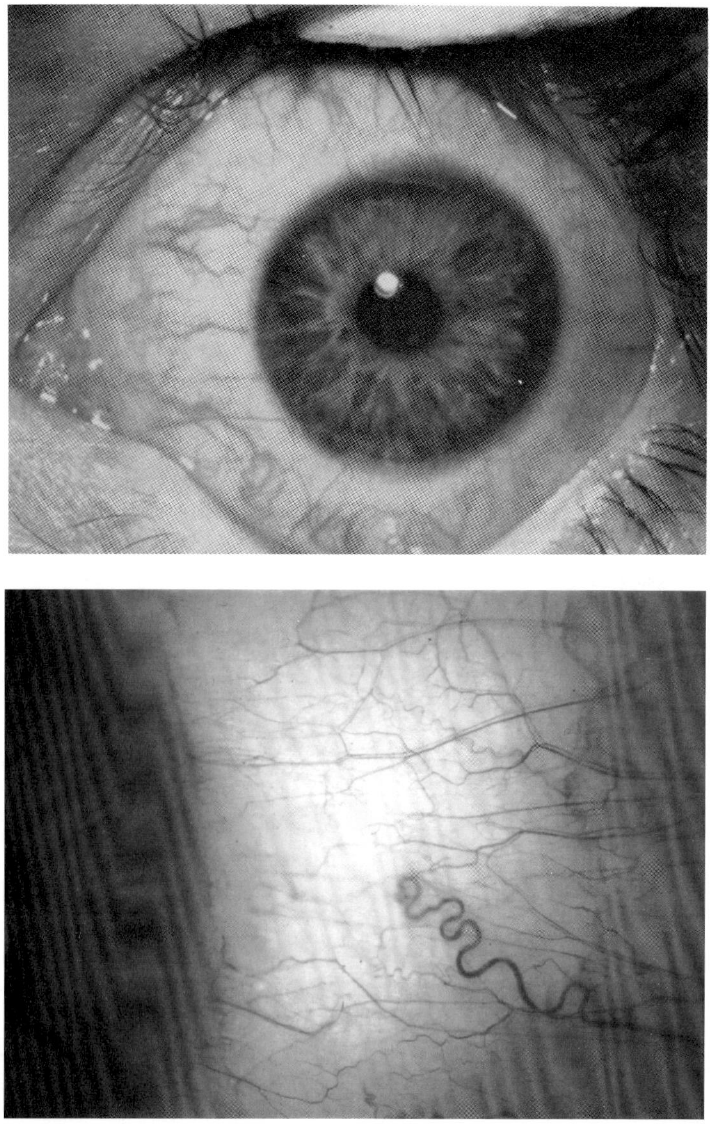

C

D

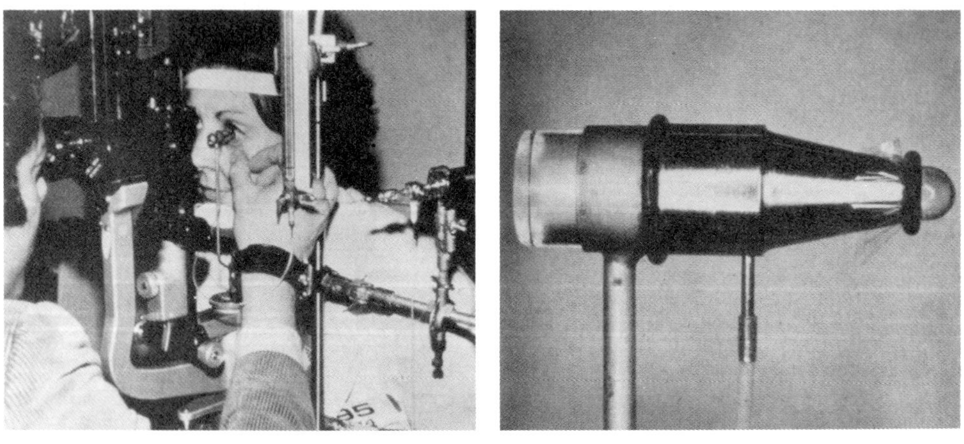

Figure 46.2. Clinical measurement of episcleral venous pressure (A). The pressure required to just compress an episcleral vein is determined. The vein is directly viewed through a fluid filled chamber (B) which is connected to a manometer. Apparatus is based on a National Eye Institute prototype and was assembled by A. Robert Bellows, MD. The membrane for the chamber is courtesy of Douglas Gaasterland, MD.

AQUEOUS HUMOR DYNAMICS: A "TRICK" QUESTION

David L. Epstein

A frequent "trick" question given to ophthalmology residents and students is: what is the tonographic outflow facility in a patient with elevated IOP due to increased episcleral venous pressure? There is a natural tendency to answer that outflow facility is abnormal because obviously the IOP is elevated. This is incorrect. Tonographic outflow facility, at least early in the disease process, can be, and is usually, normal despite the elevated IOP.

Consider the following: with a normal IOP of, e.g., 16 mm Hg, there is a resistance decrease across the trabecular meshwork (the inverse of which is mathematically termed the outflow facility or C value) to the downstream collector channel (episcleral venous) pressure of, e.g., 8 mm Hg. Assume that episcleral venous pressure is now suddenly elevated an additional 10 mm Hg to a value of 18, then the IOP would also go up 10 mm Hg to 26, even though the resistance across the trabecular meshwork is unchanged (i.e., the C value remains normal).

We have studied this phenomenon in preliminary studies using ophthalmic resident "volunteers," who in performing a Valsalva maneuver raised both measured episcleral venous pressure and IOP similarly mm for mm. For some residents, despite facial congestion during the attempted Valsalva maneuver, their episcleral venous pressure and IOP did not increase at all, whereas others did as described.

For completeness sake, the concept of pseudofacility (1) will also be described. In normal patients who had a blood pressure cuff placed around their neck and inflated, episcleral venous pressure became elevated, but IOP increased to a slightly smaller degree. IOP usually increased within 1 mm Hg of the induced episcleral venous pressure elevation. This small difference between episcleral venous and IOP elevation was termed "pseudofacility," and indicated what was believed to be an induced decrease in aqueous humor formation in response to this elevation of eye pressure. The effect is small, and the overall phenomenon actually indicated that aqueous humor formation does not, in fact, self-regulate in response to the level of IOP. There are also no known feedback loops or anatomical connections that could allow such a regulatory process (other than a direct pressure effect on the fluid secreting cells in the ciliary body).

References

1. Kupfer C: Clinical significance of pseudofacility. Sanford R. Gifford Memorial Lecture. Am J Ophthalmol 1973;75:193–204.

returns to normal. However, when the facility of outflow is abnormal (as it often is in long standing cases of increased episcleral venous pressure), glaucoma may persist even after venous pressure is normalized, as though permanent damage has been done to the aqueous outflow system by the chronic elevation of episcleral venous pressure (17). In cases of neovascularization and synechial closure of the angle, this persistent glaucoma is understandable, but the outflow system of eyes with open angles may also be affected as postulated by Weekers (18). This is a consideration that seems to us to deserve more study: why would chronic elevation of episcleral venous pressure cause trabecular meshwork dysfunction?

IDIOPATHIC ELEVATION OF EPISCLERAL VENOUS PRESSURE

To this point, we have mainly discussed elevations of IOP that are apparently secondary to abnormally high extraocular venous pressure and that can usually be relieved if the venous pressure can be reduced. There is another group of unusual cases (1–5) in which there is no recognized cause outside of the eye for elevation of venous pressure and are thus termed "idiopathic" cases, but vessels on the globe are conspicuously large, and measurement (Fig. 46.2) shows the pressure in these vessels to be elevated, to more than 30 mm Hg in some cases (Fig. 46.1C). (Patients who have primary open angle glaucoma have normal episcleral venous pressure.)

This **"idiopathic" variety** of increased episcleral venous pressure is fascinating, but poorly understood. It is underdiagnosed and **needs to be considered in the differential diagnosis of refractory cases of "open angle glaucoma."** This condition can be unilateral or bilateral. A few such patients have had intracranial scans and studies with no observed abnormality. This should now be reexamined with the latest generation of noninvasive intracranial techniques. If these tests are also negative, this entity presumably must then be caused by some orbital (4) or periocular venous abnormality with increased pressure transmitted both to the episcleral veins and also the choroidal veins. Therefore, prophylactic posterior sclerotomies (2), smaller incision/excision trabeculectomies, and anterior chamber viscoelastics or maintainers should also be used at the time of filtration surgery in such patients, as in other glaucoma patients with elevated venous pressure.

STURGE-WEBER SYNDROME

A similar set of conditions can be found unilaterally or occasionally bilaterally in cases of hemangioma (Sturge-

Weber syndrome) with open angle glaucoma (19–22). **Patients with Sturge-Weber syndrome and glaucoma fall into two categories: those with congenital mesodermal angle abnormalities and those with elevated episcleral (and orbital) venous pressure presumably due to the presence of orbital and periocular hemangiomas.**

In the first category, the onset of glaucoma is typically early in life with frequent buphthalmos, anisometropia/amblyopia, advanced disc cupping when first detected, and severe refractoriness to medical antiglaucoma therapy. Sometimes the angle abnormality (23–25) may be accompanied (perhaps later in life) by the presence of dilated episcleral vessels with increased venous pressure.

In the second category, there is no buphthalmos, etc., and, in fact, there often is a history of onset of a "red eye" and accompanying glaucoma in the teenage years, sometimes at menarche. If examined at that time, there is often high IOP but only early disc cupping, implying a later onset to the glaucoma (and perhaps also the episcleral venous prominence), as if "something new" were happening hemodynamically in the teenage years. Regardless, the glaucoma associated with Sturge-Weber, once observed, is commonly characterized by persisting high IOP, requiring filtration surgery.

TREATMENT

Standard medical antiglaucoma therapy is used first, especially the aqueous humor suppressants, which by their action can reduce the IOP downwards towards the level of the (elevated) episcleral venous pressure. When the IOP is high enough to be damaging to the optic disc and visual field despite maximal tolerated medical treatment, an operation becomes necessary. As discussed previously, tonography in these long standing cases, whether due to dural shunt, Sturge-Weber syndrome, or the idiopathic variety, shows subnormal facility of aqueous outflow, and accordingly there is little expectation that the glaucoma would be cured by reducing the venous pressure at this stage of the disease, even if we knew how to do it. Laser trabeculoplasty should be attempted and occasionally can be surprisingly effective when there is subnormal outflow facility. However, most commonly filtration surgery is required.

Filtering Surgery

A major complication of intraocular surgery in these cases is a tendency for the lens-iris diaphragm and ciliary body to push forward and flatten the anterior chamber when the anterior chamber is opened. In the postoperative period, there is a tendency for large choroidal detachments (2,23,26,27) to persist with an associated shallow or flat anterior chamber. In cases of Sturge-Weber syndrome this has been recognized for some time, but has only recently been appreciated in these other types of open angle glaucoma associated with elevated episcleral venous pressure.

Prophylactic Posterior Sclerotomy

In patients who have had open angle glaucoma and elevated episcleral venous pressure, and in certain patients with hemangioma and glaucoma, **effusion of suprachoroidal fluid begins during the filtering surgery** itself, presumably in response to rapid reduction of IOP when the anterior chamber is opened (2). The episcleral and vortex veins drain separate areas of the globe. However, we believe that the elevated episcleral venous pressure that we measure identifies an abnormal elevation of venous pressure that also affects the choroidal venous system in these patients. The effusion accounts for the pushing forward of lens, ciliary processes, and iris. **Intraoperative anterior chamber shallowing can be reduced by initially performing posterior sclerotomies before entering the eye.** This is done by making an incision through the sclera to the potential suprachoroidal space so that uveal effusion fluid can drain from the globe as it forms, rather than cause the anterior chamber to flatten (2) (Chapter 63). This also appears to reduce the extent of postoperative choroidal detachment. Although the number of cases in which this procedure has been used is still small, preliminary posterior sclerotomy has appeared so far to be of great value in reducing the complications of surgery in eyes with abnormally high episcleral venous pressure.

OTHER BASIC ASPECTS

Aside from these practical clinical points, there are some intriguing basic aspects that deserve further thought and investigation. Measurements by some of us (ARB and DLE) (Fig. 46.2) have shown that reducing the IOP by filtering operation in the syndrome of open angle glaucoma associated with elevated episcleral venous pressure does not change the episcleral venous pressure, and we conclude therefore that the pressure in these vessels must be determined by something other than the rate of outflow of aqueous humor. After successful filtration surgery the aqueous humor is no longer constrained by the regular outflow system to enter the episcleral veins against venous backpressure, but it is free to bypass this system and escape into the extravascular tissue at low IOPs.

One other intriguing aspect of the open angle glaucoma associated with elevated episcleral venous pressure of unknown origin is that in certain cases no blood has been seen gonioscopically in Schlemm's canal either before or after surgery, despite the fact that the filtration operations have made the IOP considerably lower than the pressure in the episcleral veins on the surface of the globe. This suggests obstruction within or beyond Schlemm's canal. This phenomenon may also be involved in the pathogenesis of the reduced aqueous humor outflow, which is commonly seen with chronic elevation of episcleral venous pressure.

References

1. Radius RL, Maumenee AE: Dilated episcleral vessels and open-angle glaucoma. Am J Ophthalmol 1978;86:31–5.
2. Bellows AR, Chylack LT, Epstein DL, et al: Intraoperative choroidal effusion during glaucoma surgery in patients with elevated episcleral venous pressure. Arch Ophthalmol 1979;97:493–497.
3. Talusan ED, Fishbein SL, Schwartz B: Increased pressure of dilated episcleral veins with open-angle glaucoma. Ophthalmology. 1983;90: 257–65.
4. de Keizer RJ: Secondary vascular glaucoma. Doc Ophthalmol 1983;56: 195–202.
5. Jorgensen JS, Guthoff R: The role of episcleral venous pressure in the development of secondary glaucomas. Klin Monatsbl Augenheilkd 1988; 193:471–5.
6. Comberg D, Pilz A: Der Augendruck als Funktion des Venendruckes. Ber Dtsch Ophthalmol Ges 1961;63:332–336.
7. Aron-Rosa D, Morax PV, Aron JJ, et al: Exopthalmie oedemateuses endocriniennes et blocage circulatoire veineux orbitaire. Intérêt des phlébographies. Ann Ocul (Paris) 1970;203:1–24.
8. Bettelheim H: Der episklerale Venendruck bei pulmonaler Hypertension. Ein Beitrag zur Frage des kardiogenen Glaukoms. Graefes Arch Klin Exp Ophthalmol 1969;177:108–115.
9. Aron-Rosa D, Offret G, Ramee A, et al: La phlébographie orbitaire. Bull Soc Ophthalmol Fr Numero Special 1967;1–36.
10. Blervacque A, Voillez M, Dufour D, et al: Rôle des troubles circulatoires orbito-caverneux dans la genèse du soulevement rétino-choroidien antérieur. Bull Soc Ophthalmol Fr 1968;68:1056–1058.
11. Guerry D III, Harbison JW, Wiesinger H: Bilateral choroidal detachment and fluctuating proptosis secondary to bilateral dural arteriovenous fistula treated with transcranial orbital decompression with resolution: report of a case. Trans Am Ophthalmol Soc 1975;73:64–73.
12. Fiore PM, Latina MA, Shingleton BJ, et al: The dural shunt syndrome. I. Management of glaucoma. Ophthalmology 1990;97:56–62.
13. Sanders MD, Hoyt WF: Hypoxic ocular sequelae of carotid-cavernous fistulae. Br J Ophthalmol 1969;53:82–97.
14. Spencer WH, Thompson HS, Hoyt WF: Ischaemic ocular necrosis from carotid-cavernous fistula. Br J Ophthalmol 1973;57:145–152.
15. Weiss DI, Shaffer RN, Nehrenberg TR: Neovascular glaucoma complicating carotid-cavernous fistula. Arch Ophthalmol 1963;69:304–307.
16. Grove AS Jr: The dural shunt syndrome. Pathophysiology and clinical course. Ophthalmology 1984;91:31–44.
17. Nordmann J, Lobstein A, Gerhard JP, et al: A propos de 14 cas de glaucoma par hypertension veinuse d'origine extraoculaire. Ophthalmol Suppl 1961;142:501–505.
18. Weekers R, Grieten J: Pathogenie et traitement de l'hypertension oculaire dans l'exophalmie par anévrisme arterio-veineux. Arch Ophtalmol (Paris) 1965;25:531–536.
19. Bessière E, Verin P: Le tonogramme vasculaire. Arch Ophthalmol (Paris) 1965;25:449–458.
20. Phelps CD: The pathogenesis of glaucoma in Sturge-Weber syndrome. Ophthalmology 1978;85:276–286.
21. Phelps CD, Thompson HS, Ossoinig KC: The diagnosis and prognosis of atypical carotid-cavernous fistula (red-eyed shunt syndrome). Am J Ophthalmol 1982;93:423–436.
22. Jorgensen JS, Guthoff R: Sturge-Weber syndrome: glaucoma with elevated episcleral venous pressure. Klin Monatsbl Augenheilkd 1987;191: 275–8.
23. Christensen GR, Records RE: Glaucoma and expulsive hemorrhage mechanisms in the Sturge-Weber syndrome. Ophthalmology 1979;86: 1360–6.
24. Cibis GW, Tripathi RC, Tripathi BJ: Glaucoma in Sturge-Weber syndrome. Ophthalmology 1984;91:1061–71.
25. Mwinula JH, Sagawa T, Tawara A, et al: Anterior chamber angle vascularization in Sturge-Weber syndrome. Report of a case. Graefes Arch Clin Exp Ophthalmol 1994;232:387–91.
26. Iwach AG, Hoskins HD Jr, Hetherington J Jr, et al: Analysis of surgical and medical management of glaucoma in Sturge-Weber syndrome. Ophthalmology 1990;97:904–909.
27. Bellows AR, Chylack LT Jr, Hutchinson BT: Choroidal detachment. Clinical manifestation, therapy and mechanism of formation. Ophthalmology 1981;88:1107–15.

Lens-Induced Glaucoma

47

David L. Epstein

We use the term "lens-induced" glaucoma for the secondary open-angle glaucoma associated with leakage of lens proteins into the eye, from lens particles, or from phacoanaphylaxis. Recent laboratory investigations have given insight into underlying mechanisms and offer a framework for better understanding and classification.

PHACOLYTIC GLAUCOMA

History

The term phacolytic glaucoma was first proposed by Flocks, Littwin, and Zimmerman as a secondary open-angle glaucoma of rapid onset associated with a leaking hypermature cataract (1). Subsequently, others have misused the term phacolytic as though it applied to all types of lens-induced glaucomas. Flocks, Littwin, and Zimmerman said they believed that phacolytic glaucoma was attributable to obstruction of the intertrabecular spaces by macrophages distended with engulfed lens material and Morgagnian fluid that had escaped from the lens. Goldberg popularized Millipore filtration for diagnostic identification of the macrophages in this condition, (2) but he, too, suspected that the glaucoma was caused by blockage of the angle by both proteinaceous debris and macrophages. In recent years the supposed role of macrophages in producing the glaucoma has been highlighted, and the possible obstruction of the trabecular meshwork by liberated lens material has been mentioned infrequently.

Mechanism(s) for the Glaucoma

Our laboratory investigations indicate that **soluble lens proteins that leak from hypermature cataracts cause severe obstruction of aqueous outflow and that this is likely important in the pathogenesis of phacolytic** glaucoma (3).

In these experiments, heavy-molecular-weight lens protein, infused into the anterior chamber of enucleated human eyes in amounts similar to those found clinically in the aqueous humor of patients with phacolytic glaucoma, produced a severe obstruction of fluid outflow (Fig. 47.1) that increased with the length of the perfusion time. This obstruction was not relieved by simple irrigation of the anterior chamber (Chapter 45), suggesting that dynamic mechanisms, perhaps involving macrophages, may be required in vivo to relieve such an obstruction.

Other experiments indicated that the aqueous outflow channels were also easily obstructed by particulate lens material. It was not determined what proportion of the lens particle obstruction was attributable to insoluble lens protein and what proportion to cell membrane fragments. This "lens particle glaucoma" seems likely to be the predominant mechanism in early postoperative glaucoma due to retained lens cortex and to be less often involved in spontaneous phacolytic glaucoma. In certain cases of phacolytic glaucoma, however, a hypermature lens may rupture either spontaneously or during surgery, and in such cases glaucoma of acute onset may be due to a combination of obstructing lens particles and soluble lens proteins.

Analogous to interference with outflow by lens proteins, we found that obstruction of outflow by serum proteins may be an important factor in open angle glaucoma associated with uveitis (4). In related experiments, infusion of human serum into enucleated human eyes produced a significant decrease in facility of outflow that likewise was not relieved by simple irrigation of the anterior chamber. Diluted serum caused greater obstruction upon perfusion than would be expected on the basis of viscosity alone. Lens depression, induced experimentally to simulate ciliary muscle contraction, improved the facility of outflow but did not alleviate the partial obstruction induced by serum. It is possible that normal serum components may become entrapped in the outflow channels and produce glaucoma. Such serum obstruction may be a factor in glaucoma refractory to corticosteroid therapy in eyes with chronic uveitis, especially when there is little cellular reaction but persistent flare.

In phacolytic glaucoma, the role of macrophages is unclear, but they may be present simply as scavengers of lens material in the anterior chamber, clearing lens protein from the outflow pathways. In children, macrophages have been observed in the anterior chamber in the presence of lens material without causing elevation of IOP. Yanoff and Scheie in particular described typical engorged macrophages, although perhaps fewer than in phacolytic glaucoma, in the anterior chamber fluid of children at the time of surgery for secondary cataracts, without evidence of glaucoma (5). Interestingly, Dueker has placed large numbers of rabbit macrophages, which have engulfed oil in the peritoneum, into the anterior chamber of rabbits and failed to observe any significant elevation of IOP (6).

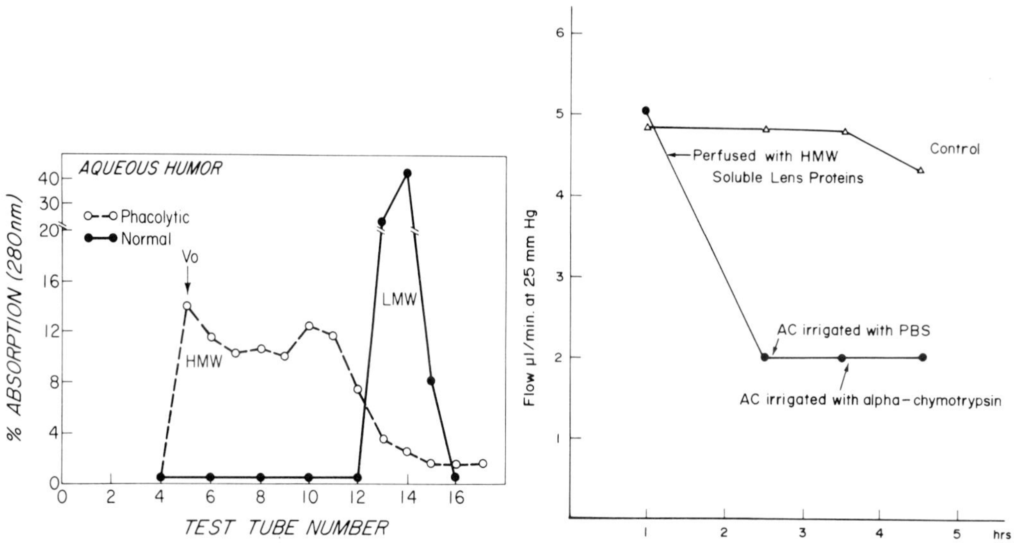

Figure 47.1. Heavy molecular weight (HMW) protein has been identified in the aqueous humor of patients with phacolytic glaucoma (A); experimental anterior chamber perfusion of similar quantities of HMW protein in excised human eyes causes a severe obstruction of aqueous humor outflow (B). Reprinted with permission from Epstein DL, Jedziniak JA, Grant WM: Identification of heavy molecular weight soluble lens protein in aqueous humor in human phacolytic glaucoma. Invest Ophthalmol Vis Sci 1978;17:398–402, and Epstein DL, Jedziniak JA, Grant WM: Obstruction of aqueous outflow by lens particles and by heavy molecular weight soluble lens proteins. Invest Ophthalmol Vis Sci 1978;17:272–277.

Clinical Findings

In phacolytic glaucoma there is rapid onset of pain and redness in the eye. IOP may become extremely high, greater than 80 mm Hg in some cases. Corneal epithelial edema is usually present. The angle remains open and without visible abnormality. The lens usually shows hypermature or mature cataract, or rarely an immature cataract in which there is liquefaction of the posterior cortex. In connection with immature cataract, the glaucoma tends to be less acute in onset and not to be associated with such high IOP at the outset. **Patches of white material, probably macrophages, may be seen on the anterior surface of the crystalline lens** (Fig. 47.2). In rare cases the cataractous lens is dislocated into the vitreous cavity, either spontaneously or as a result of trauma.

Inflammatory precipitates, such as scattered cells or conglomerate KP, may or may not be present on the corneal endothelium. Only in one case with this condition have we seen what looked like KP in the angle. Cellular reaction in the anterior chamber in some cases of phacolytic glaucoma is slight, but more often is moderate, and in rare instances is accompanied by hypopyon (7). Usually one sees circulating white particles that are significantly larger than white blood cells and that have been variously interpreted as very large cells (8,9) (such as swollen macrophages), cellular aggregates, or small particles of lens material (perhaps aggregated insoluble lens protein).

Treatment

The **eye in phacolytic glaucoma shows inadequate response to medical antiglaucoma or anti-inflammatory therapy.** The IOP may be reduced considerably, but only temporarily, with beta blockers, apraclonidine, carbonic anhydrase inhibitors and osmotic agents, but usually the IOP remains too high for adequate medical management. As a rule, patients with presumed phacolytic glaucoma should have cataract surgery fairly promptly. This may be indicated as an emergency measure if the IOP does not drop promptly from a dangerously high level in response to the initial medical treatment. The IOP usually returns to normal within a few days after cataract surgery. The relative merits and precautions of extracapsular versus intracapsular cataract surgery for phacolytic glaucoma are discussed in the subsequent section, "Understanding Lens-Induced Glaucomas."

Possible Laboratory Studies

Microscopic examination of anterior chamber fluid usually reveals engorged macrophages (8,9). They are often not numerous and their number does not correlate with the severity of the glaucoma. Occasionally there are no macrophages in the aspirated fluid, but in almost all cases there is fine amorphous material in the anterior chamber fluid. Biochemical studies have identified heavy-molecular-weight lens protein in aqueous humor from all cases of phacolytic glaucoma so far examined for this material (10).

The heavy-molecular-weight lens protein is not present in the aqueous humor of nonglaucomatous patients with ordinary cataracts or in patients with cataract and primary open angle glaucoma. Biochemical analysis of anterior chamber fluid is potentially useful in the clinical diagnosis of phacolytic glaucoma. It is now accepted practice in sus-

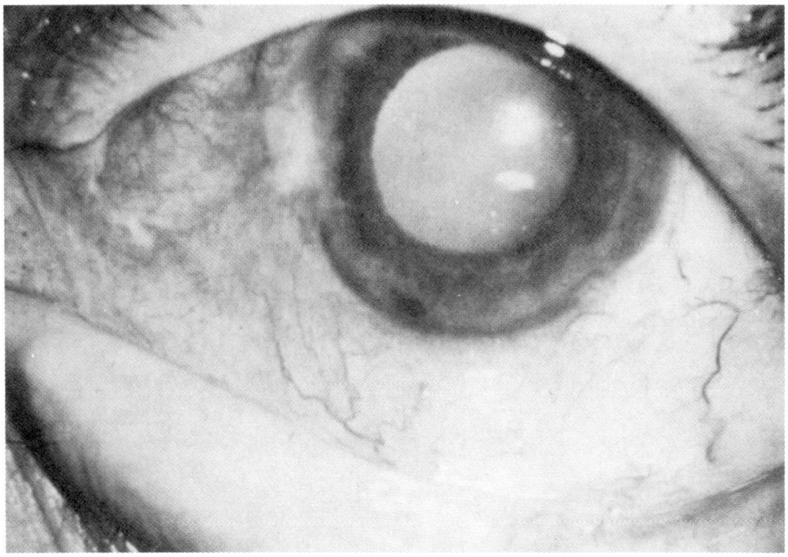

Figure 47.2. Leaking hypermature cataract with the lens nucleus suspended in a "sea" of milky white cortical fluid in a patient with phacolytic glaucoma. There are white patches present on the anterior lens capsule. Reprinted with permission from Epstein DL: Lens-induced open-angle glaucoma. In: The Secondary Glaucomas. Edited by Ritch R, Shields MB. St. Louis, C.V. Mosby Co., 1982.

pected cases to aspirate the aqueous humor and to obtain washings of the anterior chamber for microscopic search for macrophages and, if assays are available, for lens proteins. However, one can usually arrive at the correct diagnosis on purely clinical grounds.

Calcium oxalate crystals have also been found in the aqueous humor of certain patients with phacolytic glaucoma (11).

Diagnosis

Diagnosis of phacolytic glaucoma without the help of laboratory aids sometimes takes longer, but the diagnosis should not be missed. If the diagnosis for an inflamed cataractous eye with considerably elevated IOP is in doubt, the usual medical treatment for glaucoma secondary to inflammation is used: cycloplegics, topical corticosteroids, beta blockers, apraclonidine, carbonic anhydrase inhibitors, and oral osmotic agents. This treatment may bring about a temporary improvement, but if the condition is due to phacolysis we cannot cure it, and the IOP eventually becomes out of control. We then conclude that the condition is probably lens induced and proceed to perform cataract surgery.

Clinical Examples

The state of the cataract that may induce phacolytic glaucoma varies from case to case. Hypermature cataract in situ is usually responsible, but phacolytic glaucoma can be caused by an immature cataract. We will discuss the differences in these circumstances.

HYPERMATURE CATARACT: LENS IN SITU

The onset of glaucoma is usually rapid with IOP reaching very high levels, but occasionally the onset is more gradual. Unilateral severe glaucoma associated with a hypermature cataract with any or all of the signs already discussed is probably due to phacolysis and will not respond to medical measures; thus treatment should consist of removing the cataract.

In cases associated with hypermature cataract, vision may be poor, light projection may be faulty, at least in one meridian, and some eyes appear to have no more than light perception. Regardless, treatment should be cataract surgery, after the IOP has been lowered as much as possible by medical means. It is a choice of either cataract surgery or removing the eye, since medical treatment alone invariably fails to keep the IOP down. In some eyes in which light projection was extremely faulty preoperatively, useful vision has been obtained after cataract surgery. In previous decades many such eyes were unnecessarily removed when the condition could have been completely relieved by cataract surgery. In neglected cases in which the IOP has been allowed to remain high so long that no useful vision is regained after cataract removal, the eye at least remains quiet and comfortable after removal of the cataract.

The following case illustrates how poor the vision can be in lens-induced glaucoma associated with a hypermature cataract in situ, yet how much vision can be regained and how strikingly glaucoma can be cured by removal of the cataract.

Case 47-1. A 69-year-old man had an injury to the left eye 28 years previously. He stated that vision in this eye was gone within 6 months after the injury. He had had no trouble with the eye until recently, when it became red and painful. He consulted an ophthalmologist who gave him acetazolamide. When seen by us the right eye was normal in all respects. The left eye was divergent, markedly injected, cornea hazy, anterior chamber normal in depth, light projection accurate only temporally. Because of the corneal edema one could not tell much about the anterior chamber. IOP 45. He was

UNDERSTANDING LENS-INDUCED GLAUCOMAS

David L. Epstein

A simple way to view these lens-induced glaucomas is to conceptualize that with the exception of phacoanaphylaxis, these entities are mechanical glaucomas that are due to the direct obstructive properties (1) of lens proteins in the case of a leaking fairly intact crystalline lens, or lens particles in the case of a grossly disrupted lens (free lens cortical material). Hence the terms lens protein glaucoma and lens particle glaucoma. In the former it is the "viscous" (heavy molecular weight) lens proteins (2) present in advanced cataracts which leak into the anterior chamber that obstruct the trabecular meshwork, and in the latter the fragments of gross crystalline lens material (1). The inflammatory macrophage-type cellular response is not itself viewed as impairing trabecular outflow (and may actually help in clearing the liberated lens material from the outflow pathway).

With this construct the treatment is fairly straightforward and consists of removing at least the continuing source of the lens material. In lens particle glaucoma, the "free" lens material is removed from the anterior chamber, and in lens protein glaucoma where there is a relatively intact cataractous lens, treatment consists of cataract surgery. Previously we advised intracapsular cataract surgery be performed for phacolytic (lens protein) glaucoma because there was usually a friable lens capsule (through which the lens proteins were leaking), and commonly weak zonules, and there was the potential for phacoanaphylaxis or other forms of severe inflammation, should lens material containing these aggregated lens proteins be mixed with vitreous due to unexpected vitreous loss. (These heavy molecular weight lens proteins are normally concentrated in the crystalline lens nucleus and may be responsible for phacoanaphylaxis and severe complications that ensue when a nucleus is "lost" into the vitreous and allowed to remain.) However, there have been several reports (3,4) with good results of extracapsular cataract surgery in patients with phacolytic glaucoma, and probably all considered, this is now the preferred technique. In planned extracapsular cataract surgery an adequately wide incision should be employed, with attention to potentially loose zonules and a friable capsule, with an adequate cortical clean-up. (The nucleus of a phacolytic lens is usually quite "hard" and not likely suitable for current phacoemulsification techniques). Attention should be placed especially on avoiding capsular tears and thus the mixing of the offending lens contents with the vitreous.

References

1. Epstein DL, Jedziniak JA, Grant WM: Obstruction of aqueous outflow by lens particles and by heavy-molecular-weight soluble lens proteins. Invest Ophthalmol Vis Sci 1978;17:272–277.
2. Epstein DL, Jedziniak JA, Grant WM: Identification of heavy molecular weight soluble lens protein in aqueous humor in human phacolytic glaucoma. Invest Ophthalmol Vis Sci 1978;17:398–402.
3. Lane SS, Kopietz LA, Lindquist TD, et al: Treatment of phacolytic glaucoma with extracapsular cataract extraction. Ophthalmology 1988;95:749–53.
4. Singh G, Kaur J, Mall S: Phacolytic glaucoma—its treatment by planned extracapsular cataract extraction with posterior chamber intraocular lens implantation. Ind J Ophthalmol 1994;42:145–7.

admitted to the hospital at once and an operation was done. After the usual limbal incision, when the corneal flap was lifted it could be seen that the lens had ruptured posteriorly and that only the capsule was present in the pupil. Alpha chymotrypsin was injected, and after 3 minutes the capsule was removed with forceps. It then could be seen that the vitreous had a milky appearance. The vitreous chamber was irrigated and a lot of this milky material was washed out. No formed vitreous was seen. The convalescence was fairly stormy, but eventually the eye became quiet with very little vitreous opacity. The disc was found to be normal, corrected vision 20/30, IOP normal without treatment.

Because the lens had actually ruptured in situ, the glaucoma may have resulted from direct obstruction by both liberated "lens particles" and soluble lens proteins.

IMMATURE CATARACT: LENS IN SITU

Phacolytic glaucoma can occur in exceptional instances in eyes with immature cataract with the vision as good as 20/50. In these extraordinary cases there is presumably localized liquefaction of the posterior cortex. A diagnosis of phacolytic glaucoma due to immature cataract is difficult to establish. The question arises: is this a case of ordinary uveitis with an immature cataract, or are the uveitis and secondary glaucoma attributable to the lens? One cannot be sure at the initial examination. Therefore the usual treatment for glaucoma secondary to uveitis is instituted, including topical corticosteroids, cycloplegics, beta blockers, apraclonidine, and carbonic anhydrase inhibitors. Then, if in a period of weeks or months, despite vigorous treatment, the uveitis and glaucoma gradually worsen and IOP reaches high levels, one is justified in performing cataract surgery with a strong probability that the uveitis and the glaucoma will thereby be relieved. **Diagnostic paracentesis before surgery may help establish the correct diagnosis by documenting the presence of typical engorged macrophages or high-molecular-weight lens protein.**

Irvine and Irvine describe a case (their case 6) in which the cataract was clinically immature, but pathologic examination of the lens revealed that the posterior cortex was completely liquefied just as in a hypermature cataract (12). Chandler also published an example of phacolytic glaucoma induced by a clinically immature cataract and relieved by removal of the lens (13).

Biochemical analysis of the liquefied cortex of hypermature "phacolytic" lenses has indicated the presence of high levels of heavy-molecular-weight soluble lens protein. Such liquefied lens cortex contains aggregated rather than degraded lens proteins.

COMPLETELY DISLOCATED HYPERMATURE CATARACT AND GLAUCOMA

Phacolytic glaucoma may occur after complete backward dislocation of the lens into the vitreous cavity, either spontaneously or as a result of trauma. The completely backward dislocated lens may go through the stages of immature, mature, and hypermature cataract formation, just as if it were in the normal position. The diagnosis of phacolytic glaucoma in cases of completely posterior dislocation of the lens may not be obvious at first.

The glaucoma may develop acutely with a high IOP or the **glaucoma may have a gradual onset**. Even if the onset is gradual, the IOP eventually reaches high levels, despite intensive medical treatment. The diagnosis may be suspected because of the absence of any other obvious cause for such severe glaucoma, with the angle of the anterior chamber open. Also, to point to the diagnosis, one may find a few cells in the aqueous that do not circulate freely, but only tremble on motion of the eye (this clinical point may reflect the presence of "viscous" lens proteins in the aqueous humor). The vitreous in these cases is usually almost completely fluid, but if one can see vitreous strands in the vitreous cavity, one commonly sees exudates on them. Again, diagnostic paracentesis and examination of the anterior chamber fluid may be performed to help establish the correct diagnosis. If provisions for proper examination of anterior chamber fluid are not readily available, one should again be able to make the diagnosis on purely clinical grounds. Here is a glaucoma completely out of control, despite intensive medical treatment, for which we can find no other cause.

Currently, vitrectomy instrumentation is used to remove such dislocated phacolytic lenses. However, it is interesting to note Chandler's methods of treating this condition before the availability of this instrumentation. Dr. Chandler writes

> if the lens floats in the vitreous cavity and is not attached to the retina, the simplest method of removal is to make the usual incision for cataract extraction, do a sector iridectomy and inferior iridotomy, and irrigate the vitreous cavity, directing the stream of fluid toward the posterior pole of the globe as advised by Verhoeff (1). The lens may immediately float up into the wound and be removed without difficulty. If the lens floats about freely during the irrigation, but will not come out, it is because it is attached to the retina by a strand of tissue. It can be removed with forceps, but this is not a wise policy for in a case treated by PAC a hole was torn in the retina by this maneuver. Fortunately, the hole was treated and closed before the retina became detached. We have seen a safer method employed in a case in which the lens came well forward on irrigation of the vitreous chamber but would not come out. In this case, although the lens was held forward with forceps, the strand of tissue attached to the posterior surface of the lens was cut with scissors, and then the lens was removed without further complications.

Reference

1. Verhoeff FH: A simple and safe method for removing a cataract dislocated into fluid vitreous. Am J Ophthalmol 1942;25:725.

GLAUCOMA DUE TO RETAINED LENS CORTEX (LENS PARTICLE GLAUCOMA)

After planned or unplanned extracapsular cataract extraction, or after injury to the lens, a secondary open-angle glaucoma may develop (Fig. 47.3). If not much cortical material is present, the usual methods of treatment for uveitis and secondary glaucoma may be employed, such as cycloplegics, corticosteroids, a beta blocker, apraclonidine, and carbonic anhydrase inhibitors. This may suffice until the residual cortical material is completely absorbed, after which the inflammation subsides and the IOP falls. However, if by the usual treatment the inflammation is not quickly brought under control, and the IOP remains elevated, **one should proceed without delay to remove the residual lens cortex.**

If definitive treatment by removal of residual lens cortex is obviously necessary but is delayed too long, serious consequences may result, such as the following: There may be a serious persistent glaucoma due to peripheral anterior synechias, secondary to the continued inflammation. A dense inflammatory pupillary membrane may develop and may cause pupillary block. Cystic degeneration of the macula may occur, with loss of central vision. The retina may become detached as a result of inflammatory membranes that extend posteriorly and pull on the retina. Finally, there may be permanent edema of the cornea. Likewise, it is not known whether prolonged absorption of lens material, which must occur via the aqueous outflow channels, may result in outflow dysfunction and apparent open-angle glaucoma in later years. We have wondered whether this latter mechanism is not involved in the common occurrence of open angle glaucoma that can follow pediatric cataract surgery (14–18).

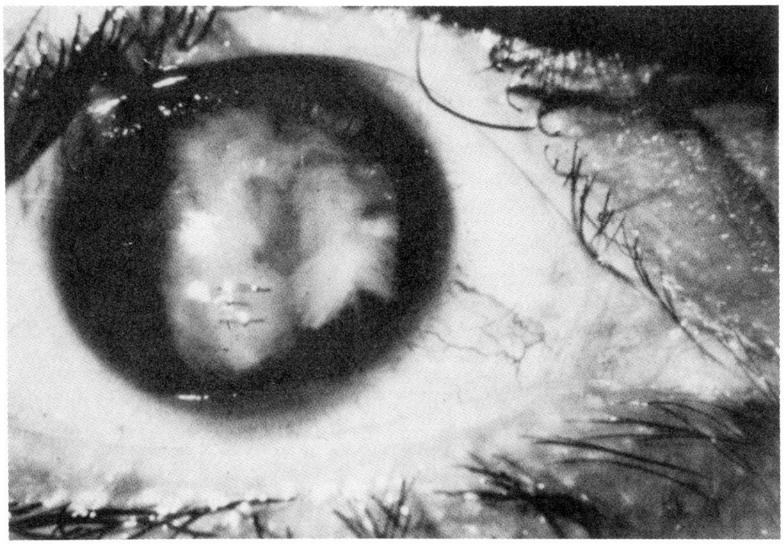

Figure 47.3. "Fluffed up" lens cortical material in the anterior chamber that may obstruct the trabecular meshwork (lens particle glaucoma). Reprinted with permission from Epstein DL: Lens-induced open-angle glaucoma. In: The Secondary Glaucomas. Edited by Ritch R, Shields MB. St. Louis, C.V. Mosby Co., 1982. Courtesy of C. Davis Belcher III, MD.

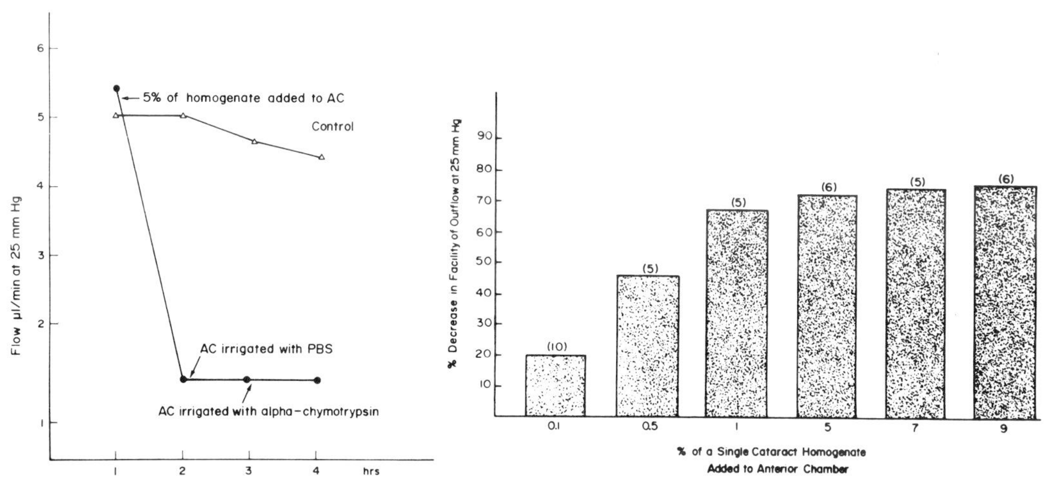

Figure 47.4. In experimental anterior chamber perfusion studies in excised human eyes only a small quantity of particulate lens material can cause substantial impairment of outflow facility. Reprinted with permission from Epstein DL, Jedziniak JA, Grant WM: Obstruction of aqueous outflow by lens particles and by heavy molecular weight soluble lens proteins. Invest Ophthalmol Vis Sci 1978;17:272–277.

In view of the seriousness of these late complications, bold measures are justified in attempting to relieve the condition. If the previous cataract operation or injury has been recent, and there is a great deal of loose cortical material in the anterior chamber, it may easily be irrigated out. If operation is undertaken weeks or months after the onset of the trouble, cortical material may be trapped between membranes, either capsular or inflammatory. Anterior segment "microvitrectomy" instrumentation is often then useful in removing such residual lens material. The use of alpha-chymotrypsin may help in removing capsular membranes that are still attached to lens zonules.

In early occurring acute cases of glaucoma due to retained lens cortex, we believe that the particles of lens material may be important in obstructing aqueous outflow (Fig. 47.4) (3). We think that early acute glaucoma due to retained lens cortex differs from the phacolytic glaucoma associated with liquefaction of lens cortex. Specifically, we postulate on the basis of our laboratory investigations that acute glaucoma associated with retained or spilled lens cortex early after operation or injury is mainly a **"lens particle" glaucoma**, whereas the "phacolytic" glaucoma that is associated with liquefaction of lens cortex without gross breaks in the lens capsule is mainly attributable to soluble proteins leaking from the lens.

In glaucoma that develops months or years after extracapsular cataract extraction or after injury of the lens, we do not yet know which of several possible mechanisms may be most important, including the role of accompanying inflammatory cells. We have yet to establish definitely whether the cells, particularly the macrophages, may be acting to clear obstructing lens material or whether they may contribute to the obstruction to aqueous outflow. We do know that severe obstruction can be produced by lens particles and by high-molecular-weight soluble lens proteins in the absence of inflammatory cells, and that clinically washing out the anterior chamber or removing retained lens matter can dramatically alleviate the glaucoma, even in these later onset cases.

We believe that the following case is an example of late lens-induced glaucoma from retained cortex, relieved by washing out the anterior chamber.

Case 47-2. A 53-year-old woman with vision of only hand movements in the right eye from old retinal detachment had an unintentional extracapsular cataract extraction in the left eye during planned intracapsular cataract surgery. Convalescence was stormy, but final corrected vision was 20/30. In the upper half of the pupil there was posterior capsule; the lower half was clear. The disc was normal. She was seen 9 years later, with a history that in recent weeks there had been episodes of profound loss of vision in the left eye. IOP in the left eye was 72, and after a gram of acetazolamide, it was 55. There was epithelial edema. Corrected vision after clearing the cornea with glycerin was 20/100, and to confrontation there was less than a 10 degree field. There were long stringy sheets of vitreous opacities that swirled around freely and obscured fundus details. They did not have the appearance of blood and did not resemble the exudative vitreous opacities that one sees in acute chorioretinitis. On gonioscopy the view was hazy but the angle seemed wide and open except for pillar synechias. On the capsular membrane in the upper half of the pupil there were many coarse whitish deposits, somewhat like KP, but irregular in size and shape. There were no deposits on the cornea.

Under treatment with acetazolamide, epinephrine, glycerin, and systemic steroids, during 3 days IOP varied from 17 to more than 60. The cornea became clearer, and through the peripheral coloboma above and temporally one could see a grayish substance that looked like lens matter. With a working diagnosis of lens-induced glaucoma, surgery was performed. Through a beveled incision in the lower cornea all the aqueous possible was aspirated. Then with another syringe filled with saline, by alternately depressing the plunger on the syringe and withdrawing it, the aqueous was thoroughly stirred up and, again, the aqueous was aspirated. Finally the anterior chamber was irrigated with 10 ml of saline solution. During the irrigation some rather coarse flecks of whitish material could be seen swirling in the anterior chamber. The two samples of fluid aspirated from the anterior chamber were examined under a glass slide within an hour by T. Kuwabara. There were isolated cells and sheets of cells that had every appearance of macrophages. All treatment, local and systemic, was discontinued. Postoperatively, the IOP remained 17 or less.

One week later corrected vision was 20/40, and by confrontation only the upper nasal field was absent. The disc showed glaucomatous cupping. Two weeks later the vitreous was practically clear except for a few fine stringy opacities; no exudates could be seen on the membrane; there were no cells or flare.

Several years after the irrigation of the anterior chamber the eye still remained quiet with no cells or KP, vitreous clear, IOP 17 without treatment.

Sometimes in patients with significant amounts of residual cortical material, many years after extracapsular cataract surgery spontaneous liberation of lens particulate material into the anterior chamber may occur associated with elevation of IOP (18–20) (Fig. 47.5). This may also be a form of lens particle glaucoma, although the inflammatory response to such liberated lens

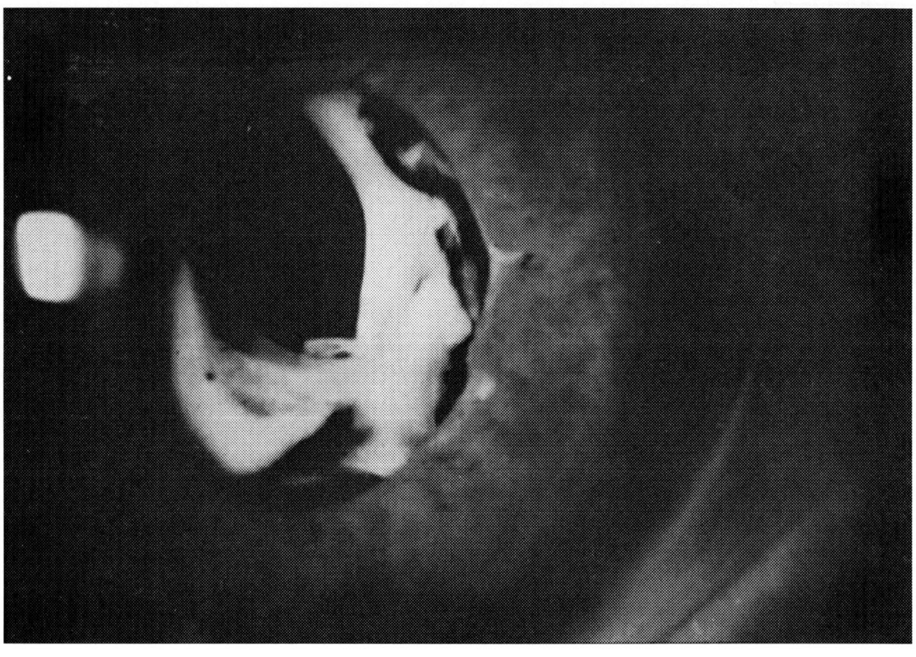

Figure 47.5. After extracapsular cataract surgery done decades previously this patient experienced episodic bouts of high IOP associated with spontaneous fragmentation and dissemination of his residual lens material into the anterior chamber. This may be a form of lens particle glaucoma.

material may also be involved. Nevertheless, these cases respond favorably to removal of the liberated lens material.

We need to keep the entity of delayed "lens particle glaucoma" in mind as the decades continue to pass for our patients who now have had modern extracapsular cataract surgery. Especially when first performed, residual cortical lens material was commonly left behind. This was the usual situation also for open angle glaucoma eyes on chronic miotic therapy. From the above observations, it seems that sometimes with the passage of time the normal sequestration barriers that the eye employs to seal off such crystalline lens material may be subject to "break down," with resulting liberation of lens material into the anterior chamber and outflow pathway. Such lens material could also be immunogenic (21). These possibilities need to be remembered when evaluating patients who have unexplained glaucoma or uveitis many years, or decades after extracapsular cataract surgery.

INTRAOCULAR PRESSURE ELEVATION FOLLOWING POSTERIOR CAPSULOTOMY WITH THE Nd:YAG LASER

Within hours after seemingly uneventful posterior capsulotomy with the Neodymium-YAG laser, a dramatic elevation of IOP can occur (22–24). IOP greater than 60 mm Hg has been observed and may persist for at least 24 to 36 hours. Needless to say, IOP needs to be carefully monitored after Nd:YAG laser capsulotomy, and significant elevations need to be treated. Based on our laboratory studies, we have wondered whether the mechanism in some of these cases involves a form of "lens-particle" or "lens protein" glaucoma due to small fragments of lens material or soluble lens proteins that are liberated into the anterior chamber and pass into the angle (25) after this procedure. Other possibilities include inflammatory (26) or mechanical (27) effects within the eye following Nd:YAG laser energy absorption, or purported vitreous factors (28). Further information is required concerning this puzzling form of transient glaucoma (which is potentially damaging to vision).

PHACOANAPHYLACTIC GLAUCOMA

This type of glaucoma is rare and has practically never been correctly diagnosed in a living eye. The pathological criteria in enucleated eye specimens that distinguish it from phacolytic glaucoma have been well defined by Zimmerman (29) and by Perlman and Albert (30). **Phacoanaphylaxis results from an immunologic response to lens protein, which involves a latent period or a previous sensitization to lens proteins.** Normally, lens proteins are isolated within the lens capsule, and they must first escape before the sensitization process can begin. We suspect that a mixture of lens material and vitreous, which may occur as a result of vitreous loss during extracapsular cataract extraction or injury, may favor development of phacoanaphylaxis by retaining and slowly releasing the sensitizing lens proteins. We believe that phacoanaphylactic reactions (with or without glaucoma) can occur especially when an intact lens nucleus is lost into the vitreous.

Two criteria must be satisfied before we would accept a diagnosis of phacoanaphylactic glaucoma: 1) polymorphonuclear leukocytes must be present in the aqueous or vitreous specimen; 2) the circulating lens protein or particle content of the aqueous humor must be insufficient by itself to explain the glaucoma.

From a practical standpoint, if this condition is suspected clinically, it is treated in the same manner as phacolytic glaucoma: by removal of the lens or lens matter.

References

1. Flocks M, Littwin CS, Zimmerman LE: Phacolytic glaucoma: Clinicopathologic study of 138 cases of glaucoma associated with hypermature cataract. Arch Ophthalmol 1955;54:37–47.
2. Goldberg MF: Cytological diagnosis of phacolytic glaucoma utilizing Millipore filtration of the aqueous. Br J Ophthalmol 1967;51:847–853.
3. Epstein DL, Jedziniak JA, Grant WM: Obstruction of aqueous outflow by lens particles and by heavy-molecular-weight soluble lens proteins. Invest Ophthalmol Vis Sci 1978;17:272–277.
4. Epstein DL, Hashimoto JM, Grant WM: Serum obstruction of aqueous outflow in enucleated human eyes. Am J Ophthalmol 1978;86: 101–105.
5. Yanoff M, Scheie HG: Cytology of human lens aspirate. Arch Ophthalmol 1968;80:166–170.
6. Dueker DK: Personal communication, 1977.
7. Bremond D, Ridings B, Devin F, et al: An uncommon clinical form of phakolytic glaucoma [French]. Bull Soc Ophtalmol Fr 1989;89:853–6.
8. Ueno H, Tamai A, Iyota K, et al: Electron microscopic observation of the cells floating in the anterior chamber in a case of phacolytic glaucoma. Jpn J Ophthalmol 1989;33:103–13.
9. Brooks AM, Grant G, Gillies WE: Comparison of specular microscopy and examination of aspirate in phacolytic glaucoma. Ophthalmology 1990;97:85–9.
10. Epstein DL, Jedziniak JA, Grant WM: Identification of heavy molecular weight soluble lens protein in aqueous humor in human phacolytic glaucoma. Invest Ophthalmol Vis Sci 1978;17:398–402.
11. Bartholomew RS, Rebello PF: Calcium oxalate crystals in the aqueous. Am J Ophthalmol 1979;88:1026–8.
12. Irvine SR, Irvine AR Jr: Lens-induced uveitis and glaucoma. II "The phacotoxic reaction." Am J Ophthalmol 1952;36:370–375.
13. Chandler PA: Problems in the diagnosis and treatment of lens-induced uveitis and glaucoma. Arch Ophthalmol 1958;60:828–841.
14. Phelps CD, Arafat NI: Open-angle glaucoma following surgery for congenital cataracts. Arch Ophthalmol 1977;95:1985–7.
15. Simon JW, et al: Glaucoma after pediatric lensectomy/vitrectomy. Ophthalmology 1991;98:670–4.
16. Parks MM, Johnson DA, Read GW: Long-term visual results and complications in children with aphakia: a function of cataract type. Ophthalmology 1993;100:826–4.
17. Munoz M, Parrish RK, Murray TG: Open-angle glaucoma after pars plicata lensectomy and vitrectomy for congenital cataracts. Am J Ophthalmol 1995;119:103–4.
18. Epstein DL: Diagnosis and management of lens-induced glaucoma. Ophthalmology 1982;89:227–230.
19. Epstein DL: Lens-induced open-angle glaucoma. In: The Secondary Glaucomas. Edited by Ritch R, Shields MB. St. Louis, C.V. Mosby Co., 1982;216–223.
20. Barnhorst D, Meyers SM, Myers T: Lens-induced glaucoma 65 years after congenital cataract surgery. Am J Ophthalmol 1994;118:807–8.

21. Rosenbaum JT, et al: Chemotactic activity of lens proteins and the pathogenesis of phacolytic glaucoma. Arch Ophthalmol 1987;105: 1582–4.
22. Terry AC, Stark WJ, Maumenee AE, et al: Neodymium-YAG laser for posterior capsulotomy. Am J Ophthalmol 1983;96:716–720.
23. Channell MM, Beckman H: Intraocular pressure changes after neodymium-YAG laser posterior capsulotomy. Arch Ophthalmol 1984;102: 1024–6.
24. Richter CU, Arzeno G, Pappas HR, et al: Intraocular pressure elevation following Nd:YAG laser posterior capsulotomy. Ophthalmology 1985; 92:636–640.
25. Flohr MJ, Robin AL, Kelley JS: Early complications following Q-switched neodymium: YAG laser posterior capsulotomy. Ophthalmology 1985;92:360–3.
26. Lynch MG, et al: The effect of neodymium: YAG laser capsulotomy on aqueous humor dynamics in the monkey eye. Ophthalmology 1986;93: 1270–5.
27. Aron-Rosa DS: Influence of picosecond and nanosecond YAG laser capsulotomy on intraocular pressure. J Am Intraocul Implant Soc 1985;11: 249–52.
28. Schubert HD, Morris WJ, Trokel SL, et al: The role of the vitreous in the intraocular pressure rise after neodymium-YAG laser capsulotomy. Arch Ophthalmol 1985;103:1538–42.
29. Zimmerman LE: Lens-induced inflammation in human eyes. In: Immunopathology of uveitis. Edited by Maumenee AE, Silverstein AM. Baltimore, Williams & Wilkins, 1964.
30. Perlman EM, Albert DM: Clinically unsuspected phacoanaphylaxis after ocular trauma. Arch Ophthalmol 1977;95:244–246.

Amyloidosis and Open Angle Glaucoma

48

David L. Epstein

Primary familial amyloidosis is a generalized systemic disease that may involve the eyes in a number of ways (Fig. 48.1). **Bilateral often severe open angle glaucoma may develop in the third, fourth, or fifth decade of life, with progressive accumulation of amyloid vitreous opacities.** These vitreous opacities may increase to the extent that vision is seriously impaired and the fundus cannot be seen. The opacities can also develop in the absence of glaucoma. Glaucoma in cases reported by Legrand (1), Limon (2), and Tsukahara (3) has been described as similar to pigmentary glaucoma or to open-angle glaucoma associated with exfoliation, in that there was pigment on the back of the cornea, **a heavy accumulation of pigment in the trabecular meshwork,** and abnormal transillumination of the iris. In all cases, there were amyloid vitreous opacities. Deposition of amyloid fibrils in the trabecular meshwork has been described by Tsukahara (3) and Segawa (4) from electron microscopy of trabeculectomy biopsy specimens. Amyloid in this location may have an important role in the obstruction of aqueous outflow.

In a case of familial amyloidosis reported by Plane, clinically there was pigment in the angle and powdery material assumed to be amyloid in the vitreous and on the front surface of the lens, yet no glaucoma (5).

In a series of 70 patients older than age 40, with lattice corneal dystrophy as a manifestation of amyloid disease, Meretoja diagnosed open-angle glaucoma in 23%, but noted no vitreous changes (6).

In a more recent report, 17% of patients with vitreous amyloidosis (requiring vitrectomy) also required filtration surgery (7).

There is a strong hereditary tendency in familial amyloidosis, and in any family in which there is hereditary glaucoma with pigment dissemination or vitreous opacities, all members of the family should be examined for amyloidosis and open-angle glaucoma. Similarly, evidence of amyloidosis and open-angle glaucoma should be looked for in patients with lattice corneal dystrophy (8).

Our experience with primary familial amyloidosis and glaucoma included the following two cases.

Case 48-1. A 55-year-old woman had a strong family history of glaucoma: mother, uncle, brother. Her brother became blind from glaucoma and was said to have a great cloud of vitreous opacities. When he died, extensive amyloidosis was found at autopsy. She herself had been under treatment for glaucoma for several months, using 4% pilocarpine every 2 hours, epinephrine twice a day, eserine ointment at bedtime, acetazolamide 250 mg tid. Despite this treatment, IOP was right and left 52. Vision was right and left 6/9. The angles were wide open, with ciliary band visible for 360 degrees. There was light brown pigment on the corneoscleral meshwork throughout, but the band was not as dark or broad as in pigmentary glaucoma. The right disc was almost totally cupped. In the right eye, the lower field was limited on the perimeter, absent entirely on the tangent screen. In the left eye the cup was wide but within physiologic limits, and the field was full.

A trephining was done on the right eye. Acetazolamide was discontinued postoperatively, and within 2 days the IOP in the left eye was 70 despite intensive local medication. A trephining was done on the left eye. For several months IOP ranged from 12 to 15 in both eyes, and there appeared to be good functioning blebs, but opacities began to appear in the vitreous. These opacities were not blood and did not resemble exudative opacities. These gradually increased until the fundi could not be seen. Nine months after operation IOP was right 24, left 32, and the bleb in each eye, though unchanged in height and extent, now had a whitish opaque appearance. Only at the borders did the blebs appear thin and succulent. At first, IOP could be lowered substantially by digital pressure from below. This was done regularly by the patient. She was given 4% pilocarpine and epinephrine. Two years after the operations, IOP was right and left 27 on pilocarpine and epinephrine, and it could not be lowered by digital pressure. An operation was done on both eyes. A thin flap was dissected to the limbus and the whitish tissue was excised, exposing the scleral opening. (The appearance of this whitened but still elevated bleb tissue was so different from the appearance of an ordinary scarred bleb that we assume that it was infiltrated by amyloid, but unfortunately histologic studies were not performed on this tissue.)

During the following 9 months IOP was 12 to 20 and could always be lowered by digital pressure. However, within 2 years, there was gradual failure of filtration, and, under the care of Richard J. Simmons, the following procedures were done in succession: cyclocryotherapy in the right eye, combined cataract extraction and cyclodialysis on both eyes, another cyclodialysis on both eyes, and then another cyclocryotherapy on both eyes.

After the cataract extraction and cyclodialysis, vision was only counting fingers at a few feet in the better left eye, due to vitreous opacities. Later a vitrectomy was done on the left eye by Robert J. Brockhurst with restoration of good vision in this eye. Examination of the material removed by vitrectomy established that it contained amyloid. When last seen, IOP was right 22, left 11. Corrected vision, left 6/12.

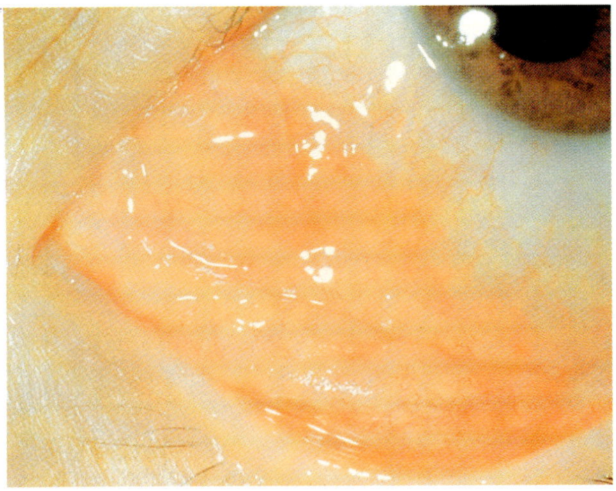

Figure 48.1. Periocular amyloid deposition in a patient with primary familial amyloidosis.

Case 48-2. A man aged 57, uncle of the patient in the preceding case, was first seen in 1944, with vision right faint hand motions, left counting fingers at 16 feet. IOP right 90, left 58. The anterior chambers were of good depth. In both eyes there were deep corneal opacities near the limbus nasally and temporally and some near the pupil, but there were no vessels in the cornea. There were also many vitreous opacities, but the fundi could be seen. The right disc was totally cupped and atrophic; the left was similarly cupped but the nasal rim was intact. The left eye on the perimeter showed loss of slightly more than the lower nasal quadrant; on the tangent screen there was a double Bjerrum scotoma isolating a small central island. With intensive miotic therapy, IOP in the left eye fell to 38. A filtering operation was done on this eye. During the next 7 months IOP was usually in the mid-to-low 20s but could always be softened by digital pressure, which the patient did regularly. Then, IOP rose to 35 and a cyclodialysis was done. During the following 7 years IOP was generally 13 to 17. The vitreous opacity gradually increased so that at the last visit in 1952 fundus details could not be seen. Last vision recorded was 6/60.

The family history of amyloidosis proved in two members of this family and the gradual increase in vitreous opacity make it probable that this patient in Case 48.2 also suffered from amyloid disease. The good control of the glaucoma for more than 7 years after filtering operation and cyclodialysis is unusual in this disease. Our experience with these patients confirms the observation of others that intraocular amyloidosis is a very serious disorder.

A relationship between ocular amyloidosis and exfoliation syndrome has been described by Meretoja and Tarkkanen, on the basis of histologic evidence, suggesting that the exfoliation syndrome may be a form of amyloid disease (9). However, clinically, we have not noted vitreous opacities to be associated with exfoliation and glaucoma.

A recent report has implicated histopathologically the deposition of a cytoskeletal modulating protein (gelsolin) product in ocular tissues in the Finnish familial form of systemic amyloidosis (Meretoja's Syndrome) (10). The authors suggest that the amyloid deposits in the optic nerve might cause an increase in susceptibility of the optic nerve to cupping.

References

1. Legrand J, Guenel J, Dubigeon Mme: Glaucome et opacification du vitre par amylose. Bull Soc Ophthalmol Fr 1986;68:13–20.
2. Limon S, Rousselie F, Joseph E: A propos d'une observation familiale d'amylose vitréenne héréditaire associée à un glaucoma. Arch Ophthalmol (Paris) 1973;33:525–528.
3. Tsukahara S, Matsuo T: Secondary glaucoma accompanied with primary familial amyloidosis. Ophthalmologica 1977;175:250–262.
4. Segawa K: The fine structure of the iridocorneal angle tissue in glaucomatous eyes (5). Glaucoma secondary to primary familial amyloidosis. Jpn J Clin Ophthalmol 1976;30:1375–1380.
5. Plane C, Maupetit J, Colnet G, et al: Manifestations oculaires de l'amylose Portugaise de Corino de Andrade. Bull Soc Ophthalmol Fr 1977; 77:123–125.
6. Meretoja J: Comparative histological and clinical findings in eyes with lattice corneal dystrophy of two different types. Ophthalmologica 1972; 165:15–37.
7. Doft BH, Machemer R, Skinner M, et al: Pars plana vitrectomy for vitreous amyloidosis. Ophthalmology 1987;94:607–11.
8. Starck T, Kenyon KR, Hanninen LA, et al. Clinical and histopathologic studies of two families with lattice corneal dystrophy and familial systemic amyloidosis (Meretoja syndrome). Ophthalmology 1991;98: 1197–206.
9. Meretoja J, Tarkkanen A: Occurrence of amyloid in eyes with exfoliation. Ophthalmic Res 1977;9:80–91.
10. Kivela T, Tarkkanen A, Frangione B, et al: Ocular amyloid deposition in familial amyloidosis, Finnish: an analysis of native and variant gelsolin in Meretoja's syndrome. Invest Opthalmol Vis Sci 1994;35:3759–69.

Glaucoma in the Phakomatoses

49

Cynthia Mattox

INTRODUCTION

The phakomatoses (Table 49.1) are a diverse group of disorders. The categorization of many disorders under the heading of the phakomatoses has created controversy and confusion since the term was first introduced in the early twentieth century. van der Hoeve originally included tuberous sclerosis (Bourneville's disease) and neurofibromatosis (von Recklinghausen's disease) as phakomatoses, and later added von Hippel-Lindau and Sturge-Weber syndrome (1,2). The common denominator seemed to be the congenital nature of multisystem tumors. He called them phakomata after the Greek name for "motherspot," indicating the congenital nature of the conditions. Others later interpreted this to mean that the phakomatoses had a "birthmark" which indicated an underlying multiorgan condition (3). In a more contemporary interpretation of the meaning behind grouping these diverse conditions, Hogan and Zimmerman described the phakomatoses as disseminated hamartomas affecting the eye, central nervous system, skin and internal organs (4). Hamartomas are tumorous masses that arise from tissue elements normally found at the site, as opposed to choristomas which are tumors derived from elements not normally found at the site. Others have proposed that the phakomatoses may be disorders of the regulation of paracrine growth factors (5).

Glaucoma is a common feature of encephalotrigeminal angiomatosis (Sturge-Weber syndrome) and is occasionally found in neurofibromatosis type 1, and von Hippel-Lindau disease. The other phakomatoses rarely have an associated glaucoma, although a secondary glaucoma may be present as a complication of the other ocular manifestations of the disease.

STURGE-WEBER SYNDROME (ENCEPHALOTRIGEMINAL ANGIOMATOSIS)

In 1860, Schirmer described a patient with glaucoma and a facial angioma. Sturge later presented a case of a child with a "port-wine stain" angioma involving half the face and head with ipsilateral buphthalmos and congenital glaucoma, and a seizure disorder in 1879. He also noticed the choroid of the involved eye was a darker red and hypothesized that the choroid was involved with a vascular lesion similar to the face. In 1922 Weber reported the characteristic intracranial calcifications seen radiographically in patients with the syndrome and suggested the parallel streaks were a result of a meningeal angioma. The syndrome became known as the Sturge-Weber syndrome and in its full presentation includes a facial hemangioma, with an ipsilateral intracranial angioma, an ipsilateral choroidal hemangioma, and congenital glaucoma (6). Incomplete forms occur, but all have the characteristic facial angioma or nevus flammeus. The syndrome has no racial or sex predilection. Unlike the other phakomatoses, Sturge-Weber does not have any identifiable hereditary pattern.

Systemic Findings

The facial angioma (Fig. 49.1) is usually unilateral, in the distribution of the first and second divisions of the trigeminal nerve. The lesion occurs bilaterally in 10–30% of cases (7–9). It appears deep burgundy in color and facial hypertrophy of varying degrees of the involved area occurs frequently. Histopathologically, the angioma is composed of dilated, telangiectatic capillaries lined by a single layer of endothelial cells in the dermis (10). Some success has been achieved using laser therapy to diminish the appearance of the lesion.

A racemose leptomeningeal hemangioma is the intracranial lesion of Sturge-Weber syndrome. It is usually ipsilateral to the facial angioma and located over the parieto-occipital region. Progressive calcification of the angioma occurs during childhood (11). Adjacent atrophy of the underlying cerebral cortex is frequent and may result in varying degrees of intellectual deficit and mental retardation in about 60% of patients (12). Contralateral focal motor seizures occur in 85% of patients and usually begin after the age of 1, but become more generalized with age (12). Permanent hemiparesis, hemiplegia, and homonymous hemianopsia may occur as a consequence of the seizures.

Ophthalmic Manifestations

The lids, orbit, episclera (Fig. 49.2), conjunctiva, iris and ciliary body may be involved with a hemangioma. Although exceptions occur, **if the upper eyelid is involved with hemangioma, the eye is involved intraocularly according to Anderson's rule** (11). The iris, if involved, will be hyperchromic in about 7% of cases (13).

Choroidal hemangiomas are the most frequent ocular manifestation of Sturge-Weber syndrome. They have been found in 40 to 50% of patients upon pathologic examina-

Table 49.1
The Phahomatoses

Disorder	Heredity/ Chromosomal abnormalities	Systemic involvement	Ocular findings	Types of glaucoma	Reference
Sturge-Weber Syndrome	Sporadic	Facial angioma Leptomeningeal hemangioma	Hemangioma of lids, orbit, conjunctiva, iris, ciliary body, choroid.	Incidence: develops in 30% of patients Congenital with buphthalmos (60%) Later onset (40%)	23
Klippel-Trenaunay-Weber Syndrome	Sporadic	Facial hemangioma. Hemangioma of extremities with hypertrophy.	Orbital varices or hypertrophy, conjunctival telangiectasias, heterochromia iridis, choroidal angiomas, retinal varicosities or vacular tumors, disc anomalies.	Incidence: less frequent than Sturge-Weber	34
Neurofibromatosis	Autosomal dominant, 100% penetrance, variable expressivity NF-1: chromosome 17 NF-2: chromosome 22	Cafe-au-lait spots, fibroma molluscum, plexiform neurofibromas. Neurofibromas of the nerve roots or spinal cord, meningiomas, intracranial or spinal cord gliomas. Acoustic neuromas in NF-2. Skeletal problems, pheochromocytomas.	Neurofibromas of eyelids, conjunctiva, or orbit. Absent greater wing of sphenoid bone. Prominent corneal nerves. Optic nerve glioma. Lisch nodules. PSC cataracts in NF-2.	incidence: ? Congenital glaucoma with buphthalmos. Childhood onset with ectropion uveae and iridogoniodysgenesis.	
von Hippel-Lindau disease	Autosomal dominant with incomplete penetrance. Chromosome 3.	Cerebellar hemangioblastoma. Polycythemia. Renal cell carcinoma.	Retinal angioma.	Incidence: low. Occasional neovascular glaucoma following exudative retinal detachment.	61
Tuberous sclerosis	Autosomal dominant with high penetrance but variable expressivity. Chromosome 9.	Ash-leaf spots. Adenoma sebaceum. Seizures; infantile spasms. Periventricular brain tumors.	Astrocytic retinal hamartoma.	Incidence: very rare. Secondary complication of total retinal detachment or neovascularization.	73; 74
Ataxia telangiectasia	Autosomal recessive. Chromosome 11.	Progressive cerebellar ataxia. Skin telangiectasias. Hypoplasia of thymus gland. Recurrent sinopulmonary infections.	Conjunctival telangiectasias. Abnormal EOMs and gaze disorders.	Incidence: none	80
Wyburn-Mason syndrome	Sporadic.	Ipsilateral facial angiomas. Intracranial, ipsilateral arteriovenous malformation.	Retinal arteriovenous malformation.	Incidence: very rare. Secondary complication of retinal ischemia.	87
Linear nevus sebaceous syndrome	Sporadic.	Congenital organoid nevi with benign and malignant transformation. Ipsilateral CNS involvement.	Coloboma or ptosis of ipsilateral upper eyelid. Epibulbar dermoids; corneal scarring/ neovascularization. Colobomas of iris; ciliary body; choroid. Optic nerve hypoplasia; pallor; cupping.	Incidence: extremely rate.	93

Table 49.1
The Phahomatoses *(continued)*

Disorder	Heredity/ Chromosomal abnormalities	Systemic involvement	Ocular findings	Types of glaucoma	Reference
Basal cell nevus syndrome	Autosomal dominant with variable penetrance.	Basal cell epitheliomas.	Orbital involvement by tumor; hypertelorism; congenital cataract; strabismus; optic nerve and choroidal coloboma; corneal leukoma.	Incidence: extremely rate.	102
Nevus of Ota	Sporadic.	Oculodermal melanosis.	Ipsilateral hyperpigmentation of sclera; conjunctiva; cornea; iris; choroid; angle structures. Uveal and orbital malignant melanoma.	Incidence: low. Associated with increased pigmentation in the angle.	106
Cutis marmorata telangiectatica congenita	Sporadic.	Congenital persistent cutis marmorata; phlebectasia; telangiectasis; superficial ulcerations of skin.	Ipsilateral congenital glaucoma.	Incidence: 6 out of 65 reported cases. Immature angle development as in primary congenital glaucoma.	110

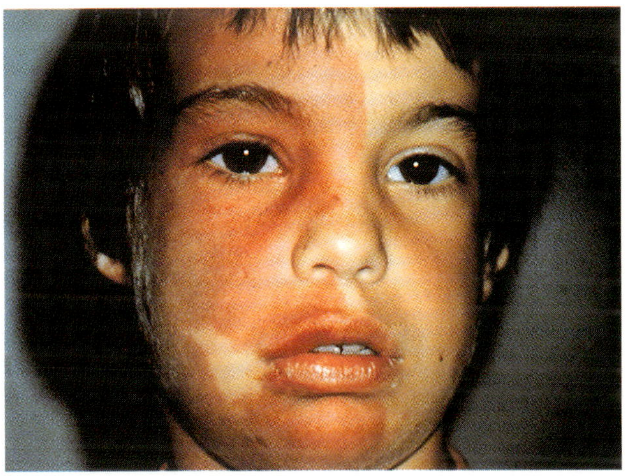

Figure 49.1. Sturge-Weber patient with characteristic "port-wine stain" facial hemangioma. (Courtesy of David S. Walton, MD).

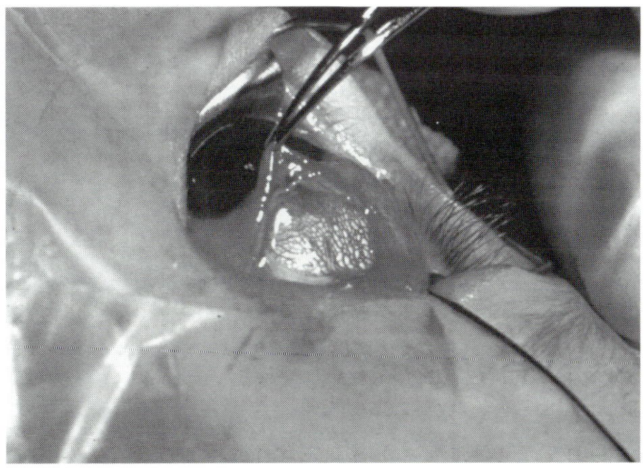

Figure 49.2. Episcleral hemangioma in a patient with glaucoma and Sturge-Weber. (Courtesy of David S. Walton, MD).

tion (14,15). In young children the lesion may simply appear as a darker red choroidal hue in the ipsilateral eye, called the "tomato catsup" fundus (16). However, as it slowly grows, it will appear as a mildly elevated, orange-yellow diffuse mass involving the posterior pole, and usually more than half the choroid. Histopathologically, the lesions are "mixed type" hemangiomas, with elements of both capillary and cavernous hemangiomas (17). Vision loss may occur in young adulthood due to a degeneration of the the overlying choriocapillaris, retinal pigment epithelium, and photoreceptors (10). Serous detachment of the retina can occur.

Glaucoma in Sturge-Weber

Glaucoma develops in a reported 30% of Sturge-Weber patients. Approximately 60% present as congenital glaucomas with buphthalmos, whereas 40% present in later childhood or adulthood (13,18). Usually, the upper eyelid is involved by the hemangioma. The most common presentation is unilateral and congenital, before the age of 2, on the side of the facial angioma. Bilateral glaucoma can occur, although usually in the presence of a bilateral facial hemangioma.

Many theories have been put forth to explain the mechanism of glaucoma in Sturge-Weber syndrome. Early theories proposed that abnormal sympathetic innervation might cause a loss of regulation of the normal uveal capillary bed which then resulted in stasis and glaucoma (19). Others proposed that transudation of fluid from the choroidal hemangioma might cause congestion of the choroid or change the composition of aqueous (13,20,21). These theories have largely been disproven or discounted.

The congenital glaucoma that is associated with Sturge-Weber syndrome is usually associated with an immature angle development, as in primary congenital glaucoma. Careful gonioscopic examination will reveal indistinct angle structures with a high iris insertion. Histopathologic specimens have shown changes consistent with developmental anomalies, such as poorly developed scleral spur, thickened uveal meshwork and an anteriorly displaced iris root (11,14,22,23,24). Others have found little structural angle abnormalities. Cibis and coworkers examined 3 trabeculectomy specimens from two patients with Sturge-Weber syndrome, both of whom had episcleral hemangiomas, and found the overall architecture of the trabecular meshwork and Schlemm's canal to be well-preserved (25). However, the individual trabecular beams were thickened, and showed signs of degeneration, which the authors proposed were primary changes associated with premature aging.

Weiss proposed that glaucoma in Sturge-Weber syndrome was a result of two mechanisms (23). In his clinical experience, the congenital glaucoma cases had anomalous appearing angles as opposed to cases with later onset glaucoma that had normal appearing angles. He also found evidence of episcleral or conjunctival angiomas in all patients examined. He proposed that **increased episcleral venous pressure from the episcleral angioma contributed to the congenital glaucoma cases, in addition to an angle abnormality; whereas juvenile and adult onset cases without angle malformations were secondary to the elevated episcleral venous pressure.** Phelps, and then Bellows and coworkers later measured episcleral venous pressure and found it elevated in patients with Sturge-Weber syndrome and glaucoma (Chapter 46) (26,27).

Management depends on the presentation of the glaucoma. Congenital cases and those with buphthalmos, implying congenital onset, are best initially managed surgically with goniotomy or trabeculotomy; however, this is frequently ineffective, and many of these eyes eventually require filtering surgery. The angle dysgenesis in Sturge-Weber is clinically indistinguishable from primary congenital glaucoma, but the surgical success rate is lower than in primary congenital glaucoma. Iwach and coworkers found the stable interval of control after a single goniotomy to be only a median of 8 months in Sturge-Weber patients presenting before age 4 (18). Interestingly, in these same patients, multiple goniotomies plus medical therapy allowed stability for almost 9 years. Older patients were more likely to receive a trabeculectomy than goniotomy; however, trabeculectomy did not afford a longer interval of successful control of the glaucoma than goniotomy. The rationale for using trabeculectomy in the older patients stems from Weiss' theory that the primary mechanism in these patients is increased episcleral venous pressure. The trabeculectomy will bypass the episcleral venous system, whereas goniotomy or trabeculotomy does not. Unfortunately, a combined surgery of trabeculotomy with trabeculectomy did not increase success in a small series (28). The results of surgical success in the era of trabeculectomy with antimetabolites such as 5-fluorouracil and mitomycin C, or with the use of aqueous drainage implants, have not yet been reported; however, **we favor filtering surgery with mitomycin C and a prophylactic posterior sclerotomy in the setting of Sturge-Weber syndrome.**

Older patients are often managed with medical therapy as long as possible, but in most cases medical therapy eventually fails. Laser trabeculoplasty was performed in 6 of 16 older onset glaucoma eyes by Iwach and coworkers, and was effective in 5 of the 6 for approximately 2 years, (18) but such efficacy has unfortunately not been our experience. Trabeculectomy, full-thickness filtration surgery, and aqueous drainage implants in patients with Sturge-Weber syndrome all carry the serious and significant risk of sudden massive intraoperative choroidal effusion or expulsive hemorrhage (14,18,27,29). The rapid transudation of fluid from the intravascular to the extravascular space in the setting of sudden hypotony and increased venous pressure is thought to be responsible for the effusion. Bellows and associates reported success in minimizing the complications from the effusion by creating a posterior sclerotomy prior to entering the anterior chamber (27). In addition, the intraocular pressure should be reduced as much as possible prior to surgery.

KLIPPEL-TRENAUNAY-WEBER SYNDROME

In 1900, Klippel and Trenaunay described a syndrome of cutaneous hemangioma of the extremities and face, with varicosities and hypertrophy of bone and soft tissues in the affected limb. Weber later described the same disorder and reported the association of arteriovenous fistulas. Seizures, mental retardation and cerebral hemangiomas may occur (30). Many features of this syndrome are similar to Sturge-Weber syndrome.

Ophthalmic Manifestations

Ophthalmic involvement is occasionally found and may include orbital varices or hypertrophy, conjunctival telangiectasias, heterochromia iridis, choroidal angiomas, retinal varicosities or vascular tumors, disc anomalies, and glaucoma with or without buphthalmos (30–33). The glaucoma is associated with an ipsilateral facial hemangioma, but the incidence appears to be less frequent than in Sturge-Weber syndrome. One eye has been examined histopathologically and found to have an anomalous development of the anterior chamber angle (34).

NEUROFIBROMATOSIS (VON RECKLINGHAUSEN'S DISEASE)

In a classic monograph by the German pathologist Freidrich Daniel von Recklinghausen in 1882, neurofibromatosis (NF) was described. NF is inherited as an autosomal dominant disease with nearly 100% penetrance but highly variable expressivity. Neuroectodermal elements of the skin, eyes, and central nervous system are involved with the development of hamartomas which grow in size and number throughout life. The hamartomas may be present at birth or later in childhood or adult life.

Two forms of NF are recognized. NF-1 is the classic form of von Recklinghausen's neurofibromatosis, and is more common. The diagnosis for NF-1 is met if the patient has 2 or more of the following: 1) 6 or more cafe-au-lait macules over 5 mm in greatest diameter in prepubertal individuals, or over 15 mm in greatest diameter in postpubertal individuals. 2) 2 or more neurofibromas of any type or 1 plexiform neurofibroma; 3) freckling in axillary or inguinal regions; 4) optic glioma; 5) 2 or more Lisch nodules; 6) a distinctive osseous lesion such as sphenoid dysplasia or thinning of long bone cortex with or without pseudoarthrosis; 7) a first-degree relative with NF-1 by the above criteria (35).

NF-1 occurs in approximately 0.05 % of the population. There is no racial or sex predilection. The NF-1 gene has been isolated on the long arm of chromosome 17, and encodes for a protein related to guanosine diphosphatase-activating protein (GAP) (36–38). GAP regulates another protein, "ras," that signals cells to grow. Mutation of the NF-1 gene is thought to inactivate the gene (38).

NF-2, also called bilateral acoustic neurofibromatosis, was first described by Henneberg and Koch in 1902. The NIH diagnostic criteria requires bilateral acoustic neuromas, or a first-degree relative with NF-2 and a unilateral acoustic neuroma; or 2 of the following: meningioma, glioma, schwannoma, neurofibroma, presenile posterior subcapsular lens opacity (35).

NF-2 is present in only 1 out of 50,000 population. The NF-2 locus has been isolated to near the center of the long arm of chromosome 22, but the molecular genetics have not been elucidated yet (39,40).

Systemic Findings

The skin is the most commonly involved organ in NF-1 (11). Cafe-au-lait spots are brown macules usually found on the trunk. Fibroma molluscum are isolated, pedunculated, pigmented nodules which are found to have enlarged cutaneous nerves, Schwann's cells, and connective tissue elements, histopathologically. Plexiform neurofibromas are groups of enlarged nerves with thickened perineural sheaths that may feel like a "bag of worms" on palpation. These lesions often appear or worsen around the age of puberty and may increase in size and number with age. Hypertrophy of the involved areas may occur. NF-2 has very little skin involvement.

CNS tumors are common in both NF-1 and NF-2. CNS tumors in NF-1 and NF-2 include neurofibromas of the nerve roots or spinal cord, meningiomas, intracranial or spinal cord gliomas. Acoustic neuromas in NF-2 usually present in the second or third decades when hearing loss, tinnitus, or balance problems are noted. In individuals with a family history of NF-2, early detection with screening tests is possible.

Skeletal problems in patients with NF-1 include rapidly progressive kyphoscoliosis and pseudoarthroses, or nonhealing fractures (10). Pheochromocytomas are 10 times more common in patients with NF than the general population (41). Other organs may be involved by hamartomas or malignant tumors.

Ophthalmic Manifestations

The eyelids are frequently involved by neurofibromas and may produce a characteristic S-shaped upper eyelid contour (Fig. 49.3). Any of the other characteristic skin lesions may present in the eyelids or surrounding periorbital area and may develop in approximately 25% of patients (42).

Rarely, the conjunctiva or orbit may develop neurofibromas, while some patients have prominent corneal nerves visible on slit lamp examination. The greater wing of the sphenoid bone at the orbital apex may be absent, allowing the frontal lobe to herniate into the orbital apex.

Optic nerve glioma has been reported to occur in 15% of NF-1 patients, although many are asymptomatic (43,44). Optic nerve gliomas tend to grow slowly and only extremely rarely develop malignant transformation, although they can be very destructive locally. **Optic nerve gliomas are the primary cause of visual loss in NF.** Tumors that invade intracranially into the chiasm have a much poorer prognosis than optic nerve gliomas that involve the orbital portion of the optic nerve. Symptoms and signs of optic nerve glioma include decreased visual acuity, proptosis, strabismus, visual field loss, and optic atrophy.

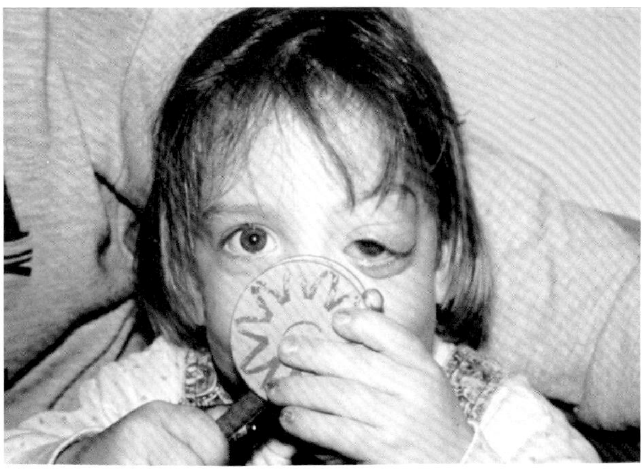

Figure 49.3. Patient with neurofibromatosis; characteristic S-shaped upper lid from neurofibroma, and buphthalmos from congenital glaucoma. (Courtesy of David S. Walton, MD).

Contrast enhanced CT scanning, or MRI will demonstrate enlargement and kinking of the optic nerve anywhere along its course and into the chiasmal region, although MRI may be able to detect intracannalicular and chiasmal masses better (45).

Lisch nodules are melanocytic hamartomas of the iris and are found in over 90% of NF-1 patients over the age of 5 (42,46). Patients younger than 2 rarely have any Lisch nodules and they are not present in unaffected first-degree relatives (42,47). Lisch nodules are avascular, smooth, dome shaped gelatinous nodules found on the iris surface. They may be mildly translucent to dark brown in color, ranging in size up to 2 mm.

NF-2 patients have a high incidence of posterior subcapsular cataract occurring at a young age (48). This association has not been seen with NF-1.

Choroidal hamartomas have been reported in a series of white NF patients but were not seen in black patients (42). Occasionally retinal astrocytic hamartomas or combined retinal and retinal pigment epithelial hamartomas have been seen in patients with NF-1.

Glaucoma in Neurofibromatosis

Congenital glaucoma and glaucoma presenting somewhat later in childhood have been reported in cases of NF-1. The actual incidence of glaucoma in neurofibromatosis is unknown. Buphthalmos in the absence of elevated intraocular pressure has been reported as a manifestation of regional giantism (49). Care must be taken to distinguish this condition from true congenital glaucoma in neurofibromatosis. Two presentations of glaucoma in neurofibromatosis are recognized. Infants and toddlers have presented with unilateral buphthalmos and elevated intraocular pressure, usually with a plexiform neurofibroma formation of the upper eyelid and hemihypertrophy of the face (Francois syndrome), and are subsequently diagnosed with NF-1 (50,51). It is reported that **glaucoma is present in 50% of eyes with a plexiform neurofibroma of the upper lid** (52). Several mechanisms for this congenital form of glaucoma have been suggested. Failure of the normal angle development, as in primary congenital glaucoma, has been implicated, and is likely the most common cause of infantile onset glaucoma in neurofibromatosis (50,53). Infiltration of the angle by neurofibroma was documented by gonioscopy by Grant and Walton, and found histopathologically by Francois (53). Closure of the angle by diffuse involvement of the ciliary body and choroid has also been recognized, and may develop as a late complication (50). Synechial angle closure from neovascularization has been reported in neurofibromatosis (54).

The other presentation of glaucoma in neurofibromatosis is usually later in childhood in association with unilateral congenital ectropion uveae (55,56) (Fig. 49.4). In a series of eight patients with congenital ectropion uveae and glaucoma, 3 were found to have neurofibromatosis (55). Congenital ectropion uveae is usually accompanied by ipsilateral ptosis, although not a palpable neurofibroma mass. The pupil may be mistakenly taken as enlarged or irregular. On careful inspection however, pigmented uveal tissue is found to overly the iris surrounding the pupil. This tissue has been identified as hyperplasia of the iris pigment epithelium, not a true ectropion, and is usually unchanged in its appearance over time (57). The mechanism for the glaucoma in these cases is an iridogoniodysgenesis. Gonioscopic findings reveal a high, or anterior, iris insertion into the trabecular meshwork (55,57).

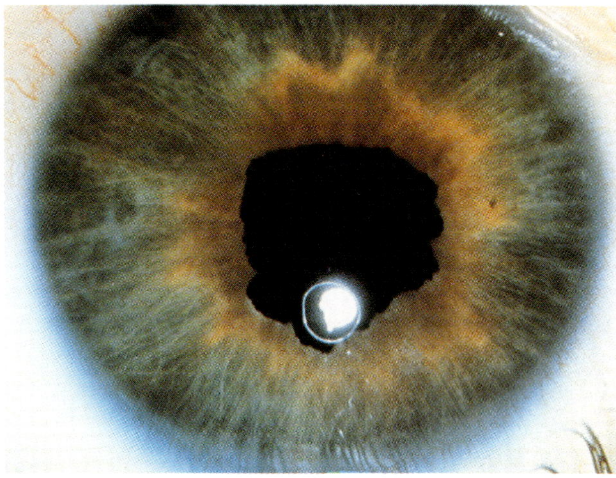

Figure 49.4. Congenital ectropion uveae in a patient with neurofibromatosis and glaucoma. (Courtesy of David S. Walton, MD).

Treatment of the glaucoma depends on the underlying mechanism. Congenital cases with abnormal angle development or infiltration are best managed by goniotomy or trabeculotomy initially, and with trabeculectomy if those procedures fail. Cases presenting later in childhood may be successfully managed medically or surgically. Since marked infiltration of the choroid or ciliary body may develop later in childhood, periodic gonioscopy is necessary to detect progressive angle closure.

VON HIPPEL-LINDAU DISEASE (RETINAL AND CEREBELLAR ANGIOMATOSIS)

In 1904, von Hippel published a seminal paper describing retinal angiomatosis in two patients. He later performed a pathologic examination and identified the lesion as a hemangioblastoma, naming the condition angiomatosis retinae. Lindau, in 1926, made the association of cerebellar hemangiomatous cysts in many patients with von Hippel's disease. The term von Hippel-Lindau disease is used when the disease involves the CNS and retina; when the retina only is involved, it is called von Hippel disease.

This rare disease is estimated to occur in 1 in 22,500 patients seen by ophthalmologists (58). About 20 to 25% of cases are familial, and in this case, it is inherited as an autosomal dominant trait with incomplete penetrance. Linkage analysis has mapped the gene for von Hippel-Lindau disease to the short arm of chromosome 3 (59).

Systemic Findings

The cerebellar hemangioblastoma tumor is the characteristic CNS lesion that occurs in an estimated ⅔ of von Hippel-Lindau cases (60,61). These tumors are often resectable but recurrences may occur. Death may ensue due to neurologic effects of the tumor. The typical presentation is of headache, vertigo, or cerebellar signs developing at an age in the mid-thirties. Medullary and spinal hemangioblastomas are uncommon (61). Polycythemia is associated with the CNS hemangioblastomas (62).

Renal cell carcinoma occurs in about ¼ of patients and may cause death from uremia or metastatic disease (60,61). It is usually diagnosed in the fifth decade of life. Pheochromocytoma is associated with von Hippel-Lindau disease in various kindreds, and therefore the reported frequency varies (61,63). Renal and pancreatic cysts may also be present.

Screening affected individuals and family members with CT or MRI of the head and abdomen may detect these lesions before the patient becomes symptomatic (61).

Ophthalmic Manifestations

The retinal angioma is usually the first feature of the syndrome to be diagnosed as it tends to present in the second or third decade of life. Retinal angiomas are detected in about ⅔ of von Hippel-Lindau patients, and are usually asymptomatic at the time of diagnosis (61,63). The capillary type angiomas are bilateral in about 50%, are multiple in about ⅓, and are usually located in the mid-periphery of the retina (64-66). The tumor develops from a lesion as small as a diabetic microaneurysm into a reddish, elevated mass of 1 to 3 disc diameters in size. A single dilated tortuous feeder artery is paired with a similar appearing vein, and there is arteriovenous shunting through the tumor (67). **If left untreated, the incompetent vascular endothelium of the tumor allows leakage and exudation to develop in the surrounding retina, and ultimately leads to an exudative retinal detachment involving the posterior pole. The neovascular glaucoma that may occur is found in this end-stage setting.**

Treatment of the angioma can be accomplished with direct photocoagulation, diathermy, or cryotherapy of the lesion (68).

The incidence of glaucoma in this condition is low, and most commonly associated with neovascularization following exudative retinal detachment. Hardwig and Robertson, in their report on 36 eyes, noted 3 of 13 eyes with poor vision due to glaucoma, and an additional 4 eyes enucleated because of pain and blindness (61).

TUBEROUS SCLEROSIS (BOURNEVILLE'S DISEASE)

Tuberous sclerosis was first described in 1880 by Bourneville. Vogt later described the triad of epilepsy, adenoma sebaceum, and mental deficiency. Tuberous sclerosis has a prevalence of 1 in 10,000 to 15,000 (69,70). The disease is transmitted as an autosomal dominant trait with high penetrance but variable expressivity. Detection of gene carriers is possible using CT scanning and an evaluation of skin lesions (71). Genetic linkage analysis has located the gene for tuberous sclerosis on the distal portion of the long arm of chromosome 9 (72).

Systemic Findings

Ash-leaf spots on the skin, detected by ultraviolet light, are usually present at birth, are found in at least 80% of affected patients and considered diagnostic of tuberous sclerosis (73,74). **Adenoma sebaceum** is the characteristic rash that appears after the age of 2, and is present in 83% of cases (74). It appears as small reddish-brown papules over the cheeks, nose, and chin, which are histologically angiofibromata (11,24). These lesions may also affect the eyelids and conjunctiva. Shagreen patches, yellow plaques, are found in about ⅓ of patients and are usually located over the lower back or the eyelids.

Seizures develop in 80–90% of patients. Infantile spasms are a common presentation of tuberous sclerosis, while later in childhood the seizures become more generalized (12,75). Mental retardation occurs in 50–60% of patients (12,74,75). The CNS effects are a result of benign periventricular brain tumors which become calcified ("brain stones") and are seen on CT scan in about half of patients (74). Renal cysts and hamartomas are also common.

Ophthalmic Manifestations

The most common associated ocular feature of tuberous sclerosis is an astrocytic retinal hamartoma, which occurs singly or multiply in half of patients (74). Multiple retinal hamartomas are diagnostic of the disease when present. The classic tumor is described as a translucent white mulberry-like lesion, calcified and located near the optic disc. These retinal tumors usually do not cause any associated visual or anatomic problems. Rarely, an exudative retinal detachment or vitreous hemorrhage may occur or the hamartoma may undergo cystic degeneration and mimic necrotizing retinitis (76–78). **The only association with glaucoma is as a rare secondary complication of a total retinal detachment or neovascularization** (73,79).

ATAXIA TELANGIECTASIA (LOUIS-BAR SYNDROME)

In 1941, Louis-Bar reported a child with progressive cerebellar ataxia and telangiectasias of the skin and conjunctiva. In 1957, Boder and Sedgwick reported seven cases and coined the name ataxia-telangiectasia (80).

This rare syndrome is inherited as an autosomal recessive trait. The search for one of the possible genes for ataxia telangiectasia has been narrowed to chromosome region 11q22 to 11q23 by linkage analysis (81).

Systemic Findings

Progressive cerebellar ataxia is usually diagnosed in the first years of life. Progression occurs so that the patient is unable to walk, and has difficulty with speech and responses by the first decade of life. Cerebellar cortical atrophy is the characteristic lesion (80).

The skin becomes involved with telangiectasias between the age of 3 and 7. These are noted on the cheeks, nose, ears, palate, and ocular adnexae. Older patients develop telangiectasias of the skin of the neck, antecubital and popliteal areas, dorsal hands and feet (80).

Hypoplasia of the thymus gland may be seen, along with an increased susceptibility to recurrent sinus and pulmonary infections in approximately 85% of patients (80). This is felt to be associated with an underlying immunological disorder (82).

Patients with ataxia telangiectasia have a greatly increased risk of developing a malignancy (81).

Ophthalmic Manifestations

Conjunctival telangiectasias are seen in childhood in all patients, usually bilaterally. Abnormal extraocular muscle movements and gaze disorders are common (83,84).

Glaucoma is not a reported feature of ataxia telangiectasia.

WYBURN-MASON SYNDROME

In 1943, Wyburn-Mason published a review of all reported cases of retinal arteriovenous (AV) communications, and emphasized the common association of intracranial arteriovenous communications in 81% of patients (85). Only a few of these patients had documented intracranial AV malformations, however. Subsequent studies have placed the incidence of intracranial AV communication in patients with retinal AV malformations at 23% to 30% (86,87). The Wyburn-Mason syndrome is not hereditary, and has no sex predilection.

Systemic Findings

Approximately half of patients have associated ipsilateral facial angiomas of variable appearance (87). The intracranial AV malformation is unilateral, ipsilateral to the involved eye and usually in the midbrain. Symptoms of headache and vomiting, often related to cerebral or subarachnoid bleeding from the lesion, develop in the second to third decades of life. Signs of hydrocephalus from obstruction of the cerebral aqueduct by an enlarging malformation may occur. Seizures are uncommon, but other neurologic deficits may result from the midbrain lesion. Treatment is generally not undertaken due to the inaccessible location of the AV malformation.

Ophthalmic Manifestations

The AV communication in the retina typically involves the vessels in the temporal midperiphery. The lesion varies from an arteriolar or capillary plexus between an artery and vein to a direct communication through large, dilated, intertwined twisting vessels (88). The retinal appearance remains stable, but vision loss may develop in the second to third decade of life, especially with the more severe malformations, and progress due to associated retinal involvement. The lesion may produce retinal or vitreous hemorrhage, nonperfusion of the retina, retinal edema and exudation (88). The vascular malformation may extend from the eye to the midbrain and cause compression of the optic nerve or visual pathway with resulting visual field defects. Symptomatic eyes may be treated with laser photocoagulation (89).

Neovascular glaucoma has been reported in a 4 year old child who developed widespread retinal and choroidal ischemia (90).

LINEAR NEVUS SEBACEOUS SYNDROME (NEVUS SEBACEOUS OF JADASSOHN)

In 1932, Robinson reported the linear nevus sebaceous syndrome, with a skin lesion as described by Jadassohn, in 4 patients (91). The syndrome consists of a triad of linear nevus sebaceous, seizure disorder and mental retardation. There is no known hereditary association.

Systemic Findings

The skin lesions consist of congenital organoid nevi which progress through stages, beginning with underdevelopment of hair and sebaceous glands, to massive development of sebaceous glands and papillomatous epidermoid hyperplasia (92). Eventually the nevus develops benign and malignant neoplasms (93). **Malignant transformation may occur in 10 to 35% of nevi** (92,94). Surgical excision is usually curative.

The syndrome may involve multiple other organ systems, including central nervous system (CNS), ophthalmic, skeletal, cardiovascular, and urogenital systems (93). Ipsilateral CNS involvement is more likely when the epidermal nevi are found on the head (95,96).

Ophthalmic Manifestations

Ophthalmic involvement is found in 68% of patients with the linear nevus sebaceous syndrome (93). Involvement of the adnexa with a coloboma or ptosis of the upper eyelid is common. Epibulbar dermoids that appear firm, flat, pink, and vascularized may involve the conjunctiva bilaterally in any location (93). The cornea may be involved with partial or total vascularization, dermoid tumor, or scarring (93). Unilateral and bilateral colobomas of the iris and ciliary body, choroid and retina have been reported (93). Optic nerve hypoplasia, optic disc pallor, and optic disc cupping also have been reported (93).

Although glaucoma has not been specifically reported, two reports have noted incomplete opening of the anterior chamber angle on pathologic examination (96,97).

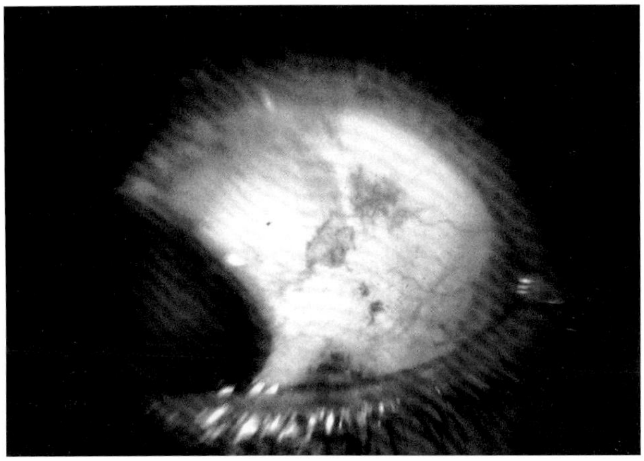

Figure 49.5. Characteristic bluish, slate gray appearance of scleral pigmentation in a patient with oculodermal melanocytosis (nevus of Ota).

BASAL CELL NEVUS SYNDROME

Basal cell nevus syndrome was described by Binkley in 1951 (98). It is inherited as an autosomal dominant trait with variable penetrance. Multiple basal cell epitheliomas, which may be present at birth and enlarge during adolescence, develop over the eyelids and face, and occasionally on the trunk and neck, and may be locally invasive (99–101). A characteristic dyskeratosis of the skin may occur, in addition to bony abnormalities, neurologic, and genital anomalies (10). Variable ocular findings occur in 30% of cases. Orbital involvement by tumor, hypertelorism, congenital cataract, strabismus, optic nerve and choroidal coloboma, corneal leukoma and glaucoma have been reported in some patients (101-104).

GLAUCOMAS ASSOCIATED WITH OTHER SKIN DISORDERS

Nevus of Ota (Oculodermal Melanocytosis, Congenital Ocular Melanosis)

The skin lesion in oculodermal melanosis or Nevus of Ota is a deeply pigmented, slate gray appearance to the skin in the distribution of the first and second divisions of the trigeminal nerve. There is no known hereditary influence. It is common in Asians and black patients.

Ophthalmic Manifestations

Most patients with the skin pigmentation have an ipsilateral hyperpigmentation of the globe, which may include the sclera (Fig. 49.5), conjunctiva, cornea, iris, and choroid. These patients are at risk for developing uveal and orbital malignant melanoma (105). The scleral pigmentation is a muted bluish or slate gray in color. **Markedly increased pigmentation may be found in the angle structures of the involved eye.** This finding may be seen without evidence of increased intraocular pressure, but open angle glaucoma has been reported in several cases (106–108). The glaucoma responds to management as a primary open angle glaucoma.

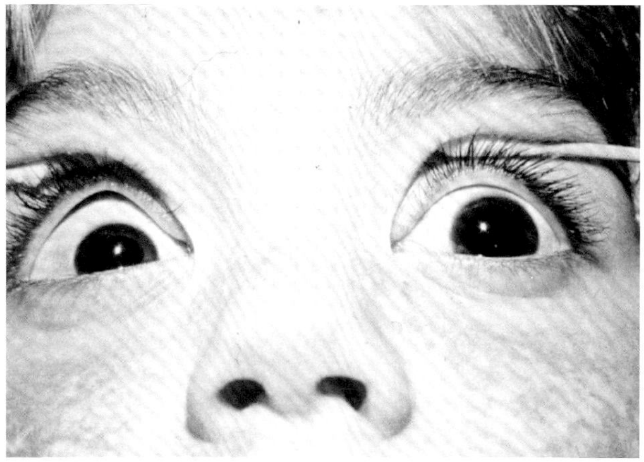

Figure 49.6. Buphthalmos and congenital glaucoma in a patient with cutis marmorata telangiectatica congenita. Note the telangiectatic, marbled appearance of the bilateral facial lesion that is more subtle than the nevus flammeus of Sturge-Weber. (Courtesy of A. Robert Bellows, MD).

CUTIS MARMORATA TELANGIECTATICA CONGENITA (CMTC)

This rare cutaneous vascular anomaly was first described in 1922 by Lohuizen. There is no known genetic pattern for CMTC. It is characterized by congenital persistent cutis marmorata, phlebectasia, telangiectasis, superficial ulcerations, with slow clinical improvement during childhood (109). The affected skin has a cutaneous marbling effect, deeper in color than in infants exposed to cold temperature (Fig. 49.6). Regional involvement of the face, trunk, or extremities occurs in about half of cases, while generalized involvement occurs in the remainder of patients (109).

Ophthalmic Manifestations

Four cases of congenital glaucoma have been reported in the literature, all associated with ipsilateral facial involvement (110). We have seen 2 additional patients with congenital glaucoma who also had facial involvement. **The associated glaucoma is related to immature angle development as in primary congenital glaucoma** (110). Increased episcleral venous pressure does not appear to occur in CMTC, as episcleral or conjunctival vascular changes were not found in the reported cases or ours, nor was blood visible in Schlemm's canal on gonioscopy (110). However, a case report describes an intraoperative suprachoroidal hemorrhage in a child with CMTC during a repeat trabeculectomy (111). The authors described the involved eye as buphthalmic with an immature angle appearance on gonioscopy, without any vascular abnormality of the eye (111). The glaucoma can be managed with goniotomy or trabeculotomy initially, adding medical therapy as needed. In the reported cases, the glaucoma has been somewhat difficult to control, with trabeculectomy required in 3 of the 6 cases.

References

1. Brouwer B, van der Hoeve J, Mahoney W: A fourth type of phakomatosis: Sturge-Weber syndrome. Verh K Akad Wet Amst 1937;36: 1.
2. van der Hoeve J: Eye diseases in tuberose sclerosis of the brain and in Recklinghausen's disease. Trans Ophthalmol Soc UK 1923;43:534.
3. Duke-Elder S: Part 2, Congenital Deformities. In: System of Ophthalmology. Normal and Abnormal Development. St. Louis, CV Mosby, 1964:1153.
4. Hogan MJ, Zimmerman LE: Ophthalmic Pathology: An Atlas and Textbook. Philadelphia: WB Saunders, 1962.
5. Kousseff BG: The phakomatoses as paracrine growth disorders (paracrinopathies). Clin Genetics 1990;37:97-105.
6. Reese AB: Tumors of the Eye. New York, Harper & Row, 1976.
7. Duke-Elder S, Jay B: System of Ophthalmology: Diseases of the Lens and Vitreous; Glaucoma and Hypotony. St. Louis, CV Mosby, 1969.
8. Shaffer RN, Weiss DI: Congenital and Pediatric Glaucomas. St. Louis: CV Mosby, 1970.
9. Peterman AF, Hayles AB, Dockerty MB, et al: Encephalotrigeminal angiomatosis: clinical study of 35 cases. JAMA 1958;167:2169–2176.
10. Ebert EM, Albert DM: Phakomatoses. In: Principles and Practice of Ophthalmology: Clinical Practice. Edited by Albert DM, Jakobiec FA. Philadelphia, WB Saunders, 1994:3298–3328.
11. Font RL, Ferry AP: The phakomatoses. Int Ophthalmol Clin 1972; 12:1.
12. Beck RW, Hanno R: The phakomatoses. Int Ophthalmol Clin 1985; 25:97.
13. Alexander GL, Norman RM: The Sturge-Weber syndrome. Bristol, England, John Wright & Sons, Ltd, 1960.
14. Christensen GR, Records RE: Glaucoma and expulsive hemorrhage mechanisms in the Sturge-Weber syndrome. Ophthalmology 1979;86: 1360-6.
15. Duke-Elder S, Perkins ES: System of Ophthalmology: Diseases of the uveal tract. St. Louis, CV Mosby, 1966.
16. Susac JO, Smith JL, Scelfo RJ: The "tomato catsup" fundus in Sturge-Weber syndrome. Arch Ophthalmol 1974;92:69.
17. Witschel H, Font RL: Hemangioma of the choroid. A clinicopathologic study of 71 cases and a review of the literature. Surv Ophthalmol 1974; 20:415.
18. Iwach AG, Hoskins HD, Hetherington J, et al: Analysis of surgical and medical management of glaucoma in Sturge-Weber syndrome. Ophthalmology 1990;97:904-909.
19. Cushing H: Cases of spontaneous intracranial hemorrhage associated with trigeminal naevi. JAMA 1906;47:178.
20. Dunphy EB: Glaucoma accompanying nevus flammeus. Trans Am Ophthalmol Soc 1934;32:143.
21. Tyson HH: Nevus flammeus of the face and globe. Arch Ophthalmol 1932;8:365.
22. Barkan O: Goniotomy for glaucoma associated with nevus flammeus. Am J Ophthalmol 1957;43:545.
23. Weiss DI: Dual origin of glaucoma in encephalotrigeminal haemangiomatosis. Trans Ophthalmol Soc UK 1973;93:477-493.
24. Gass JDM: The phakomatoses. In: Neuroophthalmology. Edited by Smith JL. St. Louis, CV Mosby, 1965:
25. Cibis GW, Tripathi RC, Tripathi BJ: Glaucoma in Sturge-Weber syndrome. Ophthalmology 1984;91:1061-1071.
26. Phelps CD: The pathogenesis of glaucoma in Sturge-Weber syndrome. Ophthalmology 1978;85:276.
27. Bellows AR, Chylack LT, Epstein DL, et al: Choroidal effusion during glaucoma surgery in patients with prominent episcleral vessels. Arch Ophthalmol 1979;97:493.
28. Board JB, Shields MB: Combined trabeculotomy-trabeculectomy for the management of glaucoma associated with Sturge-Weber syndrome. Ophthalmic Surgery 1981;12:813-817.
29. Shihab ZM, Kristan RW: Recurrent intraoperative choroidal effusion in Sturge-Weber syndrome. J Pediatric Ophthalmol Strabismus 1983; 20:250-2.
30. O'Connor PS, Smith JD: Optic nerve variant in the Klippel-Trenaunay-Weber syndrome. Ann Ophthalmol 1978;10:131.
31. Brod RD, Shields JA, Shields CL, et al: Unusual retinal and renal vascular lesions in the Klippel-Trenaunay-Weber syndrome. Retina 1992;12:355-8.
32. Limaye SR, Doyle HA, Tang RA: Retinal varicosity in Klippel-Trenaunay syndrome. J Pediatr Ophthalmol Strabismus 1979;16:371.
33. Good WV, Hoyt CS: Optic nerve shadow enlargement in the Klippel-Trenaunay-Weber syndrome. J Pediatr Ophthalmol Strabismus 1989; 26:288.
34. Reynolds JD, Johnson BL, Gloster S, et al: Glaucoma and Klippel-Trenaunay-Weber syndrome. Am J Ophthalmol 1988;106:495.
35. National Institutes of Health Consensus Development Conference Statement on Neurofibromatosis. Arch Neurol 1988;45:575.
36. Barker D, Wright E, Nguyen K, et al: Gene for von Recklinghausen neurofibromatosis is in the pericentromeric region of chromosome 17. Science 1987;236:1100.
37. Seizinger BR, Rouleau GA, Ozelius LJ, et al: Genetic linkage of von Recklinghausen neurofibromatosis to the nerve growth factor receptor gene. Cell 1987;49:589.
38. Xu G, O'Connell P, Viskochil D, et al: The neurofibromatosis type 1 gene encodes a protein related to GAP. Cell 1990;62:599.
39. Rouleau GA, Wertelecki W, Haines JL, et al: Genetic linkage of bilateral acoustic neurofibromatosis to a DNA marker on chromosome 22. Nature 1987;329:246.
40. Rouleau GA, Haines JL, Bazanowski A, et al: A genetic linkage map of the long arm of human chromosome 22. Genomics 1989;4:1-6.
41. DeAngelis LM, Kelleher MB, Post KD, et al: Multiple paragangliomas in neurofibromatosis. Neurology 1987;37:129.
42. Lewis RA, Riccardi VM: von Recklinghausen neurofibromatosis. Ophthalmology 1981;88:348.
43. Lewis RA, Gerson LP, Axelson KA, et al: von Recklinghausen neurofibromatosis: II Incidence of optic gliomata. Ophthalmology 1984;91: 929.
44. Listernick R, Charrow J, Greenwald MJ, et al: Optic gliomas in children with neurofibromatosis type 1. J Pediatrics 1989;114:788.
45. Braffman BH, Bilaniuk LT, Zimmerman RA: The central nervous system manifestations of the phakomatoses on MR. Radiol Clin North Am 1988;26:773.
46. Perry HD, Font RL: Iris nodules in von Recklinghausen's Neurofibromatosis. Electron microscopic confirmation of their melanocytic origin. Arch Ophthalmol 1982;100:1635-40.
47. Lubs ME, Bauer M, Formas ME, et al Iris hamartomas in the diagnosis of neurofibromatosis-1. Int Pediatrics 1990;5:261.
48. Pearson-Webb MA, Kaiser-Kupfer MI, Eldridge R: Eye findings in bilateral acoustic (central) neurofibromatosis: association with presenile lens opacities and cataracts but absence of Lisch nodules [letter]. N Engl J Med 1986;315:1553-4.
49. Hoyt CS, Billson FA: Buphthalmos in neurofibromatosis: is it an expression of regional giantism? J Pediatric Ophthalmol 1977;14:228-34.
50. Brownstein S, Little JM: Ocular neurofibromatosis. Ophthalmology 1983;90:1595-9.
51. Politi F, Sachs R, Barishak R: Neurofibromatosis and congenital glaucoma. A case report. Ophthalmologica 1977;176:155-9.
52. Lieb WA, Wirth WA, Geeraets WJ: Hydrophthalmos and neurofibromatosis. Confin Neurol 1958;19:230.
53. Grant WM, Walton DS: Distinctive gonioscopic findings in glaucoma due to neurofibromatosis. Arch Ophthalmol 1968;79:127.
54. Wolter JR, Butler R: Pigment spots of the iris and ectropion uveae with glaucoma in neurofibromatosis. Am J Ophthalmol 1963;56:964.
55. Ritch R, Forbes M, Hetherington J Jr, et al: Congenital ectropion uveae with glaucoma. Ophthalmology 1984;91:326–31.
56. Roth H and Shaffer RN. Neurofibromatosis and glaucoma. In: J. G.

Bellows, eds. Contemporary Ophthalmology. Baltimore: Williams and Wilkins, 1972:180-189.

57. Dowling J, Walton DS, Richardson TM, et al: Glaucoma with congenital ectropion uveae. Opthalmology 1985;92:912-921.
58. Pinkerton OD: Angioma of the retina. Am J Ophthalmol 1946;29: 711.
59. Seizinger BR, Rouleau GA, Ozelius LJ, et al: von Hippel-Lindau disease maps to the region of chromosome 3 associated with renal cell carcinoma. Nature 1988;332:268.
60. Maher ER, Yates JRW, Harries R, et al: Clinical features and natural history of von Hippel-Lindau. QJ Med 1990;66:233.
61. Hardwig P, Robertson DM: von Hippel-Lindau disease: a familial, often lethal, multisystem phakomatosis. Ophthalmology 1984;91:263-270.
62. Cramer F, Kimsey W: The cerebellar hemangioblastomas; review of 53 cases, with special reference to cerebellar cysts and the association of polycythemia. Arch Neurol Psychiatry 1952;67:237-252.
63. Melmon KL, Rosen SW: Lindau's disease: review of the literature and study of a large kindred. Am J Med 1964;36:595.
64. Welch RB: von Hippel-Lindau disease: the recognition and treatment of early angiomatosis retinae and the use of cryosurgery as an adjunct to therapy. Trans Am Ophthal Soc 1970;66:367.
65. Nicholson DH, Green WR, Kenyon KR: Light and electron microscopic study of early lesions in angiomatosis retinae. Am J Ophthalmol 1976;82:193.
66. Jakobiec F, Font RL, Johnson FB: Angiomatosis retinae: an ultrastructural study and lipid analysis. Cancer 1976;38:2042.
67. Haining WM, Zweifach PH: Fluorescein angiography in von Hippel-Lindau disease. Arch Ophthalmol 1967;78:475.
68. Gass JDM: Treatment of retinal vascular anomalies. Symposium: retinal vascular disease. Trans Am Acad Ophthalmol Otolaryngol 1977;83: 432.
69. Wiederholt WC, Gomez MR, Kurland LT: Incidence and prevalence of tuberous sclerosis in Rochester, Minnesota, 1950–1982. Neurology 1985;35:600.
70. Hunt A, Lindenbaum RH: Tuberous sclerosis: a new estimate of prevalence within the Oxford region. J Med Genet 1984;21:272.
71. Flinter FA, Neville BGR: Examining the parents of children with tuberous sclerosis. Lancet 1986;2:1167.
72. Fryer AE, Chalmers A, Connor JM, et al: Evidence that the gene for tuberous sclerosis is on chromosome 9. Lancet 1987;1:659.
73. Gomez MR: Tuberous sclerosis. New York: Raven Press, 1979.
74. Lagos JC, Gomez MR: Tuberous sclerosis: reappraisal of a clinical entity. Mayo Clin Proc 1967;42:26.
75. Williams R, Taylor D: Tuberous sclerosis. Surv Ophthalmol 1985;30: 143-54.
76. Kroll AJ, Ricker DP, Robb RM, et al: Vitreous hemorrhage complicating retinal astrocytic hamartoma. Surv Ophthalmol 1981;26:31-8.
77. Jost BF, Olk RJ: Atypical retinitis proliferans retinal telangiectasis, and vitreous hemorrhage in a patient with tuberous sclerosis. Retina 1986;6:53.
78. Coppeto JR, Lubin JR, Albert DM: Astrocytic hamartoma in tuberous sclerosis mimicking necrotizing retinochoroiditis. J Pediatr Ophthalmol Strabis 1982;19:306-13.
79. Wolter JR, Mertus JM: Exophytic retinal astrocytoma in tuberous sclerosis. J Pediatr Ophthalmol 1969;6:186.
80. Boder E, Sedgwick RP: Ataxia telangiectasia: familial syndrome of progressive cerebellar ataxia, oculocutaneous telangiectasia, and frequent pulmonary infection. Pediatrics 1958;21:526.
81. Gatti RA, Berkel I, Boder E, et al: Localization of an ataxia telangiectasia gene to chromosome 11q22-23. Nature 1988;336:577.
82. Saxon A, Stevens RH, Golde DW: Helper and suppressor T-lymphocyte leukemia in ataxia telangiectasia. N Engl J Med 1979;300:700.
83. Baloh RW, Yee RD, Boder E: Eye movements in ataxia-telangiectasia. Neurology 1978;28:1099-1104.
84. Stell R, Bronstein AM, Plant GT, et al: Ataxia telangiectasia: a reappraisal of the ocular motor features and their value in the diagnosis of atypical cases. Movement Disorders 1989;4:320-9.
85. Wyburn-Mason R: Arteriovenous aneurysm of mid-brain and retina, facial naevi, and mental changes. Brain 1943;66:163.
86. Bech K, Jenson OA: On the frequency of coexisting racemose haemangiomata of the retina and brain. Acta Psychiat Neurol 1961;36:47.
87. Theron J, Newton TH, Hoyt WF. Unilateral retinocephalic vascular malformations. Neuroradiology 1974;7:185.
88. Archer DB, Deutman A, Ernest JT, et al: Arteriovenous communication of the retina. Am J Ophthalmol 1973;75:224.
89. Hopen G, Smith JL, Hoff JT, et al: The Wyburn-Mason syndrome: concomitant chiasmal and fundus vascular malformations. J Clin Neurol Ophthalmol 1983;3:53.
90. Effron L, Zakov ZN, Tomsak RL. Neovascular glaucoma as a complication of the Wyburn-Mason syndrome. J Clin Neuro Ophthalmol 1985; 5:95.
91. Robinson S: Naevus sebaceous (Jadassohn): report of 4 cases. Arch Dermatol 1932;26:663.
92. Mehregan AH, Pinkus H: Life history of organoid nevi: special reference to the nevus sebaceous of Jadassohn. Arch Dermatol 1965;91:574.
93. Katz B, Wiley CA, Lee VW: Optic nerve hypoplasia and the syndrome of nevus sebaceous of Jadassohn. A new association. Ophthalmology 1987;94:1570-6.
94. Domingo J, Helwig EB: Malignant neoplasms associated with nevus sebaceus of Jadassohn. J Am Acad Dermatol 1979;1:545-56.
95. Baker RS, Ross PA, Baumann RJ: Neurological complications of the epidermal nevus syndrome. Arch Neurol 1987;227.
96. Wilkes SR, Campbell RJ, Waller RR: Ocular malformation in association with ipsilateral facial nevus of Jadassohn. Am J Ophthalmol 1981; 92:344-52.
97. Schochot Y, Romano A, Barishak YR: Eye findings in the linear sebaceous nevus syndrome: a possible clue to the pathogenesis. J Craniofac Genet Dev Biol 1982;2:289-294.
98. Binkley GW, Johnson HH: Epithelioma adenoides cysticum: basal cell nevi, agenesis of the corpus callosum, and dental cysts. Arch Dermatol Syph 1951;63:73.
99. Southwick GJ, Schwartz RA: The basal cell nevus syndrome: disasters occurring among a series of 36 patients. Cancer 1979;44:2294–305.
100. Nerad JA, Whitaker DC: Periocular basal cell carcinoma in adults 35 years of age and younger. Am J Ophthalmol 1988;106:723-9.
101. Markovits A, Quickert M: Basal cell nevus. Arch Ophthalmol 1972; 88:397.
102. Fehman S, Apt L, Roth A: The basal cell nevus syndrome. Am J Ophthalmol 1974;78:222.
103. Gorlin RJ, Vickers RA, Kellen E, et al: The multiple basal cell nevi syndrome. Cancer 1965;18:89.
104. Kahn LB, Gordon W: Basal cell naevus syndrome. S Afr Med J 1967; 41:832.
105. Gonder JR, Shields JA: Malignant melanoma of the choroid associated with oculodermal melanocytosis. Ophthalmology 1981;88:372.
106. Teekhasaenee C, Ritch R, Rutnin U, et al: Glaucoma in oculodermal melanocytosis. Ophthalmology 1990;97:562.
107. Foulks GN, Shields MB: Glaucoma in oculodermal melanocytosis. Ann Ophthalmol 1977;9:1299.
108. Weiss DI, Krohn DL: Benign melanocytic glaucoma complicating oculodermal melanocytosis. Ann Ophthalmol 1971;3:958.
109. South DA, Jacobs AH: Cutis marmorata telangiectatica congenita. Pediatrics 1978;93:944.
110. Sato SE, Herschler J, Lynch PJ, et al: Congenital glaucoma associated with cutis marmorata telangiectatica congenita: two case reports. J Pediatr Ophthalmol Strabismus 1988;25:13–17.
111. Kremer I, Metzker A, Yassur Y: Intraoperative suprachoroidal hemorrhage in congenital glaucoma associated with cutis marmorata telangiectatica congenita. Arch Ophthalmol 1991;109:1199.

Juvenile Open Angle Glaucoma

50

Janey L. Wiggs

Juvenile glaucoma has been defined as a form of primary open angle glaucoma that develops during the first two decades of life. **The age of onset is variable but is typically between the ages of 3 and 20.** Primary juvenile glaucoma has been previously classified as true juvenile glaucoma, neglected infantile (congenital) glaucoma, presenile glaucoma and angle-closure glaucoma. The discussion in this chapter refers to the form of juvenile glaucoma previously classified as "true juvenile glaucoma." The disease process is characterized by a severe high pressure glaucoma that can result in significant damage to the optic nerve leaving affected individuals with little useful vision early in life. There are no known associated systemic findings.

Characteristic clinical features often include a **high incidence of myopia.** Affected eyes do not show signs of buphthalmos. The cornea does not demonstrate breaks in Descemet's membrane. Gonioscopy typically shows a normal appearance to the angle structures. There is no evidence of increased pigment deposition in the angle or other findings consistent with the pigment dispersion syndrome. Some patients with juvenile open angle glaucoma may have an increased number of iris processes some of which have an anterior insertion crossing the scleral spur and posterior trabecular meshwork (Fig. 50.1). However, this is not a consistently identified finding, and these patients do not have any of the other findings associated with the Axenfeld-Rieger anomaly such as posterior embryotoxon (1). These patients do not appear to have a Barkan membrane covering the angle as is typical of patients affected by congenital glaucoma. One histopathologic study suggested that a thick compact tissue on the anterior chamber side of Schlemm's canal was present in ten cases of juvenile glaucoma. In these ten patients, the mechanism of glaucoma was postulated to be a developmental immaturity of the trabecular meshwork (2). Other specific anatomical abnormalities have not been identified in patients with juvenile glaucoma.

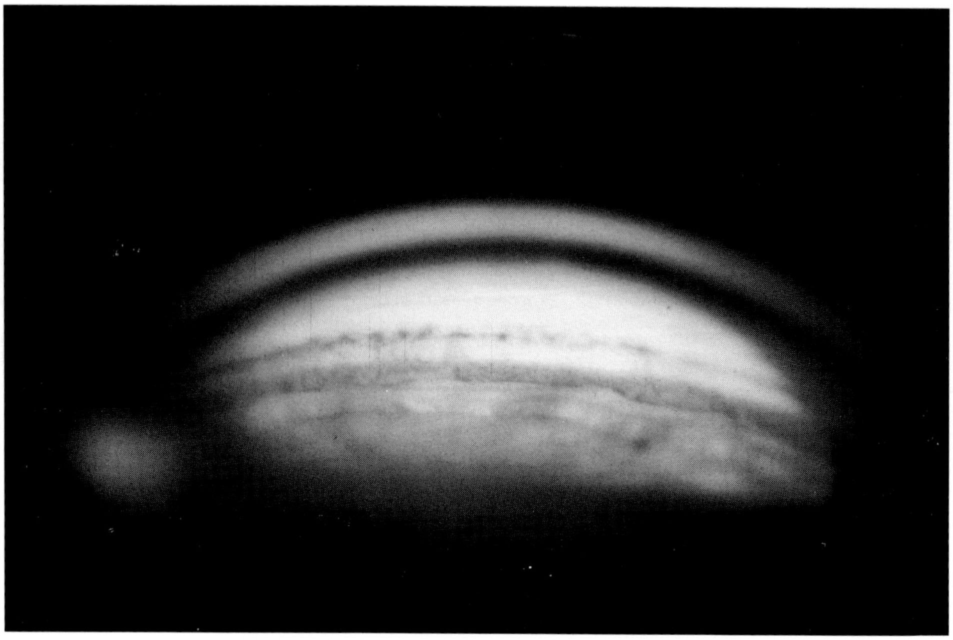

Figure 50.1. Gonioscopic appearance of a patient affected by juvenile glaucoma (individual 18 in pedigree ADG-4) showing tissue strands extending from the peripheral iris to anterior trabecular meshwork. (Photography by Kit Johnson).

AGE CUT-OFF FOR JOAG UNCERTAIN

David L. Epstein

There is an uncertain age cut-off for the entity of "juvenile open angle glaucoma" (JOAG). One of us (DLE) uses the ages between 10 and 30 years as the spectrum for JOAG. At the lower ages the condition may blend into and share common features with developmental glaucoma, and at the upper ages with "presenile" POAG. However, within any age bracket there likely is more than one distinct entity. In fact, across the whole spectrum of encompassed ages, there are cases of JOAG that behave very much like the developmental glaucomas, and others that behave like POAG.

For example, there are some patients with JOAG between the ages of 10 and 30 years that may present (apparently suddenly) with very high IOPs, corneal edema, and often minimal cupping. The glaucoma can prove to be refractory to medical antiglaucoma therapy and require early surgical intervention. In some, but not all such cases, there is an immature quality to the angle. Thus in many ways these cases share features with the developmental glaucomas of a typically younger age of onset. On the other hand, there are other cases of JOAG, with or without immature angle qualities, that respond to medical antiglaucoma therapy with apparent good control of IOP for years, as might be expected in presenile POAG (although the clinician needs to be constantly alert for the sudden loss of control of IOP in all such patients).

There are also some cases, most often with a dominant family history of JOAG (where various family members may have the onset of disease at various times within the full spectrum of ages of 10 to 30 years), in which YAG or surgical goniotomy may be beneficial for control of IOP for at least a few years, and yet there are other cases where goniotomy is without effect.

Because for all these various features there is at best only a very loose correlation with the apparent presence of immature features of the angle on gonioscopy, such as a translucent quality to the TM or forward insertion of the iris, the presence of iris processes, etc., it underscores the fact that we do not have a firm grasp of what the abnormality might be in this condition. For example, even if YAG or surgical goniotomy is successful in JOAG for a time, one does not ever see, even in the presence of definite immature features of the angle, the apparent long-term cures that characterize developmental glaucoma (between the ages 6 months to 2 years) after surgical goniotomy. There must be a different pathological mechanism in JOAG (1) than in developmental glaucoma.

Also curious is the frequent presence of disc cupping that is not far advanced despite very high IOPs at the initial presentation of JOAG at various ages. This suggests that the onset of abnormality in trabecular meshwork function might have been recent (despite the angle appearance) in some such cases.

At the upper age extreme, we suppose that whatever the abnormal mechanism is in POAG, it might occur in some individuals at a younger age (as does actually seem to occur in "adult" POAG patients with a strong family history of POAG). Some have termed this phenomenon "anticipation," and it has been postulated to occur in many other genetically determined diseases.

The clinician needs to be aware of these entities, and especially the propensity for sudden elevation of IOP to high levels that may require filtration surgery, despite a past period of apparent stability of IOP lasting years.

The fact that JOAG is uncommon but not rare, and is potentially blinding, is another strong reason to measure the IOP in patients of all ages at the time of ocular examination.

Reference

1. Tawara A, Inomata H: Developmental immaturity of the trabecular meshwork in juvenile glaucoma. Am J Ophthalmol 1984;98:82–97.

YAG (AND SURGICAL) GONIOTOMY IN JOAG

David L. Epstein

The story of the potential efficacy (for a few years) of YAG or surgical goniotomy in JOAG is of interest for several reasons. Because the trabecular meshwork is the locus of abnormal resistance in adult POAG (1), it is very rational to try to bypass this abnormality by placing one or more "holes" through the tissue (2–8). Many in the past have tried to develop such a laser "cure" for POAG, but the holes produced closed with time (which is curious in POAG where the TM is felt to be intrinsically "sick" with decreased cellularity [9]). When the YAG laser became available, one of us (DLE) wondered whether its disruptive rather than thermal properties might act to keep the laser "holes" open in POAG patients, but this proved not to happen (8). At the time there was a general feeling that surgical goniotomy was ineffective for JOAG patients, but in one desperate patient facing bilateral filtration surgery, YAG goniopuncture was very effective in the short term (8). What was also noteworthy in this particular case was the fact that the TM did not appear unequivocally abnormal until after the laser opening was made, at which time retro-illumination of the adjacent TM (by placing the slit lamp beam in the laser opening) lead to the observation that the TM was subtly abnormal in that it had a translucent, "thick" appearance.

We then gained experience with other patients with JOAG, and YAG goniopuncture was effective for some in the short-term (months) (8). Other investigators had a similar experience (10,11). In some cases, we documented definite improvement of outflow facility to normal or near normal levels with tonography. However, as the months turned into years, late failures became common, often with a fairly acute onset. In some cases this late failure was correlated with the new appearance of "webby" tissue in the laser openings into the TM. Regardless, what was curious was the fact that the YAG goniopuncture worked definitely for a while in some patients with JOAG, but not in any patient with adult POAG (8).

Melamed (12) then studied this further and had somewhat better results with a more aggressive linear YAG goniotomy technique than the simpler multiple goniopunctures that were employed earlier. He also found a correlation of success of the procedure with the presence of a dominant family history of the disease, as well as the occurrence of blood reflux from Schlemm's canal at the time of the laser goniotomy (12). At the same time, we became aware of the work of several glaucoma clinicians, such as B. Thomas Hutchinson, MD, who, in fact, had been performing surgical goniotomy on patients with JOAG and observing efficacy for a few years, especially in patients with a family history of the disease. Repeat surgical goniotomy was being performed in such patients every few years with the strategy of delaying filtration surgery until the patient was older, and there was greater chance of surgical success.

So what is the status of YAG goniotomy in JOAG today? We believe that YAG goniotomy produces the same effect as surgical goniotomy (13) in certain patients with JOAG, especially those with a dominant family history. The YAG laser is able to "cleave less tissue" than the surgical Barkan knife, and therefore the duration of the benefit is less with YAG than surgical goniotomy. But in patients with JOAG who are facing filtration surgery, we use the YAG procedure as a predictive test of whether there might be some benefit to surgical goniotomy as outlined above.

The procedure (8,12) is very straightforward and benign and basically consists of placing sharply focused YAG lesions of 4 to 6 millijoules in a linear sequence deeply into the filtration portion of the TM for one half to one hour of the circumference, at perhaps two sites in the angle. Originally because of the segmental nature of outflow through the TM and the lack of circumferential flow in Schlemm's canal (14), the technique was to place only single goniopunctures in each of four quadrants. The current linear YAG technique should be performed in two quadrants, one above and one below, and perhaps single goniopunctures in the remaining two quadrants. We would be concerned that performing the linear YAG goniotomy technique in all four quadrants initially might produce excessive damage to the angle (7) if the procedure were not successful. In our experience, limiting the linear YAG goniotomy to only two quadrants is sufficient to demonstrate efficacy.

Common mistakes are: not to be in proper focus with the YAG laser, and then to just "stir up" debris on the surface of the angle rather than penetrate deeply into the angle. The latter typically requires some superimposition of "shots" at each TM site as one progresses linearly across the TM. Commonly as pigment and other debris come forward in front of the meshwork, increasing energy levels are required to penetrate deep into the TM. It is best to place the first linear lesion inferiorly in the angle, and the second then superiorly. This is to avoid pigment debris that comes into the anterior chamber from above from interfering with proper focusing.

Likely there are some patients with JOAG who might respond to surgical goniotomy and not the YAG, but a good, albeit temporary, response to the YAG does identify those who will subsequently respond favorably to surgical goniotomy. With improved success of filtration surgery with modern techniques (Chapter 62) involving use of antimetabolites, one might argue that surgical goniotomy is just delaying the "inevitable" (with risk of high IOPs withsudden failure), and therefore one should proceed directly to filtration surgery without any type of goniotomy in all such patients. However, the risks of filtration surgery are certainly more serious than YAG goniotomy. Therefore, depending on individual patient circumstances, it is at least worthwhile for the clinician to be aware of the possibility of the time limited efficacy for both YAG and surgical goniotomy in patients with JOAG. However, the potential for sudden failure and high IOP with these goniotomy techniques needs to always be considered.

One other noteworthy observation is the fact that the ONE condition that seems to respond to YAG goniotomy with a true long-term benefit is that of glaucoma secondary to juvenile rheumatoid arthritis (Chapter 70), and one of us (DLE) would urge that this procedure be done in all such patients before filtration surgery. In fact, in this condition the YAG procedure had a direct correlate with existing (but underappreciated) clinical experience, in that a modification of a surgical goniotomy, termed trabeculodialysis (15–17), had been reported to be successful, although with a significant surgical risk of hyphema and related complications. These potential complications are actually less of a problem with the YAG procedure, and this is therefore the one circumstance where YAG goniotomy should be the surgical treatment of choice. Of course, we need further long term observations, but in a limited number of patients with glaucoma secondary to juvenile rheumatoid arthritis, one of us (DLE) has observed that YAG goniotomy has seemed at least as successful as surgical trabeculodialysis.

(An interesting anecdote in this regard is one patient, a health care professional, who had had filtration surgery for glaucoma secondary to juvenile rheumatoid arthritis, and had suffered loss of visual acuity subsequent to a late postoperative suprachoroidal hemorrhage. The patient refused a repeat filter subsequently and, as a last resort, when referred to one of us (DLE), she had a remarkably (unanticipated) successful YAG goniotomy procedure with a good result for at least 7 years. But, when DLE had cautioned the patient that the efficacy of the procedure might only last a few months, the patient stated in reply that she would prefer to come for the YAG procedure every 3 months rather than relive what she had experienced with filtration surgery. This is "food for thought" as we potentially contemplate new pharmacological or laser procedures for-glaucoma that might only be effective when given in the doctor's office, e.g., by iontophoresis, several times a year [Chapter 16]).

References

1. Grant WM: Experimental aqueous perfusion in enucleated human eyes. Arch Ophthalmol 1963;69:783–801.
2. Krasnov MM: Q-switched laser goniopuncture. Arch Ophthalmol 1974;92:37–41.
3. Ticho U: Laser application to the angle structures in animals and in human glaucomatous eyes. Adv Ophthalmol 1977;34:201–210.
4. Bonney CH, Gaasterland DE, Rodrigues MM, et al: Short-term effects of Q-switched ruby laser on monkey anterior chamber angle. Invest Ophthalmol Vis Sci 1977;22:310–318.
5. Wickham MG, Worthen DM: Argon laser trabeculotomy: long-term follow-up. Ophthalmology 1979;86:495–503.
6. Van der Zypen E, Fankhauser F: The ultrastructural features of laser trabeculopuncture and cyclodialysis; problems related to successful treatment of chronic simple glaucoma. Ophthalmologica 1979;1:109–122.
7. Melamed S, Pei J, Puliafito CA, et al: Q-switched neodymium YAG laser trabeculopuncture in monkeys. Arch Ophthalmol 1985;103: 129–133.
8. Epstein DL, Melamed S, Puliafito CA, et al: Neodymium-YAG laser trabeculopuncture in open angle glaucoma. Ophthalmology 1985;92:931–937.
9. Alvarado J, Murphy C, Juster R: Trabecular meshwork cellularity in primary open-angle glaucoma and nonglaucomatous normals. Ophthalmology 1984;91:564–579.
10. Yumita A, Shirato S, Yamamoto T, et al: Goniotomy with Q-switched Nd-YAG laser in juvenile developmental glaucoma: a preliminary report. Jpn J Ophthalmol 1984;28:349–55.
11. Mishima S, Kitazawa Y, Shirato S: Laser therapy for glaucoma. Aust NZ J Ophthalmol 1985;13:225–35.
12. Melamed S, Latina MA, Epstein DL: Neodymium:YAG laser trabeculopuncture in juvenile open angle glaucoma. Ophthalmology 1987;94:160–170.
13. Senft SH, Tomey KF, Traverso CE: Neodymium-YAG laser goniotomy vs surgical goniotomy. A preliminary study in paired eyes. Arch Ophthalmol 1989;107:1773–6.
14. Rosenquist RC, Epstein DL, Melamed S, et al: Outflow resistance of enucleated human eyes with two different perfusion pressures and different extents of trabeculotomy. Curr Eye Res 1989;8: 1233–1240.
15. Herschler J, Davis EB: Modified goniotomy for inflammatory glaucoma. Histologic evidence for the mechanism of pressure reduction. Arch Ophthalmol 1980;98:684–7.
16. Kanski JJ, McAllister JA: Trabeculodialysis for inflammatory glaucoma in children and young adults. Ophthalmology 1985;92: 927–30.
17. Williams RD, Hoskins HD, Shaffer RN: Trabeculodialysis for inflammatory glaucoma: a review of 25 cases. Ophthalmic Surg 1992;23:36–7.

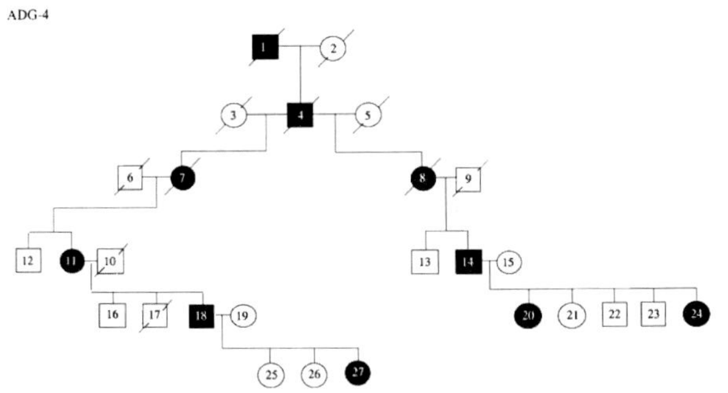

Figure 50.2. Juvenile glaucoma pedigree (ADG-4). Affected individuals are shown as solid circles (females) or squares (males). Deceased individuals not available for linkage analysis are indicated with slashes.

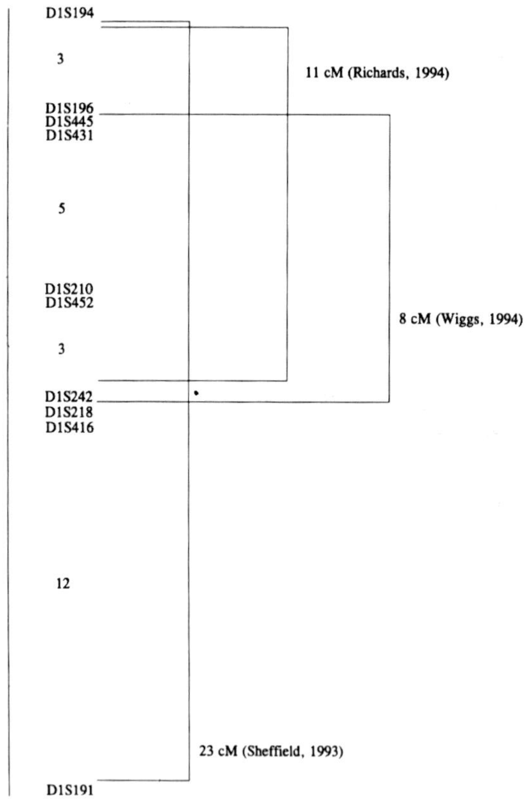

Figure 50.3. Map of the chromosome 1q21–q31 region. Map distances are from the recently published Genethon map (13). The approximate location of critical recombinants identified in previously published mapping studies are indicated by brackets (8,10,11).

Patients affected by juvenile open angle glaucoma (JOAG) develop a severe high pressure glaucoma that usually requires surgical treatment for adequate control. Patients have been treated effectively by goniotomy and trabeculectomy, although the reports of the surgical outcomes are largely anecdotal. Comparative studies designed to determine the efficacy of various surgical procedures for the treatment of juvenile glaucoma have not appeared in the recent literature.

A number of pedigrees affected with juvenile open angle glaucoma demonstrating an autosomal dominant mode of inheritance have been reported (Fig. 50.2) (3–11). Familial hypoplasia of the iris and unusually darkly pigmented irides (Ian of Blackberry Eyes) have also been reported associated with the glaucoma in pedigrees affected with autosomal dominant juvenile glaucoma (12). In the pedigrees studied, the penetrance appears to approach 100% after age 20, although formal studies of penetrance have not been performed.

In a single pedigree affected with autosomal dominant juvenile glaucoma without any associated anterior segment dysgenesis, Sheffield et al using short tandem repeat genetic markers for **genetic linkage analysis demonstrated that a gene responsible for this condition is located within a 30 cM region on the long arm of chromosome** 1 (1q21–q31) (8). This result has subsequently been confirmed by similar studies (10–11).

Current data places the putative gene within an 8 cM interval on chromosome 1 between markers D1S196 and D1S218 (Fig. 50.3) which are within the initial 30 cM region (8,10,11). It is likely that a single locus in this region contains a gene responsible for juvenile open angle glaucoma. However, this region is large enough (13) that a second locus can not be completely ruled out by the current data. The clinical presentation of the pedigrees demonstrating linkage to this region have in common an autosomal dominant form of glaucoma with a characteristic juvenile onset. There are some differences, however, in the clinical presentation that could support the possibility of two separate loci in this region of chromosome 1. These clinical differences include an apparent difference in the susceptibility of the optic nerve to high pressure, and subtle differences in the anatomy of the anterior segment of the eye (1,9). These issues of genetic and clinical heterogeneity will not be completely resolved until the gene (s) responsible for this disorder are isolated and specific mutations are defined.

A number of genes reside in this defined area on chromosome 1. Most of these genes code for proteins whose functions would appear to be unrelated to any mechanism that could result in glaucoma (14). One gene located in this region that has been entertained as a candidate for juvenile autosomal dominant glaucoma is the gene for atrial natriuretic peptide receptor (ANPR-A) (8). This protein has been speculated to play a role in the pathogenesis of glaucoma because a high density of receptors are located on the epithelial side of the ciliary body (15), and the concentration of atrial natriuretic peptide is elevated in the anterior chamber of glaucomatous eyes in rabbits (16). It is unlikely however that this protein-receptor system could result in a reduction in outflow facility through the trabecular meshwork, which is the probable cause of the disease in humans (17).

Juvenile glaucoma may be more frequent among Americans of African ancestry (18). To date, all the pedigrees demonstrating linkage to the chromosome 1q21–q31 locus are white. The clinical and genetic heterogeneity of this condition remains to be defined.

The identification of one locus containing a gene responsible for juvenile glaucoma allows the investigation of the role of that gene in other forms of glaucoma. Like juvenile glaucoma, pigmentary glaucoma affects young individuals. Several investigators have speculated that pigmentary glaucoma may be related to primary open angle glaucoma and may be a form of primary juvenile glaucoma (19). To investigate the role of the juvenile glaucoma gene in the pigment dispersion syndrome, three pedigrees affected by the pigment dispersion syndrome and pigmentary glaucoma were identified and analyzed for genetic linkage to markers located in the chromosome 1q21–q31 region. The results of these experiments indicate that the gene responsible for the pigment dispersion syndrome is not located in this region of the human genome and that the pigment dispersion syndrome is genetically distinct from the form of juvenile glaucoma caused by the gene mapped to chromosome 1q21–q31. Current studies are underway to identify and isolate the gene responsible for the pigment dispersion syndrome (20).

References

1. Wiggs JL, et al: Autosomal dominant glaucoma: clinical features of three pedigrees demonstrating genetic linkage to chromosome 1q21-q31. Submitted (1996).
2. Tawara A, Inomata H: Developmental immaturity of the trabecular meshwork in juvenile glaucoma. Am J Ophthalmol 1984;98:82–97.
3. Allen TD, Ackerman WG: Hereditary glaucoma in a pedigree of three generations. Arch Ophthal 1942:27:139–157.
4. Courtney RH, Hill E: Hereditary juvenile glaucoma simplex. JAMA 1931;97:1602–1609.
5. Martin JP, Zorab EC. Familial glaucoma in nine generations of South Hampshire family. Br J Ophthalmol 1974;58:536–542.
6. Stokes WH: Hereditary primary glaucoma. Arch Ophthalmol 1940;24: 885–909
7. Dorozynski A: Privacy rules blindside French glaucoma effort. Nature 1991;252:369.
8. Sheffield VC, et al: Genetic linkage of familial open angle glaucoma to chromosome 1q21-q31. Nature Genetics 1993;4:47.
9. Johnson AT, et al: Clinical features and linkage analysis of a family with autosomal dominant juvenile glaucoma. Ophthalmology 1993;100: 524–529.
10. Richards JE, et al: Mapping of a gene for autosomal dominant juvenile-onset open-angle glaucoma to chromosome 1q. Am J Hum Genet 1994; 54:5462–70.
11. Wiggs JL, et al: Genetic linkage of autosomal dominant juvenile glaucoma to 1q21-q31 in three affected pedigrees. Genomics 1994;21: 299–303.
12. Weatherill JR, Hart CT: Familial hypoplasia of the iris stroma associated with glaucoma. Br J Ophthalmol 1969;53:433–438.
13. Gyapay G, et al: The 1993-1994 Généthon human genetic linkage map. Nature Genetics 1994;7:246–339.
14. Dracopoli NC, et al: The CEPH consortium linkage map of human chromosome 1. Genomics 1991;9:686–700.
15. Bianchi C, et al: Localization and characterization of specific receptors for atrial natriuretic factor in the ciliary processes in the eye. Curr Eye Res 1986;5:283–293.
16. Fernandez-Durango R, et al: Immunoreactive atrial natriuretic factor in aqueous humor: Its concentration is increased with high intraocular pressure in rabbit eyes. Vision Res 1990;30:1305–1310.
17. Rohen JW, Lutjen-Drecoll E: Biology of the trabecular meshwork. In: Lutjen-Drecoll E (ed.) Basic Aspects of Glaucoma Research. Schattauer Verlag, Stuttgart, 1982.
18. Lotufo D, Ritch R, Szmyd L, et al: Juvenile glaucoma, race and refraction. JAMA 1989;261:249–252.
19. Becker B, Podos SM: Krukenberg's spindles and primary open-angle glaucoma. Arch Ophthalmol 1966;76:635.
20. Paglinauan CM, et al: Exclusion of chromosome 1q21-q31 from linkage to three pedigrees affected by the pigment dispersion syndrome. Am J Hum Genet 1995;56:1240–1243.

Laser Methods in Glaucoma VIII

Glaucoma Laser Surgery

51

Overview

Joel S. Schuman

Since the previous editions of this book, glaucoma laser surgery has progressed in several areas. Advances have occurred in laser trabeculoplasty, laser iridectomy, laser cyclophotocoagulation, and laser sclerectomy. Additionally, lasers have been useful for gonioplasty, to shrink the iris away from the trabecular meshwork in cases of early peripheral anterior synechia or plateau iris; laser suture lysis, to titrate intraocular pressure (IOP) after trabeculectomy; for treatment of failing blebs, to incise areas of episcleral or subconjunctival fibrosis; in instances of hypotony, to coagulate, scar and induce inflammation in the conjunctiva, or to cause adhesion of the conjunctiva to the underlying episclera. Lasers continue to be used, although infrequently, for goniophotocoagulation, to ablate new blood vessels growing in the trabecular meshwork while waiting for panretinal photocoagulation to take effect; and for goniopuncture, in which the Nd:YAG laser is aimed at the trabecular meshwork to open channels into Schlemm's canal, in cases such as juvenile open angle glaucoma (JOAG) and angle recession glaucoma, in which a hyaline-membrane is thought to obstruct outflow (1–3).

Each of these applications are covered in turn. Laser trabeculoplasty (LTP), which has proven effective in postponing trabeculectomy, or in some cases eliminating the need for filtering surgery entirely, has been studied extensively since the third edition of this book (4–24). Although the exact mechanism by which this procedure functions is still not known, insight has been gained into its workings and effects. In this way, realistic expectations allow the clinician to apply this technique in the appropriate settings, and to anticipate the outcome of such treatment. Additionally, various wavelengths are available for performing LTP, the effects of which are relatively wavelength independent. Nearly any photocoagulator, including the argon, diode, krypton and continous wave Nd:YAG laser (different from the Q-switched, pulsed Nd:YAG laser used for photodisruption), can be successfully employed for LTP.

When the previous edition was published, the argon laser was still the preferred instrument for performing laser peripheral iridectomy (LPI); use of the pulsed Nd:YAG laser for this procedure was still experimental and thought to be excessively hazardous. Modern LPI, of course, is routinely performed preferentially with the Nd:YAG laser, and we have learned that such iridectomies are, in fact, more likely to retain their patency than those created with the argon laser (25–37). Photocoagulators, such as those mentioned for LTP, have their place in LPI, as they coagulate blood vessels, thin the iris and do not induce bleeding at the time of LPI; however, LPI is more efficient and long lasting when done with the Nd:YAG laser, or with a combination of a photocoagulator and photodisruptor (33,35).

Laser cyclophotocoagulation was investigational when the third edition was published, but now has supplanted cyclocryotherapy as the cyclodestructive procedure of choice in advanced glaucoma uncontrolled by maximal tolerated medical therapy. This modality gained popularity rapidly as a more gentle means to reduce aqueous production, and perhaps slightly increase outflow, as compared with cyclocryotherapy. Contact transscleral Nd:YAG or diode laser cyclophotocoagulation causes little postoperative discomfort, but carries with it the same risks for hypotony and visual loss as cyclocryotherapy; therefore, laser cyclophotocoagulation remains a procedure of last resort.

Laser sclerectomy is a technique in evolution. Although a variety of lasers have been investigated for this purpose, results remain disappointing to date. The prospect for this procedure is tantilizing: a minimally invasive means by which to perform filtering surgery, with little or no conjunctival manipulation, perhaps even performed in the office. Unfortunately, we have so far been unable to adapt this technology to safely and effectively perform filtering surgery with long lasting success and limited complications.

The list of miscellaneous procedures continues to grow as our experience with lasers increases. Gonioplasty is useful in eyes with angle closure despite a patent iridectomy, either to break PAS formed within the previous 6 months (38) or to thin the peripheral iris. Laser suture lysis allows titration of IOP in the early postoperative period, but carries with it the risks of hypotony and conjunctival bleb

Table 51.1
Glaucoma Laser Therapy

Procedure	Laser	Settings
Laser Trabeculoplasty	Argon Green	50 μm spot; 0.1 s; 300–1000 mW; 35–50 spots over 180 ; Goldmann or Ritch lens.
	Diode	50–75 μm spot; 0.1 s; 750–1250 mW; 35–50 spots over 180 ; Goldmann or Ritch lens.
Laser Iridectomy	Nd:YAG	4–6 mJ; 1–3 bursts of 3 pulses per burst; Abraham lens
	Argon Green	Short Pulse Technique (Dark Brown Iris): 50 μm spot; 0.02–0.05 s; 1000–1500 mW; 20–50 spots; Abraham or Wise lens. Long Pulse Technique (Blue; Hazel or Light Brown Iris): 50 μm spot; 0.2 s; 1000 m W; 20–30 spots; Abraham or Wise lens.
	Diode	50–75 μm spot; 0.05–0.1 s; 750–1250 mW; 20–50 spots; Abraham or Wise lens.
Combined Argon or Diode and Nd:YAG laser iridectomy	Argon/Diode: Nd:YAG:	50 μm spot; 0.02–0.05 s; 1000 mW; 5–10 spots. 4–6 mJ; 1–3 bursts of 3 pulses per burst; Abraham lens.
Laser Cyclophotocoagulation	Contact cwNd:YAG	7 W; 0.7 s; 24–32 spots; probe centered 1.5–2 mm posterior to limbus; sapphire tipped probe.
	Contact diode	3 W; 1.3–1.5 s; 18 spots; probe with automatic offset of 1.2 mm from limbus (Iris Medical Instruments "G-Probe").
Laser Sclerectomy	Holmium	100 mJ/pulse; 20–30 pulses to perforate; Side-firing fiberoptic.
	cwNd:YAG	10–12 W; 1.0 s; 2–5 spots to penetrate; synthetic sapphire tip.
Laser Gonioplasty	Argon; Diode	200–500 μm spot; 0.2–0.5 s; 200–400 mW; 24–32 spots in far periphery; Goldmann lens.
Laser Suture Lysis	Argon; Diode	50 μm spot; 0.02 s; 300–800 mW; 1 or more spots; Hoskins lens.
Laser to Failing Bleb	Nd:YAG	1–2 mJ; single pulse mode; aim deep into tissues; avoiding conjunctiva; follow with digital pressure and 5-FU.
Laser to Conjunctiva (Hypotony)	Argon; Diode	Paint bleb with 2% fluorescein or methylene blue for argon; indocyanine green for diode laser. 200 μm spot; 0.5 s; 200–300 mW; 30–50 spots or more covering as much conjunctiva as possible.
Laser Goniophotocoagulation	Argon	50 μm spot; 0.1 s; 1000 mW; sufficient spots to blanch vessel trunks.
Laser Goniopuncture	Nd:YAG	5–7 mJ; 3 pulses per burst; fire through TM until bright white of outer wall of Schlemm's canal is seen. Begin inferiorly; as may get blood reflux. Open 1–2 clock hours.

Table 51.2
Perioperative Care

Procedure	Preop	Postop
Laser Trabeculoplasty	Apraclonidine 0.5–1%	Prednisolone acetate 1% hourly for one day; then qid for four days; then stop. Check IOP at 1 hour; 1 day; 1 week and 4–6 weeks.
Laser Iridectomy	Apraclonidine 0.5–1%; Pilocarpine 2% × 3	Prednisolone acetate 1% hourly for one day; then qid for four days; then stop. Check IOP at 1 hour; 1 day; 1 week and 4 weeks. Gonioscopy at 1 and 4 weeks and dilation at 4 weeks.
Laser Cyclophotocoagulation	Apraclonidine 0.5–1% Retrobulbar Lidocaine 2%/Marcaine 0.75%/Wydase 150 units	Prednisolone acetate 1% qid and Atropine 1% bid until inflammation subsides. Continue all preoperative antiglaucoma medications; with exception of miotics (may resume when eye quiet).
Laser Sclerectomy	Retrobulbar or Subconjunctival Lidocaine 2%/Marcaine 0.75%/Wydase 150 units	Prednisolone acetate 1% qid; Atropine 1% bid; Polymixin-Bacitracin and dexamethasone 0.05% ointments nightly.
Laser Gonioplasty	Apraclonidine 0.5–1%; Pilocarpine 2% × 3	Prednisolone acetate 1% hourly for one day; then qid for four days; then stop. Check IOP at 1 hour; 1 day and 1 week. Gonioscopy and dilation at 1 week.
Laser Suture Lysis	Proparacaine 0.5%	Check IOP 1 hour & 1 day after LSL. Do not cut more than one suture per day.
Laser to Failing Bleb	Proparacaine 0.5%	Check IOP 1 hour & 1 day after; follow with digital pressure and 5-FU.
Laser to Conjunctiva (Hypotony)	Proparacaine 0.5%	Check IOP 1 hour; 1 day and 1 week after procedure. If ineffective; may require repeat treatment or other intervention.
Laser Goniophotocoagulation	Apraclonidine 0.5–1%	Prednisolone acetate 1% hourly for one day; then qid for four days; then stop. Follow carefully for regression of vessels; or regrowth.
Laser Goniopuncture	Apraclonidine 0.5–1%	Prednisolone acetate 1% hourly for one day; then qid for four days; then stop.

leak (due to an inadvertent conjunctival burn). Laser treatment of the bleb tissue, using an absorbing dye such as 2% fluorescein, methylene blue or indocyanine green, is effective in some cases of overfiltration with hypotony, inducing conjunctival contraction, scarring and adhesion to the underlying sclera. Goniophotocoagulation, now rarely performed, can treat blood vessels encroaching on the trabecular meshwork in the post-panretinal photocoagulation period of neovascular glaucoma.

Each of these "miscellaneous" procedures requires the use of a photocoagulator, and each can be done with an argon or diode laser (or others). To incise tissue, such as is necessary when treating a failing bleb or for goniopuncture, the pulsed Nd:YAG laser is needed. This is the same laser used for LPI or capsulotomy. Other pulsed lasers, such as the picosecond laser, although not widely available, can also be used for this task.

An overview of glaucoma laser therapy is presented in Tables 51.1 and 51.2.

References

1. Melamed S, Latina MA, Epstein DL: Neodymium:YAG laser trabeculopuncture in juvenile open angle glaucoma. Ophthalmology 1987;94: 160–170.
2. Melamed S, Pei J, Puliafito CA, et al: Q-switched neodymium-YAG laser trabeculopuncture in monkeys. Arch Ophthalmol 1985;103: 129–133.
3. Epstein DL, Melamed S, Puliafito CA, et al: Neodymium-YAG laser trabeculopuncture in open-angle glaucoma. Ophthalmology 1985;92: 931–937.
4. Dreyer EB, Gorla M: Laser trabeculoplasty in the pseudophakic patient. J Glaucoma 1993;2:313–315.
5. Feldman RM, Katz LJ, Spaeth GL, et al: Long-term efficacy of repeat argon laser trabeculoplasty. Ophthalmology 1991;98:1061–5.
6. Gross RL, Wilson RP, Feldman RM: Encapsulated bleb after trabeculectomy: a frequent complication. Clin Signs Ophthalmol 1987;9:2–16.
7. The GLT Group: The Glaucoma Laser Trial 1. Acute effects of argon laser trabeculoplasty on intraocular pressure. Arch Ophthalmol 1989; 107:1135–1142.
8. The GLT Group: The Glaucoma Laser Trial (GLT). 2. Results of argon laser trabeculoplasty versus topical medicines. Ophthalmology 1990;97: 1403–13.
9. Higginbotham EJ, Richardson TM: Response of exfoliation glaucoma to laser trabeculoplasty. Br J Ophthalmol 1986;70:837–839.
10. Juhas T: Argon laser trabeculoplasty in the treatment of primary closed-angle glaucoma. Cesk Oftalmol 1989;45:197–205.
11. Richter CU, Shingleton BJ, Bellows AR, et al: Retreatment with argon laser trabeculoplasty. Ophthalmology 1987;94:1085–1089.
12. Runderman JM, Zweig KO, Wilensky JT, et al: Effects of corticosteroid pretreatment on argon laser trabeculoplasty. Am J Ophthalmol 1983; 96:84–89.
13. Schwartz AL: Argon laser trabeculoplasty in glaucoma: what's happening (surgery results of American Glaucoma Society members). J Glaucoma 1993;2:329–335.
14. Shingleton BJ, Richter CU, Bellows AR, et al: Long-term efficacy of argon laser trabeculoplasty. Ophthalmology 1987;94:1513–1518.
15. Swartz AL, Whitten ME, Bleiman B, et al: Argon laser trabecular surgery in uncontrolled phakic open-angle glaucoma. Ophthalmology 1981;88: 203–212.
16. Thomas JV, Simmons RJ, Belcher CD: Argon laser trabeculoplasty in the management of the surgical glaucoma patient. Ophthalmology 1982;89: 187–197.
17. Thomas JV, Simmons RJ, Belcher CD: Argon laser trabeculoplasty in the pre-surgical glaucoma patient. Ophthalmology 1982;89:187–197.
18. Thomas JV, Simmons RJ, Belcher CD: Complications of argon laser trabeculoplasty. Glaucoma 1982;4:250–5.
19. Wickham MG, Worthen DM: Argon laser trabeculoplasty: long term follow-up. Ophthalmology 1979;86:495–503.
20. Wilensky JT, Jampol LM: Laser therapy for open-angle glaucoma. Ophthalmology 1981;88:213–217.
21. Wise JB: Ten year results of laser trabeculoplasty. Does the laser avoid glaucoma surgery or merely defeat it? Eye 1987;1:45–50.
22. Wise JB, Witter SL: Argon laser therapy for open-angle glaucoma: A pilot study. Arch Ophthalmol 1979;97:319–322.
23. Wise JB: Long-term control of adult open-angle glaucoma by argon laser treatment. Opthalmology 1981;88:197–202.
24. Richter C, Shingleton B, Bellows A, et al: The development of encapsulated filtering blebs. Ophthalmology 1988;95:1163–1168.
25. Beckman H, Barraco R, Sugar S, et al: Laser iridectomites. Am J Ophthalmol Soc 1971;77:674–706.
26. Beckman H, Sugar HS: Laser iridectomy therapy of glaucoma. Arch Ophthalmol 1973;90:453.
27. Khuri CH: Argon laser iridectomies. Am J Ophthalmol 1973;76: 490–495.
28. Klapper RM: Argon laser iridectomies. Ophthalmology 1984;91: 1017–21.
29. Latina MA, Puliafito CA, Steinert RR, et al: Experimental iridotomy with the Q-switched neodymium:YAG laser. Arch Ophthalmol 1984; 102:1211–3.
30. Moster MR, Schwartz LW, Spaeth GL, et al: Laser iridectomy. A controlled study comparing argon and neodymium:YAG. Ophthalmology 1986;93:20–4.
31. Pollack IP, Robin AL, Dragon DM, et al: Use of the neodymium:YAG laser to create iridotomies in monkeys and humans. Trans Am Ophthalmol Soc 1984;82:307–28.
32. Richardson TM, Brown SV, Thomas JV, et al: Shock-wave effect on anterior segment structures following experimental neodymium:YAG laser iridectomy. Ophthalmology 1985;(92):1387–95.
33. Robin AL, Pollack IP: A comparison of neodymium:YAG and argon laser iridotomies. Ophthalmology 1984;91:1011–6.
34. Schuman JS, Jacobson JJ, Puliafito CA: Semiconductor diode laser peripheral iridotomy. Arch Ophthalmol 1990;108:1207–1208.
35. Striga M, Curkovic T, Vukas Z: Combined technique of argon-laser and neodymium:YAG laser photocoagulation for narrow or closed angle glaucoma. Acta Med Iugosl 1990;44:521–32.
36. Weaver YK, Lin CP, Schuman JS, et al: Experimental iridotomy with a picosecond Nd:YAG laser. Invest Ophthalmol Vis Sci 1992;(suppl) 33):1265.
37. Frangie JP, Park SB, Aquavella JV: Peripheral iridotomy using Nd:YLF laser. Ophthalmic Surg 1992;23:220–221.
38. Weiss HS, Shingleton BJ, Goode SM, et al: Argon laser gonioplasty in the treatment of angle-closure glaucoma. Am J Ophthalmol 1992;114: 14–18.

Laser Trabeculoplasty

52

Joel S. Schuman

ARGON LASER TRABECULOPLASTY (LTP)

Since the tissue between the anterior chamber and Schlemm's canal is the site of both normal resistance to aqueous humor outflow and abnormal resistance, (1) it was natural to attempt to penetrate this tissue with the laser, and thus bypass the abnormality. However, similar to the results of Barkan's surgical goniotomy in adult open-angle glaucoma, only temporary lowering of IOP was achieved with laser applications that attempted to penetrate to Schlemm's canal. Gaasterland and Kupfer then demonstrated that heavy applications of argon laser energy to the trabecular meshwork can actually produce glaucoma in animals (2). After this demonstration, enthusiasm for laser therapy to the trabecular meshwork in glaucomatous eyes diminished.

We owe a great debt to Wise and Witter (3) for reintroducing laser treatment to the trabecular meshwork. Instead of attempting to penetrate the trabecular meshwork, they popularized circumferential, non-penetrating applications to the tissue to produce small superficial scars. They hypothesized that this corrected a supposed mechanical "sag" of the tissue, which they felt to be the basic defect in open-angle glaucoma. One can debate whether these authors were the first to apply such a laser method, and whether this hypothesis is correct. It is clear, however, that they deserve much credit for advocating and promulgating this technique in the face of adverse laboratory data, and for introducing the modern laser era of open-angle glaucoma therapy.

The results of Wise and Witter have been confirmed by many authors (4–7). It is remarkable how consistent the results have been. Depending on the pretreatment intraocular pressure (IOP) and type of glaucoma, an average 6–10 mm Hg, or approximately 20%, pressure reduction can be expected. The best response is obtained in pseudoexfoliation glaucoma, whereas the poorest results tend to be in young patients with glaucoma. Certain secondary glaucomas such as uveitic glaucoma also respond poorly, although occasional successes are reported. It seems worthwhile now to attempt LTP in almost all forms of open-angle glaucoma before embarking on filtration surgery, although for those with poor prognosis and potential for worsening of IOP with laser, lesser amounts of the angle are treated initially.

Depending on the indications for LTP, most patients who are uncontrolled before laser treatment need to maintain maximally tolerated medical therapy after laser treatment. For less severe glaucoma or in eyes with dramatic responses, some medications can be discontinued. **The efficacy of LTP should be assessed 4–6 weeks after treatment.** Shorter term IOP measurements may be misleading.

The major risk of the procedure is acute IOP elevation, which can be severe and can compromise vision. This should be monitored and treated appropriately. The magnitude of IOP elevation also has been reduced by the tendency to divide the sessions into two or three, using 35–50 spots per session, with lower power settings than originally described, as well as by the use of alpha-2 agonists, such as apraclonidine (8,9).

Mechanistically it is unclear how LTP works. It is possible that Wise's hypothesis is correct, but there are certain inconsistencies with this mechanical hypothesis. Treating smaller portions of the angle than 360 often produces a disproportionally greater effect than would be anticipated mechanically. Also the type of glaucoma that responds best to LTP, pseudoexfoliation glaucoma, is the one type of glaucoma in which mechanical trabecular collapse is not believed to be involved, but rather it seems that accumulation of extracellular pseudoexfoliation material in the juxtacanalicular tissue is responsible for the increase in outflow resistance (10).

The effects of LTP on IOP seem to persist for years in most patients, although occasional patients demonstrate drift of IOP upward after 6 months. This seems especially common in exfoliation glaucoma. (Is more material being deposited?) As a general rule, **LTP maintains IOP control in 80% of eyes for one year, 50% for five years and 30% for 10 years** (11). Roughly 30% of eyes respond to retreatment with LTP (12), and we have observed some success with retreatment in some patients who initially demonstrated a good, but not long-lasting response. (In contrast, no success has been observed with retreatment in those who failed to respond initially.) More importantly, no dramatic worsening of the glaucoma has been demonstrated in those who failed to respond to retreatment on half the angle (with less than 50 applications), and subsequently, filtration surgery has been performed uneventfully.

There are many unanswered questions about LTP. In open-angle glaucoma it is not certain what the basic abnormality may be (nor even is it known precisely how aqueous

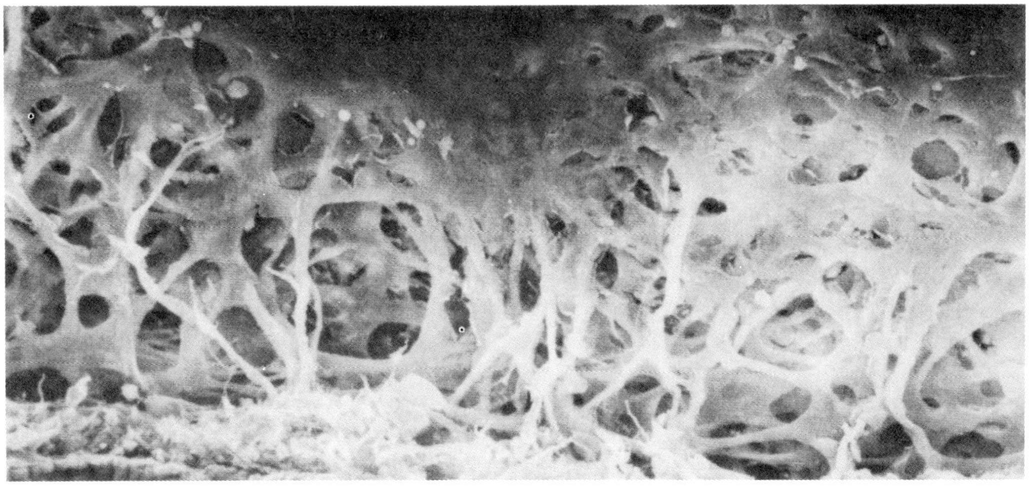

Figure 52.1. Argon laser trabeculoplasty performed in a cynomolgus monkey. The treated area of trabecular meshwork occupies the right half of the photograph. Note the destructive aspect of the lesion with scarring and collapse of trabecular beams in the treated area. Courtesy of Shlomo Melamed, MD.

humor normally makes its way through the aqueous outflow system). Yet it is clear that LTP works, at least for several years. Just as clear is the fact that we are destroying trabecular meshwork tissue with this method (Fig. 52.1), and there is still the potential for long term adverse effects, e.g., downgrowth of endothelial cells from the cornea and hyalinization of the angle. (Some have hypothesized that trabecular meshwork cells may normally act by contact inhibition to prevent this endothelial downgrowth). It is obvious that because of the initial good results of LTP, it is now being applied to earlier stages of open-angle glaucoma, for instance in place of pilocarpine. Some have in fact raised the question whether LTP should be a substitute for all medical glaucoma therapy (see the discussion of the Glaucoma Laser Trial, below). This is a thought-provoking question, but considering all the uncertainties, continued caution and further long-term, systematic study are called for.

It is interesting to compare the dose of laser energy utilized in LTP with the dose required to produce glaucoma in monkeys. Quigley has demonstrated that these differ by an approximate factor of 6 (13). It is noteworthy that this fact seems to increase the enthusiasm of some surgeons for the procedure and diminish the enthusiasm of others!

Wise has stressed the importance of precise focusing of the laser and proper alignment of the instrument, both of which are quite appropriate (14). It is likewise important that the actual power output of the laser be checked and calibrated periodically. Care and caution are necessary to avoid errors in LTP (Table 52.1).

HOW DO WE DO LASER TRABECULOPLASTY?

We are frequently questioned regarding our technique for this commonly performed procedure.

Following informed consent, the patient receives a drop of apraclonidine 0.5% or 1% in the eye to be treated. Proparacaine 0.5% is placed in both eyes, to anesthetize the treated eye, but also to decrease blinking in the contralateral eye, which can disrupt the treatment. A Goldmann 3-mirror lens is applied, using methylcellulose as a coupling solution. The angle, which was evaluated preoperatively, is again examined. If the angle is judged to be narrow preoperatively to an extent that would preclude LTP, laser iridectomy, and gonioplasty, if necessary, are performed at least one week prior to LTP. A week is allowed to intervene between treatments, to minimize the effect of inflammatory material and debris on scattering of the laser energy during LTP.

If this is the first treatment, the temporal angle is treated. The rationale is that if the LTP is ineffective, and the patient requires filtering surgery, then the nasal angle is not directly involved by the LTP, and the filtering surgery may be less likely to suffer bleb encapsulation from the prior LTP (15). Alternately, the nasal angle may be treated first, for the same reason, as the completion of the LTP (the second 180) then involves the temporal 180 . If then the completion of the LTP is not successful, filtering surgery can ensue shortly after, without the nasal angle having recent exposure to laser energy.

Still others suggest treatment of the inferior angle as the initial site, as it is generally the widest area of the angle. This is acceptable, but is not our practice. The single most important factor in deciding where to treat is consistency: if one treats the temporal angle first, one should always treat this area first. In this way, errors are avoided, and when the patient's chart cannot be found, but the patient is to have their second LTP, one knows that the temporal angle was the part treated previously.

The area to receive LTP is visualized in the goniolens,

Table 52.1
Common Mistakes in Laser Trabeculoplasty

Error	Solution
Treatment too anterior	This results in ineffective LTP, and is more common in the setting of Sampaolesi's line and a narrow angle (eg. pseudoexfoliation). Take care to perform gonioscopy prior to LTP, to identify landmarks that can be used during the surgery.
Treatment too posterior	Posterior burns predispose to postoperative uveitis and PAS formation. Careful gonioscopy, with identification of landmarks, avoids this problem.
Treatment too intense	Bursting bubbles during treatment indicate explosive tissue damage. The desired endpoint is just a blanching of the tissue. Excessive energy during LTP incites unwanted postoperative inflammation and PAS formation.
Treatment too light	If there is no tissue response with argon LTP, it is unlikely that there will be an IOP response. A blanching of the tissue should be seen with each spot, and the power titrated to produce this effect. The diode laser is an exception, as there is generally no tissue response, regardless of the parameters employed.
Retreatment of previously treated angle	Unless procedure is the third LTP on a given eye, that is, 360 have already been treated, virgin angle is prefered for the treatment. This complication can be avoided by always recording the location and parameters for the LTP, and by always treating the same portion of the angle first.
Difficulty treating the horizontal angle, or when the angle appear too narrow	A simple means to gain access to a narrow appearing angle, or to the horizontal angle, is to have the patient look towards the goniomirror. This will have the effect of opening the angle for treatment.
Treating with an elliptical spot	It is important that the spot be round and sharp in order to deliver laser energy with maximum efficiency. A round spot can be achieved by keeping the goniolens perpendicular to the laser beam at all times; this will also achieve the sharpest focus on the tissue.

and the 6:00 position is treated first. Additional burns are then made moving temporally in the mirror, treating more temporally inferiorly. It **is crucial to remember that the mirror does not cross the image of the angle**, and that the more temporal portion in the mirror is indeed the more temporal part of the angle (Figs. 52.2, 52.3). The goniolens is rotated clockwise in the right eye, or counterclockwise in the left eye, in order to keep the beam in the center of the goniomirror, to keep the spot round, and to deliver the most effective treatment with the least possible energy.

Approximately **50 spots are applied over 180°, 8–9 spots per clock hour. The laser settings are a 50 μm spot, 0.1 second duration, and the starting power is generally 600 mW. The surgical endpoint is a blanch or small bubble.** If the bubble bursts, then the power setting is too high; if there is no blanch, the power is too low. Burns are placed at the junction of the anterior third and posterior two-thirds of the trabecular meshwork, in an effort to avoid injury to the filtering portion of the TM (Fig. 52.4). Also, **the more posterior the burn, the more likely inflammation and peripheral anterior synechias (PAS) are to occur postoperatively.**

Following treatment, the patient is given prednisolone acetate 1% every hour for the first day, then four times a day for four days, and then this drug is discontinued. The patient is examined at one hour, one day, one week and 4-6 weeks; the efficacy is judged at the 4–6 week follow-up examination.

IMMEDIATE POST-LASER TREATMENT

Immediately after LTP the patient may experience minor photophobia and irritation, and examination shows conjunctival injection and often some ciliary flush and anterior chamber cellular reaction. Topical steroids are prescribed and then tapered over a five day period (see Chapter 51, Table 51.2). The patient is free to ambulate without restriction. As mentioned previously, the principal short term risk is acute IOP elevation, which should be monitored. Additional antiglaucoma therapy with carbonic anyhdrase inhibitors (CAI) or osmotics may be prescribed. Data show that neither pretreatment with corticosteroids nor antiprostaglandin drugs reduces the magnitude of this acute post-LTP IOP elevation.

POST-LASER VISITS

Following the patient's first LTP treatment in his first eye, it is wise to have the patient return 24 hours after treatment for evaluation. **At all post-LTP visits, in addition to routine ophthalmological examination in which applanation tonometry is performed, the anterior chamber should be examined carefully for inflammatory signs, and gonioscopy should be performed.** For this purpose the Zeiss lens is convenient. The angle should be carefully examined for signs of inflammatory exudates and beginning PAS formation. Such synechias are not always benign, and when observed to be forming, steroid dosage should be increased. On the first day after LTP occasionally we have seen true inflammatory precipitates, KPs, on the trabecular meshwork (17). At these sites subsequent PAS to the trabecular meshwork have evolved, similar to organization of KP in the angle in certain inflammatory glaucomas (Chapter 42). (These must be differentiated, of course, from mere blanched areas, which are often still visible 24 hours after LTP, but soon disappear.) After all, one is actually "burning" the trabecular meshwork and initiating an inflammatory reaction, which may be part of

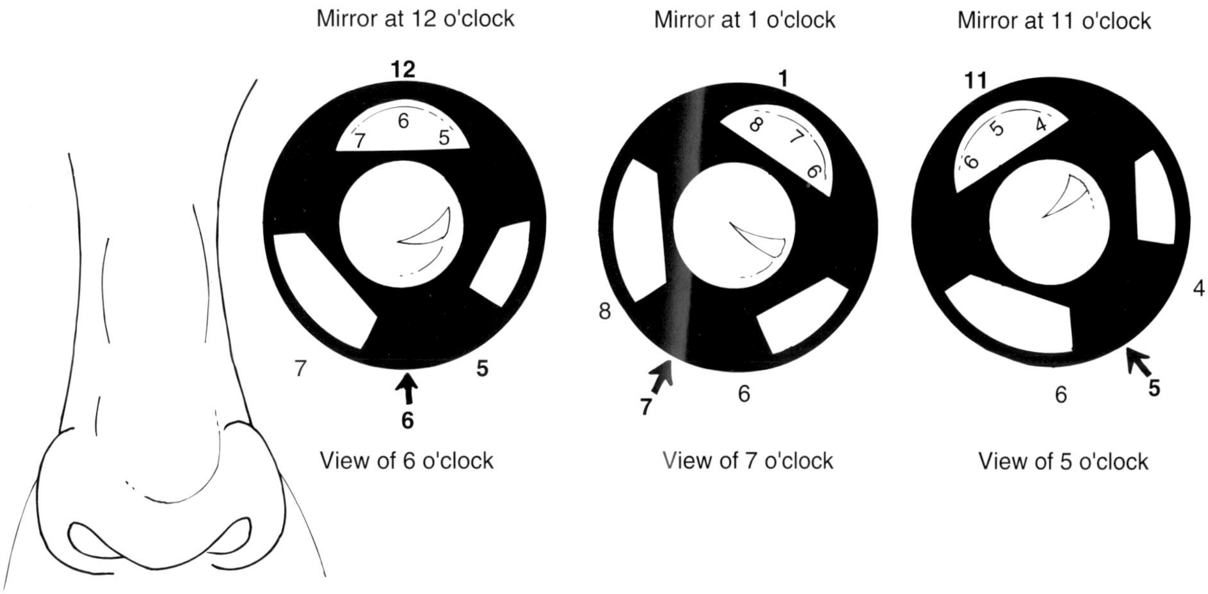

Figure 52.2. The mirrored goniolens does not invert the image of the angle. If the mirror is centered at 12:00, the 12:00 position of the mirror represents 6:00 in the angle, the 11:00 position of the mirror represents 7:00 in the angle, and the 1:00 position of the mirror represents 5:00 in the angle. Knowledge of the position in the angle relative to the image in the mirror is essential, particularly in laser treatment of the angle.

the mechanism for its efficacy. It is important to detect these inflammatory changes in the meshwork at an early stage in order to increase steroid therapy and attempt to prevent PAS, which when extending up to the meshwork in a substantial portion of the circumference can result in impairment of outflow and in poorer glaucoma control.

Depending on the findings at the first post-LTP visit, the interval for the next visit is determined. For example, if IOP is elevated or if there are inflammatory signs in the angle, the patient should be seen in a few days. Otherwise, if this is the first laser treatment, the patient is seen within a week, at which time the above examination is repeated, including gonioscopy. Often there is some IOP elevation at this time, which might relate to the laser "healing process" or to the steroid therapy, which is being tapered and discontinued. If nothing adverse is detected, the patient is usually next seen 3 weeks later, at which time the efficacy of LTP for the first time is truly assessed.

At this 1 month post-LTP visit, some IOP lowering is to be expected, usually more than half the ultimate total effect on "outflow pressure," i.e., IOP minus episcleral venous pressure. It is to be expected that the lower the starting IOP before the treatment, the less the absolute reduction in mm Hg for an equivalent effect. For example, with an episcleral venous pressure of 10 mm, an IOP reduction from 20 to 15 mm is equivalent to that from 30 to 20 mm. Both represent a 50% decrease in "outflow pressure." If no IOP reduction is manifest, it is unlikely that completing the remaining half of the angle will result in substantial IOP reduction, but there are notable exceptions to this. Unless there has been actual worsening of IOP from the first half of LTP, or extensive PAS formation, the second half of the angle is treated with LTP. For the second half treatment one is tempted in such non-responsive cases to alter the laser parameters somewhat, e.g., in a pale meshwork to increase the power to higher levels to try to achieve bubble formation, or if fewer than 50 applications were made for the first half, to apply a full 50 applications to the second half. It is not certain that these maneuvers result in any improvement in efficacy, however.

If the first half of LTP results in an adequate IOP decrease, it is justifiable not to perform the second half of treatment until a time when IOP drifts higher. In some patients this has not yet happened and only one half of the angle has been treated. Especially if some PAS formation has occurred, even if not to meshwork but only to scleral spur, one should pause in patients with good responses before completing LTP therapy. **Gonioscopy should, thus, always be performed at this one month post-LTP visit.**

It is curious that there is little correlation between the acute effects of LTP on IOP and the long-term efficacy. Patients with acute IOP elevation seem, at first glance, just as likely to show a long-term IOP improvement as those without such acute IOP elevation. If the current trend toward lesser number and power of laser applications continues, it will be interesting to see whether some correlation between short-term and long-term IOP effects does, however, emerge.

It is important to state that when some IOP decrease occurs with full LTP treatment, it is still necessary for the ophthalmologist to judge whether there has been sufficient

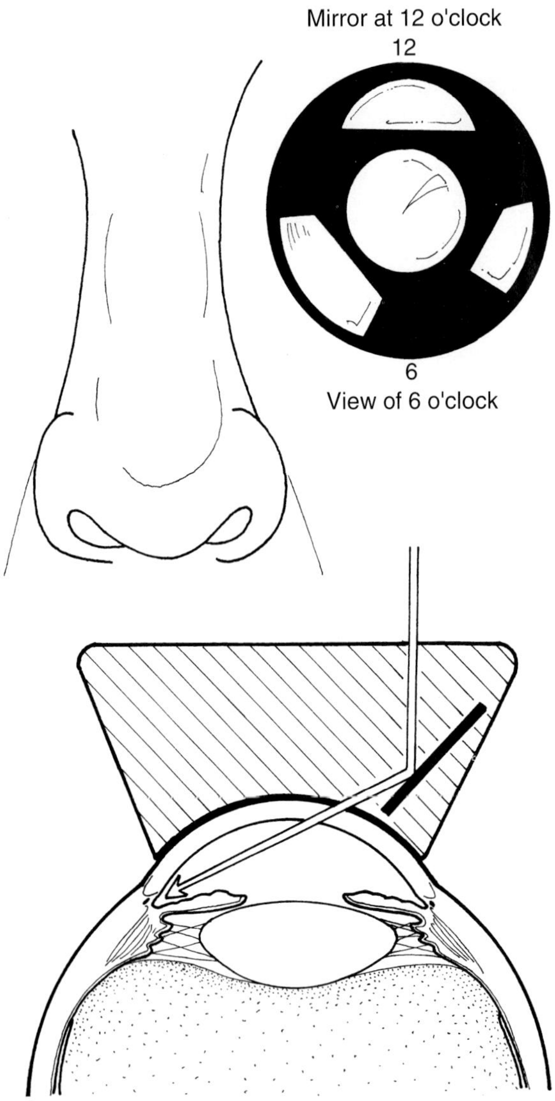

Figure 52.3. The parabola shaped mirror at 12:00, used to view and treat the angle, produces a view of the trabecular meshwork at 6:00. The 12:00 position of the mirror permits treatment of the inferior trabecular meshwork with laser trabeculoplasty.

lowering of IOP to obviate the need for filtration surgery. There seems to be a tendency, which to us is not at all justified, not to proceed with filtration surgery in patients with advanced glaucoma who have had LTP with minimal IOP lowering. For example, in a patient with a central island of vision due to glaucoma and an IOP of 30, if LTP lowers the IOP to only 25 one month after full treatment, filtration surgery should be performed. A pressure of 25 is clearly too high for such a patient (an IOP in the teens is required), and if such an IOP were encountered on maximum medical therapy, filtration surgery would have been proposed.

INDICATIONS

In almost all forms of open-angle glaucoma, LTP should be performed before embarking on filtration surgery. In young patients with juvenile open-angle glaucoma, or those with secondary inflammatory glaucomas, it is rare for LTP to be effective, but there are noteworthy exceptions. The risk/benefit ratio of LTP versus filtration surgery is such that it always seems justifiable to perform LTP in at least a portion of the angle prior to performing filtration surgery. For those with unfavorable prognosis in whom there seems to be some potential for actual worsening of the glaucoma with LTP (such as in inflammatory glaucomas or young patients), it seems prudent not to attempt LTP. Some would argue that full LTP treatment in the whole angle should be performed prior to filtration surgery in all open-angle glaucoma patients; however, especially in cases with poor prognosis and definite chronic elevation of IOP after initial LTP, this does not seem warranted to us.

In aphakic and many pseudophakic eyes, the response to LTP, although often significant, seems clearly less than in the phakic eye. (The reason for this is obscure; there does not seem to be any "mechanical" basis for this). Pseudophakic eyes may behave no differently with respect to LTP response than do phakic eyes, although this point remains controversial (18). Dreyer and colleagues studied the effectiveness of LTP in pseudophakic eyes in a retrospective fashion using historical controls. While their data suggest no difference in the effectiveness of LTP in pseudophakic and phakic eyes with POAG, this problem deserves further investigation in a prospective study.

In patients with chronic angle-closure glaucoma with synechias in the angle, we will always treat the open portions of the angle (if 3 or more hours are open) with LTP prior to embarking on filtration surgery. This is most often unsuccessful, but there are occasional gratifying exceptions.

All these discussions have concerned patients on maximum tolerated medical therapy who are facing filtration surgery. What is the role of LTP in replacing medical therapy for glaucoma? Should LTP be used in place of pilocarpine? In place of medical therapy entirely?

The Glaucoma Laser Trial, a study of 271 patients with POAG, attempted to answer these questions (19,20). In this experiment, one eye received 360 LTP divided into two sessions separated by one month, while the other eye was treated with timolol. There was a series of medical steps that the "medication first" eye could undergo for IOP control, from timolol to dipivefrin, to low dose pilocarpine, to high dose pilocarpine, to timolol and high dose pilocarpine, to dipivefrin and high dose pilocarpine, thence to the ophthalmologist's discretion. The "laser first" eye initially received no medications, but was medically treated if necessary for IOP control.

Of the eyes treated with LTP, 44% were controlled on no medications, 70% were controlled with the addition of timolol, and 89% were controlled with LTP and medications, but no surgery. The "medication first" eyes showed

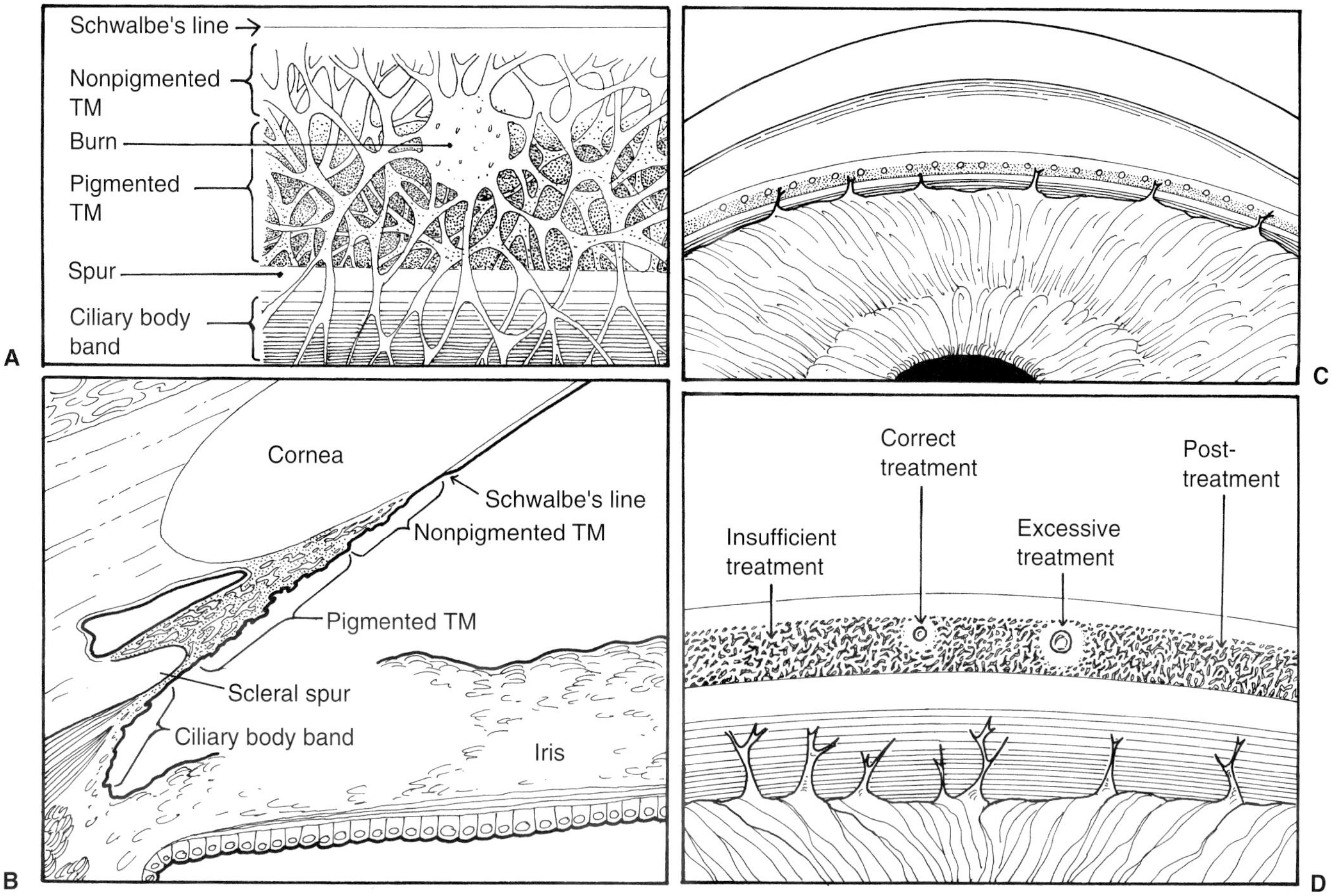

Figure 52.4. Laser trabeculoplasty lesions are placed at the junction of the anterior ⅓ and posterior ⅔ of the trabecular meshwork (A). This minimizes damage to the more posterior trabecular meshwork, which is the filtering portion, with access to Schlemm's canal (B). Spots are placed 100-150 microns apart, such that 50 spots cover 180 of the angle (C). The endpoint is a blanch or small bubble. If a large bubble is seen, or if the bubble bursts, then excessive energy is being delivered to the trabecular meshwork, and the treatment power should be decreased (D).

30% controlled on timolol alone, 51% controlled on a single medication, and 66% controlled on multiple medications.

These short-term, two year results, indicate that LTP is efficacious in lowering IOP, but that it is not a panacea (19,20). Indeed, more than half the eyes treated with LTP first later required some sort of medical or surgical therapy. A further follow-up of three and a half years examining visual field progression found little difference between the "laser first" and "medicine first" groups, although the "laser first" eyes performed slightly better on some measures of visual field function (21).

As noted above, LTP is a destructive procedure (22), eliminating a portion of an already marginally functional trabecular meshwork. It may make future filtering surgery less likely to succeed, and may predispose to bleb encapsulation following trabeculectomy (15). For these reasons, **we place LTP in our armamentarium after miotics, but before systemic CAIs and trabeculectomy**. Still, in those patients unable to take miotics due to lens opacity or other side effects, LTP is commonly used as the third line of therapy, following beta-blockers and topical carbonic anyhdrase inhibitors or alpha-2 agonists. LTP may fall further back in the medical regimen with the introduction of latanaprost. Additionally, in those individuals with poor or borderline compliance, LTP is a useful option for initial therapy.

CONTRAINDICATIONS

Except for corneal opacification or total synechial closure of the angle, LTP should be attempted in at least a portion of the angle for uncontrolled glaucoma, as already discussed. We believe that documented long-term worsening of the glaucoma after the initial half-angle treatment is at least a relative contraindication to the completion of the treatment, as discussed in the previous section.

COMPLICATIONS

Long-Term Worsening of the Glaucoma

It must be remembered that approximately 3% of patients with open-angle glaucoma actually get worse following

LTP (23). This, of course, does not specifically refer to or include patients with acute IOP elevation shortly after the procedure. The mechanism for this sustained worsening is not known, but it possibly may relate to the destruction of meshwork tissue with the laser, with possible scar formation (22).

Acute Pressure Elevation

Cases with resulting visual loss have been documented. The IOP shortly after LTP needs to be monitored and treated.

Uveitis

Occasionally this is severe and needs to be vigorously treated to prevent synechia formation.

Peripheral Anterior Synechias

These are often described as being "benign" and extending only up to scleral spur. However, **cases of extensive functional angle closure due to PAS have been documented following LTP.** The appearance of the angle post-LTP needs to be carefully monitored and steroid dosage appropriately adjusted.

Corneal Burns

Occasionally corneal epithelial opacities are encountered (Fig. 52.5) but these heal within a few days without sequelae. Corneal endothelial burns are rare.

Hyphema

This is an uncommon complication, but has been observed. There seem to be two causes. Occasionally there are meandering normal vessels in the angle which are inadvertently disrupted by the laser energy. **Treatment immediately consists of pressing the goniolens against the cornea to raise IOP and thus achieve hemostasis,** or, if the vessel is visible through the goniolens, to treat it directly with further laser applications in order to coagulate it as in goniophotocoagulation. The other cause of hyphema is encountered when there is blood in Schlemm's canal and the laser energy penetrates deeply into the meshwork to the canal. Most patients with open-angle glaucoma do not have blood in Schlemm's canal (it is important to contemplate why this is so), but occasionally it is found, especially in patients with abnormally elevated episcleral venous pressure, e.g., in association with a dural shunt. Treatment consists of raising IOP with goniolens pressure and/or tilting the lens to relieve compression at the limbus in the involved portion of the angle. It is this initial compression of limbal episcleral vessels with the goniolens that promotes blood reflux into the canal. One should avoid the temptation to increase the laser power further and treat the bleeding portion of the angle further (unless a blood vessel can be identified), for this simply may allow further penetration into the blood filled canal. If hemostasis is obtained by these means, one can proceed to complete the LTP, but lower power settings should be chosen for the remaining portions of the angle.

Usually only a small amount of bleeding is encountered in such cases, but rarely significant hyphema has been observed with associated elevation of IOP.

The Unknown

In any procedure whose optimal parameters and long term biological effects are not clearly known, we must all be diligent in looking for and documenting unexpected long-term consequences of our treatment.

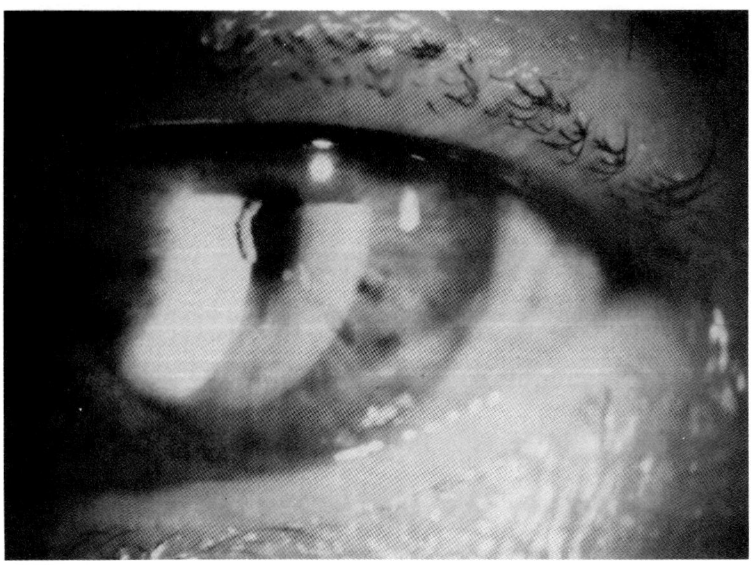

Figure 52.5. Corneal epithelial "paint-drop" type opacity that occurred during laser trabeculoplasty. This condition resolved within a few days.

A discussion of the mechanisms of action of LTP and the treatment of acute IOP elevation are covered in the following chapters.

References

1. Grant WM: Further studies on facility of flow through the trabecular meshwork. Arch Ophthalmol 1958;102:1211–1213.
2. Gaasterland D, Kupfer C: Experimental glaucoma in the rhesus monkey. Invest Ophthalmol 1974;13:455–457.
3. Wise JB, Witter SL: Argon laser therapy for open-angle glaucoma: A pilot study. Arch Ophthalmol 1979;97:319–322.
4. Swartz AL, Whitten ME, Bleiman B, et al: Argon laser trabecular surgery in uncontrolled phakic open-angle glaucoma. Ophthalmology 1981;88: 203–212.
5. Wilensky JT, Jampol LM: Laser therapy for open-angle glaucoma. Ophthalmology 1981;88:213–217.
6. Thomas JV, Simmons RJ, Belcher CD: Argon laser trabeculoplasty in the management of the surgical glaucoma patient. Ophthalmology 1982;89: 187–197.
7. Wise JB: Long-term control of adult open-angle glaucoma by argon laser treatment. Ophthalmology 1981;88:197–202.
8. Coleman AL, Robin AL, Pollack IP: Apraclonidine hydrochloride. Ophthalmol Clin North Am 1989;2:97–108.
9. Robin AL: The role of apraclonidine hydrochloride in laser therapy for glaucoma. Trans Am Ophthalmol Soc 1989;87:729–761.
10. Richardson TM, Epstein DL: Exfoliation glaucoma: a quantitative perfusion and ultrastructural study. Ophthalmology 1981;88:968–980.
11. Shingleton BJ, Richter CU, Bellows AR, et al: Long-term efficacy of argon laser trabeculoplasty. Ophthalmology 1987;94::1513–1518.
12. Richter CU, Shingleton BJ, Bellows AR, et al: Retreatment with argon laser trabeculoplasty. Ophthalmology 1987;94:1085–1089.
13. Quigley HA, Holman RM: Laser energy levels for trabecular meshwork damage in the primate eye. Invest Ophthalmol Vis Sci 1983;24: 1305–1307.
14. Wise JB: Errors in laser spot size in laser trabeculoplasty. Ophthalmology 1984;91:186–190.
15. Richter C, Shingleton B, Bellows A, et al: The development of encapsulated filtering blebs. Ophthalmology 1988;95:1163–1168.
16. Pappas HR, Berry DP, Partamian L, et al: Topical indomethacin before argon laser trabeculoplasty. Am J Ophthalmol 1985;99:571–575.
17. Fiore PM, Melamed S, Epstein DL: Trabecular precipitates and elevated intraocular pressure following argon laser trabeculoplasty. Ophthalmic Surg 1989;20:697–701.
18. Dreyer EB, Gorla M: Laser trabeculoplasty in the pseudophakic patient. J Glaucoma 1993;2:313–315.
19. The Glaucoma Laser Trial Research Group: The Glaucoma Laser Trial 1. Acute effects of argon laser trabeculoplasty on intraocular pressure. Arch Ophthalmol 1989;107:1135–1142.
20. The Glaucoma Laser Trial Research Group: The Glaucoma Laser Trial (GLT). 2. Results of argon laser trabeculoplasty versus topical medicines. Ophthalmology 1990;97:1403–13.
21. The Glaucoma Laser Trial Research Group: The Glaucoma Laser Trial (GLT): 6. Treatment group differences in visual field changes. Am J Ophthalmol 1995;120:10–22.
22. Melamed S, Pei J, Epstein DL: Delayed response to argon laser trabeculoplasty in monkeys: Morphological study and morphometric analysis. Arch Ophthalmol 1986;104:1078–1083.
23. Thomas JV, Simmons RJ, Belcher CD: Argon laser trabeculoplasty in the pre-surgical glaucoma patient. Ophthalmology 1982;89:187–197.

How I Do Laser Trabeculoplasty

53

Claudia U. Richter

Once the decision to lower intraocular pressure (IOP) by laser trabeculoplasty (LTP) has been made, careful prelaser evaluation and preparation of the patient (Table 53.1) is necessary to be certain that LTP may be effective and to minimize postlaser complications. Preoperative evaluation includes slit-lamp examination to determine corneal clarity, gonioscopy to determine the status of the angle, and IOP measurement. Preoperative preparation includes informed consent, topical apraclonidine, topical anesthesia, and laser adjustment.

Prelaser evaluation should first assess the clarity of the cornea. Opacification of the cornea from edema, scarring, or dystrophy prevents delivery of laser energy to the trabecular meshwork, impairing the efficacy of the LTP. If corneal opacification is from corneal edema, topical glycerin may be used to temporarily clear the cornea. Additionally, if the corneal edema is caused by elevated IOP, the IOP can be acutely lowered by topical apraclonidine, topical beta-adrenergic antagonists, oral or intravenous acetazolamide, and/or oral or intravenous hyperosmotic agents.

Gonioscopy should be performed before the LTP to determine the status of the angle. If the angle is closed, a laser iridectomy should be performed and the IOP and angle status reevaluated. If the angle is narrow so that visualization of the trabecular meshwork is difficult, a laser iridectomy can deepen the angle and facilitate the LTP. If the angle remains narrow and visualization of the trabecular meshwork is difficult after an iridectomy has been placed, laser gonioplasty to the peripheral iris can deepen the angle, allowing the LTP to be performed. **If laser iridectomy or gonioplasty is performed, at least 1 week should elapse before LTP**, to allow for clearing of debris and inflammatory material from the anterior chamber. This permits the use of lower energy levels for LTP than if the two procedures were performed simultaneously.

The angle should also be evaluated for evidence of neovascularization, peripheral anterior synechias from previous angle closure glaucoma, surgery or trauma, or an iridocorneal endothelial syndrome. Extensive angle closure will prevent effective IOP reduction by the LTP.

The IOP should be measured using applanation tonometry. A prelaser measurement is necessary to compare with a postlaser measurement and to detect any increase in IOP.

The procedure is explained to the patient and informed consent obtained. Potential complications to be discussed with the patient include a postlaser IOP elevation, loss of vision, peripheral anterior synechias, uveitis, hyphema, corneal burns, syncope, inadequate effect on IOP, and a possible adverse effect on future filtration surgery. Once informed consent has been obtained, topical apraclonidine is administered just before the LTP to minimize a postlaser IOP elevation (1). Topical anesthesia, such as proparacaine, is given immediately before the procedure. Rarely retrobulbar anesthesia may be required, such as in a patient with nystagmus. A mirrored contact lens with an antireflective coating is filled with goniosolution and placed on the eye. Either the Goldmannn 3-mirror lens or the Ritch lens (2) may be used. The Ritch lens has four mirrors, two with buttons that magnify the target and minify the spot, increasing the efficiency of the laser delivery. The mirrors are placed at two different angles, to allow access to angles of varying configuration. If the diode laser is used, the Ritch lens is preferred.

The argon blue-green laser provides the most commonly used laser wavelength for LTP, although the diode laser is also effective (Table 53.2). **The argon laser is set at 50 micron spot size and 0.1 second spot duration. Laser treatment is initiated at laser power of 600 milliwatts, adjusting the power to achieve slight blanching or small bubble formation on the anterior trabecular meshwork.** If large bubbles or cracking of the trabecular meshwork is noted, the power should be lowered. If no reaction occurs in the meshwork, the power should be increased to a maximum of 1200 milliwatts. **The diode laser is set at 50 to 75 micron spot size, 0.1 second duration, and power 750 to 1250 milliwatts** (3,4). Tissue reaction is uncommonly seen with the diode laser and power alterations are not necessary. With either laser, treatment is aimed toward the anterior trabecular meshwork, at the junction of the pigmented and nonpigmented trabecular meshwork.

The laser treatment consists of 35 to 50 spots over 180 degrees of the trabecular meshwork. The **laser spots are placed with a space equal to three laser spots between them.** Treatment is conveniently begun at 6 o'clock by placing the contact lens mirror at 12 o'clock and rotating the lens as necessary to treat the necessary extent of the angle (Table 53.3). To treat the nasal trabecular meshwork of the right eye the contact lens is rotated counterclock-

Table 53.1
Preoperative Preparation

1. Preoperative evaluation of corneal clarity and angle status
2. Informed consent
3. Intraocular pressure measurement
4. Topical apraclonidine 1 hour prior to LTP
5. Topical proparacaine 5 minutes prior to LTP
6. Adjustment of the patient at laser slit-lamp
7. Placement of mirrored contact lens with goniosolution

Table 53.2
Laser Parameters

	Argon	Diode
Spot size	50 Microns	50–75 Microns
Duration	0.1 Second	0.1 Second
Power	600 milliWatts	750–1250 milliWatts
Reaction Endpoint	Minimal blanching or small bubble formation	None or minimal blanching

Table 53.3
How Not to Get Lost in the Angle During Laser Trabeculoplasty

1. Perform prelaser gonioscopy on every patient and note any variations in the angle appearance, such as synechias, pigment, and prominent blood vessels, to use as landmarks. Be certain to distinguish Schwalbe's line, the pigmented trabecular meshwork, scleral spur, and the ciliary body band before beginning treatment.
2. Always begin laser trabeculoplasty at the same position in every patient so you always know where the starting point and, therefore, the endpoint will be.
3. Remember, and write down nearby if necessary, which way the contact lens will be rotated during the procedure, so that the direction is not inadvertently reversed and the same area retreated. Directions which may be useful:

Right eye	Nasal meshwork	Counterclockwise rotation
Right eye	Temporal meshwork	Clockwise rotation
Left eye	Nasal meshwork	Clockwise rotation
Left eye	Temporal meshwork	Counterclockwise rotation

4. When the contact lens must be rotated to treat additional portions of the trabecular meshwork, rotate the mirror so that both treated and untreated trabecular meshwork are visible in the mirror and you can begin treatment again adjacent to the last treated spot.

wise. To treat the nasal meshwork of the left eye the contact lens is rotated clockwise. Treatment with only 50 spots over 180 degrees reduces the maximum increase in IOP in the immediate postlaser period (5) and many patients

Table 53.4
Postoperative Management

1. Topical apraclonidine
2. Measure intraocular pressure at 1 hour and 3–4 hours following LTP
3. Topical steroids QID for 5 days
4. Measure intraocular pressure at 1 and 4 to 6 weeks
5. Decision on further treatment at 4 to 6 weeks

will have adequate IOP reduction with this amount of treatment. (6–9)

After the LTP (Table 53.4), patients should be given topical apraclonidine, if they did not receive it preoperatively. The IOP should be measured 1 hour and 3 hours later to detect and treat any IOP elevations. Topical steroids are prescribed four times a day for five days to treat the transient iritis, which is common after LTP. The IOP should be reassessed at 1 week and again at 4 to 6 weeks, earlier if clinically indicated. Effective IOP reduction may not be fully apparent until 4 to 6 weeks after LTP. Routine examination of the patient at that time allows the clinician to determine if the laser has been effective. If the IOP has reached the target level, no further treatment is indicated. If adequate IOP reduction has not occurred, the untreated half of the trabecular meshwork may be treated using the same technique.

References

1. Robin AL, Pollack IP, House B, et al: Effects of ALO 2145 on intraocular pressure following argon laser trabeculoplasty. Arch Ophthalmol 1987;105:646–650.
2. Ritch R: A new lens for argon laser trabeculoplasty. Ophthalmic Surg 1985;16:331–2.
3. Brancato R, Carassa R, Trabucchi G: Diode laser compared with argon laser trabeculoplasty. Am J Ophthalmol 1991;112:50–55.
4. McHugh D, Marshall J, Ffytche TJ, et al: Diode laser trabeculoplasty (DLT) for primary open-angle glaucoma and ocular hypertension. Br J Ophthalmol 1990;74:743–7.
5. Weinreb RN, Ruderman J, Juster R, et al: Immediate intraocular pressure response to argon laser trabeculoplasty. Am J Ophthalmol 1983;95:279–286.
6. Horns DJ, Bellows AR, Hutchinson BT, et al: Argon laser trabeculoplasty for open angle glaucoma. A retrospective study of 380 eyes. Trans Ophthalmol Soc UK 1983;103:288–295.
7. Weinreb EB, Wilensky JT: Clinical aspects of argon laser trabeculoplasty. Int Ophthalmol Clin 1984;29:79–96.
8. Heijl A, Bengtsson B: The short-term effect of laser trabeculoplasty on the glaucomatous visual field. A prospective study using computerized perimetry. Acta Ophthalmol 1984;62:705–714.
9. Lustgarden J, Podos SM, Ritch R, et al: Laser trabeculoplasty. A prospective study of treatment variables. Arch Ophthalmol 1984;102:517–519.

Argon Laser Trabeculoplasty—How Does It Work?

54

Shlomo Melamed

INTRODUCTION

Argon Laser Trabeculoplasty (ALT) is currently used in the treatment of various types of open angle glaucoma (1–4), and it is usually applied after maximally tolerated medical therapy has failed to control the intraocular pressure (IOP) (4). Although ALT is considered a very safe and effective method, its exact mechanism of action still remains unclear. Important clinical observations along with several basic research studies reported in the last 10 years may shed some light on its mode of action.

CLINICAL OBSERVATIONS RELATED TO THE MECHANISM OF ALT

Since 1979, when Wise and Witter originally described ALT in glaucoma patients (1), its efficacy and safety has been repeatedly confirmed by numerous studies (5–12). Today, it is widely accepted that ALT reduces IOP in uncontrolled open angle glaucoma patients, with success rate ranging from 97% in the first year to 55% in the 10th year after treatment (4,13). Several observations reported in clinical studies of ALT may give some hints as to the mode of action of this procedure:

1. Increased outflow facility—tonography was performed in patients before and after ALT and C values were substantially increased after treatment (9). A fluorophotometric study disclosed no effect on aqueous humor inflow (14). From these studies, it is concluded that ALT mainly affects outflow facility, most probably through the trabecular meshwork—Schlemm's Canal region.
2. Complete (entire circumference) and partial (180 and 90 degrees) ALT may be equally effective in IOP control. Interestingly, different patterns of ALT which are associated with various degrees of direct involvement of the angle may result in similar IOP reduction. Low dose (11) and low power (15) ALT have also been observed to effectively control IOP in glaucoma patients. Such successful results of only minimal or partial treatment of the outflow system may suggest that triggered biological processes could be involved, affecting nonlasered regions as well.
3. Some subtypes of open angle glaucoma are more responsive to ALT than others. Pseudoexfoliative glaucoma (PXF), primary open angle glaucoma (POAG) and pigmentary dispersion glaucoma (PDG) are the subtypes of glaucoma in which ALT is most beneficial (4). The common feature of these three diseases may be the "wear and tear" phenomenon. In this concept, particulate matter (PXF material, pigment or some unknown protein or proteoglycan) is blocking the trabecular spaces and is associated with a diminished number of trabecular cells (16). Reduction in trabecular cellularity may subsequently result in adherence of trabecular beams and total collapse of the trabecular meshwork, with increased resistance to aqueous flow. It is conceivable, then, that ALT may affect vital cellular processes related to this "wear and tear" phenomenon, and indeed several studies confirmed such an effect of ALT and will be described later (17–22).

   In contrast, other types of open angle glaucoma are poorly responsive to ALT, such as aphakic/pseudophakic glaucoma, uveitic glaucoma and juvenile glaucoma (4).

THE MECHANICAL THEORY OF ALT

Wise and Witter (1), initially proposing this treatment, suggested that mechanical shrinkage of the trabecular ring following ALT causes widening of the trabecular spaces with subsequent decrease in resistance to aqueous outflow and reduction of IOP. However, up to now, no proof for such mechanical stretching of the trabecular sheets has been reported. It has been speculated that in glaucomatous eyes, where the trabecular beams are collapsed, the pattern of ALT may result in scarring of the lasered areas with widening of the trabecular spaces and Schlemm's canal due to traction of the beams in adjacent regions. However, in a study of 23 pairs of enucleated human eyes, no significant change in the cross-sectional area of Schlemm's canal could be demonstrated after ALT (23).

Because no accurate morphometric analysis has been done in glaucomatous eyes after ALT, the mechanical explanation for its effect still remains theoretical.

THE BIOLOGICAL EFFECT OF ALT

ALT may be associated with triggering of a cascade of complex biological processes in the outflow system

(17–22). Such cellular and biological processes may play an important role in the therapeutic efficacy of ALT.

Histopathology of ALT

In a series of electron-microscopic experiments performed in non-glaucomatous monkeys (17,18,21), Melamed et al described the acute and long term cellular changes in the trabecular meshwork and Schlemm's canal in the treated eyes. Immediately after ALT, the common features of laser effect were coagulative necrosis, disruption of trabecular beams and dispersion of tissue debris. Small fragments of tissue could be found throughout the trabecular spaces, accumulating in the juxtacanalicular region. **This accumulation of debris might explain the IOP spike sometimes detected immediately after ALT** (in up to 31% of ALT cases) (24).

Many trabecular cells were rounded up, dislodged from their supportive beams and some were very actively phagocytic, containing large phagosomes with an excessive amount of fibrillar material.

After 4 weeks, the treated, lasered spots were detected as scarred regions with flattened beams. A cellular layer continuous with the corneal endothelium was found to cover these regions. The inner wall beneath these areas was flat, with no giant vacuoles present. Rodrigues et al (25) and Weber et al (26) found similar changes in their studies of trabeculectomy specimens. Early changes consisted of disrupted trabecular beams and accumulation of fibrinous debris. Six months later, scarred treated regions with a corneal endothelial sheet covering its surface could be detected, whereas nontreated regions appeared normal (26).

In human eyes, ALT reduces IOP despite scarring of the lasered regions. In a tracer study performed in monkeys by using the molecule cationized ferritin, the scarred lasered sites were observed to be impermeable to aqueous flow (21). Gaasterland (27) has shown that confluent ALT results in chronic IOP elevation due to trabecular scarring (in fact, it is the best available method still in practice to create a model for glaucoma in monkeys).

How is it, then, that despite all this damage to and scarring of the trabecular meshwork, IOP is reduced after ALT? Several studies may help in resolving this intriguing puzzle by suggesting some biological processes which might be initiated or enhanced by this therapy.

ENHANCED BIOLOGICAL AND PHAGOCYTIC ACTIVITY OF TRABECULAR CELLS

One of the main tasks of the trabecular cells is to act as the "biological filter" of the eye. Particles or materials obliterating the trabecular spaces are usually phagocytosed by these cells, which later leave the beams and the outflow system. After ALT, trabecular cells were detected in various stages of enhanced biological and phagocytic activity (17). This increased activity might have resulted from the absorption of laser energy itself or have been triggered by the debris of lasered tissue. It is conceivable that such an effect of ALT might explain its high success rate in the previously mentioned "wear and tear" glaucomas, where the presumed particulate matter blocking the trabecular spaces may be more efficiently removed by trabecular cells activated by ALT, with subsequent reduction of resistance to aqueous flow.

STRUCTURAL CHANGES OF REGIONS ADJACENT TO LASERED SITES

Four weeks and after ALT, non-lasered regions adjacent to lasered spots demonstrated an array of significant structural changes (18). These regions had wide open intertrabecular spaces with herniations of the juxtacanalicular meshwork and inner wall of Schlemm's canal into and across its lumen. These herniations contained more vacuoles than in the control eyes, suggesting increased flow of aqueous humor. A tracer study with cationized ferritin also suggested this with the demonstration of excessive decoration of all trabecular spaces, in contrast to its non-penetration into adjacent scarred, treated areas. It was suggested that these changes are a compensatory response to ALT, allowing the aqueous blocked by the scarred spots to be shifted into less resistant trabecular routes, with the net effect of IOP reduction (Figure 54.1).

INFLAMMATORY RESPONSE INITIATED BY ALT

In humans, ALT usually stimulates an inflammatory response in the eye, requiring the use of anti-inflammatory agents (7,8).

In addition, the trabecular meshwork in monkeys was found to contain an abundance of inflammatory cells such as lymphocytes, pigment-laden macrophages and plasma cells (18). Such trabeculitis may also be associated with decreased IOP, through the release of mediators affecting aqueous outflow.

INCREASED CELL DIVISION AFTER ALT

Further support for the importance of **the biological response of the trabecular meshwork to ALT** was given by a series of experiments evaluating cellular division after this treatment (19,20,22).

Increased trabecular cell division after ALT has been shown in organ cultured human eyes (19) as well as living cats (22) and monkeys (28).

In organ cultured human eyes, trabecular cell division and migration were studied by exposure to tritiated thymidine. Two days after ALT, non-treated areas of the trabecular meshwork disclosed a marked incorporation of thymidine into the nuclei's DNA, indicating increased cellular division (19,20).

In the organ cultured human eyes, thymidine incorpora-

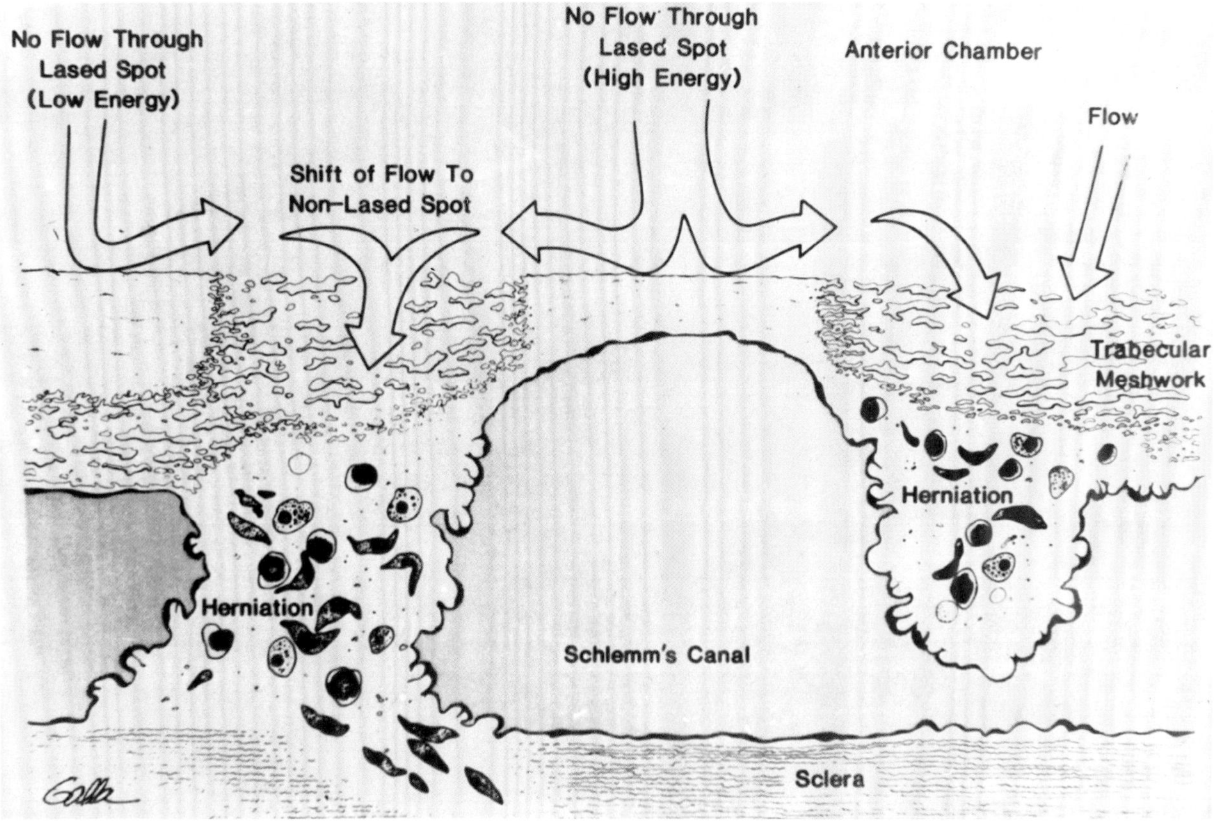

Figure 54.1. Laser trabeculoplasty results in regions of decreased flow where the actual laser lesions occur, and areas of increased flow visible as locations where the trabecular meshwork is herniated into Schlemm's canal. Reprinted with permission from Melamed S, Epstein DL Br J Ophthalmol 1989;71:776.

tion occurred predominantly in the anterior, non-filtering region of the trabecular meshwork (which might represent "Schwalbe's line cells"). Two weeks later, the labeled cells were more concentrated in the lasered regions, suggesting active migration from the anterior trabeculum into the treated area. In the living cat model, DNA replication in the trabecular meshwork was also demonstrated in response to ALT (22), although no accurate localization to the anterior trabecular region could be made. A significant increase in the mitotic index of trabecular cells in response to ALT was also confirmed by Dueker et al in the monkey model (28).

Enhanced DNA synthesis, cell replication, and migration comprise a fundamental biological response of trabecular cells to ALT.

ALTERATION IN TURNOVER OR SYNTHESIS OF GLYCOSAMINOGLYCANS AFTER ALT

The hypothesis that ALT causes the release of a factor that induces trabecular cell division or other cellular and extracellular actions away from the lasered site was tested by Ruddat et al (29). In this study, the levels of mRNAs for a family of matrix metalloproteinases (MMPs) were measured in response to ALT. These enzymes are synthesized and secreted to release cells from their extracellular matrix, allowing their increased mobility. After ALT, the levels of these mRNAs were significantly increased, suggesting the release of a media-borne signal by ALT, biologically affecting remote, non-treated trabecular regions. In addition, evidence for alteration of turnover or synthesis of glycosaminoglycans after ALT has been reported (19).

SUMMARY

Argon laser trabeculoplasty (ALT) is a widely accepted treatment modality for open angle glaucoma. Despite its widespread use, we still lack a thorough understanding of its mode of action.

With the support of numerous studies reported so far, the mechanical explanation for IOP reduction in glaucomatous eyes cannot be ruled out, but it may be too simplistic and awaits scientific confirmation.

In contrast, several biological processes are triggered by ALT and may play an important role in altering outflow pathway conductivity. These biological processes in the trabecular meshwork include: early increase in cell division, migration, and phagocytic activity; release of media-borne factors and alteration of glycosaminoglycans; structural changes in lasered and adjacent non-treated regions affect-

Table 54.1
Argon Laser Trabeculoplasty (ALT): How Does It Work?

Clinical Facts Related to ALT Pathophysiology
- ALT reduces intraocular pressure (IOP) in glaucoma patients
- ALT causes an increase in outflow facility in glaucoma patients
- ALT has no effect on inflow of aqueous humor
- ALT of both 180 and 360 of the angle are effective
- It takes 4–6 weeks for ALT to reach its maximal effect
- Low dose and low power ALT are equally effective
- "Wear and tear" glaucoma, (pseudoexfoliative, primary open angle and pigmentary glaucoma) respond better to ALT than other types of open angle glaucoma).

Mechanism of Action of ALT
- Two main mechanisms of IOP reduction by ALT may be involved:
  - The mechanical theory
  - The biological effect of ALT

Indications for the Mechanical Theory	Indications for the Biological Effect
1. Shrinkage of the inner trabecular ring.	1. Signs of increased biological and phagocytic activity of some trabecular cells
2. Separation of trabecular sheets and opening of aqueous channels.	2. Lasered regions are flat, with cellular sheet extending from corneal endothelium covering them. Inner wall of Schlemm's canal is flat with no vacuoles present.
3. Traction on collapsing Schlemm's canal (not proven in enucleated human eyes).	3. Adjacent non-lasered regions disclosed herniations of juxtacanalicular meshwork into Schlemm's canal, containing an abundance of vacuoles.
	4. Tracer studies with cationized ferritin demonstrated no aqueous flow through lasered areas, with probable shift of flow through adjacent herniations.
	5. Alteration in turnover or synthesis of glycosaminoglycans.
	6. Increased trabecular cell division after ALT.
	7. Signs for release of media-borne factor affecting remote, non-treated trabecular areas.
	8. Induced inflammatory response (trabeculitis).

ing aqueous flow patterns; and the trabecular inflammatory response. These concepts are summarized in Table 54.1.

References

1. Wise JB, Witter SL: Argon laser therapy for open angle glaucoma: A pilot study. Arch Ophthalmol 1979;13:455.
2. Thomas JV, El-Mofty A, Hamdy EE, et al: Argon laser trabeculoplasty as initial therapy for glaucoma. Arch Ophthalmol 1984;102:702.
3. Horns DJ, Bellows AR, Hutchinson BT, et al: Argon laser trabeculoplasty for open angle glaucoma: A retrospective study of 380 eyes. Trans Ophthalmol Soc 1983;103:288.
4. Thomas JV, Simmons RJ, Belcher CD: Argon laser trabeculoplasty in the pre-surgical glaucoma patient. Ophthalmology 1982;89:187.
5. Wise JB: Long term control of adult open-angle glaucoma by argon laser treatment. Ophthalmology 1981;8:157.
6. Ruderman JM, Zweig KO, Wilensky JT, et al: Effects of corticosteroid pretreatment on argon laser trabeculoplasty. Am J Ophthalmol 1983;96:84.
7. Pappas HR, Berry DP, Partamian L, et al: Topical indomethacin therapy before argon laser trabeculoplasty. Am J Ophthalmol 1985;99:571.
8. Weinreb RN, Robin AL, Baerveldt G, et al: Flurbiprofen pretreatment in argon laser trabeculoplasty for primary open angle glaucoma. Arch Ophthalmol 1984;102:1629.
9. Wilensky JT, Jampol LM: Laser therapy for open angle glaucoma. Ophthalmology 1981;88:213.
10. Rouhiainen H, Terasvirta ME, Tuolinen EJ: The effect of some treatment variables on the results of trabeculoplasty. Arch Ophthalmol 1988;106:611.
11. Wilensky JT, Weinreb RN: Low-dose trabeculoplasty. Am J Ophthalmol 1983;95:423.
12. Klein HZ, Shields MB, Ernest JT: Two-stage argon laser trabeculoplasty in open angle glaucoma. Am J Ophthalmol 1985;99:392.
13. Ticho V, Nesher R: Laser trabeculoplasty in glaucoma: ten years evaluation. Arch Ophthalmol 1989;107:844.
14. Yablonski ME, Cook DJ, Gray J: A fluorophotometric study of the effect of argon laser trabeculoplasty on aqueous humor dynamics. Am J Ophthalmol 1985;99:579.
15. Shirakashi M, Iwatak NT: Long term efficacy of low power argon laser trabeculoplasty. Arch Ophthalmol 1990;68:23–28.
16. Alvarado J, Murphy C, Juster R, et al.: Trabecular meshwork cellularlity in primary open angle glaucoma and non-glaucomatous normals. Ophthalmology 1984;91:564–579.
17. Melamed S, Pei J, Epstein DL: Short-term effect of argon laser trabeculoplasty in monkeys. Arch Ophthalmol 1985;103:1546.
18. Melamed S, Pei J, Epstein DL: Delayed response to argon laser trabeculoplasty in monkeys. Arch Ophthalmol 1986;104:1078.
19. Bylsma SS, Samples JR, Acott TS, et al: Trabecular cell division after argon laser trabeculoplasty. Arch Ophthalmol 1988;106:544.
20. Acott TS, Samples JR, Bradley JMB, et al: Trabecular repopulation by anterior trabecular meshwork cells after laser trabeculoplasty. Am J Ophthalmol 1989;107:1.
21. Melamed S, Pei J, Epstein DL: Alteration of aqueous humor outflow following Argon Laser Trabeculoplasty in monkeys. Br J Ophthalmol 1987;71:776–781.
22. Bylsma SS, Samples JR, Acott TS, et al: DNA replication in the cat trabecular meshwork after laser trabeculoplasty in vivo. J Glaucoma 1994;3:36–43.
23. Van-Buskirk EM, Pond V, Rosenquist EC, et al.: Argon laser trabeculoplasty: studies on mechanism of action. Ophthalmology 1984;91:1005.
24. Glaucoma Laser Trial Research Group: The Glaucoma Laser Trial. I: Acute effects of argon laser trabeculoplasty on intraocular pressure. Arch Ophthalmol 1989;107:1135.
25. Rodrigues MM, Spaeth GL, Donahoo P, et al: Electron microscopy of argon laser therapy in phakic open angle glaucoma. Ophthalmology 1982;89:198.
26. Weber PA, Davidoff FH, McDonald C: Scanning electron microscopy of argon laser trabeculoplasty. Ophthalmol Forum 1983;1:26–29.
27. Gaasterland D, Kupfer C: Experimental glaucoma in the Rhesus monkey. Invest Ophthalmol Vis Sci 1974;14:455–457.
28. Dueker DK, Norberg M, Johnson DH, et al: Stimulation of cell division by argon and Nd-YAG laser trabeculoplasty in cynomologous monkeys. Invest Ophthalmol Vis Sci 1990;31:115–124.
29. Ruddat MS, Alexander JR, Samples JR, et al.: Early changes in trabecular metalloproteinase mRNA levels in response to laser trabeculoplasty are induced by media borne factors. Invest Ophthalmol Vis Sci (Suppl) 1989;30:280.

Postlaser Elevation of Intraocular Pressure 55

Marshall N. Cyrlin

Anterior segment laser surgery for glaucoma and for post-cataract extraction capsulotomy has eliminated many of the complications that can occur with traditional incisional surgery. Laser surgery does, however, have its substantial risks. These include inflammation, hemorrhage, synechia formation, and transient or prolonged intraocular pressure (IOP) elevation. Postlaser IOP elevations may be significant, particularly in the patient with preexisting advanced glaucoma. IOP spikes, if undetected or untreated, can result in further visual loss or blindness.

MECHANISMS OF IOP ELEVATION

Argon laser, employed for iridectomy or trabeculoplasty, interacts with pigmented tissue through its coagulative effect which either contracts collagen (lower energies) or vaporizes tissue with explosive force (higher energies). Laser treatment can result in the formation of vapor bubbles, pigment debris, and the release of prostaglandins, plasma, or fibrin that can reduce facility of outflow through the trabecular meshwork by mechanical obstruction or by inciting inflammation. Neodymium:YAG laser employed for iridectomy or capsulotomy exerts its physical effect on pigmented or nonpigmented tissue by photodisruption with the creation of an explosive, expanding plasma shockwave. IOP elevation may result from the previously noted mechanisms as well as from hemorrhage or hyphema in the case of iridectomy, or from capsular or cortical debris in the case of capsulotomy.

INCIDENCE OF IOP ELEVATION

Postoperative elevation of IOP may commonly follow either argon laser or Nd:YAG laser iridectomy (1,2). IOP elevation, which occurs within two hours postlaser in 96% of the cases, has been reported to have an incidence from 60% to 65%, and a range of 1 to 38 mm Hg over pretreatment levels, with no significant difference found between the type of laser used, total energy employed or the amount of resulting inflammation (3,4).

IOP elevation after argon laser trabeculoplasty may occur in approximately one third (5) to one half (6) of patients, is dependent on the treatment variables, and can be visually threatening if the optic nerve is already compromised by advanced glaucomatous optic atrophy (7,8). The Glaucoma Laser Trial evaluated the immediate postlaser IOP elevation in 271 eyes of patients with primary open angle glaucoma who were assigned to argon laser trabeculoplasty as an initial treatment. The patients received two treatments, 1 month apart, to 180 degrees of the trabecular meshwork. The treatments were standardized as to power intensity (threshold of bubble formation) and to location (straddling the pigmented and nonpigmented anterior trabecular meshwork). Intraocular pressures were measured at 1 hour and 4 hours after each treatment session. **Increases of IOP greater than 5 mm Hg occurred in 34% of eyes after one or both treatment sessions and increases of greater than 10 mm Hg occurred in 12%.** Only a small percentage of eyes had IOP rises greater than 5 mm Hg 4 hours after laser treatment without an elevation 1 hour after treatment. Eyes with increases of IOP after the first treatment were more likely to have increases after the second treatment. Of all of the parameters evaluated, **only pigmentation of the trabecular meshwork was associated with IOP increases** (9). Other studies have found a greater incidence and severity of postlaser elevations of IOP from treatments of 100 burns delivered to 360 degrees than from 50 burns delivered to 180 degrees (5,10).

After Nd:YAG laser capsulotomy, IOP can also rise within the first few hours and rarely may last for weeks or months (11–14). The amount of laser energy delivered, preexisting glaucoma, prelaser elevated IOP, absence of an intraocular lens, or the sulcus fixation of a posterior chamber lens are additional risk factors.

MANAGEMENT

Management of IOP elevations after anterior segment laser surgery as described, entails preoperative IOP measurement, prophylactic medical therapy and appropriate postlaser IOP monitoring and treatment. Patients currently taking glaucoma medication should be instructed to take their medication before arriving for laser or it should be administered on arrival. Baseline IOP measurements are taken before the laser treatment is performed. Routinely measure the IOP of the fellow eye to use as a control. Historically, pilocarpine, beta blockers, oral carbonic anhydrase inhibitors, oral osmotic agents, topical steroids, and nonsteroidal anti-inflammatory agents have been used with little or variable success for either preoperative prophylaxis or postlaser treatment of IOP elevations (7,15–21).

Apraclonidine hydrochloride, an alpha-2 adrenergic agonist which reduces the rate of aqueous formation, was the first medication to be significantly and reliably effective in reducing postoperative elevations of IOP following laser iridectomy, argon laser trabeculoplasty or Nd:YAG laser capsulotomy (7,22–25). In a study of 261 eyes assigned to receive either apraclonidine 1%, pilocarpine 4%, timolol maleate 0.5%, dipivifrin 0.1%, or acetazolamide 250 mg both 1 hour before and immediately after 360 degree argon laser trabeculoplasty, apraclonidine was the only medication to reduce the mean IOP siginificantly from baseline (26). Only 3% of the apraclonidine eyes had elevations of IOP greater than 5 mm Hg, compared with 39% for acetazolamide, 38% for dipivifrin, 33% for pilocarpine, and 32% for timolol. Brimonidine 0.5%, another alpha-2 adrenergic agonist under clinical investigation, also reduces the incidence of postlaser IOP elevation when administered either before or after argon laser trabeculoplasty (27,28).

Treat prophylactically the eye that is to receive laser with a drop of apraclonidine hydrochloride 1%, either 30 to 60 minutes preoperatively or immediately postoperatively. Apraclonidine 0.5% solution may be an acceptable substitute if the 1% is not readily available. The IOP should be measured again in both eyes 1 and 2 hours after the laser. **In cases of advanced glaucoma a 3- or 4-hour postlaser evaluation may be beneficial**. Should the IOP become elevated 5 mm Hg or more from the baseline, or should it reach a clinically unacceptable level, an additional drop of apraclonidine should be administered as well as any other topical miotic, beta blocker or carbonic anhydrase inhibitors that the patient is able to take (29). For eyes unresponsive to the previous regimen or for more marked elevations of IOP in patients with advanced glaucoma, consider administering oral osmotic agents at a dose of at least 1 g per kg. Patients with significant elevations of postlaser IOP should be monitored until the IOP is reduced to a clinically acceptable level; they should be examined again the following day.

References

1. Krupin T, Stone RA, Cohen BH, et al: Acute intraocular pressure response to argon laser iridotomy. Ophthalmology 1985;92:922.
2. Taniguchi T, Rho SH, Gotoh Y, et al: Intraocular pressure rise following Q-switched neodymium:YAG laser iridotomy. Ophthal Laser Ther 1987;2:99.
3. Robin AL, Pollack IP: A comparison of neodymium:YAG and argon laser iridotomies. Ophthalmology 1984;91:1011.
4. Moster MR, Schwartz LW, Spaeth GL, et al: Laser iridectomy: a controlled study comparing argon and neodymium:YAG. Ophthalmology 1986;93:20.
5. Weinreb RN, Ruderman J, Juster R, et al: Immediate intraocular pressure response to argon laser trabeculoplasty. Am J Ophthalmol 1983; 95:279.
6. Krupin T, Kolker AE, Kass MA, et al: Intraocular pressure the day of argon laser trabeculoplasty in primary open angle glaucoma. Ophthalmology 1984;91:361.
7. Robin AL: Medical management of acute post-operative intraocular pressure rises associated with anterior segment ophthalmic laser surgery. Int Ophthalmol 1990;30:102.
8. Thomas JV, Simmons RJ, Belcher CD III: Complications of argon laser trabeculoplasty. Glaucoma 1982;4:50.
9. Glaucoma Laser Trial Research Group. I: Acute effects of argon laser trabeculoplasty on intraocular pressure. Arch Ophthalmol 1989;107: 1135.
10. Weinreb RN, Ruderman J, Juster R, et al: Influence of the number of laser burns administered on the early results of argon laser trabeculoplasty. Am J Ophthalmol 1983;95:287.
11. Channell MM, Beckman H: Intraocular pressure changes after neodymium-YAG laser posterior capsulotomy. Arch Ophthalmol 1984;102: 1024.
12. Richter CU, Arzeno G, Pappas HR, et al: Intraocular pressure elevation following Nd:YAG laser posterior capsulotomy. Ophthalmology 1985; 92:636.
13. Keates RH, Steinert RF, Puliafito CA, et al: Long term follow-up of Nd:YAG laser posterior capsulotomy. Ophthalmology 1985;92:636.
14. Demer JL, Koch DD, Smith JA, et al: Persistent elevation in intraocular pressure after Nd:YAG laser treatment. Ophthal Surg 1986;17:465.
15. Ruderman JM, Zweig KO, Wilensky JT, et al: Effects of corticosteroid pretreatment on argon laser trabeculoplasty. Am J Ophthalmol 1983; 96:84.
16. Ofner S, Samples JR, Van Buskirk EM: Pilocarpine and the increase in intraocular pressure after trabeculoplasty. Am J Ophthalmol 1984;97: 647.
17. Hotchkiss ML, Robin AL, Pollack IP, et al: Nonsteroidal anti-inflammatory agents after argon laser trabeculoplasty. A trial with flurbiprofen and indomethacin. Ophthalmology 1984;91:969.
18. Pappas HR, Berry DP, Partamian L, et al: Topical indomethacin therapy before argon laser trabeculoplasty. Am J Ophthal 1985;99:571.
19. Cyrlin MN, Beckman H. Low-dose oral glycerin for the prevention of post-laser IOP elevation. Invest Ophthalmol Vis Sci (suppl) 1987;28: 272.
20. Metcalfe TW, Etchells DE: Prevention of the immediate intraocular pressure rise following argon laser trabeculoplasty. Br J Ophthalmol 1989;73:612.
21. Migliori ME, Beckman H, Channell MM: Intraocular pressure changes after neodymium-YAG laser capsulotomy in eyes pretreated with timolol. Arch Ophthalmol 1987;105:473.
22. Robin AL, Pollack, IP, House B, et al: Effect of ALO 2145 on intraocular pressure following argon laser trabeculoplasty. Arch Ophthalmol 1987; 105:646.
23. Robin AL, Pollack IP, DeFaller JM: Effects of topical ALO 2145 (p-aminoclonidine hydrochloride) on acute intraocular pressure rise following argon laser iridotomy. Arch Ophthalmol 1987;105:1208.
24. Brown RH, Stewart RH, Lynch MG, et al: ALO 2145 reduces the intraocular pressure elevation after anterior segment laser surgery. Ophthalmology 1988;95:378.
25. Pollack IP, Brown RH, Crandall AS, et al: Prevention of the rise in intraocular pressure following neodymium-YAG posterior capsulotomy using topical 1% ALO 2145. Arch Ophthalmol 1988;106:754.
26. Robin AL: Argon laser trabeculoplasty medical therapy to prevent the intraocular pressure rise associated with argon laser trabeculoplasty. Ophthal Surg 1991;22:31.
27. Barnebey HS, et al: The efficacy of brimonidine in decreasing elevations in intraocular pressure after laser trabeculoplasty. Ophthalmol 1993; 100:1083.
28. David R, Spaeth GL, Clevenger CE, et al: Brimonidine in the prevention of intraocular pressure elevation following argon laser trabeculoplasty. Arch Ophthalmol 1993;111:1387.
29. Dapling RB, Cunliffe IA, Longstaff S: Influence of apraclonidine and pilocarpine alone and in combination on postlaser trabeculoplasty pressure rise. Br J Ophthalmol 1994;78:30.

Laser Peripheral Iridectomy

56

Joel S. Schuman

In angle-closure glaucoma, where the goal is to allow communication between the posterior and anterior chamber through the peripheral iris and thus alleviate pupillary block, the laser has allowed iridectomy to be performed as an outpatient procedure with great safety and low morbidity. All ophthalmologists routinely learn and master this technique.

It is still a matter of debate whether this technique should be called laser "iridotomy" or "iridectomy," depending on whether one feels that the laser is simply penetrating the iris or actually destroying (and removing) a portion of it. Due to local custom we have utilized the term "iridectomy" in this book.

Laser iridectomy (LPI) has, except in the most extreme cases (eg., severe uveitis with a plasmoid aqueous and recurrent closure of LPI), replaced surgical peripheral iridectomy (Chapter 67). Many deserve credit for early work on laser techniques for iridectomy (1–5), but two major developments have contributed to the current application and efficacy of this method: 1) the development of lasers with good optics, capable of delivering sufficient energy and 2) the development of a corneal contact lens with a plano-convex "button," such as that developed by Robert Abraham (Fig. 56.1), or that of James Wise, which improve energy delivery to the iris (Table 56.1).

INDICATIONS

While LPI is clearly indicated in acute angle closure glaucoma, there are several other situations where this procedure is beneficial as well. These settings include pupillary block with narrow, occludable angles, chronic angle closure glaucoma, combined mechanism glaucoma, imperforate surgical iridectomy, suspected malignant glaucoma, pupillary block after cataract surgery, and nanophthalmos (Table 56.2).

In acute angle-closure glaucoma, if IOP can be reduced by osmotics, timolol and carbonic anhydrase inhibitors (CAIs), and if topical glycerin is used to clear the cornea, LPI is almost always successful in relieving pupillary block. Sometimes without even penetrating the iris, the pupillary distortion induced by a photocoagulative laser resolves the attack. Gonioplasty (Chapter 60) can also be utilized to open the angle if iris penetration cannot be achieved. LPI can usually be easily accomplished, even in postoperative eyes or those with dilated pupils. In inflamed eyes, laser openings in the iris may close subsequently, necessitating a second treatment session.

Even if it is suspected preoperatively that the angle is extensively involved with PAS, LPI should be done initially rather than filtration surgery, and the IOP and angle should be assessed after treatment. In combined-mechanism glaucoma it eliminates the angle-closure component. LPI should always be done initially in preference to filtering surgery for acute angle closure.

Has the apparent efficacy and safety of laser iridectomy changed or softened our indications for an iridectomy procedure? Should LPI be done as a diagnostic test? These are difficult questions which every ophthalmic surgeon should ask himself. Our answer to the first question is "probably yes" and to the second "probably no." Previously we always advocated surgical iridectomy (rather than medical therapy) to treat eyes with angle closure and eyes with suspected combined-mechanism glaucoma. In fact, Paul Chandler had surgical peripheral iridectomy himself for the latter condition. However, it is for the eye with a very narrow angle but normal IOP that we seem to be more aggressive applying LPI at the present time. Presently, even with an equivocal identification of PAS with Zeiss indentation gonioscopy we would go ahead with LPI, whereas in the past we would have required an unequivocal finding to justify surgical iridectomy.

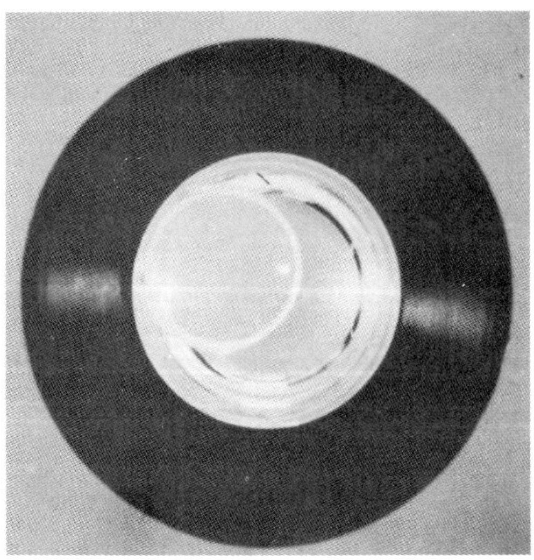

Figure 56.1. Abraham lens used for laser iridectomy (Ocular Instruments, Inc., Redmond, WA).

THE CHOICE OF IRIDECTOMY LENS

Joel S. Schuman

We tend to favor the Nd:YAG laser Abraham iridectomy lens, as it has a 66 diopter plano-convex button which is both larger and easier to focus through than either the argon laser Abraham lens or the Wise iridectomy lens. The argon Abraham lens also has a 66 diopter button, but the button is smaller than the Nd:YAG laser version. This is because the cone angle of the argon laser is smaller than that of the Nd:YAG laser. (The cone angle is the angle created by the laser beam coming together to focus into a spot, which is the waist, or narrowest point of the beam. The smaller the cone angle, the easier it is to focus the laser, as the waist of the beam is present for a greater distance in space. This is why focus is so critical with the Nd:YAG laser, as there is only a very small area where the waist of the beam is present). Because of the larger cone angle of the Nd:YAG laser, the Abraham lens for this instrument requires a bigger button. While this enables use of the lens with the Nd:YAG laser, it also facilitates its use with the argon or diode lasers.

The Wise lens, with its 103 diopter button, minifies the spot and magnifies the target to a greater extent than the Abraham lens, which is an advantage, as it concentrates the laser energy more; however, because of the higher power of the button, focus is more difficult with the Wise lens than with the Abraham. Many surgeons prefer the Wise lens because of its optical properties, while others favor the Abraham for its ease of use.

Table 56.1
Advantages of Therapeutic Contact Lens Use in the Performance of a Laser Iridectomy

1. Lens creates concentration of energy at the iris level.
2. Lens acts as heat sink, decreasing corneal epithelial and endothelial burns.
3. Lens acts as speculum, keeping lids apart.
4. Lens provides limited control of ocular movement.
5. Lens provides magnification of target site.

Table 56.2
Indications for Laser Peripheral Iridectomy

1. Pupillary block with angle closure
2. Pupillary block with narrow, occludable angle
3. Chronic angle closure glaucoma
4. Combined mechanism glaucoma
5. Imperforate surgical iridectomy
6. Suspected malignant glaucoma
7. Fellow eye in acute angle closure glaucoma
8. Pupillary block after cataract operation
9. Nanophthalmos

However, what about the eye with a narrow angle with normal IOP and definitely no PAS identified on Zeiss indentation gonioscopy? In prior times we would follow such patients with repetitive dark-room tests, and if the results were negative, no iridectomy would be performed. Nowadays, if the angle appears occludable, and hardly any angle structures can be seen, we would advocate LPI. The risk/benefit ratio of LPI is such that, **if an experienced observer were concerned that an angle appeared occludable, LPI is recommended**. In this context one should treat the patient as one would wish one's own eye treated. What should act as a restraint is that, at the present time, we do not know if there will be long-term adverse effects from LPI that will be demonstrated, perhaps in low incidence, in future years, (e.g., lens changes, that are not apparent now) (Chapter 22). Perhaps, this stated "aggressive" posture towards LPI in occludable angles will have to be revised in future years. It is seldom in medicine that any procedure is without risk, and the art and science of medicine involve balancing the benefits and risk of the disease with those of the treatment.

CONTRAINDICATIONS

Are there any absolute contraindications to LPI? In addition to the inability to position the patient at the slit lamp, one should also be concerned about the presence of various corneal diseases and of a totally flat anterior chamber with the iris up to the cornea. Nevertheless, we would recommend that consideration always be given to trying LPI initially, at least in one circumscribed area. We have successfully performed LPI in patients with interstitial keratitis and with posterior crocodile shagreen, although some endothelial damage (Fig. 56.2) did occur in the latter condition.

TECHNIQUE OF LASER IRIDECTOMY

There are several techniques that have been utilized to penetrate the iris and perform the procedure. Our favored technique is described in the box on page 477, and involves the use of the Nd:YAG laser.

TECHNIQUE OF LASER IRIDECTOMY

C. Davis Belcher III

The concept behind a laser iridectomy is straightforward. A hole is put in the iris to relieve relative or absolute pupillary block and thus relieve iris bombé and angle closure glaucoma. The hole can be made with any number of laser sources but most commonly argon, diode, Nd:YAG, or a combination of argon or diode and Nd:YAG lasers are used.

With all techniques, miotics should be used to constrict the pupil and thin the target tissue and anti-glaucoma medications should be used to prevent a post-laser pressure spike. An iridectomy lens should be used. The Nd:YAG laser Abraham type iridectomy lens by Ocular Instruments (Bellvue, WA) is an excellent choice. The contact lens increases the power density at the target site and additionally gives limited control over ocular movement. While the argon laser can be used for iridectomies in light or dark eyes, the Nd:YAG laser used alone is best with lighter eyes. The combined argon or diode and Nd:YAG laser technique can be used in almost all situations, but is excellent for dark eyes and in special situations, such as angle closure attack eyes or pseudophakic pupillary block.

Pre-Treatment Regimen

- Miotics (eg. pilocarpine 1–4%) every 5 minutes × 3 (pupil must be immobile at beginning of iridectomy).
- Apraclonidine (½ hour before laser).
- Beta blocker if no medical contraindication.
- Carbonic anhydrase inhibitor—if visual field deficit is present.
- Oral osmotic agent—in presence of advanced glaucomatous visual field loss to prevent pressure spike.
- Topical anesthetic (eg. proparacaine).
- The patient is seated at the laser, and a contact lens with methylcellulose is applied.

Argon Laser Technique

The technique with the argon laser, whether the long pulse technique in the lighter eye, or the short pulse technique in the darker eye, is the same. The aiming beam is brought into focus at an appropriate spot on the iris surface at either 11 o'clock or 1 o'clock (12 o'clock is avoided to elude bubbles obstructing the view) and the laser is fired with the shots superimposed until a pigment flume is seen coming forward ("smoke signal"). When the anterior lens capsule is visible in the aiming beam the iridectomy is complete.

ARGON PARAMETERS

Long pulse technique (for blue, hazel, or light brown eyes)

TIME: **0.2 seconds**
POWER: **1000mW**
SPOT SIZE: **50 microns**
NUMBER OF APPLICATIONS: 1–30

Short pulse technique (for dark brown eyes)

TIME: **0.02–0.05 seconds**
POWER: **1000–1500mW**
SPOT SIZE: **50 microns**
NUMBER OF APPLICATIONS: 25–100

Nd:YAG Laser Technique

The iridectomy can be placed anywhere between 11 and 1 o'clock as bubbles are less of an issue. Try to avoid visible blood vessels. The spots of the aiming beam are brought into single, crisp focus aiming through the center of the contact lens button. The red aiming beams are then separated slightly, by advancing focus forward, to ensure focus into the iris stroma. The laser is fired; frequently the iridectomy will be complete after the first burst. If not, sequential bursts are applied, taking care to avoid any injury to the anterior lens capsule.

Nd:YAG PARAMETERS
ENERGY: 4–6mJ
NUMBER OF APPLICATIONS: 1–10 bursts; of 1–3 pulses per burst

Argon/Nd:YAG Technique

The argon laser is used to thin the iris so that approximately 20% of the tissue remains. It is done in identical fashion to the argon technique mentioned above using the 0.02–0.05 time settings. When this is accomplished, the laser is changed to the Nd:YAG mode or the patient is moved to the Nd:YAG laser. The contact lens can usually be left in place and will not fall out. The Nd:YAG laser beam is then focused into the depth of the crater and one shot will usually complete the iridectomy.

ARGON/Nd:YAG PARAMETERS (for dark brown eyes, pseudophakic eyes, patients on anti-coagulant therapy, etc)

Argon thinning of the iris:

TIME: **0.02–0.05 seconds**
POWER: **1000mW**
SPOT SIZE: **50 microns**
NUMBER OF APPLICATIONS: 5–25.

Nd:YAG perforation of the iris:

ENERGY: 4–6mJ
NUMBER OF APPLICATIONS: 1 or more bursts of 1–3 pulses per burst.

Postoperative Management

Following laser iridectomy, the intraocular pressure should be checked sometime during the first postoperative hour to be sure there is no IOP elevation. Depending on the risk to the optic nerve, the IOP should then be checked again at one day to one week and gonioscopy should be performed to assess the success in opening the drainage angle. Topical steroids are routinely used four times a day for three days. It is important to try to avoid the formation of posterior synechia between the iris and the crystalline lens.

Postoperative Medications

- Apraclondine
- Topical steroids QID × 3 days
- Avoid miotics post laser if possible to avoid posterior synechias
- Others prn

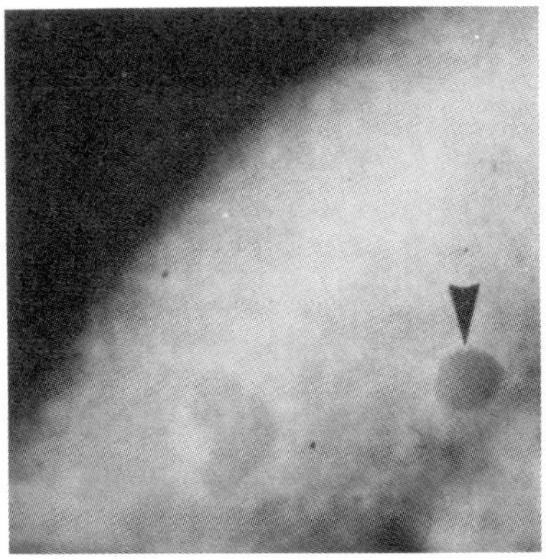

Figure 56.2. Corneal endothelial clear "blister-like" areas (arrowhead) after argon laser iridectomy in a patient who has posterior crocodile shagreen.

This differs from the description of this procedure in the previous edition of this book, in which we advocated the use of the argon laser, as the use of the Nd:YAG laser for LPI was still experimental at that point. Time and experience, however, have shown the value of photodisruption in LPI, and while the argon (or diode) laser is a useful photocoagulator, and may be used to thin the iris or coagulate blood vessels to prevent bleeding, the Nd:YAG laser is superior for the purpose of LPI. Iridectomies so created are both simpler to perform and longer lasting than those made by photocoagulation (Fig. 56.3) (5–7).

ENLARGEMENT OF ARGON OR DIODE LASER IRIDECTOMY

It is also important that careful attention be given to this detail when enlarging the iris opening. One should attempt to **treat the circumference of the opening rather than residual tissue or debris in the center of the opening** (Figs. 56.4, 56.5). One often encounters, especially in blue irides, thin strands that bridge an iris opening but are resistant to coagulation. These are easy to sever with the Nd:YAG laser, but considerably more difficult to remove with a photocoagulator. If there is a patent iridectomy on either side of the strand, it should be left alone (Fig. 56.6). If the strand is thinner than 50 microns, the center of the strand should be avoided, lest there be energy absorption by the crystalline lens, but instead the ends of the strand merging into the circumference of the opening can be treated if it is deemed important to break the strand. Again, if there is an adequate opening in the iris to relieve pupillary block, even if it is irregular in shape or contains bridging strands, it is best left alone without additional (excessive) laser applications. On the other hand, one wants an opening sufficient in size to be able to see the underlying lens capsule before concluding the laser session.

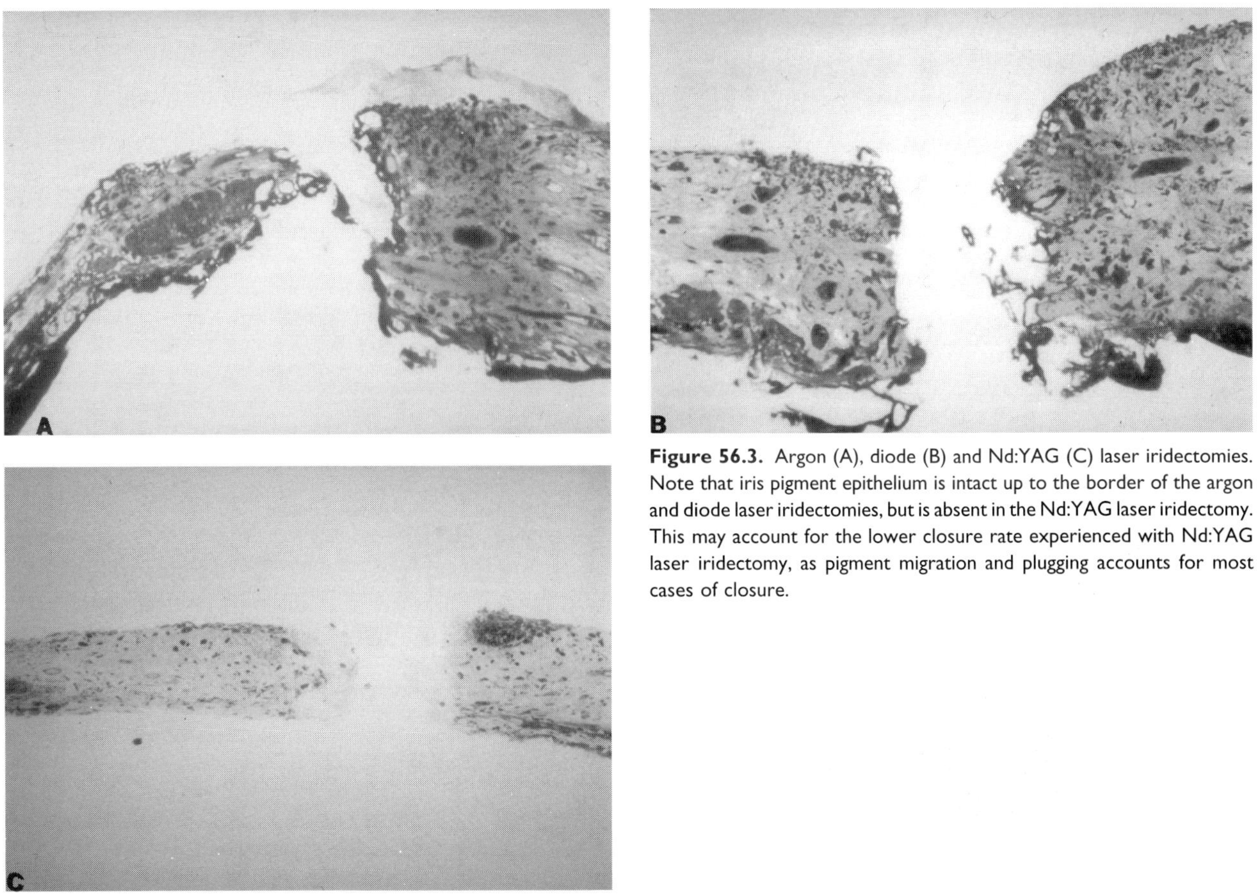

Figure 56.3. Argon (A), diode (B) and Nd:YAG (C) laser iridectomies. Note that iris pigment epithelium is intact up to the border of the argon and diode laser iridectomies, but is absent in the Nd:YAG laser iridectomy. This may account for the lower closure rate experienced with Nd:YAG laser iridectomy, as pigment migration and plugging accounts for most cases of closure.

WHICH LASER SHOULD I USE?

Joel S. Schuman

For almost any iris, the Nd:YAG laser is preferable to the argon or diode laser for the creation of a laser peripheral iridectomy. It is only in the unusual instances of a thick brown iris or an unusually vascular iris (e.g., in the setting of inflammation) that an argon or diode laser can be used to advantage to thin the iris tissue and to prevent bleeding by coagulating the vasculature. In these cases, the combined argon or diode plus Nd:YAG laser is the preferred technique. Otherwise, the Nd:YAG laser alone can be used with great efficiency, and an iridectomy made with this laser is less likely to close than one made with the argon or diode laser alone.

INDICATION FOR ARGON OR DIODE VERSUS Nd:YAG LASER IN IRIDECTOMY

Nd:YAG Laser

Almost all LPIs, except thick brown iris or vascular congestion.

Argon or Diode Laser

Useful for thinning iris in combined argon or diode and Nd:YAG laser iridectomy, or in coagulating vessels in vascular congestion. Can be used for LPI in nearly any iris; however, "ice blue" iris photocoagulation is difficult to achieve.

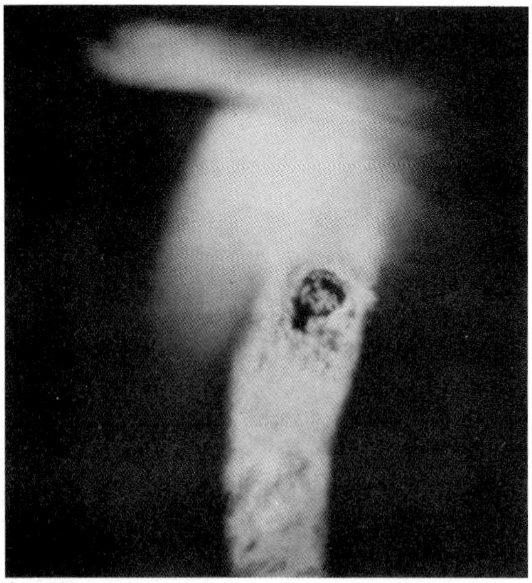

Figure 56.4. Pigment debris in the center of a patent laser iridectomy. It is difficult to remove this debris with the argon or diode laser (although possible with the Nd:YAG laser) without the occurrence of some energy absorption by the crystalline lens. Such pigment debris most often clears spontaneously. The iris opening is already adequate.

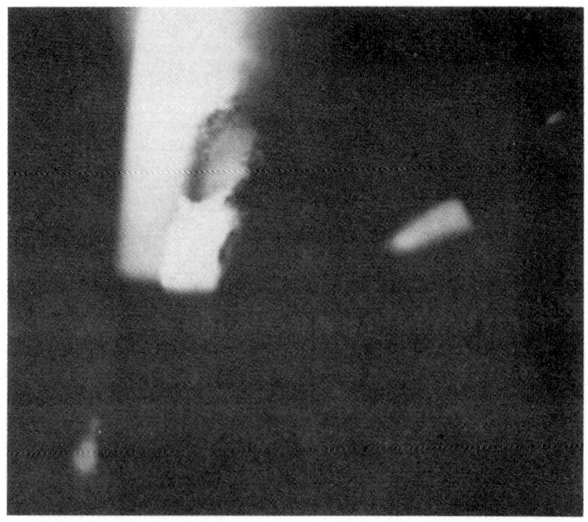

Figure 56.5. During a laser iridectomy, pigment can be deposited on the anterior lens capsule, which is easily seen in this large iridectomy. This occurrence is quite common. Obviously, the laser should never be erroneously applied to such areas on the crystalline lens.

ENLARGEMENT OF ND:YAG LASER IRIDECTOMY

Frequently, one or two bursts of three pulses per burst are all that is required to create a patent Nd:YAG laser iridectomy. If the LPI is patent, but the opening is small, the surgeon may wish to enlarge the opening. This is done by treating the edges of the iridectomy, using the same energy settings employed initially, but switching to only one pulse per shot. The edges of the iridectomy are chipped away, until the iridectomy is of a sufficient size to allow visualization of the underlying lens capsule, such that it is unlikely to close in the future. Intervening strands are easily severed with the Nd:YAG laser, but care should be taken to avoid blood vessels traversing the opening. **Should a blood vessel be ruptured, gentle pressure applied through the goniolens is usually sufficient to arrest any bleeding.** Such bleeding tends to be inconsequential and self-limited in any event.

A SECOND IRIDECTOMY

After completing one iridectomy, or while waiting for pigment and debris from the first opening to clear from the overlying aqueous humor, a second iridectomy is some-

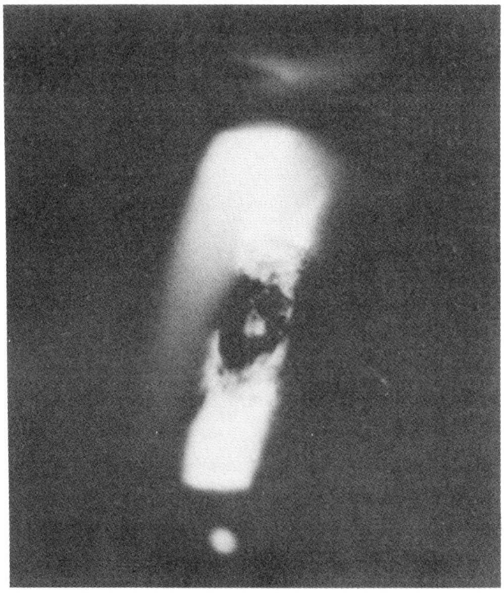

Figure 56.6. Lens capsular epithelial burn and opacity that occurred during an argon laser iridectomy. The opacity was beneath an iris strand that was difficult to separate with the argon laser. The iridectomy was subsequently observed to increase spontaneously in size. In retrospect, it was not necessary to separate the bridging strand. Such complications are uncommon with the Nd:YAG laser.

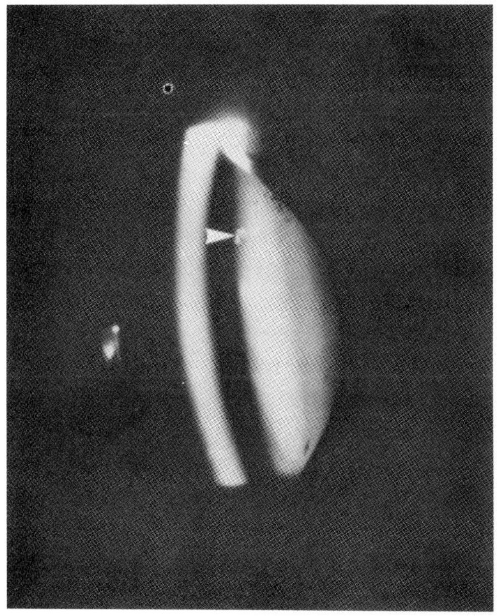

Figure 56.7. Small lens capsular epithelial opacity (arrowhead) from argon laser iridectomy.

times initiated in the other upper quadrant, particularly in iris bombé or inflammatory pupillary block. Since only one iridectomy is required to cure pupillary block, if one of the two openings should close during the ensuing weeks, no further laser sessions will be required. This offers convenience to the patient, but must be weighed against the effect of additional applications of laser energy during the second iridectomy. After all, one is injuring iris tissue, and possibly exposing the lens to injury or depriving it of nourishment (aqueous can now travel through the iridectomy directly into the anterior chamber, without bathing the crystalline lens). It can be argued that this should be kept to a minimum. As described below, occasionally iritis can develop after LPI, although this has resolved without sequelae in our experience. At the present time, **we do two iridectomies only when one is likely to close, such as in iris bombé or inflammatory pupillary block.**

LENS OPACITIES

One risk of this procedure is possible lens injury, either direct, from the laser itself, or indirect, due to reduced nourishment of the lens by circulating aqueous. The procedure should be planned with the purpose of avoiding any whitening of, or damage to, the lens underlying the treatment site (Fig. 56.7). Sometimes, with the argon or diode laser, a small capsular whitening cannot be avoided but one should strive to avoid this. Such capsular white areas do not appear to progress, but the implication that these are harmless may be misleading. The lens epithelium is the permeability barrier of the lens, and if there is epithelial-capsular injury, one would expect fluid shifts within the whole lens (possibly increasing nuclear sclerosis or posterior subcapsular changes) rather than merely a progression locally in the whitened areas of the lens epithelium. This potential for lens injury must be remembered and is to us the major long term uncertainty of the procedure.

It is extremely unusual to induce lens injury with the Nd:YAG laser; such injury manifests as a rupture in the lens capsule, and should be avoided at all costs.

In argon or diode laser iridectomies, localized lens whitening occurs about one-third of the time, after the initial penetration through the iris pigment epithelium when the iris opening is enlarged (4,8,9). When the lens capsule is exposed by opening the iris it is vulnerable to laser injury if the subsequent applications are not fully absorbed by iris tissue. Another mechanism for lens whitening with photocoagulation is posterior displacement of pigment from the iris onto the anterior lens capsule during the iridectomy, with subsequent absorption of laser energy by this pigment through a patent iridectomy. It is therefore imperative that the surgeon recognize when the iridectomy is patent, in order to avoid thermal injury to the lens capsule in this manner (Fig. 56.9).

IMMEDIATE POST-TREATMENT MANAGEMENT

The patient is immediately ambulatory without restriction, although vision is often decreased for an hour or so due to a sensation of "dazzling" light and also blurred vision from the methylcellulose solution. A small amount of photophobia and irritation is to be expected, for which mild topical steroids are applied. One may choose to dilate the patient's pupil immediately with a weak mydriatic, such as phenylephrine, which often serves also to expel

ONE TECHNIQUE FOR LASER PERIPHERAL IRIDECTOMY

Joel S. Schuman

We are often asked for our technique for LPI, which is outlined in the text and tables above and below; however, what follows is a brief synopsis of our LPI method.

Following informed consent, the patient receives a drop of apraclonidine just prior to the procedure, and two or three drops of pilocarpine 2%, each drop separated by five minutes from the next. When adequate miosis and akinesia of the pupil are achieved, the patient is seated at the laser. The Nd:YAG laser is set at 6 mJ, 3 pulses per burst. A drop of proparacaine 0.5% is instilled, and the Nd:YAG laser Abraham goniolens is placed on the eye, using methylcellulose as the coupling solution. The patient is instructed to look straight ahead, and the lens is held perpendicular to the laser beam. The two or four spots of the Nd:YAG laser aiming beam are brought into a single spot by focusing the laser. If the spots cannot be brought together, it is due to malposition of the lens, which is moved slightly to join the beams.

The laser is then moved *slightly* towards the patient, to defocus the beam just the smallest amount (Fig. 56.8). The patient is told that he may see a flash or hear a "pop," but should feel no pain, and should not move. The laser is fired, and an iridectomy is often achieved with the first burst. If an iridectomy is not achieved, the focussing and firing procedure are repeated until a patent iridectomy is present.

If the iridectomy is small, it is enlarged by changing the laser setting to the single pulse mode, and the laser is aimed at the edges of the opening. The laser is fired until the iridectomy is of adequate size, generally about 200 μm.

The lens is removed, a drop of prednisolone acetate 1% is placed in the patient's eye, and the patient is asked to wait one hour. Following this the IOP is checked, and the patient is told to instill prednisolone acetate 1% hourly until bedtime, and to return the next day. If the IOP is greatly elevated, for example, 35 mm Hg or higher, or too high for a compromised optic nerve, additional apraclonidine, timolol 1/2%, two 250 mg acetazolamide tablets, and oral osmotic (if necessary), are given to the patient, and the patient is checked again in another hour. This is generally adequate to bring the IOP to a safe level; if not, ocular hypotensive agents are employed and the patient is followed until the IOP is controlled.

The above measures are specific for Nd:YAG laser iri-

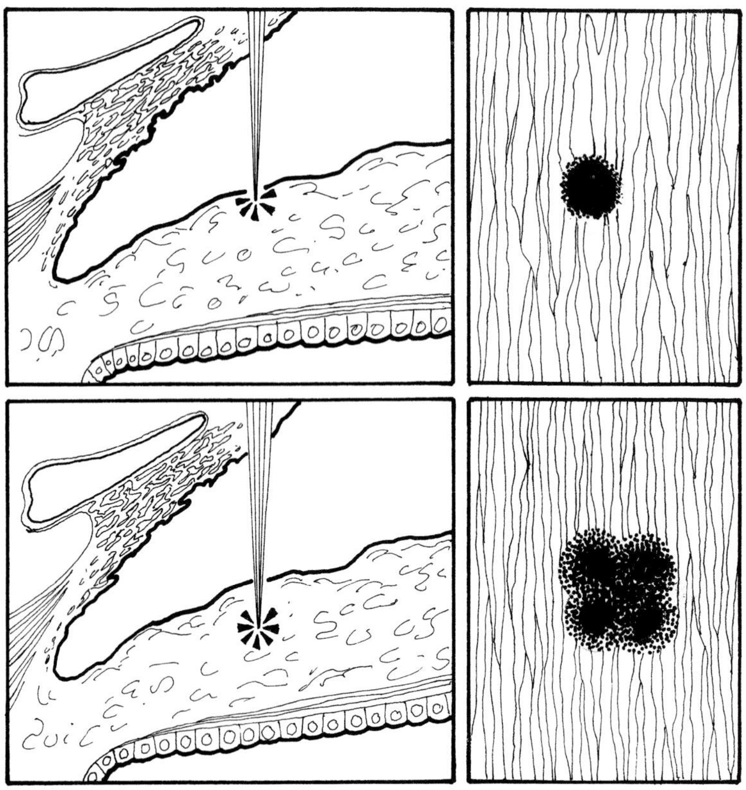

Figure 56.8. The top panel demonstrates sharp focus of the laser, with the four aiming beams joining to form a single spot when the laser is focused on the surface of the iris. The laser is defocused slightly posteriorly by moving it towards the patient, and the beams separate minimally (below panel). This is the optimal condition for Nd:YAG laser iridectomy, as it makes maximal use of the shock wave generated by the laser, by focusing the laser slightly below the surface of the iris. Subsequent exposures are treated in the same manner, focusing slightly deep to the surface of the tissue, to maximize laser effect and minimize the number of shots necessary to create a patent iridectomy.

dectomy, but the same principles apply for argon or diode laser iridectomy, or for combined argon or diode and Nd: YAG laser iridectomy. If a photocoagulator is used, either the short pulse technique, for dark brown irides (50 μm spot, 0.02-0.05 s, 1000–1500 mW, 20–50 spots, Abraham or Wise lens), or the long pulse technique, for blue, hazel, or light brown irides (50 μm spot, 0.2 s, 1000 mW, 20–30 spots, Abraham or Wise lens) is utilized. The laser is focussed to a tight spot, and fired repeatedly into the crater, creating an iridectomy. The LPI is complete only when the anterior lens capsule can be seen through the opening; a plume of pigment is not a signal that the procedure is finished.

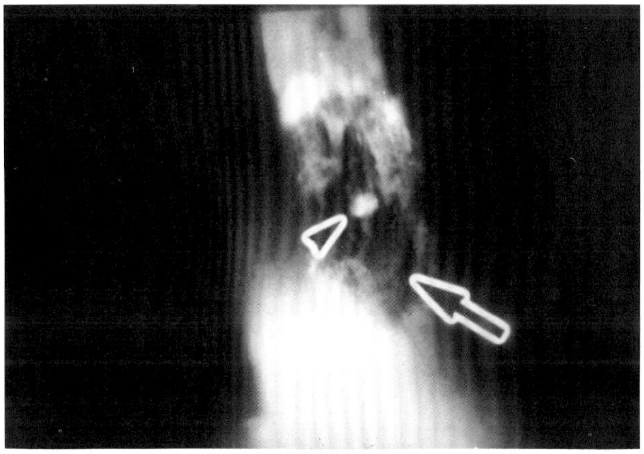

Figure 56.9. One month following diode laser peripheral iridectomy. Note the thinning of the stroma and the underlying anterior capsular opacity (arrowhead) (From Schuman JS, Jacobson JJ, Puliafito, CA: Semiconductor Diode Laser Peripheral Iridectomy. Archives of Ophthalmology 1990; 108:1207-1208).

pigment debris from the iridectomy site. However, since the laser opening can close anytime within a 6-week period, long acting cycloplegics are avoided.

IOP can be elevated shortly after the procedure and this should be monitored closely in patients with damaged optic nerves. This can usually be managed by use of timolol, apraclonidine or a CAI, although occasionally very high IOP can be encountered.

POSTOPERATIVE VISITS

The patient is usually seen at 1 hour, 1 day, 1 week, and 4 weeks after the LPI procedure (Table 56.3). At each visit, in addition to the routine ophthalmologic examination including measurement of visual acuity and applanation IOP, the status of the overlying corneal endothelium, anterior chamber reaction, and iridectomy patency are evaluated. Can the lens capsule be definitely seen through the iris opening?

Table 56.3
Perioperative Care: Laser Iridectomy

Preop	Postop
Apraclonidine 0.5–1%, Pilocarpine 2% × 3	Prednisolone acetate 1% hourly for 1 day, then qid for 4 days, then stop. Check IOP at 1 hour, 1 day, 1 week and 4 weeks. Gonioscopy at 1 week and dilation at 4 weeks.

In addition, **gonioscopy is always performed to be sure pupillary block has been relieved and to determine the extent of PAS.** With a patent iridectomy and relative pupillary block now relieved, the iris should no longer be convex, but rather flat in contour. In particular, the iris and angle in the quadrants *away* from the iridectomy site are assessed. In the quadrant of direct argon or diode laser application, iris contraction, flattening and angle openings can result, being present simply from the effects of focal laser burns on the iris, even without a full thickness iris opening. In fact, this is the basis of the gonioplasty technique (Chapter 60) for breaking recent PAS in the angle. Therefore, it is important to assess the angle in all quadrants to be sure pupillary block has been eliminated.

If there is an adequate iridectomy and the angle has opened, the patient is followed at intervals of several months. Topical steroids are discontinued after the fifth day of use, if inflammation has resolved. If the iridectomy seems to be decreasing in size but is still patent, this is simply kept under observation. Often an iridectomy created with the argon or diode laser, due to thermal coagulation necrosis in the adjacent tissue, will increase in size spontaneously after several weeks (Figs. 56.9, 56.10). If the iridectomy has closed, then an additional laser application should be performed. (If two LPIs were performed and one subsequently closes, however, no retreatment is required). Such retreatments are often easily accomplished (Fig. 56.11).

Occasionally one observes an apparently patent LPI, but pupillary block seems not to have been relieved. In such a case, one should suspect posterior sequestration of the iridectomy by adherence of the iris to the lens capsule. An additional LPI should then be performed. By performing the LPI as far peripherally as possible one can usually avoid this situation.

We are often asked what is the smallest sized iris opening that is acceptable for following LPI. We suppose that the answer is 60 microns or greater. More importantly, however, one must be able to see the lens capsule through

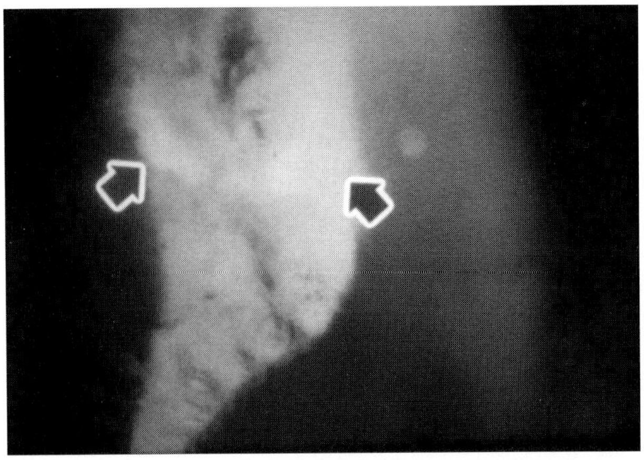

Figure 56.10. Patient on day 1 following diode laser peripheral iridectomy. Note the zone of hyperpigmentation surrounding the iridectomy (arrows). Figure 56.9 demonstrates the same iridectomy one month later. Note the dramatic loss of tissue in that interval. (From Schuman JS, Jacobson JJ, Puliafito, CA: Semiconductor Diode Laser Peripheral Iridectomy. Archives of Ophthalmology 1990; 108:1207-1208).

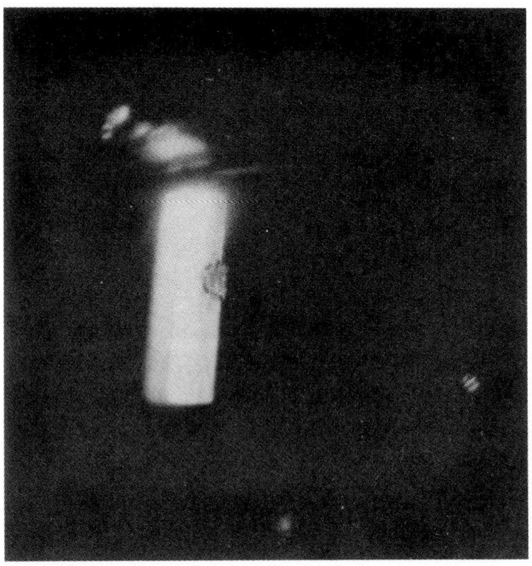

Figure 56.11. Closure of a previously patent laser iridectomy by pigment epithelial-like tissue. Such closure can occur anytime within a 6-week period after iridectomy. It was easily reopened during a second laser session.

the iris opening and document relief of pupillary block by gonioscopy. Failing this, repeat treatment is indicated.

FOUR TO SIX WEEK VISIT

If an LPI is patent 4–6 weeks after treatment, then, barring an unusual occurrence such as (unrelated) uveitis or neovascularization, the opening should remain patent indefinitely. At this visit, gonioscopy should always be performed prior to and after pupillary dilation with a weak mydriatic to rule out the rare condition of plateau iris (Chapters 25 and 26). Also the crystalline lens should be carefully inspected with the pupil dilated (Figs. 56.7, 56.9), and routine retinal examination (including indirect ophthalmoscopy) should be performed.

If the iridectomy is irregular, but pupillary block has been relieved, nothing further needs to be done. Needless "touch ups" should be avoided. Performed in the aforementioned manner, a retreatment rate of approximately 20% with the argon or diode laser should be expected. The retreatment rate for Nd:YAG laser or combined argon or diode and Nd:YAG laser iridectomies is considerably lower (2,4,8,10–14).

We recommend that patients without residual glaucoma be next examined in 6 months and then yearly. More commonly than expected, some type of open-angle glaucoma seems to develop in patients with previous angle-closure glaucoma (Chapter 22), for which such patients should always be followed.

RESIDUAL GLAUCOMA

In patients with residual PAS or combined-mechanism glaucoma, IOP may, of course, continue to be uncontrolled after LPI. However, in addition to the almost immediate elevation of IOP that may occur following LPI, due to the open-angle mechanism described above, the IOP may be moderately elevated for several weeks to months due to a second ill-defined open-angle mechanism. Perhaps this relates to liberation of pigment or other debris, for often the inferior angle especially contains much more pigment after LPI. In any case, this is usually a temporary phenomenon. Therefore, for borderline or moderately uncontrolled "residual" open-angle glaucoma, **it is best to wait if possible at least a month after LPI before deciding on further intervention, such as LTP or filtration surgery.**

For residual PAS, especially if these are of suspected recent onset (less than six months or so), one may elect to perform gonioplasty to separate these adhesions from the angle wall and open up potentially functional trabecular tissue. This is described in the introduction to the laser section (Chapter 51), and again in the chapter on miscellaneous laser procedures (Chapter 60). In brief, after pretreatment with pilocarpine, low-energy argon laser applications are made to the peripheral iris under direct view (200–500 μm spot, 0.2-0.5 s, 200–400 mW, 24–32 spots in the far periphery, Goldmann contact lens). Some PAS are easily separated, but others, presumably older, do not break. Dramatic improvement in glaucoma control has followed this procedure, but we are not yet sure of the exact incidence of success, nor how often PAS older than six months may respond to this treatment (15). However, if more than half of the angle is involved with PAS, then, in the presence of residual glaucoma, we recommend that gonioplasty be performed. Often moderate inflammation is noted following this procedure, for which a brief course of topical steroids is prescribed.

COMPLICATIONS

While any serious complication of laser peripheral iridectomy is rare, a number of complications can occur, as described below and listed in Tables 56.4 and 56.5.

CORNEA

As mentioned previously, corneal endothelial whitening (Fig. 56.12) can occur with photocoagulation (argon, diode) due to energy absorption by the endothelium, necessitating prompt discontinuation of laser applications through this area. When so discontinued, these clouded endothelial areas disappear with time without residue, but we have heard of unusual cases in which permanent corneal edema has resulted. Corneal endothelial burns can be responsible for patient discomfort following the procedures. As already mentioned, we have observed endothelial blister formation (Fig. 56.2) in a patient with pre-existing posterior crocodile shagreen, which has so far persisted without apparent adverse effects on corneal clarity and function.

With the Nd:YAG laser, localized corneal edema can occur, due to disruption of the corneal endothelium overlying the site of the LPI, especially in eyes with very little space between the iris and the posterior surface of the cornea. These lesions tend to be small and self-limited, and resolve over time with adjacent corneal endothelial cells spreading to cover the defect.

Rarely, corneal epithelial burns can occur as with laser trabeculoplasty (Chapter 52), but these clear without sequelae.

Table 56.4
Common Errors and Problems in LPI

Error or Problem	Solution
• Iridectomy not patent	• Make sure lens capsule is visible through iridectomy site at conclusion of procedure. "Smoke signal" is not enough!
• Pupil distorted at conclusion of LPI	• Inadequate miosis prior to procedure. Much more common with argon or diode LPI than with Nd:YAG laser. Will likely resolve with time.
• Diplopia	• Iridectomy made in palpebral fissure, or so peripheral that tear meniscus acts as prism, creating second image. If intolerable, patient can wear cosmetic contact lens, blocking light from LPI, but not pupil.
• Bleeding	• Choose correct laser; use argon, diode or argon or diode plus Nd:YAG in patients on anti-coagulants, with iris neovascularization, etc.
• Difficulty in perforating the iris	• Use correct techniques for eye color and situation. • Use adequate miotics to thin and stabilize target. • Use contact lens.
• Closure of initially patent iridectomy	• Use Argon or diode plus Nd:YAG or Nd:YAG to prevent closure and use Nd:YAG to reopen to prevent repeat occurrence.
• Pressure spike	• Use aggressive pre-medication to prevent pressure spikes, especially in eyes with compromised optic nerves and visual field deficits.

Table 56.5
Complications of Laser Iridectomy

Corneal burns
Uveitis
Transient elevation of the intraocular pressure
Lenticular opacities
Pigment dispersion
Retinal burns
Corectopia
Diplopia
Iris atrophy
Precipitation of malignant glaucoma
Failure to obtain iridectomy
Late closure of iridectomy
Posterior synechia formation
Hemorrhage

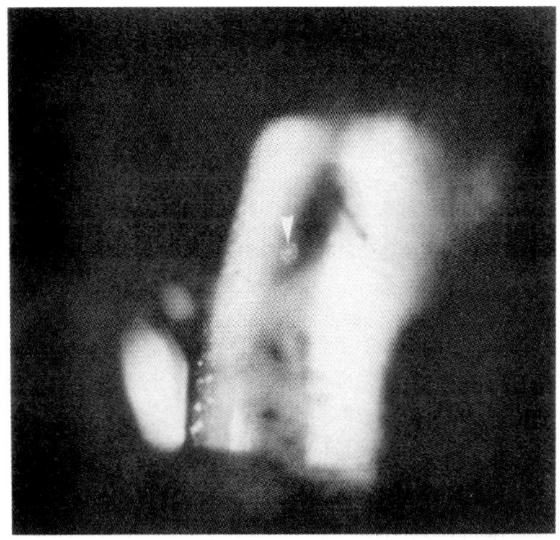

Figure 56.12. Corneal endothelial burn (arrows) that occurred during laser iridectomy. When a burn is observed, laser applications must cease through this area of the cornea. The lesions resolved without apparent sequelae.

UVEITIS

A small amount of inflammation is to be expected following LPI, for which a few days' tapering course of topical steroids is routinely prescribed. Our routine regimen is prednisolone acetate 1% hourly on the day of the LPI, followed by four times a day administration for four days, and then discontinuation of the drop. Occasionally, substantial iritis can occur, but this has always responded well to increased steroid therapy and has been short-lived in our experience. Nevertheless, one should always remember that, after all, we are ablating iris tissue with this procedure and varying amounts of inflammation are to be expected.

ELEVATED INTRAOCULAR PRESSURE

This has been discussed previously. On the day of the procedure additional antiglaucoma therapy may be prescribed, and the IOP should be monitored. A moderate, although often temporary, IOP elevation may persist for a month or so, which must be remembered when considering additional surgical intervention.

LENS INJURY

This has been discussed above. Although the white epithelial capsular opacity often seen following argon or diode LPI (Figs. 56.6, 56.7, and 56.9) may not progress, evidence of fluid movement into the crystalline lens must be watched for. Lens injury represents the main unknown long-term potential complication of this procedure.

PIGMENT DISSEMINATION

The trabecular meshwork in the open portions of the angle frequently contains additional pigment after LPI. Possibly this relates to the moderate IOP elevation that may occur for several weeks to months after the procedure. The long-term consequences of this pigment dissemination on the outflow pathways is not known.

RETINAL BURN

We have not observed this complication of photocoagulation of the iris, but it has been reported by others. Some protection may be gained by performing LPI far peripherally beyond the lens equator and by aiming obliquely rather than perpendicularly, through the cornea.

CORECTOPIA

The pupil often becomes irregularly dilated towards the lasered quadrant when photocoagulation is used during the LPI procedure, but most often this returns to normal in a few days. Rarely has it persisted.

DIPLOPIA

Occasionally patients will complain of diplopia or "ghost imaging" after LPI. It has been more commonly observed when LPI has been performed in the horizontal meridians or more centrally, but it is also surprising how many patients with such "exposed" laser openings do not notice such symptoms. By performing LPI in the upper quadrants and far peripherally where the iris openings are covered by the upper lid, such patient complaints can be minimized. Interestingly, some patients have diplopia despite an iridectomy well covered by the upper lid, which disappears when the lid is lifted away from the eye. This is presumably due to the prism effect of the tear meniscus of the upper lid (16).

IRIS ATROPHY

This complication is rare with modern LPI techniques. In the early days of LPI, when only low power photocoagulators were available, a method called "hump and burn" was used to create the iridectomy. This resulted in a large area of collateral thermal damage to the iris surrounding the actual iridectomy. This area appeared intact at the time of the procedure, but several weeks later would thin and develop a lacy appearance, finally becoming atrophic and eventually resulting in a large iridectomy, often two to three times the size of the original opening (Figs. 56.9 and 56.10).

MALIGNANT GLAUCOMA

This complication has been reported following LPI (17). Perhaps not surprisingly, as the eyes most susceptible to malignant glaucoma are those eyes requiring LPI, the process of LPI itself can apparently precipitate an attack of malignant glaucoma. It is easy to differentiate malignant glaucoma from pupillary block, on the basis of lens position and axial anterior chamber depth (Chapter 29).

FAILURE TO OBTAIN AN IRIDECTOMY

It is essential to always ensure that the iridectomy is patent, if possible through direct visualization of the anterior lens capsule. If the iridectomy is not patent, it is often a simple task, using the Nd:YAG laser, to perforate the iris through the partial thickness iridectomy.

LATE CLOSURE OF IRIDECTOMY

Occasionally, especially in the case of iridectomies created with the argon or diode laser, the iridectomy will close late, after the first four to six weeks. In these cases, it is relatively easy to reopen the LPI with the Nd:YAG laser; or, if the occluding material is pigmented, the argon or diode laser can be used. As the Nd:YAG laser creates a large zone of iris pigment epithelial loss surrounding the iridectomy (Fig. 56.3), presumably due to its shock wave effect, and because pigment migration is the most common cause of late iridectomy closure, the Nd:YAG laser is preferred for this task.

POSTERIOR SYNECHIA

Inflammation in the anterior segment can result in the formation of posterior synechias. These are best avoided after LPI by dilating the pupil, when certain that the iridectomy is patent, at the one or four week follow-up visit.

HEMORRHAGE

This problem is almost unique to LPIs created using the Nd:YAG laser. Since the argon and diode lasers are photocoagulators, they function by absorption of the light energy, and conversion of the energy to heat. This heat cauterizes the tissue as it burns a hole through the iris. The Nd:YAG laser creates optical breakdown of tissue, inducing a plasma that results in a cavitation bubble and shock wave, which tears the tissue apart. The photodisruption does not heat the tissue, and any blood vessels ruptured therefore bleed. This **bleeding is generally minimal and self-limited, but can be treated by gentle pressure on the eye applied through the contact lens.** Once the bleeding has stopped, the contact lens is slowly removed from the eye, and no special precautions are necessary other than the usual postoperative regimen.

References

1. Abraham RK: Procedure for outpatient argon laser iridectomies for angle closure glaucoma. Ophthalmol Clin 1976;16:1.
2. Beckman H, Barraco R, Sugar S, et al: Laser iridectomies. Am J Ophthalmol Soc 1971;77:674–706.
3. Khuri CH: Argon laser iridectomies. Am J Ophthalmol 1973;76: 490–495.
4. Pollack IP: Use of argon laser energy to produce iridotomies. Trans Am Ophthalmol Soc 1979;77:674–706.
5. Latina MA, Puliafito CA, Steinert RR, et al: Experimental iridotomy with the Q-switched neodymium-YAG laser. Arch Ophthalmol 1984; 102:1211–1213.
6. Robin AL, Pollack IP: A comparison of neodymium:YAG and argon laser iridotomies. Ophthalmology 1984;91:1011–1016.
7. Pollack IP, Robin AL, Dragon DM, et al: Use of the neodymium:YAG laser to create iridotomies in monkeys and humans. Trans Am Ophthalmol Soc 1984;82:307–328.
8. Pollack IP: Use of argon laser energy to produce iridotomies. Ophthalmic Surg 1980;11:506–515.
9. Schuman JS, Jacobson JJ, Puliafito CA: Semiconductor diode laser peripheral iridotomy. Arch Ophthalmol 1990;108:1207–1208.
10. Ritch R, Liebmann J, Solomon IS: Laser iridectomy and iridoplasty. In: Ritch R, Shields MB, Krupin T (eds.), Glaucomas. St. Louis: CV Mosby, 1989;581–603.
11. Ritch R, Podos SM: Argon laser treatment of angle-closure glaucoma. Perspect Ophthalmol 1980;4:129.
12. Moster MR, Schwartz LW, Spaeth GL, et al: Laser iridectomy. A controlled study comparing argon and neodymium:YAG. Ophthalmology 1986;93:20–24.
13. Jacobson JJ, Schuman JS, El Khoumy H, et al: Diode laser peripheral iridectomy. Int Ophthalmol Clin 1990;30:120–122.
14. Beckman H, Sugar HS: Laser iridectomy therapy of glaucoma. Arch Ophthalmol 1973;90:453.
15. Weiss HS, Shingleton BJ, Goode SM, et al: Argon laser gonioplasty in the treatment of angle-closure glaucoma. Am J Ophthalmol 1992;114: 14–18.
16. Weintraub J, Berke SJ: Blurring after iridotomy. Ophthalmology 1992; 99:479–480.
17. Cashwell LF, Martin TJ: Malignant glaucoma after laser iridectomy. Ophthalmology 1992;99:651.

Cyclodestruction

57

Joel S. Schuman

Cyclodestructive surgery is a procedure of last resort. It is a means by which to lower intraocular pressure (IOP) by decreasing aqueous production. Glaucoma occasionally is refractory to conventional medical and surgical treatment, and requires destruction of the ciliary body to bring the IOP to a level adequate for the preservation of optic nerve tissue and vision. Filtration surgery is usually preferable to cyclodestructive procedures, as filtration surgery attacks the cause of the glaucoma, lowering the IOP by improving aqueous outflow, while cyclodestructive procedures tend to have more complications than filtering surgery and do not treat the root of the problem. Several techniques have been used to destroy the ciliary processes.

HISTORICAL PERSPECTIVE

The first reports of destruction of the ciliary body in order to lower IOP were by Weve in 1933 (1), using diathermy. Penetrating diathermy was used by Vogt in 1936 (2), and reported again by Stocker in 1945 (3), by Lachman in 1953 (4), and by Nesterov in 1983 (5). The principle was the ablation of the ciliary body by the heat caused by the diathermy procedure (6). A report by Walton and Grant in 1970 revealed low success rates for this procedure, as well as significant hypotony, and led to the gradual abandonment of cyclodiathermy (7). Non-penetrating diathermy has been investigated by several investigators; however, both penetrating and non-penetrating diathermy appear to cause significant scleral damage in addition to the effect on the ciliary body (4,8–14). Haik used beta irradiation to induce ciliary ablation, but this is cataractogenic (15). Cyclolelectrolysis was described in 1949 by Berens and associates, but did not gain favor, as the technique did not represent a significant advantage over cyclodiathermy (6,16).

Freezing to destroy the ciliary body was suggested in 1950 by Bietti (17), and in 1964, Polack and de Roetth (18) and McLean and Lincoff (19) reported on the use of this technique in rabbits and in humans. This procedure was called cyclocryotherapy (CCT), and de Roetth later showed long-term effectiveness of CCT in lowering IOP (20,21). CCT was adopted quickly, as it was felt to be less destructive and more predictable then penetrating cyclodiathermy (22). Bellows and Grant reported that CCT was especially useful in advanced, inadequately controlled glaucoma, particularly in aphakic eyes (23,24). CCT had limited success in treating neovascular glaucoma; however, this glaucoma subtype was notoriously difficult to manage with any means, and reports of IOP control using CCT were variable (25,26). A major complication noted with CCT was phthisis, rates of which varied from 0 to 12% or more. Visual loss was also a significant complication, with rates up to 67% of treated eyes (23–29). The use of xenon arc panretinal photocoagulation in combination with CCT resulted in good IOP control and no phthisis after 2.5 years, according to Nissen and colleagues; there was no control group in this study (30).

Ultrasound has been used to cause focal ciliary body destruction since its description by Purnell and associates in 1964 for that purpose (31). Perhaps the greatest proponent of this technique has been Coleman, who has reported significant pressure lowering with ultrasound, proposing a mechanism of ciliary body destruction, thinning of scleral collagen, and separation of the ciliary body from the sclera (32–35). Several reports have supported these findings, both clinically (36) and in animal models (37–39).

Finally, Freyler and Scheimbauer noted that partial cyclectomy could control end-stage glaucoma in some cases, although the phthisis rate was 10 to 15% (40).

CYCLOPHOTOCOAGULATION

The first form of cyclophotocoagulation was performed not with a laser, but with the xenon arc photocoagulator. Transscleral xenon arc cyclophotocoagulation was reported by Weekers in 1961 (41). Unfortunately, this technique offered no clear advantage over other treatment modalities, and it was not until 1971 that the use of the laser for cyclophotocoagulation was introduced. Lee and Pomarantzeff suggested transpupillary cyclophotocoagulation, (42) but Shields showed that this procedure produced only limited success, due to the small amount of ciliary process that could be visualized through the pupil (22). Shields found that the argon laser could be used for laser endocyclophotocoagulation with good results (22,43). Uram has shown excellent results for endocyclophotocoagulation using a diode laser coupled to a fiberoptic endoscope (44–46).

A less invasive means of cyclophotocoagulation is via the transscleral route, and in 1972, Beckman described transscleral cyclophotocoagulation using a ruby laser (47). One year later, he discussed the use of the neodymium laser for this procedure, and in a 10 year follow-up of 241 patients treated with transscleral cyclophotocoagulation with the ruby laser, Beckman found 62% with an IOP of 5 to 22 mm Hg (48,49). His greatest success was in aphakic eyes, and the highest phthisis rates were in neovascular glaucoma patients (10% compared to 7% overall and a 17% incidence of hypotony overall).

Until recently, despite good results with cyclophotocoagulation, the cyclodestructive treatment of choice in patients with glaucoma refractory to medical and surgical treatment has been cyclocyrotherapy. This was due to the limited availability of the ruby laser; however, the excellent results shown for Nd:YAG and diode laser cyclophotocoagulation have revolutionized this therapeutic modality. The Nd:YAG and diode lasers have several advantages over the ruby and neodymium lasers. Longer wavelengths provide good scleral penetration with less backscatter than shorter wavelengths (50–52). Both the Nd:YAG and diode lasers have excellent absorption by melanin within the ciliary body. Nd:YAG and diode lasers are present in many medical centers, and contact Nd:YAG lasers may be found in many general hospitals, as they have many uses outside of ophthalmology. Diode lasers can be used as photocoagulators for laser trabeculoplasty (53–55), laser iridectomy (56–58), retinal photocoagulation, endophotocoagulation and transscleral retinopexy (59–68). Diode lasers are compact, portable, lightweight, are air or electrically cooled, and use standard current. Finally, the Nd:YAG and diode lasers offer an inexpensive means by which to perform cyclophotocoagulation compared to the ruby laser.

INDICATIONS AND CASE SELECTION FOR TRANSSCLERAL LASER CYCLOPHOTOCOAGULATION

Laser cyclophotocoagulation is a destructive procedure. It is a therapeutic modality of last resort, useful in advanced glaucoma, in which the IOP is uncontrolled despite maximum tolerated medical treatment, in eyes that have failed filtering surgery, or are likely to fail future filtering surgery. This includes eyes in which filtering surgery has a high risk, such as aphakic glaucoma, neovascular glaucoma, glaucoma after penetrating keratoplasty, or in eyes with very low visual potential. **Cyclophotocoagulation destroys tissue, lowering IOP by the destruction of the ciliary body, decreasing the amount of aqueous humor produced.** Hypotony can result from overly aggressive treatment, because inadequate functional ciliary body remains, while an insufficient treatment will not produce adequate lowering of IOP. The therapeutic window is relatively narrow in cyclodestructive procedures, especially in light of the fact that aqueous outflow tends to be compromised in eyes undergoing this type of surgery.

Other possible risks of cyclodestructive surgery include pain, inflammation, chronic hypotony with macular edema, vitreous hemorrhage and phthisis. While cyclophotocoagulation may produce fewer side effects than other cyclodestructive procedures, these risks persist, and tend to make cyclophotocoagulation a treatment of last resort in the management of advanced glaucoma.

Table 57.1
Indications for Cyclophotocoagulation

1. Failed prior filtration surgery, or the expectation that further glaucoma filtering surgery will fail

or

2. Glaucoma that is likely to fail filtering surgery (neovascular, inflammatory, post-penetrating keratoplasty, post-scleral buckling) or is a high risk for complications of filtering surgery (vitrectomized aphakic eye)

or

3. Poor visual acuity, such that the eye is being treated with cyclophotocoagulation to maintain comfort and prevent visual loss

or

4. The patient is not a surgical candidate for filtering surgery for general medical reasons.

A patient to undergo cyclophotocoagulation (Table 57.1) should have IOP that is uncontrolled despite maximum tolerated treatment and:

1. failed prior filtration surgery, or the expectation that further glaucoma filtering surgery will fail

or

2. glaucoma that is likely to fail filtering surgery (neovascular, inflammatory, post-penetrating keratoplasty, post scleral buckling) or is a high risk for complications of filtering surgery (vitrectomized aphakic eye)

or

3. poor visual acuity, such that the eye is being treated with cyclophotocoagulation to maintain comfort and prevent visual loss

or

4. the patient is not a surgical candidate for filtering surgery for general medical reasons.

TRANSSCLERAL LASER CYCLOPHOTOCOAGULATION

Transscleral laser cyclophotocoagulation may be performed either through the air (non-contact) or with a fiberoptic touching the eye (contact).

CONTACT

Laboratory Studies

Contact transscleral Nd:YAG laser cyclophotocoagulation (CYC) was first reported by Brancato in 1987 (69). He studied the effects of CYC on Chinchilla rabbits. Federman and coworkers (70), that same year, as well as Peyman in 1987 (71) and Schubert and Federman in 1989 (72,73), in addition to Latina and coauthors in 1989 (74), each studied CYC lesions in rabbit ciliary bodies. The lesions appeared on post-operative day number one to be 1 mm white well demarcated spots (69,74). Thermal injury occurred in the ciliary body stroma, with coagulation necrosis of the ciliary pigmented and non-pigmented epithelia; there was no significant scleral damage (69,74). Four week follow-up demonstrated atrophy, fusion, and fibrosis of the ciliary processes (73,74). In some cases, the ciliary process was covered with a fibrous membrane, with abnormal ciliary epithelium, pigment epithelial proliferation and focal epithelial interruptions (69,73,74). Areas of scleral compression and hypercellularity occurred, but there was no scleral thermal damage present (73). Epithelial regeneration following CYC did not occur, according to Van der Zypen, indicating that the vascular network remained atrophic in the ciliary body (75,76). Similar lesions have been noted using the diode laser in the contact mode in rabbit eyes (Figs. 57.1, 57.2, 57.3) (77,78).

Pulsed contact Nd:YAG laser transscleral cyclophotocoagulation results in lesions similar to non-contact transscleral Nd:YAG laser cyclophotocoagulation (NCYC) (79). The coagulative lesions seen with CYC do not occur in this setting; rather, blistering lesions are noted.

CYC performed in human cadaver eyes causes coagulation to occur in the ciliary body, with disruption of the ciliary pigmented and non-pigmented epithelium (80). Allingham showed that **optimal probe placement is with the anterior edge of the contact probe 1/2 to 1 mm posterior to the limbus.** More posterior placement results in lesions in the pars plana, while more anterior placement causes iris burns. The optimal power setting was found to be 7 to 9 watts, with 5 watts creating only minimal coagulation necrosis of the ciliary body and 11 watts causing a striking loss of anatomic integrity of the ciliary process. No scleral damage was noted at this power setting. Exposure time was optimized at 0.7 seconds (80). Brancato and co-authors showed *in vivo* in eyes destined for enucleation due to choroidal melanoma that only two joules of energy were needed to create lesions in the ciliary body using placement similar to that described above; (81) however, in another paper, Brancato showed that higher energy levels produce better clinical results (82).

Contact diode laser cyclophotocoagulation (CDC) in human cadaver eyes induced similar epithelial coagulation necrosis and thermal coagulation of the ciliary stroma and vasculature. Energy levels were 3 to 5 joules (83).

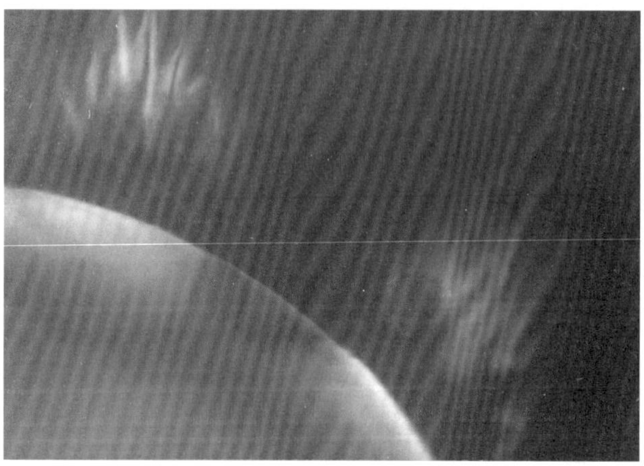

Figure 57.1. Acute effect of contact transscleral diode laser cyclophotocoagulation in a rabbit ciliary body. Note whitening of ciliary processes. From Schuman JS, Jacobson JJ, Puliafito CA, et al. Experimental use of semiconductor diode laser in contact transscleral cyclophotocoagulation in rabbits. Arch Ophthalmol 1990; 108(8):1152–1157.

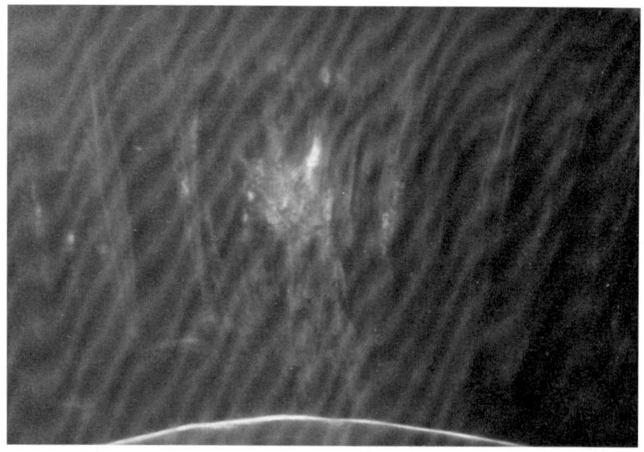

Figure 57.2. Gross photograph demonstrating atrophy, fusion and fibrosis of ciliary processes in rabbit ciliary body 6 weeks after contact transscleral diode laser cyclophotocoagulation. From Schuman JS, Jacobson JJ, Puliafito CA, et al. Experimental use of semiconductor diode laser in contact transscleral cyclophotocoagulation in rabbits. Arch Ophthalmol 1990; 108(8):1152–1157.

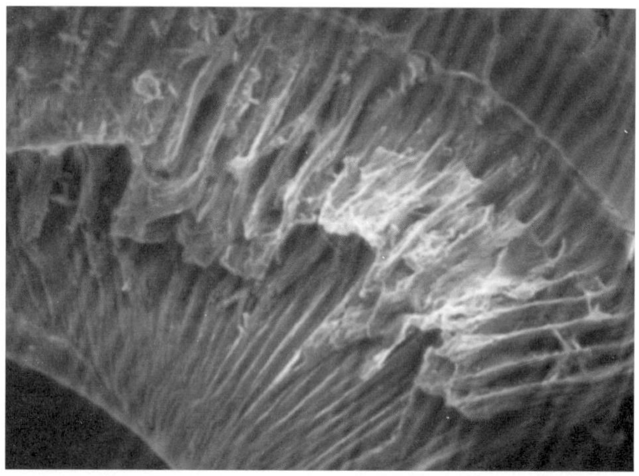

Figure 57.3. Scanning electron micrograph showing atrophy, fusion and fibrosis of rabbbit ciliary processes 6 weeks following contact transscleral diode laser cyclophotocoagulation. From Schuman JS, Jacobson JJ, Puliafito CA, et al. Experimental use of semiconductor diode laser in contact transscleral cyclophotocoagulation in rabbits. Arch Ophthalmol 1990; 108(8):1152–1157.

Clinical Studies

In 116 eyes of 114 patients followed for a minimum of one year after treatment with CYC, Schuman and coworkers in 1992 found that 3/4 of eyes achieved an average final IOP of 25 mm Hg or less, 2/3 22 mm or less, and over 1/2 of the eyes treated achieved a final IOP of 19 mm Hg or less (Table 57.2, Figs. 57.4, 57.5). **The major complications noted were hypotony and visual loss.** Nine eyes (8%) had a final IOP less than 3 mm Hg, with an IOP of 0 mm Hg in 6 eyes. Seventeen of 36 eyes (47%) with an initial visual acuity of 20/200 or better lost 2 or more Snellen lines. Nineteen eyes, all with an initial visual acuity of counting fingers or worse, progressed to no light perception. Retreatment was required in 31 eyes (27%) (84). The findings were similar to that group's earlier report in 1990, studying 160 treatments in 140 eyes of 136 patients (85). The interesting finding in comparing these two studies was that the success rates remained similar, but the rate of complications increased over time (84,85).

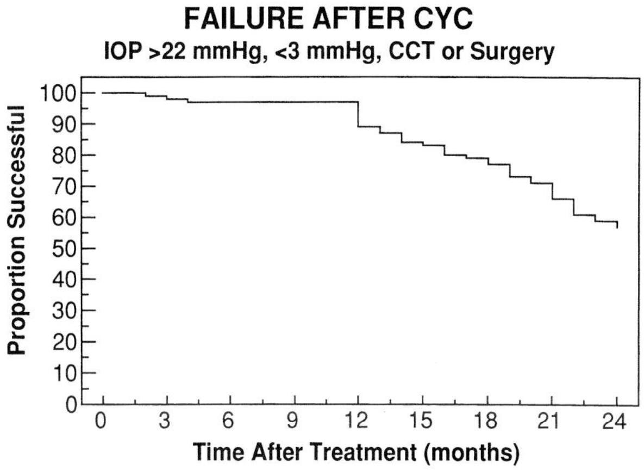

Figure 57.5. Kaplan-Meier survival curve for contact transscleral continuous wave Nd:YAG laser cyclophotocoagulation. From Schuman JS, Bellows AR, Shingleton BJ, Latina MA, Allingham RR, Belcher CD, Puliafito CA: Contact Transscleral Nd:YAG Laser Cyclophotocoagulation: Midterm Results. Ophthalmology 1992; 99 (7):1089-1094.

Table 57.2
Success Rates by Glaucoma Subtypes

	Ranges in mm Hg		
	3–25	3–22	3–19
Primary open angle glaucoma	78% (35/45)	68% (32/47)	60% (28/47)
Neovascular glaucoma	43% (10/23)	39% (9/23)	39% (9/23)
Glaucoma in aphakia or pseudophakia	76% (52/69)	69% (49/71)	63% (45/71)
Post penetrating keratoplasty	70% (7/10)	60% (6/10)	50% (5/10)

Success rates in four subtypes of glaucoma present in patients treated with contact transscleral Nd:YAG laser cyclophotocoagulation. Reprinted with permission from Schuman JS, Bellows AR, Shingleton BJ, et al. Contact Transscleral Nd:YAG Laser Cyclophotocoagulation: Midterm Results. Ophthalmology 1992; 99:1089–1094.

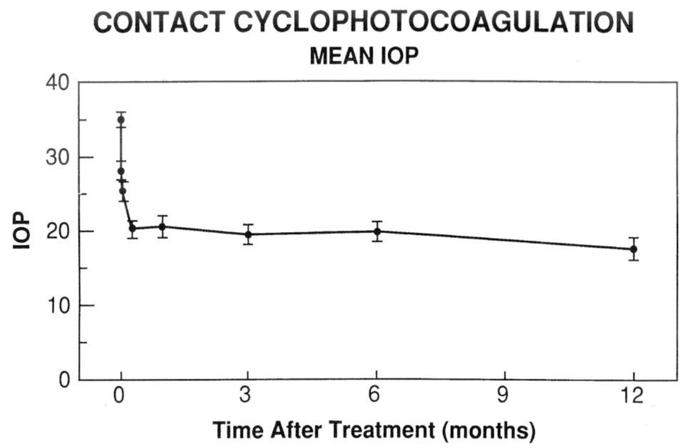

Figure 57.4. Intraocular pressure response to contact transscleral continuous wave Nd:YAG laser cyclophotocoagulation. IOP falls rapidly within first 1 to 4 weeks after treatment. From Schuman JS, Bellows AR, Shingleton BJ, Latina MA, Allingham RR, Belcher CD, Puliafito CA: Contact Transscleral Nd:YAG Laser Cyclophotocoagulation: Midterm Results. Ophthalmology 1992; 99 (7):1089-1094.

Brancato reported on CYC in 23 patients, using less energy and fewer spots. The success rate in this case was somewhat lower than that reported by Schuman, and retreatment was required in 57% of eyes (82).

The **contact diode laser** has been used clinically for cyclophotocoagulation (CDC), and was approved for this procedure by the US Food and Drug Administration in 1994. Gaasterland headed a multi-center clinical study of 30 eyes in 30 patients, and noted **results nearly identical to those encountered with CYC** (86). The treatment parameters for CDC, however, called for less energy and fewer spots than CYC, and the fact that similar clinical results could be achieved using these parameters suggested that CDC resulted in a larger area of tissue destruction per spot. Further, Carassa, using CDC, noted a 50% IOP lowering in 12 eyes of 12 patients, with 16 spots over 360 , using 2.5 watts for 1.5 seconds (3.75 J) (87).

NON-CONTACT CYCLOPHOTOCOAGULATION

Laboratory Studies

Non-contact Nd:YAG laser cyclophotocoagulation (NCYC) preceded CYC historically; however, it has proven to be a modality resulting in more inflammation and pain post-operatively than CYC. **CYC, therefore, is generally preferred to NCYC in treating patients.** Wilensky reported NCYC in rabbits in 1985 (88). Reports on histopathology of the laser lesions and the use of the technique in patients soon followed (52, 89–94).

Fankhauser demonstrated NCYC lesions in the ciliary body of human cadaver eyes using 6 to 7 joules aiming the spot ½ to 1 mm posterior to the limbus with maximum defocusing and a 20 millisecond pulse (95). Hampton and Shields showed that optimum parameters for treatment were an energy level of 8 joules delivered 1½ mm posterior to the limbus with maximum defocusing (96). They showed histologic damage to the iris when the beam was aimed more anteriorly, and pars plana lesions when the beam was aimed more posteriorly. No differences were seen when the energy was delivered tangentially versus perpendicular to the sclera. In a later study, Shields noted that a specialized contact lens could increase the efficiency and accuracy of laser delivery (97,98). Hampton and Shields found that tissue damage with NCYC differed from that seen with CYC: the destruction of the ciliary epithelium was accompanied by the creation of a blister-like space, and coagulation necrosis was not present (96). Similar findings have been seen *in vivo* in blind human eyes treated with NCYC just prior to enucleation for pain. In these cases, the blister-like space was filled with eosinophilic material (99).

NCYC in rabbits resulted in the acute destruction of the ciliary epithelium and the associated vessels, with subsequent atrophy of the ciliary processes one to two months after injury (52,89,90). The laser energy was absorbed by melanin; no histopathologic changes were seen in albino rabbits (100).

Unlike the effects seen with NCYC, non-contact transscleral diode laser cyclophotocoagulation (NCDC) resulted in a thermal ciliary body lesion (101). Hennis demonstrated thermal effects in the ciliary body with as little as 900 mJ energy with NCDC, using a spot size of 100 to 500 microns, with the beam 0.5 mm posterior to the limbus, defocused 1 mm posteriorly (102). In a study comparing CDC and NCDC in living rabbits using the same laser for both treatments, Shepps reported that 50% more energy was needed to create the same lesion with NCDC as compared to CDC (101). This is consistent with the findings on scleral light scattering presented by Vogel (51). In comparing NCDC to NCYC and CCT in cadaver eyes, Assia found that all were effective in ciliary body destruction, and none damaged the crystalline lens (103).

Clinical Studies

Cyrlin reported in 1985 that 60 to 70% of patients treated with NCYC had an IOP between 5 and 22 mm Hg at 6 to 12 months follow-up, using 8 J of energy, with 32 spots (93). In 1986, Schwartz and Moster found that 20 of 29 treated eyes (69%) had final IOPs of 22 mm Hg or less, and noted one questionable case of phthisis, with an average 32 week follow-up (104). Devenyi, using 40 spots at 1.8 to 3.0 J for 20 millisecond placed 2 to 3 mm posterior to the limbus with maximum defocusing, found that 11 of 24 eyes developed an IOP of 21 mm Hg or less, and that neovascular glaucoma eyes did somewhat worse than others (94). While Devenyi, with 8.8 months average follow-up, had no cases of phthisis, in a subsequent study on the same patient population, Trope and Ma reported a phthisis rate of 10.7%, and a 30% rate of visual loss, when the patients were followed for average of 21.9 months (105).

Klapper reported that 86% of treated eyes achieved an IOP between 5 and 22 mm Hg, with a mean decrease in IOP of 68%, with an average follow-up of 6 months. Klapper used 32 spots at 3.5 to 4.5 J for 20 milliseconds placed 2 to 3 mm posterior to the limbus with maximum defocusing (106).

Hampton reported on 100 NCYC treatments, and noted severe pain in 13.5%, severe inflammation in 28%, a retreatment rate of 25%, and visual loss in 50% (107). Wright noted that a majority of 35 eyes treated required further intervention, or lost vision if followed long enough, and that 31% of eyes lost two or more lines of vision or light perception over the three year follow-up period of their study (108).

Hennis and Stewart found a 30% reduction in IOP over a six month follow-up with a single NCDC treatment in 14 eyes, using 1.2 watts for 0.99 seconds (1.2 J) with 40 to 45 applications of a 100 micron spot placed 1 mm posterior to the limbus and defocused 1 mm posteriorly. Similar to NCYC, conjunctival burns occurred with NCDC, as well as anterior chamber inflammation (109).

Maus and Katz found severe hypotony, flat anterior chamber and serous choroidal detachment after NCYC in three patients, all of whom had previous filtering surgery; two of the patients were black (110). Fiore and co-workers reported focal scleral thinning following NCYC in one patient (111). Hardten and Brown reported malignant glaucoma following NCYC in one eye, (112) as did Wand, Schuman and Puliafito (113). Blomquist showed that NCYC could damage intraocular lens haptics in cadaver eyes at energy levels higher than those used clinically (114); Lim failed to damage intraocular lens haptics with CYC (115). Subretinal fibrosis and lens subluxation, while reported with cyclocryotherapy, (116,117) have not been found with Nd:YAG or diode laser cyclophotocoagulation.

Sympathetic ophthalmia is a controversial finding in association with cyclophotocoagulation. Reports of this complication have been in eyes having previous trauma or other ocular procedures, (118,119) and the relationship between cyclophotocoagulation and sympathetic ophthalmia is uncertain (120). Sympathetic ophthalmia has been described following cyclocryotherapy, (121) as well as after helium ion irradiation followed by cyclocryotherapy (122).

CYCLOPHOTOCOAGULATION VERSUS OTHER CYCLODESTRUCTIVE PROCEDURES

As a treatment of last resort, cyclocryotherapy (CCT) was an effective means to control IOP in eyes refractory to all other forms of treatment. Bellows and Grant showed that the IOP could be lowered in advanced, uncontrolled glaucoma, especially in aphakia, with CCT (23,24). Nevertheless, phthisis occurred in up to 12% of patients and visual loss in two-thirds of CCT treated eyes; this relegated CCT to the role of a treatment of last resort (23–27). **Transscleral laser cyclophotocoagulation destroys less tissue than CCT**, with similar effects on IOP in rabbits, as demonstrated by Higginbotham (124). NCYC may be as effective as CCT clinically, but produces fewer complications, as shown by Suzuki (125). Further, NCYC was demonstrated by Noureddin, in an uncontrolled retrospective study, to be superior to drainage implant surgery (126). Noureddin found that while both procedures lowered IOP, serious complications such as retinal detachment, expulsive hemorrhage, phthisis, and endophthalmitis were much more common in the tube treated group. In addition, the incidence of visual loss among tube treated eyes was higher than in eyes treated with NCYC. Both groups had similar post-operative IOPs in Noureddin's report.

CONTACT VERSUS NONCONTACT CYCLOPHOTOCOAGULATION

There are several differences between CYC and NCYC. CYC is performed with the patient supine, while NCYC is done with the patient at the slit lamp. The contact laser is portable, and can be used in remote locations, such as the operating room with the patient under general anesthesia, with relative ease. NCYC utilizes more energy, and significantly more power, than CYC, and results in more inflammation and pain post-operatively than CYC (52,82, 85,94,104,106,107).

CYC, NCYC, CDC, and NCDC all center the laser beam approximately 1.5 mm to the limbus (52,80,83,96). With the laser delivered via fiberoptic, as in CYC and CDC, the anterior edge of the probe is offset from the limbus to achieve beam placement. With the non-contact techniques, the laser is aimed approximately 1.5 mm posterior to the limbus. Schuman did not find any clinical differences in CYC treatments performed with the beam centered 1.5, 2.0 or 2.5 mm posterior to the limbus (84, 85, 123). Schubert, however, showed that NCYC and CYC lesions performed with the beam centered 3.0 mm posterior to the limbus caused lesions in the pars plana (127). He demonstrated that these lesions resulted in an increase in outflow facility (128), and this report was supported by Pham-Duy, who also showed that CCT increased outflow facility while transiently reducing aqueous flow (129). These studies, however, were limited by blood aqueous barrier disruption following CCT. Higginbotham demonstrated ciliary epithelial destruction in proportion to the degree of CCT, with consequent proportional effects on IOP and aqueous flow; however, Higginbotham did not study outflow facility (130). CYC has been shown to increase uveoscleral outflow in rabbits by Schmidt, possibly by an effect mediated by prostaglandins (131). In Schmidt's work, when IOP returned to normal, uveoscleral flow returned to baseline as well.

Contact cyclophotocoagulation appears to have several advantages over the non-contact modality. A longer exposure time is used for CYC as compared to NCYC. The histopathological change in CYC is coagulative necrosis, whereas explosive damage is seen with NCYC (73,80,96,97). With regard to the diode laser, both modalities use long exposure times; however, 50% more energy is required with NCDC to achieve the same lesion seen with CDC (101). In comparing the diode and Nd:YAG lasers, the diode laser has the advantage of greater absorption by melanin, and nearly equivalent scleral transmission when the sclera is compressed as it is for contact cyclophotocoagulation (51). The diode laser offers greater convenience and economy compared to the Nd:YAG laser. Anecdotally, there is less pain and inflammation with CYC as opposed to NCYC, which is most likely related to the histopathological changes noted above. The CYC unit is portable, and is present in many general hospitals, and is therefore more available than the NCYC unit. The diode unit, with its multitude of uses in ophthalmology, affords even greater flexibility to the ophthalmologist, as well as potentially greater availability. Any of the above cyclophotocoagulation techniques offer a titratable treatment that is generally well tolerated by the appropriately selected patient.

GLAUCOMA SUBTYPE AND THE PIGMENT EFFECT

Glaucoma subtype may be important in the response to cyclophotocoagulation. **Neovascular glaucoma, difficult to treat with any modality, responds least well of the glaucoma subtypes to cyclodestruction** (23,26), and eyes with neovascular glaucoma have the most severe and greatest number of complications (inflammation, pain, and visual loss). Neovascular glaucoma eyes have less IOP response to cyclophotocoagulation as well, although the difference in IOP response does not achieve statistical significance (84,85).

While aphakic eyes respond better to CCT than phakic eyes, this is not seen with CYC (24,84). Aphakic eyes do have less inflammation than others. **Cyclophotocoagulation seems to be an effective means of controlling IOP in eyes following penetrating keratoplasty** (85, 123–134).

Intraocular pigment is a significant factor in the response to cyclodestruction, and in subsequent complications. This has been seen with CCT, as noted by De Roetth, (21) and Cantor noted this in studying NCYC in pigmented and albino rabbits (100). Schubert and Federman reported this phenomenon in relation to cyclophotocoagulation, as well (73). Coleman found the pigment effect in cadaver eyes and in monkeys (135), and Schuman described this finding in relation to CYC (85). **Eyes with more pigment may require less energy for the same level of cyclodestruction than less heavily pigmented eyes,** as the pigment acts as a chromophore, absorbing the light energy and converting it to heat, with greater tissue damage at the same energy level in eyes with more pigment.

OPERATIVE TECHNIQUE

The treatment technique for laser cyclophotocoagulation is shown in Table 57.3, and the lasers in Figs. 57.6 and 57–7. All glaucoma medications are continued prior to laser treatment. Written informed consent is obtained, and retrobulbar or peribulbar anesthesia is administered. The contralateral eye is patched and the patient lies supine. A lid speculum is placed upon the eye receiving treatment, and surgeon and assistants wear protective eye glasses (blocking 1064 nanometers for the Nd:YAG laser, 800 nanometers for the diode laser). **Patients with neovascular glaucoma and non-white patients may develop fewer complications if treated with less power than that called for in the standard protocol** (5 to 6 watts instead of 7 watts for CYC, 2 to 2½ watts instead of 3 watts for CDC); however, this has not been systematically evaluated to date. For CYC, studies have evaluated the use of 32 spots (8 spots per quadrant), sparing the 3 and 9 o'clock meridians (Fig. 57.8). CDC has used 18 spots over 270 degrees. Fewer spots may be used, and Schuman and co-workers found no difference in the results of CYC with 24 versus 32 spots, either for IOP effects or for complications. The probe is centered 1½ mm posterior to the limbus (for CYC, the anterior edge of the probe is placed ½ to 1 mm posterior to the limbus) (Fig. 57.9). The offset from the limbus may be measured with calipers. The probe

Table 57.3
Laser Cyclophotocoagulation Technique

1. Continue all preoperative glaucoma medications prior to treatment.
2. Informed consent
3. Laser operational
4. Retrobulbar or peribulbar anesthesia
5. Patient recumbant for contact cyclophotocoagulation; sitting for non-contact treatment.
6. Laser settings:

Contact Nd:YAG: 7 watts, 0.7 seconds
Contact Diode: 3 watts, 1.3 seconds
With contact treatment, if pops are heard with three consecutive spots, decrease power by 0.5 watts.
Non-Contact Nd:YAG: 4–8 Joules; 20 millisecond exposure (thermal mode); maximum offset (9).

7. Treatment parameters

Nd:YAG: 32 spots over 360 ; 8 spots per quadrant, sparing 3 and 9 o'clock.
Diode: 18 spots over 270 , sparing inferonasal quadrant.

8. Spot location

Contact Nd:YAG: Anterior edge of probe 0.5–1.0 mm posterior to limbus. Measure with calipers. Press gently with probe during treatment throughout exposure, keeping the handpiece perpendicular to the sclera. Maintain contact throughout energy delivery.
Contact Diode: With G-Probe, place edge of handpiece at limbus, which centers fiberoptic 1.2 mm posterior to limbus. With each subsequent spot, the radial edge of the handpiece overlaps the previous spot, producing 18 spots over 270 . Press gently with probe during treatment throughout exposure, keeping the handpiece perpendicular to the sclera. Maintain contact throughout energy delivery.
Non-Contact Nd:YAG: Center beam 1.0–1.5 mm posterior to limbus, using calipers to measure for each spot; alternately, keeping the aiming beam in the center of a 3.0 mm slit beam placed with one edge on the limbus produces a displacement of 1.5 mm from the limbus.

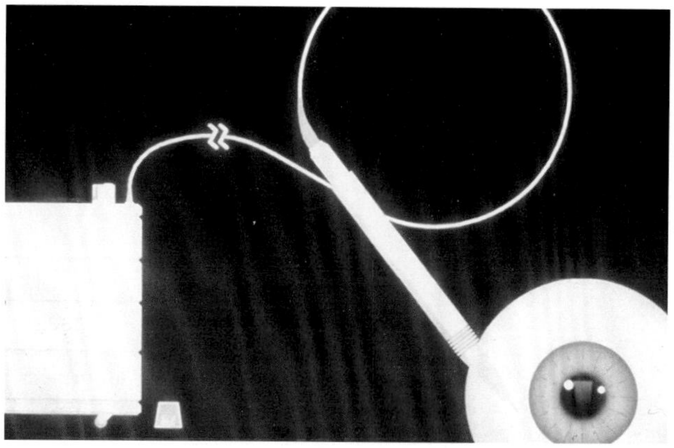

Figure 57.6. Schematic of contact transscleral Nd:YAG cyclophotocoagulation delivery system (Surgical Laser Technologies, Inc., Malvern, PA). Laser unit is portable. From Schuman JS, Puliafito CA: Laser Cyclophotocoagulation. International Ophthalmology Clinics 1990; 30:111-119.

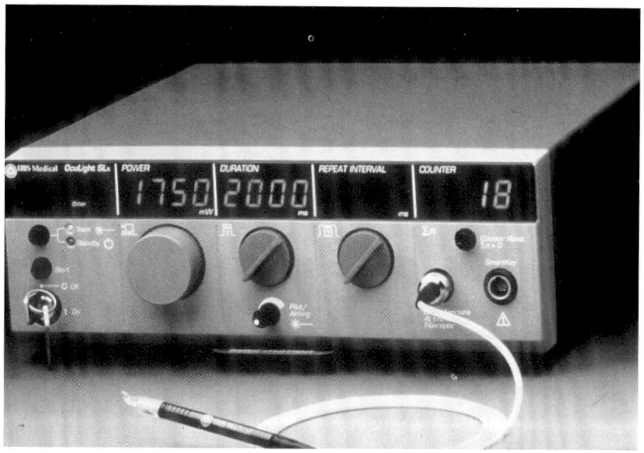

Figure 57.7. Diode laser unit (Oculight[R] SLx, Iris Medical Instruments, Mountain View, CA). Laser is small, lightweight, portable, air cooled, uses standard current and may be used for contact cyclophotocoagulation, transscleral retinopexy, adapted to a slit lamp or indirect ophthalmoscope or used as an endophotocoagulator. From Schuman JS, Puliafito CA: Laser Cyclophotocoagulation. International Ophthalmology Clinics 1990; 30: 111-119.

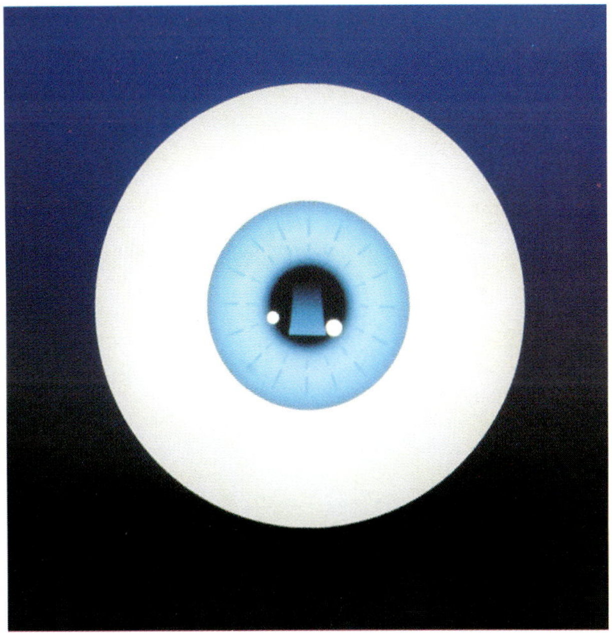

Figure 57.8. Pattern for non-contact or contact cyclophotocoagulation. Note that 3 and 9 o'clock meridians are spared treatment. From Schuman JS, Puliafito CA: Laser Cyclophotocoagulation. International Ophthalmology Clinics 1990; 30:111-119.

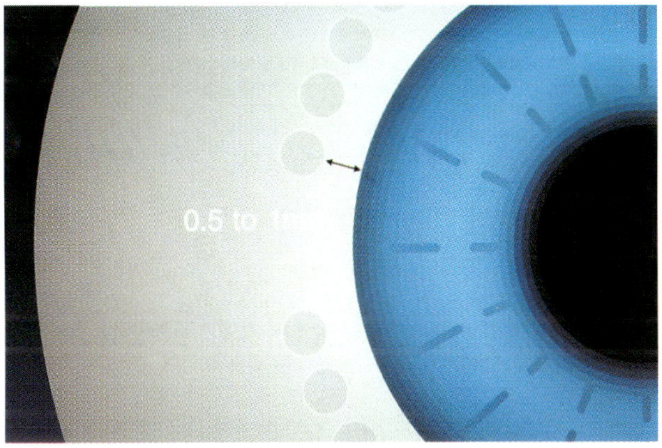

Figure 57.9. Distance of application from limbus for cyclophotocoagulation. Non-contact spots should be centered **1.0 to 1.5 mm** posterior to limbus (not shown). With contact transscleral Nd:YAG cyclophotocoagulation, the anterior edge of the probe should be placed **0.5 to 1.0 mm** posterior to the limbus (as illustrated). From Schuman JS, Puliafito CA: Laser Cyclophotocoagulation. International Ophthalmology Clinics 1990; 30:111-119.

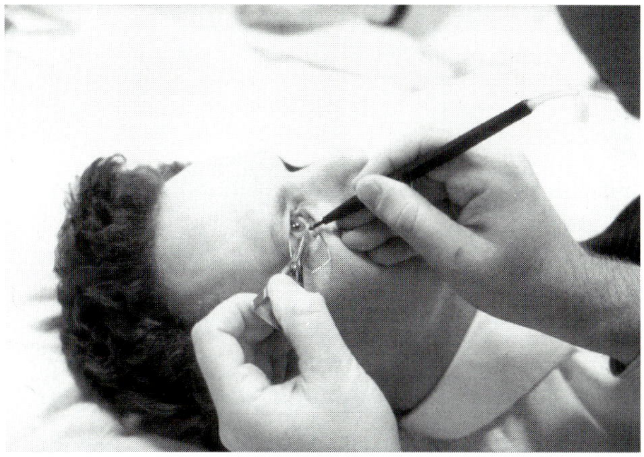

Figure 57.10. Patient is supine for treatment. A lid speculum is placed in the eye to be treated, and the probe is held perpendicular to the sclera. Contact between the probe and the eye is maintained throughout energy delivery. From Schuman JS, Puliafito CA: Laser Cyclophotocoagulation. International Ophthalmology Clinics 1990; 30:111-119.

is gently pressed against the eye, and kept perpendicular to the sclera, and contact with the eye is maintained throughout laser energy delivery (Fig. 57.10).

Power, duration, number of applications, distance from the limbus and the total energy delivered and treatment pattern are documented.

POSTOPERATIVE CARE

The treated eye is patched for six hours after cyclophotocoagulation following the instillation of prednisolone acetate 1% and atropine sulfate 1%. Prednisolone acetate 1% is applied four times a day and atropine sulfate 1% is given twice a day; both are tapered as the inflammation subsides. All preoperative glaucoma medications are continued with the exception of miotics, which may be reinstituted as the inflammation is reduced. The IOP should be checked postoperatively at one day and one week, and thereafter depending on the patient's clinical response.

RETREATMENT

At times, patients require **retreatment** due to inadequate response to cyclophotocoagulation. This **may be performed at one month postoperatively** (123). All parameters are identical to that for the initial treatment. There is no limit to the number of times that retreatment may be performed; however, each retreatment increases the possibility of phthisis.

CONCLUSIONS

Laser cyclophotocoagulation offers the opportunity to control IOP in eyes refractory to other forms of medical and surgical treatment. While cyclophotocoagulation is restricted to patients with the most advanced glaucoma, this therapeutic modality is the current state-of-the-art in cyclodestructive procedures, a treatment that has moved from cyclodiathermy through cyclocryotherapy to cyclophotocoagulation.

References

1. Weve H: Die Zyklodiatermie das Corpus ciliare bei Glaukom. Zentralbl Ophthalmol 1933;29:562–569.
2. Vogt A: Versuche zur intraokularen Druckherabsetzung mittels Diatermieschadigung des Corpus cilare (Zyklodiatermiestichelung). Klin Monatsbl Augenheilkd 1936;97:672–677.

3. Stocker F: Response of chronic simple glaucoma to treatment with cyclodiathermy puncture. Arch Ophthalmol 1945;34:181–189.
4. Lachman B, Rochwell P. Follow-up study of 39 patients with glaucoma treated with cyclodiathermy. Arch Ophthalmol 1953;50:265–266.
5. Nesterov A, Egorov E. Transconjunctival penetrating cyclodiathermy in glaucoma. J Ocular Ther Surg 1983;216–217.
6. Sheppard L: Retrociliary cyclodiathermy versus retrociliary cycloelectrolysis: Effects on the normal rabbit eye. Am J Ophthalmol 1958;46: 27–37.
7. Walton D, Grant W: Penetrating cyclodiathermy for filtration. Arch Ophthalmol 1970;83:47–48.
8. Pham L, Wang Y, Wang N, et al: Experimental nonpenetrating transscleral cyclodiathermy in rabbits. Ophthalmic Surg Lasers 1996;27: 301–307.
9. Berens C: Glaucoma surgery. Arch Ophthalmol 1955;54:548–563.
10. Oosterhuie J, Brihaye M, De Haan A: A comparative study of experimental transscleral cryocoagulation by solid carbon dioxide and diathermocoagulation of the retina. Ophthalmologica 1968;156:38–76.
11. Swan D, Christensen L: Ocular changes induced by diathermy in the treatment of retinal detachment. Trans Am Ophthalmol Soc 1954;52: 65.
12. deGuillebon H, Eng D, Ishii Y: Scleral changes during diathermy application. Arch Ophthalmol 1970;83:752–759.
13. deGuillebon H, Eng D, and Elzeneiny I: Electrical impedance of ocular coats during diathermy applications, voltage and time of application. Arch Ophthalmol 1970;83:489–503.
14. Elzeneiny I, deGuillebon H, Eng D: Scleral damage in diathermy. Am J Ophthalmol 1970;69:754–762.
15. Haik G, Breffeilh L, Barbar A: Beta irradiation as a possible therapeutic agent in glaucoma: An experimental study with the report of a clinical case. Am J Ophthalmol 1948;31:945–952.
16. Berens C, Sheppard L, Duel A, Jr: Cycloelectrolysis for glaucoma. Trans Am Ophthalmol Soc 1949;47:364–380.
17. Bietti G: Surgical intervention on the ciliary body: New trends for the relief of glaucoma. JAMA 1950;142:889–897.
18. Polack F, de Roetth A: Effect of freezing on the ciliary body (cyclocryotherapy). Invest Ophthalmol 1964;3:164.
19. McLean J, Lincoff H: Cryosurgery of the ciliary body. Trans Am Ophthalmol Soc 1964;62:385.
20. de Roetth A: Cryosurgery for the treatment of glaucoma. Trans Am Ophthalmol Soc 1965;63:189.
21. de Roetth A: Cryosurgery for the treatment of advanced simple glaucoma. Am J Ophthalmol 1968;66:1034.
22. Shields MB: Cyclodestructive surgery for glaucoma: past, present, and future. Transactions of the American Ophthalmological Society 1985; 83:285–303.
23. Bellows AR, Grant WM: Cyclocryotherapy in advanced inadequately controlled glaucoma. Am J Ophthalmol 1973;75:679.
24. Bellows AR, Grant WM: Cyclocryotherapy of chronic open-angle glaucoma in aphakic eyes. Am J Ophthalmol 1978;85:615–621.
25. Feibel R, Bigger J: Rubeosis iridis and neovascular glaucoma: Evaluation of cyclocryotherapy. Am J Ophthalmol 1972;74:862–867.
26. Krupin T, Mitchell K, Becker B: Cyclocryotherapy in neovascular glaucoma. Am J Ophthalmol 1978;86:24–26.
27. Brindley G and Shields M: Values and limitations of cyclocryotherapy. Graefe's Arch Clin Exp Ophthalmol 1986;224:545–548.
28. Benson M and Nelson M: Cyclocryotherapy: A review of cases over a 10-year period. Br J Ophthalmol 1990;74:103–105.
29. Gross R, Feldman R, Spaeth G, et al: Surgical therapy of chronic glaucoma in aphakia and pseudophakia. Ophthalmology 1988;95: 1195–1201.
30. Nissen O, Schiodte S, and Kessing S: Panretinal xenonphotocoagulation combined with cyclocryotherapy in the treatment of severe glaucoma. Acta Ophthalmol (Copenh) 1989;67:652–656.
31. Purnell E, Sokollu A, Torchia R, et al: Focal chorioretinitis produced by ultrasound. Invest Ophthalmol 1964;3:657–664.
32. Coleman D, Lizzi F, Driller J, et al: Therapeutic ultrasound in the treatment of glaucoma: I. Experimental model. Ophthalmology 1985; 92:339–346.
33. Coleman D, Lizzi F, Driller J, et al: Therapeutic ultrasound in the treatment of glaucoma: II. Clinical applications. Ophthalmology 1985; 92:347–353.
34. Coleman D, Lizzi F, Silverman R, et al: Treatment of glaucoma with high-intensity focused ultrasound. Ophthalmology 1986;93:831.
35. Margo C: Therapeutic ultrasound. Light and electron microscopic findings in an eye treated for glaucoma. Arch Ophthalmol 1986;104: 735–738.
36. Haut J, Colliac JP, Falque L, et al: Indications and results of Sonocare (ultrasound) in the treatment of ocular hypertension. A preliminary study of 395 cases. Ophtalmologie 1990;4(2):138–141.
37. Finger P, Smith P, Paglione R, et al: Transscleral microwave cyclodestruction. Invest Ophthalmol Vis Sci 1990;31:2151–2155.
38. Finger P, Moshfeghi D, Smith P, et al: Microwave cyclodestruction for glaucoma in a rabbit model. Arch Ophthalmol 1991;109:1001–1004.
39. Valtot F, Kopel J, and Le M: Principles and histologic effects of the treatment of hypertension with focused high-intensity ultrasound. Ophtalmologie 1990;4:135–137.
40. Freyler H and Scheimbauer I: Excision of the ciliary body (Sautter Procedure) as a last resort in secondary glaucoma. Klin Monatsbl Augenhielkd 1981;179:473–477.
41. Weekers R, Lavergne G, Watillion M, et al: Effects of photocoagulation of ciliary body upon ocular tension. Am J Ophthalmol 1961;52: 156–163.
42. Lee P-F and Pomerantzeff O: Transpupillary cylclophotocoagulation of rabbit eyes: An experimental approach to glaucoma surgery. Am J Ophthalmol 1971;71:911–920.
43. Shields MB: Intraocular cyclophotocoagulation. Transactions of the Ophthalmological Societies of the United Kingdom 1986;105 (Pt 2): 237–241.
44. Uram M: Ophthalmic laser microendoscope ciliary process ablation in the management of neovascular glaucoma. Ophthalmology 1992; 99(12):1823–1828.
45. Uram M: Laser endoscope in the management of proliferative vitreoretinopathy. Ophthalmology 1994;101(8):1404–1408.
46. Uram M. Diode laser endocyclodestruction [letter]. Ophthalmic Surgery 1994;25(4):268–269.
47. Beckman H, Kinoshita A, Rota AN, et al: Transscleral ruby laser irradiation of the ciliary body in the treatment of intractable glaucoma. Transactions—American Academy of Ophthalmology & Otolaryngology 1972;76(2):423–436.
48. Beckman H and Sugar HS: Neodymium laser cyclocoagulation. Archives of Ophthalmology 1973;90(1):27–28.
49. Beckman H and Waelterman J. Transscleral ruby laser cyclocoagulation. Am J Ophthalmol 1984;98:788–795.
50. Rol P, Niederer P, Durr P, et al: Experimental investigations on the light scattering properties of the human sclera. Lasers and Light in Ophthalmology 1990;3:201–221.
51. Vogel A, Dlugos C, Nuffer R, et al: Optical properties of human sclera and their significance for trans-scleral laser use. Fortschritte der Ophthalmologie 1991;88(6):754–761.
52. Fankhauser F, van der Zypen E, Kwasniewska S, et al: Transscleral cyclophotocoagulation using a neodymium YAG laser. Ophthalmic Surgery 1986;17(2):94–100.
53. Schuman J, Puliafito C, Allingham R, et al: A controlled clinical trial of diode versus argon laser trabeculoplasty. Ophthalmology 1990; 97(suppl):143.
54. Brancato R, Carassa R, Trabucchi G: Diode laser compared with argon laser for trabeculoplasty. Am J Ophthalmol 1991;112:50–55.
55. McHugh D, Marshall J, Ffytche J, et al: Diode laser trabeculoplasty for primary open angle glaucoma and ocular hypertension. Br J Ophthalmol 1990;74:743.

56. Jacobson J, Schuman J, el Khoumy H, et al: Diode laser peripheral iridectomy. Int Ophthalmol Clin 1990;30:120–122.
57. Schuman J, Jacobson J, and Puliafito C: Semiconductor diode laser peripheral iridotomy. Arch Ophthalmol 1990;108:1207–1208.
58. Emoto I, Okisaka S, and Nakajima A. Diode laser iridotomy in rabbit and human eyes. Am J Ophthalmol 1992;113:321–327.
59. Balles M, Puliafito C, D'Amico D, et al: Semiconductor diode laser photocoagulation in retinal vascular disease. Ophthalmology 1990; 97: 1553–1561.
60. Brancato R, Pratesi R, Leoni G, et al: Histopathology of diode and argon laser lesions in rabbit retina. A comparative study. Invest Ophthalmol Vis Sci 1989;30:1504–1510.
61. Duker J, Federman J, Schubert H, et al: Semiconductor diode laser endophotocoagulation. Ophthalmic Surg 1989;20:717–719.
62. Jennings T, Fuller T, Vukich J, et al. Transscleral contact retinal photocoagulation with an 810-nm semiconductor diode laser. Ophthalmic Surg 1990;21:492–496.
63. McHugh J, Marshall J, Ffytche T, et al: Initial clinical experience using a diode laser in the treatment of retinal vascular disease. Eye 1989.
64. Peyman G, Naguib K, and Gaasterland D: Trans-scleral application of a semiconductor diode laser. Lasers Surg Med 1990;10:569–575.
65. Puliafito C, Deutsch T, Boll J, et al: Semiconductor laser endophotocoagulation of the retina. Arch Ophthalmol 1987;105:424–427.
66. Sato Y, Berkowitz B, Wilson C, et al: Blood-retinal barrier breakdown caused by diode vs argon laser endophotocoagulation. Arch Ophthalmol 1992;110:277–281.
67. Suh J, Miki T, Obana A, et al: Effects of indocyanine green dye enhanced diode laser photocoagulation in non-pigmented rabbit eyes. Osaka City Med J 1991;37:89–106.
68. Wallow I, Sponsel W, and Stevens T: Clinicopathologic correlation of diode laser burns in monkeys. Arch Ophthalmol 1991;109:648–653.
69. Brancato R, Leoni G, Trabucchi G, et al: Transscleral contact cyclophotocoagulation with Nd:YAG laser CW: experimental study on rabbit eyes. International Journal of Tissue Reactions 1987;9 (6):493–498.
70. Federman J, Ando F, Schubert H, et al: Contact laser for transscleral photocoagulation. Ophthalmic Surg 1987;18:183–184.
71. Peyman GA, Katoh N, Tawakol M, et al: Transscleral and intravitreal contact Nd:YAG laser application. An experimental study. Retina 1987;7(3):190–197.
72. Schubert HD and Federman JL: The role of inflammation in CW Nd:YAG contact transscleral photocoagulation and cryopexy. Investigative Ophthalmology & Visual Science 1989;30(3):543–549.
73. Schubert HD and Federman JL: A comparison of CW Nd:YAG contact transscleral cyclophotocoagulation with cyclocryopexy. Invest Ophthalmol Vis Sci 1989;30(3):536–542.
74. Latina MA, Patel S, de Kater AW, et al: Transscleral cyclophotocoagulation using a contact laser probe: a histologic and clinical study in rabbits. Lasers in Surgery & Medicine 1989;9(5):465–470.
75. van der Zypen E, England C, Fankhauser F, et al: Cyclophotocoagulation in glaucoma therapy. International Ophthalmology 1989;13(1–2): 163–166.
76. van der Zypen E, England C, Fankhauser F, et al: The effect of transscleral laser cyclophotocoagulation on rabbit ciliary body vascularization. Graefes Archive for Clin Exp Ophthalmol 1989;227(2):172–179.
77. Brancato R, Leoni G, Trabucchi G, et al: Histopathology of continuous wave neodymium: yttrium aluminum garnet and diode laser contact transscleral lesions in rabbit ciliary body. A comparative study. Invest Ophthalmol Vis Sci 1991;32(5):1586–1592.
78. Schuman JS, Jacobson JJ, Puliafito CA, et al: Experimental use of semiconductor diode laser in contact transscleral cyclophotocoagulation in rabbits. Arch Ophthalmol 1990;108(8):1152–1157.
79. Iwach AG, Drake MV, Hoskins HD, Jr., et al: A new contact neodymium:YAG laser for cyclophotocoagulation. Ophthalmic Surgery 1991; 22 (6):345–348.
80. Allingham RR, de Kater AW, Bellows AR, et al: Probe placement and power levels in contact transscleral neodymium:YAG cyclophotocoagulation. Archives of Ophthalmology 1990;108(5):738–742.
81. Brancato R, Leoni G, Trabucchi G, et al: Probe placement and energy levels in continuous wave neodymium-YAG contact transscleral cyclophotocoagulation. Arch Ophthalmol 1990;108(5):679–683.
82. Brancato R, Giovanni L, Trabbuchi G, et al: Contact transscleral cyclophotocoagulation with Nd:YAG laser in uncontrolled glaucoma. Ophthalmic Surg 1989;20:547–551.
83. Schuman JS, Noecker RJ, Puliafito CA, et al: Energy levels and probe placement in contact transscleral semiconductor diode laser cyclophotocoagulation in human cadaver eyes. Arch Ophthalmol 1991;109(11): 1534–1538.
84. Schuman JS, Bellows AR, Shingleton BJ, et al: Contact transscleral Nd:YAG laser cyclophotocoagulation. Midterm results. Ophthalmology 1992;99(7):1089–1094; discussion 1095.
85. Schuman JS, Puliafito CA, Allingham RR, et al: Contact transscleral continuous wave neodymium:YAG laser cyclophotocoagulation. Ophthalmology 1990;97(5):571–580.
86. Gaasterland D, Abrams D, Belcher C, et al: A multicenter study of contact diode laser transscleral cyclophotocoagulation in glaucoma patients. Invest Ophthalmol Vis Sci 1992;33(suppl):1019.
87. Carassa R, Trabucchi G, Bettin P, et al: Contact transscleral cyclophotocoagulation (CTCP) with diode laser: a pilot clinical study. Invest Ophthalmol Vis Sci 1992;33 (suppl):1019.
88. Wilensky JT, Welch D, and Mirolovich M: Transscleral cyclocoagulation using a neodymium:YAG laser. Ophthalmic Surg 1985;16(2): 95–98.
89. England C, van der Zypen E, Fankhauser F, et al: Ultrastructure of the rabbit ciliary body following transscleral cyclophotocoagulation with the free-running Nd:YAG laser: Preliminary findings. Lasers Ophthalmol 1986;1:61–72.
90. Gross R, Smith J, Font R, et al: Transscleral Nd:YAG laser cycloablation in rabbits. Invest Ophthalmol Vis Sci 1986;27(suppl):253.
91. Devenyi RG, Trope GE, and Hunter WH: Neodymium-YAG transscleral cyclocoagulation in rabbit eyes. Br J Ophthalmol 1987;71 (6): 441–444.
92. Moster M, Schwartz L, Cantor L, et al: Treatment of advanced glaucoma with Nd:YAG laser cyclodiathermy. Invest Ophthalmol Vis Sci 1986; 27(Suppl):253.
93. Cyrlin M, Beckman H, and Czedik C: Neodymium:YAG transscleral cyclocoagulation for severe glaucoma. Invest Ophthalmol Vis Sci 1985; 26(suppl):253.
94. Devenyi R, Trope G, Hunter W, et al: Neodymium:YAG transscleral cyclocoagulation in human eyes. Ophthalmology 1987;94:1519–1522.
95. Fankhauser F, Kwasniewska S, and Van der Zypen E: Experimental and clinical use of the thermal mode neodymium:YAG laser. Klin Monatsbl Augenheilkd 1987;191:169–173.
96. Hampton C and Shields MB: Transscleral neodymium-YAG cyclophotocoagulation. A histologic study of human autopsy eyes. Arch Ophthalmol 1988;106(8):1121–1123.
97. Shields M, Blasini M, Simmons R, et al: A contact lens for transscleral Nd:YAG cyclophotocoagulation. Am J Ophthalmol 1989;08: 457–458.
98. Simmons RB, Blasini M, Shields MB, et al: Comparison of transscleral neodymium:YAG cyclophotocoagulation with and without a contact lens in human autopsy eyes. Am J Ophthalmol 1990;109(2):174–179.
99. Blasini M, Simmons R, and Shields MB: Early tissue response to transscleral neodymium: YAG cyclophotocoagulation. Investigative Ophthalmol Vis Sci 1990;31 (6):1114–1118.
100. Cantor L, Nichols D, Katz J, et al: Neodymium-YAG transscleral cyclophotocoagulation. The role of pigmentation. Invest Ophthalmol Vis Sci 1989;30:1834–1837.
101. Shepps G, Schuman J, Wang N, et al: Non-contact Versus Contact Semiconductor Diode Laser Transscleral Cyclophotocoagulation in Rabbits. Invest Ophthalmol Vis Sci 1991;32 (suppl):861.
102. Hennis HL, Assia E, Stewart WC, et al: Transscleral cyclophotocoagu-

lation using a semiconductor diode laser in cadaver eyes. Ophthalmic Surgery 1991;22(5):274–278.

103. Assia EI, Hennis HL, Stewart WC, et al: A comparison of neodymium: yttrium aluminum garnet and diode laser transscleral cyclophotocoagulation and cyclocryotherapy. Invest Ophthalmol Vis Sci 1991;32 (10): 2774–2778.

104. Schwartz L and Moster M: Neodymium:YAG laser transscleral cyclodiathermy. Ophthalmic Laser Ther 1986;1:135–141.

105. Trope G and Ma S: Mid term effects of Nd:YAG transscleral cyclocoagulation in glaucoma. Ophthalmology 1990;97:73–75.

106. Klapper R, Wandel T, Donnenfeld E, et al: Transscleral neodymium: YAG thermal cyclophotocoagulation in refractory glaucoma, a preliminary report. Ophthalmology 1988;95:719–722.

107. Hampton C, Shields M, Miller K, et al: Evaluation of a protocol for transscleral cyclophotocoagulation in 100 consecutive patients. Ophthalmology 1990;97:910–917.

108. Wright M, Grajewski A, and Feuer W: Nd:YAG cyclophotocoagulation: Outcome of treatment for uncontrolled glaucoma. Ophthalmic Surg 1991;22:279–283.

109. Hennis HL and Stewart WC: Semiconductor diode laser transscleral cyclophotocoagulation in patients with glaucoma. Am J Ophthalmol 1992;113(1):81–85.

110. Maus M and Katz L: Choroidal detachment, flat anterior chamber and hypotony as complications of Nd:YAG laser cyclophotocoagulation. Ophthalmology 1990;97:69–72.

111. Fiore P, Melamed S, Krug J: Focal scleral thinning after transscleral Nd:YAG cyclophotocoagulation. Ophthalmic Surg 1989;20:215–216.

112. Hardten D and Brown J: Malignant glaucoma after Nd:YAG cyclophotocoagulation [letter]. Am J Ophthalmol 1991;111:245–247.

113. Wand M, Schuman J, and Puliafito C: Malignant Glaucoma After Contact Transscleral Nd:YAG Laser Cyclophotocoagulation. Journal of Glaucoma 1993;2(2):110–111.

114. Blomquist P, Gross R, Koch D: Effect of transscleral neodymium: YAG cyclophotocoagulation on intraocular lenses. Ophthalmic Surg 1990; 21:223–226.

115. Lim E, Solomon K, Van Meter W, et al: Continuous wave transscleral Nd:YAG laser: A postmortem study of probe placement and destructive effects on tissue, transscleral sutured lenses and capsular bag fixated lenses. Invest Ophthalmol Vis Sci 1992;33(suppl):1268.

116. Kao S, Morgan C, Bergstrom T: Subretinal fibrosis following cyclocryotherapy. Case report. Arch Ophthalmol 1987;105:1175–1176.

117. Pearson P, Baldwin L, Smith T: Lens subluxation as a complication of cyclocryotherapy. Ophthalmic Surg 1989;20:445–446.

118. Bechrakis NE, Muller-Stolzenburg NW, Helbig H, et al: Sympathetic ophthalmia following laser cyclocoagulation. Arch Ophthalmol 1994; 112:80–84.

119. Edward D, Brown S, Higginbotham E, et al: Sympathetic ophthalmia following Nd:YAG cyclotherapy. Ophthalmic Surg 1989;20: 544–546.

120. Minckler D: Does Nd:YAG cyclotherapy cause sympathetic ophthalmia? Ophthalmic Surg 1989;20:543.

121. Sabates R: Choroiditis compatible with the histopathologic diagnosis of sympathetic ophthalmia following cyclocryotherapy of neovascular glaucoma. Ophthalmic Surg 1988;19:176–182.

122. Fries P, Char D, Crawford J, et al: Sympathetic ophthalmia complicating helium ion irradiation of a choroidal melanoma. Arch Ophthalmol 1987;105:1561–1564.

123. Schuman JS, Puliafito CA: Laser cyclophotocoagulation. Int Ophthalmol Clin 1990;30:111–119.

124. Higginbotham EJ, Harrison M, Zou XL: Cyclophotocoagulation with the transscleral contact neodymium: YAG laser versus cyclocryotherapy in rabbits. Ophthalmic Surg 1991;22:27–30.

125. Suzuki Y, Araie M, Yumita A, et al: Transscleral Nd: YAG laser cyclophotocoagulation versus cyclocryotherapy. Graefes Arch Clin Exp Ophthalmol 1991;229:33–36.

126. Noureddin B, Wilson-Holt N, Lavin M, et al: Advanced uncontrolled glaucoma: Nd:YAG cyclophotocoagulation or tube surgery. Ophthalmology 1992;99:430–437.

127. Schubert HD: Noncontact and contact pars plana transscleral neodymium: YAG laser cyclophotocoagulation in postmortem eyes. Ophthalmology 1989;96:1471–1475.

128. Schubert HD, Agarwala A, Arbizo V: Changes in aqueous outflow after in vitro neodymium: yttrium aluminum garnet laser cyclophotocoagulation. Invest Ophthalmol Vis Sci 1990;31:1834–1838.

129. Pham-Duy T: Cyclocryotherapy in chronic glaucoma. Fortschr Ophthalmol 1989;86:214–220.

130. Higginbotham E, Lee D, Bartels S, et al: Effects of cyclocryotherapy on aqueous humor dynamics in cats. Arch Ophthalmol 1988;106: 396–403.

131. Schmidt K, Lee P, Bhuyan D, et al: The role of prostaglandins (PGs) and uveoscleral outflow (Fu) in the reduction of intraocular pressure (IOP) after contact transscleral Nd:YAG laser cyclophotocoagulation (CYC) in pigmented rabbits. Invest Ophthalmol Vis Sci 1992; 33(suppl):1269.

132. Zaidman G, Wandel T: Transscleral YAG laser photocoagulation for uncontrollable glaucoma in corneal patients. Cornea 1988;112–114.

133. Levy NS, Bonney RC: Transscleral YAG cyclocoagulation of the ciliary body for persistently high intraocular pressure following penetrating keratoplasty. Cornea 1989;8:178–181.

134. Cohen EJ, Schwartz LW, Luskind RD, et al: Neodymium: YAG laser transscleral cyclophotocoagulation for glaucoma after penetrating keratoplasty. Ophthalmic Surg 1989;20:713–716.

135. Coleman A, Jampel H, Javitt J, et al; Transscleral cyclophotocoagulation of human autopsy and monkey eyes. Ophthalmic Surg 1991;22: 638–643.

Laser Sclerectomy

58

Joel S. Schuman

PRINCIPLES OF LASER SCLERECTOMY

Filtration surgery has been performed for nearly 100 years. The objective is to create a fistula between the anterior chamber and the subconjunctival space, thereby decreasing resistance to aqueous outflow, and lowering the intraocular pressure (IOP). The ultimate goal has always been the preservation of visual function.

In the early 1900s, an operation was described by Major Robert Elliot (1) using a trephine to create a full thickness sclerectomy. This procedure was modified by Scheie; he introduced the use of a thermal cautery in an effort to enhance the success of filtration surgery. The thermal sclerotomy was also a full thickness procedure. Posterior lip sclerectomy was introduced to simplify the sclerectomy procedure, by allowing the filtration surgery to be performed by a slit incision into the eye, with subsequent removal of the posterior scleral lip, minimizing the risk of incision into the ciliary body.

Perhaps the greatest advance in conventional filtration surgery was the introduction of the trabeculectomy, which is a guarded filtration procedure. In this operation, a partial thickness scleral flap is dissected anteriorly, and a block of corneoscleral tissue is removed underneath this flap. The flap is then sutured into place, providing some resistance to outflow, and helping to reduce hypotony, with its attendant risks.

All of these operations have potential complications. Leaks can occur at the conjunctival wound, or if the conjunctiva is inadvertently buttonholed during the dissection. Shallow or flat anterior chambers can occur, especially with the full thickness procedures. Hypotony is a serious problem, not in and of itself, but because it can lead to choroidal effusion and cataract. Choroidal effusion can lead to suprachoroidal hemorrhage, which may have disastrous results. In addition, any of these procedures can fail, primarily because of subconjunctival fibrosis, but also because of occlusion or closure of the scleral ostium, or due to episcleral fibrosis, especially with the trabeculectomy procedure.

Laser sclerectomy offers an alternative to conventional filtration surgery. When judging any alternative to what exists, one must assess the advantage of the new procedure over the existing one. Some laser sclerectomy techniques offer the advantage of fistulizing surgery with no conjunctival incision. Other techniques offer the advantage of minimal conjunctival manipulation. All of the laser sclerectomy procedures are in their youth, and long-term results are not yet available.

Laser sclerectomy may be performed either ab interno, from the inside out, or ab externo, from the outside in. Ab interno lasers include the continuous wave Nd:YAG laser (2–5), the Nd:YLF picosecond laser (6,7), the dye enhanced, flash lamp-pumped microsecond pulsed dye laser (8–10), the excimer laser (11), the diode laser, the erbium:YAG and erbium:YSGG lasers (12,13), the holmium:YAG (12,13), and the argon laser (14,15). Only the continuous wave Nd:YAG laser is approved by the United States Food and Drug Administration for ab interno laser sclerectomy. Ab externo lasers include the holmium:YAG (16–18), the erbium:YAG and erbium:YSGG lasers (12,13), the excimer laser (19,20), and the diode laser. In this group, only the holmium:YAG laser is approved by the United States Food and Drug Administration for laser sclerectomy.

These lasers offer the potential for little or no conjunctival manipulation, through the lack of a conjunctival incision with the ab interno techniques, or a small conjunctival incision with the holmium, erbium, and diode laser ab externo techniques. The small or absent conjunctival incision minimizes or eliminates the risks of a conjunctival wound leak, perhaps permitting the earlier use of 5-fluorouracil or other antimetabolites. In addition, these lasers offer access to surgically difficult areas for conventional surgery, and the procedures are often technically simpler than conventional surgery.

On the downside, **the laser sclerectomy techniques represent a return to full thickness filtration surgery, with all of the risks attendant, including flat chambers, hypotony, suprachoroidal hemorrhage and cataract formation.** Additionally, the ab externo techniques often do not permit an iridectomy at the time of surgery, resulting in a potential for occlusion of the sclerectomy site by iris.

HOLMIUM LASER SCLERECTOMY

The holmium laser has a 2.1 micron wavelength, which is highly absorbed in water, within 330 microns. One instrument that has been approved by the United States Food and Drug Administration is the Sunrise gLase 210 (Sunrise Technologies, Fremont, CA), which has a side firing fiberoptic, with the diameter of a 22 gauge needle. This is a portable, solid state laser that has self-contained cooling, and uses standard current. In addition, the set up is menu driven.

For this procedure, a retrobulbar or peribulbar anesthetic is required. The surgical site is sterilely prepared, and a lid speculum is used. A bridle suture may be used if needed. A paracentesis is always performed, so as to inflate the eye after sclerectomy, and to ensure patency of the sclerectomy site. The conjunctiva is ballooned with viscoelastic, and the laser fiberoptic is inserted through a 1 to 2 mm conjunctival opening, which has been made 10 to 15 mm posterior to the proposed sclerectomy site. The fiberoptic is advanced subconjunctivally to the fistula site. It is important to be as anterior as possible without compromising the conjunctival insertion, and care should be taken not to buttonhole the conjunctiva while advancing the probe. With the side-firing probe tip tangential to the limbus, **the probe is rotated so that the aiming beam is as parallel as possible to the iris.** The laser is set at 100 mJ per pulse; the instrument fires at 5 pulses per second. The laser will stop firing after 20 pulses, and the foot pedal must be depressed again if more shots are required. In most cases, the sclerectomy can be performed with 20 to 30 shots.

The surgeon will know that the sclerectomy is patent by three signs. Small bubbles will appear in the anterior chamber. The sound of the laser will change from dull to sharp, and upon removal of the probe, a good bleb will be seen to form. In addition, on inflation of the eye with balanced salt solution through the paracentesis, the bleb will enlarge.

The wound is closed with 10-0 nylon or 9-0 vicryl. Usually, just one stitch is necessary. The wound should be checked for leaks with balanced salt solution through the paracentesis site and 2% fluorescein at the conjunctival wound. Antibiotic and steroid ointments are used on the eye, the eye is patched, and the patient is followed as for full-thickness filtering surgery.

Holmium laser sclerectomy has the advantages of a small conjunctival wound and minimal conjunctival manipulation making wound leaks less likely (Table 58.1). This may result in less episcleral and subconjunctival fibrosis, with less risk of failure. In addition, easier access than with conventional surgery is possible in previously operated areas, as the conjunctiva is elevated with viscoelastic, without the need for dissection. The side-firing fiberoptic allows access to areas otherwise difficult to operate in, including the inferior and inferonasal areas. Surgical time is short with the holmium laser, and this procedure may be performed in a minor operating room, although patients still require close monitoring and minimal activity postoperatively.

The risks of this procedure include hypotony, shallow or flat anterior chamber, choroidal effusion, suprachoroidal hemorrhage, occlusion of the sclerectomy site by iris, cataract, and conjunctival buttonhole at the time of sclerectomy (Table 58.2). Should the iris occlude the ostium, it may be possible to retract the iris from the fistula site with the argon laser, or to cut the iris with the Nd:YAG laser.

In a study of holmium YAG laser sclerectomy (18) on 49 eyes of 46 patients with a 1 year follow-up, the mean preoperative IOP was approximately 27 mm Hg and the mean postoperative IOP was 19.7 mm Hg (Figs. 58.1 and 58.2). Nearly ⅔ of the eyes achieved a final IOP of 5 to 22 mm Hg, and 73% of the eyes treated adjunctively with 5-fluorouracil achieved a final IOP of 21 mm Hg or less, which is identical to the results found by the 5-fluorouracil surgery study group (21). No median change in visual acuity was noted. **Suprachoroidal hemorrhage occurred in 14% of all eyes; in aphakic eyes, suprachoroidal hemorrhage occurred in 33%.**

We are currently investigating the use of mitomycin C applied at the time of holmium YAG laser sclerectomy, randomized against the use of 5-fluorouracil postoperatively with this procedure (Fig. 58.3), and a new guarded technique for laser sclerectomy (Table 58.3). The results to date are encouraging (22).

CONTINUOUS WAVE ND:YAG LASER SCLERECTOMY

The continuous wave Nd:YAG laser has multiple uses in ophthalmology, including laser sclerectomy and laser cyclophotocoagulation. In addition, it is useful in several surgical disciplines, including plastic surgery, general surgery, obstetrics and gynecology and urology. The Nd:YAG

Table 58.1
Advantages of Laser Sclerectomy

Little or no conjunctival manipulation theoretically means less stimulation for subconjunctival fibrosis and bleb failure.
A small or absent conjunctival incision minimizes the risk of wound leak.
Lasers provide access to surgically difficult areas.
Laser sclerectomy is often simpler than conventional surgery.
Surgical time is rapid.

Table 58.2
Disadvantages of Laser Sclerectomy

A return to full thickness filtration surgery, with risks of flat chamber, hypotomy, suprachoroidal hemorrhage and cataract formation.
Success rate lower than trabeculectomy with mitomycin C.
It is difficult, if not impossible, to perform an iridectomy with most of these procedures, introducing the risk of occlusion of the sclerectomy site.
At 50–200 microns, the sclerectomy may be small enough to allow closure by scleral fibroblasts, which is rarely a problem with conventional surgery where the ostium is often greater than 1 mm in size.

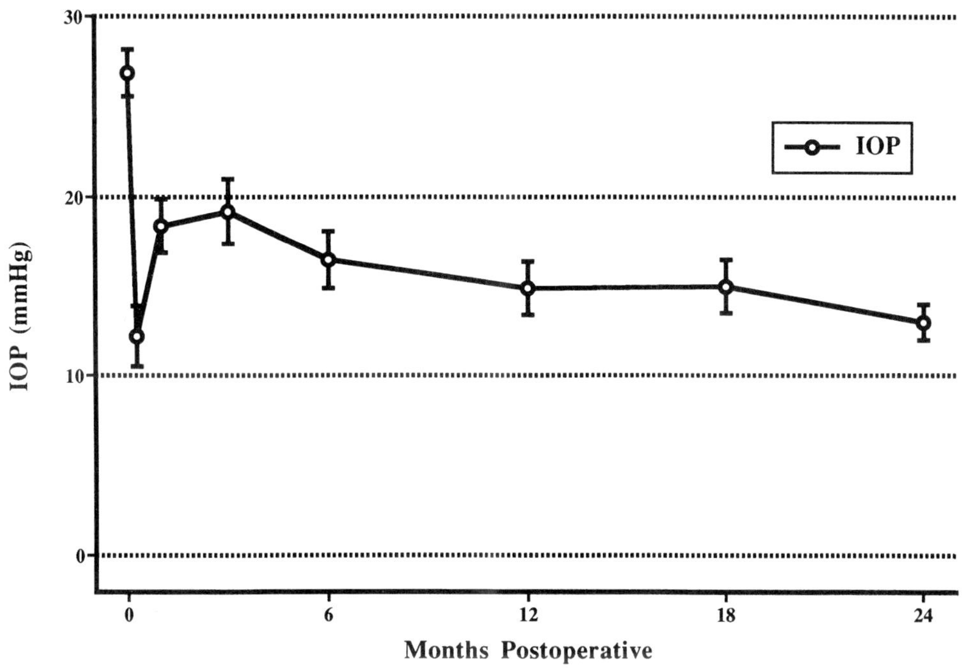

Figure 58.1. Intraocular pressure (IOP) response to holmium YAG laser sclerectomy. Notice the rapid fall in IOP with stabilization over 3 to 6 months. From Schuman JS, Stinson WG, Hutchinson BT, Bellows AR, Puliafito CA, Lytle R: Holmium Laser Sclerectomy: Success and Complications. Ophthalmology 1993;100:1060–1065.

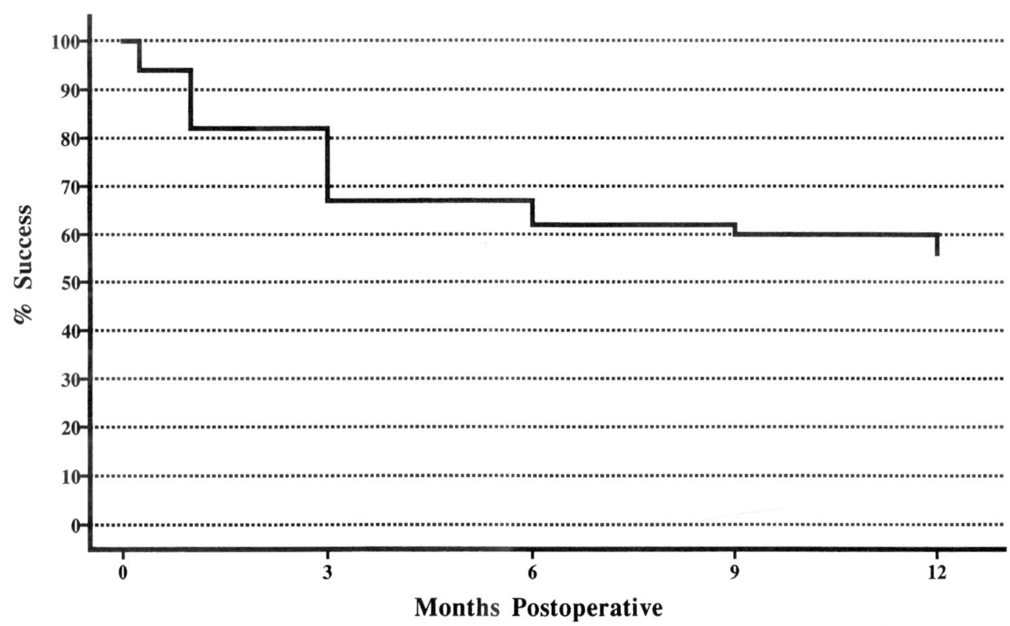

Figure 58.2. Kaplan-Meier survival curve demonstrates success of holmium YAG laser sclerectomy with final IOP of 5 to 19 mm Hg. Most failures occur within the first 3 months postoperatively. From Schuman JS, Stinson WG, Hutchinson BT, Bellows AR, Puliafito CA, Lytle R: Holmium Laser Sclerectomy: Success and Complications. Ophthalmology 1993;100:1060–1065.

laser has a wavelength of 1064 nanometers, which is well absorbed by water. Sclerectomy with the continuous wave YAG laser, as with the holmium laser, is thermal.

Continuous wave Nd:YAG laser sclerectomy ab interno is described in detail in the following chapter, as is ab interno gonioscopic laser sclerectomy. Results with the continuous wave Nd:YAG laser have indicated a success rate of 50 to 70% (5). The risks and benefits of the procedure are similar to those outlined for holmium YAG laser sclerectomy outlined.

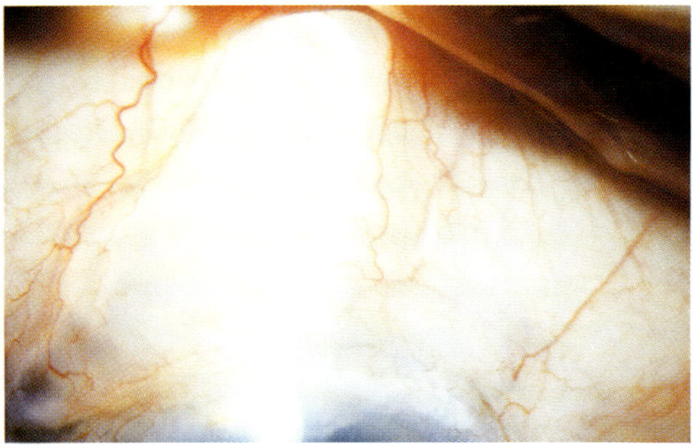

Figure 58.3. Appearance of eye one year after holmium laser sclerectomy with transconjunctival mitomycin C. This eye sustained successful control of IOP on no medications. Sausage shaped bleb is in the shape of the tract created by viscoelastic used to expand conjunctiva at the time of surgery.

Table 58.3
Goals for the Future

A guarded laser sclerectomy procedure, one that will minimize or eliminate the problems of full thickness filtering surgery.
A laser procedure that is analogous to trabeculectomy with laser suture lysis, one where the intraocular pressure can be titrated postoperatively.
Appropiate selection of antimetabolites and their delivery. The postoperative use of 5-fluorouracil and the intraoperative use of mitomycin C (MMC) enhance the success of laser sclerectomy, but subconjunctival delivery of MMC with laser sclerectomy is difficult. We and others have investigated transconjunctival application and found it useful in animals and humans; however, there may be other, better antimetabolites to be discovered that will further enhance the success of this procedure, and reduce the complications attendant to their use.

EXPERIMENTAL TECHNIQUES

Ab Interno Techniques

The pulsed dye laser has been investigated for ab interno laser sclerectomy through a goniolens (8–10). The advantage of this procedure is that no incision is made in the eye at all. Successful sclerectomy is performed in 50% of eyes undergoing this procedure, and 50% of those eyes have IOP control at 9 months; 25% of eyes have adequate IOP control with this technique at 15 months (10). This technique is described in the next chapter.

The picosecond Nd:YLF laser is currently under investigation for ab interno sclerectomy through a gonioscopic lens. The primary advantage of this laser is that by using a very short pulse length, very little energy is required to achieve optical breakdown in tissue, and the cavitation bubble created is on the order of 100 μm. No dye is required with the picosecond laser (6,7). Preliminary studies are encouraging; however, this procedure is still in its infancy.

Ab Externo Techniques

The excimer laser is currently being studied for sclerectomy (19,20). This laser offers the advantage of performing a partial thickness sclerectomy, as the excimer laser wavelength of 193 nanometers causes the ablation of tissue to essentially stop once aqueous is reached. This means that when a sclerectomy is performed, the ablation stops once the surgeon enters the trabecular meshwork. The theoretical advantage is that some trabecular tissue remains, perhaps providing some additional resistance to outflow, and decreasing the risk of hypotony. Unfortunately, these potential advantages have not been borne out in clinical studies.

The picosecond Nd:YLF may also be used for ab externo sclerectomy, and readily ablates scleral tissue (7). Ab externo approaches with both the picosecond and excimer lasers require the creation of a conjunctival flap, as they cannot ablate scleral tissue beneath conjunctiva without damaging the overlying conjunctiva itself.

CONCLUSIONS

Laser sclerectomy may represent the next step in glaucoma filtration surgery, from trephination through thermal sclerostomy to posterior lip sclerectomy to trabeculectomy. Laser sclerectomy offers several advantages. That there is little or no conjunctival manipulation theoretically means less stimulation for subconjunctival fibrosis and bleb failure. A small or absent conjunctival incision minimizes the risk of wound leak. Lasers provide access to surgically difficult areas. Laser sclerectomy is often simpler than conventional surgery, and the surgical time is rapid.

Despite this, laser sclerectomy is a step backwards to full-thickness filtering surgery, with all of its attendant risks. It is difficult, if not impossible, to perform an iridectomy with most of these procedures, introducing the risk of occlusion of the sclerectomy site. Finally, at 50–200 microns, the sclerectomy may be small enough to allow closure by scleral fibroblasts, rarely a problem with conventional surgery, where the ostium is often greater than 1 mm in size.

Work remains to be done in refining laser sclerectomy techniques (Table 58.3). **We no longer perform full-thickness laser sclerectomy for any indication.** For laser sclerectomy to become a procedure in which the benefit of surgery outweighs the risks, several advances are required. We must develop a guarded laser sclerectomy procedure that is analogous to trabeculectomy with laser suture lysis, one where the IOP can be titrated postoperatively, one that will minimize or eliminate the problems of full thickness filtering surgery. Antimetabolite selection and delivery must be refined. The postoperative use of 5-Fluorouracil and the intraoperative use of mitomycin C (MMC) enhance the success of laser sclerectomy, but subconjunctival delivery of MMC with laser sclerectomy is difficult. We and others have investigated transconjunctival application and found it useful in animals and humans (22); however, there may be other, better antimetabolites to be discovered that will further enhance the success of this procedure, and reduce the complications attendant to their use.

Perhaps some day all filtering surgery will be done with a laser. For now, however, conventional surgery offers superior success rates with fewer complications than laser sclerectomy.

References

1. Elliot RH: Preliminary note on a new operative procedure for the establishment of a filtering cicatrix in the treatment of glaucoma. Ophthalmoscope 1909;7:804.
2. Federman JL, Wilson RP, Anso F, et al: Contact laser thermal sclerostomy ab interna. Ophthalmic Surg 1987;18:726–727.
3. Higginbotham EJ, Kao G, Peyman G: Internal sclerostomy with the Nd:YAG contact laser versus thermal sclerostomy in rabbits. Ophthalmology 1988;95:385–390.
4. Javitt JC, O'Connor SS, Wilson RP, et al: Laser sclerostomy ab interno using a continuous wave Nd:YAG laser. Ophthalmic Surg 1989;20: 552–556.
5. Wilson RP, Javitt JC: Ab interno laser sclerostomy in aphakic patients with glaucoma and chronic inflammation. Am J Ophthalmol 1990;110: 178–184.
6. Zysset B, Fujimoto JG, Puliafito CA, et al: Picosecond optical breakdown: tissue effects and reduction of collateral damage. Lasers Surg Med 1989;9:193–204.
7. Cooper HM, Schuman JS, Puliafito CA, et al: Picosecond Nd:YLF sclerectomy. Am J Ophthalmol 1993;115:221–224.
8. Latina MA, Goode S, de Kater AW, et al: Experimental ab interno sclerotomies using a pulsed-dye laser. Lasers Surg Med 1988;8:233–240.
9. Latina MA, Dobrogowski M, March WF, et al: Laser sclerostomy by pulsed-dye laser and goniolens. Arch Ophthalmol 1990;108: 1745–1750.
10. Latina MA, Melamed S, March WF, et al: Gonioscopic ab-interno laser sclerostomy: a pilot study in glaucoma patients. Ophthalmology 1992; 99:1736–1744.
11. Muller-Stolzenburg M, Muller GJ: Transmission of 308 nm excimer laser radiation for ophthalmic microsurgery—medical, technical and safety aspects. Biomed-Tech (Berlin) 1989;34:131–138.
12. Ozler SA, Hill RA, Andrews JJ, et al: Infrared laser sclerostomies. Invest Ophthalmol Vis Sci 1991;32:498–503.
13. Gaasterland DE, Hennings DR, Boutacoff TA, et al: Ab interno and ab externo filtering operations by laser contact surgery. Ophthalmic Surg 1987;18:254.
14. Jaffe GJ, Williams GA, Mieler WF, et al: Ab interno sclerostomy with a high-powered argon endolaser. Am J Ophthalmol 1988;106:391–396.
15. Jaffe GJ, Mieler WF, Radius RL, et al: Ab interno sclerostomy with a high-powered argon endolaser. Clinicopathologic correlation. Arch Ophthalmol 1989;107:1183–1185.
16. Hoskins HD, Iwach AG, Drake MV, et al: Subconjunctival THC:YAG laser limbal sclerostomy ab externo in the rabbit. Ophthalmic Surg 1990; 21:589–592.
17. Hoskins HD, Iwach AG, Vassiliadis A, et al: Subconjunctival THC: YAG laser thermal sclerostomy. Ophthalmology 1991;98:1394–9.
18. Schuman JS, Stinson WG, Hutchinson BT, et al: Holmium Laser Sclerectomy: Success and Complications. Ophthalmology 1993;100: 1060–1065.
19. Seiler T, Kriegerowski M, Bende T, et al: Partial external trabeculectomy. Klin Monatsbl Augenheilkd 1989;195:216–220.
20. Aron-Rosa D, Maden A, Ganem S, et al: Preliminary study of argon fluoride (193 nm) excimer laser trabeculectomy. Scanning electron microscopy at five months. J Cataract Refract Surg 1990;16:617–620.
21. Fluorouracil Filtering Surgery Study Group: Fluorouracil filtering surgery study one-year follow-up. Am J Ophthalmol 1989;108:625–635.
22. Schuman JS, Namazi N, Wang N, et al: Transconjunctival mitomycin C with holmium laser sclerectomy in rabbits and humans. Invest Ophthalmol Vis Sci 1993(suppl),:1808.

Ab Interno Laser Sclerectomy

59

Eve J. Higginbotham

The most common cause of failure following filtration surgery has been demonstrated to be episcleral scarring due to fibroblastic proliferation (1). There have been several approaches which have been described to circumvent this problem. Two recent approaches are 1) the use of antimetabolites as a method of modulating the fibroblastic response following surgery (2) and 2) minimization or elimination of conjunctival dissection at the time of surgery in order to diminish the effects of one possible stimulus for fibroblastic proliferation, excessive dissection and handling of the conjunctiva and Tenon's fascia (3). Techniques which aim to minimize conjunctival manipulation also offer the advantage of facilitating access to otherwise unreachable areas of conjunctiva which are still virgin, such as the nasal conjunctiva. This section will describe those techniques which utilize an *ab interno* approach as a method for using these latter advantages.

LASER *AB INTERNO* TECHNIQUES

Noninvasive

This approach (4–8) has the advantage of being noninvasive and can be accomplished in an outpatient setting. However, the disadvantage is that excellent clarity of the media is required to clearly identify the target tissue. In those eyes which have undergone several previous surgical procedures, the media may not be clear enough to perform this procedure. Initial investigations were reported by March and colleagues (4) who indicated that high levels of energy were required to penetrate the sclera. Using the Microrupter Nd:YAG laser (LASAG), one may need to use as much as 27 joules to create the sclerectomy, which often results in damage to surrounding tissues. The technique was improved by Latina and coworkers (5) who described a dye-enhanced sclerectomy technique. The details of this technique are described in the following clinical panel.

Invasive

Invasive laser sclerostomy has been evaluated in an animal model using the Nd:YAG (3), the diode (9), argon (10), and excimer (11) lasers. The advantage of this approach compared to conventional filtration surgery has been evaluated with both Nd:YAG and diode lasers. The laser technique was superior to the conventional technique in certain laboratory studies. In the case of the Nd:YAG laser, fifteen rabbits underwent internal laser sclerectomy, requiring 9 to 15 joules each, while twelve underwent conventional external thermal sclerectomy. The procedures were done in one eye of each animal and the fellow eyes remained as unoperated controls. When intraocular pressure (IOP) differed by 3 mm Hg or less between the operated and fellow unoperated eye, digital compression was applied twice to both eyes. If this failed to produce a difference of more than 3 mm Hg between the two eyes on two occasions within two days, the filter was considered failed. None of the laser treated eyes required digital compression during the first week; however, 75% of the standard thermal sclerostomy eyes did require digital compression. By the thirteenth day postoperatively, all of the thermal sclerectomy eyes had failed, whereas 80% of the laser sclerectomy eyes were still functioning at 21 days and two at 28 days. Histologically, there was greater cellular reaction within the conjunctiva of the thermal sclerectomy group versus the laser group (3).

Although animal studies have been encouraging, clinical use of this technique has not proven to be as successful as conventional surgery. Wilson and Javitt (12) reported a series of five aphakic patients with glaucoma who underwent successful Nd:YAG laser *ab interno* sclerectomy. At a mean follow-up of 25 months, three of five patients demonstrated a successful outcome with an average IOP of 15 mm Hg. Liu and Higginbotham (13) also reported their experience with Nd:YAG laser *ab interno* sclerotomy using a synthetic sapphire-tipped laser scalpel in four aphakic human eyes. An average decrease in IOP measuring 14 mm Hg was noted at a mean postoperative interval of 4.5 months. One patient with a history of uveitis developed hypotony and was excluded from the analysis of IOP; two patients without blebs were successfully managed medically. One patient remained well controlled off medications with a functioning bleb.

Indications

Based on the only fair results of Nd:YAG laser sclerectomy, the indications for *ab interno* laser sclerectomy are conservative. Patients who have failed previous filtration surgery with antimetabolites may be considered candidates. Also, patients who may be under consideration for shunt placement, such as Molteno or Baerveldt, may be candidates. This procedure may be considered prior to cycloablative

GONIOSCOPIC AB INTERNO SCLEROSTOMY

Mark A. Latina

Gonioscopic laser sclerostomy was developed to perform glaucoma filtration surgery in an outpatient setting with the patient at a slit-lamp. A laser has been used so that no instruments or devices entered the eye. It has been the goal of many ophthalmologists and glaucoma specialists to improve the success and reduce the risks and complications of filtration surgery. Therefore, the ability to perform filtration surgery using only laser light to penetrate the eye is very appealing because the risks of entering the eye with instruments is eliminated, and many of the sequelae associated with conjunctival incisions and conjunctival manipulation should be minimized.

To create a fistula or channel connecting the anterior chamber to the subconjunctival space using laser energy delivered gonioscopically requires removal (ablation) of sclera. The optical requirements for the technique are: 1) the wavelength of laser light must be transmitted by the cornea, 2) the laser energy can be delivered to the angle of the anterior chamber with a gonioscopy-type lens, 3) the sclera absorbs sufficient laser energy to result in ablation.

To meet the requirements stated above and to maximize the efficiency and effectiveness of scleral ablation, Latina and associates (1) introduced the concept of "dye-enhanced scleral ablation" using a flashlamp pumped dye laser, also called a pulsed dye laser. This laser emits visible light which is readily transmitted by the cornea and can be tuned to various wavelengths. However, visible light is poorly absorbed by the sclera. To enhance the optical absorption of sclera, methylene blue dye, a water soluble dye with an absorption peak of 688 nm, was non-invasively deposited into the sclera using iontophoresis. By matching the output of the pulsed dye laser to the absorption peak of the methylene blue dye (668 nm) and by utilizing a short pulse duration (7 microseconds), ablation of sclera and formation of a full-thickness fistula can be achieved in less than 20 pulses. Utilizing a short pulse duration also minimizes thermal damage to the surrounding sclera. The technique is schematically shown in Figure 59.1.

The safety and efficacy of gonioscopic *ab interno* laser sclerostomy was studied in 35 glaucoma patients (2). Briefly, patients who would normally be eligible for glaucoma filtration surgery were considered eligible for inclusion into the study. Iontophoresis of methlyene blue dye (1%) into the sclera at the limbus was performed at the slit-lamp following instillation of topical proparacaine and application of topical cocaine 4% to the site where the sclerotomy was to be performed. Penetration of dye

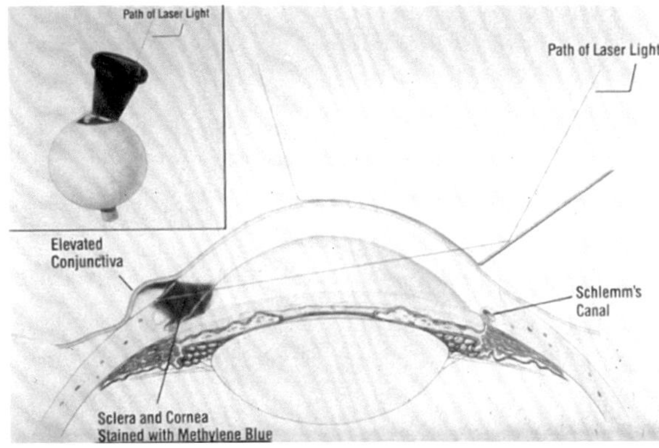

Figure 59.1. Schematic representation of gonioscopic *ab interno* laser sclerostomy. The laser beam emitted from a pulsed dye laser (688 nm, 7 μsec pulse duration) is directed through a goniolens onto the region of dyed sclera to create a fistula.

throughout the full-thickness of sclera was required. The output of a pulsed dye-laser (Candela Corp., Wayland, MA) emitting at 660 nm with a pulse duration of 7 microseconds, coupled to a slit-lamp delivery system was then focused onto dyed sclera aiming at the level of Schwalbe's line. Pulse energies were typically between 200 mJ and 300 mJ per pulse and an average of 9 pulses were required for complete perforation.

While no significant adverse effects resulted from the procedure, complete fistula formation could be achieved in only 55% of eyes. With a criterion for clinical success of 22 mm Hg or lower, at 3 months 74% of eyes with complete fistulas were successful, by 9 months 53% of eyes were successful but by 15 months only 25% of eyes were successful. Kaplan-Meier survival estimates indicated an 84% failure rate over 15 months.

Thus, gonioscopic laser sclerostomy has the potential to advance the outpatient treatment of glaucoma by providing a slit-lamp approach to filtration surgery. However, in its present form, long-term control of intraocular pressure is unacceptable. Hopefully, future research will continue to lead us in the right direction and provide an acceptable alternative to conventional filtration surgery.

References

1. Latina MA, Dobrogowski M, March WF, et al: Laser sclerostomy by pulsed dye-laser and goniolens. Arch Ophthalmol 1990;108: 1745–1750.
2. Latina MA, Melamed S, March WF, et al: Gonioscopic *ab interno* laser sclerostomy: A pilot study in glaucoma patients. Ophthalmology 1992;99:1736–1744.

Table 59.1
Indications for Ab Interno Laser Sclerectomy

Patients who have failed previous filtration surgery with antimetabolites
Patients under consideration for shunt placement, such as Molteno or Baerveldt
Prior to cycloablative procedures
Must have mobile conjunctiva adjacent to the limbus in the area that is planned for procedure

Table 59.2
Requirements for Widespread Use of Ab Interno Laser Sclerectomy

Enhanced success rate
Reduced complication rate
Refined delivery of antimetabolites
Titratable postoperative intraocular pressure

procedures. Patients, however, should have mobile conjunctiva, particularly adjacent to the limbus in the area that is planned for the procedure (Table 59.1).

Technique—ND:YAG

The procedure is performed with a synthetic sapphire-tipped laser probe connected to a continuous wave Nd: YAG laser (Surgical Laser Technologies, Malvern, PA). A retrobulbar anesthetic is administered and the conjunctiva which will incorporate the bleb is ballooned with balanced salt solution. A paracentesis tract is created and Healon is injected in the anterior chamber. The laser scalpel (probe size, 200–400 microns) is inserted into the eye, the scalpel is positioned adjacent to the angle, and using a pulsed mode, a power of 10–12 joules is required to create a sclerectomy. The author generally creates two to three sclerectomies and also applies short laser bursts of energy to the adjacent iris to create an effect similar to iridoplasty. This last application diminishes the likelihood that the iris will become incarcerated in the sclerectomy site. The scalpel is then removed and the corneal wound is closed with a 10-0 nylon suture. Subconjunctival dexamethasone is given, an antibiotic-steroid ointment is applied and the eye is patched. Postoperatively, patients have been given 5-fluorouracil injections as required by their high risk status.

Complications

Observed complications have included inflammation, hyphema, hypotony, choroidal detachment, and choroidal hemorrhage.

FUTURE CONSIDERATIONS

Based on early clinical experience with Nd:YAG ab interno laser sclerectomy, this procedure needs further refinement prior to expanding its indications beyond high risk patients (Table 59.2). The pulsed mode of the Nd:YAG laser is preferred over the continuous wave mode and the 400 micron probe results in a sclerectomy which persists for a longer period than that created by the 200 micron probe. Experiments in animals have been performed which suggest that a transconjunctival application of mitomycin C may be beneficial in enhancing the rate of success following this procedure (14).

AUTOMATED TREPHINE

Brown and associates have described an automated trephine for performing an internal sclerectomy in patients with advanced glaucoma. This instrument, alternatively termed trabecuphine, is a 19 gauge automated trephine with a tapered cutting blade (15). The procedure is performed in a similar fashion to the *ab interno* laser sclerectomy technique. Prior to the procedure, an anterior vitrectomy is performed if vitreous is present and an iridectomy is completed. The trephine is inserted through a paracentesis tract into the anterior chamber and positioned against the area which will later serve as the site of the sclerectomy.

In an early series reported by Brown and coworkers (16), this procedure was performed in seven patients. In five patients, there was a functional bleb postoperatively, over a follow-up period extending 4 to 24 months.

GONIODIATHERMY

As early as 1950 Scheie (17) described a goniopuncture technique and reported only limited success in juvenile glaucoma patients. Following this report, in 1976 Kozart and Cameron (18) described a technique which was performed in two steps. First a Barkan knife was used to incise the trabecular meshwork. Then a diathermy probe was passed to cauterize the site. However, considering the difficulty encountered when attempting to relocate the exact site following the initial incision, this procedure has received little support.

Brown and colleagues (19) reported little success using a goniodiathermy probe which consisted of a 23 mm long stainless steel probe which was cased in Teflon material and subsequently inserted into a diathermy handpiece. This procedure was performed in four patients and was successful in only two patients.

CONCLUSION

Ab interno sclerectomy has been only moderately successful and requires additional refinement prior to its use in virgin eyes. **Conventional filtration surgery performed adjunctively with antimetabolites is more successful and should be performed prior to considering the *ab interno* procedure.** The clinician needs to consider the risk of inserting instrumentation into the eye, as well as the full thickness nature of this approach. Future refinement will undoubtedly use more effective antimetabolites or antifibrotic agents. On the positive side, this technique can be useful in reopening failed sclerectomies and may be considered prior to shunts in some patients and cycloablative procedures in many other patients.

References

1. Addicks EM, et al: Histologic characteristics of filtering blebs in glaucomatous eyes. Arch Ophthalmol 1983;101:795.
2. Skuta GL, Parrish RK: II. Wound healing in glaucoma filtering surgery. Surv Ophthalmol 1987;32:149.
3. Higginbotham EJ, Kao G, Peyman G: Internal sclerostomy with the Nd:YAG contact laser versus thermal sclerostomy in rabbits. Ophthalmology 1988;95:385.
4. March WF, et al: Experimental YAG laser sclerostomy. Arch Ophthalmol 1984;102:1834.
5. Latina M, et al. Experimental ab interno sclerostomies using a pulsed-dye laser. Lasers Surg Med 1988;8:233.
6. Melamed S, et al. Internal sclerostomy using laser ablation of dyed sclera in glaucoma patients: a pilot study. Br J Ophthalmol 1993;77:139.
7. March WF, Shaber RP: Fluorescein in laser sclerostomy. Am J Ophthalmol 1987;104:432.
8. March WF, et al. Silver oxide in YAG sclerostomy. Lasers Surg Med 1987;7:353.
9. Karp CL, et al: Diode laser surgery: ab interno and ab externo versus conventional surgery in rabbits. Ophthalmology 1993;100:1567.
10. Jaffe GJ, et al: Ab interno sclerostomy with a high-powered argon endolaser. Am J Ophthalmol 1988;106:391.
11. Berlin MS, et al: Goniophotoablation: Excimer laser glaucoma filtering surgery. Lasers Light Ophthalmol 1988;2:17.
12. Wilson RP, Javitt JC: Ab interno laser sclerostomy in aphakic patients with glaucoma and chronic inflammation. Am J Ophthalmol 1990;110:178.
13. Liu SJ, Higginbotham EJ: Contact Nd:YAG laser internal sclerostomy in aphakic eyes: initial experience. Ophthalmology (Suppl) 1989;96:125.
14. Karp CL, Higginbotham EJ, Griffin EO: Adjunctive use of transconjunctival mitomycin-C in ab externo diode laser sclerostomy surgery in rabbits. Ophthalmic Surg 1994;25:22.
15. Brown RH, et al: Internal sclerostomy for glaucoma filtering surgery with an automated trephine. Arch Ophthalmol 1987;105:133.
16. Brown RH, et al: Internal sclerectomy with an automated trephine for advanced glaucoma. Ophthalmology 1988;95:728.
17. Scheie HG: Goniopuncture—a new filtering operation for glaucoma. Arch Ophthalmol 1950;44:761.
18. Kozart DM, Cameron JD: Goniodiathermy; experimental studies on ab interno filtration. Ann Ophthalmol 1978;14:1597.
19. Brown SVL, et al: Ab-Interno sclerostomy using a goniodiathermy instrument. Arch Ophthalmol 1994;25:112.

Miscellaneous Laser Procedures

60

Joel S. Schuman

LASER GONIOPLASTY

This procedure is useful in opening an angle closed despite the presence of a patent iridectomy. Gonioplasty can be performed to break peripheral anterior synechia (PAS), or to thin the iris, retracting it from the angle, in the presence of plateau iris syndrome, or angle closure syndromes with "posterior pushing" mechanisms (1–5).

The technique for this procedure is outlined in Table 60.1 (see also Chapters 25 and 51). An important consideration is when to perform gonioplasty. **This procedure is most effective if done within 6 months of the formation of PAS, (4) and is seldom successful if PAS have been present for longer than 1 year.** Laser gonioplasty is also not helpful and may be harmful (due to inflammation subsequent to the procedure) if PAS are secondary to membranes pulling the iris into the angle, such as in neovascular glaucoma or the iridocorneal endothelial (ICE) syndromes.

Laser gonioplasty may be done either without a lens, through the clear center of the Goldmann or other contact lens, or through a goniomirror. The goniomirror allows more peripheral (and therefore often more effective) treatment, but is more difficult to use, and usually necessitates higher energy levels (Fig. 60.1). We recommend treating through the clear center of the lens initially, as far peripherally as possible, using just enough energy to achieve contraction of the iris, but not enough to cause bubble formation, and placing approximately 30–40 spots 360 around the iris. After completion of the procedure, the goniomirror is used to inspect the angle, and if PAS remain, they can be attacked through the mirror at that point.

LASER SUTURE LYSIS

This technique is described in Table 60.2 (Fig. 60.2), and in detail in the surgical chapters (Chapters 62, 63, see also Chapter 51). By permitting selective cutting of subconjunctival sutures, without disturbing the overlying tissues, laser suture lysis allows postoperative titration of intraocular pressure (IOP). In this way, hypotony and bleb failure can both be avoided, and the glaucoma surgeon is given an extra measure of control over the operation.

Laser suture lysis should be used wisely because it is a powerful technique. Cut one suture too many, and the surgeon is dealing with hypotony, rather than glaucoma, and hypotony can be much more difficult to manage. Laser suture lysis should rarely be performed on the first postoperative day following filtration surgery with mitomycin C (MMC), especially in combined cataract and glaucoma surgery using this antimetabolite. **Never cut more than one suture a day.** Even with MMC, it is unlikely that cutting a suture will release the trabeculectomy flap after the first postoperative month, although anecdotal reports of hypotony following laser suture lysis at 6 months exist.

If blood is present under the conjunctiva obscuring the suture, either choose a different suture to cut, or use a longer wavelength laser, as there is less absorption by hemoglobin, and therefore less risk of a conjunctival burn. Use of a short exposure time (0.02 seconds) also decreases the chance of a conjunctival burn. Visualization is maximized with use of a contact lens. Several lenses are on the market, including the Hoskins, Ritch and Mandelkorn; the Hoskins lens has been available longest, and is the easiest to use.

LASER REVISION OF THE FAILING BLEB

The Nd:YAG laser can revive a failing filter by cutting through episcleral and Tenon's fascial tissue transconjunctivally. In addition, a gonioscopic approach can be used to ablate transparent (or pigmented) membranes occluding the sclerotomy site.

For the transconjunctival approach to be used, the bleb must be relatively transparent, and the laser is aimed deep to the tissues, to avoid injuring the overlying conjunctiva with either the shock wave or spark of the Nd:YAG laser (Fig. 60.3). The procedure is described in Table 60.3.

LASER TREATMENT OF BLEB TISSUE FOR HYPOTONY

By inciting inflammation and scarring, and through the use of an absorbing dye, the laser is used to elevate the IOP in cases of hypotony. The peak absorption of the dye is matched to the laser wavelength used, as the conjunctiva and sclera absorb little energy in the blue-green to near-infrared spectrum. The technique of this procedure is described in Table 60.4.

LASER GONIOPHOTOCOAGULATION

This procedure is rarely performed, but can be helpful in ablating new blood vessels growing across the trabecular meshwork while waiting for panretinal photocoagulation

Table 60.1
Laser Gonioplasty

Procedure	Laser	Settings
Laser gonioplasty	Argon, Diode	200–500 μm spot; 0.2–0.5 s; 200–400 mW; 24–32 spots in far periphery; Goldmann lens.

Perioperative Care

Procedure	Preop	Postop
Laser gonioplasty	Apraclonidine 0.5–1%, Pilocarpine 2% × 3	Prednisolone acetate 1% hourly for 1 day, then qid for 4 days, then stop. Check IOP at 1 hour, 1 day and 1 week. Gonioscopy and dilation at 1 week.

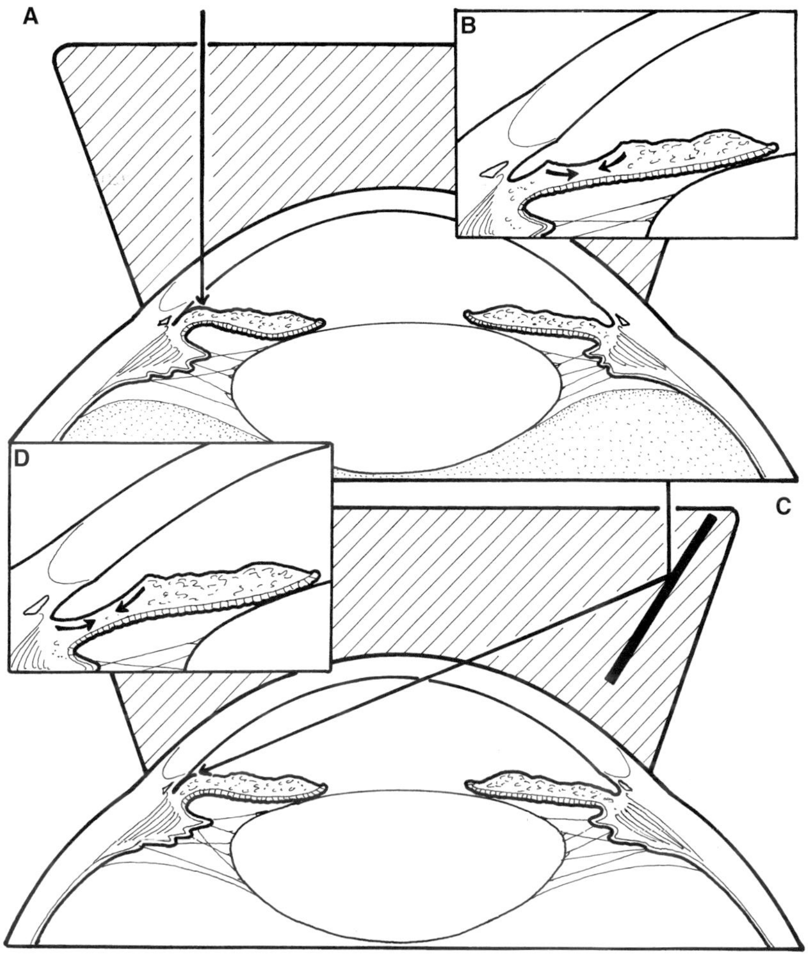

Figure 60.1. A. Laser gonioplasty, with treatment through the center of the Goldmann 3-mirror lens, as far peripheral as possible, in order to shrink the iris from the angle, thinning the iris tissue and relieving appositional closure despite a patent peripheral iridectomy (e.g., plateau iris syndrome) or early peripheral anterior synechias (PAS). B. Thinning of the iris occurs in the periphery using this technique, with contraction from all directions towards the laser lesion. C. An alternate method of laser gonioplasty calls for use of the goniomirror. This is somewhat more technically challenging, but results in a more peripheral contraction and thinning of the iris, often producing a wider, more open angle (D).

Table 60.2
Laser Suture Lysis

Procedure	Laser	Settings
Laser suture lysis	Argon; Diode	50 μm spot; 0.02 s; 300–800 mW; 1 or more spots; Hoskins lens.

Perioperative Care

Procedure	Preop	Postop
Laser suture lysis (LSL)	Proparacaine 0.5%	Check IOP 1 hour & 1 day after LSL. Do not cut more than one suture per day.

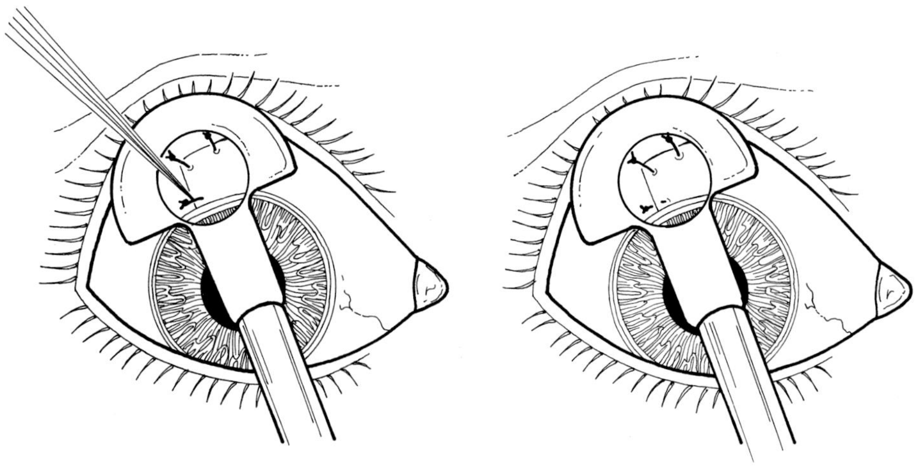

Figure 60.2. Laser suture lysis (LSL) using the Hoskins lens. Good visualization is essential, and gentle pressure on the lens will improve the view. Time (a minute or more) may be needed for the suture to become visible. Always cut the side flap sutures first, and the apical suture last, to avoid hypotony. After LSL, the Traverso maneuver can be employed, pushing on the eye adjacent to the trabeculectomy flap margin with a moistened cotton tipped swab or a muscle hook, to separate the trabeculectomy flap from the underlying scleral bed.

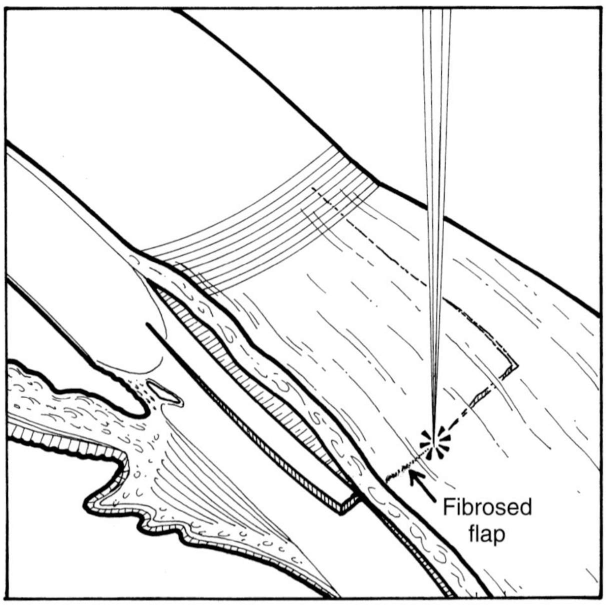

Figure 60.3. When applying laser to the trabeculectomy flap wound, focus down below the conjunctiva, use low energies, and outline the scleral flap. Following this, apply gentle digital pressure to elevate the bleb.

to take effect. The important pearl for this procedure is to treat the branch point of the vessel at its trunk, and to insure that the vessel is photocoagulated, and not still perfused, at the completion of treatment (Fig. 60.4). Treatment parameters are listed in Table 60.5.

LASER GONIOPUNCTURE

In living monkey eyes it is very easy to penetrate through the trabecular meshwork into Schlemm's canal and lower IOP (6). Unfortunately these openings close with time and IOP returns to baseline levels. We have observed similar closure of Nd:YAG trabecular punctures in human adults with open-angle glaucoma (7). We have also used the Nd:YAG laser as an alternative to surgical goniotomy in treating patients with juvenile open-angle glaucoma (see Chapter 50) in whom a pretrabecular membrane or abnormality in uveal meshwork seemed to be involved in the pathogenesis (Table 60.6, Fig. 60.5) (7,8). Dramatic lowering of IOP has occurred in a few such patients following Nd:YAG penetration of the trabecular meshwork associated with improvement in tonographic outflow facility, but with time, healing of the Nd:YAG lesion has usually occurred associated with elevation of IOP. Goniopuncture appears to be particularly useful in certain types of inflammatory glaucomas, most notably the glaucoma associated with juvenile rheumatoid arthritis, again, probably related to membrane formation across the trabecular meshwork,

Table 60.3
Laser Revision of The Failing Bleb

Procedure	Laser	Settings
Laser to failing bleb	Nd:YAG	1–2 mJ, single pulse mode; aim deep into tissues, avoiding conjunctiva; follow with digital pressure and 5-FU.

Perioperative Care

Procedure	Preop	Postop
Laser to failing bleb	Proparacaine 0.5%	Check IOP 1 hour & 1 day after; follow with digital pressure and 5-FU.

Table 60.4
Laser Treatment of Bleb Tissue for Hypotony

Procedure	Laser	Settings
Laser to conjunctiva (Hypotony)	Argon; Diode	Paint bleb with 2% fluorescein or methylene blue for argon, indocyanine green for diode laser. 200 μm spot; 0.5 s, 200–300 mW; 30–50 spots or more covering conjunctiva as much as possible.

Perioperative Care

Procedure	Preop	Postop
Laser to conjunctiva (Hypotony)	Proparacaine 0.5%	Check IOP 1 hour, 1 day and 1 week after procedure. If ineffective, may require repeat treatment or other intervention.

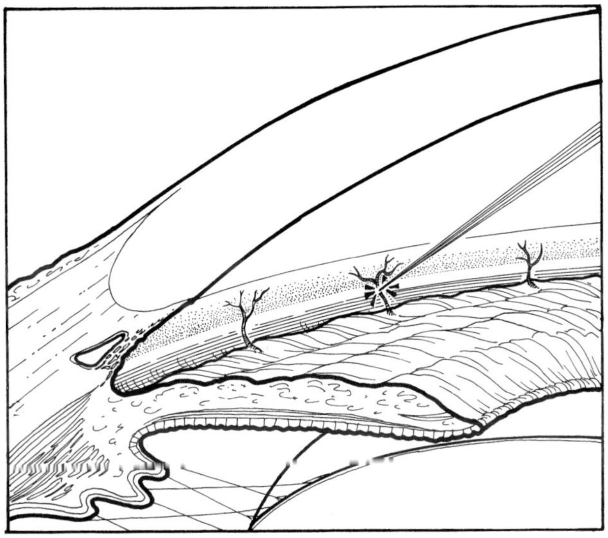

Figure 60.4. In performing laser goniophotocoagulation, the laser beam is aimed at the trunk of the arborizing new vessel, and sufficient energy is used, usually 1 watt or more, to completely blanch the trunk. The optimal spot is frequently just over the scleral spur.

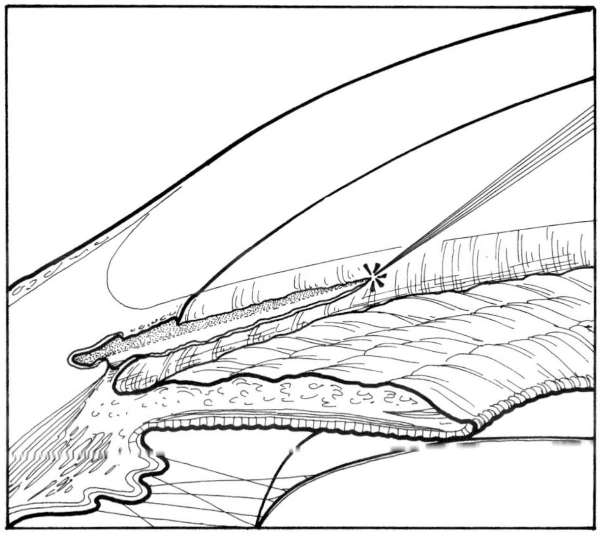

Figure 60.5. Laser goniopuncture is a relatively noninvasive means of performing a partial goniotomy. The laser is aimed into the inferior angle first, so that if bleeding occurs, as is common, another less dependent portion of the angle can be treated next. The laser is aimed into the trabecular meshwork, and fired until the white of the outer wall of Schlemm's canal is seen. Approximately 1 clock hour is opened in one session.

Table 60.5
Laser Goniophotocoagulation

Procedure	Laser	Settings
Laser goniophotocoagulation	Argon	50 μm spot; 0.1 s; 1000 mW; sufficient spots to blanch vessel trunks.

Perioperative Care

Procedure	Preop	Postop
Laser goniophotocoagulation	Apraclonidine 0.5–1%	Prednisolone acetate 1% hourly for one day, then qid for four days, then stop. Follow carefully for regression of vessels, or regrowth.

and disruption of the membrane by the Nd:YAG laser. Whether the Nd:YAG laser may be effective in other cases of juvenile glaucoma or in true congenital glaucoma, in which healing of the meshwork lesion might (for unknown reasons) not occur, is uncertain at this time. A successful, albeit temporary, response to Nd:YAG laser-angle treatment in juvenile open-angle glaucoma may help identify the potential benefit of a surgically performed goniotomy (7,8).

Regardless, the potential usefulness of the Nd:YAG laser on the trabecular meshwork is currently limited by our lack of understanding of basic biological processes

Table 60.6
Laser Goniopuncture

Procedure	Laser	Settings
Laser goniopuncture	Nd:YAG	5–7 mJ; 3 pulses per burst; fire through TM until bright white of outer wall of Schlemm's canal is seen. Begin inferiorly, as may get blood reflux. Open 1–2 clock hours.
Perioperative Care		
Procedure	Preop	Postop
Laser goniopuncture	Apraclonidine 0.5–1%	Prednisolone acetate 1% hourly for one day, then qid for four days, then stop.

within this tissue, which is a major site of abnormality in glaucoma. One can only hope that with further research this situation will change in the future. Investigational studies such as those involving erbium:YAG laser trabecular ablation may be fruitful both therapeutically, in permitting true laser goniotomy, and from a basic science perspective, in helping to unlock some of the mysteries of the trabecular meshwork.

References

1. Walker JD: A suggested role for argon laser iridoplasty in management of pigmentary glaucoma. Ophthalmic Surg 1986;17:762–763.
2. Verma N, Fromberg G: Combined argon laser iridoplasty and trabeculoplasty in the management of open angle glaucomas. Indian J Ophthalmol 1986;34:221–223.
3. Wand M: Argon laser gonioplasty for synechial angle closure. Arch Ophthalmol 1992;110:363–367.
4. Weiss HS, Shingleton BJ, Goode SM, et al: Argon laser gonioplasty in the treatment of angle-closure glaucoma. Am J Ophthalmol 1992;114: 14–18.
5. Tanihara H, Nagata M: Argon-laser gonioplasty following goniosynechialysis. Graefes Arch Clin Exp Ophthalmol 1991;229:505–507.
6. Melamed S, Pei J, Puliafito CA, et al: Q-switched neodymium-YAG laser trabeculopuncture in monkeys. Arch Ophthalmol 1985;103:129–133.
7. Epstein DL, Melamed S, Puliafito CA, et al: Neodymium-YAG laser trabeculopuncture in open-angle glaucoma. Ophthalmology 1985;92: 931–937.
8. Melamed S, Latina MA, Epstein DL: Neodymium:YAG laser trabeculopuncture in juvenile open angle glaucoma. Ophthalmology 1987;94: 160–170.

Glaucoma Surgery

IX

What I Say to Glaucoma Patients Prior to Filtration Surgery

61

David P. Berry

Patients who face glaucoma filtering surgery often have a variety of questions regarding the need for surgery, goals of the operation, and likely outcome (Table 61.1). **Since the main goal of filtering surgery is to reduce IOP and preserve vision rather than improve vision, this should be carefully discussed preoperatively.** Not infrequently, it may be necessary to briefly review glaucoma and how it causes vision loss. New therapies such as the use of anti-metabolites, including their indications and use should be discussed. Additionally, if indicated, whether cataract surgery should be performed as a staged procedure or as a combined operation.

What follows is a stylized exchange between a patient and her ophthalmologist regarding planned glaucoma filtering surgery. Although it is not practical to address all of the questions raised in this discussion with each patient prior to filtering surgery, we strongly feel that it is in the best interests of all concerned to have a well informed and prepared patient prior to embarking on the surgical management of glaucoma.

Mrs. Smith is a 67 year old Caucasian female with exfoliative glaucoma OU having been diagnosed approximately 4–5 years previously. Despite maximally tolerated medical and laser therapy, the patient's IOP is 25 mm Hg OD and 18 mm Hg OS. The patient's visual acuity is 20/50–2 OD with -1.00 -1.00×170 and 20/30–2 OS with $-.50$ -1.25×10. Relevant family history includes a sister who has undergone laser treatment for glaucoma and Mrs. Smith's mother was on drops for glaucoma in the 2 years just prior to her death at age 74. Mrs. Smith is also being treated for mild essential hypertension which is presently controlled with one drug therapy.

Dr. B.: "Mrs. Smith, as we have discussed on many occasions, glaucoma is a very serious and chronic condition which is a leading cause of blindness."

Mrs. S.: "Yes, Dr. Berry, I have been so afraid of losing my vision. I have tried very hard to use the medicines as you have prescribed, and I still can see to sew, to drive, and to do most things."

Dr. B.: "Fortunately, glaucoma does not affect the central vision until the very end stages of the disease; yet you do appear to have damage in both eyes. Actually from the time of diagnosis the right eye has evidenced rather significant damage from the appearance of the optic nerve and as well from the visual field which you know is the test that evaluates the function of the optic nerve."

Mrs. S.: "Is my left eye also damaged?"

Dr. B.: "At least from the appearance of the optic nerve and a suggestion of early changes on the visual field, it also evidences damage. Fortunately, however, there have been no advanced changes or threatening findings on the visual field. The concern presently is with the pressure being too high in the right eye."

Mrs. S.: "But I thought that the pressures had come down significantly! How low does the pressure need to be?"

Dr. B.: "Actually your pressure had responded and initially for a year or so was adequately reduced. We don't really know exactly what the safe pressure level is for people in general. It is a very individual consideration with the pressure goal for each patient's glaucoma being different and perhaps even different for each eye of each patient. Since the damage in your right eye is significantly greater than would appear in the left eye, it would be reasonable to understand that the right eye pressure must be reduced to a much lower level than the left eye pressure. In some patients with pressures at even 20–22 mmHg or lower which is considered 'normal,' glaucoma type damage to the optic nerves has still occurred. Such patients are felt to have 'normal' or 'low pressure' glaucoma in that the optic nerve has some peculiar sensitivity to even 'normal' levels of pressure. It would seem that we need your pressures at a very low level in the right eye, perhaps at 10–15 on a continuous basis, and at 18 or so in the left eye."

Mrs. S.: "But I thought that we had gotten the pressure to a safe level! The pressure in the right eye had been in the teens after the laser. Has the laser stopped working again? We seem to have gotten a really good effect from the original laser and some help from the one re-treatment two years later. Can't we try the laser again?"

Dr. B.: "Oftentimes laser will work very well, especially in certain types of glaucoma. We have talked many times about exfoliation, an interesting type of glaucoma with extra pigment and material which somehow plugs up the filter or drain that normally drains the fluid from your eye, and the laser can be highly effective especially initially

Table 61.1
Points to Discuss Before Filtration Surgery

Glaucoma
How it causes vision loss
Why reducing IOP is beneficial
Treatment alternatives
Combined cataract surgery
Goals of filtering surgery
Reduce IOP
Preserve vision
Potential for vision improvement (if any)
Reduce medications
Risks and benefits
Filtering surgery
Anesthesia
Description of surgery
Length of surgery
Antimetabolites
Postoperative course
Medications
Eye shield
Activity restrictions
Vision changes
Frequency of eye exams
Common complications
Hypotony
Elevated IOP (post-operative)
Choroidal effusion or hemorrhage
Cataract
Cosmetic factors (eyelid, bleb)
Success rate
Risk of endophtalmitis
Preoperative instructions
Discontinue aspirin and NSAIDs
Glaucoma medications (discontinue prior to surgery)

and even with a re-treatment. Yet, over time exfoliative glaucoma tends to be progressive and ultimately the laser has no significant sustained effect that would warrant an additional treatment."

Mrs. S.: "Well is there any alternative other than surgery?"

Dr. B.: "As you know we have had to use Neptazane and previously Iopidine in order to achieve adequate control of the pressures. Unfortunately, the Iopidine caused you irritation and you have had difficulty with the higher doses of Neptazane."

Mrs. S.: "Yes, I felt awful on the two tablets twice a day and still seem to have no energy. I just don't feel like myself."

Dr. B.: "Well, obviously it is unlikely that you would be able to continue on oral medication and this is why we have evolved to the point of needing to discuss surgery. The surgery is designed to create an opening or to establish a filter so as to allow fluid to drain externally from the eye under a protective layer of tissue and thus to provide lowering of the eye pressure."

Mrs. S.: "Yes, we have talked about surgery in the past. But, what exactly is a filter? Do you place a device in my eye? It seems that I have heard or read about filtering devices being placed in an eye."

Dr. B.: "There are devices such as small valves that are used and inserted in some eyes that have glaucoma. Typically, however, valve surgery or the insertion of a small seton is used in patients with more advanced forms of glaucoma, in patients who have not responded to conventional filtering surgery or have certain significant risk factors such as inflammation in the eye or scar tissue from previous surgery, or active scar tissue formation as in African Americans and young people."

Mrs. S.: "What actually do you do? Do you put me to sleep? Will the surgery be painful?"

Dr. B.: "Actually, the surgery is performed under local anesthesia. You will be given preoperative sedation to relax you and you will be kept sedated and comfortable for the procedure. A member of the anesthesia staff will be monitoring your vital systems, and it is unlikely that you will have any life threatening problems. It will be necessary to use a Novocaine-like local anesthetic to inject medicine around your eye to put the pain and motor fibers to sleep so that your eye will not move, and you will have no discomfort during the surgery. The method for using local anesthesia to put the eye to sleep is quite similar to that which is performed for a dental procedure.

The surgery is very delicate and involves creating a controlled opening which will allow fluid to escape from the eye. It is somewhat like creating a manhole cover with stitches around the edges of the cover so that fluid can flow out around the edges of the cover and as well through the thin layer of tissue that covers the small opening that is made. An additional outer layer of tissue known as the conjunctiva will then be sewn over this cover which will help allow the fluid to diffuse out and away from the eye."

Mrs. S.: "Will I feel this filter or be able to see it?"

Dr. B.: "Yes, often times there will be a small raised, localized area of tissue, like a little bubble or bleb, that will be hidden under the upper lid. It is likely that you could see it in a mirror with the lid elevated, and it may be that you will have an awareness or sensation of a raised area under your lid with blinking and lid movement."

Mrs. S.: "How long will the surgery take?"

Dr. B.: "The time required for the surgery will vary with each patient. Sometimes the tissue dissection can be more difficult due the conjunctiva being thinner or there can be prominent blood vessels and a bit more localized bleeding in certain patients, thus requiring more cautery and prolonging the time required for the surgery. So do not let the time be a concern, though usually the surgery lasts approximately 40–50 minutes once the eye has been put to sleep."

Mrs. S.: "Will I see better or differently after the surgery?"

Dr. B.: "It's good that you inquired about your vision as there are several important considerations. As you have commented on several occasions, your vision has been variable and at times somewhat blurred."

Mrs. S.: "Yes, and my night vision has been poor for some time. I have even stopped driving at all after sunset because things are so dark."

Dr. B.: "These symptoms, as we have discussed before, are related to the use of pilocarpine which narrows your pupils, thus letting in less light and making it more difficult for you to see in low light conditions. Also, the pilocarpine causes variable effects on your refractive error causing intermittent blurring. My hope is that you will be able permanently to remain off of the pilocarpine which should allow improved vision. You also have developed a cataract which is typical for patients who have exfoliation. Cataracts frequently develop earlier in the more involved eye. During the first several weeks after surgery the vision will be quite variable as the pilocarpine gradually loses its effect. You have been on the drug for several years and, it will take some time for your refraction possibly to shift in a less near-sighted direction. Also, you will be on a red top drop for a while post-operatively. The red top drop is a cycloplegic which will dilate your pupil and may blur your vision. This drop will be used to relax your pupil and to quiet your eye during the immediate post-operative period when there can be more inflammation. It is the same type of medicine that has been used to dilate your pupil in the office for evaluating your retina. After 2–4 weeks it is hoped that you will be tapered off of the cycloplegic and will not have to be back on the pilocarpine. It is anticipated that you might have improved visual function. Thus it is likely that the prescription for your glasses may shift more in the direction of your original prescription prior to having been placed on the pilocarpine. You may recall that we changed your glasses prescription several months after being placed on the stronger concentration of pilocarpine."

Mrs. S.: "Is the surgery reasonably safe? Could my vision be worse or even possibly could I go blind?"

Dr. B.: "In every way I would want to reassure you that the chances are very minimal that you would have any major problem that would affect your vision significantly. Patients who undergo any type of intraocular surgery can experience some degree of accelerated cataract formation. Since you already have a cataract related to your age as well as the exfoliative condition, it is likely that your cataract could significantly progress over time requiring removal of the cataract. And, one must acknowledge that, however small the risk, you could develop an infection or have a hemorrhage that could result in catastrophic consequences in which you could lose all vision in your eye and possibly even have to have the eye removed. Since glaucoma patients typically have variable eye pressures which affects the retinal vasculature, they are at greater risk for developing spontaneous hemorrhages of one of the layers under the retina, the choroid, than are patients who do not have glaucoma and are merely undergoing cataract surgery."

Mrs. S.: "Are there any other complications or problems that may occur and that I need to know about?"

Dr. B.: "During the early post-operative period it can happen that the filter could drain too much fluid from the eye and the chamber in the front part of the eye may shallow resulting in the lens moving forward and possibly even touching the back surface of the cornea. Occasionally it happens that this type of over-filtration does occur resulting in fluid accumulating under the choroid. If the process does not respond to tight patching of the eye or other attempts at retarding filtration, then an additional surgical procedure may be required."

Mrs. S.: "What type of surgical procedure and would it be very risky to have this surgery?"

Dr. B: "Yes, unfortunately there is rather moderate risk with each additional surgical intervention; yet, the procedure is usually able to be performed without significant additional complications. Should there be over-filtration in the early postoperative period that warrants correction then we would need to return to surgery again under local anesthesia to perform a procedure in which the fluid is drained from the choroid and the chamber is deepened. A small incision will have been placed into the anterior chamber through the cornea in the original procedure and this incision site will be used for filling the chamber with fluid or perhaps air or even a thick jelly-like material which will allow deepening of the chamber and thus normalizing the distance between the cornea and the lens. At the same time a small incision will be made just back from the edge of the cornea over the site of fluid accumulation which will allow drainage of the fluid from the choroid and thus will also assist with deepening the chamber and reducing the excessive filtration of fluid. It can happen that the incision in the tissue overlying the choroid could result in a significant hemorrhage or possibly even a tear of the retina. There could also be more accelerated cataract formation which develops over several days or perhaps over several months thus necessitating removal of the cataract."

Mrs. S.: "Well, you have indicated that I already have a cataract. Why aren't we removing the cataract at the same time I'm to undergo the glaucoma surgery so that all is done at one time?"

Dr. B.: "It certainly is possible that a combined cataract-glaucoma procedure could be performed with insertion of an implant and often this type of combined procedure is performed very successfully. Your pressure is just at a borderline level for allowing consideration of a combined procedure since surgical procedures that are more complicated such as combining cataract and filtering surgery have less chance of providing the very low pressure that would be needed to protect your optic nerve. In patients who have advanced optic nerve damage and pressures at the mid-20 range one often proceeds with a staged approach to the surgery with the initial procedure being a filtering procedure which hopefully will achieve low pressures. Subsequently after the filter has become well established and has matured, a second procedure, a cataract procedure, will be performed from the side or from below so as to avoid the area of filtration. As mentioned to you earlier, it is hoped that you will be able to be off of the pilocarpine and, with the pupil wider, perhaps you will have sufficiently improved vision to allow adequate function; at the same time, the pressure will be reduced to a protective level.

Mrs. S.: "Could I choose to have the combined procedure just because I really don't think I would want to go through the second operation if it could be avoided? Yet, I do want to have the pressure reduced to a level that is safe for my optic nerve."

Dr. B.: "A consideration would be that of proceeding with a combined procedure and perhaps using a chemo-therapeutic agent at the time of surgery which would enhance the filtration and allow the cataract surgery to be performed."

Mrs. S.: "You mentioned chemo-therapeutic agent. Is this some type of cancer drug? I thought that such drugs could be dangerous or life-threatening."

Dr. B.: "In certain types of high-risk glaucoma procedures and also now increasingly in combined cataract-glaucoma operations, studies have indicated a significant benefit in using certain chemo-therapeutic drugs such as 5-fluorouracil and mitomycin C, which can have local effects in preventing scar formation and enhancing filtration without having any significant generalized side effects as are often encountered when used for combating cancer throughout the body. 5-fluorouracil has been used for a longer period of time; yet, it requires multiple injections around the eye, often given multiple times following the surgery. The injections can be uncomfortable. Certain toxic changes of the cornea and conjunctiva can develop which temporarily result in discomfort and irritation. More recently, mitomycin C is being used more frequently because it can be applied at the time of surgery to a very localized area and thus produce its effect from a simple application. Usually, no injections are required."

Mrs. S.: "Then there are no dangers with using these drugs? Are both drugs considered to be safe to use in the eye? I do believe that I would rather not have the injections."

Dr. B.: "Both drugs are very powerful agents which interfere with the activity of fibroblastic cells and help to minimize scar tissue formation. Yet, these drugs can also result in defective healing with resultant separation of the wound, defects in the filter site itself with leakage and flattening of the bleb, and can be dangerous to the internal aspects of the eye if inadvertently getting into the interior of the eye. Yet, much information has been gathered about these drugs, and we have become very skilled at using them in appropriate doses for our desired effect. It also must be mentioned that a very thin filtering bleb may develop after use of these drugs and with time the eye can over-filter with the pressure becoming too low. The filtering bleb itself can become too thin resulting in leakage and prompting the need to have the area re-sutured and possibly patched with some type of eye-bank tissue. If indeed the pressure becomes too low on an extended basis then the eye can become soft with stretch marks developing in the central retina or the macular area with some damaging effect from the hypotony.

If the pressure is not adequately reduced or is too high in the early post-operative period, whether a primary filtering procedure is done or a combined cataract-filtering procedure, then the laser can be used to cut one of the stitches in the edge of the 'manhole cover' to allow more fluid to be released from the eye, thus lowering the pressure. Usually there are no problems with performing the laser. If one of the chemo-therapeutic drugs is used, one must be aware that the laser's being performed through the conjunctiva or outer layer of tissue could result in a hole being created which would leak and thus require suturing or patching."

Mrs. S.: "So it does seem to be quite complicated; yet, I do believe that the only alternative at this time for my eye is surgery to lower the pressure. I really would have to defer to your recommendation regarding the need for performing the filtering procedure alone or in combination with the cataract procedure."

Dr. B.: "It would seem that you are in a borderline situation in which almost either procedure could be performed. With your vision being at the 20/50 level while on pilocarpine and with the need to achieve very low pressures to protect your damaged optic nerve, I would recommend proceeding with the filtering surgery alone. Since you do not have any significant risk factors and have never undergone an operative procedure of the eye, then I would think that a trabeculectomy or a type of filtering procedure with a small flap as described with regard to the manhole cover example would be the appropriate procedure. I do not think there would be a need for the use of chemo-therapeutic agents. Should it be, however, that there is sluggish filtration in the first several days after the surgery, then the laser would be used possibly to cut sutures along the edge of the flap to improve filtration. It may even be that several injections of 5-fluorouracil could be used as well.

Mrs. S.: "Well, it seems that we have decided what to do about the right eye. Do you feel comfortable that my left eye is in a stable situation"?

Dr. B.: "Actually, I have some concern that there has been damage of the optic nerve. There also are early changes on the visual field and the pressure is at a borderline level even now while on oral medication which we will be needing to discontinue for the filtering surgery."

Mrs. S.: "As I indicated to you, I do think that I will

be able to tolerate the Neptazane if I only have to take one twice daily."

Dr. B.: "Once the decision is made to proceed with surgery in one eye, it is our usual practice to discontinue the oral medication. Systemic medicine affects both eyes, and the effect is that of reducing flow in the eye which results in lower pressures. Once the filter is created, it is necessary that fluid flow through the opening in order to maintain the patency and to assist with the filter's becoming established and reducing the eye pressure. Thus it would be potentially harmful to the success of the surgery to be on the oral medication."

Mrs. S.: "But what about the pressure in my left eye?"

Dr. B.: "It is likely that the pressure will increase once you are off of the Neptazane, and the pressure would then be at a level that would be unsafe. We can add Trusopt to the fellow eye to avoid this problem. Trusopt is a topical drug which functions like Neptazane but would not lower the eye pressure in your operated eye. Another consideration would be that of proceeding now with at least one treatment with the laser hopefully to reduce the pressure to a safer level in the left eye by the time of the surgery for the right eye, which is to be done in the next few weeks. Should it be that the pressure is not at an adequately low level in the left eye, then a second laser procedure could be performed at some time during the time that we are following the post-operative course of your right eye. Also, it should be mentioned that a certain percentage of glaucoma patients will experience pressure rises if placed on steroids for an extended period. Topical steroids will be needed on a somewhat frequent basis in the right eye during the postoperative period in order to quiet the inflammation from the surgery to prevent scarring of the filter, and at times even oral steroids may be required in the form of prednisone for controlling the inflammation. Although you will be using the topical steroid in the right eye there can be sufficient absorption of the steroid through the tear system and into the blood stream so as to produce a significant rise in the pressure in the non-operated left eye. Thus this presents an additional reason to consider laser trabeculoplasty in the left eye at this time, with the goal of providing a safer level of pressure should it be that steroid responsiveness does occur."

Mrs. S.: "Thank you for discussing this surgery and my various options and the risks of this procedure as I have had great concern about my vision. Actually I should tell you that a good friend of mine who lives in Ohio underwent some type of glaucoma procedure last year and had a most difficult time and lost all of the vision in one eye. She is now faced with having laser and possibly even surgery on her only remaining eye and I have been scared to death."

Dr. B.: "Mrs. Smith there is risk with everything that we do. The greatest risk in glaucoma is not controlling the pressure and not being appropriately aggressive since untreated glaucoma and inadequately reduced pressure results in loss of all vision. What I would want you and your family to know and to understand is that we are partners in this process and that no matter what may occur we will deal with problems and situations as they come up. Meanwhile we will be confident that things will go well and that we can achieve control of your pressure and preserve your vision."

Filtering Surgery in the Management of Glaucoma

62

R. Rand Allingham

The rationale for performing glaucoma filtration surgery is simple. It is to provide for aqueous humor a pathway that has a resistance to outflow that is lower than the failing or irreversibly obstructed trabecular meshwork. The desired result is to lower intraocular pressure (IOP) to a level compatible with normal function of the optic nerve.

Embarking on incisional surgery for the treatment of glaucoma is a major decision made between patient and physician (Table 62.1). Typically, this becomes a realistic management alternative after medical and laser treatment has failed to reduce IOP to the desired level. Indications for advancing therapy are progressive glaucomatous optic nerve cupping or visual field loss or uncontrolled IOP which has a high likelihood of producing the same type of damage. Whether this treatment paradigm is the optimal approach is a point of ongoing debate (1).

Many techniques and procedural variations have been employed to bypass the trabecular meshwork. Procedures that are of historical interest include cyclodialysis (2) (Chapter 66) and iridencleisis. In the past, unguarded or full-thickness surgery was primarily used (3). However, the incidence of postoperative hypotony, with its associated complications, was extremely high. Today, guarded filtering surgery or trabeculectomy is the primary operation almost exclusively performed for the surgical (non-laser) management of glaucoma. A renewed interest in full-thickness (unguarded) glaucoma surgery in the form of laser sclerectomy procedures are being investigated. However, as in traditional full-thickness surgery, postoperative hypotony is still frequent (Chapters 58 and 59).

PREOPERATIVE ASSESSMENT

Many factors contribute to the final outcome of filtration surgery. In some cases, the risk factors for failure can be modified or reduced by taking specific courses of action before and during filtration surgery.

With the exception of highly myopic patients, younger patients are at increased risk for filtration failure. The younger the patient, the greater the risk. A concerted effort to reduce pre- and postoperative scarring and inflammation is imperative. Intra- and/or postoperative anti-metabolite therapy may promote success in those patients under the age of 20 years and is advisable for all of those undergoing filtration surgery under 40 years of age. Older patients are at decreased risk for surgical failure. However, compliance with the postoperative medical regimen may be an important issue to address in those with memory deficits or physical handicaps. Discussing the perioperative process with family or other support persons or occasionally consulting with social services may be necessary. It is crucial to establish that the patient will be able to care for him- or herself or be cared for before surgery is undertaken.

It is not clear whether patients with greater skin pigmentation are more or less likely to experience glaucoma filtration failure (4). However, many surgeons feel that there is at least some increased risk of surgical failure which warrants the routine use of anti-metabolites.

MEDICATIONS

Factors that increase pre- and postoperative inflammation should be reduced. One of these factors is the use of preoperative glaucoma medications. Generally speaking, topical and oral glaucoma medications may be continued until the day of surgery. Regarding topical medications, it is best to substitute direct miotics (pilocarpine) for indirect acting agents (echothiophate iodide) in order to decrease postoperative inflammation associated with the latter. Frequently, in patients on both topical epinephrine compounds and beta blockers, epinephrine or dipivefrin may be stopped pre-operatively. Particularly when combined with non-selective beta blockers, the epinephrine compounds may produce little effect on IOP while contributing to unwanted conjunctival inflammation. Topical beta blockers may be stopped 24–48 hours before filtration surgery. In patients taking timolol it has been shown that aqueous humor production begins to increase to baseline levels only after 3–4 days (5). It may be advantageous to try to promote aqueous humor production in patients undergoing filtration surgery to reduce the incidence of postoperative hypotony.

Preoperative steroids may be useful in those patients with uveitic glaucoma where inflammation poses an increased risk for surgical failure. The use of topical steroids such as prednisolone acetate 1% every 2 hours 24–48 hours before filtration surgery may be useful. However, in those patients without preoperative inflammation, the advan-

Table 62.1
Indications for Filtering Surgery

Progressive visual field loss or optic nerve cupping despite maximally tolerated medical and laser therapy
Chronically elevated IOP greater than 40 mm Hg
Inability to achieve IOP (usually low teens) in patients with visual field loss approaching fixation (unable to follow for progression)

tage of using prolonged and frequent steroids is less clear, and in fact may cause elevated IOP in those patients at risk. This is a particular problem in the unoperated fellow eye which will not have the benefit of filtering surgery. Preoperative systemic steroids can produce a wide variety of serious adverse effects and should only be used in selected cases and after consultation with an internist.

Systemic medications may also influence the outcome of filtration surgery. Anticoagulants can add significantly to complications during and after filtration surgery. Excessive bleeding encountered during surgery may produce increased postoperative scarring and make laser suture lysis of the trabeculectomy flap more difficult if not impossible. Whether these medications increase the risk of suprachoroidal hemorrhage is unknown. However, they might make bleeding worse. **Stopping all use of aspirin, aspirin-containing compounds, and non-steroidal anti-inflammatory agents 3–6 weeks before surgery is desirable if possible.** It may be helpful to instruct the patient to use only acetaminophen compounds only for the time prior to and immediately after surgery. Where aspirin is being used long term for prophylaxis for specific medical conditions it is advisable to consult with the patient's internist before changing or withholding these medications. In many cases it is possible to stop these for a 4–6 week period. Coumadin is another commonly encountered anticoagulant. This medication has not been associated with excessive intraoperative bleeding in the experience of this author. In general, we recommend that Coumadin not be discontinued for filtration surgery.

The interventions described should always be considered within their clinical context. Adjusting systemic medications should only be entertained after consultation with the patient's internist. In patients with far advanced optic nerve disease, where even short term elevations of IOP may be hazardous to the patient, caution should be used when altering the medical regimen. On the other hand, reducing intraoperative and postoperative bleeding, inflammation and hypotony are important to long term surgical success.

Other considerations relate to the preoperative ocular status (Table 62.2). Hyperopic eyes, particularly those which are very small (axial length <21 mm) frequently have an axially shallow anterior chamber. There may be a history of chronic angle closure. These eyes are prone to postoperative shallow or flat chambers or, more rarely, malignant glaucoma. The risk of this can be reduced by using a tighter scleral flap closure to guard against postoperative

Table 62.2
Special Considerations

Hyperopic eyes
1. More prone to shallow or flat anterior chambers postoperatively
2. In chronic angle closure eyes there is an increased risk of malignant glaucoma
3. Consider tighter scleral flap closure to avoid postoperative hypotony and shallow/flat anterior chamber

Pseudophakic (postoperative) eyes
1. Check conjunctival mobility prior to choosing a filter site
2. Use caution when creating scleral flap through old cataract wound incision (risk of avulsion of scleral flap)
3. Perform anterior vitrectomy for vitreous in the anterior chamber
4. Use antimetabolites (mitomycin C or 5-FU)

hypotony. This is discussed more fully in Chapter 29. **Pseudophakic or other eyes where conjunctiva has been disturbed should be evaluated for conjunctival mobility preoperatively.** Special care should be taken in the vicinity of scleral incisions or where vitreous may be present near the planned sclerectomy site. In the former case the scleral flap may be avulsed if too much tension is placed on the flap. Vitreous should be thoroughly removed prior to making the sclerectomy to avoid obstruction of the sclerectomy by vitreous postoperatively.

SURGICAL TECHNIQUE

Glaucoma filtration surgery is typically performed in either the superotemporal or superonasal quadrant. This approach leaves a relatively undisturbed quadrant if additional procedures, such as cataract extraction or repeat filtration surgery, are required.

What follows is a view of the step by step approach to modern guarded filtration surgery. It should become apparent that each step in the process of performing this surgery must be carefully considered.

Anesthesia

Retrobulbar anesthesia with lidocaine 4%, bupivacaine 0.75%, and hyaluronidase is effective for the majority of cases. Additional blocks which are used to obtain lid akinesia such as the modified van Lint are not necessary for filtering surgery. Retrobulbar anesthesia is preferred over peribulbar anesthesia which inflates the conjunctiva, rendering surgical dissection more difficult.

In cases in which extensive and/or numerous previous surgeries have been performed, obtaining satisfactory local anesthesia may prove problematic and general anesthesia may be required. This is particularly true where prior scleral buckling surgery has been performed. In these cases peribulbar scarring may prevent adequate anesthesia despite multiple injections. **If a patient is going to require general anesthesia it is important to inform the anesthesiologist if indirect acting cholinergic acting agents such as echothiophate iodide have been used recently.**

Bridle Sutures

Retracting the eye inferiorly is useful since surgery is usually performed in a superior quadrant. Many surgeons prefer the traditional superior rectus bridle suture for surgical exposure (Fig. 62.1). The assistant gently sweeps the superior conjunctiva toward the limbus as the surgeon grasps the superior rectus muscle with 0.5 mm forceps. Using a 4-0 silk suture on a tapered needle, the surgeon places the suture beneath the superior rectus tendon. The suture is drawn superiorly and clamped to the drape.

An alternative approach is to use a superior corneal bridle suture (Fig. 62.2). In this case a 6-0 or 7-0 silk or Vicryl suture on a spatulated needle is passed through clear, midstromal cornea approximately 1 mm from the limbus for approximately 2–2.5 mm. Gentle traction on the suture assures its integrity prior to taping or clamping the suture to the inferior drape. An alternative approach is to place an inferior corneal bridle suture. In this instance the midstromal corneal suture is placed 1 mm above the inferior limbal margin. The suture is then placed beneath the inferior lid speculum. Gentle traction on the suture depresses the eye. In either case, **it is essential that the suture does not pass into the anterior chamber**, which produces a persistent aqueous leak at the suture site, hypotony and a shallow anterior chamber during surgery, increasing the difficulty of the procedure and making mitomycin C application hazardous.

Corneal bridle sutures produce wide exposure of the superior conjunctiva. Additionally, inflammation or bleeding from manipulating the superior rectus and tenting of the conjunctiva in this region is avoided, making closure of the conjunctival flap easier. A potential disadvantage is the small area of corneal epithelial disruption at the suture site. This may delay use of 5-FU in the early postoperative period. In actuality this area is usually re-epithelialized within 24–48 hours after surgery in the vast majority of patients.

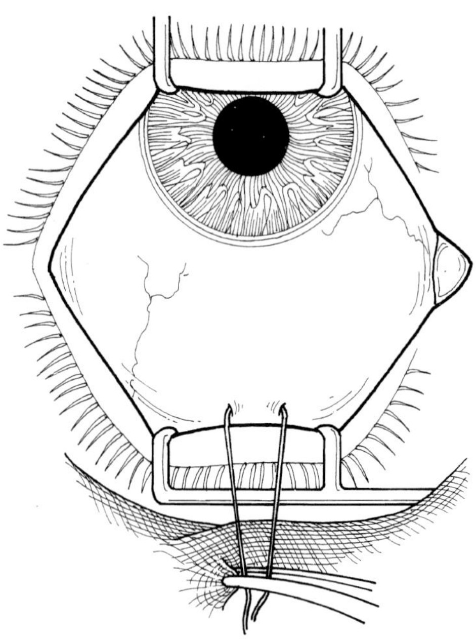

Figure 62.1. A 4-0 silk bridle suture can provide excellent exposure of the superior fornix but can bunch up conjunctiva.

Paracentesis

Placement of a paracentesis during filtration surgery is essential (Fig. 62.3). A paracentesis permits the surgeon to gain access to the anterior chamber throughout the procedure. **The paracentesis allows the surgeon to reform the anterior chamber, test the function of the sclerectomy, check the relative seal of the scleral flap, and fill the conjunctival bleb to test for leaks at the end of the procedure.** In cases where the IOP is very high the paracentesis can be used early in the case to bring the IOP down "gently," which prevents the eye pressure from rapidly plummeting when the sclerectomy is performed later in the procedure. Avoiding rapid decompression of the eye may help prevent the development of intraoperative suprachoroidal hemorrhage.

The paracentesis is typically placed temporally. It should be beveled which makes the wound self sealing. A 15 degree sharp blade or a Wheeler knife can be used. The knife is oriented tangential to the pupil to reduce the chance of lens injury. The orientation of the paracentesis and location should be carefully kept in mind by the surgeon. A frustrating and not infrequent occurrence is the inability of the surgeon to locate the entrance or to successfully cannulate the paracentesis. This problem is compounded in the presence of a soft eye. The inclination to "force" a cannula through the paracentesis is tempting but futile. Suffice it to say, this approach does not work. **Gently cannulating the paracentesis site in the correct orientation is essential to gain access to the anterior chamber.** Additionally, it is important that the internal opening (endothelial side) is of adequate size. It is wise to cannulate the paracentesis immediately after it is made to ensure its patency rather than discover later that it is nonfunctional when it is needed and the eye is hypotonous. Although the paracentesis wound is usually self sealing, it is important to check for a persistent leak with fluorescein at the end of the case. Occasionally a 10-0 nylon suture will be required to close the wound.

Conjunctival Flap

The surgical management of the conjunctiva in filtering surgery is crucial to the long-term surgical outcome. This tissue will ultimately function as a fluid flow resistor. If IOP is to be in the normal range postoperatively, subconjunctival fibrosis, the most common cause of filtration failure, must be minimized. Therefore, excessive tissue manipulation should be avoided. Only non-toothed forceps should be used on this tissue.

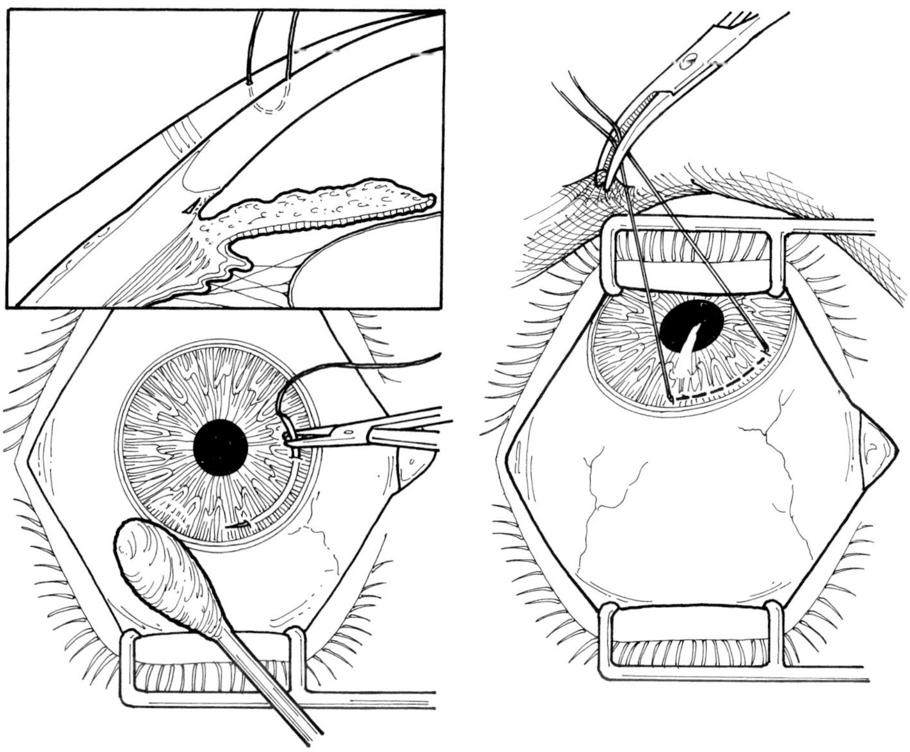

A

B

Figure 62.2. A superior corneal bridle suture can provide excellent exposure of the superior fornix without disturbing conjunctiva. A 7-0 Vicryl or silk suture on a spatulated, non-cutting needle is used. The eye can be held in place with a cotton swab (A) while passing the needle through mid corneal stroma (inset). The suture is taped or clamped to the inferior drape (B).

The conjunctival flap may be either limbus or fornix based. It is felt by some of us that a limbus based flap produces a lower postoperative IOP and is preferred in cases where a low postoperative IOP is necessary (i.e. advanced glaucoma or normal tension glaucoma). Fornix based flaps are surgically easier to perform. They are often used in cases where IOP is high but the optic nerve is otherwise healthy. Fornix based flaps may also be necessary in cases where there is significant perilimbal scarring from previous surgical procedures.

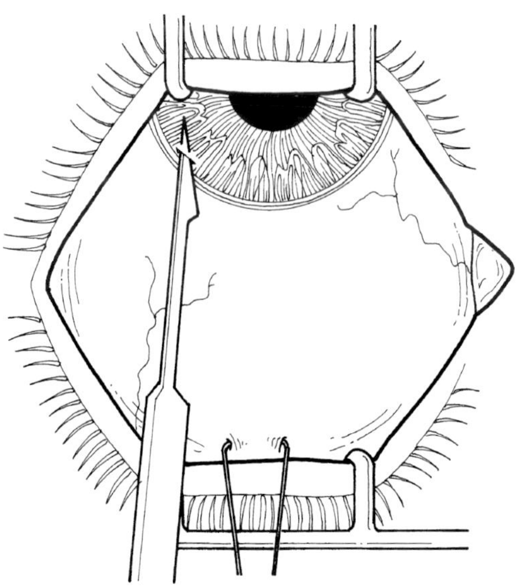

Figure 62.3. A beveled paracentesis is made with a super sharp blade. Entry of the blade should be over the iris and adjacent to the pupil. The specific location and direction of the paracentesis should be kept in mind for later use.

Limbus-based conjunctival flaps are less likely to leak postoperatively and therefore are less likely to flatten and scar down. The postoperative posterior limit of the filtering bleb is usually demarcated by the conjunctival closure site. Therefore **it is necessary to make the initial incision through the conjunctiva as posterior as possible.** A minimum of 8 mm is advisable. A Castroviejo caliper can be used to ensure that one does not enter the conjunctiva too anteriorly, because once done, the surgeon is committed. Once the conjunctiva is incised, Tenon's fascia in turn is grasped and incised (Fig. 62.4). This process continues until the episclera is visualized. The conjunctival wound should be lengthened to 1–1.5 clock hours. The conjunctiva and Tenon's tissue should only be incised when in the grasp of a forceps and while they are raised over the episclera. This precaution reduces the likelihood of accidentally incorporating a rectus muscle with these tissues, which is more likely to occur in cases where scarring from previous surgery is present.

The conjunctival flap is bluntly dissected to the limbus. The flap may incorporate conjunctiva alone or Tenon's fascia and conjunctiva. In either case, meticulous hemostasis using pinpoint cautery is essential to prevent blood from collecting in the subconjunctival space where it can create adhesions between conjunctiva and episclera postopera-

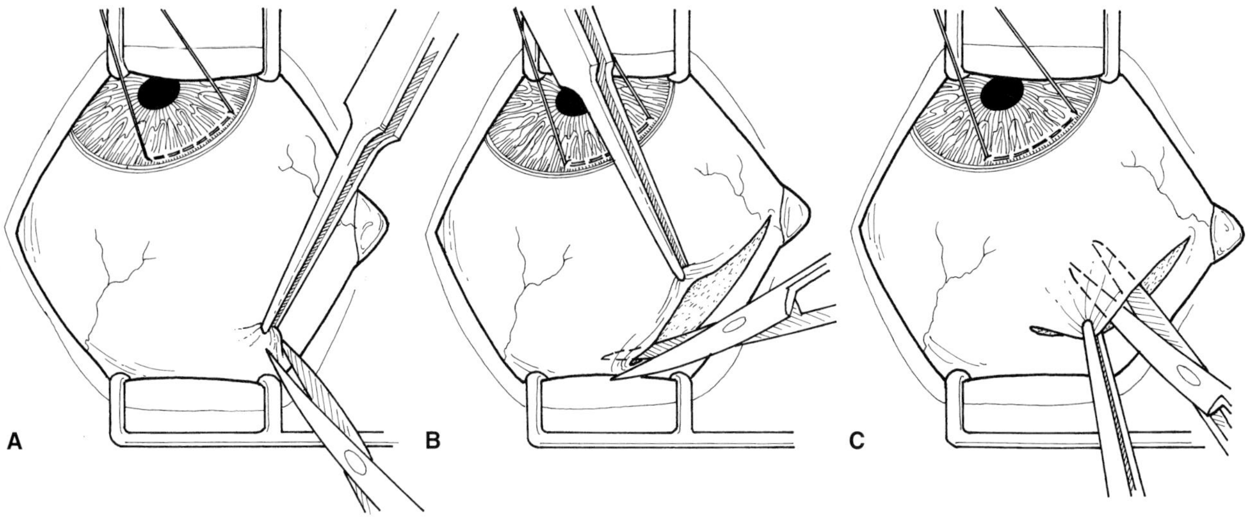

Figure 62.4. Limbus-based conjunctival flap: The conjunctival incision is made 8–10 mm from the limbus (A). When incised, the conjunctiva is tented over the episcleral surface (B) in order to avoid injuring rectus muscles. A conjunctival flap is dissected anteriorly with a combination of blunt and sharp dissection (C).

tively. Hydrodissection can be employed in cases where postoperative scarring is present from prior surgery. Hydrodissection helps define regions of conjunctival adhesion to the episclera. These sites are particularly prone to the development of buttonholes during blunt dissection and require gentle, deliberate sharp dissection. **A blunt tipped Westcott scissors and/or Took knife is used to carry the dissection through the insertion of Tenon's fascia (approximately 0.5-0.75 mm posterior to the limbus) to the insertion of the conjunctiva, which is about 0.5 mm onto clear cornea** (Fig. 62.5). Surgical success does not appear to be influenced by the presence or absence of Tenon's fascia. It is useful to have it in place while the conjunctival flap is being manipulated. It can be excised prior to conjunctival closure if desired. **Removal of Tenon's tissue does permit improved visualization of sutures if laser suture lysis is required postoperatively.** Otherwise, the bleb appearance or stability does not appear to be affected in the long term (author's opinion).

Fornix based conjunctival flaps are initiated with a 2 clock hour limbal peritomy (Fig. 62.6). Blunt dissection is carried posteriorly using a blunt tipped Westcott scissors through the insertion of Tenon's fascia. As described above, hydrodissection may be useful to define areas of subconjunctival scarring when present. Although performing a tenonectomy is difficult with a fornix based flap, it can be accomplished in many cases. It is useful to remove at least the leading edge of Tenon's fascia prior to suturing the flap to the limbus postoperatively. This helps prevent "wicking" of aqueous through the flap and aids the conjunctival epithelium in its effort to anchor to limbal stroma. Another technique which promotes adhesion of the epithelium of the conjunctival flap to the limbus is to gently cauterize or scrape away a 1–1.5 mm band of the

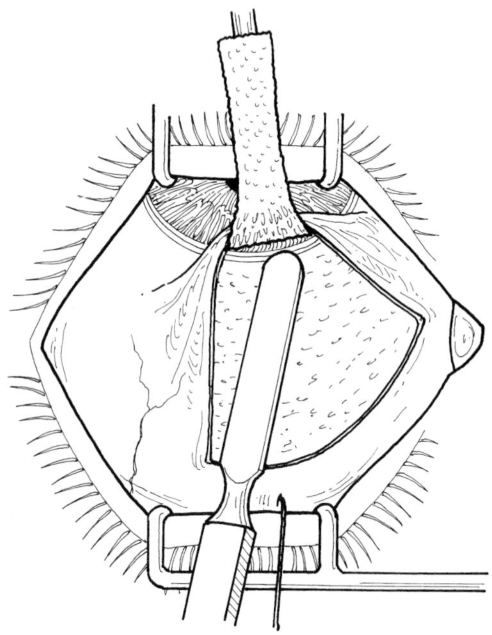

Figure 62.5. A Took knife permits fine dissection of the anterior most conjunctival flap through the insertion of Tenon's fascia. A Weck cell sponge is used to retract the conjunctival flap.

peripheral corneal epithelium where the conjunctival flap is to be sutured. This helps limit the posterior migration of corneal epithelium between the conjunctiva and limbus.

The intraoperative application of mitomycin C or 5-FU to the sclera to prevent postoperative subconjunctival fibrosis in high risk cases has become an important adjunct in glaucoma filtration surgery. **This is typically performed after conjunctival dissection, but prior to entering the eye.**

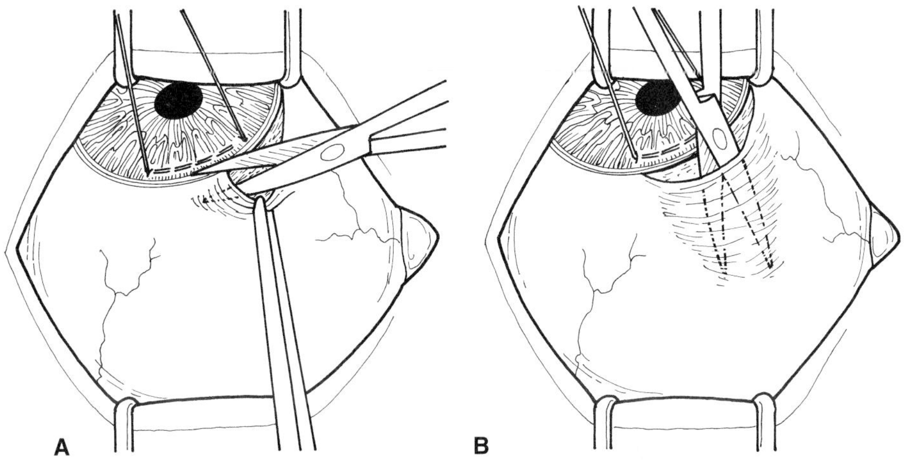

Figure 62.6. Fornix-based conjunctival flap: After the peritomy is made (A), a conjunctival flap is formed with a combination of blunt and sharp dissection (B).

Creating A Scleral Flap

The sclera is an excellent barrier to fluid flow, and therefore the scleral flap should not be considered a porous tissue which will function as a fluid filter in the mature bleb. Rather, **the scleral flap, if adequately sutured, is a temporary resistor in the early postoperative period which reduces the incidence of hypotony.** Ultimately, aqueous humor will flow around the scleral flap. The shape of the scleral flap is of little consequence as long as the flap completely covers the sclerectomy. It is preferable for the scleral flap to be at least twice the size of the sclerectomy. A Beaver 75 or diamond blade can be used to create the margins of the flap as the globe is held in place with a 0.12 mm forceps. The flap is dissected anteriorly with a Beaver No. 57 or 69 blade in a lamellar fashion (Fig. 62.7).

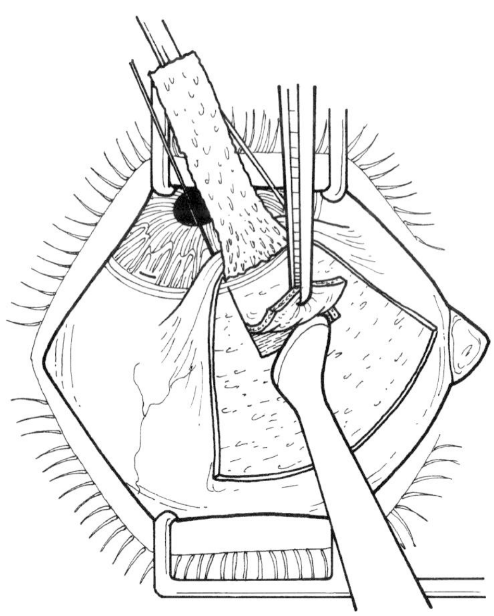

Figure 62.7. Scleral flap: A super sharp blade or diamond knife is used to create the margins of the scleral flap. A Beaver No. 57 blade (shown) or 69 blade is used to create the scleral flap.

The flap thickness should be at least one-half to two-thirds of the scleral thickness (Fig. 62.8). Otherwise the flap may be difficult to close or may avulse or tear during manipulation. The dissection is carried forward well beyond the gray line and into clear cornea, if possible. It is important

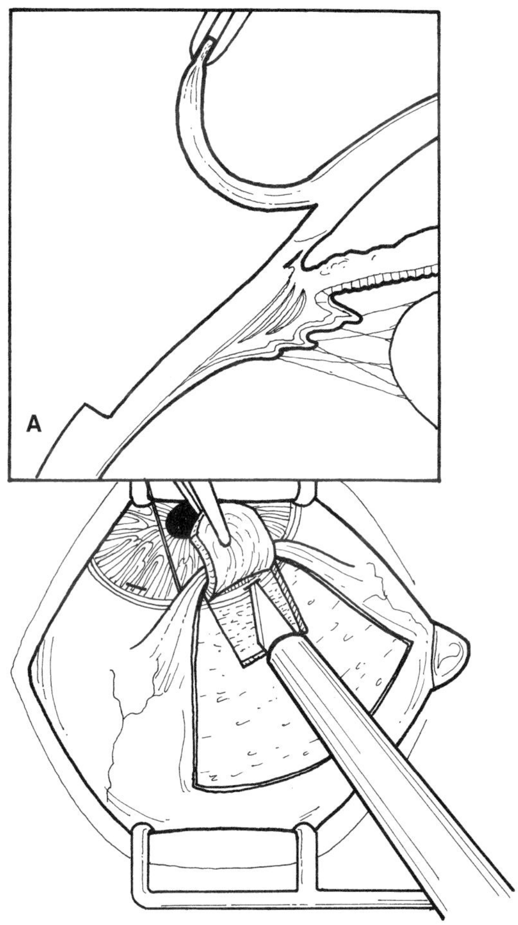

B

Figure 62.8. Scleral flap: The scleral flap is 1/2 to 2/3 scleral thickness and should extend into clear cornea (A). A Beaver No. 75 blade is used to enter the anterior chamber (B).

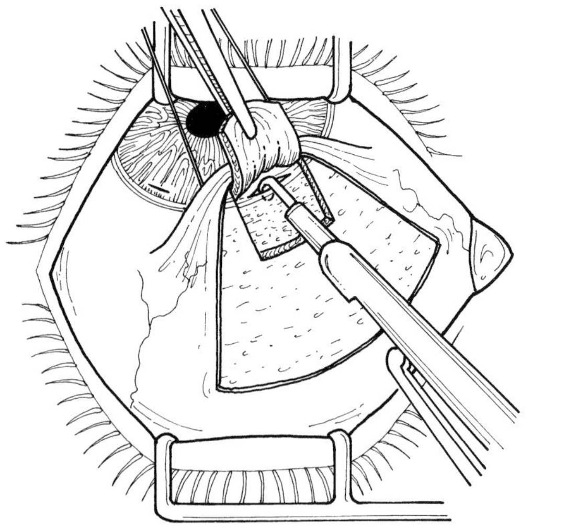

Figure 62.9. A Descemet's punch is used to create a $1\frac{1}{2}$ mm sclerectomy. The sclerectomy should extend to the scleral spur.

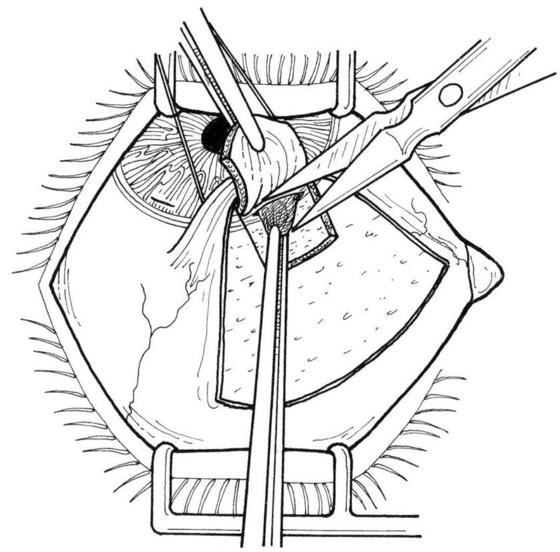

Figure 62.10. Iridectomy: A Vannas scissors is used to cut the iris as it is gently retracted through the sclerectomy.

to create a flap which is hinged as far forward as possible to ensure that the entry site for the sclerectomy is well anterior of the scleral spur and ciliary body.

The Sclerectomy

The sclerectomy is created by excising a block of tissue at the corneoscleral junction with scissors or with a punch; each approach has its advocates. In either case, the anterior chamber is entered at the anterior most point adjacent to the scleral flap with a Beaver No. 75 blade or other suitable sharp knife. If a block of tissue is to be excised, two radial incisions are made approximately 1.5–2 mm apart using Vannas scissors centered under the scleral flap. The block, now hinged posteriorly, is retracted posteriorly and excised with Vannas scissors. Frequently, the trabecular meshwork can be viewed directly while employing this procedure, which reduces the likelihood of bleeding as a result of inadvertent cutting into the ciliary body. Alternatively, a sclerectomy can be made with a Kelly-Descemet punch (Fig. 62.9). Two to three punches may be required to make a sclerectomy of adequate size. The punch is technically easier to use. However, bleeding from small vessels in the angle is more common. Gentle cautery of small bleeders can be performed under direct visualization and preferably prior to making the iridectomy. In order to stop persistent bleeding, epinephrine 1:100,000 solution (sterile and unpreserved) can be used.

The Iridectomy

A peripheral iridectomy is performed to prevent obstruction of the sclerectomy by the iris. It should be larger than the sclerectomy in all dimensions. Performing an iridectomy in a deliberate and careful manner is essential to prevent the undesired challenge of revising an inadequate iridectomy which is difficult to do and can be hazardous. **The iridectomy should be wide at its base but should not extend too far anteriorly, since this can result in monocular diplopia.** The assistant should gently retract the scleral flap to permit an unobstructed view of the sclerectomy. The surgeon grasps the iris 0.5 mm from its root with a 0.12 mm or non-toothed forceps in the surgeon's nondominant hand (Fig. 62.10). The iris is retracted through the sclerectomy toward the same side (e.g. the left side if the surgeon's nondominant hand is left). The Vannas scissors, in the surgeon's dominant hand cuts approximately half of the iris; aqueous humor may be released through the partial iridectomy. The jaws of the Vannas scissors are reopened, and the iris; is retracted to the opposite side (toward the surgeon's dominant hand) and the remaining iris is resected. The iris is reposited with a stream of balanced salt or by closing and gently massaging over the scleral flap. Forceps are never used as they may cause lens injury or vitreous loss. Upon completion of the iridectomy, the surgeon should have a view of the ciliary processes and occasionally the lens equator. **If iris remnants or ciliary processes occlude the sclerectomy these should be excised only with great caution. It is exceedingly easy to damage the lens or hyaloid face.** Redeepening the anterior chamber adjacent to the sclerectomy with viscoelastic material through the paracentesis is a useful maneuver to give the surgeon working space in these situations.

SCLERAL FLAP CLOSURE

The scleral flap is closed tightly enough to prevent postoperative hypotony. It is generally easier to cut or release sutures when the IOP is higher than desired than to deal with the complications related to prolonged low postoperative IOP. The flap is closed with interrupted 10-0 nylon sutures. A 2-1-1 knot buries well and secures the flap

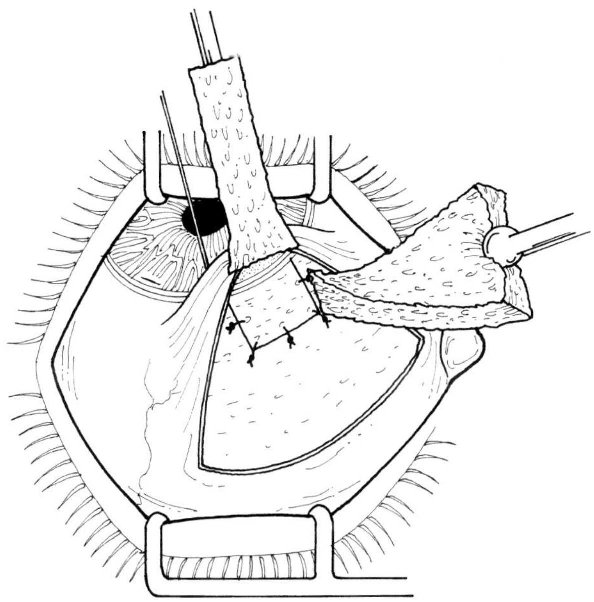

Figure 62.11. The scleral flap is closed with 10-0 nylon sutures. Scleral flap function is assessed with a Weck-cell sponge after the anterior chamber is filled with balanced salt solution.

adequately. Usually 3 sutures are used to close a triangular flap and 3–5 sutures for a rectangular flap. Once the flap is secured, it is wise to reform the anterior chamber through the paracentesis with balanced salt solution and bring the eye up to an adequate intraocular pressure. In this way the integrity and function of the scleral flap can be assessed using a Weck-cell sponge (Fig. 62.11). **If the IOP and anterior chamber depth are maintained with slow oozing of aqueous humor, then scleral flap closure is usually adequate.** However, if aqueous humor flows freely and the anterior chamber shallows, additional sutures are required. On the other hand, if the IOP is high and aqueous does not flow through the flap, sutures should be loosened. If aqueous humor still does not flow, it may be necessary to reopen the scleral flap and inspect the sclerectomy to ensure it is not obstructed.

Conjunctival Closure

Hydrodissection can be performed prior to conjunctival closure on either side of the bleb (Fig. 62.12). A strong stream of balanced salt solution is directed into the subconjunctival space using a blunt tipped cannula along the perilimbal region in both directions. Westcott scissors are used to bluntly dissect Tenon's fascia from the conjunctiva to promote filtration over a wide circumlinear area (Fig. 62.13).

Watertight conjunctival closure using non-toothed forceps is necessary to create an elevated filtering bleb. Tissues should be brought to apposition only. Tight sutures "cheesewire" postoperatively creating a leaky, inflamed wound. **Meticulous closure of the conjunctiva can save**

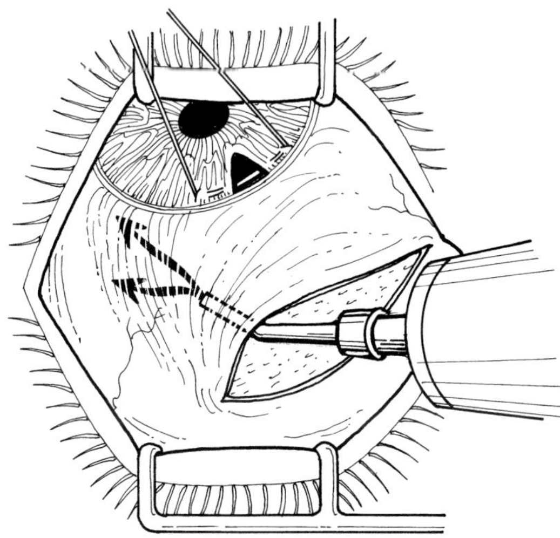

Figure 62.12. Hydrodissection of the subconjunctival tissues adjacent to the filter site with balanced salt solution prior to closing the conjunctival wound.

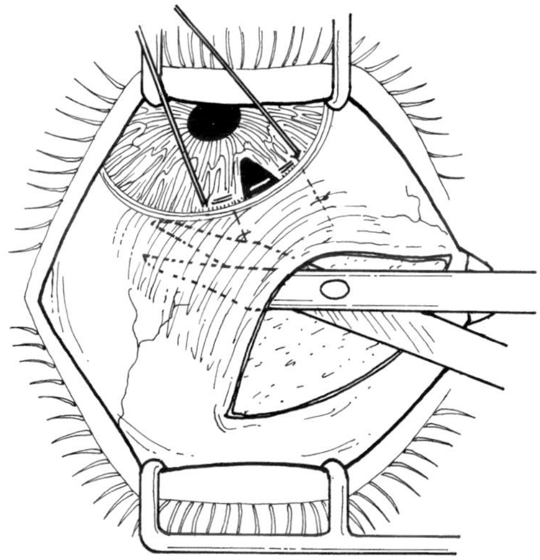

Figure 62.13. Blunt dissection of subconjunctival tissue adjacent to filter site promotes a wider area of filtration.

many postoperative hours dealing with the complications related to poorly closed wounds.

Limbus based flaps are closed in a variety of ways. However, most surgeons currently favor the use of running conjunctival closures with 9-0 or 10-0 absorbable suture (e.g. Vicryl or Dexon) on a tapered vascular needle. Where Tenon's fascia has been preserved, a double running closure can be used. In this case Tenon's fascia is closed in one direction and the conjunctiva is closed in the opposite direction. In cases where a tenonectomy has been performed, approximating the wound with 2–3 interrupted sutures reduces the tension across the wound and makes the running closure simpler to perform. **Including a small amount of posterior Tenon's fascia in the interrupted sutures may reduce the tendency for the wound to**

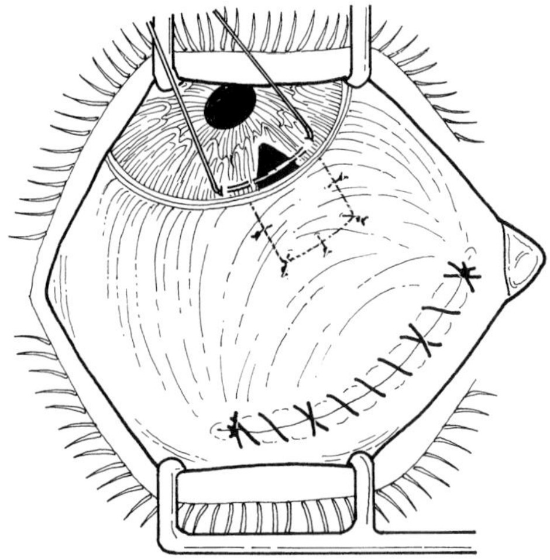

Figure 62.14. Running closure of conjunctival wound with absorbable 10-0 suture on a tapered needle. Locking every third or fourth suture increases wound integrity.

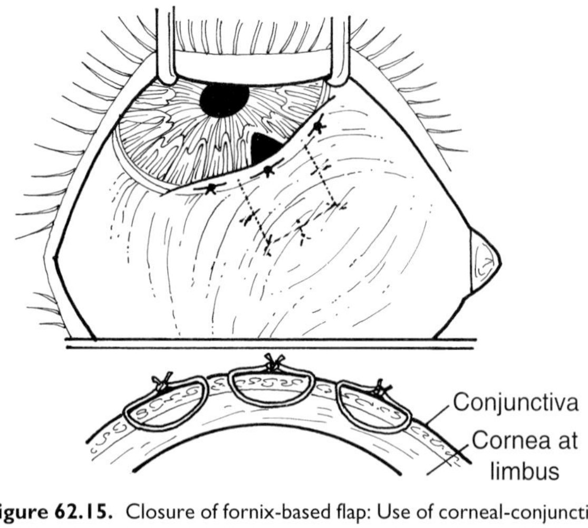

Figure 62.15. Closure of fornix-based flap: Use of corneal-conjunctival horizontal mattress sutures creates a watertight closure of a fornix based flap.

migrate anteriorly in the postoperative period. The conjunctiva is then closed in a running manner. It may be useful to lock the running suture periodically to prevent unraveling (Fig. 62.14).

Fornix based flaps can be closed in a watertight manner as well. Closure with winged sutures using nylon or Vicryl at either end of the conjunctival flap may position the leading edge of the flap over the limbus but may not offer a watertight closure in the early postoperative period. This can produce a lower, more circumscribed bleb postoperatively and delay the use of 5-FU if it is needed. If conjunctival wing sutures prove inadequate for watertight closure of a fornix based flap, 3–4 long mattress sutures are placed at the limbus using 10-0 nylon or 8-0 to 10-0 Vicryl on a spatulated needle (Fig. 62.15). The suture should be placed through midstromal cornea. In order to avoid cheesewiring the sutures should not be tied too tightly. Typically the sutures become buried in conjunctival tissues and cause no postoperative discomfort. Exposed non-absorbable sutures are removed after wound healing has occurred.

There are other techniques which may help decrease the incidence of early postoperative bleb leaks in fornix based flaps. Debriding a 1–1.5 mm zone of limbal corneal epithelium by gentle abrasion with a knife or by using cautery promotes adhesion of the conjunctival flap to the corneal stroma. Trimming Tenon's fascia from beneath the leading edge of the conjunctival flap may help to prevent "wicking" of aqueous humor under the anterior flap edge.

Fluorescein testing for bleb leaks should be performed at the conclusion of filtration surgery. This can be done after the anterior chamber has been reformed with balanced salt solution and the bleb has been inflated. Either 2% fluorescein sodium solution or a saturated fluorescein strip is placed on the conjunctival closure and paracentesis site, covering them in dense orange. A leak is readily apparent as an area of greenish flow in a "sea of orange." If a bleb leak is detected it should be closed with a single suture or a horizontal mattress suture and the wound rechecked with fluorescein. A beveled paracentesis site rarely leaks; however, if a persistent leak does occur, a single interrupted 10-0 nylon suture should be placed.

Conjunctival Buttonholes

Buttonholes can generally be avoided by meticulous handling of the conjunctiva with non-toothed forceps. Where they are more likely to occur is where there is conjunctival scarring from previous surgery or trauma, or where excessive traction has been used in an attempt to improve exposure of the surgical site. If a large buttonhole is found which overlies the filter site early in the case, the surgeon should consider relocating the filter to the adjacent quadrant.

It is frequently best to repair buttonholes after completing the planned filtration surgery. By delaying it to the end of operation, it is less likely that the conjunctival repair will be weakened. However, where there is a buttonhole, the surgeon must be especially cautious not to extend it during the operative procedure.

The manner of repair depends on the location of the buttonhole. If the edges of the buttonhole are within the conjunctiva, a horizontal mattress suture which includes both conjunctival margins and Tenons fascia is effective (Fig. 62.16). Absorbable 10-0 Vicryl or Dexon suture on a tapered vascular needle is preferred. When closed, the inner conjunctival wound margins should be well apposed.

If the buttonhole is located at the limbus where no conjunctiva is available on the corneal side of the buttonhole, a horizontal mattress suture is placed which includes peripheral cornea and the edges of the conjunctiva. Prior to closing the buttonhole the peripheral corneal epithelium is abraded or removed by gentle cautery to promote adhesion of the conjunctiva to the cornea (Fig. 62.17). A 10-0

A
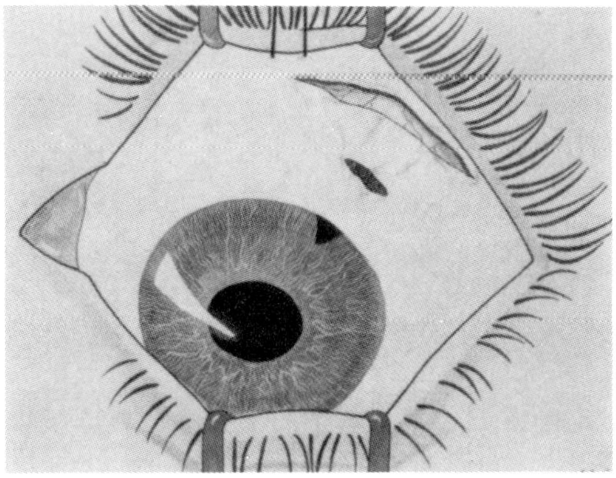

B
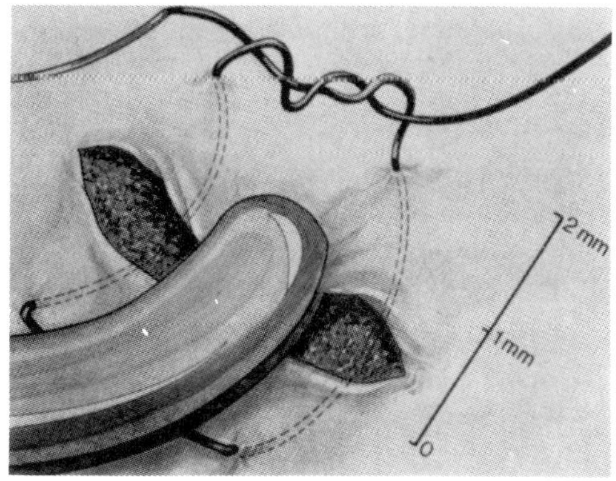

C
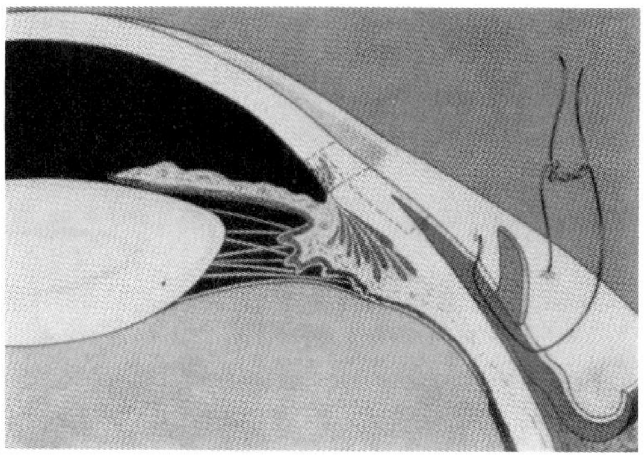

Figure 62.16. Conjunctival buttonhole occurring away from the limbus, surrounded by conjunctiva (A). Mattress suture with 10-0 Vicryl or Dexon suture with tapered needle incorporating Tenon's capsule (B). Side view of suture depth (C).

A
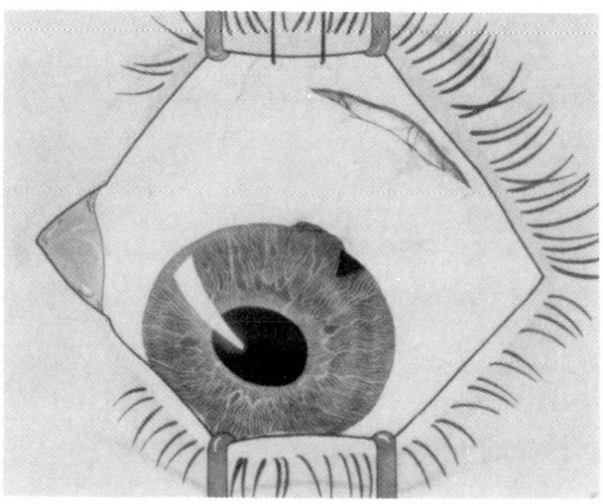

B
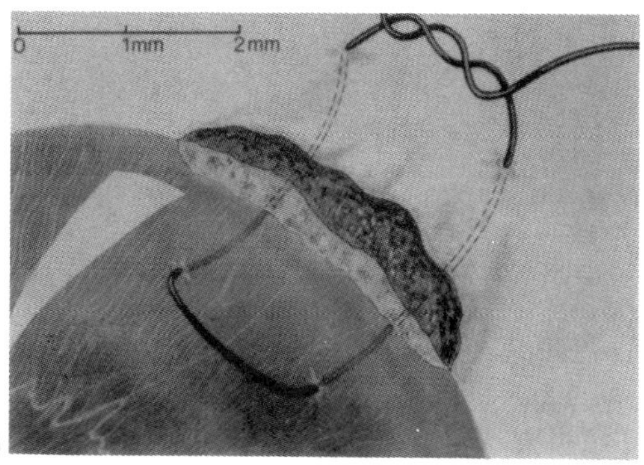

C
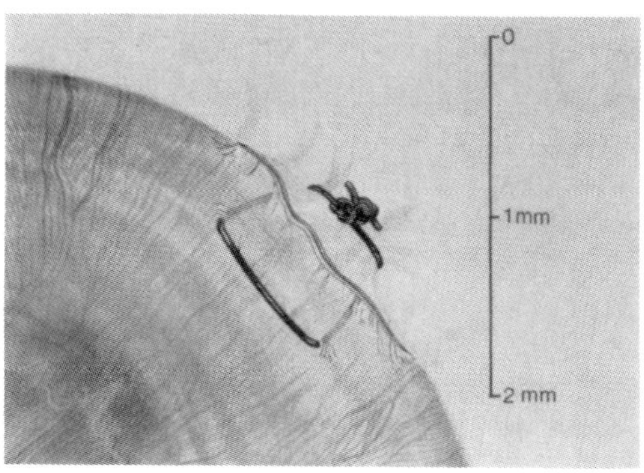

Figure 62.17. Conjunctival buttonhole occurring at the limbus. In this case, conjunctiva is only available on one side of the defect (A). After the surgical conjunctival wound is closed, attention is turned to repair of the limbal buttonhole. Suture placement and abraded corneal surface at desired site of adhesion (B). Watertight limbal closure of buttonhole (C).

nylon suture on a tapered needle or an absorbable suture (as above) can be used. Tapered needles are fragile and bend easily. However, if the needle is grasped closer to the point it is usually possible to pass the needle through the superficial cornea.

Once the conjunctival flap closure is complete, the anterior chamber is filled with balanced salt solution and the bleb is elevated. Water tight closure of the buttonhole repair and the conjunctival wound is tested with fluorescein.

Conclusion

At the conclusion of filtering surgery, subconjunctival dexamethasone phosphate 6–12 mg. is injected opposite the filtering bleb. Injectable antibiotics are not needed in uncomplicated cases and may increase postoperative inflammation. Cycloplegics (e.g. atropine 1% or scopolamine 0.25%) followed by an antibiotic ointment (e.g. Bacitracin or erythromycin) can then be applied. The eye is then gently patched and an eye shield applied.

IMMEDIATE POSTOPERATIVE MANAGEMENT

The postoperative period following glaucoma filtering surgery is frequently challenging (Chapter 63). This is largely because surgery is only the initial step in a long process which culminates in a functional drain for aqueous humor. In order to be successful, the surgeon must frustrate the natural healing process while attending to wide fluctuations of IOP in the operated eye and not infrequently the fellow eye as well. Due to the number of events transpiring in this period, frequent examinations are required.

The Fellow Eye

Postoperatively there are many changes in the patient's medical regimen which may affect the fellow eye. In order to promote normal outflow of aqueous humor after filtering surgery, it is common practice to discontinue oral carbonic anhydrase inhibitors (CAI). Frequently, however, the fellow eye suffers from glaucoma as well and benefits from oral agents. In these cases, the use of the topical CAI dorzolomide 2% in the fellow eye should be initiated once oral CAIs are stopped.

Unintentional non-compliance may occur due to major changes in the patient's drug regimen. **A medication chart is very useful for patients who may be taking half a dozen different drops with varying dosing schedules** (see Figure 18.4). Having the patient describe how they are actually taking their medication can be illuminating as well. On rare occasion, topical steroids in the operated eye may produce a "crossover" effect on IOP in the fellow eye. Therefore, **it is essential to monitor postoperative IOP in both eyes following surgery.**

If the IOP reaches unsafe levels in the fellow eye, the surgeon must advance therapy accordingly. The introduction of additional topical medications may be useful. Laser intervention or filtration surgery may ultimately be necessary. Although the prospect of additional surgery is stressful to the patient, it is important to prevent progressive optic nerve damage from occurring in the fellow eye during this time period.

Postoperative Medications

Topical steroids improve intermediate and long term postoperative IOP control after filtering surgery, although no additional benefit has been demonstrated with the use of systemic prednisone (6). Prednisolone acetate 1%, is administered every 2–4 hours to reduce postoperative inflammation and scarring. Steroids are tapered over 8–12 weeks according to the patient's clinical response, although occasionally they are continued for longer periods of time for persistent inflammation.

Cycloplegics (atropine 1% or scopolamine 0.25%) can be used twice a day for 2–3 weeks after surgery to help maintain anterior chamber depth in phakic eyes. These medications are long acting. Therefore, if the IOP is greater than 5 mm Hg and the anterior chamber is deep, administration once daily is adequate.

Antibiotics are given and tapered over a time course which is similar to that for topical steroids. An antibiotic ointment at bedtime is all that is necessary. Whether antibiotics should be given for long-term prophylaxis is a source of continuing debate. Prophylactic antibiotics may be warranted in cases where filtering blebs are thin or are placed in an inferior quadrant (7). If prophylactic antibiotics are used, medications should be replaced every 2 months and refrigerated to reduce the likelihood of bacterial contamination.

INTRAOPERATIVE AND POSTOPERATIVE ADJUNCTS

Antimetabolites

Antimetabolites, primarily five-fluorouracil (5-FU) and mitomycin C (MMC), are playing an increasingly important role as an adjunct to improve postoperative surgical success in both primary and high risk glaucoma cases. Although many chemotherapeutic agents have been or currently are being investigated for this purpose, others have not gained widespread clinical acceptance (8–10).

5-FU and MMC act by decreasing postoperative subconjunctival fibrosis, the most common cause of filtration surgery failure. 5-FU, a pyrimidine base analog, is incorporated into replicating strands of RNA and DNA. MMC, an antineoplastic antibiotic, acts as an alkylating agent which blocks DNA and protein synthesis leading to cell death. MMC is approximately 100 times more potent than 5-FU on a weight-for weight basis (11). Mitomycin is very toxic and should be handled with great care.

ANTIPROLIFERATIVE THERAPY FOR FILTRATION SURGERY

David A. Lee

The purpose of glaucoma filtration surgery is to bypass the pathological obstruction of the outflow channels of the eye in order to decrease the intraocular pressure (IOP) to a level low enough to prevent progressive damage to the optic nerve. Glaucoma filtration surgery does not directly address the causes of the abnormalities in aqueous humor outflow and "cure" glaucoma. However, it does lower the IOP by a more physiological mechanism than by decreasing the inflow of aqueous humor into the eye as is done by many of the topical and systemic antiglaucoma medications. It is arguable whether glaucoma filtration surgery should be performed early in the treatment of glaucoma, even before the use of antiglaucoma medications. The surgical treatment of glaucoma does have its risks which may be greater than those from medical therapy.

A major risk of glaucoma filtration surgery is failure due to obstruction of drainage of aqueous humor through the surgical site. This obstruction is most commonly due to the normal ocular wound healing response to surgical injury. The end result is formation of scar tissue which blocks the passage of aqueous humor from the surgical area. Conditions which may increase the risk of failure of glaucoma filtration surgery include previously failed glaucoma surgery, aphakia or pseudophakia, uveitis, neovascularization, youth, or an African-American ethnic background.

To improve the success of glaucoma filtration surgery and limit scar tissue formation it is important to understand the basic mechanisms of the wound healing response. The wound healing response is essential to the survival of all living organisms and has evolved over millions of years. It is a complex and time-limited series of events which begin when tissue is injured (1). The initial event is coagulation and vasoconstriction to stop the bleeding. This is immediately followed by inflammation with the entry of white blood cells into the injured area and the release of enzymes and cytokines to prevent infection and initiate the wound healing process. Epithelial cells, macrophages, and fibroblasts migrate into the injured area to begin closure of the wound and tissue repair. Granulation tissue forms and is composed of vascular endothelial cells which deliver a new blood supply to nourish the rapidly dividing fibroblasts. These events occur within the first several days following injury. Over the following weeks as the inflammatory process subsides, the fibroblasts produce and secrete collagens and other extracellular matrix proteins which are the major components of scar tissue. The collagen becomes cross-linked and remodeling occurs as the scar tissue matures over the following months and the wound healing process concludes. The remaining scar tissue that is impermeable to aqueous humor causes failure of glaucoma filtration surgery.

Tissue culture and animal models have been used to better understand and control the complex wound healing process. Tissue culture models can quantitatively study isolated aspects of fibroblastic activity (attachment, migration, proliferation, and extracellular matrix protein synthesis) relatively rapidly and inexpensively. However, the immune and vascular systems important to wound healing cannot be accurately duplicated in tissue culture. The most commonly used animals to model glaucoma filtration surgery and ocular wound healing are monkeys and rabbits because of similarities in ocular size and anatomy to human eyes. However, both of these animal species have a more rapid and aggressive ocular scarring reaction following glaucoma filtration surgery than humans, and the results in an animal model may not be totally applicable to humans. Both tissue culture and animal models have been used to test the efficacy, safety, and proper concentrations of wound healing inhibitory agents before their use in human eyes.

Many attempts have been made to minimize the scarring and improve the success of glaucoma filtration surgery including modifications of surgical technique, drainage devices, and medications. Various medications can affect the different stages of the wound healing process. Some of the earliest and most commonly used agents were topical corticosteroids which inhibit the initial ocular inflammatory response following surgery. These agents are very efficacious, but are frequently not sufficient to prevent the scar tissue growth that causes surgical failure. Antiproliferative agents which inhibit the growth of living cells have been used for the treatment of cancer for many years and for the prevention of ocular scar formation for over 10 years. They have been used to treat proliferative vitreoretinopathy as well as to prevent scarring after glaucoma filtration surgery.

The first antiproliferative agent used following glaucoma filtration surgery was 5-FU (2). This agent acts selectively during the synthesis phase of the cell cycle to inhibit DNA synthesis. The metabolites of 5-FU are even more potent than the original drug in inhibiting cell proliferation. This agent was originally administered as a subconjunctival injection following surgery at a dose of 5 mg. in 0.5 ml. twice daily in the first postoperative week and once a day in the second postoperative week, for a maximum total dose of 105 mg. The subconjunctival injections were given with a 30 gauge needle 180 from the surgical site after local anesthesia was induced using a cotton pledget soaked with proparacaine or cocaine. This regimen was found to significantly improve the success rate of glaucoma filtration surgery in eyes at high risk for failure from 26% in the standard treatment group to 51% in the 5-FU treatment group after 3 years of follow up. Complications from this treatment include corneal epithelial defects, conjunctival wound leaks, and bleb ruptures. The frequency and amounts of 5-FU have been titrated according to clinical response and lower doses (ranging from a total amount of 17.5 to 62.5 mg., given in 2 to 12 injections) may be as effective as the original regimen with fewer adverse side effects.

Mitomycin C is almost 100 times more potent than 5-FU in inhibiting fibroblast proliferation and is not cell cycle specific, inhibiting DNA-dependent RNA synthesis. It may also have antiangiogenic effects on blood vessels and toxicity to the ciliary epithelium and its nerve supply. These effects may account for the conjunctival avascularity and hypotony seen after mitomycin C is used during glaucoma filtration surgery. This agent is usually administered at the time of surgery using a Weck sponge saturated with 0.2 to 0.5 mg./ml. of mitomycin C and placed between the sclera and conjunctival flap for 1–5 minutes (3). The sponge is then removed and the exposed area is irrigated with 15 to 250 ml. of balanced salt solution to minimize toxic effects. Complications from mitomycin C are similar to 5-FU and also include chronic hypotony and maculopathy.

Other antiproliferative agents are currently under investigation which may be safer, more potent, or more specific for the cells actively involved in the wound healing process. A key challenge is to find an agent, or more likely a group of agents, which selectively acts on those cells which produce or assist in the production of scar tissue and physiologically regulates their behavior. Perhaps the most promising agents are cytokines or antibodies to cytokine receptors which are able to affect collagen synthesis without interfering with other normal cellular activities (4). After these agents are identified, there is the further challenge of delivering them to their intended site of action at the most effective concentration and at the proper duration. Novel drug delivery systems include liposomes and synthetic polymers of various shapes and sizes. An ideal system would provide nontoxic, localized, and sustained delivery of the agent(s) of choice in a properly timed sequence, and it would eventually disappear to avoid any foreign body complications.

Understanding and addressing the basic mechanisms of the ocular wound healing response are the best ways to improve the success and safety of glaucoma filtration surgery.

References

1. Tahery MM, Lee DA: Pharmacologic control of wound healing in glaucoma filtration surgery. J Ocul Pharmacol 1989;5:155–179.
2. The Fluorouracil Filtering Surgery Study Group: Three-year follow-up of the fluorouracil filtering surgery study. Am J Ophthalmol 1993;115:82–92.
3. Chen CW, Huang HT, Bair JS, et al: Trabeculectomy with topical application of mitomycin-C in refractory glaucoma. J Ocul Pharmacol 1990;6:175–182.
4. Nguyen KD, Hoang AT, Lee DA: Transcriptional control of human Tenon's capsule fibroblast collagen synthesis in vitro by gamma-interferon. Invest Ophthalmol Vis Sci 1994;35:3064–3070.

5-FU was the first chemotherapeutic agent to be successfully used to reduce filter failure in high risk surgical cases. The original regimen consisted of 5-mg subconjunctival injections (0.5 ml) twice daily for 1 week followed by once daily injections for an additional week (12). Complications of 5-FU use include corneal toxicity, bleb leaks, and postoperative hypotony. An increased incidence of postoperative endophthalmitis may also occur (7,13). Fewer injections maintain surgical success while decreasing the incidence of toxic side effects (14,15). In high-risk cases (e.g., neovascular glaucoma, re-operations, uveitic glaucoma) the decision to use 5-FU is usually straight forward in the absence of conjunctival wound leaks or significant pathology of the corneal epithelium. The use of 5-FU in primary filtration surgery increases operative success as well (16,17).

Regardless of risk status, initiating the use of adjunctive 5-FU is clearly indicated when there are signs of impending bleb failure. These include increased vascularization around the bleb site, particularly in those cases where the bleb is becoming marginated and "cystic," or there is decreasing microcyst formation, or flattening of the bleb. Daily injections of 5-FU are needed when these signs appear to be increasing. Injections two to three times a week may suffice if initiated early in the course of bleb failure.

If frequent injections of 5-FU are anticipated or there are concerns about corneal toxicity, a large diameter therapeutic contact lens can reduce toxic effects of this drug and promote patient comfort (18). Pain from 5-FU injections are of brief duration but can be substantial; therefore, it is important to apply adequate topical anesthesia when injecting 5-FU. Placing a small rolled pledget of cotton which has been saturated with proparacaine 0.5% into the inferior or superior fornix works well. Applying a drop of phenylephrine 2.5—5% to the eye prior to the injection will constrict conjunctival vessels and reduce subconjunctival bleeding, which can be brisk.

5-FU can also be used intraoperatively in a manner similar to MMC (19). In this case, after conjunctival dissection, a sponge saturated with 5-FU solution (50 mg/ml) is placed on bare sclera for 3–5 minutes. The surgical site is then irrigated with balanced salt solution (10–20 ml) and the operation completed in the usual manner. How this use of intraoperative 5-FU compares with that of MMC is not yet known.

MMC is used intraoperatively to reduce postoperative subconjunctival scarring, thus reducing the need for or eliminating multiple postoperative subconjunctival injections of 5-FU. It is used primarily in cases at high risk for failure; however, its use in primary filters is being explored (20). When compared to 5-FU, MMC may produce less corneal toxicity (21,22). However, a severe dose-dependent complication from MMC administration is long term postoperative hypotony with associated maculopathy (23–25). The hypotony is usually due to overfiltration through avascular thin walled filtering blebs. However, aqueous hyposecretion secondary to ciliary body toxicity may play a role in some cases (26).

The concentration of MMC employed and the duration of application during glaucoma filtration surgery varies in the literature (20,21,23–25,27). **The concentration of MMC used in clinical studies to date varies from 0.2–0.5 mg/ml. The duration of exposure varies from 2–5 minutes in most studies.** In order to reduce the risk of long term hypotony with maculopathy a protocol has been reported which adjusts the duration of MMC exposure according to risk factors of the individual patient (28).

Because MMC can be highly toxic to the corneal endothelium and tissues of the anterior segment (29,30), it should be applied in a controlled manner to bare sclera prior to entering the eye. **A cellulose or Merocel sponge which has been saturated with MMC is applied to bare sclera.** After the exposure period, the sponge is removed and the surgical site is thoroughly irrigated with balanced salt solution (15–50 ml). The remainder of the surgical procedure is completed in the usual manner.

It is not necessary to alter the suture material used for conjunctival closure when using MMC. Absorbable 10-0 sutures (Dexon, Vicryl) perform well whether 5-FU or MMC is employed. Conjunctival closure, as usual, must always be meticulous to avoid postoperative bleb leaks.

Scleral Flap Suture Release

Laser suture lysis is a technique which allows the surgeon to modify scleral flap aqueous humor outflow resistance postoperatively (31–33). By so doing, the scleral flap can be closed more tightly intraoperatively, thus reducing the occurrence of postoperative hypotony and its attendant complications.

Suture lysis is performed sequentially, that is, one suture at a time. The time interval between cutting sutures can be from hours to days, depending on the response. **Suture lysis is most effective if performed within 2 weeks of filtering surgery.** After this time period the scleral flap is frequently fibrosed in place. An exception to this rule is in cases where intraoperative MMC has been used. Some investigators have noted substantial IOP reduction from suture lysis months after surgery, and in some cases hypotony resulted (34). The time frame for suture lysis with the use of postoperative 5-FU does not seem to be substantially altered from that where no 5-FU has been used.

After application of topical anesthesia, a Zeiss or Hoskins lens is used to flatten the bleb overlying the scleral flap (Fig. 62.18). By placing the lens over the peripheral cornea first and gently sliding the lens toward the scleral flap there is less stress on the conjunctival wound (for fornix based conjunctival flaps the approach is reversed). **The lens may need to be held in place for a short period of time (up to 1–2 minutes) to compress the bleb tissues and improve the view of the suture before lasering** (Fig. 62.19). Usually, an argon green or comparable wavelength is used with settings of 300–1000 mW, 0.02—0.2 seconds, and a 50 μm spot size. **If subconjunctival hemorrhage is present a krypton laser (wavelength 640 nm) or a diode laser may reduce absorption by surrounding blood products.** The suture should clearly separate when successfully cut (Fig. 62.20). If there is no clear separation of the suture, it wasn't cut or it was not functionally closing the scleral flap. Additional sutures may need to be cut in the latter situation. Occasionally, a cut end stands vertically inside the bleb after lysis. If this occurs it is wise to cut the base of the vertical segment to prevent it from later puncturing the bleb.

Releasable sutures, a method to remove scleral flap sutures at the slit lamp, can be used to circumvent the need for a laser. Blood, Tenon's fascia, conjunctival pigmentation, or fibrovascular tissue can obstruct the view of the suture and frustrate the surgeon's ability to release the flap by laser suture lysis. Additionally, the conjunctiva can be buttonholed by the laser, or stresses to the bleb can create wound leaks both of which may produce hypotony. Sometimes there may not be ready availability of a laser.

Methods have been developed for sutures which can be released at the slit lamp. The main advantages of these techniques are the relative ease of suture removal and the lack of bleb manipulation. One or more sutures can be placed to produce a watertight scleral flap. The time frame for suture removal is similar to that described above for laser suture lysis. However, scar tissue may be incorporated within the releasable knot after 10–14 days, thus preventing its removal. If the suture breaks or cannot be released, the suture can still usually be cut with a laser.

THE FAILED FILTER

Unfortunately, even surgery performed and followed in the most meticulous manner may fail. Failure occurs when aqueous humor meets elevated resistance between the sclerectomy and the conjunctival epithelium. **The most common cause of filter failure is subconjunctival fibrosis.** If intervention is made early, filter failure can be avoided in many instances. **This includes digital pressure and the late use of 5-FU injections.** In some cases the sclerec-

HOW TO HANDLE MITOMYCIN C

David P. Tingey

The use of mitomycin C (MMC) intraoperatively for glaucoma filtration procedures requires a relatively small volume of a very potent and expensive chemotherapeutic agent. This raises issues of safety and cost.

MMC is packaged as 5 milligrams of powder contained in a 10 cc amber glass vial. It must be reconstituted by adding the necessary amount of sterile water for the desired concentration. The vial is then shaken and allowed to stand at room temperature until the powder is dissolved completely. The concentration of mitomycin used by most surgeons during filtration surgery ranges from 0.2 mg/ml to 0.5 mg/ml. Adding 10 cc of sterile water to the vial gives a final concentration of 0.5 mg/ml. For lower concentrations of mitomycin the solution must be removed and further diluted to the desired concentration. Reconstitution may be carried out in the operating room for immediate use or it may be done preoperatively in the pharmacy.

The stability of MMC is pH dependent (1). Acidic pH will rapidly inactivate MMC. Sterile water or sterile 0.9% sodium chloride solution diluents can range in pH from 4 to 7. Diluents having a pH in the lower range may contribute to instability (2). During and after reconstitution the solution must be handled with great care in the operating room. Direct exposure to skin or eyes as well as inhalation of aerosolized solution is to be avoided. All personnel handling MMC must have appropriate protective eyewear, operating room mask and gloves. If the MMC is being reconstituted in the operating room, a specialized vial cap such as the Oncoline (Chemo Pin) may be used to prevent aerosolization. The desired quantity of reconstituted MMC (e.g., 1 or 2 cc) is placed in a sterile container within the sterile field. Mitomycin degrades after prolonged exposure to light and it should be covered from light once it is out of the vial awaiting use. After use, all materials must be handled as biohazardous waste and disposed of via the appropriate institutional biohazardous waste methods.

One vial of MMC yields 10 cc of a 0.5 mg/ml solution for an approximate cost of $90 (1995). Only a fraction of this is required for each case and it would be most cost effective to get several uses out of a single vial. For centers performing a large volume of surgery with MMC a single reconstituted vial may be used on consecutive cases over a short period of time. Reconstituted MMC is stable for 7 days if stored at room temperature (25 degrees C) and for 14 days under refrigeration (4 degrees C) (3).

For less frequent use it would be ideal to store the reconstituted solution for some time. It has been shown that MMC 0.5 mg/ml demonstrates greater than 85% inhibition of fibroblast proliferation measured by tritiated thymidine uptake even after being stored at room temperature for 6 weeks (4). McMenemy et al. studied the effect of lower concentrations of MMC (0.1 mg/ml and 0.2 mg/ml) on fibroblast proliferation after storage using a Coulter counter method. They suggested that it is feasible to store MMC at 0 to −5 degrees centigrade for up to 4 weeks with negligible loss of activity (5). A comparison of the effect of fresh MMC versus stored mitomycin on bleb survival in rabbits suggested that MMC that has been stored for up to two months is as effective as fresh mitomycin-C in prolonging bleb life and lowering intraocular pressure (6).

There is thus preliminary evidence that storage beyond the manufacturer's recommended duration still affords effectiveness, but this is unproven in human subjects. In addition, issues of sterility with prolonged storage at room temperature and 4 degrees centigrade have not been addressed. However, prolonged storage at room temperature might be the only option for some remote third world settings without refrigeration. MMC 0.5 mg/ml in sterile water for injection, USP has less than a 10% loss of potency for up to 52 weeks when stored at −20 degrees C in amber glass vials. It may be frozen and thawed for up to 17 cycles and still retain its potency (2). Another study indicated that MMC reconstituted at 0.6 mg/ml in normal saline and stored in plastic bags at −20 degrees centigrade showed a significant loss of potency which the authors felt was due to crystallization. At −30 degrees centigrade there was no significant loss of potency over a four week period (7). Some authors have recommended that, after reconstitution with sterile water, small aliquots of MMC in the desired concentrations be aseptically transferred in a laminar-airflow hood to sterile vials or syringes, appropriately sealed, and frozen at −20 degrees C for single use (1). This approach appears to be safe and cost effective.

References

1. Fiscella RG, Proffitt DF, Weisbacker CA: Stability of mitomycin for ophthalmic use. Am J Hosp Pharm 1994;49:2438.
2. Dorr RT: University of Arizona. Unpublished report provided by Bristol-Myers Squibb Medical Information Services, 1994.
3. Bristol Laboratories: Mitomycin for injection package insert. Evansville, IN: May, 1990.
4. Tingey DP, Hooper PL, Woo E, et al: Stability of Mitomycin C after reconstitution. Poster Presentation, American Academy of Ophthalmology, Annual Meeting, October 1994.
5. McMenemy MG, Lahiri-Munir D, King RT, et al: Effect of storage on antifibroblastic activity of mitomycin C. Invest Ophthal Vis Sci 1994;35:1425.
6. Henderson PR, Karp K, Higginbotham EJ, et al: Evaluation of the efficacy of stored mitomycin-C as adjunctive therapy in glaucoma filtration surgery in rabbits. Invest Ophthal Vis Sci 1994;35:1425.
7. Stolk et al: Stability after freezing and thawing of solutions of mitomycin C in plastic minibags for intravesical use. Pharmaceutisch Weekblad Scientific Edition 1996;8:286–288.

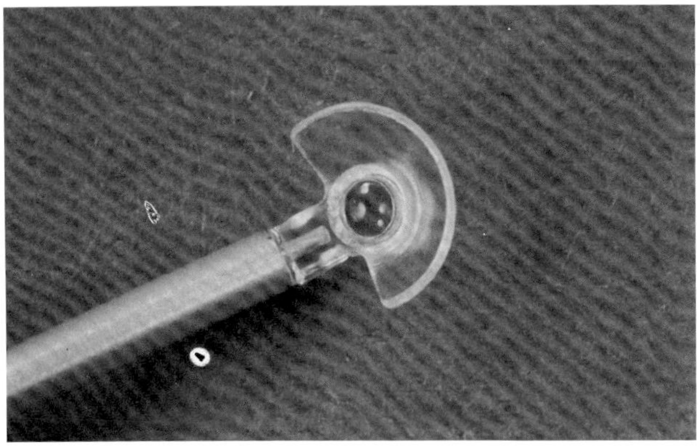

Figure 62.18. Hoskins lens used for laser suture lysis. (Courtesy of Richard J. Simmons, MD.)

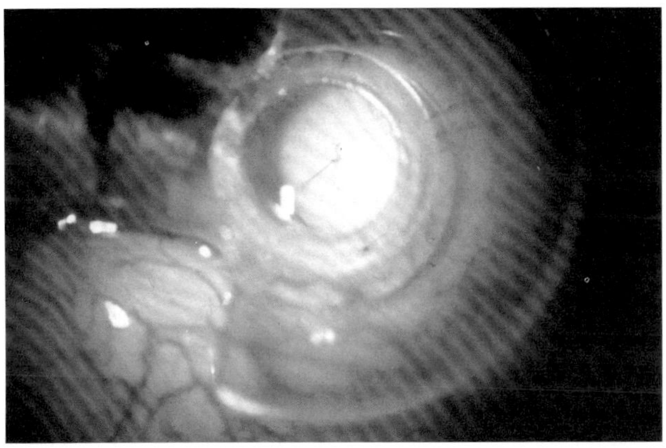

Figure 62.19. Scleral flap suture seen through Hoskins lens. (Courtesy of Richard J. Simmons, MD.)

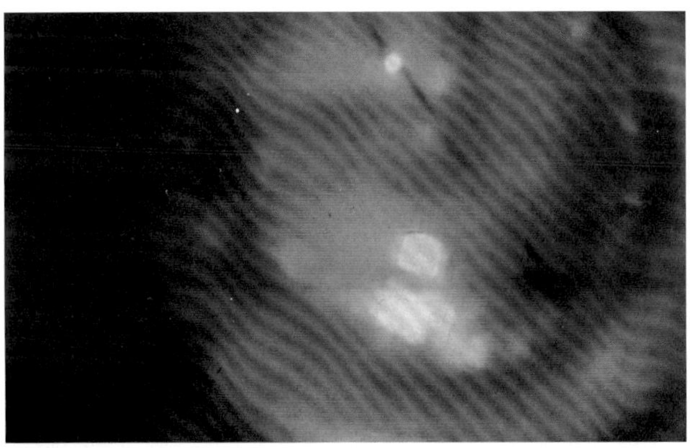

Figure 62.20. Scleral flap suture lysis: Note how scleral flap opens after the suture is cut. (Courtesy of Richard J. Simmons, MD.)

tomy is blocked by iris, vitreous, or lens material. In others, the scleral flap may become fibrosed. A "Tenon's cyst" can form which is a fluid filled cavity lined internally by fibrous tissue.

Revision filtration surgery can be successful in selected cases. **Revision surgery is especially likely to succeed when a filtering bleb was functional for months or years prior to failure.** In many cases the filtration site is quiet and the procedure can be performed without producing the usual amount of postoperative inflammation. Additionally, revision surgery conserves conjunctiva for future filtration surgery if it should become necessary. In any case, the failed filter requires careful examination prior to embarking on revision surgery in order to define the cause of failure. Once the cause of failure is known, the optimal surgical approach can be determined.

Conjunctival mobility can be assessed with a sterile moistened cotton tip swab after topical anesthesia has been applied. In regions where the conjunctiva is tightly adherent to the episclera and little conjunctival movement can be demonstrated, it is unlikely that revision surgery will succeed. **If the conjunctiva overlying the previous filter site is mobile, surgical revision is more likely to be successful.** This technique should always be used in the initial evaluation to examine the conjunctiva prior to embarking on filtration surgery in cases where there has been previous surgery or trauma.

Gonioscopy is performed to assess patency of the sclerectomy. Membranes, iris, or lens remnants may cover or occlude the internal sclerectomy. It is possible to reopen the sclerectomy with Nd:YAG or argon laser in selected cases (35–39).

Anesthesia considerations are identical to primary filtration surgery.

Internal Surgical Revisions

Internal revision of the failed filter is most likely to succeed in cases where the filtering bleb was functional for a period of months or years. The bleb conjunctiva is freely mobile. The site of the obstruction is at the level of the sclerectomy and/or scleral flap. This approach entails opening the sclerectomy and scleral flap with the use of a cyclodialysis spatula, needle knife, or cautery.

A beveled paracentesis is made through clear cornea. The paracentesis is angled toward the sclerectomy site (Fig. 62.23). The anterior chamber is then filled with viscoelastic in order to maintain the chamber and protect the lens in phakic eyes. **Under gonioscopic visualization, a 0.5 mm cyclodialysis spatula is guided through the sclerectomy into the subconjunctival space** (Fig. 62.24). The goniolens is removed when the tip of the instrument is visualized in the subconjunctival space. Episcleral attachments are broken by forcefully sweeping the spatula in an arc-like fashion. Aqueous humor typically fills the bleb during this maneuver demonstrating restored patency of the sclerectomy.

In some cases a needle knife or thermal cautery may be required to restore patency of the sclerectomy (Fig. 62.25) (40). In order to avoid perforating the conjunctiva, balanced salt solution is injected subconjunctivally to elevate the bleb

EXTERNALIZED RELEASABLE SUTURES IN FILTERING SURGERY

Murray A. Johnstone

Externalized releasable sutures have several benefits in comparison with laser suture lysis. The first is avoidance of need for laser access, scheduling and cost. The second is the lack of a need for compression of the conjunctiva with a lens; this avoids issues of pain, inflammation and the risk of disrupting the limbal adhesion of fornix based flaps. A third benefit is lack of a need for suture visualization. Inability to visualize the suture is common with laser suture lysis when the overlying conjunctiva is thickened, edematous or contains blood; these are situations where the ability to release the suture early is of special importance. A fourth benefit is the absence of the risk of perforation of the conjunctival flap, a special concern with laser suture lysis in the presence of blood. Conjunctival perforations are of greater significance after mitomycin treatment because of the tendency of perforations to be persistent in tissue devoid of the normal fibroblast population.

EXTERNALIZED RELEASABLE SUTURE TECHNIQUES

Surgeons have described alternative types of externalized releasable sutures to close the scleral flap in trabeculectomy. The first, described by Wilson (1), involved use of a horizontal mattress suture that passes from the edge of the rectangular scleral flap, beneath the conjunctival reflection, to the surface of the cornea. Another technique described by Shin (2), utilizes a slip knot at the apex of a triangular scleral flap, with the suture end then brought to the surface of the conjunctiva. Cohen (3) reported the use of a slip knot at the apex of the triangular flap, with the suture end then passed beneath the corneal reflection to rest on the surface of the cornea (Fig. 62.21A-B). A modification uses two of the same type of slip knot sutures in the corners of a rectangular scleral flap (Fig. 62.21C).

A technique that I have used in more than 1500 trabeculectomies since 1984 involves placement of compression sutures directly over the scleral flap (Fig. 62.22). The compression or tamponading effect occurs because the scleral flap is not pinned down at its corners by short interrupted sutures. The flap is anchored posteriorly by a single, horizontal mattress suture that passes through the posterior corners of the flap. This mattress suture combines with the releasable suture to create a web of nylon over the anterior surface of the flap and a V-shaped area of compression just behind the sclerotomy site. The surface arrangement allows the flap to function as a valve-like device. The long runs of nylon in the web are free to stretch as IOP increases, permitting the flap to elevate slightly and release aqueous into the bleb. As the IOP decreases, the active elastic recoil in the nylon sutures pushes the flap back to its position in the scleral bed, preventing excessive filtration.

This technique generally provides satisfactory filtration while preventing a substantial reduction in chamber depth (4). In a recent series (5) of primary trabeculectomies mean first day postoperative IOP grouped by week varied from 8.3–11.2 mm Hg during the first six weeks after surgery. Sufficient anterior chamber shallowing to cause iridocorneal apposition was seen in 8/230 (3.4%) of eyes. No anterior chambers had persistent shallowing beyond the first two weeks and there were no axially flat chambers.

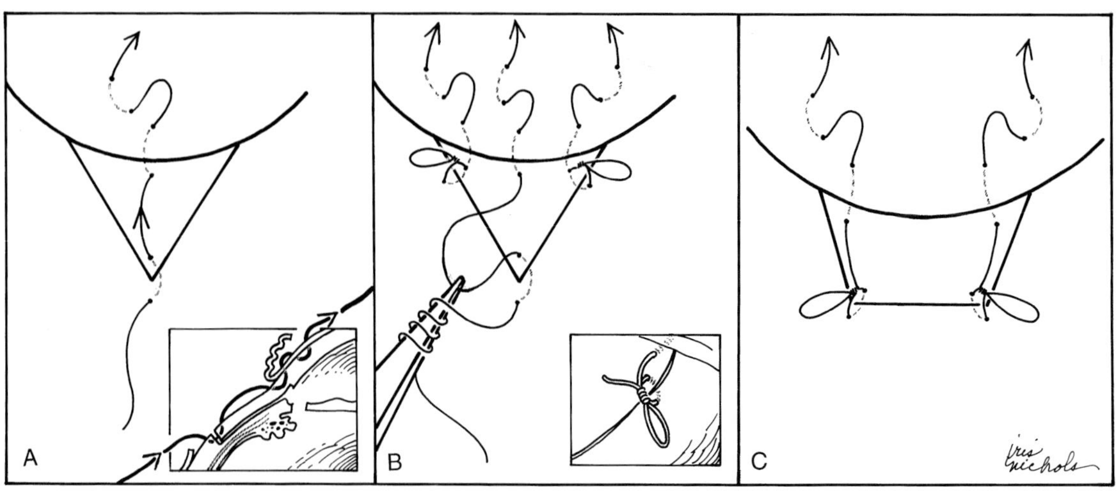

Figure 62.21. Externalized releasable suture employing a slip knot at the apex of a triangular flap (A,B) and at the corners of a rectangular flap (C). Modified from Cohen J, Osler RH: Releasable suture in filtering and combined surgery. Ophthalmol Clin North Am 1988;1:187–197.

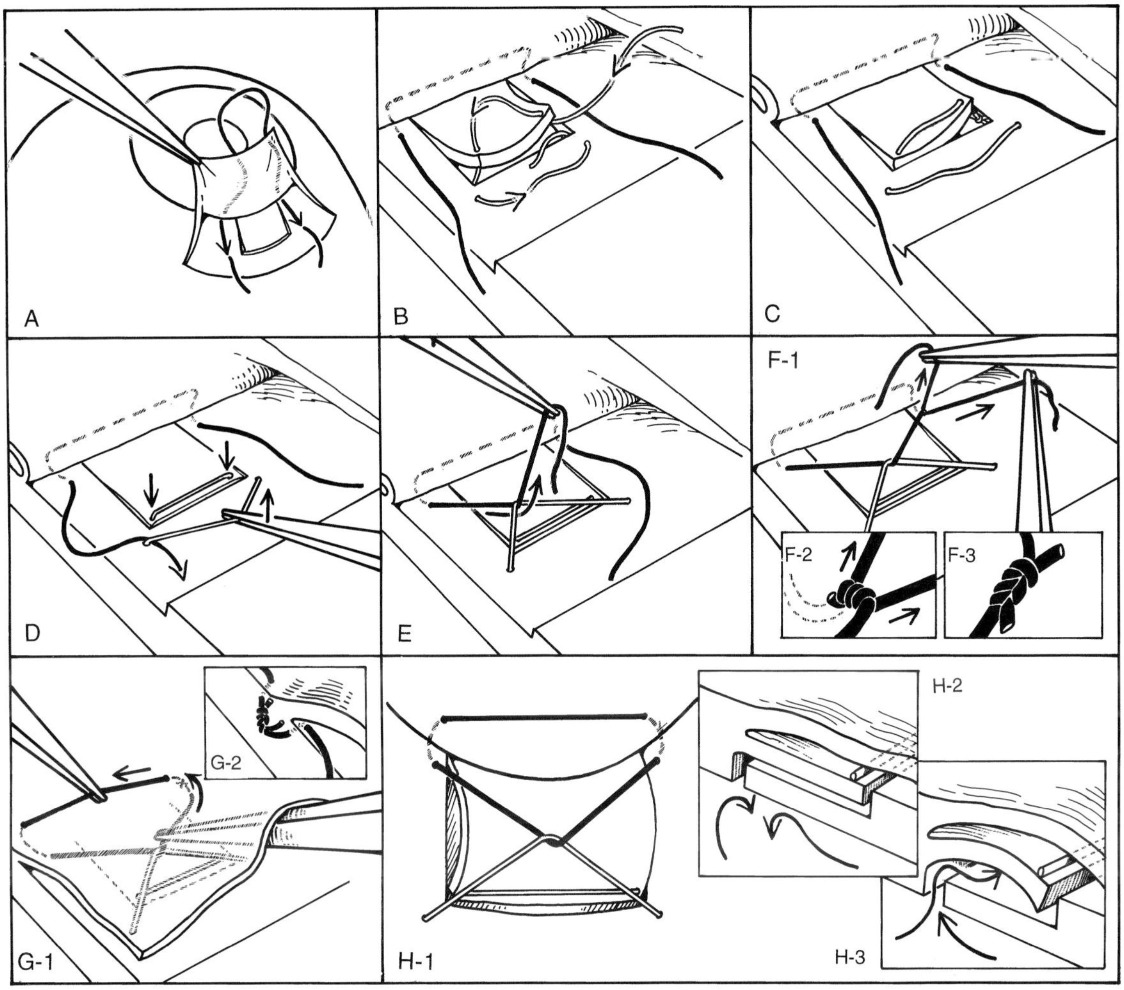

Figure 62.22. (A-H) Externalized releasable suture employing a compression suture technique. This technique produces a tamponade effect over the scleral flap (see text).

Suture Release Timing

Suture release is generally delayed for 2–6 weeks or longer after surgery in eyes with an acceptably low IOP or if IOP can be lowered easily with digital pressure. Early suture release may increase the incidence of complications and does not generally appear to improve the long-term results in eyes with acceptable initial control.

In patients who have received antimetabolites, the interval in which suture release increases the risk of hypotony is extended and should be delayed beyond two weeks whenever possible. In a recent study involving antimetabolites, with use of the scleral flap tamponade suture and digital pressure, only 6% of eyes required suture release within the first two weeks after surgery.

The concept of placing multiple sutures with subsequent control of IOP by incremental suture release is appealing. However, tight closure with multiple short sutures at the incision edges tends to force earlier suture release. In addition, there is often a single key or cardinal suture that causes most of the IOP lowering effect. It is not possible to know whether the key or cardinal suture will be the first, an intermediate, or the last suture cut. Because of the unpredictability of the effect of releasing any individual suture, it is appropriate to be cautious with suture release whether one or multiple sutures have been placed.

Beyond the first two weeks after surgery, suture release is generally done if IOP remains elevated after digital pressure. Valuable indicators of the ability to release sutures without causing persistent hypotony are the need for progressively more digital pressure to cause distention of the bleb, clearly defined margins limiting the extent of lateral dissection and elevation of the bleb with digital pressure, and a subtle line of finely arborizing vessels completely outlining the margins of the bleb. Recurrent bleb flattening despite repeated digital pressure and generalized bleb vascularity are additional useful factors in deciding the timing of suture release.

In summary, releasable suture techniques increase our ability to avoid the profound hypotony and aqueous runoff associated with shallow and flat anterior chambers. The use of releasable sutures raises new questions related to optimizing suture placement techniques and finding additional clinical clues to assist in the safe timing of suture release.

References

1. Wilson R: Technical advances in filtration surgery In: McAllister JA, ed. Glaucoma 1986:243–250.
2. Shin DH: Removable-suture closure of the lamellar scleral flap in trabeculectomy. Ann Ophthalmol 1987;19:51–53, 55.
3. Cohen J, Osher RH: Releasable suture in filtering and combined surgery. Ophthalmol Clin North Am 1988;1:187–197.
4. Johnstone MA, Wellington DP, Ziel CJ: A releasable scleral-flap tamponade suture for guarded filtration surgery. Arch Ophthalmol 1993;111(3):398–403
5. Johnstone MA, Ziel CJ. Releasable scleral flap tamponade suture to control IOP and chamber depth after filtering surgery. Invest Ophthalmol Vis Sci 1995;36(4):411.

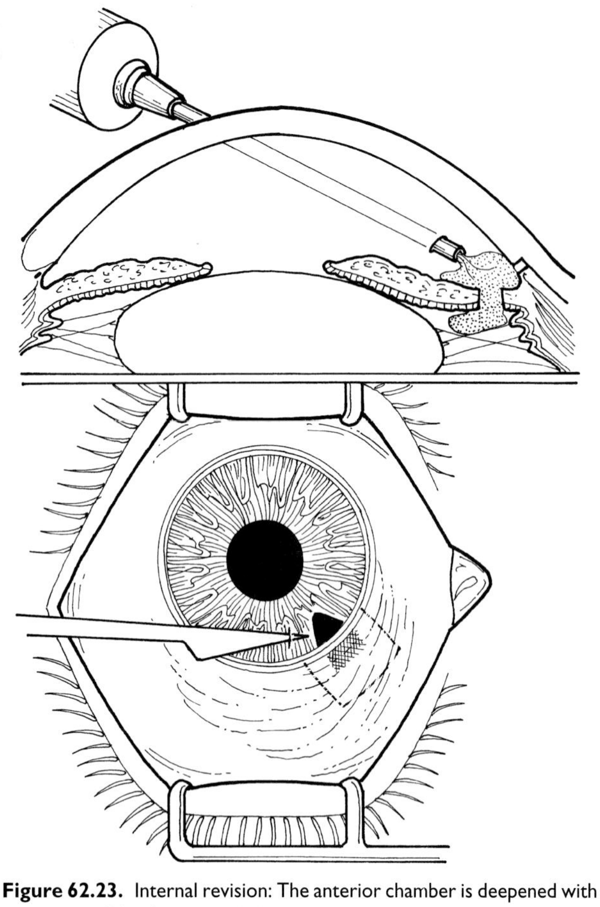

Figure 62.23. Internal revision: The anterior chamber is deepened with viscoelastic (A), after a beveled paracentesis is made in the direction of the sclerectomy (B).

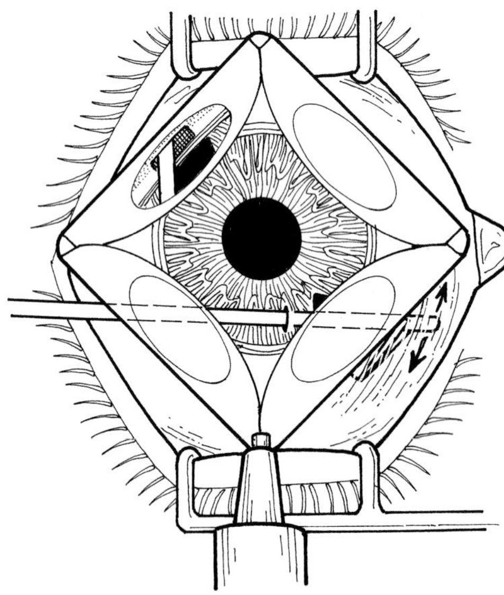

Figure 62.24. Internal revision: A gonioscope is used to direct the cyclodialysis spatula or needle knife toward the sclerectomy. Once the instrument tip is visualized in the subconjunctical space the goniolens is removed. Adhesions are broken by a "to and fro" movement with the spatula.

prior to probing the sclerectomy site. A coaxial endodiathermy (Mira) unit (25.5 gauge, angulated) probe or 23 gauge blunt tipped cautery (Mentor) can be used to recanulate obstructed sclerectomies. A needle knife can restore patency of the sclerectomy. However, cautery enlarges the sclerectomy by producing collagen shrinkage around and away from the probe. This may prevent recurrent closure of the sclerectomy.

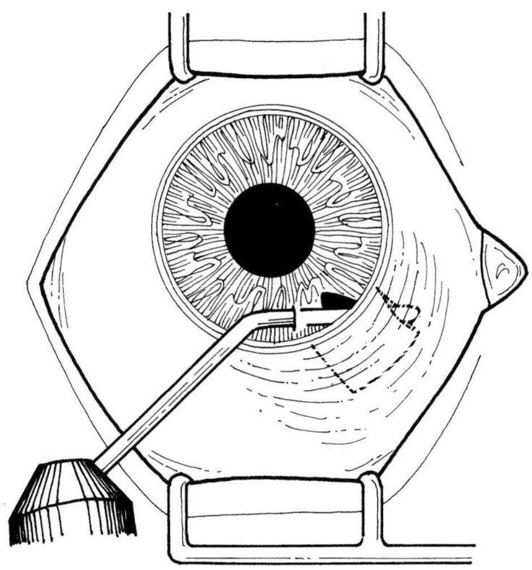

Figure 62.25. Internal revision: The scleral opening can be opened with coaxial diathermy or cautery. The conjunctiva is elevated with balanced salt solution prior to diathermy or cautery to avoid perforating the bleb.

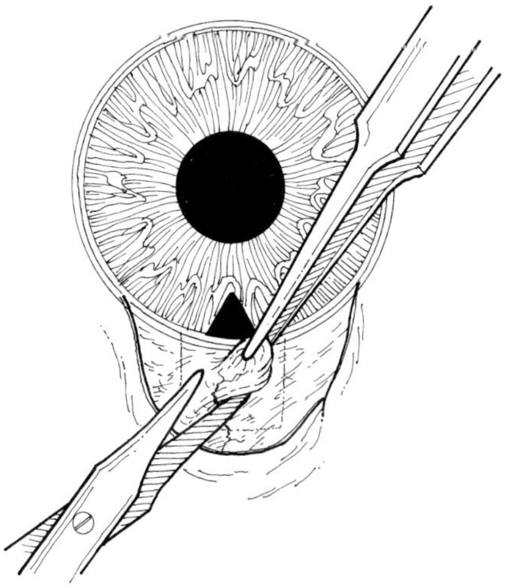

Figure 62.26. External revision: After the conjunctiva is retracted, the underlying episcleral scar tissue is dissected from the scleral flap.

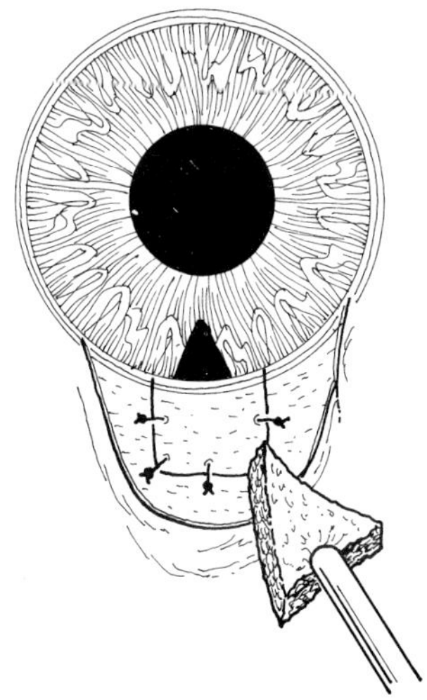

Figure 62.27. External revision: The scleral flap is closed with 10-0 nylon suture. Aqueous flow is evaluated using a Weck-cell sponge.

Table 62.3
Common Errors and Problems in Filtering Surgery

Short conjunctival flap (limbus-based flap)	Reduces potential filtration area and increases likelihood of postoperative failure. Initiate conjunctival flap **at least 8 mm** from the limbus.
Toothed forceps for conjunctival manipulation	Use of **non-toothed forceps** and gentle handling of tissues reduces buttonholes and post operative inflammation.
Thin or small scleral flap	The scleral flap should be **at least half total scleral thickness** and large enough to functionally cover the sclerectomy site to prevent prolonged postoperative hypotony.
Paracentesis too small, can't be found, or can't be cannulated	To cannulate easily, a paracentesis must have a **large internal (endothelial) opening** and **known location and orientation** (test paracentesis before continuing case).
Iridectomy imperforate or too small	The iridectomy must be patent and extend to the posterior sclerectomy margins (so one can see the red reflex or ciliary processes). Extreme caution must be used to enlarge a small iridectomy to avoid vitreous loss.
Sclerectomy site too far posterior	Excessive bleeding or occlusion of the sclerectomy by the ciliary body can be avoided by making the initial anterior chamber entry site as far **anterior** as possible (well into the limbal gray-blue zone). **Cautery** should be performed cautiously for bleeding.
Sclerectomy site too close to lateral scleral flap margin	The scleral flap must **completely cover the sclerectomy,** otherwise resistance to aqueous flow will be low and hypotony will result.
Occlusion of the sclerectomy by ciliary processes	Particularly seen in small hyperopic eyes. An anterior sclerectomy site is helpful. **Ciliary processes can be gently cauterized**, grasped with .12 forceps **and excised** with Vannas scissors if necessary.
Vitreous loss through sclerectomy site	Fortunately a rare complication. A meticulous Weck cell vitrectomy can salvage the bleb. **Postoperative hypotony with a shallow anterior chamber must be avoided** (to prevent posterior vitreous from entering the sclerectomy site).
Scleral flap closure (too tight or too loose)	With irrigation through the paracentesis, fluid should flow slowly with a **maintained anterior chamber** depth.
Conjunctival wound leak	Wound leaks can be reduced by meticulous wound closure and testing with fluorescein.

External Surgical Revision

Not uncommonly, the overlying filtering bleb is well elevated but thick walled ("Tenon's cyst"). The thickness of this subconjunctival collagenous tissue can be equivalent to that of the cornea (41), and frequently produces great resistance to aqueous humor outflow. Surgical dissection of all or a portion of the scar tissue can relieve this barrier. In other cases because revision may be required despite adequate function, but high elevation or overall size may produce difficulties with corneal exposure, dellen formation, or offer an unacceptable cosmetic appearance.

A paracentesis is performed in the usual manner. A fornix-based or limbus-based conjunctival flap is created. Utilizing sharp and blunt dissection, the conjunctiva is freed from underlying scar tissue. Gentle cautery is required to control bleeding, avoiding cautery to the conjunctiva itself. The scar tissue overlying the scleral flap is excised (Fig. 62.26). The scleral flap is recanalized and balanced salt solution is instilled into the anterior chamber to demonstrate patency of the sclerectomy. Viscoelastic can be used to maintain the anterior chamber if necessary. The flap is closed (if possible) with 10-0 nylon suture (Fig. 62.27). If visualization of the flap sutures is expected to be a problem in the postoperative period, releasable sutures may be used. Closure of the limbus-based or fornix-based conjunctival flap is performed as described above.

Postoperatively, the patient is treated in essentially the same manner as a primary filtration surgery. Frequent topical steroids, cycloplegics, and antibiotics are used. Adjunctive 5-FU is used where necessary to prevent the recurrence of a cystic bleb. A full course of 5-FU may be required. **The use of MMC is not advisable during bleb revisions.** Severe toxicity may occur if MMC enters the anterior chamber through the scleral flap (29).

CONCLUSION

The process of glaucoma filtration surgery is a challenge (Table 62.3) to the ophthalmic surgeon. Meticulous technique combined with careful and close observation are required throughout the peri-operative period. Managing and supporting the patient through this process can be a daunting task at times; however, a successful outcome is highly gratifying to both the patient and the surgeon.

References

1. Sherwood MB, Migdal CS, Hitchings RA, et al: Initial treatment of glaucoma: surgery or medications. (Review). Surv Ophthalmol 1993; 37:293–305.
2. Cyclodialysis. In: Chandler and Grant's Glaucoma, Epstein DL (editor), 3rd Edition, Lea & Febiger, 1986;451–457.
3. Simmons RJ: Filtering operations. In: Chandler and Grant's Glaucoma, Epstein DL (editor), 3rd Edition, Lea & Febiger, 1986;425–426.
4. Wilson MR, Baker R: Prognostic factors for glaucoma filtration surgery. J Glaucoma 1993;2:223–226.
5. Schlect LP, Brubaker RF: The effects of withdrawal of timolol in chronically treated glaucoma patients. Ophthalmology 1988;95:1212–1216.
6. Starita RJ, Fellman RL, Spaeth GL, et al: Short and long-term effects of postoperative corticosteroids on trabeculectomy. Ophthalmology 1985;92:938–946.
7. Wolner B, Liebmann JM, Sassani JW, et al: Late bleb-related endophthalmitis after trabeculectomy with adjunctive 5-fluorouracil. Ophthalmology 1991;98:1053–1060.
8. Jampel HD: Impact of adjuvant chemotherapy on glaucoma filtration surgery. J Glaucoma 1993;2:58–63.
9. Lee DA: Antifibrosis agents and glaucoma surgery. Invest Ophthalmol Vis Sci 1994;35:3789–3791.
10. Parrish RK II: Who should receive antimetabolites after filtering surgery? Arch Ophthalmol 1992;110:1069–1071.
11. Yamamoto T, Varani J, Soong KH, et al: Effects of 5-fluorouracil and MMC on cultured rabbit subconjunctival fibroblasts. Ophthalmology 1990;97:1204–1210.
12. The Fluorouracil Filtering Surgery Study Group. Three-year follow-up of the Fluorouracil Filtering Surgery Study. Am J Ophthalmol 1993; 115:82–92.
13. Rockwood EJ, Parrish RK II, Heuer DK, et al: Glaucoma filtering surgery with 5-fluorouracil. Ophthalmology 1987;94:1071–1078.
14. Weinreb RN: Adjusting the dose of 5-fluorouracil after glaucoma filtering surgery to minimize the side effects. Ophthalmology 1987;94:564.
15. Krug JH, Melamed S: Adjunctive use of delayed and adjustable low-dose 5-fluorouracil in refractory glaucoma. Am J Ophthalmol 1990;109: 412.
16. Ophir A, Ticho U: A randomized study of trabeculectomy and subconjunctival administration of fluorouracil in primary glaucomas. Arch Ophthalmol 1992;110:1072–1075.
17. Liebmann JM, Ritch R, Marmor M, et al: Initial 5-fluorouracil trabeculectomy in uncomplicated glaucoma. Ophthalmology 1991;98: 1036–1041.
18. Beckman RL, Sofinski SJ, Greff LJ, et al: Bandage contact lens augmentation of 5-fluorouracil treatment in glaucoma filtration surgery. Ophthalmic Surg 1991;22:563–564.
19. Dietze PJ, Feldman RM, Gross RL: Intraoperative application of 5-fluorouracil during trabeculectomy. Ophthalmic Surg 1992;23: 662–665.
20. Kitazawa Y, Suemori-Matsushita H, Yamamoto T, et al: Low-dose and high-dose mitomycin trabeculectomy as an initial surgery in primary open-angle glaucoma. Ophthalmology 1993;100:1624–1628.
21. Skuta GL, Beeson CC, Higginbotham EJ, et al: Intraoperative mitomycin versus postoperative 5-fluorouracil in high-risk glaucoma filtering surgery. Ophthalmology 1992;99:438–444.
22. Lee DA, Hersh P, Kersten D, et al: Complications of subconjunctival 5-fluorouracil following glaucoma filtering surgery. Ophthalmic Surg 1987;18:187–190.
23. Chen C-W: Enhanced intraocular pressure controlling effectiveness of trabeculectomy by local application of MMC. Trans Asia-Pacific Acad Ophthalmol 1983;9:172–177.
24. Chen C-W, Huang H-T, Sheu M-M: Enhancement of IOP control effect of trabeculectomy by local application of anticancer drug. Acta XXV Concilium Ophthalmologicum (Rome) 1986;2:1487–1491.
25. Chen C-W, Huang H-T, Bair JS, et al: Trabeculectomy with simultaneous topical applications of mitomycin C in refractory glaucomas. J Ocul Pharmacol 1990;6:175–182.
26. Kirchhof B, Diestelhorst M: The effect of mitomycin C on the aqueous humor dynamics in glaucomatous eyes. Invest Ophthalmol Vis Sci (Suppl) 1993;34:815.
27. Neelakantan A, Rao BS, Vijaya L, et al: Effect of the concentration and duration of application of mitomycin C in trabeculectomy. Ophthalmic Surg 1994;25:612–615.
28. Shields MB, Scroggs MW, Sloop CM, et al: Clinical and histopathologic observations concerning hypotony after trabeculectomy with adjunctive mitomycin C. Am J Ophthalmol 1993;116:673–683.
29. Derick RJ, Pasquale L, Quigley HA, et al: Potential toxicity of mitomycin C. Arch Ophthalmol 1991;109:1635.
30. Seah SK, Prata JA Jr, Minckler DS, et al: Mitomycin-C concentration in human aqueous humour following trabeculectomy. Eye 1993;7: 652–655.
31. Hoskins HD Jr, Migliazzo C: Management of failing filtering blebs with the argon laser. Ophthalmic Surg 1984;15:731.
32. Savage JA, Simmons RJ: Staged glaucoma filtration surgery with planned early conversion from scleral flap to full-thickness operation using the argon laser. Ophthalmic Laser Therapy 1986;1:201.
33. Savage JA, Condon GP, Lytle RA, et al: Laser suture lysis after trabeculectomy. Ophthalmology 1988;95:1631.
34. Pappa KS, Derick RJ, Weber PA, et al: Late argon suture lysis after mitomycin C trabeculectomy. Ophthalmology 1993;100:1268–1271.
35. Ticho U, Irvy M: Reopening of occluded filtering blebs by argon laser photocoagulation. Am J Ophthalmol 1977;84:413.
36. Van Buskirk EM: Reopening filtration fistulas with the argon laser. Am J Ophthalmol 1982;94:1.
37. Cohn HC, Aron-Rosa D: Reopening blocked trabeculectomy sites with the YAG laser. Am J Ophthalmol 1983;95:293.
38. Kurata F, Krupin T, Kolker AE: Reopening filtration fistulas with trans-

conjunctival argon laser photocoagulation. Am J Ophthalmol 1984;98: 340.
39. Latina MA, Rankin GA: Internal and transconjunctival neodymium: YAG laser revision of late failing filters. Ophthalmology 1991;98:215.
40. Lytle RA, Simmons RJ: Internal revision in glaucoma filtration surgery. Scientific Poster 79, American Academy of Ophthalmology Annual Meeting, Las Vegas, NV, October 8–12, 1988.
41. Addicks EM, Quigley HA, Green WR, et al. Histologic characteristics of filtering blebs in glaucomatous eyes. Arch Ophthalmol 1983;101: 795–798.

Postoperative Management Following Filtration Surgery

63

A. Robert Bellows

Management of the patient following filtration surgery for glaucoma is the most important step in obtaining long-term success in control of intraocular pressure (IOP) and preservation of vision. Advances in surgical techniques, careful patient selection, recognition of high-risk patients, introduction of antimetabolites that are used both intra- and postoperatively, and new awareness of the early signs of bleb compromise have all improved long-term surgical success rates. The role of trabeculectomy in achieving control of glaucoma is well established (1). Early surgical intervention before the use of medicines has been proposed (2).

The intraoperative advances that have evolved since the introduction of the operating microscope for almost all glaucoma surgery have clearly enhanced the exact technique of tissue manipulation and alignment. Serious problems, such as failure to recognize a thin fragment of Descemet's membrane, which were not easily assessed with loupes, are more easily recognized using the operating microscope. The advent of microsurgical instrumentation, extremely sharp blades and scissors, precise cautery or diathermy, delicate tissue handling, and fine suture materials has resulted in improved surgical techniques that enhance the possibility of surgical success.

The recognition and management of early postoperative complications, including wound leaks, choroidal detachment, flat chambers and compromised blebs, have been facilitated by the absolute necessity of examining patients with the slit-lamp biomicroscope with attention to the finest details of recently operated eyes.

Recognizing a satisfactory postoperative bleb appearance and overall ocular course is essential. **Recognizing impending bleb failure and ultimate loss of IOP control is critical to successful postoperative management following filtration surgery.** The early observations of bleb compromise with vascular injection and inflammation of Tenon's capsule and the episclera are important. Observing a diffusely quiet and noninflamed bleb with tiny microcysts and obvious succulence and an IOP in the high single digits or low teens is the ultimate goal of all glaucoma surgeons. However, recognizing a slight but definitive vascular ingrowth into the base of the bleb, decreased size and evidence of flattening of a previously functioning bleb, and a gradual IOP increase alerts the surgeon that bleb failure is occurring. Intervention at this stage is absolutely critical to long-term bleb survival. There are many techniques and options available to the surgeon at this time; frequent postoperative visits are necessary to institute the appropriate techniques to shepherd the bleb through this critical time.

In the late stages of bleb evolution when the ocular condition is stable and the IOP is controlled, **the risk of infection and late aqueous leaks must be adequately conveyed to the patient and the patient's family.** A delay in follow-up examination when early bleb infection or early endophthalmitis is present could result in blindness. Alerting the patient to the symptoms and signs of infection and/or leak is an absolute necessity and the surgeon's responsibility. The symptoms and signs of ocular infection should be reviewed at all patient visits, and the patient encouraged to seek ophthalmic assessment at the earliest suggestion of ocular infection.

PREVENTION OF COMPLICATIONS

The discontinuation of topical agents that may create vascular congestion and ocular inflammatory reactions should be considered three to five days preoperatively. In particular, Phospholine Iodide and topical epinephrine can cause alterations in vascular permeability that persist intraoperatively. Evidence of lid infection or inflammation should be treated before filtration surgery is contemplated. Patients with underlying uveitis should be receiving corticosteroids preoperatively, and those with neovascular glaucoma should have undergone an adequate course of panretinal photocoagulation to decrease the fibrovascular reactive state and enhance the chances of successful filtration surgery.

Gentle handling of ocular tissues is an integral part of the surgical management of glaucoma patients. Using smooth or cusped forceps when handling conjunctiva and Tenon's capsule prevents multiple tiny perforations and crushed tissue that occur with toothed or serrated forceps, both of which can promote the release of inflammatory mediators that increase scarring (3).

The immediate use of hemostasis with unipolar diathermy or underwater bipolar cautery is essential to prevent blood and blood products which stimulate inflammation from permeating the periocular space. When blood is absorbed by Tenon's tissue, it often can be removed only by excision. **Immediate cautery is advised to minimize blood in the subconjunctival space when bleeding occurs.**

Additional intraoperative therapeutic modalities have become an essential part of filtration surgery to minimize postoperative complications, particularly fibrosis, scarring and bleb failure. The use of intraoperative mitomycin C in concentrations ranging from 0.2 to 0.5 mg/cc for one to five minutes has been advocated by many authors in patients with complex glaucoma (4,5). The use of postoperative 5-fluorouracil (5-FU) has also decreased the failure rate of patients when used in a standard protocol (6) or with modifications (7). The long-term complications of antimetabolite usage are not presently known, although many express concern regarding late bleb thinning resulting in chronic leaks, an increased incidence of endophthalmitis and the potential of bleb necrosis and sloughing. Efforts to minimize these potential complications are being made.

Efforts to achieve tight trabeculectomy flap closure with subsequent laser suture lysis or a releasable suture that provides firm flap apposition and better control of aqueous egress result in a high proportion of well formed anterior chambers and reasonable early postoperative IOPs. This suturing technique combined with conjunctival closure (single running-locking closure or double closure involving Tenon's capsule first and a conjunctival closure second) has been facilitated with fine tapered needles and absorbable suture material (Vicryl). The capacity to reduce wound leaks with tight conjunctival closure has resulted in significantly fewer flat anterior chambers with hypotony and subsequent choroidal detachment, and fewer prolonged flat anterior chambers.

EARLY POSTOPERATIVE MANAGEMENT

The critical period of postoperative management of filtration surgery occurs in three phases: the early postoperative course of approximately one to seven days; the mid-postoperative course, between one week and three months; and the late postoperative course, three months and longer. On the first postoperative day, routine assessments are made of the anterior chamber depth; the character, extent, and elevation of the bleb; conjunctival wound closure and integrity; IOP; and the posterior pole.

Assessment of Flat Anterior Chamber (Table 63.1)

Wound Leaks

When a shallow or flat anterior chamber is present during the first postoperative week, wound leaks are often responsible. The wound leak is almost always accompanied by a low IOP (0–6 mm Hg) and must be evaluated by assessing the conjunctiva and the conjunctival wound with a 2% solution of fluorescein (Fig. 63.1) to detect small bleb leaks that can be overlooked when a fluorescein strip is used. With the patient looking down, the 2% fluorescein is applied to the conjunctival surface in the region of the conjunctival incision and the entire surface of the bleb. The physician must immediately examine this region with a cobalt blue filter on a standard biomicroscope. A leak is present if cascading darker aqueous with fluorescent edges is observed as the fluid runs from the wound leak. This is popularly called a positive Seidel test. However, Seidel originally described the phenomenon of aqueous fluorescence with transconjunctival bulk flow as a characteristic "watering can" appearance with evidence of multiple tiny areas of aqueous leaks distributed on the bleb surface. The entire bleb surface should then be methodically examined, with particular attention to the area of the conjunctival wound and the area over the sclerectomy. A large buttonhole or a very tiny bleb perforation can result in significant aqueous flow and profound anterior chamber shallowing. Because wound leaks can be subtle, 2% fluorescein solution should be used to detect func-

Table 63.1
Indications for Choroidal Tap

Lens-cornea touch (axially flat anterior chamber)	Choroidal tap should be performed within 24 hours of lens-cornea touch.
Corneal edema	Associated with very shallow anterior chamber.
Prolonged peripherally flat anterior chamber (>5 days)	In the absence of anterior chamber deepening.
Appositional or "kissing" choroidals	Choroidal tap should be performed within 24–48 hours.
Prolonged hypotony, low bleb (>7days) with a moderate to large choroidal effusion	

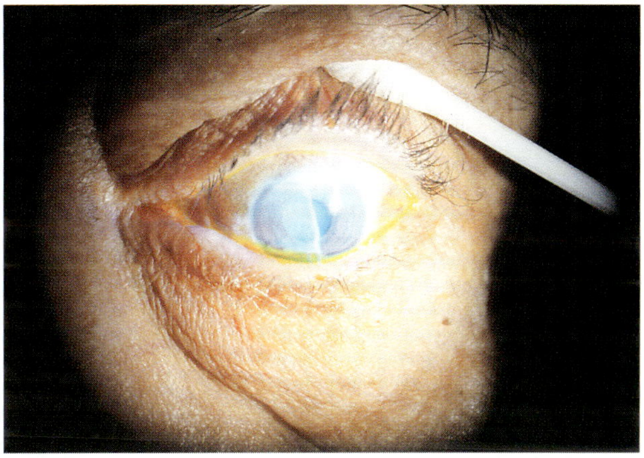

Figure 63.1. Demonstration of a conjunctival wound leak with 2% fluorescein.

PRESSURE PATCHING AND THE SIMMONS SHELL

R. Rand Allingham

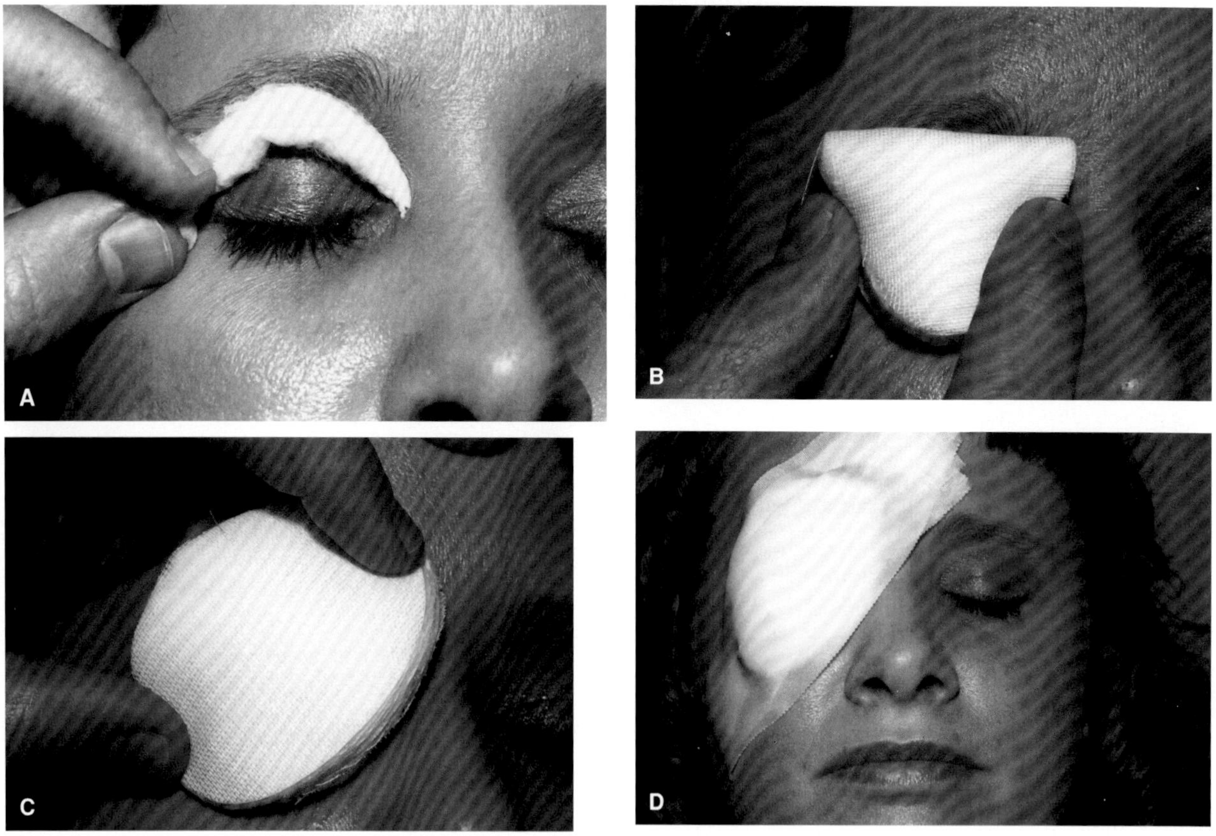

Figure 63.2. Pressure patching. A slightly damp torpedo-shaped cotton ball is placed over the upper lid (A) where it will exert pressure on the trabeculectomy site. A folded eye pad is placed over the cotton ball as shown (B) followed by an additional open eye pad (C). The eye pads and cotton ball are tightly opposed with tape (D). The patient should be reexamined in 1 hour before being sent home.

Pressure patching (Fig. 63.2) may be used in cases of postoperative hypotony-associated shallow anterior chamber due to excess aqueous humor run off through the scleral flap. Moist cotton is rolled into long rolls ("torpedo" shaped). The patient looks down as the cotton rolls are placed into the superior and (with use of the Simmons shell) inferior orbital sulcus. One or two eye pads are taped tightly over the cotton rolls. The superior roll exerts pressure over the scleral flap. The patient should be checked in one hour to assess the response to pressure patching. When correctly placed, this method of tamponade reduces aqueous outflow and thereby assists in reforming the anterior chamber. If there is an increase in anterior chamber depth, the patch can be replaced and the patient seen on a daily basis till the anterior chamber stabilizes. Topical cycloplegics, steroid and antibiotic ointments should be used concurrently.

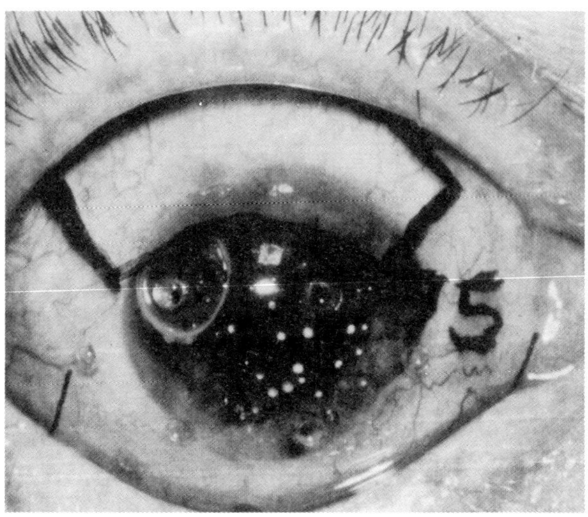

Figure 63.3. Simmons shell in place following filtering surgery. Note the platform (outlined in black) is centered over the superiorly placed filtering site.

The Simmons shell is a contact lens designed with a smooth raised platform at its periphery and vent holes centrally, which is placed over the eye to tamponade aqueous humor flow (Fig. 63.3). After topical proparacaine is instilled, antibiotic ointment is applied to the concave surface of the Simmons shell, and while grasped with forceps through the vent holes on the convex side, it is placed on the eye. The platform is oriented over the scleral flap. The eyelids are closed and the eye is pressure-patched as described above. The patient is re-examined in 1–2 hours and daily thereafter. The use of medications and follow up is the same as that for pressure-patching.

tional leaks because fluorescein strips are not sufficiently concentrated to be effective.

When a leak is detected, aqueous suppressants, beta-blockers and/or carbonic anhydrase inhibitors (CAI), are initially prescribed. These agents decrease aqueous flow and allow conjunctival epithelial cells to slide to seal or diminish the leak. The use of a firm pressure patch is a time-honored remedy for a flat anterior chamber associated with a wound leak. However, this therapy can exacerbate lenticular-corneal touch and even precipitate the active development of lens opacification.

If the leak is still present after one or two days of aqueous suppressant therapy and the chamber remains shallow, suturing the leak under biomicroscopic observation with the appropriate microvascular needle (Ethicon 2850-BV-75 10-0 nylon) can effectively close the leak and re-establish the normal anterior chamber architecture. If a wound leak persists despite these efforts, and no improvement is observed, a definitive operating room procedure involving deepening of the anterior chamber, choroidal tap, and wound repair is indicated.

Management of Wound Leaks

Wound leaks that develop in thin conjunctival tissue close to the limbus and sclerectomy site can be effectively managed with a large, soft contact lens (18 to 22 mm) that serves to tamponade the leak. The contact lens may be left in place for up to ten days. The rigid glaucoma (Simmons) shell (Fig. 62.3) is most effective when used early in managing friable conjunctival tissue with multiple holes. The use of tissue glues in conjunction with a soft contact lens can be helpful if a dry surface is present and suture ends support the adhesive capacity of the glue.

Choroidal Detachment

If the anterior chamber is shallow (Fig. 63.4) or flat with a normal or low IOP and no demonstrable wound leak, choroidal detachment should be considered. Fluid collects in the suprachoroidal space and results in forward movement of the lens iris diaphragm with anterior chamber shallowing and flattening (8,9). The serous effusion is easily recognized when the pupil is dilated and mound-like elevations of the peripheral retina and choroid are seen.

The most common clinical scenario is an IOP reading

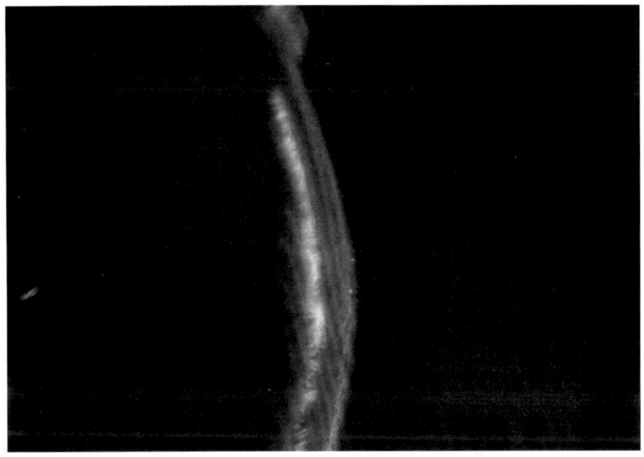

Figure 63.4. Peripherally flat anterior chamber in patient with hypotony following filtering surgery.

below 6 mm Hg, a shallow anterior chamber, no lenticular corneal touch, and large choroidal effusions. In the absence of a significant indication to perform surgical drainage (choroidal tap), choroidal detachment can be treated with cycloplegic-mydriatics, topical steroids and observation. **If there is evidence of corneal edema and lenticular-corneal touch as well as a failing bleb, increasing inflammation, rising IOP, retinal apposition (kissing choroidals), then drainage of the suprachoroidal space and anterior chamber reformation are advised (8).**

In the absence of indications to drain the suprachoroidal space, the anterior chamber gradually deepens as the suprachoroidal fluid is absorbed when the IOP rises to more normal levels. Observation and medical management are usually effective in treating this disorder.

Suprachoroidal Hemorrhage

A much more serious complication of filtration surgery is the development of a suprachoroidal hemorrhage. This often dramatic complication usually occurs within the first week after filtration surgery and is usually associated with postoperative hypotony. **A suprachoroidal hemorrhage is heralded by the sudden onset of severe pain that is diagnostic when associated with profound choroidal detachment, a shallow anterior chamber, and a highly elevated IOP** (10,11). After the acute event, the eye frequently becomes inflamed. The patient may have an inordinant amount of pain before the blood is drained from

PERFORMING A CHOROIDAL TAP

R. Rand Allingham

A choroidal tap is performed to reform the anterior chamber and drain suprachoroidal fluid (effusion or blood in the case of a suprachoroidal hemorrhage). If the eye is extremely soft, we prefer to use a peribulbar block. Local anesthetic is placed subconjunctivally in the quadrants to either side and the furthest away from the filtering bleb.

If the original paracentesis cannot be found or cannulated, a new beveled paracentesis is made. The paracentesis should be made slowly with a very sharp blade in order to avoid a rapid entry into the anterior chamber which could result in damage to the iris or lens. Grasping the horizontal rectus muscle on the same side as the paracentesis with a 0.5 mm forcep can help stabilize the eye and reduce corneal wrinkling while performing the paracentesis. Using a 27 gauge cannula, the anterior chamber is reformed with balanced salt solution. The cannula tip must be through the cornea and in the anterior chamber before infusing fluid to prevent the stripping of Descemet's membrane.

A horizontal conjunctival incision is made 3–6 mm from the limbus in the inferonasal or inferotemporal quadrant (away from the filtering bleb). Small blood vessels are gently cauterized prior to making the sclerotomy. The 2–3 mm radial sclerotomy is centered 3–4 mm from the limbus (Fig. 63.5). We prefer to use a No. 15 Bard-Parker or No. 67 Beaver blade to make the sclerotomy because they are sharp enough to incise the sclera, but not so extremely sharp as to cut through the choroid on contact. Sharper blades can be used, but there is increased risk of penetrating the choroid and inadvertently entering the vitreous cavity. Clear to yellowish-tinged fluid often drains spontaneously once the incision is carried into the suprachoroidal space. Once the fluid flow slows, the tip of a 0.5—1.0 mm

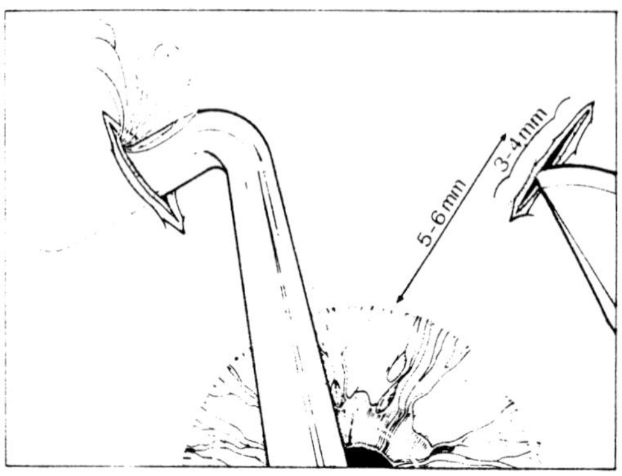

Figure 63.5. Sclerotomy sites in the inferior quadrants, 2 to 3 mm in length and centered 3 to 4 mm from the limbus. A No. 15 Bard-Parker or No. 67 Beaver scalpel blade is used because they are not extremely sharp and thus there is less danger of inadvertently penetrating into the vitreous cavity.

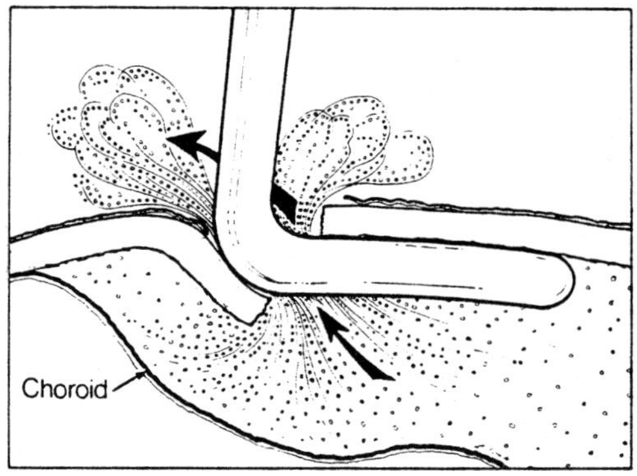

Figure 63.6. Side view of sclerotomy. The heel of the cyclodialysis spatula is used to depress the lip of the wound to aid the escape of suprachoroidal fluid.

cyclodialysis spatula can be carefully inserted into the suprachoroidal space in a circumferential direction (parallel to the limbus) (Fig. 63.6). The spatula is removed and reinserted in the opposite direction. The anterior chamber is reformed periodically when the eye softens. The eye should not be allowed to become too soft in order to reduce the possibility of suprachoroidal hemorrhage. This cycle of anterior chamber reformation and fluid drainage is repeated until no further fluid drains from the sclerotomy. The anterior chamber is then reformed with special emphasis on reforming the filtering bleb (Fig. 63.7). The eye pressure required to elevate the filtering bleb may be quite high to break conjunctival adhesions to episclera.

Once the anterior chamber has been reformed and the choroidal effusions have been drained, the sclerotomy openings are left open and the conjunctiva is closed with 10-0 absorbable suture. Subconjunctival dexamethasone phosphate 8–12 mg is injected inferiorly. Atropine and antibiotic ointment are applied to the eye. The eye is gently patched and an eye shield placed.

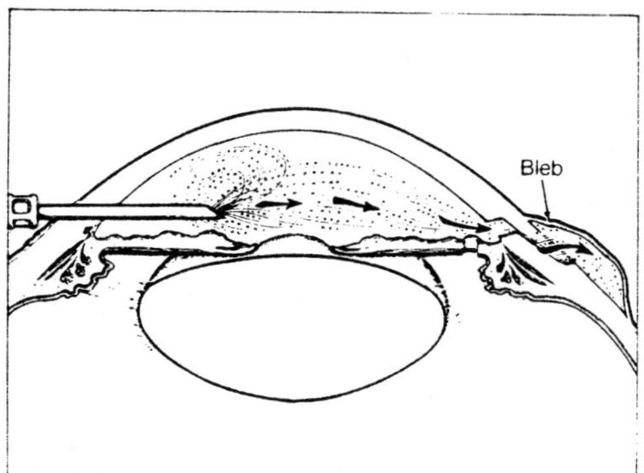

Figure 63.7. Injection of balanced salt solution deepens the anterior chamber and elevates the filtration bleb.

the suprachoroidal space. A waiting period of 7 to 10 days following a suprachoroidal hemorrhage is advised for the fibrinolytic response of fluid to liquify the clot and allow for more effective evacuation of the suprachoroidal space and retinal and choroidal flattening (12). **The risk of suprachoroidal hemorrhage is greater in patients with high myopia, aphakia or pseudophakia, in vitrectomized patients, in the presence of elevated blood pressure, advanced arteriosclerosis, bleeding disorders, and following the hypotony associated with tube-shunt surgery.** At the time of suprachoroidal fluid drainage, using vitrectomy techniques with the instillation of intraocular expandable gases can effectively decrease the incidence of rebleeding and tamponade the choroid and retina in their anatomic positions so that reoperation is less likely. Inflation of the bleb and evaluation of wound leaks should be performed during evacuation of the suprachoroidal space.

Pupillary Block

Pupillary block is another cause for formation of a peripherally shallow or flat anterior chamber in the early postoperative period. **Pupillary block may occur in the presence of normal or elevated IOP.** The inability of aqueous to pass from the posterior to anterior chamber results in the forward movement of the peripheral iris and closure of the drainage channel. Pupillary block occurs when there is a peripheral iridectomy which is not patent, when there are adhesions of the iris to the lens (posterior synechiae) with resultant iris bombé, or with an anterior chamber lens (without a peripheral iridectomy) that prevents aqueous movement into the anterior chamber. Therapy with cycloplegic-mydriatics sometimes resolves pupillary block. However, a laser iridectomy is curative and advisable. In the presence of localized compartments of block, multiple iridectomies are suggested.

Elevated IOP and Flat AC

The final differential diagnostic category of a shallow to flat anterior chamber during the early postoperative period is characterized by an IOP elevated to the high-normal or much higher levels and is associated with aqueous diversion or malignant glaucoma (13) (Chapter 29). Aqueous diversion results from posterior movement of aqueous into the vitreous cavity that forces the vitreous forward with resultant lens-iris diaphragm displacement and closure of the drainage channel angle. Hyperopic eyes with chronic angle closure following filtration surgery are most at risk. However, pseudophakic or aphakic eyes with an impermeable anterior hyaloid face are also at risk of developing this uncommon symptom complex (14).

Aqueous diversion often responds to medical management with CAIs, mydriatic-cycloplegics and beta-blocking agents with re-establishment of the anterior chamber and an IOP decrease. If medical management is not successful, YAG laser disruption of the anterior hyaloid face and posterior capsule can immediately and effectively deepen the anterior chamber and lower the IOP (15). If phakic patients do not respond to medical therapy, the Nd:YAG laser may be attempted if a view of the ciliary processes can be obtained through a peripheral iridectomy or dilated pupil. This view is often difficult to obtain and injury to the crystalline lens can occur. Surgical therapy for aqueous diversion is penetration or removal of the anterior hyaloid face and penetration of the posterior vitreous with aspiration of liquid vitreous with a needle or vitreous cutting instrument. In patients at risk, pilocarpine can precipitate aqueous misdirection.

Early Bleb Evaluation

Careful observation of the bleb in the early postoperative period is extremely important (Fig. 63.8). **A diffuse nonvascular, slightly elevated bleb with diffuse microcysts and an appearance of succulence that involves a superior portion of the globe, and may even extend 360°, is an encouraging observation following filtration surgery.** Recognizing blood under the bleb, a flat vascularized bleb, or a very localized elevated bleb (16) during the early postoperative period is a very poor prognostic sign and requires aggressive management. Little can be done for blood under the bleb, but blood and blood products that seal the trabeculectomy flap or hyphema and a blood clot in the sclerectomy respond dramatically to an intracameral or subconjunctival injection of 10—20 μg of tissue plasminogen activator (tPA) (10 μg/0.1 cc). This procedure can be done at the biomicroscope through a paracentesis and can be repeated if necessary (17). The frequent use of topical steroids, cycloplegics, and nonsteroidal anti-inflammatory agents can minimize the inflammatory response that occurs when blood is present in the subconjunctival or intraocular space.

If the bleb is flat and vascularized and the anterior chamber is formed with a normal or elevated IOP, obstruction to aqueous flow into the bleb is likely. Determining the site of obstruction is essential, and gonioscopy is the most effective method of evaluating the internal structures that are obstructed. **Gonioscopy is essential for evaluating all postoperative bleb complications because the obstruction site can only be determined by careful examination.** If there is evidence of obstruction by a Descemet's flap, iris, ciliary body, or vitreous, laser intervention is often helpful. The argon laser can remove pigmented uveal tissue or blood products from the sclerectomy site. In other situations, a Nd:YAG laser can remove clear membranes or cut adherent uveal tissue that is not amenable to argon laser therapy.

When the sclerectomy site is patent, attention needs to be directed to the episcleral ocular surface. **The most**

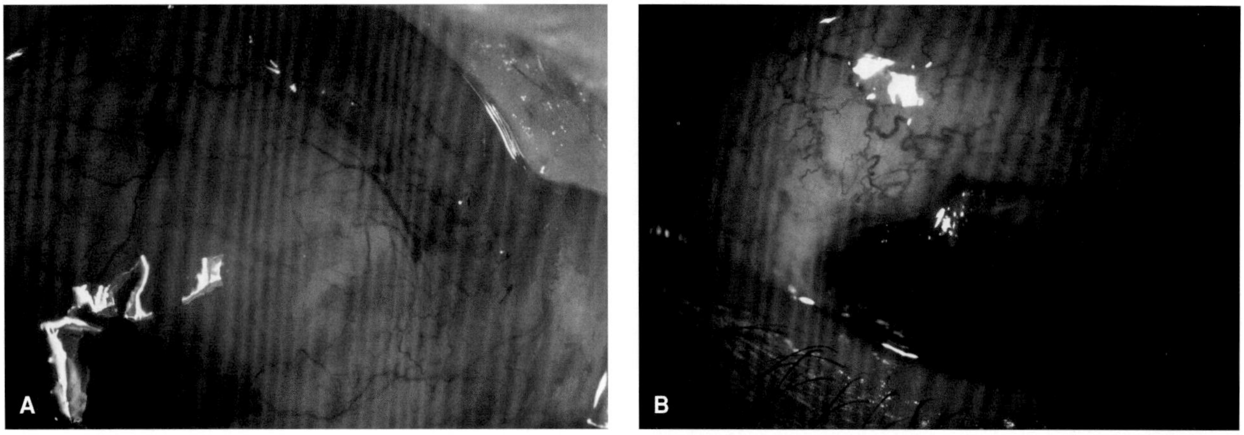

Figure 63.8. Quiet elevated bleb one week after uncomplicated filtering surgery (A). Early bleb failure; note increased vascularity surrounding and overlying bleb (B).

common site of obstruction to aqueous outflow is at the level of the episclera in the region of the trabeculectomy flap. Gentle digital pressure can result in the bleb filling with aqueous and adequate aqueous flow into the bleb. If digital pressure does not result in bleb elevation, laser suture lysis is the next step (Chapter 62).

Cutting a single radial suture with the argon laser using the Hoskins lens encourages flow. With the advent of intraoperative antimetabolites, it is advisable to cut only one suture at a time, because overfiltration can result when multiple sutures are released. Some physicians are hesitant to do laser suture lysis on the first or second postoperative days and instead treat the patient medically to establish more stability in the region of the wound, reserving laser suture lysis for a later therapeutic option. The utility of laser suture lysis diminishes with time. Generally, if it is to be effective, laser suture lysis should be performed within 2 weeks unless adjunctive mitomycin C was employed. If the IOP is very high and the optic nerve integrity is threatened, immediate suture lysis is advised. Releasable sutures with more than one arm can be effectively altered by performing laser suture lysis on the posterior extent of the releasable suture, thus elevating the back of the flap while maintaining tension on the anterior portion of the flap (Fig. 63.9). This gradual release of the flap helps prevent a sudden decrease in IOP and helps maintain anterior chamber depth. It should be kept in mind that laser suture lysis may produce complications such as hypotony, conjunctival wound leaks, or hyphemas (Fig. 63.10).

In the early postoperative period focal pressure with a cotton-tipped swab or muscle hook adjacent to the scleral flap can sometimes "gape" the scleral flap and allow aqueous to dissect and elevate the bleb. This technique is less useful after actual subconjunctival fibrosis has occurred.

MID-POSTOPERTIVE COURSE FOLLOWING FILTRATION SURGERY (1 Week to 3 Months)

Following filtration surgery it is ideal to maintain the IOP between 8 to 14 mm Hg with a diffuse, pale, succulent, superiorly placed bleb. Multiple fine microcysts with an opalescent, multichambered, non thin-walled conjunctiva are the hallmarks of a well-functioning and long-lived filtration bleb. It is advisable to observe the bleb and peribleb region critically throughout this time period. **Subtle vascular ingrowth patterns, flattening of a previously elevated bleb, development of a Tenon's cyst, subtle thickening of the bleb, and a rising IOP should alert the surgeon to potential problems.** It is important for the patient to continue taking anti-inflammatory medications during this mid-postoperative period until all signs of inflammation have disappeared. The use of topical steroids must be predicated upon the inflammatory response of the episclera, not the anterior chamber.

In addition to topical anti-inflammatory agents, subconjunctivally injected 5-FU can help diminish post-filtration inflammation. The daily or alternate day administration of 5 mg of 5-FU into the subconjunctival space can decrease the vascular proliferative process and result in a quiet functioning bleb (Chapter 62).

Recognizing a Failing Bleb

Recognizing a failing bleb during the mid-postoperative period following filtration surgery is key to salvaging the operative results. Progressive management of a compromised or failing bleb is essential to long-term success. Occasionally, the bleb may appear to be unchanged from week to week. However, if the IOP is gradually rising from single digits to the mid-teens and higher, bleb failure is in progress. The signs of impending bleb failure are often subtle and identified late in the course so that therapy is less effective. An inflamed, flat bleb that has lost its succulence and is surrounded by blood vessels has a very grim prognosis. The high, thick-walled, highly domed elevation of a Tenon's cyst is also a problematic prognostic sign.

Managing a failing bleb should begin the moment failure is suspected. If there is evidence of iris, Descem-

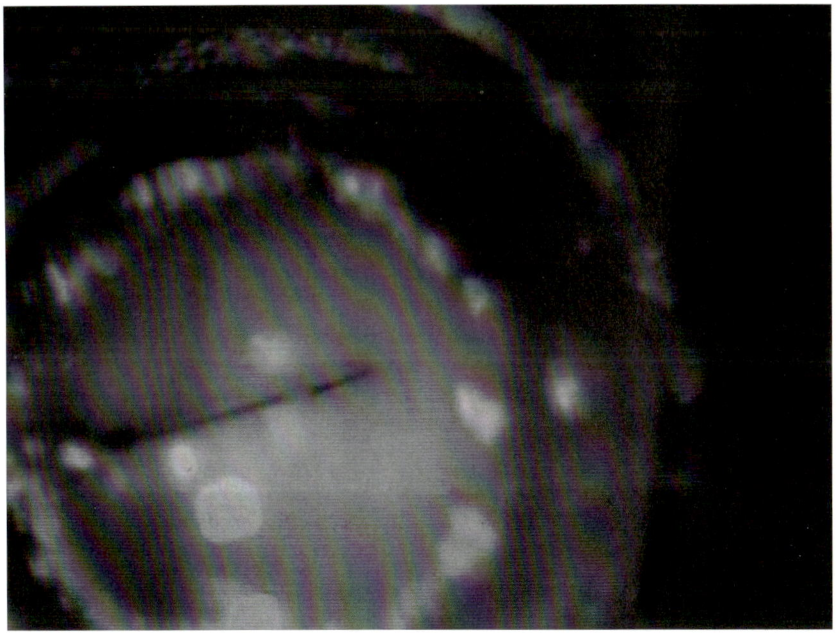

Figure 63.9. Scleral flap suture status post laser suture lysis. Laser energy is applied to either the posterior or anterior end of the suture. (Courtesy of Richard J. Simmons, M.D.)

et's membrane, fibrin, or vitreous blocking the sclerectomy, laser intervention or even surgical removal of the obstruction may be necessary. Suture lysis, especially in those patients where intraoperative adjunctive mitomycin C has been used, may be effective even months after filtration surgery. Repeat gonioscopy at this time is essential to assess the patency of the sclerectomy.

Topical anti-inflammatory medications including steroids, nonsteroidal anti-inflammatories, and cycloplegic-mydriatic agents should be prescribed in increased frequencies. (Of course, steroids may increase IOP.)

Frequent application of topical steroids (every two hours) is advised during this period involving the maturation of the filtration bleb. In some cases, systemic steroids may be beneficial, although the patient must be followed closely for systemic side effects.

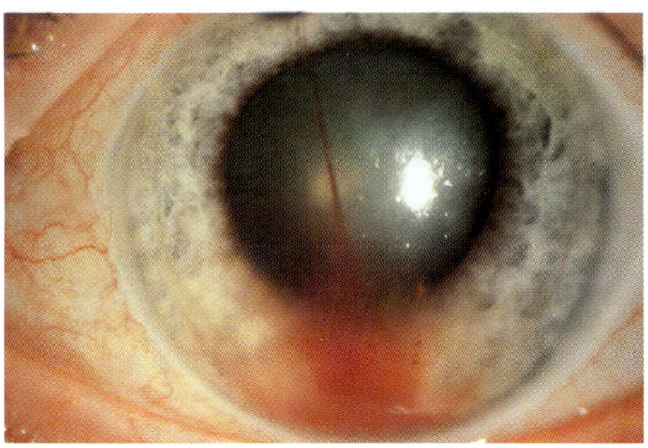

Figure 63.10. Hyphema originating from the sclerectomy site immediately following "uneventful" laser suture lysis.

Needling the Bleb

Where there is early bleb failure in the early postoperative period, through the first few weeks, needling the bleb can be a useful intervention in addition to medical treatment. A short, sharp needle should be used (27 or 30 gauge) on a tuberculin syringe with either lidocaine 1% alone or combined with 5-FU (5 mg total). The patient is seated at the slit lamp and is instructed to remain perfectly still. An assistant should be available to hold the patient's head if needed. After topical proparacaine is applied the needle is inserted into the subconjunctival space approximately 5—8 mm from the scleral flap and a small amount of solution is injected elevating the conjunctiva to provide anesthesia. Then, as the conjunctiva elevates, the needle is advanced until the tip of the needle is inside the filtering bleb. **No further fluid is injected once the needle is within the bleb.** If there is a fibrous capsule the needle can be used to create several openings. The location of the needle tip must be kept in mind at all times to prevent cutting blood vessels or perforating the globe or bleb. This procedure can be remarkably effective when used within a few days of the conjunctiva adhering to the episclera. However, it is less effective after the bleb capsule has become thick and adherent.

Digital Pressure

Digital pressure should be instituted by the physician at this time and if possible the technique taught to the patient. There are many techniques that have been developed for applying digital pressure, but it is essential to evaluate the pressure response following the application of digital pressure to a recently filtered eye. The surgeon is advised to

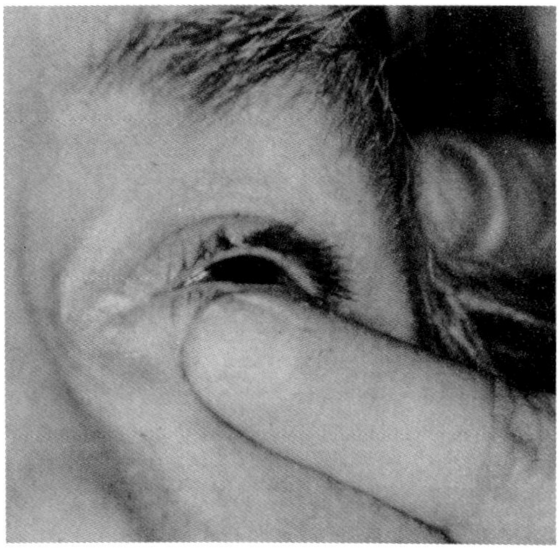

Figure 63.11. Digital pressure technique.

apply digital pressure with the index finger to the inferior portion of the globe while observing the anterior chamber and appearance of the bleb at the slit-lamp. With these precautions, exact, effective properly applied pressure can be evaluated. **If the IOP decreases and the patient can master this maneuver, the digital pressure technique should be taught to the patient or a person available to perform this technique at home.**

The technique generally used is as follows. Instruct the patient to look up and nasal and then to identify the infraorbital rim with his or her index finger. The patient should place the soft fingerprint portion of the index finger against the inferior aspect of the globe through the lower lid with pressure directed inward and upward for a count of 5 to 10 seconds (Fig. 63.11). A rest period of 5 seconds is encouraged and then repeat digital pressure is applied 2 to 10 times sequentially, alternating with a 5-second rest period each time. The patient is encouraged to keep his or her index finger in the digital pressure position so that the orbital landmarks are maintained. If this maneuver results in a lowering of the IOP by 3 mmHg or more, the patient is encouraged to perform this maneuver three to five times daily depending on individual needs.

Each time the patient is examined, the IOP should be measured and the patient should be requested to perform digital pressure in the manner in which he or she performs at home. Not infrequently, a refresher course is necessary. When digital pressure effectively lowers the IOP acutely, the surgeon should establish how long after the procedure the pressure remains in an acceptable range. Once the bleb has been salvaged, the patient can gradually taper the daily repetitions of the technique.

Tenon's Cyst

When Tenon's capsule adheres to the episclera near the operative site, a high-domed, smooth, two-layered bleb forms that is impervious to aqueous humor and is an extension of the anterior chamber, with a resultant IOP elevation. With time and IOP management, this barrier often becomes less dense and the IOP stabilizes at a safe level. However, not infrequently, when IOP elevation associated with a Tenon's cyst cannot be tolerated by a severely compromised optic nerve, additional therapy is necessary (18–20). As stated earlier, repeated needling of Tenon's cysts at the slit-lamp can effectively penetrate the fibrous barrier and encourage filtration. A more extensive surgical revision, i.e., excising the fibrovascular membrane, also may be necessary (19,20).

When a Tenon's cyst is identified, introducing CAIs, apraclonidine, and beta-blockers may lower the IOP. Adding digital pressure can break the cicatrix responsible for the pressure elevation. If the noninvasive techniques are ineffective, a Wheeler knife or a 25-gauge needle may be used at the slit-lamp after applying topical anesthestic. The knife can be passed through distant conjunctiva, advanced to the Tenon's cyst area, and the cyst wall penetrated. Repeated needling may be indicated if the IOP rises and the cyst opening seals. If there is persistent IOP elevation or if a delle develops, surgical revision of the Tenon's cyst with excision of the fibrovascular cyst wall may be necessary. Assessment of the patency of the sclerectomy is performed at the same time.

Progressive Bleb Failure

If all efforts at medical and minimally invasive surgical management are unsuccessful, the possibility of bleb revision or re-operation in an adjacent site should be considered (Chapter 62). Internal bleb revision may be effective if a blunt spatula is passed into the sclerectomy and used to break any adhesions present. This technique is most effective during the first two to three months following filtration surgery. It is also most effective and least likely to cause problems when blood vessels in this area are minimal. Topical vasoconstrictors can be very important in decreasing the chance of bleeding during manipulation of the bleb associated with internal revision. Underwater diathermy to coagulate bleeding vessels intraoperatively has been helpful.

If there is marked scarring and a thick-walled, highly vascularized bleb is present, external revision may be more effective. An incision posterior to the original conjunctival incision should be made and careful dissection carried forward utilizing immediate cautery for hemostasis. The use of antimetabolites can be considered if there is no communication with the anterior chamber. **When there is significant inflammation, extremely friable conjunctiva, or densely bound down tissues, an adjacent, nonoperated site should be used to create a new area for filtration.** The use of intra- and postoperative 5-FU should be instituted immediately to establish successful filtration.

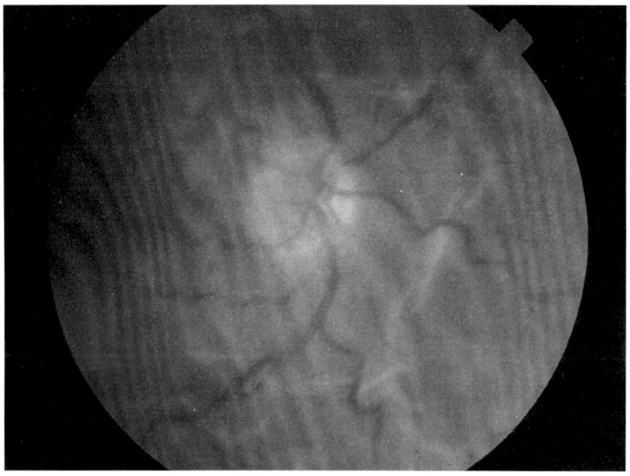

Figure 63.12. Hypotonous maculopathy after filtering surgery. This has become increasingly common after use of adjunctive mitomycin C.

Hypotonous Maculopathy

One of the most serious, newly recognized complications primarily associated with the use of 5-FU and MMC is the development of hypotonous maculopathy (Fig. 63.12) (21–23). This complication is characterized by an IOP less than 6 mm Hg with associated swelling of the macula often accompanied by choroidal and retinal folds. There is a dose and time-related component, but the high-risk patient is often young and highly myopic. Early interventions which have been suggested include pressure patching and laser and cautery application to the bleb. Resuturing the flap and obliterating the bleb has also been suggested. In addition, the use of autologous blood injected into the bleb has been advocated (23).

LATE POSTOPERATIVE MANAGEMENT AFTER FILTRATION SURGERY

The ideal course following filtration surgery is to control the IOP below the anticipated target pressure. In phakic patients, the bleb that is identified with successful control of IOP often is diffuse, low-lying, avascular, succulent, slightly elevated, and superiorly placed with no visible boundaries. Also the bleb manifests delicate microcysts and is not particularly thin-walled. Unfortunately, the development of the ideal bleb is not common and all permutations of this bleb description are possible. Adequate IOP can even be established and maintained in the absence of a visible filtering bleb, especially in pseudophakia or aphakia.

Since the introduction of antimetabolites, particularly intraoperative MMC, a "cadaveric," avascular, localized, often rectangular-shaped bleb that mimics the size of the cellulose sponge used to apply the antimetabolite is commonly seen. Reports exist of postoperative melting and persistent chronic leaks with expectations that later complications of bleb sloughing and necrosis will occur. The early evidence of a definitive increase in success rates, particularly in difficult cases, has led to the use of antimetabolites in almost all filtration operations. However, **recognizing that late bleb infections are often associated with bleb leaks, and the fact that they are usually observed in thin-walled blebs, has dampened enthusiasm for the universal use of antimetabolites.**

Infection

Bleb infection "blebitis" and bleb infection with endophthalmitis are the most serious complications following successful filtration surgery (Fig. 63.13). The surgeon must instruct his or her patients about the symptoms and signs of bleb infection and insist that the patient be seen immediately if these symptoms develop. The incidence of bleb infection was not well established before the advent of antimetabolites, but may range between 2% and 5%. There is certainly a higher incidence of bleb-related endophthalmitis when a full-thickness, thin-walled bleb is present. In the antimetabolite era, bleb infection with endophthalmitis may be increasing in frequency.

We instruct our patients and members of the patient's family that ocular inflammation characterized by a red eye with purulent discharge, localized discomfort, and even subtle alterations of vision may be the earliest signs of a bleb infection and the patient must be examined promptly. It is not uncommon to have a bleb leak precede a definitive infection, so that the onset of profound tearing or ocular discharge should be reported to an ophthalmologist. There is clinical evidence to suggest that blebs placed inferiorly have a higher incidence of endophthalmitis than blebs placed under the upper lid (24). Attention and therapy should be directed toward treating blepharitis and recurrent conjunctivitis in patients with filtering blebs.

When a patient with a suspected bleb infection is examined, there is often a definitive vascular response at the base of the bleb that creates a "peribleb" halo of blood vessels, which may be the earliest sign of bleb infection (Fig. 63.14). It is helpful to use 2% fluorescein to stain the bleb to recognize subtle leaks and visible epithelial defects that may be the site of bacterial penetration. An increase in the haziness of a previously clear bleb or frank pus in the bleb may be the extremes noted when evaluating the bleb for infection. The anterior chamber may have a significant cellular response and even hypopyon indicating endophthalmitis. In phakic or pseudophakic eyes, the vitreous cavity may not be involved and drastic surgical intervention may not be necessary. However, with visualization of white cells in the vitreous cavity or ultrasonographic evidence (25) to indicate vitreous involvement, immediate vitrectomy and administration of intravitreal antibiotics is advised.

When "blebitis" or bleb involvement with anterior chamber reaction is recognized, the aggressive use of topical antibiotics, topical steroids, and cycloplegics is indicated. A culture of the bleb surface, conjunctiva, and aqueous leak should be obtained prior to the use of antibiotics. An aggressive course of topical antibiotics should be introduced with vancomycin, gentamicin and the quinolones administered hourly as well as a bacteriocidal ointment applied at bedtime. Following 24–48 hours of intensive topical antibiotic therapy, dexamethasone or prednisolone acetate can be prescribed every three to four hours if improvement is noted.

When an infected bleb is associated with hypopyon in a phakic patient, systemic antibiotics, e.g., vancomycin 500 mg every 8 hours and gentamicin 80 mg every 8 hours, can be introduced. When there is obvious or suspected vitreous involvement, a vitreous tap and often pars plana vitrectomy should be performed with intravitreous administration of vancomycin 1 mg/cc and amikacin 400 μg. The most common and most devastating organisms involved with bleb infections are Streptococcus and Haemophilus influenzae (26). However, many other organisms, including gram-negative organisms, have been identified (27). The use of prophylactic antibiotics has not been generally accepted. However, some centers advocate the use of topical sulfa drugs or erythromycin ointment as long-term bleb antibiotic treatment. (Although a minority of glaucoma surgeons routinely use prophylactic antibiotics following filtration surgery, one of us (DLE) feels that this use significantly reduces the incidence of postoperative blebitis and endophthalmitis. This may be particularly true in those cases where a thin bleb is present after full thickness or antimetabolite surgery.)

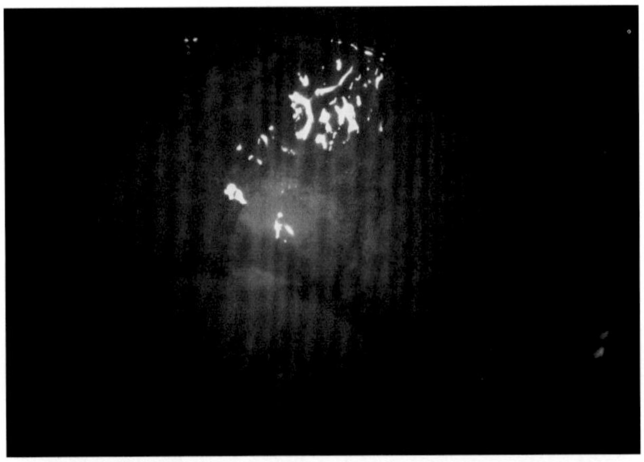

Figure 63.13. Patient with acute "blebitis." Note intense vascular reaction around the white bleb. A hypopyon was also present.

With early intervention and aggressive antibiotic and topical steroid therapy, particularly with nonvirulent pathogens, filtering blebs can be salvaged. The critical elements are the immediate examination of the patient and institution of appropriate therapy.

Cataract Formation

When the development of a flat anterior chamber and early profound hypotony were common, the incidence of cataract formation was thought to be between 20% and 30% (28). More recently, with adoption of trabeculectomy and laser suture lysis, the development and progression of cataract formation may be less. However, despite these improved surgical techniques, cataract formation remains a significant problem. **Cataracts develop in 22 to 47% of patients after trabeculectomy surgery** (28–30). The risk of cataract formation increases with age, presence of exfoliation, when air is used to reform the anterior chamber, and in cases where hypotony occurs postoperatively (31,32).

When a cataract becomes visually significant, the use of an intraocular lens (IOL) at the time of cataract surgery and the less traumatic techniques associated with phacoemulsification through small incisions has resulted in more effective visual rehabilitation and preservation of functioning filtering blebs (33–36). **A controversy surrounding placement of the cataract incision in an eye with a functioning filter has been more or less resolved by the adoption of a temporal incision for phacoemulsification and by the use of a foldable IOL.** In the past, there had been a preference to operate as far from the bleb as possi-

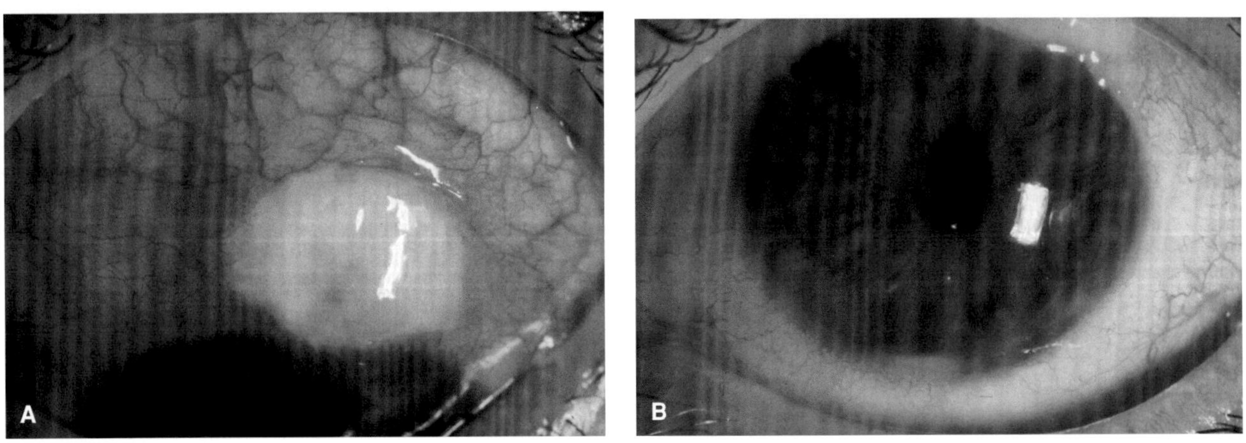

Figure 63.14. Patient with an early bleb infection. There is only minimal injection surrounding the bleb (A) despite the presence of a hypopyon (B).

TREATMENT OF HYPOTONOUS MACULOPATHY

R. Rand Allingham

Hypotonous maculopathy secondary to antifibrotic therapy in the glaucoma filter patient should be treated in a step-wise fashion.

1. Medications: Medications should be reviewed with the patient. Unbeknownst to the physician, the patient may still be taking glaucoma medications in the hypotonous eye. If the patient is taking systemic carbonic anhydrase inhibitors for the fellow eye, it may be possible to switch to topical dorzolamide instead. Topical steroids should be stopped. The use of medications which "irritate" the bleb (e.g. gentamicin) are of little benefit.

2. Contact lens trial: The use of large diameter contact lenses, in our experience, has not been effective where a large diffuse bleb is present. In cases where there is a single leaking site they can be used effectively.

3. Autologous blood injection into the bleb can be successful (Fig. 63.15). We use an approach similar to that described by Nuyts et al. (1). This procedure can be performed at the slit lamp or in a minor operating room. Gentamicin is placed in the eye prior to injection. The anterior chamber is filled with viscoelastic, in order to prevent blood from flowing through the sclerectomy and entering the anterior chamber. One cc of blood is drawn from the patient's arm in a sterile manner. A sterile 27 gauge needle is used to inject the blood. The needle enters the subconjunctival space approximately 7–8 mm away and is carefully moved to the center of the bleb. The bleb is inflated with blood (approximately 0.1–0.2 cc). Postoperatively, the patient is seen the next day. Elevated IOP is reduced by paracentesis, if necessary. The patient is then seen weekly. The procedure can be repeated.

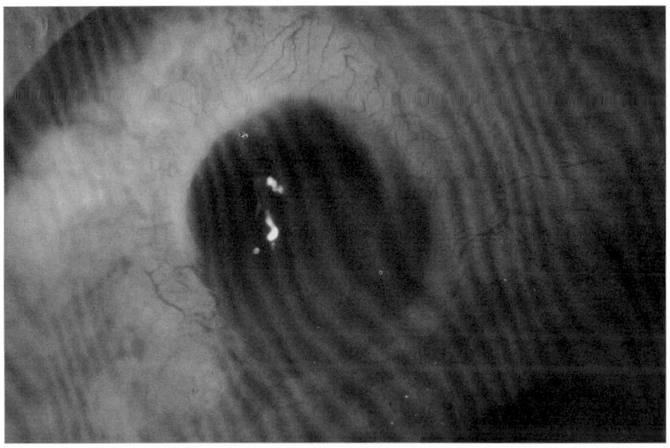

Figure 63.15. Appearance of filtering bleb following autologous blood injection in a patient with hypotonous maculopathy after a trabeculectomy with adjunctive mitomycin C.

4. Surgical management: In patients where autologous blood injection has failed, we revise the bleb. If possible, we attempt to close the scleral flap with interrupted 10-0 nylon sutures. If this is not possible, we use donor sclera to close the sclerectomy site. Usually, the conjunctiva is so fragile that it must be resected in its entirety. In these cases, surrounding conjunctiva is mobilized and brought over the filter site and sutured to the limbus with horizontal mattress sutures. Vicryl (8-0) on a spatulated needle has been effective. In rare cases, conjunctiva must be harvested from the inferior fornix. Despite extensive tissue manipulation, many of these patients do well with long term functioning blebs. Postoperatively, patients are treated in the same manner as other filter patients. 5-FU should be used cautiously, if at all.

5. Co-existing cataract: In patients with hypotonous maculopathy who have a cataract (pre-existing or one which developed postoperatively), inflammation from cataract surgery alone often increases IOP and improves visual acuity. In general, the bleb should not be revised in conjunction with cataract surgery in these cases.

Reference

1. Nuyts RMMA, et al: Treatment of hypotonous maculopathy after trabeculectomy with mitomycin-C. Am J Ophthalmol 1994;118: 322.

ble, but even with this technique, some surgeons experienced a 50% bleb failure rate. Although this has not been our experience, the use of a small temporal wound with a foldable IOL hopefully will result in longer bleb survival. With the diminution of intra- and postoperative complications, the use of phacoemulsification combined with glaucoma surgery has improved vision and controlled the IOP with a reduction or discontinuation of medication. The gratitude expressed by a patient who has improved vision and a diminished need for long-term antiglaucoma medications has been a recognized benefit of these newer surgical advances with improvement in the patient's quality of life.

Late Bleb Failure

Despite a perfect operation and a very successful early and late courses with a functioning filtering bleb and low IOP, the attrition to constant wound modification results in a definite incidence of late failed filtration operations. When the IOP is elevated in the presence of a failed filter, introducing aqueous suppressants such as a topical beta-blockers or carbonic anhydrase inhibitors can result in profound hypotony or the development of large choroidal detachments (37,38). Cessation of aqueous suppressants results in disappearance of the choroidal detachment and elevation of the

IOP in two to three weeks. Occasionally, a beta-blocker used in a fellow eye presumably causes this unusual complication.

When a failing bleb no longer responds to maximum medical therapy, either bleb revision or filtration in an area with virgin conjunctiva is considered. In noninflamed, non-injected eyes with thin, obstructing adhesions, an internal revision may be attempted (Chapter 62). **Late external revisions with excision of the fibrovascular tissue have been disappointing. The most effective approach is filtration in an area that has not undergone previous surgery.** The use of antimetabolites and releasable sutures is advised. Following one or two failed filtering operations, most surgeons suggest the use of a tube-shunt (Chapter 65) as the next step. Finally, when the visual acuity is severely compromised and all methods have failed, cyclodestructive procedures (Chapter 57) may be used.

CONCLUSION

Intensive observation after filtering operations is possibly the most important insurance for long term success. Recognition of early, mid and late changes in the status of the bleb can prevent failure of the bleb and impending serious complications. Anticipating bleb failure by treating leaks and evaluation for endophthalmitis are the most obvious preventive measures. **The judgment involved in increasing topical steroid dosages, performing laser suture lysis, and introducing digital pressure may be the determining factors for long-term success following filtering operations.**

References

1. Watson PG, Grierson I: The place of trabeculectomy in the treatment of glaucoma. Ophthalmology 1981;88:175.
2. Migdal C, Hitchings R: Control of chronic simple glaucoma with primary, medical, surgery and laser treatment. Trans Ophthalmol Soc UK 1986;105:653.
3. Skuta GL, Parrish RK: Wound healing in glaucoma filtering surgery. Surv Ophthalmol 1987;32:149.
4. Chen C-W: Enhanced intraocular pressure controlling effectiveness of trabeculectomy by local application of mitomycin-C. Trans Asia-Pacific Acad Ophthalmol 1983;9:172.
5. Skuta GL, et al: Intraoperative mitomycin vs. postoperative 5-FU in high risk glaucoma filtering surgery. Ophthalmology 1992;99:438.
6. Rockwood EJ, et al: Glaucoma filtering surgery with 5-fluorouracil. Ophthalmology 1984;91:831.
7. Weinreb RN: Adjusting the dose of 5-fluorouracil after filtration surgery to minimize side effects. Ophthalmology 1987;94:564.
8. Bellows AR, Chylack LT, Hutchinson BT: Choroidal detachment: Clinical manifestation, therapy and mechanism of formation. Ophthalmology 1981;88:1107.
9. Brubaker RF, Peterson JE: Ciliochoroidal detachments. Surv Ophthalmol 1983;27:281.
10. Gressel MG, Parrish RK, Heuer DK: Delayed non-expulsive suprachoroidal hemorrhage. Arch Ophthalmol 1984;102:1757.
11. Givens K, Shields MB: Suprachoroidal hemorrhage after glaucoma filtering surgery. Am J Ophthalmol 1987;103:689.
12. Lambrou FH, Meredith TA, Kaplan HG: Secondary surgical management of expulsive choroidal hemorrhage. Arch Ophthalmol 1987;105:1195.
13. Chandler PA, Simmons RJ, Grant WM: Malignant glaucoma, medical and surgical treatment. Am J Ophthalmol 1968;66:492.
14. Dueker D: Ciliary-block glaucoma: Differential diagnosis and management. J Glaucoma 1994;3:167.
15. Epstein DL, Steinert RF, Puliafito CA: Nd:YAG therapy to the anterior hyaloid in aphakic malignant (ciliovitreal block) glaucoma. Am J Ophthalmol 1984;98:137.
16. Scott DR, Quigley HJ: Medical management of a high bleb phase after trabeculectomies. Ophthalmology 1988;95:1169.
17. Tripathi RC, Tripathi BJ, Bornstein S, et al: Use of tissue plasminogen activator for rapid dissolution of fibrin and blood clots in the eye after surgery for glaucoma and cataract in humans. Drug Dev Res 1992;27:147–159.
18. Richter CU, et al: The development of encapsulated filtering blebs. Ophthalmology 1988;95:1163.
19. Peterson JE, Smith SG: Surgical management of encapsulated filtering blebs. Ophthalmology 1985;92:955.
20. Shingleton BJ, Richter CU, Bellows AR, et al: Management of encapsulated filtration blebs. Ophthalmology 1990;97:63.
21. Stampfer RL, McMenemy MG, Lieberman MF: Hypotonous maculopathy after trabeculectomy with subconjunctival 5-fluorouracil. Am J Ophthalmol 1992;114:544.
22. Shields MB, et al: Clinical and histopathologic observations concerning hypotony after trabeculectomy with adjunctive mitomycin-C. Am J Ophthalmol 1993;116:673.
23. Nuyts RMMA, et al: Treatment of hypotonous maculopathy after trabeculectomy with mitomycin-C. Am J Ophthalmol 1994;118:322.
24. Wolner B, et al: Late bleb-related endophthalmitis after trabeculectomy with adjunctive 5-fluorouracil. Ophthalmology 1991;98:1053.
25. Dacey MP, et al: Echographic findings in infectious endophthalmitis. Arch Ophthalmol 1994;112:1325.
26. Mandelbaum S, et al: Late-onset endophthalmitis associated with filtering blebs. Ophthalmology 1985;92:964.
27. Brown RH, et al: Treatment of bleb infection after glaucoma surgery. Arch Ophthalmol 1994;112:57.
28. Lamping K, et al: Long-term evaluation of initial filtration surgery. Ophthalmology 1986;93:931.
29. Vesti E: Development of cataract after trabeculectomy. Acta Ophthalmologica 1993;71:777–781.
30. Asamoto A, Yablonski ME: Post-trabeculectomy anterior subcapsular cataract formation induced by anterior chamber air. Ophthalmic Surg 1993;24:314–319.
31. Akato SK, Goulstine DB, Rosenthal AR: Long-term post trabeculectomy intraocular pressures. Acta Ophthalmol 1992;70:312–316.
32. Tornquest G, Drolsum LK: Trabeculectomies. A long-term study. Acta Ophthalmol 1991;69:450–454.
33. Popovic V, Sjostrand J: Long-term outcome following trabeculectomy: I. Retrospective analysis of intraocular pressure regulation and cataract formation. Acta Ophthalmol 1991;69:299–304.
34. Stewart WC, Krinkley CMC, Carlson AN: Results of trabeculectomy combined with phacoemulsification vs. trabeculectomy combined with extracapsular cataract extraction in patients with advanced glaucoma. Ophthalmic Surg 1994;25:621.
35. Wishart PK, Austin MW: Combined cataract extraction with trabeculectomy: Phacoemulsification compared with extracapsular technique. Ophthalmic Surg 1993;24:814.
36. Lyle WA, Jin JC: Comparison of 3 and 6mm incision in a combined phacoemulsification and trabeculectomy. Am J Ophthalmol 1991;111:189.
37. Vela MA, Campbell DG: Hypotony in ciliochoroidal detachment following pharmacologic aqueous suppressant therapy in previously filtered patients. Ophthalmology 1985;92:50.
38. Berke SJ, et al: Chronic and recurrent choroidal detachment after glaucoma filtration surgery. Ophthalmology 1987;94:154.

The Management of Coexisting Cataract and Glaucoma

64

Joel S. Schuman

INTRODUCTION

Cataract and glaucoma are common entities that frequently coexist, especially in older individuals. The management of either requires consideration of both, particularly when surgical intervention is contemplated. The decision for cataract or filtration surgery, or combined cataract and glaucoma surgery, necessitates evaluation of the need for visual rehabilitation and the urgency of intraocular pressure (IOP) control.

Cataract surgery is considered when the patient complains of deterioration of vision to a point where it interferes with the ability to read, write, and perform other activities of daily living, and when examination of the patient's eye reveals cataract as the source of some or all of these visual complaints. A complete history determines the onset and course of visual loss, previous ocular history, and any history of systemic illness. Refraction is essential in any consideration of cataract surgery. **One critical aspect of the examination of the patient with cataract is assessment of the surgeon's view into the eye**; this will often mimic the patient's view out. For this maneuver, the eye should be examined with a direct ophthalmoscope. The surgeon must recall, however, when determining the cataract's functional effect, that a small cataract may have a disproportionately large effect in the glaucomatous eye, especially in the presence of compromised visual field.

The examination may also include evaluation of visual acuity in high and low contrast settings, potential acuity testing as well as the routine examination of the pupil, anterior segment, including gonioscopy, and dilated fundus examination. Ultrasonography may be required in patients with very dense cataracts in whom media opacity precludes examination of the fundus. In such cases, cataract extraction may be indicated to permit management of retinal disease.

Glaucoma subtype, IOP control, current ocular hypotensive therapy, and the severity of glaucomatous optic nerve damage each have impact on the decision regarding the role of filtering surgery in the patient with cataract. History of prior laser trabeculoplasty, laser iridectomy, or incisional glaucoma surgery, are factors involved in the surgical management of these patients. Any history of intolerance or allergy to anti-glaucoma medications must be considered.

The preoperative examination includes assessment of IOP, anterior segment evaluation with gonioscopy, stereoscopic biomicroscopy of the optic nerve and fundus, and visual field examination. Extremely miotic eyes may require pupillary dilation prior to visual field testing. The contribution of cataract is considered in visual field interpretation. Previous visual fields, changes in optic nerve head appearance by direct observation and stereoscopic disc photography, and IOP determination are all important factors in the decision making process.

SPECIAL CONSIDERATIONS

Surgery in glaucomatous eyes involves special considerations. Conjunctival scarring from previous surgery increases the difficulty of conjunctival dissection, and increases the risk of conjunctival tear or buttonhole. A small pupil due to long-term use of miotics increases the difficulty of capsulorhexis and phacoemulsification. Clinically, significant anterior synechias preclude anterior chamber intraocular lens insertion. Eyes with exfoliation have weak zonular attachments, which increase the risk of zonular dialysis and vitreous loss during surgery. If zonular weakness is prominent, as manifest by phacodonesis, extracapsular cataract surgery is difficult, and intracapsular cataract extraction can be considered; however, it is only rarely necessary to stray from extracapsular extraction or phacoemulsification, especially with the use of viscoelastic materials and sulcus fixated intraocular lenses. A high preoperative IOP, with a rapid reduction in IOP at the time of surgical entry into the eye, predisposes to suprachoroidal hemorrhage; preoperative reduction of IOP with topical and intravenous agents and compression of the globe may reduce this risk.

SURGICAL OPTIONS

The presence of a visually significant cataract in a glaucomatous eye presents three options: combined cataract and glaucoma surgery, cataract surgery alone, or filtering sur-

Table 64.1
Clinical Decision Making in Eyes With Coexisting Cataract and Glaucoma

Well Controlled IOP
Controlled on a single medication, cataract visually significant
- Little or no visual field loss or disc change: Cataract Surgery Alone
- Mild to moderate visual field loss or disc change: Combined Filtering Surgery and Cataract Extraction

Controlled on two or more medications, cataract visually significant
- Combined Filtering Surgery and Cataract Extraction

Uncontrolled IOP; cataract visually significant
- Mild to moderate visual field loss or disc change: Combined Filtering Surgery and Cataract Extraction
- Moderate to severe visual field loss or disc change: Two-Stage Procedure, ***Unless*** Urgent Need to Restore Vision or Two-Stage Procedure not Feasible, then Combined Filtering Surgery and Cataract Extraction

gery followed by cataract surgery at some future time (Table 64.1).

Combined Cataract and Glaucoma Surgery

Cataract and glaucoma surgery performed in the same session is considered in those eyes with visually significant cataract where two or more medications are required for IOP control. Combined surgery can also be performed to reduce the risk of IOP spike following cataract surgery in eyes with compromised optic nerves in which there is good IOP control, but in which an IOP spike presents a high risk for further loss of visual field. The combined procedure offers the advantage of rapid visual recovery and good control of IOP. Visual rehabilitation is generally faster than with a two-stage procedure, and control of IOP, especially with the use of antimetabolites, can equal that of filtering surgery alone.

Combined surgery, however, can be technically more challenging than cataract surgery alone, with greater potential complications, and requiring closer postoperative monitoring.

Classically, two-stage filtering surgery followed by cataract extraction has been thought to offer better control of IOP than the combined procedure; however, the use of antimetabolites such as mitomycin C (MMC) and the advent of phacoemulsification surgery with small incision intraocular lenses, has changed the outlook on this issue. Combined procedures, as mentioned above, can provide IOP control as good as filtering surgery alone.

Cataract Surgery Alone

Glaucomatous eyes with visually significant cataract in which the IOP is well controlled on one or two medications can be considered for cataract extraction alone, especially in patients unable to use miotics because of their lens opacity. Eyes dependent on adrenergic agents should not be considered in this category; cystoid macular edema is a significant risk in aphakic and pseudophakic eyes treated with epinephrine compounds (Chapter 12).

Laser trabeculoplasty (LTP) can be considered prior to cataract extraction in eyes with borderline control of IOP undergoing cataract surgery alone. LTP is less effective in aphakic eyes, but the efficacy of LTP in pseudophakia may equal that in phakic eyes.

Cataract surgery alone is technically simpler than combined cataract and glaucoma surgery, or even filtration surgery followed by cataract extraction, with fewer attendant complications. **If cataract surgery alone is contemplated, it should be performed temporally, in order to preserve superior conjunctiva for future filtration surgery.** In some situations, such as phacomorphic angle closure or phacolytic glaucoma, cataract extraction alone may eradicate the glaucomatous state. On the other hand, cataract extraction rarely has a long-lasting IOP-lowering effect in primary open angle glaucoma (1,2).

Two-Stage: Filtering Surgery Followed by Cataract Extraction

In eyes with advanced glaucomatous damage with profound cupping of the optic nerve and dramatic visual field loss, where the IOP is poorly controlled despite maximum tolerated medical treatment, where there is an urgent need to control the IOP, filtering surgery alone, followed at a later date by cataract extraction, may be the best option. While antimetabolites have altered the success rate associated with combined procedures, certain precarious eyes deserve filtering surgery first, with cataract extraction reserved for a later date. This is especially true in eyes with severely compromised optic nerves that are at high risk for filter failure, e.g., eyes that have undergone prior intraocular surgery, eyes with neovascular or inflammatory glaucoma, eyes of young individuals and African-Americans.

There are disadvantages to the two-stage approach. This technique subjects the patient to two surgical procedures with two recovery periods, each requiring frequent office visits. The patient has poor vision for a prolonged time period while waiting for the second stage of cataract surgery. Finally, the cataract surgery may cause the filter to fail. **Cataract extraction after filtering surgery can be expected to elevate IOP by an average of approximately 5 mm Hg.** The use of MMC at the time of filtering surgery in such a situation may guard the filter against future failure; such eyes tend to experience an average IOP increase of only about 3 mm Hg following cataract extraction (3).

Filtering surgery preceding cataract extraction may obviate the need for cataract surgery itself, if the patient's lens opacities are visually significant only because of miotic use. The discontinuation of miotics, in such instances, will often lead to a marked improvement in visual function;

however, the frequent progression of cataract following filtering surgery may negate this beneficial effect. This situation can be determined prior to surgery with a dilated examination.

Important technical points in surgery for coexisting cataract and glaucoma are discussed later and are highlighted in Table 64.2 (also see Chapter 62).

SURGICAL TECHNIQUE: COMBINED SURGERY

General Preoperative Technique

Preoperatively, miotics can be discontinued the day prior to surgery to allow maximal pupillary dilation. If IOP control is an issue, apraclonidine or carbonic anhydrase inhibitors can be instituted for the short term, if not otherwise contraindicated. To dilate the pupil, three applications each of tropicamide 1%, cyclopentolate 1%, phenylephrine 2.5% and flurbiprofen are administered just prior to surgery.

Anesthesia can be topical, local or general. Retrobulbar or peribulbar local anesthesia, with sedation if possible, provides the greatest patient comfort while producing akinesia, facilitating the surgical procedure. General anesthesia introduces, among many other risks, the possibility of postoperative suprachoroidal hemorrhage due to coughing during the recovery from anesthesia. For retrobulbar or peribulbar anesthesia, a 1:1 mixture of 2% lidocaine and 0.75% bupivicaine, together with 150 units of hyaluronidase in 10 cc of this mixture, are injected. This mixture is also administered to the facial nerve as either a Van Lint or O'Brien block, if desired. Gentle digital pressure is applied through the lids to soften the globe, intermittently for approximately five minutes following injection of anesthetic. **A mechanical device such as a Honan balloon can be used in lieu of digital pressure if desired, but caution is required with this device in the glaucomatous eye.** If the preoperative IOP is extremely high, 25% mannitol in 250–500 cc saline can be given intravenously to avoid suprachoroidal hemorrhage on sudden decompression of the globe.

The eye is sterilized with a single drop of 5% povidone iodine, followed by cleaning of the lids, lashes and surrounding facial quadrant with 10% povidone iodine. Irrigation of the face or eye with water or saline is not necessary.

Choice of Cataract Surgical Technique

Trabeculectomy can be performed together with either phacoemulsification, phacosection or extracapsular cataract extraction, depending on the surgeon's preference; however, the smaller the incision the better, (e.g. phacoemulsification or phacosection), since less conjunctival dissection results in less postoperative inflammation, and a greater likelihood of successful filtration surgery. Phacoemulsification in glaucomatous eyes can be especially challenging due to poor pupillary dilation which frequently accompanies dense nuclear sclerosis. The small pupil and hard lens nucleus are important to consider when deciding on the surgical approach to such an eye. The surgeon with limited experience in phacoemulsification usually favors an extracapsular approach.

Bridle Suture

A Barraquer open loop wire speculum is used to provide adequate exposure while allowing passage of the phacoemulsification handpiece without impedance. Jaffee lid specula may be substituted. A 7-0 silk suture on a tapered needle is used as a traction suture through peripheral clear cornea in the area of the trabeculectomy incision. **A long, deep sweep through the perilimbal cornea** (but not into the AC) is required to prevent tearing of the suture through the cornea. A cotton tipped swab is used to oppose the needle during insertion; the eye is not grasped during this procedure.

Conjunctival Flap

Either a limbus based or fornix based conjunctival flap can be used, and either one with adjunctive MMC. A fornix based flap is faster and technically easier, but a limbus based flap is less likely to leak, and may provide better long-term IOP control. The flap is created in either the superotemporal or superonasal quadrant, leaving the other quadrant free for future filtering surgery, should it be necessary. By performing phacoemulsification or phacosection instead of extracapsular cataract extraction (ECCE), it is possible to allow future filtering surgery in virgin conjunctiva in a superior quadrant, even in an eye with prior cataract extraction.

In a fornix based flap, a five to seven mm chord-length peritomy is performed at the limbus, and Tenon's fascia is incised at its insertion and dissected free. Once Tenon's fascia is free, only Tenon's is grasped during manipulation of the conjunctival-Tenon's flap. Conjunctiva is handled only with non-toothed, non-serrated forceps, such as Max Fine forceps, to avoid tearing of the conjunctiva. The sub-Tenon's dissection is extended posteriorly and laterally using a spreading action with the Wescott scissors. The limbus is treated with diathermy to denude the corneal epithelium in the area of the peritomy, and the coagulum is removed with a Weck-Cel.

For a limbus based flap, a conjunctival incision of approximately two to three clock hours is made 10 mm posterior to the limbus. The incision is carried through Tenon's fascia, and meticulous dissection is extended to the limbus, through Tenon's insertion, using rounded tip Wescott scissors. Similar to the fornix based flap, **the conjunctiva**

Table 64.2
Important Technical Points in Surgery for Coexisting Cataract and Glaucoma

Technique

- A. Combined Cataract and Glaucoma Surgery
  - 1. Basic premise - minimize changes from standard phaco (phaco-emulsification) and trabeculectomy techniques
  - 2. Choose your best operation - Phaco (Phacoemulsification) or ECCE with PC IOL. Minimize manipulation, be atraumatic to tissues. Phaco/small IOL may have advantage for enhanced bleb development and improved IOP control over ECCE combined procedure
  - 3. Pre-Op
    - a. Dilation-stop miotics 1 week pre-op, consider Ocufen with usual dilation regimen
    - b. Soft eye-post injection compression (Honan balloon)
    - c. Consider pre-op CAI, beta-blocker if post-op IOP spike a concern
  - 4. Paracentesis - mandatory for testing filter outflow
  - 5. Location - superonasal or superotemporal: spare virgin conjunctiva for future filtration surgery if needed. Phaco with small IOL an advantage
  - 6. Conjunctival flaps
    - a. Fornix - faster, more anterior leaks
    - b. Limbal - more tedious, better early IOP control, may permit earlier 5-FU and laser suture lysis
    - c. Tenon's excision - facilitates laser suture lysis
  - 7. Scleral flap and sclerectomy
    - a. Any shape flap - mobilize anteriorly into clear cornea
    - b. Base of flap equals size required for IOL
    - c. Generally perform sclerectomy after IOL implantation; consider sclerectomy before foldable IOL implantation to permit smaller incision
    - d. Tightness of closure-strive for slow, spontaneous flow under flap with maintenance of anterior chamber
    - e. Scleral flap can be modified: conventional phaco scleral pocket with stitch or no stitch—modified scleral pocket with relaxing incision—conventional trabeculectomy flap
    - f. Mitomycin C
  - 8. Management of miotic pupils and iris - achieve adequate size (4–5 mm), preserve pupillary reactivity, preserve pupillary shape
    - a. Avoid excessive iris manipulation
    - b. Epinephrine in infusion
    - c. Strip peripupillary membranes
    - d. Sweep and release synechias
    - e. Stretching
    - f. Iris hooks
    - g. Sphincterotomies
      - 1. Few (1–3)
        - a. Short or long
        - b. 1 quadrant - oval; 2 quadrants - hammock
        - c. Aid inferior exposure
        - d. Couple with superior sphincterectomy to aid superior exposure
        - e. Beware iris tags - "magnetic" atraction to phaco tip
      - 2. Multiple (Fine technique)
        - a. 8
        - b. Short cuts
        - c. Rapazzo scissors
        - d. Stretch with hook to break fibrotic adhesions
        - e. Preserve function and pupillary contour
    - h. Superior Sphincterectomy
      - 1. Two instrument technique - hook and long angled Vannas scissors
      - 2. Aids superior exposure
      - 3. Pupillary reactivity preserved with near normal iris contour
    - i. Keyhole/sector iredectomy
      - 1. Maintain sector for diabetics/patients with retinal disease minimizes inflammation and maximizes posterior segment view
      - 2. Iris suture
        - a. 10–0 prolene or nylon
        - b. Pre or Post-place: tie after IOL implantation
        - c. Utilize paracentesis to enhance needle passage
        - d. Form chamber with viscoelastic
        - e. Ethicon CIF-4, TG-160, STC-6 (straight); Alcon PC7
        - f. Facilitates restoration of taught iris diaphragm
    - j. Use second instrument (Kuglen hook) to move iris and facilitate exposure for capsulorhexis and phacoemulsification
  - 9. Capsule - small capsulorhexis
    - a. Keeps iris away from phaco tip in endocapsular techniques
    - b. Facilitates separation of IOL from the iris - reduces pupillary capture of IOL and posterior migration of iris
    - c. Small opening does not preclude large optic implantation
  - 10. Phacoemulsification
    - a. Two instrument technique
    - b. Hydrodisection/delineation
    - c. Control of nucleus is critical - free rotation in the bag
    - d. Divide and conquer
    - e. Stabilize AC depth - avoid flux
  - 11. IOL
    - a. Foldable silicone IOL
    - b. 7 mm - no holes - best with enlarged pupil
    - c. Small IOL - reduces incision size, inflammation
    - d. If oval IOL, orient long axis in direction of greatest pupillary dimension
    - e. All IOL's in bag - reduce pigment dispersion
    - f. Beware exfoliation - zonular weakness - check intra-op
    - g. Avoid AC IOL if angle compromise; open loop (tripod, quadripod) lenses okay
  - 12. Assess Pupil after IOL implantation
    - a. Intra-op carbachol (Miostat) may induce greater miosis than acetylcholine (Miochol) - helpful to bring iris over IOL; may also enhance post-op IOP
    - b. Minimal iris manipulation
    - c. Suture iris prn
    - d. Remove viscoelastic after iris suturing
  - 13. Conjunctival closure - tight. If fornix-based flap, bring flap well anterior to base of scleral flap to minimize leaks. Closure with wing overlapping sutures using Ethicon 9–0 monofilament Vicryl or 10-0 nylon TG-160-4 7707G four-wire cutting needle anchoring to episclera. If limbal based flap, use Ethicon 9-0 monofilament Vicryl, or 10–0 nylon BV-75 four-wire taper needle or Ethicon TG-160-4 7707G four-wire cutting needle.
  - 14. Test filtration and bleb elevation via paracentesis at completion of procedure
  - 15. Post-op
    - a. Early compression at edge of flap (Traverso maneuver)
    - b. Early laser suture lysis (delay as long as possible if mitomycin C used) - days 3–10 (longer stitch easier to cut with laser)
    - c. Consider contact lens tamponade of early, anterior, fornix-based conjunctival flap leak to facilitate bleb development
    - d. Consider 5-FU if bleb failure
    - e. Frequently fail to develop bleb on long term follow-up
- B. Cataract Surgery Alone
  - 1. Same considerations as combined cataract and glaucoma surgery - see text for technical details
  - 2. Location - superonasal or superotemporal. Preserve virgin conjunctiva for future filtration surgery if needed
  - 3. Post-op
    - a. Monitor IOP closely
    - b. Consider post-op CAI, beta-blocker, alpha-agonist (apraclonidine)
    - c. Avoid injection of long acting steroid—beware of steroid response
- C. Two Stage: filter first, cataract second
  - 1. Filter first
    - a. Superonasal
    - b. Favor full-thickness sclerectomy or trabeculectomy with mitomycin C - less compromise with subsequent cataract operation; cataract progression not a concern
    - c. Tube procedures (i.e. Molteno or Baerveldt tube) not excluded
  - 2. Cataract extraction
    - a. Same considerations as cataract extraction alone; no Honan balloon if filter effective
    - b. Timing - as long as possible after cataract extraction, preferably 4–6 months
    - c. Location
      - 1. Inferotemporal (180 degrees from bleb) - incision greatest distance from bleb; easy access for phaco and nuclear expression; can add glaucoma procedure prn; standard scleral tunnel incision possible
      - 2. Clear cornea (anterior to bleb) - no conjunctival manipulation; anterior incision - more difficult phaco and nuclear expression; increase astigmatism; pocket incision possible
    - d. No PI required - already present with filter
    - e. Wound closure - extra sutures to permit earlier digital pressure; no stitch with scleral tunnel
    - f. Confirm sclerectomy patency and bleb elevation at end of case. Internal revision of bleb with spatula possible, if obstruction present
    - g. Post-Op
      - 1. Vigorous topical steroids
      - 2. 5-FU
      - 3. Expect some loss of long-term IOP control

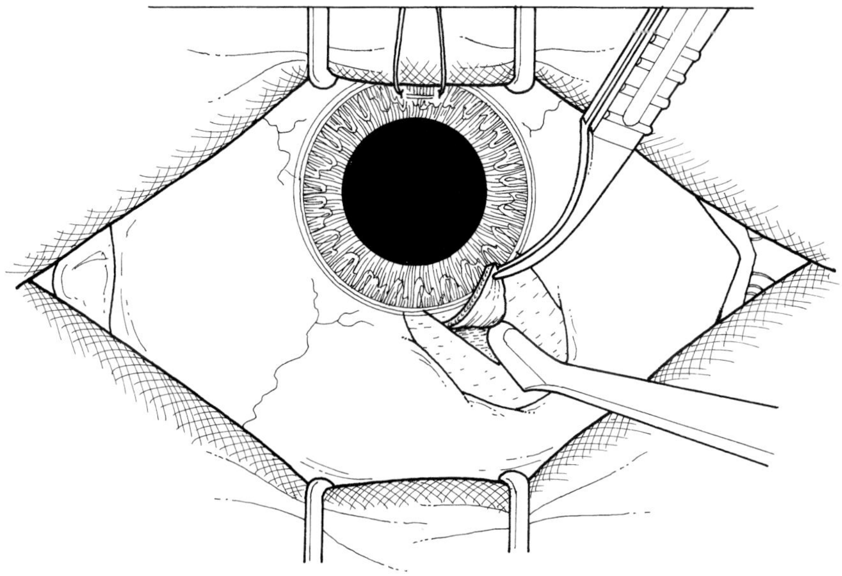

Figure 64.1. A half thickness scleral flap constructed with width at its base to match the intraocular lens diameter.

is handled with non-toothed, non-serrated forceps to minimize trauma and avoid tearing of the tissue.

Hemostasis

Excellent hemostasis is achieved with underwater diathermy (MIRA, Waltham, MA). This is preferable to bipolar cautery, as diathermy causes less tissue shrinkage and charring. Diathermy is applied selectively because not all vessels require closure, and only bleeding vessels or those likely to bleed are treated. Prior to scleral flap construction, the planned area of the flap is outlined with diathermy.

Scleral Flap

A half thickness triangular or rectangular scleral flap is created, with dimensions equivalent to the width of the intraocular lens to be inserted (Fig. 64.1). A 3.2 mm wide base is adequate for foldable IOLs; a larger flap is required for rigid lenses. The scleral flap is outlined with either a Grieshaber 681.01 blade or a Beaver 69 blade. A 0.12 toothed forceps, such as a Maumenee-Calibri, is used to grasp one corner of the scleral flap, and the dissection is carried forward at one-half thickness into clear cornea. **Care is taken to maintain a constant plane of depth in creating the scleral flap**, to avoid inadvertent early entry into the anterior chamber (dissection too deep) or amputation of the flap (dissection too superficial). Additionally, the dissection must proceed sufficiently anterior to avoid entry over the ciliary body.

Mitomycin C (MMC)

Following creation of the scleral flap, MMC is applied on a pledget fashioned from a section of Weck-Cel soaked in 0.2–0.4 mg/cc MMC. This pledget is placed under the scleral flap and the conjunctiva is draped over the pledget (Fig. 64.2). The cut edge of the conjunctiva is not permitted to contact the pledget. The pledget is left in place for two to three and a half minutes, depending on whether or not the eye has had prior surgery. The pledget is then removed, and the area is irrigated with 15 cc balanced salt solution. It is important to avoid accidental inoculation of MMC into the eye. To this end, **no entry into the anterior chamber is made prior to application of MMC, and any instruments in contact with MMC are rinsed prior to reuse.** The MMC solution is kept covered in the operating room, and handling and disposal are in accordance with the Occupational Safety and Health Administration guidelines to avoid exposing operating room personnel to

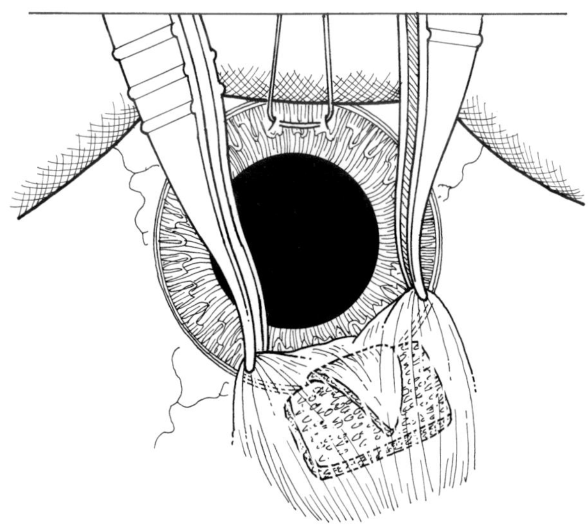

Figure 64.2. After a pledget saturated with mitomycin C solution is placed beneath the scleral flap, the fornix-based conjunctival flap is pulled anteriorly so that its edges will not be exposed to the mitomycin C.

undue risk (Chapter 62). The optimal concentration of MMC to be used and time of exposure are still under investigation, but 0.2–0.4 mg/cc MMC for 2–4 minutes appears to provide adequate success with acceptable risks.

Paracentesis

Following irrigation of MMC from the surgical field, a Beaver 75 blade is used to make a paracentesis incision at the 1:30 position to allow reformation of the anterior chamber and the insertion of a second instrument for phacoemulsification or phacosection. **The internal opening is made larger than the external by pivoting the blade around the corneal entry site toward the sharp edge;** this facilitates insertion of instruments through the wound.

Anterior Chamber Entry

A 3.0 mm keratome is used to enter the eye at the anterior most point beneath the scleral flap. The keratome is positioned parallel to the iris plane to avoid dissection into the corneal stroma or stripping of Descemet's membrane. Viscoelastic is injected into the anterior chamber prior to capsulorhexis or pupillary enlargement.

Management of the Pupil

If posterior synechias are present, they are broken with a cyclodialysis spatula. A small pupil can be enlarged adequately by a simple stretching technique. A Kuglen, Sinskey or Hunkler hook is placed through the paracentesis and a collar-button hook is placed through the keratome incision. The pupil is stretched limbus to limbus with the two hooks at each clock hour, the hooks are removed, and the anterior chamber filled with viscoelastic, further enlarging the pupil. In almost every case, this technique produces sufficient exposure to proceed with phacoemulsification, yet the pupil regains near normal function postoperatively.

Another technique is the use of multiple small sphincterotomies performed using long Gills-Vannas scissors or Rappozzo scissors, as described by I. Howard Fine of Eugene, Oregon and Howard Gimbel of Calgary, Alberta, Canada (Fig. 64.3). The sphincterotomies are each approximately 1 mm in length and do not extend across the full width of the sphincter muscle, in order to preserve pupillary function postoperatively. For the sphincterotomy near 12 o'clock, a Sinskey hook is used to elevate and stabilize the iris prior to cutting. Alternatively, a peripheral iridectomy can be performed and extended into a sector iridectomy with long Gills-Vannas scissors. This sector, or keyhole, iridectomy can be left as is or reapproximated at the conclusion of the case, using 10-0 prolene suture.

After surgical pupilloplasty, viscoelastic is injected into the anterior chamber to enlarge the pupil further. An adequate pupil size of at least 4 to 5 mm is generally required for phacoemulsification.

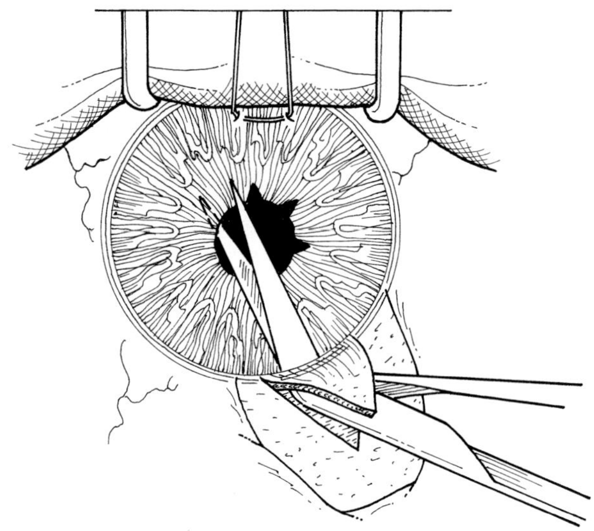

Figure 64.3. In eyes with small pupils, multiple partial sphincterotomies can be created with the Gills-Vannas scissors to enlarge the pupil. A Rappazzo scissors can be used as well.

The pupil can also be enlarged by the use of iris hooks. Four of these disposable devices, constructed of prolene with silicone sleeves, are inserted through limbal corneal stab incisions made in each of four quadrants with a Grieshaber 681.05 blade. The hooks catch the edge of the pupil, and then are drawn toward the limbus, stretching the pupil. The end result is a large, square pupil, through which capsulotomy and lens extraction can be performed. The hooks are removed at the conclusion of the surgery; the stab wounds are self-sealing.

Capsulotomy and Hydrodissection

For phacoemulsification, capsulorhexis is the preferred capsulotomy technique. The capsulorhexis is started with the cystotome and continued with either the cystotome or Utrata forceps. Hydrodissection is performed with balanced salt solution and a 27 gauge cannula, injecting the BSS between the lens capsule and lens cortex, and then between the lens cortex and lens nucleus.

Phacoemulsification

The lens nucleus is divided into quadrants and each is phacoemulsified, in turn (Fig. 64.4). The epinucleus is left for last, so that this layer can offer protection to the capsule from sharp edges of lens nuclear material during phacoemulsification. Cortex is removed with an automated irrigation/aspiration unit. Cortex near the keratome site is removed with a curved irrigation/aspiration tip, or with a Simcoe cannula through the paracentesis site, or simply with gentle aspiration on a 25 or 27 gauge cannula on a saline filled syringe inserted through the paracentesis. If the cortex is recalcitrant, it may be removed following

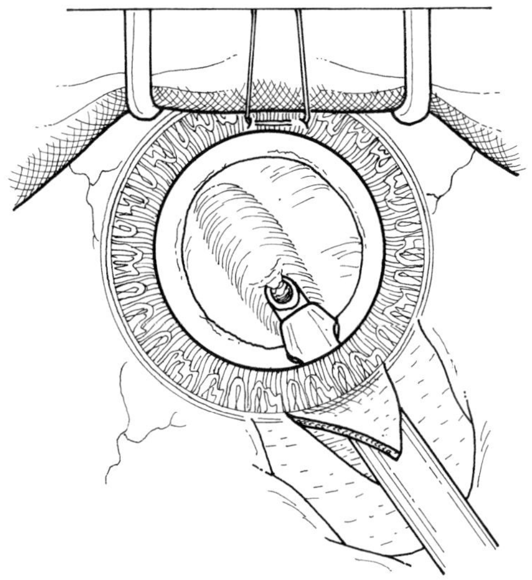

Figure 64.4. The nucleus is phacoemulsified through an incision made beneath the scleral flap.

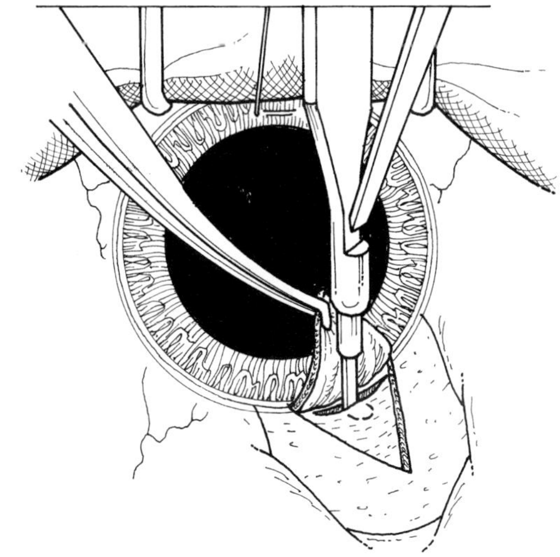

Figure 64.5. After intraocular lens implantation, a sclerectomy is done using the Kelly Descemet's punch.

insertion of the posterior chamber IOL, which will protect the posterior capsule during aspiration.

IOL Insertion

Following cortical clean-up, the capsular bag and anterior chamber are filled with viscoelastic. The scleral incision is enlarged to an appropriate size for the IOL to be used. The IOL is inserted in the capsular bag to prevent chafing of the iris pigment epithelium by the lens.

If a capsular rent is noted, and it is small, it may still be possible to place an IOL in the capsular bag; however, if the rent is large, this is not feasible. In such cases, given adequate anterior capsular support, a posterior chamber IOL is placed in the ciliary sulcus. Such a lens should have PMMA haptics to reduce the risk of inflammation postoperatively; IOL's with prolene haptics should not be placed in the sulcus.

If capsular support does not exist, an anterior chamber IOL can be positioned. The anterior chamber is filled with viscoelastic following careful vitrectomy and inspection to insure that no vitreous is present in the anterior chamber. **The lens is placed so that the superior haptic rests at least one clock hour from the sclerectomy site,** to minimize the risk of prolapse of the IOL into the trabeculectomy. Intraoperative gonioscopy confirms the haptic position.

Sclerectomy

Following IOL placement, viscoelastic is aspirated from the eye, and carbachol is injected into the anterior chamber to constrict the pupil for iridectomy. The assistant retracts the scleral flap, and the Kelly-Descemet's punch is used to remove a block of sclera, approximately two by two mm

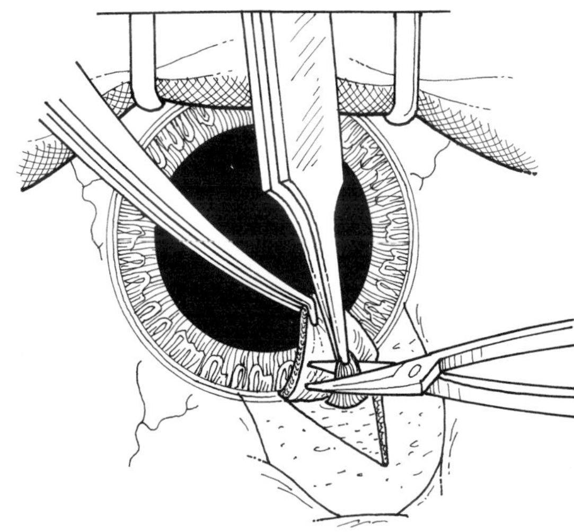

Figure 64.6. An iridectomy is performed using Vannas scissors, taking care not to cut the scleral flap.

in width (Fig. 64.5). Alternatively, the Beaver 75 blade can be used to cut two radial incisions perpendicular to the scleral incision. In this way a rectangular flap is created beneath the scleral guard flap. The deep flap can then be grasped with 0.12 mm toothed forceps, reflected posteriorly, and excised with Vannas scissors. Care is taken not to excise sclera excessively posteriorly, in order to avoid encountering the ciliary body, which would result in bleeding.

Iridectomy

As an assistant continues to retract the scleral flap, the iris is grasped with non-toothed forceps (to avoid damage to the zonules, lens haptic and ciliary processes), and the peripheral iris is gently withdrawn from the eye (Fig. 64.6).

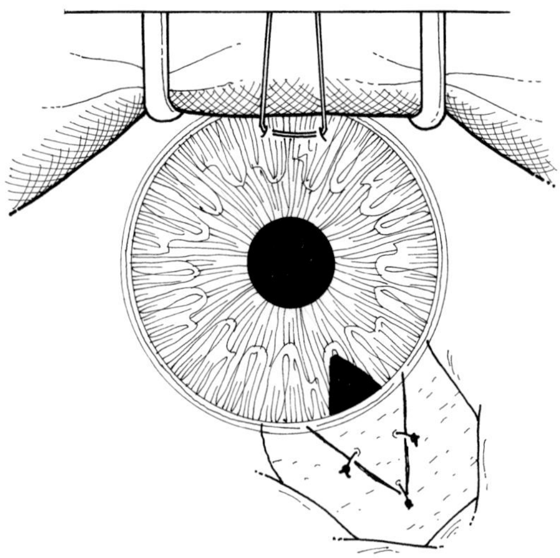

Figure 64.7. The scleral flap is closed with interrupted 10-0 nylon sutures.

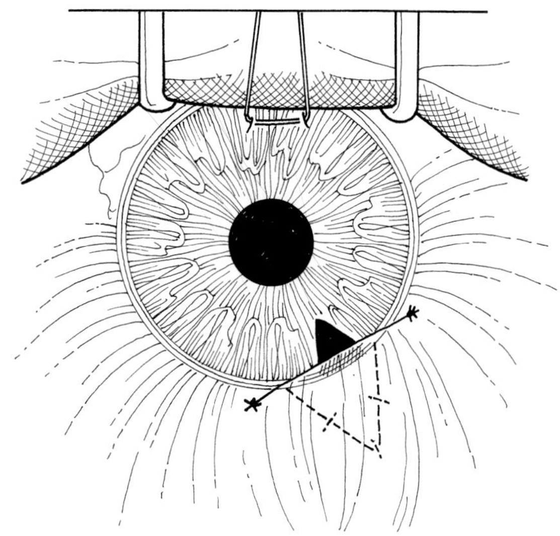

Figure 64.8. The conjunctiva is closed with interrupted sutures, after which the bleb is expanded by filling the eye with balanced salt solution injected through the paracentesis site.

The Vannas scissors are positioned horizontally, and the iris is drawn away and then towards the scissors as the incision is made. This maneuver creates a broad, basilar iridectomy, reducing the risk of occlusion of the sclerectomy site.

Closure of the Scleral Flap

The scleral flap is closed tightly with 10-0 nylon sutures. Three sutures are used for a triangular flap (Fig. 64.7), five for a rectangular flap. The use of multiple sutures allows titration of the IOP postoperatively with laser suture lysis. **The number of sutures may be adjusted as necessary intraoperatively in order to keep the anterior chamber deep while allowing a slow flow of aqueous from the edges of the scleral flap.** The flow rate is tested by injecting balanced salt solution through the paracentesis while holding a Weck-Cel sponge at the scleral flap to observe how quickly fluid is absorbed from the filtration site.

Closure of the Conjunctiva

With fornix based flap: The conjunctiva is closed with 9-0 monofilament Vicryl on a taper needle. A bite is taken through cornea and episclera, exiting just inside the edge of the conjunctival wound at the limbus. The needle is then passed through the underside of the cut edge of the conjunctiva, then through the conjunctiva from the external side to the internal side, and repeatedly from internal to external, then external to internal, leaving approximately ½ mm between bites, incorporating loose conjunctiva, until the conjunctiva can be pulled taut across the limbus, slightly indenting the cornea. In this fashion, dog-ears are avoided, and a watertight closure is achieved. The excess conjunctiva at the limbus is imbricated into the wound by the over-under suture technique (Fig. 64.8).

With limbus based flap: The conjunctiva is closed with 9-0 monofilament Vicryl on a taper needle, the same as used with fornix based flaps. A running, locking closure is used, and **a bite of posterior Tenon's is taken with every second or third pass** of the suture.

With either technique, a tenonectomy is performed if there is excessive Tenon's fascia which will obscure the scleral flap sutures for laser suture lysis.

Following closure of the conjunctiva, balanced salt solution is injected through the paracentesis to reform the anterior chamber and elevate the conjunctiva. The wound is tested for water tightness with 2% fluorescein solution; fluorescein strips may be used if the solution is not available, but the strips do not show leakage as readily as the solution. Leaks are closed with either the 9-0 monofilament Vicryl or 10-0 nylon on a BV-75 tapered vascular needle. Testing is repeated until no leaks are found.

Cefazolin (50 mg in 0.5 cc) and dexamethasone (2 mg in 0.5 cc) are administered subconjunctivally in the inferonasal quadrant, as this is the area least likely to undergo filtering surgery in the future. Dexamethasone and polymixin-bacitracin ointments are applied, followed by a patch and shield.

MODIFICATIONS FOR ECCE OR PHACOSECTION

For ECCE or phacosection, certain aspects of the surgical technique differ from those described for phacoemulsification. The width of the scleral flap need not be based on the size of the IOL. After creating the scleral flap, scleral incisions are made to the right and left, in order to create a wound large enough for expression or extraction of the lens. Corneoscleral scissors are used to create this scleral wound. After cataract removal and lens implantation, the limbal incisions to the sides of the trabeculectomy flap are closed with interrupted 10-0 nylon sutures. Sufficient sutures are used in the closure of this wound to allow for digital pressure, should it be necessary postoperatively.

CATARACT SURGERY ALONE

Cataract surgery in the glaucomatous eye is performed in either the temporal clear cornea or the superonasal or superotemporal quadrant **to preserve conjunctiva for future filtration surgery**, should it be necessary. Once again, procedures such as phacoemulsification or phacosection are preferable to ECCE, as they require less conjunctival manipulation, and preserve virgin tissue for future surgery. ECCE may be done from an inferior limbal approach or through clear cornea in order to preserve conjunctiva for possible filtering surgery.

TWO STAGE SURGERY—TRABECULECTOMY FOLLOWED BY CATARACT EXTRACTION

A two-stage approach may be indicated in eyes in which the optic nerve is severely compromised, where a single digit IOP is the desired surgical outcome. In this case, the filtering surgery is performed several months prior to cataract extraction. This could be trabeculectomy or a seton procedure; **if trabeculectomy, antimetabolites at the time of surgery are recommended.** The trabeculectomy is done in a superonasal quadrant if possible, to allow for a limbal cataract extraction inferotemporally in the future, at the furthest possible site from the filter. If the performed filter is of borderline function, a combined cataract extraction and trabeculectomy can be performed superotemporally. Again, the adjunctive use of MMC is highly valuable in this setting. Another approach for the cataract extraction is a clear corneal incision, especially with phacoemulsification. This has the disadvantage of greater postoperative astigmatism, and is more challenging technically. **The closure of the cataract wound should be strong enough to allow for use of digital pressure in the early postoperative period.**

CATARACT EXTRACTION FOLLOWING FILTERING SURGERY: THE EYE WITH A PRE-EXISTING BLEB

This situation is nearly exactly analogous to the two-stage filter-followed-by-cataract-extraction, except that in this case, the cataract surgery was not planned at the time of trabeculectomy. Still, in a previously unoperated eye, one hopes that the trabeculectomy was made superonasal, in order to facilitate future cataract surgery. In this case, the cataract is removed from an infero-temporal approach. If the bleb is elsewhere, it is important to operate as far from it as possible when removing the cataract, or to use a clear-corneal technique. **All efforts are made to avoid conjunctival manipulation, in order to preserve bleb function.** At the conclusion of the case, a cyclodialysis spatula may be passed through the sclerectomy and into the bleb, with the intention of freeing any adhesions that might have formed in the subconjunctival space. Gonioscopy can be helpful in locating the sclerectomy site, and perhaps surprisingly, subconjunctival hemorrhage is uncommon with this procedure.

Despite the best and most careful procedures, a rise in IOP is expected postoperatively (see below). Care must be taken, as in the two-stage approach, to close the scleral wound tightly (to allow postoperative digital pressure) as well as the conjunctival wound (to avoid leaks). Postoperatively, inflammation is managed aggressively, with topical steroids and 5-fluorouracil, if necessary, no matter how old the filter. Even needling of the bleb is required to restore function in rare cases.

POSTOPERATIVE CARE

Combined Surgery for Cataract and Glaucoma

In the immediate postoperative period frequent use is made of topical steroids, such as prednisolone acetate 1% six or more times daily, in addition to antibiotic (polymixin bacitracin) and steroid (dexamethasone) ointments at bedtime. Topical glaucoma medications are continued in the unoperated eye. Oral carbonic anhydrase inhibitors are discontinued, as they decrease aqueous flow through the bleb. Should additional IOP control be required for the unoperated eye, apraclonidine 0.5% two or three times daily can be of value.

Laser Suture Lysis

Laser suture lysis (LSL) is performed if the IOP is too high postoperatively (Chapters 60 and 63). Topical anesthesia with proparacaine 0.5% is used, and a Hoskins, Ritch, or Mandelkorn lens is applied to the bleb. **Especially in fornix-based conjunctival flaps, care is taken to avoid putting stress on the wound; the lens is placed on the bleb and drawn towards the conjunctival wound.** The scleral flap sutures are generally readily seen beneath the lens. The argon green (514 nm) laser is used to perform LSL, with a 0.02-second pulse, 50 μm spot size, beginning at 300 mW, and increasing power as needed. If subconjunctival blood obscures the sutures, a longer wavelength laser, such as the diode laser (800 nm) is used. This wavelength penetrates blood better than the argon laser, and is well absorbed by black nylon sutures. Care is taken to avoid conjunctival burns, even with the diode laser.

The surgeon must be extremely cautious in the early postoperative period in performing LSL on eyes in which

MMC was used intraoperatively. Early LSL can result in severe, sometimes intractable, postoperative hypotony. **Early IOP rises related to residual viscoelastic material, inflammation, fibrin, or other transient causes should be treated with observation, digital pressure, or even paracentesis, rather than LSL in the first postoperative week in the setting of intraoperative MMC use.**

Consideration is given to the effects of LSL on IOP and astigmatism. If postoperative astigmatism is a problem, but the eye is hypotonous, astigmatic keratotomy can be a better option than LSL.

Digital Pressure

Should the IOP rise to potentially unsafe levels, the patient is instructed in the use of digital pressure postoperatively (see Fig. 63.11). The patient is told to press through the upper or lower eyelid while looking down or up, respectively, for three ten second counts, with intervals of ten seconds between each count. The patient is asked to perform this exercise four to six times per day, depending on the degree of IOP lowering desired. The technique is demonstrated to the patient while in the office, and the IOP is measured before and after digital pressure.

Digital pressure can also be useful on an intermittent basis for use by the surgeon in the early postoperative period. It can be used to break adhesions forming between the trabeculectomy flap and the underlying sclera, or between the episclera and conjunctiva. In this case, the surgeon may elect to use a muscle hook or moistened cotton-tipped swab, which is placed just adjacent to the trabeculectomy flap. Gentle, but firm, pressure is applied to the sclera, in an effort to separate the trabeculectomy flap from its scleral bed. This is also known as the Traverso maneuver.

5-Fluorouracil

5-fluorouracil is employed in cases where the bleb appears injected, shallow or localizing, when failure of the filtering surgery appears possible, even if MMC was used intraoperatively. 5-fluorouracil is administered under topical anesthesia (proparacaine or tetracaine), injected through a 30 gauge needle subconjunctivally 180 from the bleb. A volume of 0.1 cc of 5-FU 50 mg/cc is given.

5-fluorouracil can be given once or twice a week, or even more frequently, usually with a total of seven to ten doses (35–50 mg total dose). **It can be used even weeks, months or years postoperatively, and can be combined with needling of the bleb in order to revive a failing filter.**

Bleb Leaks

Leakage at the wound margin is more common in association with fornix based flaps than with limbus based flaps. Should a leak occur, it is managed with aqueous suppressants, a bandage contact lens and aminoglycoside antibiotics to stimulate wound healing. Autologous blood can be injected into the bleb. If these approaches fail, the leak is closed surgically.

Inadvertent Cyclodialysis Cleft

An uncommon complication of combined cataract and glaucoma surgery, or of cataract surgery alone, is the formation of an inadvertent cyclodialysis cleft (see Chapter 66). This should be suspected in the presence of persistent postoperative hypotony, and must be located gonioscopically or by ultrasound biomicroscopy. Once located, the cleft can be closed either with laser to the wall of the cleft, if small, or by cryopexy or conventional surgical technique if larger. If left untreated, the very low IOP resulting from such a cleft can cause hypotonous maculopathy, which can be irreversible.

Cataract Surgery Alone

If cataract surgery alone is performed in glaucomatous eyes, a combination topical antibiotic and steroid drop is used four times a day postoperatively (e.g. prednisolone acetate 1% and gentamicin sulfate or dexamethasone and tobramycin). All anti-glaucoma medications used preoperatively are resumed postoperatively, with the exception of adrenergic agents, which may induce cystoid macular edema in aphakia or pseudophakia. Following cataract surgery, glaucomatous eyes have early elevations of IOP more often than non-glaucomatous eyes, especially in the first two postoperative days (4). If long term IOP control is an issue, laser trabeculoplasty may be useful, even in pseudophakia (5).

Glaucoma Filtering Surgery Followed by Cataract Extraction

The care of the eye following trabeculectomy alone is similar to that for the eye following combined cataract extraction and trabeculectomy, except that topical atropine 1% twice daily is used in the former setting, to aid in maintaining a deep anterior chamber. Following subsequent cataract surgery, frequent topical steroids (prednisolone acetate 1% six or more times daily) and topical antibiotic and steroid ointments (bacitracin-polymixin and dexamethasone ointments) are used at bedtime. 5-fluorouracil injections are given if the bleb appears inflamed or shows any signs of impending failure. Digital pressure is used after the cataract extraction if needed, with special attention to any indication of wound dehiscence.

ALTERNATIVE TECHNIQUES

While this chapter describes techniques for cataract extraction and trabeculectomy in the setting of coexisting cataract and glaucoma, other approaches used in the past include intracapsular cataract extraction (ICCE), cyclodialysis and full-thickness filtering surgery, albeit using a "guarded" technique. Guarded sclerectomy in combination with ECCE or ICCE requires the creation of a highly beveled corneoscleral wound, in which the fistula is created by removing tissue from the posterior lip with a sclerectomy punch (1,6,7). A Pearce trabeculectomy combined with phacoemulsification is similar; a smaller beveled incision is created, from which tissue is excised from the posterior lip of the wound (8). Posterior lip sclerectomy may be combined with ECCE (9) or may be used before cataract extraction in a two-stage procedure (1); however, the advent of MMC has diminished the use of posterior lip sclerectomy. A clear corneal incision can be used for cataract extraction either combined with trabeculectomy or in the second stage of two-stage surgery (1,10,11). Phacoemulsification can be combined with holmium laser sclerectomy ab interno (12) or ab externo (13). Cyclodialysis can be performed at the time of cataract extraction (14,15). In this case, miotics are used postoperatively to maintain a patent cyclodialysis cleft (15). Cyclodialysis, however, carries with it a multitude of possible complications, including hyphema, hypotony and sudden failure (Chapter 66); therefore, most surgeons prefer trabeculectomy to cyclodialysis.

SURGICAL OUTCOMES

IOP Control

CATARACT EXTRACTION ALONE

Cataract extraction alone does not effect a long term reduction in IOP in the glaucomatous eye; about the most that can be expected is one to two mm Hg IOP drop at one to two years postoperatively following cataract surgery (1,4). Still, eyes undergoing ECCE with posterior chamber intraocular lens implantation, or even ICCE, may require fewer postoperative anti-glaucoma medications (2). **Although long term IOP control is generally not diminished by cataract surgery, early postoperative IOP elevations can be troublesome,** especially in glaucomatous eyes (1,2,4,9). As many as 20% of glaucomatous eyes can have IOP rises of 20 mm Hg or more following ECCE and 12% after ICCE (2). Glaucomatous eyes have IOP elevations in the early postoperative period at a significantly higher rate than non-glaucomatous eyes (4). The implantation of a posterior chamber IOL does not affect the incidence of the early postoperative IOP rise. In one study, an IOP elevation occurred in 23% of eyes with IOP medically controlled before surgery, in 39% of eyes with prior laser trabeculoplasty, but in only 3% of nonglaucomatous eyes. In eyes with splitting of fixation or constriction of the visual field to within 10 of fixation, 10% had worsening of the visual field postoperatively (4).

TWO-STAGE: FILTERING SURGERY FOLLOWED BY CATARACT EXTRACTION

In comparing the various surgical techniques for the management of coexisting cataract and glaucoma, care must be taken in interpretation of data from retrospective studies, as a profound selection bias exists for which eyes are chosen for which procedure. One study found that the two-stage approach offered the greatest reduction of IOP. Trabeculectomy or posterior lip sclerectomy resulted in an average fall of 11.7 mm Hg; however, following the second stage, in which ECCE was done through a clear corneal incision, the overall reduction of IOP was only 7.7 mm Hg. This same study observed only a 2 mm Hg drop following ECCE with posterior chamber intraocular lens implantation or combined ECCE and guarded sclerectomy. The combined procedure, in this study, as well as the two stage surgery, had fewer early postoperative IOP elevations than cataract extraction alone (1).

COMBINED FILTERING SURGERY AND CATARACT EXTRACTION

Trabeculectomy appears more efficacious in long-term IOP control than guarded sclerectomy when combined with cataract extraction. Combined trabeculectomy and ECCE result in an average 6 mm Hg IOP reduction 17 months postoperatively, and 10 mm Hg with two years follow-up (16,17). In comparing trabeculectomy alone to combined trabeculectomy with ECCE, trabeculectomy alone predictably fares better, lowering IOP 12.1 mm Hg, but with the combined procedure IOP drops 9.8 mm Hg, with two years follow-up (17). The authors did not report IOP following cataract extraction in eyes undergoing trabeculectomy alone.

The way in which cataract extraction is done in eyes with trabeculectomy does not appear to affect control of IOP. A similar magnitude of pressure reduction is seen with limbal or clear corneal ECCE, with phacoemulsification through limbal or clear corneal approaches, or post-phacosection. With clear corneal ECCE combined with limbal trabeculectomy, IOP reductions of 9 mm Hg are seen after a mean follow-up of 12 months (11) and 6 mm Hg after two years (10). In combined trabeculectomy and phacoemulsification with a foldable posterior chamber intraocular lens, a mean fall of 7.7 mm Hg is reported, with 13 months follow-up (18). A study comparing the use of rigid and foldable IOLs in combined trabeculectomy and phacoemulsification finds that the surgery with the rigid lens, requiring a 6 mm incision, results in a 6.8 mm Hg drop, while the operation with the foldable lens, with a 3 mm incision, is accompanied by a fall in IOP of 8.9 mm Hg at six months follow-up (19). In comparing ECCE combined with trabeculectomy to phacoemulsification combined with trabeculectomy, at a mean follow-up of 16 months, there is no significant difference between eyes,

WHEN TO FILTER THE PSEUDOPHAKIC EYE

Joel S. Schuman

Pseudophakia presents special problems and opportunities to the ophthalmic surgeon. The fact that the eye has undergone prior surgery in and of itself predisposes it to filtering surgery failure. Pseudophakia, however, allows the use of strong miotics, drugs that cannot be used in the presence of the crystalline lens.

The pseudophakic eye with uncontrolled glaucoma, with progressive loss of nerve fiber layer and cupping and visual field loss, should be treated first with a non-selective beta-blocker, then with dorzolamide, and next with a weak concentration of Phospholine Iodide. This drug is available at 0.03%, which is approximately equivalent to pilocarpine 2–4%, and has twice daily, or even once a day, dosing.

If the IOP is still uncontrolled, and laser trabeculoplasty has not been previously performed, or if only 180 were treated (and that treatment was successful), or even if 360 were treated successfully, then LTP should be tried, using 50 spots over 360 if 360 were previously treated, or else 35–50 spots over an untreated 180 .

Should the glaucoma remain uncontrolled, either chronic oral CAI therapy or filtering surgery should be pursued. The choice is one made by the surgeon and the patient, and if the patient chooses surgery, trabeculectomy should be performed. A full-thickness procedure is inadvisable in this setting, due to the risk of flat anterior chamber, lens-corneal touch, and suprachoroidal hemorrhage, especially in an aphakic or pseudophakic eye. Despite previous manipulation of the superior conjunctiva, this area should be used for the filter, due to the risk of endophthalmitis with inferior blebs. If conjunctival scarring precludes the creation of a conjunctival flap for trabeculectomy, a glaucoma drainage implant, such as a Baerveldt, Krupin, Ahmed, Molteno, or other tube-shunt device (Chapter 65), should be placed. If trabeculectomy is possible, mitomycin C, 0.2–0.4 mg/cc for 3.5 minutes, is applied intraoperatively, as described elsewhere in this text. Although a limbus-based conjunctival flap is preferred, it is not required, and a fornix-based flap can be utilized even with MMC.

If the conjunctiva is so scarred over 360 that neither filtering surgery nor glaucoma drainage implant is possible, or if the eye has extremely poor vision and has been vitrectomized, cyclophotocoagulation can be considered. This is a treatment of last resort, and results in a 50% incidence of visual loss, with nearly 20% of those with visual acuities of counting fingers or worse progressing to no light perception (Chapter 57). For these reasons, surgery to improve aqueous outflow is always preferable to that for decreasing aqueous inflow.

although the mean fall in IOP in the phacoemulsification group is 5 mm Hg, compared with 2.9 mm Hg in the ECCE group (20). This study does not utilize LSL or antimetabolites.

A recent study indicates that with one year follow-up, 73% of eyes (54/74) achieve IOPs of 15 mm Hg or less following combined trabeculectomy with MMC, and ECCE. Symptomatic hypotony occurred in 4% of eyes (21). Another recent work finds an average reduction of 6.4 mm Hg following combined trabeculectomy with MMC and phacoemulsification with posterior chamber intraocular lens implantation, for an average postoperative IOP of 13.2 mm Hg, with no need for glaucoma medications in any eye in this series (22). (Fig. 64.9)

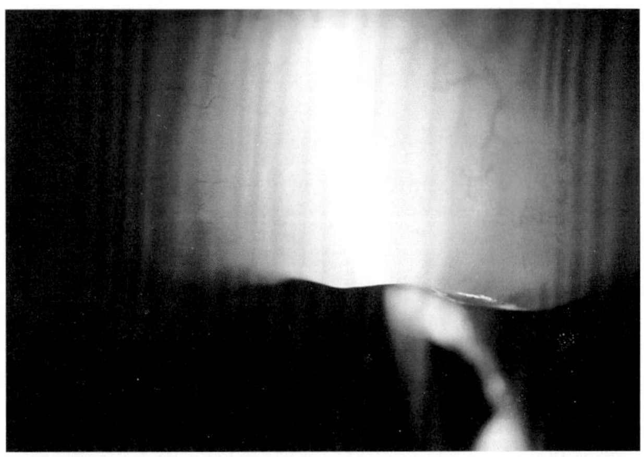

Figure 64.9. The appearance of an eye following combined trabeculectomy with mitomycin C and phacoemulsification. Note the typical diffuse pale, avascular bleb. This procedure, in contrast to combined extracapsular cataract extraction and trabeculectomy, tends to behave and appear more like a trabeculectomy alone than the traditional combined cataract and glaucoma surgery.

COMBINED CYCLODIALYSIS AND CATARACT EXTRACTION

Cyclodialysis combined with cataract extraction is reported to control IOP in 87% of eyes in one study, but control is not defined. This study found that 54% of eyes required no IOP lowering medications postoperatively (14). Another study reports that 87% of eyes with cyclodialysis and ECCE had significant IOP reduction, but that all eyes were maintained on miotic therapy to prevent closure of the cleft. In this work, 39% of eyes had IOP of 0 to 14 mm Hg, and 44% had IOP from 15 to 20 mm Hg postoperatively (15).

CATARACT SURGERY AFTER FILTERING SURGERY

Cataract surgery in eyes with pre-existing blebs will almost certainly result in some elevation in IOP. We found that cataract extraction after filtering surgery caused an IOP rise on average of approximately 5 mm Hg. Although antimetabolite use at the time of filtering surgery seemed to improve these results somewhat, it did not produce a statistically significant protective effect. Even in eyes with MMC trabeculectomies there was an average IOP increase of about 3 mm Hg after cataract extraction; eyes treated with no antimetabolite sustained an IOP increase of about 6 mm Hg (3).

Visual Acuity

According to one study, following ECCE with posterior chamber intraocular lens (ECCE/PCIOL) alone, 79% of glaucomatous eyes achieve visual acuity of 20/40 or better, while combined ECCE/PCIOL and guarded sclerectomy results in 20/40 or better vision in 59% of eyes; however, the patients in this study differ preoperatively as well (1). Another study finds that 89% of eyes without macular disease reach 20/40 vision or better following combined trabeculectomy and ECCE/PCIOL (16). The combined procedure, however, is associated with more postoperative against-the-rule astigmatism than ECCE/PCIOL alone (16,23,24). Combined trabeculectomy and ECCE through a clear corneal incision and trabeculectomy with phacoemulsification have similar postoperative visual results. One study finds that after clear cornea incision combined surgery, (10) 86% of eyes have 20/40 or better visual acuity, while another investigation finds that 87% of eyes undergoing combined trabeculectomy and phacoemulsification have 20/40 or better vision postoperatively, with no difference between 6 and 3 mm incisions (19).

Complications

Cataract extraction alone is associated with fewer complications than combined cataract and filtering surgery (1,9). Combined procedures can be complicated by choroidal effusion, suprachoroidal hemorrhage, shallow or flat anterior chamber, conjunctival wound leak, hyphema, cystoid macular edema, retinal detachment, IOL decentration, hypotony and postoperative visual field loss (1,9,11,16,19,22). Complications occurring with trabeculectomy or posterior lip sclerectomy followed by cataract extraction include malignant glaucoma, choroidal effusion, and flat anterior chamber (1). Cyclodialysis combined with cataract extraction is associated with hyphema in nearly 50% of cases (14).

Wound leak can be a significant and troubling complication associated with filtering surgery. One study found no difference in long term IOP control between limbus and fornix based conjunctival flaps in eyes undergoing ECCE/PCIOL combined with guarded sclerectomy (6). In this study, vitreous loss was much more frequent in eyes with limbus based flaps (18%) compared to fornix based flaps (0%).

CONCLUSIONS

Cataract and glaucoma are each common conditions that frequently coexist. Surgical techniques for management of visually significant cataract in glaucomatous eyes are constantly evolving. The increased utilization of phacoemulsification and phacosection, as well as the continued development of antimetabolites with which to modulate wound healing, continue to enhance the success of simultaneous management of cataract and glaucoma. Advances in technology and techniques provide the means by which ophthalmic surgeons may produce earlier restoration of good visual acuity and can more effectively control the IOP postoperatively.

References

1. Murchison JF, Shields MB: An evaluation of three surgical approaches for coexisting cataract and glaucoma. Ophthalmic Surg 1989;20:393–398.
2. Vu MT, Shields MB: The early postoperative pressure course in glaucoma patients following cataract surgery. Ophthalmic Surg 1988;19(7): 467–470.
3. Zaltas M, Schuman J, Shingleton B, et al: Cataract extraction following filtering surgery. Invest Ophthalmol Vis Sci 1994;35(ARVO suppl): 1420.
4. Savage JA, Thomas JV, Belcher CDI, et al: Extracapsular cataract extraction and posterior chamber intraocular lens implantation in glaucomatous eyes. Ophthalmology 1985;92:1506–1516.
5. Thomas JV, Simmons RJ, Belcher CDI: Argon laser trabeculoplasty in the presurgical glaucoma patient. Ophthalmology 1982;89:187–197.
6. Murchison JF, Jr, Shields MB: Limbal-based vs fornix-based conjunctival flaps in combined extracapsular cataract surgery and glaucoma filtering procedure. Am J Ophthalmol 1990;109(6):709–715.
7. Shields MB: Combined cataract extraction and guarded sclerectomy. Reevaluation in the extracapsular era. Ophthalmology 1986;93(3): 366–370.
8. Pasquale LR, Smith SG: Surgical outcome of phacoemulsification combined with the Pearce trabeculectomy in patients with glaucoma. J Cataract Refract Surg 1992;18(3):301–305.
9. Krupin T, Feitl ME, Bishop KI: Postoperative intraocular pressure rise in open-angle glaucoma patients after cataract or combined cataract-filtration surgery. Ophthalmology 1989;96:579–584.
10. Longstaff S, Wormald RPL, Mazover A, et al: Glaucoma triple procedure: Efficacy of intraocular pressure control and visual outcome. Ophthalmic Surg 1990;21:786–793.
11. Williamson TH, Bacon AS, Flanagan DW, et al. Combined extracapsular cataract extraction and trabeculectomy using a separated corneal section. Eye 1989;3:547–552.
12. Terry S: Combined no-stitch phacoemulsification cataract extraction with foldable silicone intraocular implant and holmium laser sclerostomy followed by 5-FU injections. Ophthalmic Surg 1992;23:218–219.

13. Kendrick RM, Kollarits CR: Combined cataract-glaucoma surgery using the THC:YAG (holmium) laser ab interno without gonioscopy. Ophthalmic Surg 1992;23(10):697–699.
14. Montgomery D, Gills JP: Extracapsular cataract extraction, lens implantation and cyclodialysis. Ophthalmic Surg 1988;11:343–347.
15. Shields MB, Simmons RJ: Combined cyclodialysis and cataract extraction. Ophthalmic Surg 1976;7(2):62–73.
16. McCartney DL, Memmen JE, Start WJ, et al: The efficacy and safety of combined trabeculectomy, cataract extraction, and intraocular lens implantation. Ophthalmology 1988;95:754–763.
17. Naveh N, Kottas R, Glovinsky J, et al: The long-term effect on intraocular pressure of a procedure combining trabeculectomy and cataract surgery, as compared with trabeculectomy alone. Ophthalmic Surg 1990; 21:339–345.
18. Wedrich A, Menapace R, Radax U, et al: Combined small-incision surgery and trabeculectomy—technique and results. Int Ophthalmol 1992; 16:409–414.
19. Lyle WA, Jin JC: Comparison of a 3- and 6-mm incision in combined phacoemulsification and trabeculectomy. Am J Ophthalmol 1991;111: 189–196.
20. Shingleton BJ, Jacobson LM, Kuperwaser MC: Comparison of combined cataract and glaucoma surgery by the planned extracapsular and phacoemulsification techniques [personal communication].
21. Joos KM, Bueche MJ, Palmberg PF, et al: One-year follow-up results of combined mitomycin C, trabeculectomy and extracapsular cataract extraction. Ophthalmology 1995;102:76–83.
22. Zacharia P, Zaltas M, Schuman J: Combined phacoemulsification and trabeculectomy with mitomycin C. Invest Ophthalmol Vis Sci 1994; 35(ARVO suppl):1431.
23. Choplin NT, Monroe JF: Surgically-induced astigmatism in combined ECCE with filtering procedures compared to ECCE alone. Ophthalmic Surg 1992;23:81–84.
24. Fusco R, Guacci P, Ambrosio G, et al: Trabeculectomy and extracapsular cataract extraction with posterior chamber lens implantation: A long term study. Documenta Ophthalmol 1990;74:303–308.

Aqueous Shunting Procedures

65

Frederic J. Gross

HISTORY

Aqueous shunting procedures were introduced by Molteno in 1968 to treat refractory glaucomas (1). In the initial design, Molteno used an 8.5 mm acrylic plate attached to an acrylic tube which he hoped would allow the formation of a bleb, with free communication to the anterior chamber, which could not shrink to an area less than that of the plate. Molteno found that this device was successful in controlling intraocular pressure (IOP) in many patients who were otherwise poor surgical candidates. However, problems related to early postoperative hypotony from overfiltration and late IOP increases resulting from fibrous encapsulation of the filtering bleb limited the usefulness of this procedure. Over the past twenty-five years, design modifications and improvements in surgical technique have led to greater success and lower complication rates using the Molteno implant. In addition, other aqueous shunting devices have been introduced which offer unique features designed to facilitate implantation, improve IOP control, and reduce the acute postoperative hypotony associated with implant procedures.

PATIENT SELECTION

Aqueous shunting procedures are typically reserved for patients with severe uncontrolled glaucoma who have failed previous glaucoma surgery (Table 65.1). In addition, they appear to be advantageous as a primary procedure in patients with neovascular glaucoma (2,3). Recent studies suggest an increasing role for seton procedures in the management of advanced congenital and juvenile glaucoma, traumatic glaucoma, aphakic and pseudophakic glaucoma, post-keratoplasty glaucoma, and other secondary glaucomas (4,5,6). In eyes with useful remaining vision, setons may be preferable to cyclodestructive procedures which are associated with a high rate of visual loss and phthisis bulbi.

DIFFERENT IMPLANT DESIGNS (Fig. 65.1)

Molteno Implant

The Molteno implant consists of a silicone tube with internal diameter of 0.63 mm connected to a rigid polypropylene plate which is 13 mm in diameter (surface area: 270 mm)(Fig. 65.1A). Single or double plate implants (Fig. 65.1B) are available. A dual-chamber single-plate implant which incorporates a pressure ridge on the upper surface of the episcleral plate has been introduced in an effort to reduce immediate postoperative hypotony and its related complications.

Anterior Chamber Tube to Encircling Band (ACTEB)

The ACTEB implant consists of a silastic tube with internal diameter of 0.64 mm connected to a #20 band 360 degrees in length (surface area: 350–450 mm). The band is placed under three or four rectus muscles creating a reservoir for aqueous drainage.

Ahmed Glaucoma Valve

The Ahmed Glaucoma Valve consists of a silastic tube which is connected to an elliptical polypropylene body and plate with an anterior surface area of 184 mm (13 mm by 16 mm) (Fig. 65.1C). The valve body contains a pressure sensitive membrane valve which consists of two opposed silastic sheets which separate to allow aqueous flow at an intraocular pressure of between 8–12 mm Hg.

Baerveldt Implant

The Baerveldt implant consists of a silicone tube with an internal diameter of 0.3 mm connected to a Barium-impregnated plate which is 1 mm thick (Fig. 65.1D). The implant plates are made with surfaces areas of 200 mm (20 × 13 mm), 350 mm (32 × 14 mm) and 500 mm (36 × 17.5).

Krupin Valve with Disc

The Krupin Valve with Disc consists of a silastic tube with an internal diameter of 0.38 mm connected to an oval silicone plate measuring 13 mm × 18 mm which is 1.75 mm thick (Fig. 65.1E). The tube incorporates a unidirectional and pressure sensitive slit valve (opening pressure 11 mm Hg; closing pressure 9 mm Hg) which serves to maintain the anterior chamber depth and IOP in the immediate post-operative period.

SURGICAL TECHNIQUE

Implantation of aqueous shunting devices requires careful attention to detail at every step of the procedure to improve

Table 65.1
Patient Selection for Glaucoma Implant Surgery

Primary Procedure
Patients with neovascular glaucoma
Secondary Procedure: Usually after failed anti-metabolite filter
Aphakic/pseudophakic glaucoma
Traumatic glaucoma
Uveitic glaucoma
Congenital/juvenile glaucoma
Other secondary glaucomas

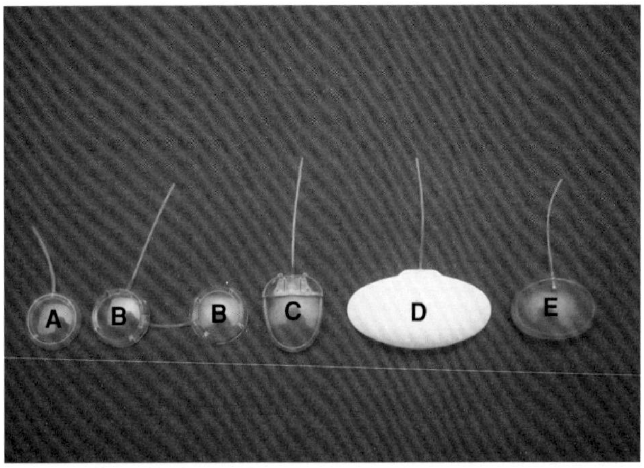

Figure 65.1. (A) Single plate Molteno implant, (B) double plate Molteno implant, (C) Ahmed Glaucoma Valve, (D) Baerveldt implant, (E) and Krupin Valve with Disc.

Table 65.2
Insertion of Implants

100 degree peritomy with radial relaxing incision
Sub-Tenon's dissection of muscle free quadrant
Attachment of plate to sclera 8–10 mm posterior to limbus
Entry into anterior chamber with 23 gauge needle
Paracentesis and fill anterior chamber (AC) with viscoelastic
Cut tube with anterior bevel to allow 2–3 mm of tube in AC
Insert tube into AC and examine position (avoid tube-cornea touch)
Fashion 6 × 6 mm scleral graft
Attach graft at limbal edge to cover tube insertion site
Thin limbal edge of scleral graft to avoid Dellen formation
Close conjunctiva with absorbable suture

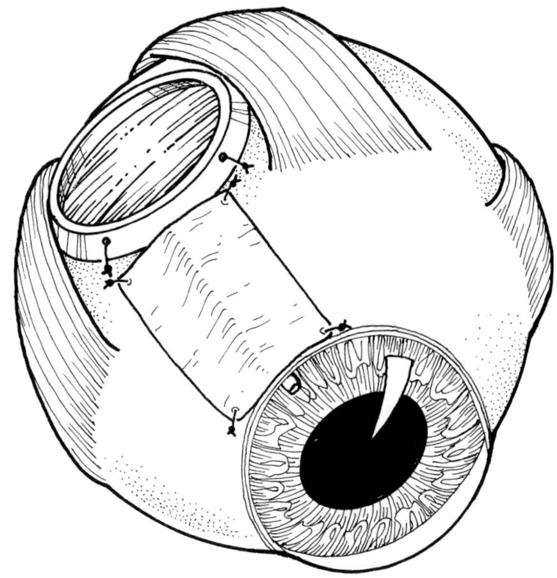

Figure 65.2. Proper placement of the implant plate in a muscle free quadrant with the leading edge 10 mm posterior to the limbus.

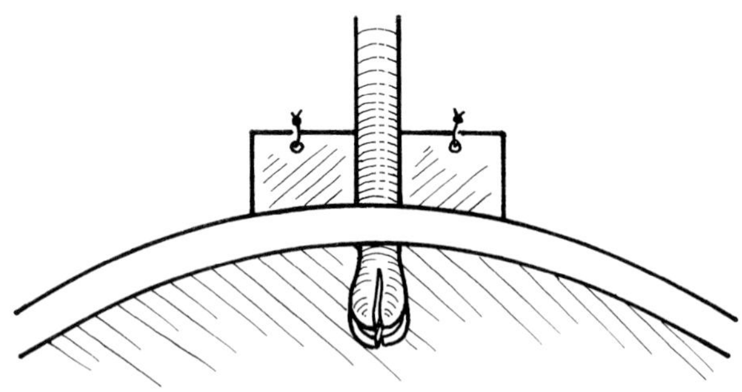

Figure 65.3. Plate sutured to sclera using 5-0 to 8-0 nonabsorbable suture.

results and minimize post-operative complications (Table 65.2). Surgery can usually be performed under local anesthesia with a retrobulbar or peribulbar block. For a one-plate implant, a fornix-based or limbus-based conjunctival incision is created extending for 90 to 110 degrees centered between two rectus muscles. Implantation of the plate is slightly easier with a fornix-based flap; however, the conjunctival closure is more involved. If a fornix-based flap is created, one or two radial relaxing incisions are usually required to allow adequate exposure for insertion of the plate. With the conjunctiva and Tenons retracted away from the globe to expose bare sclera, the implant is positioned between two rectus muscles so that the anterior edge is approximately 8 to 10 mm posterior to the limbus (Fig. 65.2). With larger and oval shaped implants (Krupin, Baerveldt), the implant is inserted with its long axis directed toward the apex of the orbit and then rotated horizontally so that the tube points directly toward the anterior chamber. If a two plate implant is used, one plate is positioned in each of two quadrants. The tube connecting the two plates may be passed under or over the intervening rectus muscle.

Once the implant has been appropriately positioned, each plate is secured to the globe with two non-absorbable sutures (5-0 to 8-0) (Figs. 65.2 and 65.3). Secure attachment to the underlying sclera is essential to prevent anterior to posterior or lateral migration of the implant during the post-operative period. **Inadequate scleral fixation may also lead to retraction of the tube from the anterior chamber or expulsion of the entire plate from the subconjunctival space.**

After the plate is attached to the globe, the tube is laid across the cornea and cut with a sharp scissors to create a beveled edge with the opening toward the cornea. **The tube should extend approximately 2.5 to 3 mm into the anterior chamber in order to minimize the risk of tube cornea touch or retraction out of the anterior chamber.** A 23-gauge needle is used to create a track into the anterior chamber just anterior and parallel to the iris through which the tube is inserted (Fig. 65.4). Occasionally insertion of the tube through the scleral track is difficult. A well-beveled tube end (30 to 45 degrees, bevel up) simplifies this procedure; however, a metallic insertion forceps which surrounds the distal end of the tube is available to facilitate this maneuver (Fig. 65.5). After the tube has been inserted into the anterior chamber, its position is checked carefully to insure that there is no tube-cornea touch or iris incarceration. If the tube is malpositioned a new entry track should be created 2 mm to the side of the original track through which the tube should be reinserted. If the original entry site is leaking, the scleral opening should be sutured closed to avoid postoperative overfiltration and hypotony. If a two stage procedure is planned, the tube is sutured to the sclera and covered with Tenons and conjunctiva. Five to six weeks later, the conjunctiva is opened to expose the tube which is then inserted into the anterior chamber as previously described.

A 6 mm by 6 mm scleral patch graft is then prepared from banked sclera. The thinnest available piece of sclera should be chosen since it will be easier to handle and secure to the globe. The graft is positioned to overly the tube insertion site into the anterior chamber and the limbal edge is thinned in order to avoid an overhanging bleb which can lead to Dellen formation (Fig. 65.6). The scleral graft may be secured to the globe using two vertical mattress sutures placed on either side of the tube. Alternatively, four interrupted 8-0 nylon sutures may be placed

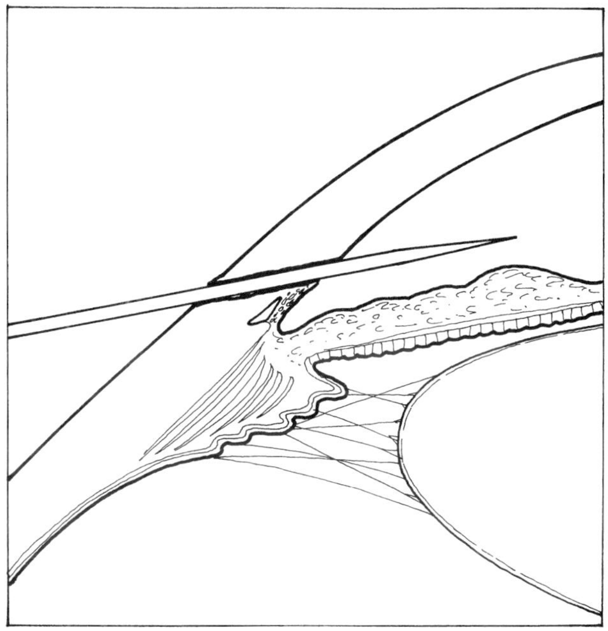

Figure 65.4. Entry into the anterior chamber with a 23-gauge needle should create an entry track just anterior and parallel to the iris plane.

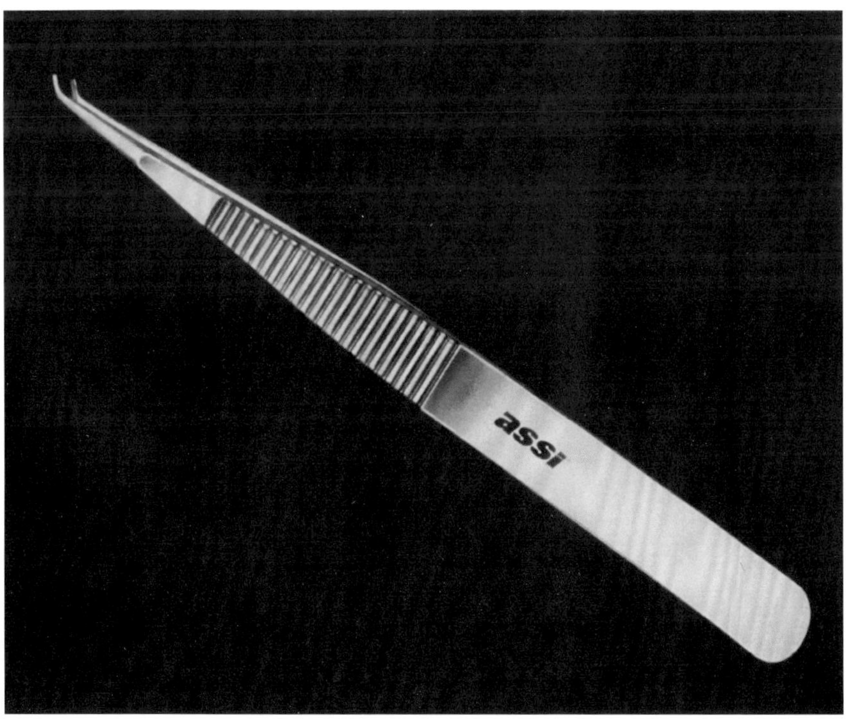

Figure 65.5. Insertion forceps may aid in the placement of the shunt tube into the anterior chamber.

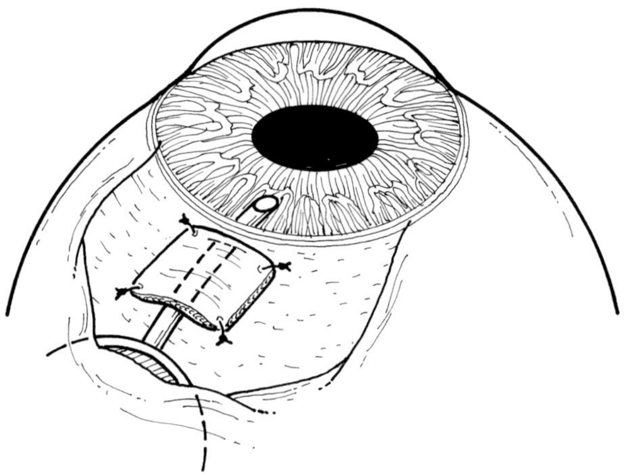

Figure 65.6. Placement of the 6 mm × 6 mm scleral graft over the tube entry site just posterior to the limbus.

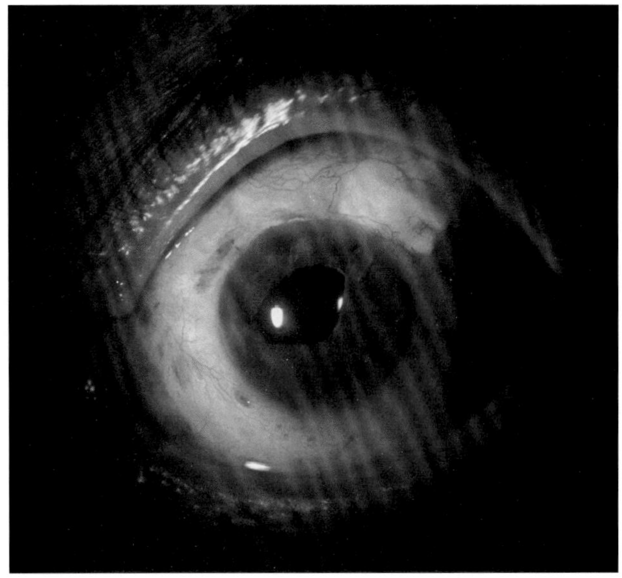

Figure 65.7. Well positioned implant in the superotemporal quadrant.

at the corners of the graft. All suture ends should be buried beneath the scleral graft to prevent them from later eroding through the conjunctiva.

Recently some surgeons have begun to use banked dura to cover the tube because of its greater availability, reduced cost, and easier handling in comparison to preserved donor sclera.

After the graft has been placed, the conjunctiva and Tenons are pulled over the plate, tube, and graft and secured into place with 8-0 Vicryl sutures. Prior to conjunctival closure, the limbal margin of the cornea may be cauterized in order to remove the epithelium and provide a bed to facilitate the attachment of the conjunctiva during the healing process. Wing sutures at both ends of the peritomy are recommended to approximate the conjunctiva at the limbus. A locked running Vicryl suture is useful in closing the radial relaxing incision.

At the end of the operation, the eye should be inspected to assure that the implant plate, scleral graft, and intraocular portion of the tube are in good position (Fig. 65.7). **If a valved implant is used, balanced salt solution should be injected through the paracentesis track in order to confirm that the implant is functioning.** Fluorescein drops can be used to inspect the conjunctiva for leaks. Any buttonholes which are found in the conjunctiva should be closed with 9-0 Vicryl suture on a vascular needle in a water tight fashion. At the conclusion of the procedure, atropine sulfate 1% drops are instilled topically and the surgeon's preferred antibiotic and steroid regimen is administered.

POSTOPERATIVE COURSE

Following glaucoma implant surgery, the IOP follows a typical course. During the early postoperative period (one to two weeks), the IOP is typically low which may lead to shallowing of the anterior chamber, choroidal effusions, and other complications of hypotony. This is followed by a period of elevated IOP (hypertensive phase) which may last from two to seven weeks corresponding to the development of fibrous encapsulation around the plate. During the hypertensive phase, digital massage and anti-glaucoma medications may be needed to control the IOP. The hypertensive phase is followed by a gradual decline in IOP over the ensuing weeks to months providing long term IOP reduction. The duration and magnitude of the early postoperative hypotony and hypertensive phases are influenced by the surgical technique and implant selected as well as the use of adjunctive anti-metabolites.

MODIFICATIONS TO PREVENT HYPOTONY

Internal Tube Occlusion (stent)

Aqueous drainage through a seton can be regulated in the early postoperative period by passing a 3-0 or 4-0 Prolene suture through the lumen of the implant tube (7,8). The stent suture is brought out through the tube, over the implant plate, and placed with its free end in an adjacent sub-conjunctival quadrant (Fig. 65.8). One to two weeks after the initial operation, the stent suture is removed at the slit lamp under local anesthesia allowing the free flow of aqueous into the fibrous bleb which has formed around the implant plate. Although this technique is effective in preventing early post-operative hypotony, immediate post-operative IOP elevations from tube occlusion may make early suture removal necessary, increasing the risk of hypotony, shallow chamber, and related complications.

External Tube Occlusion (Ligature)

The flow of aqueous through a seton can be restricted by placing a suture ligature around the external aspect of the tube (7,9). The external occlusion may be accomplished

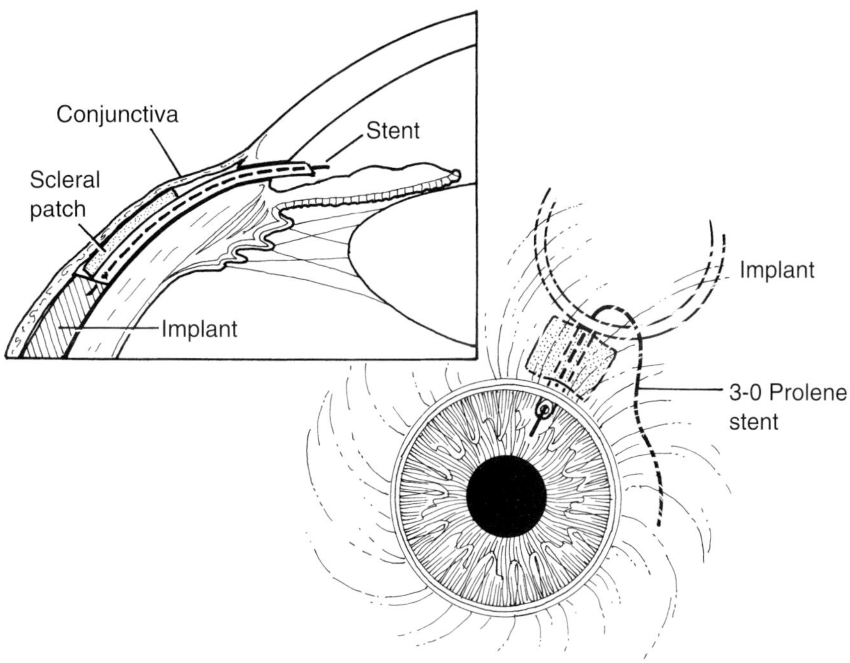

Figure 65.8. Placement of a stent suture through the tube reduces the risk of post-operative hypotony when using non-valved implants.

using a non-absorbable 7-0 suture with a releasable knot or a 7-0 or 8-0 absorbable Vicryl suture tied around the tube. Alternatively, a 9-0 nylon suture may be used to ligate the tube inside the anterior chamber allowing later suture lysis with the argon laser. The remnant of the 9-0 suture remains in the anterior chamber. Similar to an internal occluding suture, release of an external ligating suture is usually performed at one to two weeks postoperatively which allows time for a fibrous bleb to form around the plate providing resistance to aqueous flow when the suture is released. If a Vicryl suture ligature is used, IOP control may continue to be difficult for 3–4 weeks until the Vicryl suture dissolves. Due to this prolonged delay before the IOP is reduced, this technique is poorly suited for patients with exceedingly high pressures during the preoperative period. Attempts to tie the ligature at different tensions to create a titrated aqueous flow rate are unpredictable and may result in under- or overfiltration.

Two Stage Procedure

In order to prevent postoperative hypotony, a shunt procedure may be performed in two stages. In the first stage of the procedure, the plate is attached to the globe and the tube is left in the subconjunctival space without entering the eye. Four to six weeks later after a capsule has formed around the implant, the conjunctiva is opened and the tube is inserted into the anterior chamber completing the procedure. A major disadvantage of this procedure is that it does not reduce IOP until the second stage is complete making it poorly suited for eyes with extremely high IOP in the preoperative period. Combining the first stage of the operation with a trabeculectomy in an adjacent quadrant allows for immediate IOP control and provides a time interval for plate encapsulation. In this procedure, the second stage of the valve is performed when the trabeculectomy fails and IOP increases.

Device Modifications

Hypotony may also be prevented by using devices with design modifications to prevent postoperative hypotony. **The Krupin Valve with Disc and Ahmed Glaucoma Valve incorporate pressure sensitive valves which regulate the flow of aqueous and maintain anterior chamber depth in the early postoperative period** (10). Results of studies using this device have been encouraging, demonstrating less early postoperative hypotony and chamber collapse than with unregulated devices. The dual chamber Molteno incorporates a pressure ridge on the upper surface of the episcleral plate which is designed to serve as a pressure-sensitive valve in the early post-operative period. Clinical experience with this device also suggests that it produces less anterior chamber shallowing and hypotony than the standard Molteno implant.

SITE OF IMPLANTATION

With the exception of the two plate Molteno implant, most glaucoma implants are placed in a single muscle-free quadrant. **Whenever possible, single plate implants should be placed in the supero-temporal quadrant.** This area provides the easiest access for the surgeon to implant the plate and is least likely to produce motility disturbances. Implantation of large plate aqueous shunts in the superonasal quadrant have been associated with a Brown's superior oblique tendon syndrome (11). Substantial hypertropias and limitations of down gaze have been reported with inferior implantation of two-plate Moltenos and the Krupin Valve with Disc (12). If severe conjunctival scarring necessitates the placement of an inferior or superonasal shunt, the possibility of ocular motility disturbance and diplopia should be discussed with the patient. Use of a smaller plate implant (Molteno or Baerveldt) may be less likely to cause a muscle imbalance; however, the risk of strabismus must be weighed against the better IOP control which is often achieved with a larger or multiple plate implant.

ADJUNCTIVE MEDICAL THERAPY

Molteno was the first to suggest that the success rate of aqueous shunting procedures could be improved by the addition of anti-fibrosis therapy (1). Molteno used a combination of epinephrine, atropine, topical steroids, oral steroids and colchicine to reduce postoperative scarring and bleb fibrosis in an attempt to increase the success rate of his procedure. Because of the high frequency of systemic side-effects associated with this regimen, it is rarely used today.

The success of anti-metabolites in improving the success of high risk glaucoma procedures has led to considerable interest in the use of these agents in seton procedures. Early studies have indicated that patients receiving mitomycin-C at the time of a seton procedure have lower final IOPs, require fewer post-operative medications, and have less pronounced hypertensive phases; however, the duration of the post-operative hypotensive phase is prolonged and is associated with an increase in choroidal effusions, flat anterior chambers, and other post-operative complications (13). Further research is required to determine the exact role of anti-metabolites in aqueous shunting procedures. At the current time, they should be used judiciously in glaucoma implant surgery.

RESULTS

Aqueous shunting procedures are effective in controlling IOP in eyes which have failed prior surgery or have a poor prognosis for standard filtration surgery (3,4,5,14,15,16). At two years of follow-up most studies indicated overall success rates of seton procedures from 50 to 80% with the outcome depending on the type of glaucoma present and type of implant selected. Several studies have indicated that devices with larger surface areas provide better IOP control (10,15,16). For example, the double-plate Molteno implant has been shown to produce better long-term IOP control and was associated with a less pronounced hypertensive phase than a single plate Molteno implant (15). Similarly, in a study comparing the results of the 350 and 500 mm Baerveldt implants, patients who received the larger implant required significantly fewer post-operative medications to maintain an adequate IOP (16). Both the Krupin Valve with Disc and Baerveldt implants which have large surface area plates appear to provide equivalent IOP control to a two-plate Molteno implant while allowing implantation in a single quadrant. As an isolated procedure, larger surface area implants are associated with an increased risk of suprachoroidal hemorrhage or effusion, flat anterior chambers, and corneal decompensation (15); however, in the long-term, their complication rate compares favorably to the overall complication rate in patients treated with single-plate implants who are more likely to require subsequent glaucoma procedures.

After glaucoma implant surgery, visual acuity is maintained within one line of preoperative acuity in 60 to 80% of patients at two year follow-up (10,15). Even in patients with neovascular glaucoma, IOP control is usually adequate to keep the eye comfortable and preserve the remaining vision (3). The visual outcome of patients with neovascular glaucoma is primarily determined by underlying disease process with diabetic patients doing significantly better than patients with a central retinal vein occlusion (3). In eyes with neovascular glaucoma and diabetic vitreous hemorrhage, vision may be stabilized or in certain cases improved by timely intervention with a combination of vitreo-retinal surgery, endolaser, and glaucoma shunt implant surgery.

COMPLICATIONS

Aqueous shunting procedures are associated with a significant risk of postoperative complications. The surgeon should be aware of the common complications and their management before undertaking these procedures. Careful attention to plate and tube placement, use of an

Table 65.3
Avoiding Complications with Glaucoma Implant Procedures

Complication	Preventive Step
Hypotony, shallow chamber	Tube stent Ligate tube Use valved implant
Migration or expulsion	Avoid anterior plate placement Attach plate with 5–0 to 8–0 nonabsorbable suture
Conjunctival melts	Use scleral graft to cover tube for 6 mm from limbus Avoid buttonholes Bury all suture knots
Corneal edema	Avoid tube-cornea touch Prevent hypotony and flat AC
Diplopia	Avoid inferior placement Avoid superonasal placement Avoid muscle/plate contact
Elevated IOP	Check for tube occlusion Needle bleb Subconjunctival 5-FU

appropriately fashioned scleral graft, careful conjunctival closure, and use of a hypotony preventing surgical modification or implant will minimize these problems (Table 65.3). The early postoperative complications of aqueous shunt procedures are similar to other filtration procedures including flat chambers, hypotony, and suprachoroidal hemorrhage (1,2,15,16) (Table 65.4). Hyphema is a relatively common complication following procedures performed on eyes with neovascular glaucoma. However, the hyphema is typically small and clears spontaneously with no adverse effect on the outcome of surgery (Fig. 65.9). Tube block from blood, vitreous, fibrin, or iris incarceration in the early post-operative period can occasionally be treated with laser; however, in some instances, a return trip to the operating room to clear the tube end may be required (Table 65.5).

Endophthalmitis and intra-operative scleral perforation are rare but serious complications of seton procedures which require rapid identification and treatment to preserve the remaining vision. Intermediate and long-term complications of aqueous shunting procedures include conjunctival melting, tube migration, plate migration, tube-cornea touch, corneal decompensation, and retinal detachment. **Conjunctival melting usually occurs near the limbus overlying the tube and may be related to poor graft preparation or placement**; however, even without these factors, in some cases melting of the conjunctiva and scleral patch graft occur resulting in tube exposure (Fig. 65.10). Replacement of the scleral graft and mobilization of a conjunctival sliding graft may be useful in repairing these defects. Migration or expulsion of the plate most commonly results from placement of the plate too anteriorly. Poor tube placement with lens–cornea touch or persistent flat chamber from

Table 65.4
Treatment of Early Postoperative Hypotony

Most early postoperative hypotony is self-limited and will resolve spontaneously without treatment. However, intervention is warranted when there is lens-cornea touch or when there is evidence that the hypotony will be prolonged if no intervention is made.
Identify and repair any bleb leaks which result in significant hypotony associated with a flat chamber. A small leak may be observed if the chamber is adequately maintained allowing time for spontaneous closure.
Deepen the chamber with viscoelastic through the paracentesis if there is lens-cornea touch. This procedure can be repeated daily until the IOP begins to rise and the chamber stabilizes (usually at the end of week two).
Drain large choroidals if there is lens-cornea touch. This will deepen the chamber and expedite the return to a normal IOP.

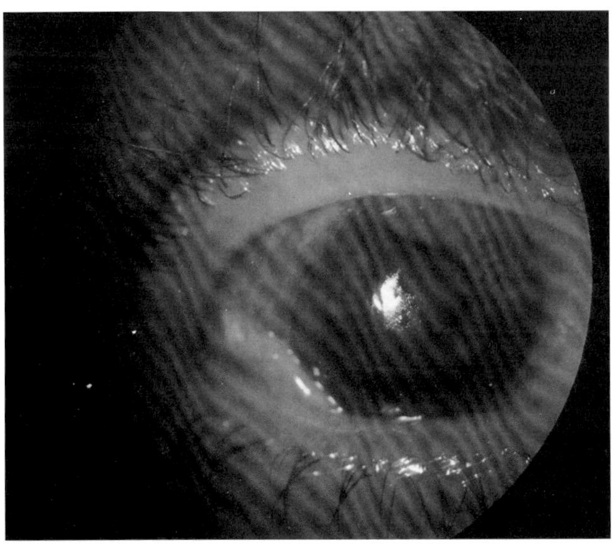

Figure 65.9. Hyphema following shunt placement in an eye with neovascular glaucoma.

Table 65.5
Treatment of Early PostOperative Hypertension

Observation for first 48 hours if not severe. The IOP will frequently come down spontaneously as viscoelastic, blood, fibrin, or other occlusive material is cleared from the anterior chamber.
If the IOP is unacceptably high, the addition of digital massage or anti-glaucomatous medications may be useful. This will allow time for an absorbable suture ligature to dissolve or for bleb encapsulation to occur allowing removal of the tube occluding (stent) suture.
Remove the occluding (stent) suture. If this is done during the first week, the chance of severe hypotony, shallow chamber, and related complications is increased.
If the end of the tube is occluded by vitreous, iris, or fibrin, the Nd:Yag laser may be used to clear the obstruction. In some cases, a return trip to the operating room may be necessary. This is particularly common if there is a large anterior hyphema in the early post-operative period which is associated with significant IOP elevation.

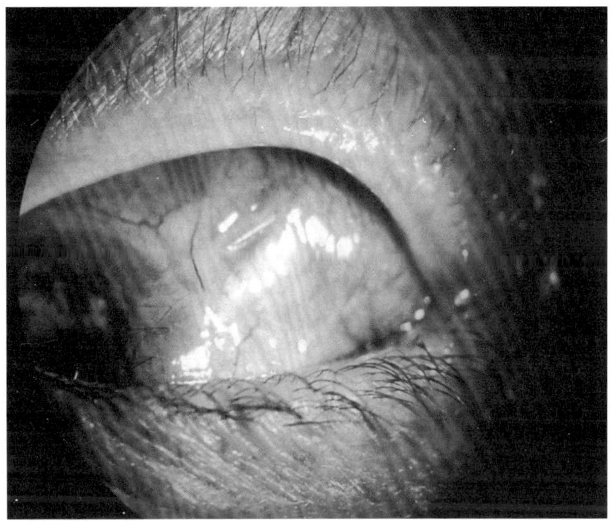

Figure 65.10. Conjunctival melt several months following an uncomplicated shunting procedure. Note exposed tube.

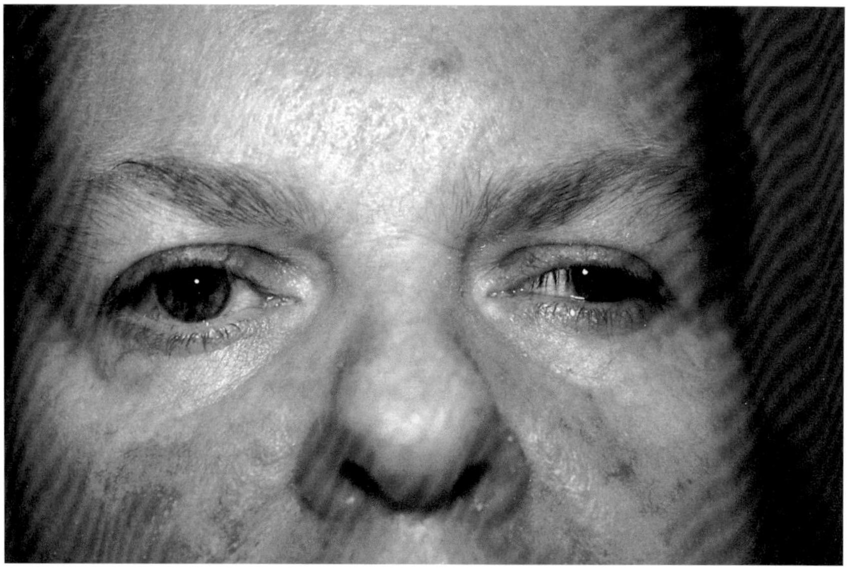

Figure 65.11. Exotropia following superotemporal placement of a shunt in the left eye.

hypotony may result in corneal edema. **In eyes which have undergone penetrating keratoplasty, the risk of graft failure in eyes which develop a flat chamber post-operatively is high** (17–20). The use of valved and stented implants which better maintain the anterior chamber depth have reduced this complication to an acceptable level. If the scleral graft is too thick or the plate is too anterior, an overhanging bleb may be created resulting in chronic Dellen formation and ocular irritation. This complication is best prevented by appropriate plate and graft placement during surgery.

Extraocular muscle imbalance (Fig. 65.11) with devastating diplopia may also occur and is particularly common in cases of inferior valve placement. This complication appears to be more common in valves with larger diameter plates which impinge on the adjacent rectus muscles.

References

1. Molteno ACB: New implant for drainage in glaucoma: clinical trial. Br J Ophthalmol 1979;53:606–615.
2. Brown RD, Cairns JE: Experience with the Molteno long tube implant. Trans Ophthalmol Soc UK 1983;103:297–312.
3. Mermoud A, Salmon JF, Alexander P, et al: Molteno tube implantation for neovascular glaucoma: long term results and factors influencing outcome. Ophthalmology 1993;100:897–902.
4. Munoz M, Tomey KF, Traverso C, et al: Clinical experience with the Molteno implant in advanced infantile glaucoma. J Ped Ophthalmol Strabismus 1991;28:68–72.
5. Beebe WE, Starita RJ, Fellman RL: The use of the Molteno implant and anterior chamber tube shunt to encircling band for the treatment of glaucoma in keratoplasty patients. Ophthalmology 1990;97:1414–22.
6. Hill RA, Nguyen QH, Baerveldt G, et al: Trabeculectomy and Molteno implantation for glaucomas associated with uveitis. Ophthalmology 1993;100:903–908.
7. Hoare Nairne JE, Sherwood D, Jacob JSH, et al: Single stage insertion of the Molteno tube for glaucoma and modifications to reduce postoperative hypotony. Br J Ophthalmol 1988;72:846–851.
8. Egbert PR, Lieberman MF: Internal suture occlusion of the Molteno glaucoma implant for the prevention of postoperative hypotony. Ophthalmic Surg 1989;20:53–56.
9. El-Sayyad F, El-Maghraby A, Helal M, et al: The use of releasable sutures in Molteno glaucoma implant procedures to reduce postoperative hypotony. Ophthalmic Surg 1991;22:82–84.
10. Krupin Eye Valve Filtering Surgery Study Group: Krupin Eye Valve with Disc for filtration surgery. Ophthalmology 1994;101:651–658.
11. Ball SF, Ellis GS, Herrington RG, et al: Browns superior oblique tendon syndrome after Baerveldt implant. Arch Ophthalmol 1992;110:1368.
12. Christman LM, Wilson ME: Motility disturbances after Molteno implants. J Ped Ophthalmol Strabismus 1992;29:44–48.
13. Gross FJ: Six month success of Krupin Valve with and without Mitomycin-C in the treatment of complicated glaucomas. Invest Ophthalmol Vis Sci 1994 (Suppl);35:1422.
14. Freedman J: Clinical Experience with the Molteno dual-chamber single-plate implant. Ophthalmic Surg 1992;23:238–241.
15. Heuer DK, Lloyd MA, Abrams DA, et al: Which is better? One or two? A randomized clinical trial of single-plate versus double-plate Molteno implantation for glaucomas in aphakia and pseudophakia. Ophthalmology 1992;99:1512–1519.
16. Lloyd MA, Baerveldt G, Fellenbaum PS, et al: Intermediate-term results of randomized clinical trial of the 350 versus 500 mm Baerveldt Implant. Ophthalmology 1994;101:1456–1464.
17. Sherwood MB, Smith MF, Driebe WT Jr., et al: Drainage tube implants in the treatment of glaucoma following penetrating keratoplasty. Ophthalmic Surg 1993;24(3):185–189.
18. Beebe WE, Starita RJ, Fellman RL, et al: The use of Molteno implant and anterior chamber tube shunt to encircling band for the treatment of glaucoma in keratoplasty patients. Ophthalmology 1990;97(11):1414–1422.
19. McDonell PJ, Robin JB, Schanzlin DJ, et al: Molteno implant for control of glaucoma in eyes after penetrating keratoplasty. Ophthalmology 1988;95(3):364–369.
20. Lloyd MA, Sedlak T, Heuer DK, et al: Clinical experience with the single-plate Molteno implant in complicated glaucomas. Update of a pilot study. Ophthalmology 1992;99(5):679–687.

Cyclodialysis

66

David L. Epstein

INTRODUCTION

Cyclodialysis (1) performed in an eye rendered previously aphakic or as part of a combined intracapsular cataract operation (2), used to be a frequently performed glaucoma procedure. Although the success was only in the 30–40% range, it was a fairly quick procedure with a rapid postoperative recovery. It has fallen into disuse with the advancement in techniques of combined cataract/filtration surgery (Chapter 64), but perhaps it deserves further evaluation in pseudophakic eyes with good central visual acuity, that are not suitable for filtration surgery, prior to consideration of a laser ciliodestructive procedure (which has some risk of inducing cystoid macular edema and decreased central acuity). Some have proposed combination surgery of cyclodialysis with extracapsular cataract surgery (3).

The mechanism of intraocular pressure (IOP) lowering with cyclodialysis to likely due to increased outflow into the nonconventional outflow pathway (4,5) via the surgically created cleft, as has previously been described (Chapters 2 and 3), although some have thought that the procedure also acts to decrease the rate of aqueous humor formation (6). The technique of the surgical procedure will be described later in this chapter.

SYNDROME OF SUDDEN CLOSURE OF A CYCLODIALYSIS CLEFT

One of the unfortunate complications that sometimes occurred in some of the "successes" with the cyclodialysis surgical procedure was ocular hypotony (7). But in addition, what was occasionally also observed was **a syndrome of a sudden "high IOP" if the cyclodialysis cleft should suddenly close.** Often the IOP observed in this syndrome would far exceed the preoperative IOP levels for a day or so. The mechanism for this phenomenon was believed to involve the fact that when the cyclodialysis cleft was functioning, aqueous humor was flowing not into the trabecular meshwork, but into the cleft. When the cleft closed, the trabecular meshwork, having been previously underperfused and underutilized, temporarily offered substantially more resistance to aqueous outflow than prior to surgery. It is noteworthy that an early explanation of this phenomenon was made by Hans Goldmann (8). **There have been histological studies of experimentally produced "hypoperfusion" of the trabecular meshwork, which demonstrated increased proteinaceous material extracellularly in the outflow pathway**, as well as other structural changes (9). Such an acute "underperfusion syndrome" of the trabecular meshwork theoretically might also occur after filtration surgery, if the fistula were to suddenly close due to iris incarceration or blood, for example. Clinically, this sudden cleft closure syndrome lasted only 1–2 days, after which there was return to baseline glaucoma status (likely continued poor control).

Patients who were postoperative from cyclodialysis procedures would routinely be maintained on miotics indefinitely, in order to cause ciliary muscle contraction, and therefore both to pull the ciliary body further away from the separated scleral spur and to narrow the ciliary body ring (Chapter 29) and thus expand the potential fluid space beneath the sclera. Sometimes sympathomimetic drugs such as phenylephrine were used in addition to miotics to contract the iris dilator muscle, since it was felt that this action might, by increasing iris tone, act with co-existing cholinergic miotics to move the iris away from the cleft. Also sympathomimetic drugs may cause weak contraction of the ciliary muscle (10).

A common situation that precipitated the sudden cleft closure syndrome was when the patient was dilated for fundoscopy with a cycloplegic drug. Presumably, the cycloplegic drug caused relaxation of ciliary muscle tone and dilatation of the ciliary body ring (Chapter 29), and this outward movement of the ciliary body could close the space between the ciliary body and sclera, which represented the cleft.

INADVERTENT CYCLODIALYSIS CLEFTS

Nowadays one encounters cyclodialysis clefts mostly as inadvertent complications, resulting from trauma (Chapter 43) or after anterior segment surgery (11–16). Sometimes some of the newer scleral tunneling techniques (16) in cataract surgery may inadvertently cause this separation of the ciliary body from the scleral wall.

How should such inadvertent cyclodialyses be treated? Building upon what we have learned from the above, a trial of cycloplegics, initially short acting agents, but later daily atropine or scopolamine, should be attempted first. This failing, the cleft, if small, may be therapeutically closed sometimes by applying argon laser gonioplasty type applications (Chapters 51 and 60) to the visible scleral

"MYSTERY" DIAGNOSIS

David L. Epstein

One of us (DLE) was once presented with the following case: A patient had just undergone trabeculectomy, performed elsewhere, for uncontrolled IOP in the 20s. On the first postoperative day, the IOP was 6, but there was no obvious bleb. On day 2, the IOP had suddenly increased to 60 mm Hg, which was much higher than it ever had been before. The angle was described as being open. One drop of 1% pilocarpine was placed in the eye, and the IOP decreased to 9 mm Hg.

This patient proved to have an inadvertent cyclodialysis cleft as a result of the "trabeculectomy," but it is important for the reader to realize that when trabeculectomy was first introduced as a surgical technique, it was common to extend the sclerectomy posteriorly and excise the scleral spur (1). If one reads the early literature after the development of the procedure of "trabeculectomy," there is often much confusion about the absence of blebs despite good IOP results in many patients (we believe now that this was likely due to having produced a cyclodialysis rather than a filter in such patients; maybe cyclodialysis is not such a bad operation after all!). Trabeculectomy originally was conceptualized to remove "diseased" trabecular meshwork and allow aqueous humor to flow into the cut ends of Schlemm's canal (2). This does not, in fact, happen as the cut ends of the canal collapse (3). Regardless, there would be little potential anyway for resulting circumferential flow of aqueous humor in Schlemm's canal, as the outflow pathway functions in a segmental manner (4,5) (Chapter 3). Thus, this was not the first, nor likely the last time, that a procedure designed to work by one mechanism, actually works by another! Trabeculectomy functions really as a guarded filtering procedure in which, under a scleral flap, a fistula is created to the subconjunctival space (6).

The key to the "mystery diagnosis" in this case was the sudden occurrence of a high IOP far above baseline postoperatively despite an open angle, and the "super" response to pilocarpine that actually resulted in the reopening of the cleft, rather than a mechanical tension on the trabecular meshwork. (The first suspicion from the history of course was that, with such a pilocarpine effect, the patient might have developed angle closure that was relieved with this weak miotic therapy or perhaps suffered a miotic-related retinal detachment, but this proved not to be the case). Likely in this case (and others), the routine use of a cycloplegic drug post-"trabeculectomy" may have precipitated the sudden cleft closure syndrome.

References

1. Watson PG: Surgery of the glaucomas. Br J Ophthalmol 1972;56: 299.
2. Cairns JE: Trabeculectomy. Preliminary report of a new method. Am J Ophthalmol 1968;66:673.
3. Spencer WH: Histologic evaluation of microsurgical glaucoma techniques. Trans Am Acad Ophthal Otol 1972;76:389.
4. Van Buskirk EM, Grant WM: Lens depression and aqueous outflow in enucleated primate eyes. Am J Ophthalmol 1973;76:632–640.
5. Rosenquist RC, et al: Outflow resistance of enucleated human eyes with two different perfusion pressures and different extents of trabeculotomy. Curr Eye Res 1989;8:1233–1240.
6. Grant WM: Symposium: Microsurgery of the outflow channels. Trans Am Acad Ophthalmol Otolaryngol 1972;76(2):398–404.

wall of the cleft, with perhaps a few applications to the peripheral iris in the same area (17–20). What one is really trying to do is to cause inflammation to potentially encourage adhesion of the ciliary body back to the sclera. Therefore, minimal to no steroids should be used and cycloplegics maintained after argon laser treatment. Because the sclera is white and does not absorb the energy well (which is why the peripheral iris is sometimes also treated nonspecifically to encourage inflammation), and because there are likely nerves in the sclera, **this is an uncomfortable procedure for the patient, and likely it should be performed in multiple smaller sessions**. This argon laser procedure is not ideal and often fails. It probably is fruitless to attempt this procedure in the presence of a large cleft.

(It is noteworthy in contemplating the limited efficacy of laser applications in closing clefts to realize that Nd: YAG laser applications have been reported to reopen a cleft! (21))

The next alternative, which one of us (DLE) has had good success with, is to treat the sclera external to the cleft with two rows of cyclocryotherapy (full freeze applications for 30–60 seconds each). One's goal is to totally overlap the circumferential extent of the cleft (e.g. one to three hours of the limbus). The efficacy of this modality is felt to be by the induced inflammation that the procedure causes. Retrobulbar anesthesia is necessary, but the postoperative morbidity is much less than after the standard 6 clock hour cyclocryotherapy for antiglaucoma therapy. However, one must also be prepared to deal with the high IOP of the sudden cleft closure syndrome, should this procedure be successful.

Finally, as a last resort, some have described direct su-

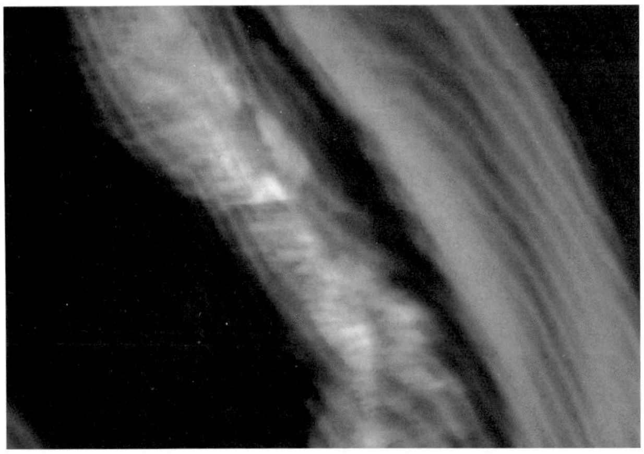

A

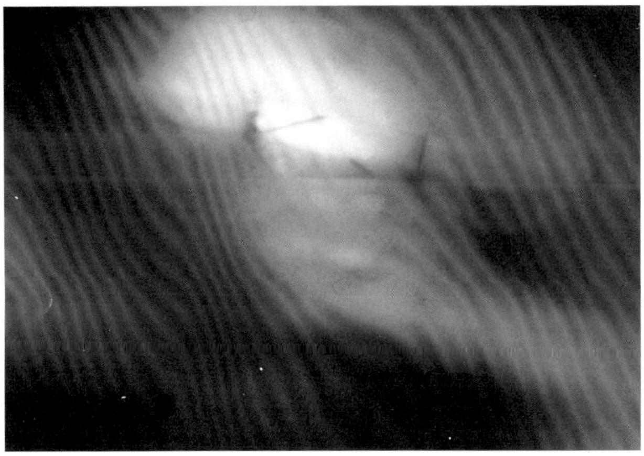

B

Figure 66.1. A, Large cyclodialysis cleft visible gonioscopically, which occurred following blunt trauma from a handball. Patient developed an IOP of 0–2 and hypotonous maculopathy. B, After cycloplegics and laser failed to close the cleft, the ciliary body was resutured to the sclera. IOP was maintained in the mid-teens following 1–2 days of IOPs in the 40s in the immediate postoperative period. Visual acuity was restored to a level of 20/25.

turing (22–26) of the ciliary body back to the sclera, preferably under a scleral flap (Fig. 66.1). Laser endophotocoagulation has also been described (27).

One of the major problems in treating an inadvertent cleft is the difficulty in identifying the exact location of the cleft gonioscopically. In these cases the anterior chamber is usually somewhat shallow because of the accumulating suprachoroidal fluid, and the iris therefore can hide the area of the cleft. In this situation, **one can deepen the anterior chamber with viscoelastic to identify the site of the cleft**, and then perform one's therapy. We recommend always looking carefully at the 12 o'clock meridian, since this is a common site of occurrence. An excellent non-invasive technique for identification and assessment of the cleft is the use of the ultrasound biomicroscope. The size and location of the cleft can thus be clearly mapped (Fig. 66.2).

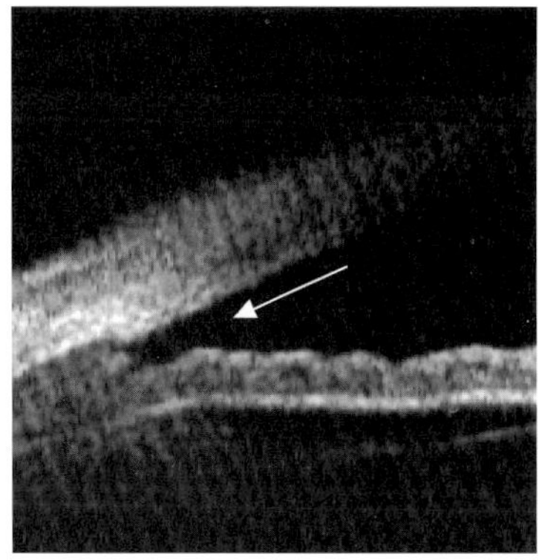

Figure 66.2. Ultrasound biomicroscopy clearly demonstrates the presence of a cyclodialysis cleft (arrow). Note the separation of the ciliary muscle from the scleral spur.

SURGICAL TECHNIQUE OF CYCLODIALYSIS FOR INTENDED ANTIGLAUCOMA THERAPY (FIG. 66.3)

The technique of cyclodialysis is simple. The first step in the operation should be to make a beveled paracentesis incision in the lower cornea with a Wheeler-type knife (Fig. 66.4). A conjunctival incision is made radially in one quadrant centered equidistant between rectus muscles 4 or 5 mm from the limbus. A circumferential scleral incision 4 to 5 mm from the limbus is made with a blunt tipped knife such as a 67 Beaver or 15 Bard Parker, separating scleral fibers fully down to ciliary body but being careful not to penetrate it. A blunt tipped cyclodialysis spatula (28) is then introduced into the suprachoroidal space with the dorsal surface of the spatula hugging the inner surface of the sclera. It is then passed towards the anterior chamber at the horizontal or vertical meridian. It is often useful to grasp the scleral wound with a Colibri forceps and elevate it as the spatula passes hugging the inner (elevated) aspect of sclera, until the tip of the spatula is seen in the anterior chamber (as it passes just below the scleral spur). The spatula is then "swept" from the extreme position with the tip at the horizontal (or vertical) meridian to a position with the tip straight ahead in the anterior chamber, being careful to avoid the corneal endothelium. The spatula is then withdrawn, staying within the suprachoroidal space, towards the scleral wound. It is then passed again as previously but towards the other extreme position, i.e., the vertical (or horizontal) meridian, and the process is repeated.

For example, in a right eye, if the scleral incision is made inferonasally at 4:30, the spatula is initially introduced into the anterior chamber at 3 o'clock, then swept to 4:30, partially withdrawn, then reintroduced into the anterior chamber at 6 o'clock with sweeping to 4:30. **With the spatula passed in this way from extreme toward the center, rather than vice versa, false passages in the ciliary body are avoided.** Following removal of the

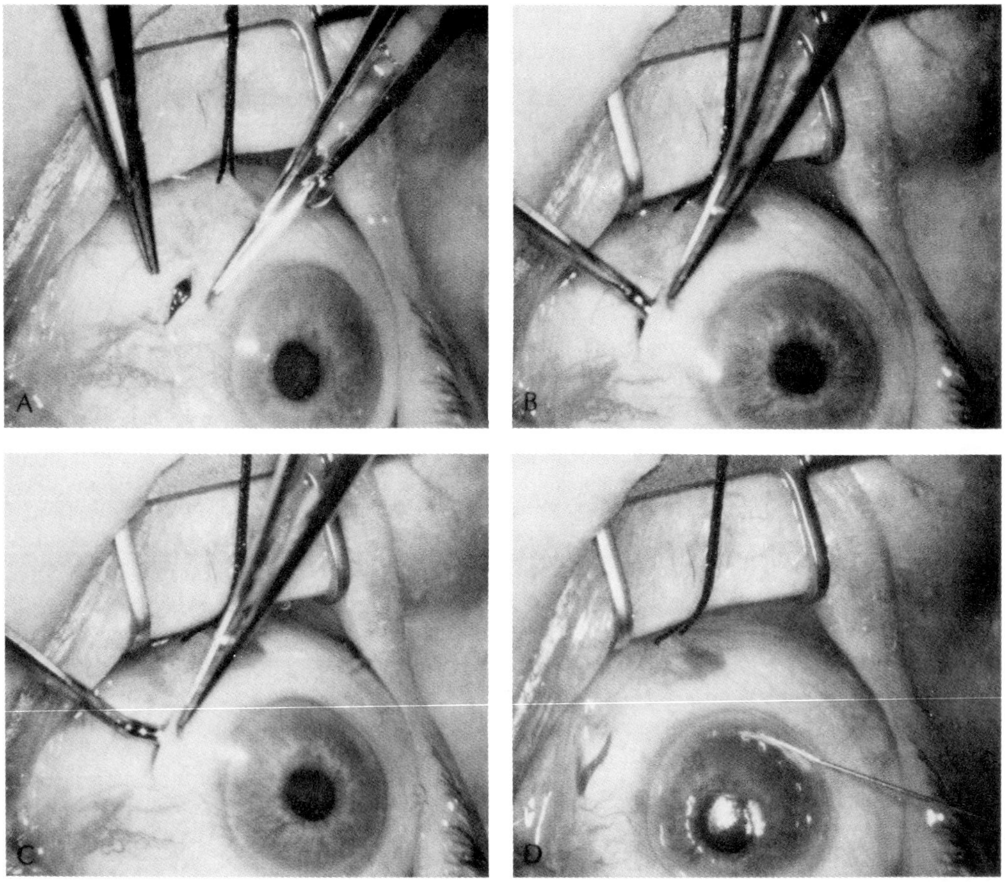

Figure 66.3. Surgical technique of cyclodialysis. A, A sclerotomy is made down to the level of the ciliary body. B, The cyclodialysis spatula is introduced into the suprachoroidal space "hugging" the inner surface of sclera and is directed to the extreme position of the operated quadrant. The tip is just seen in the anterior chamber. C, The spatula is swept from the extreme position to the central "straight ahead" position, not vice versa. D, After a similar maneuver to the other extreme position in the operated quadrant, the spatula is removed and air is introduced into the anterior chamber through the previously made paracentesis site to achieve hemostasis.

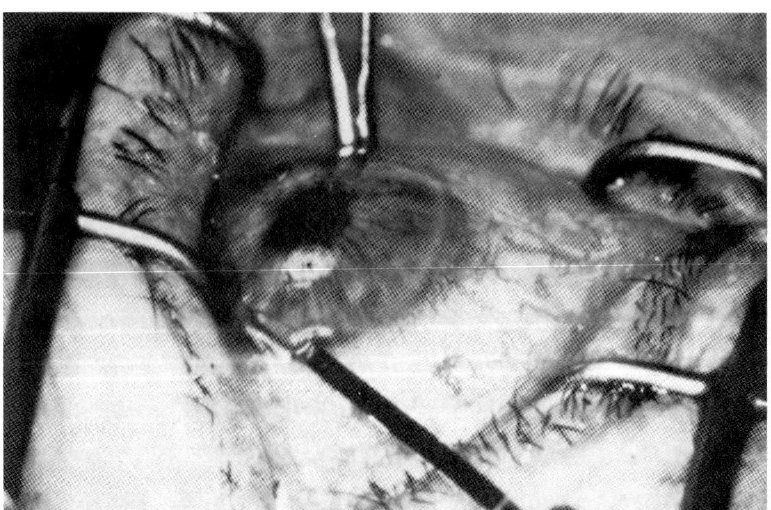

Figure 66.4. Paracentesis incision made using a Wheeler knife for access to the anterior chamber following cyclodialysis.

spatula, the anterior chamber should be entered via the paracentesis site and the chamber filled with an air bubble to firm the eye and achieve hemostasis. Hemorrhage frequently occurs, but unless it is massive it apparently does not materially influence the result of the operation. Cyclodialysis is especially risky from the standpoint of hemorrhage if the eye is considerably inflamed at the time of operation. If hemorrhage is severe during operation, it can nearly always be stopped by quickly filling the anterior chamber with a large bubble of air. When it is apparent that the hemorrhage has stopped, the air can be removed and at least some of the blood can be irrigated out of the anterior chamber. Then, at the end of the operation the anterior chamber can be filled with saline solution or a bubble of air.

Hemorrhage can be reduced by use of viscoelastic (29) in the anterior chamber and possibly in the cleft space, but the potential for a severe postoperative secondary trabecular open angle glaucoma needs to be remembered (30) should the cleft not function.

COMPLICATIONS

Damage to Angle Structures and Closure of the Cleft

In the region of the dialysis, the ciliary muscle is torn from the corneoscleral meshwork and from the scleral spur, and if a cleft does not form, the situation may be similar to what is seen after severe contusion of the globe with angle deformity (Chapter 43). The portion of the angle where the cyclodialysis has been done may not function as well as other portions of the angle due to the absence of ciliary muscle tension in the affected segment. Cholinergic miotics should not be effective on (open angle) trabecular meshwork function in the affected segment, and similar to the action of cycloplegics to elevate IOP on an open angle mechanism in some primary open angle glaucoma patients (Chapters 3 and 25), intrinsic outflow function also may be adversely affected. However, it is important to realize that traumatic angle recession results in secondary open angle glaucoma more from the direct contusion and damage to the trabecular meshwork (31) at the time of injury, rather than the loss of ciliary muscle tone.

Thus, if the cleft closes, or fails to form, the glaucoma is usually more difficult to control medically postoperatively than it was preoperatively. For this reason it is wise not to dialyze too large an area. If 3 or 4 hours of the clock are dialyzed, the chances of success are as good as if 6 to 12 hours are dialyzed. If the cleft closes and the operation has to be repeated, it had best be done in the same area so as not to injure other portions of the angle if the cleft again closes. Cases have been observed in which half the circumference was dialyzed at the first operation, and when no cleft formed the operation was repeated, dialyzing the remaining half. Then, when the cleft closed, the IOP reached high levels, as much as 80 mm Hg, with all the symptoms of acute glaucoma.

The continued use of miotics after cyclodialysis, especially the stronger miotics plus 5% phenylephrine, favors the formation and maintenance of an open cleft. Strong miotics should be used routinely and indefinitely in aphakic or pseudoaphakic eyes. In the uncommon circumstance when cyclodialysis is performed in a phakic eye, however, one must be more cautious because of the possibility of extensive formation of posterior synechias. In phakic eyes it is best not to begin miotic treatment until slit lamp examination indicates that the anterior segment is entirely quiet, with the possible exception of eyes with a sector coloboma of the iris.

Eyes have been observed in which, after cyclodialysis, there was an adequate cleft with a low IOP, then weeks or months later the cleft suddenly closed and IOP rose to very high levels. This situation was discussed above.

Corneal Damage

Descemet's membrane can be injured by the cyclodialysis spatula (Fig. 66.5), but this is usually without sequelae.

Postoperative Hemorrhage

Severe hemorrhage occurring in the postoperative period may be a serious complication. In the first place it greatly lessens the chance of ultimate success of the operation.

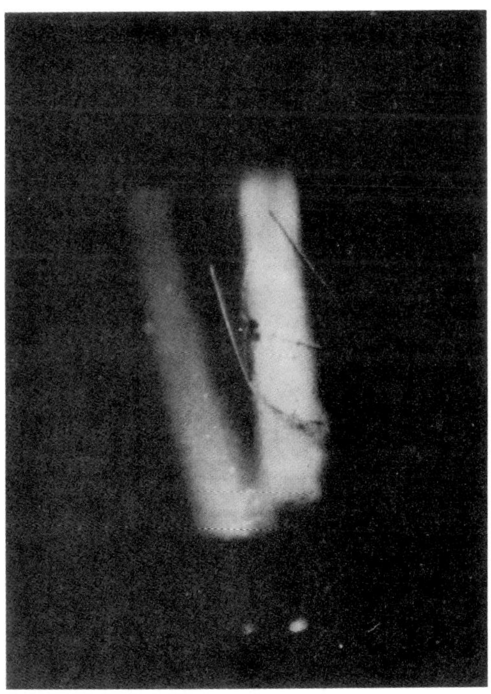

Figure 66.5. Large scroll of Descemet's membrane that inadvertently occurred from too anterior a placement of the cyclodialysis spatula tip during surgery. Resultant corneal edema cleared up completely.

Furthermore, the hemorrhage itself may cause an acute rise in IOP. It may be controlled with aqueous humor suppressants, but in some cases oral glycerin or I.V. mannitol is necessary. In some cases one must open the eye and irrigate the blood from the anterior chamber. The redder the eye at the time of surgery, the greater is the risk of hemorrhage at the time of operation or later. In any case in which cyclodialysis is planned, the operation should be deferred if at all possible until the eye is reasonably quiet. As mentioned above viscoelastic can be injected into the anterior chamber at the time of the procedure to minimize hyphema, but viscoelastics, themselves, commonly produce a temporary severe secondary open angle glaucoma (30) (Chapter 39).

Hypotony

One of the most unfortunate and undesirable complications of cyclodialysis is extreme hypotony. IOP may be too low to register. There may be extensive separation of the ciliary body and the choroid, which may reach the macula and impair visual acuity. Papilledema is sometimes seen. Furthermore, very soft, phakic eyes often develop cataract within a year or two after cyclodialysis.

When a cyclodialysis cleft is open there is always some separation of the ciliary body with a layer of fluid between ciliary body and sclera. Apparently it is the circumferential extent of this separation of the ciliary body that determines the level of IOP. In one case of Chandler and Maumenee (6), after a weak solution of fluorescein was injected into the anterior chamber, the sclera was opened 180 away from the site of operation where presumably the cleft was. Fluorescein-stained fluid escaped through the wound, proving that a 360 separation of the ciliary body was present. The eye in this case was mushy soft.

In eyes in which the extent of separation of the ciliary body is limited to a small area there is little or no reduction of IOP. In one of Chandler and Maumenee's cases there was a wide-open cleft from 11 to 1 o'clock. When the sclera was opened at 3 o'clock and a cyclodialysis spatula was passed upward, fluid was encountered only when the tip of the spatula reached the region of the cleft, demonstrating a limited separation of the ciliary body confined to the region of the cleft itself, insufficient to lower the IOP significantly.

In cases in which IOP is not unusually low after cyclodialysis, i.e., of the order of 15, 20, or 25 mm Hg, but considerably lower than before operation, it is presumed that there is separation of the ciliary body of a considerably lesser extent than 360 . The extent of separation of the ciliary body necessary to give the ideal level of IOP is unknown, but it is probably of the order of one-half the circumference.

The degree of hypotony and separation of the ciliary body and choroid apparently bears no relation to the length or width of the cleft in the angle that is observed gonioscopically. In some cases no sign of a cleft can be seen gonioscopically, but IOP is low and we know that there is in fact a cleft even if we cannot see it.

We know of no technique of doing cyclodialysis to prevent the extreme hypotony that occurs in certain cases. Theoretically one might partially close the cleft by penetrating cyclodiathermy or cyclocryotherapy in cases with extreme hypotony, but again one has little control over this procedure. It may be completely ineffective on the one hand, or completely effective on the other hand, closing the cleft and bringing about a return of high IOP.

Flat Anterior Chamber

In the immediate postoperative period following cyclodialysis, the anterior chamber may shallow, especially peripherally, associated with the induced choroidal separation. This can result in peripheral anterior synechia formation and ultimate worsening of the glaucoma, should there be late failure of the cleft. This usually transient shallowing of the chamber is not rare but it may be unsuspected because of the lowering of IOP from the cleft formation.

Special attention to this possibility should be made postoperatively and gonioscopy should be performed if peripheral anterior chamber shallowing is observed. Frequent topical steroids may retard synechia formation, but drainage of suprachoroidal fluid and reformation of the anterior chamber may be required, especially in combined cataract surgery (in which the potential for permanent PAS is even greater because of the presence of the fresh cataract wound).

Of all operations for the relief of glaucoma, cyclodialysis yields the least predictable results, and it is the least amenable to improvement by variations in surgical technique. For these reasons we believe cyclodialysis should be employed only in aphakic eyes or in eyes in which two or more conventional filtering operations have failed. Due to the unpredictability of the results, we believe cyclodialysis is not a good choice as a primary procedure in open-angle glaucoma.

References

1. Boke H: Zur Geschichte der Zyklodialyse. Klin Monatsbl Augenheilkd 1990;197(4):340–8.
2. Shields MB, Simmons RJ: Combined cyclodialysis and cataract extraction. Ophthalmic Surg 1976;7(2):62–73.
3. Montgomery D, Gills JP: Extracapsular cataract extraction, lens implantation and cyclodialysis. Ophthalmic Surg 1980;11(5):343–7.
4. Toris CB, Pederson JE: Effect of intraocular pressure on uveoscleral outflow following cyclodialysis in the monkey eye. Invest Ophthalmol Vis Sci 1985;26(12):1745–9.
5. Pederson JE: Ocular hypotony (review). Trans Ophthalmol Soc UK 1986;105(Pt2)220–6.
6. Chandler PA, Maumenee AE: A major cause of hypotony. Trans Am Acad Ophthalmol Otolaryngol 1961;2:609–618.
7. Shaffer RN, Weiss DL: Concerning cyclodialysis and hypotony. Arch Ophthalmol 1962:25–31.

8. Goldmann H: Klinische Studien zum Glaucom-problem. Ophthalmologica 1953;125:16–21.
9. Lütjen-Drecoll E: Functional and electron microscopic changes in the trabecular meshwork remaining after trabeculectomy in cynomolgus monkeys. Invest Ophthalmol 1974;13(7):511–524.
10. Garner LF, Brown B, Baker R, et al: The effect of phenylephrine hydrochloride on the resting point of accommodation. Invest Ophthalmol Vis Sci 1983;24(4):393–5.
11. Meislik J, Herschler J: Hypotony due to inadvertent cyclodialysis after intraocular lens implantation. Arch Ophthalmol 1979;97(7):1297–9.
12. Davenport WH, Brown RH, Lynch MG: Hypotony after rotation of an intraocular lens haptic into a cyclodialysis cleft. Am J Ophthalmol 1986; 101(6):736–7.
13. Terry SA: Cyclodialysis cleft following holmium laser sclerostomy, treated by argon laser photocoagulation. Ophthalmic Surg 1992;23(12): 825–6.
14. Aminlari A: Inadvertent cyclodialysis cleft. Ophthalmic Surg 1993; 24(5):331–5.
15. Small EA, Solomon JM, Prince AM: Hypotonous cyclodialysis cleft following suture fixation of a posterior chamber intraocular lens. Ophthalmic Surg 1994;25(2):107–9.
16. Maffett MJ, O'Day DM: Cyclodialysis cleft following a scleral tunnel incision. Ophthalmic Surg 1994;25(6):387–8.
17. Joondeph HC: Management of postoperative and post-traumatic cyclodialysis clefts with argon laser photocoagulation. Ophthalmic Surg 1980; 11(3):186–8.
18. Harbin TS, Jr: Treatment of cyclodialysis clefts with argon laser photocoagulation. Ophthalmology 1982;89(9):1082–1083.
19. Partamian LG: Treatment of a cyclodialysis cleft with argon laser photocoagulation in a patient with a shallow anterior chamber. Am J Ophthalmol 1985;99(1):5–7.
20. Ormerod LD, Baerveldt G, Sunalp MA, et al: Management of the hypotonous cyclodialysis cleft. Ophthalmology 1991;98(9):1384–93.
21. Fellman RL, Starita RJ, Spaeth GL: Reopening cyclodialysis cleft with Nd:YAG laser following trabeculectomy. Ophthalmic Surg 1984;15(4): 285–8.
22. Shea M, Mednick EB: Ciliary body reattachment in ocular hypotony. Arch Ophthalmol 1981;99(2):278–81.
23. Demeler U: Refixation of the ciliary body after traumatic cyclodialysis. Dev Ophthalmol 1987;14:199–201.
24. Kuchle M, Naumann GO: Direkte Zyklopexie bei Zyklodialyse mit persistierendem Hypotonie-syndrom. Fortschr Ophthalmol 1990;87(3): 247–51.
25. Metrikin DC, Allinson RW, Snyder RW: Transscleral repair of recalcitrant, inadvertent, postoperative cyclodialysis cleft. Ophthalmic Surg 1994;25(6):406–8.
26. Klemm M, Winter R: Reversible translimbal suture fixation of the ciliary body in treatment of ocular persistent hypotonia after surgical cyclodialysis. Ophthalmologie 1994;91(5):694–6.
27. Alward WL, Hodapp EA, Parel JM, et al: Argon laser endophotocoagulator closure of cyclodialysis clefts. Am J Ophthalmol 1988;106(6):748–9.
28. Simmons RJ, Kimbrough RL: A modified cyclodialysis spatula. Ophthalmic Surg 1979;10(2):67–68.
29. Alpar JJ: Sodium hyaluronate (Healon) in cyclodialysis. CLAO J 1985; 11(3):201–4.
30. Berson FG, Patterson MM, Epstein DL: Obstruction of aqueous outflow by sodium hyaluronate in enucleated human eyes. Am J Ophthalmol 1983;95:668–672.
31. Herschler J: Trabecular damage due to blunt anterior segment injury and its relationship to traumatic glaucoma. Trans Am Acad Ophthalmol Otolaryngol 1977;83(2):239–48.

Surgical Peripheral Iridectomy

67

David L. Epstein

The second edition of Glaucoma makes the following statement: "The first edition of Lectures on Glaucoma contained a detailed description of our preferred technique for doing a peripheral iridectomy. Peripheral iridectomy has become one of the commonly used operations for angle-closure glaucoma. All ophthalmic surgeons are capable of performing the operation well and have developed their own preferred technique. Suturing the wound is now almost universally practiced. For these reasons we have decided to omit a detailed discussion of technique of iridectomy in this edition."

Since the advent of laser iridectomy, it is now rare for ophthalmology residents to perform a surgical peripheral iridectomy. Yet, as alluded to previously, there are certain situations when it is not possible to employ a laser technique, e.g., cloudy cornea, when the ophthalmologist should be able to perform a surgical iridectomy. We should also not forget that there are areas of the world where lasers are not yet available.

We would therefore like to mention here a few aspects of this surgical technique which was often known as the "most underrated operation in ophthalmology."

TECHNIQUE OF SURGICAL PERIPHERAL IRIDECTOMY (FIG. 67.1)

Either a limbal or fornix based flap is prepared over approximately $1\frac{1}{2}$ clock hours in one of the upper quadrants, in order to save the other quadrant for possible future filtration surgery. The superotemporal quadrant is usually preferred for iridectomy, so that, if cataract formation were to occur after a subsequent superonasal quadrant filtering operation, the cataract could be removed more easily from the side rather than from below. We usually prefer a fornix based flap due to its better limbal exposure.

The key to the operation is the incision. For this purpose a somewhat rounded knife blade, such as a Beaver No. 67 or Bard-Parker No. 15, is preferred to enter the eye so that it will slide over iris without perforating it. A sharp blade is best avoided, since it is apt to make a small hole in the iris and the iris will then not spontaneously prolapse. The incision must be perpendicular and "clean" and wide enough so that the iris will spontaneously prolapse and will easily reposit. An irregular incision will catch iris tissue and prevent repositioning. In making the incision, when one gets the first "gush" of aqueous humor, one should not immediately withdraw the knife (as is one's instinct), but should continue to enlarge the opening to a full clock hour. One is more confident in doing this with a rounded rather than a sharp blade.

It is important to do this operation outside the eye, rather than to reach inside to grasp the iris. If the incision is wide enough (and the iris not penetrated by the knife), gentle pressure on the posterior lip of the wound will allow the pressure in the posterior chamber to spontaneously prolapse the iris into the wound, where it should be firmly grasped and cleanly cut. The cut iris tissue is inspected for pigment epithelium to ensure that full thickness of the iris has been excised. Then the iris is reposited by exerting a sweeping motion with the irrigator tip across the limbal incision. **No instrument is placed into the eye.** Repositing the iris is often the most difficult part of the procedure. Preoperative pilocarpine will often aid in this.

After the iridectomy is performed, iris is often present in the wound. **The gentle sweeping pressure of the irrigating tip allows some aqueous humor to escape and the iris to fall back inside the eye.** Sometimes this can also be accomplished by applying a small amount of pressure directly on the posterior lip of the wound or by gently separating the anterior and posterior lips with forceps. The iris is often "boggy" in eyes with acute angle closure and tends to get "hung up" in irregular incisions, especially if they are not of adequate size.

At the end of the procedure the pupil should be round and the iridectomy opening visualized inside the eye. Otherwise, if the iridectomy is caught in the wound, pupillary block will not be relieved. The flap may be closed by a variety of methods. A useful closure approach is to incorporate conjunctiva in the single suture used to close the limbal incision (Fig. 67.1 F,G).

Surgical peripheral iridectomy is often a quick, straightforward procedure. However, there are numerous pitfalls that often relate to a suboptimal incision and subsequent problems with iris prolapse and repositioning.

POSTOPERATIVE CARE

A single dressing may be used, but in most cases no dressing is required. A combination of local steroid and antibiotic drops 3 or 4 times a day, and 5% phenylephrine drops twice a day are begun on the day of operation, and continued until there are no inflammatory signs in the anterior segment, usually 2 to 3 weeks. One must make sure that

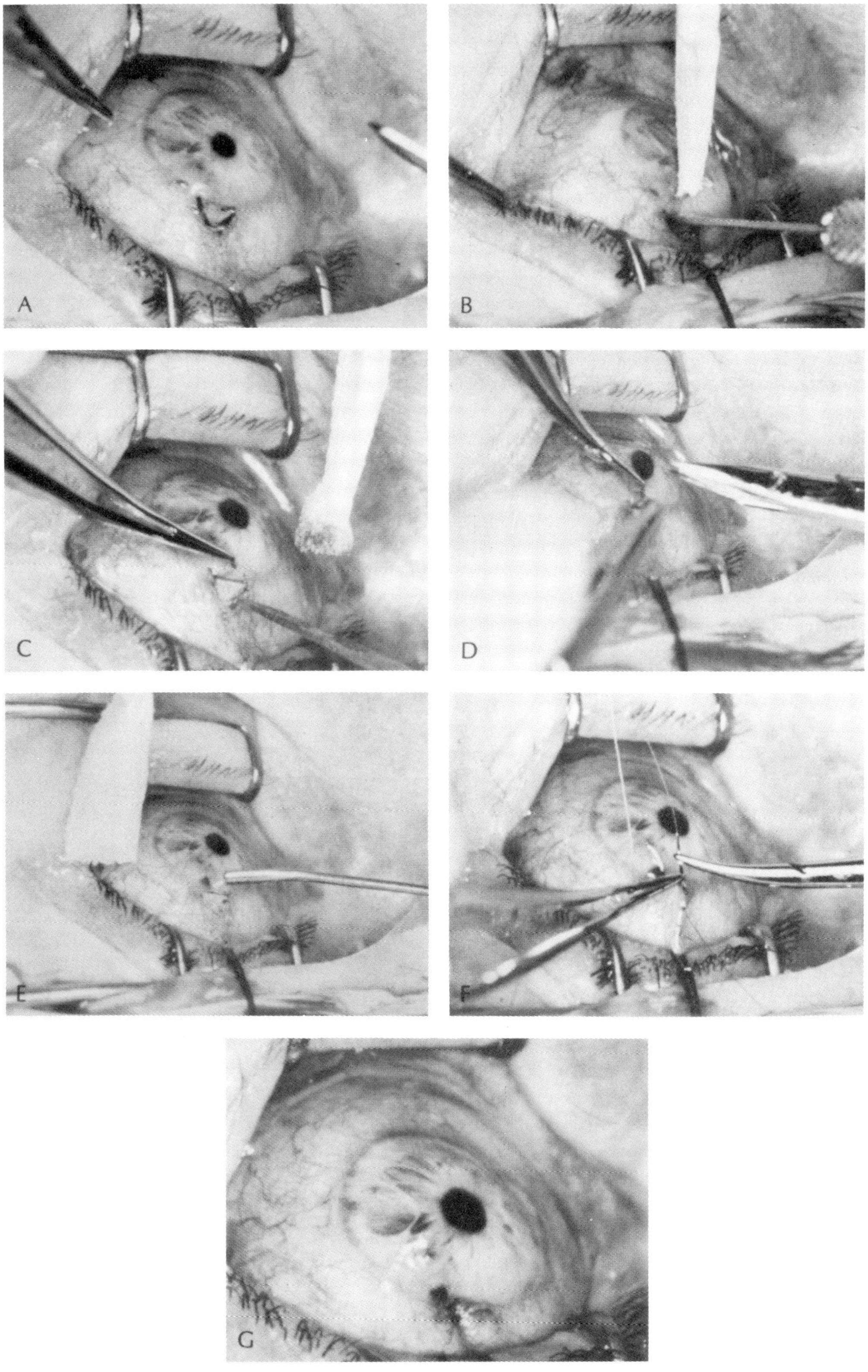

Figure 67.1. Technique of surgical peripheral iridectomy. A, A fornix-based conjunctival flap is prepared with scissors. A knife with a rounded tip is brought forward to make the incision (B) which is perpendicular, "clean," and accomplished by a slight rolling motion. After the first "gush" of aqueous the incision is slightly extended and is then inspected (C). The anterior lip may be grasped with Colibri forceps, while the iris forceps gently depresses the posterior lip (D) so that iris is spontaneously prolapsed into the wound where it is grasped with the iris forceps and is smoothly cut with fine scissors at the wound margin. No instruments should be placed inside the eye. The iris is reposited by a sweeping motion of the irrigator tip across the limbal incision (E). The pupil is observed to be round and the iridectomy patent. The wound and conjunctiva may be then closed by a variety of methods. Shown in (F) and (G) is the technique of "incorporating the flap" in which the posterior arm of a double armed suture, having already been placed through the limbal wound, is passed a few millimeters posterior to the edge of the conjunctiva, and then the anterior arm of the same suture is placed (F) through the anterior edge and is then tied (G).

the pupil dilates readily. If there is evidence of iritis, short-acting cycloplegics, such as cyclopentolate or tropicamide, are employed.

COMPLICATIONS

A flat or very shallow anterior chamber without elevation of IOP is probably always due to a wound leak. The suture may have been placed too deeply, or it may not have been tied tightly. Of course a wound leak is more apt to occur if no suture is used. **A shallow or flat anterior chamber after peripheral iridectomy calls for prompt intervention.** Iridectomy was chosen instead of some other operation because preoperatively the angle was in large part capable of opening, and one must not allow the previously open angle to become closed by peripheral anterior synechias as a result of prolonged absence of the anterior chamber. There is much more urgency in the prompt reformation of the anterior chamber after a peripheral iridectomy than after a filtering operation. The wound should be promptly explored. The original suture or sutures should be removed, since they may have been improperly placed. Then new sutures are placed until one can be sure that the wound is tight. **After peripheral iridectomy, a flat or shallow anterior chamber and elevated IOP most likely indicates the development of malignant glaucoma** (Chapter 29).

If the iridectomy includes only the stroma of the iris, and the pigment epithelium is left behind, then of course the operation will be completely without effect. When the iridectomy is done, one must make sure that there is posterior pigment epithelium on the piece of iris excised. If, in the postoperative period, it is discovered that the pigment epithelium in the peripheral coloboma is intact, it can generally be easily opened with an argon laser.

The incision should never be more than 1.5 mm from the limbus. If it is too posterior, a piece of ciliary body may be excised instead of iris. **One cannot be sure that the operation has been properly performed unless a peripheral iris coloboma is clearly visible at the end of the operation.** If some uveal tissue has been excised, but at the end of the operation, with the pupil round and central, no iris coloboma can be seen, one may think of reopening the wound, introducing forceps, grasping the peripheral iris, and doing a proper iridectomy. However, this entails significant risk of injury to the lens. It is better in such cases to suture the original wound and repeat the operation in another area.

Elevated intraocular pressure (IOP) and haziness of the cornea may be noted in the immediate postoperative period. This need cause no great concern if the anterior chamber is of normal depth and a definite coloboma of the iris is present. Gonioscopy should be performed to determine whether the angle is, in fact, open or closed. The Zeiss lens is readily utilized in such postoperative eyes. If the angle is closed, then in the presence of a normal axial anterior chamber depth, plateau iris syndrome needs to be considered. Routine mydriatic/cycloplegic drops should be discontinued and weak pilocarpine therapy initiated. It is curious that in the immediate postoperative period, certain cases of apparent plateau iris syndrome (Chapter 26) that demonstrate angle closure with cycloplegic therapy will fail to do so again when rechallenged several months later. Such patients need to be followed long term, but it seems as if certain patients may demonstrate angle closure with pupillary dilatation only as a temporary postoperative phenomenon, perhaps due to iris swelling.

Another cause of IOP elevation postoperatively is the presence of extensive pre-existing peripheral anterior synechias.

Sometimes IOP is temporarily elevated after surgical iridectomy due to an ill-defined open-angle glaucoma mechanism which may relate to cycloplegic therapy, inflammation, or other unknown factors, but which can be managed conservatively with aqueous humor suppressants.

Posterior synechias can be avoided in most cases by the routine use of phenylephrine along with local steroids beginning on the day of operation, but cycloplegics should be used where iritis develops.

Chandler wrote: Within a day or two after surgical iridectomy, when the eye is being treated with topical corticosteroid and periodic dilation of the pupil with phenylephrine to prevent formation of posterior synechias, in rare instances there is a recurrence of acute glaucoma. This has happened in cases in which the attempt at iridectomy failed to produce a functional hole through the iris, owing to inadvertently leaving the pigment layer of the iris intact or to unintentionally incarcerating the iridectomy coloboma in the wound. The usual solution is to perform a laser iridectomy or, failing this, to go back promptly and do a proper iridectomy at a different site. However, if the intact iris pigment layer is visible in an easily accessible location and is bulging forward because of unrelieved pupillary block, it can usually be easily disrupted with the argon laser.

In doing a surgical peripheral iridectomy for angle closure glaucoma we may feel sure that we have excised uveal tissue, but in some cases no coloboma is visible. Did we really excise a piece of iris in the extreme periphery, or a piece of ciliary body? What should we do at this point? We cannot be certain that there is a real coloboma. One alternative is to introduce forceps that are toothless and without sharp points to grasp the iris, pull it out of the wound, and excise a piece. This is risky; however, suppose there is, in fact, a small peripheral coloboma of the iris. When forceps are introduced there is great danger of injuring the lens. In one case the lens was injured by this maneuver by one of us (PAC), with rapid development of cataract. It was decided that never again would we introduce forceps in such a case. Instead we have used the following course in patients in whom at the end of the operation no coloboma was visible. The anterior chamber is formed with saline solution, the suture is tied, and the entire operation is repeated, then and there, at another site.

One of us (PAC) recalls the case of a physician on whom a peripheral iridectomy was being done. At the end of the procedure no coloboma was visible, and the operation was promptly repeated at another site. There was then a visible coloboma. At the end of the procedure the physician patient inquired how the operation had gone. The answer had to be, "The operation went very well, but I had to do it twice!"

Diagnosis and Treatment of Glaucoma in Children

X

Approach to Infants and Children with Glaucoma

68

Sharon F. Freedman
David S. Walton

The glaucomas of childhood constitute a rare, but sight-threatening and heterogeneous group of diseases. It has been estimated that a busy ophthalmologist in general practice will encounter a new case of childhood glaucoma about once every five years. While patients with childhood glaucomas make up less than 0.1% of ophthalmic patients, they constitute 2–15% of populations in institutions for the blind (1). Intraocular pressure (IOP) control is only a small part of the battle to preserve vision in children with glaucoma. **Visual loss may result not only from optic nerve damage, but also from associated corneal scarring, irregular astigmatism, and anisometropic and strabismic amblyopia.**

The pathogenesis of glaucoma in childhood, and the responses of the child's eye to this disorder, are often very different from those seen in older patients. Specialized information and techniques for the evaluation and care of children with glaucoma are therefore required. In addition, successful management of the childhood glaucoma patient requires cooperation and support from the entire family, not only from the patient. Since systemic disorders not infrequently coexist with glaucoma in children, and since most of these patients will require one or more general anesthesias during the management of their glaucomas, the ophthalmologist should work closely with his pediatric colleagues in the care of children with glaucoma.

CLASSIFICATION

Although many classification schemes have been devised to categorize the various childhood glaucomas, their subdivision into primary and secondary mechanisms can be clinically useful. Primary glaucomas are those resulting from an intrinsic disease of the aqueous outflow pathways, and are often genetic in origin. Secondary glaucomas, by contrast, result from disease originating in other regions of the eye or body (Table 68.1) (2). Both primary and secondary glaucomas may be associated with significant systemic conditions; astute assessment of the ocular signs of glaucoma may aid in appropriate classification and systemic evaluation of these patients.

CLINICAL MANIFESTATIONS

Symptoms and Signs

Infants and young children with glaucoma usually present for ophthalmologic evaluation because the pediatrician or parents have noted something unusual about the appearance of the patient's eyes or behavior. Often corneal opacification and/or enlargement (a response to elevated IOP) are the signs which signal glaucoma in the infant (Fig. 68.1). At other times, **the child's glaucoma may manifest itself as one or more of the "classic triad" of findings: epiphora, photophobia, and blepharospasm.** Photophobia and epiphora result from corneal edema (often with associated breaks in Descemet's membrane). The baby may be noted to withdraw from light or to bury his head against his parent or bedding to prevent exposure to light. Even indoors, the infant may show an apparent reluctance to face upward, and may mistakenly be considered shy (Fig. 68.2). Blepharospasm may be yet another manifestation of photophobia, often accompanying epiphora, but without the mucoid discharge so often seen in congenital nasolacrimal duct obstruction (3,4).

In children older than one year of age, glaucoma usually induces fewer overt signs and symptoms. Children with glaucoma developing between one and four years of age may not be correctly diagnosed unless glaucoma is suspected from other accompanying ocular or systemic abnormalities.

Children older than four years of age with glaucoma most frequently seek examination for decreased distance acuity related to myopia. Significant astigmatism and anisometropia are often also present. An exception to the relatively asymptomatic presentation of glaucoma in older children is secondary glaucoma presenting with an acute rise in IOP to levels sufficient to cause nauseating eye pain, headaches, and even colored haloes around lights (as seen with adults having angle-closure glaucoma). In these children, sudden-onset glaucoma may be the result of traumatic hyphema or of angle-closure glaucoma from lens dislocation or cicatricial retinopathy of prematurity. Less frequently acute glaucoma develops secondary to other processes (Table 68.1, see also Chapter 71) (4).

Table 68.1
Childhood Glaucomas—A Classification Scheme

I. Primary glaucoma
- A. Congenital open-angle glaucoma
- B. Congenital glaucoma associated with iris defects
- C. Juvenile glaucoma
- D. Primary glaucomas associated with systemic or ocular abnormalities
  - 1. Associated with systemic abnormalities
    - a. Axenfeld-Rieger syndrome (iridocorneal goniodysgenesis)
    - b. Chromosomal disorders
      - i) Trisomy 13 (13–15 Trisomy)
      - ii) Trisomy and partial deletions of chromosome 18
      - iii) Turner syndrome
      - iv) Chromosome 6 (ring syndrome and translocations)
    - c. Congenital Rubella
    - d. Cutis marmorarta telangiectasia congenita
    - e. Fetal alcohol syndrome
    - f. Hepatocerebrorenal (Zellweger) syndrome
    - g. Infantile glaucoma associated with mental retardation and paralysis
    - h. Kniest syndrome
    - i. Marfan syndrome
    - j. Michel syndrome
    - k. Mucopolysaccharidosis
    - l. Neurofibromatosis (NF-1)
    - m. Nonprogressive hemiatrophy
    - n. Oculocerebrorenal (Lowe) syndrome
    - o. Oculodentodigital syndrome
    - p. Open-angle glaucoma associated with microcornea and absent frontal sinuses
    - q. Prader-Willi syndrome
    - r. Rubinstein-Taybi (broad-thumb) syndrome
    - s. Stickler syndrome
    - t. Sturge-Weber syndrome
    - u. Warburg syndrome (skeletal dysplasia)
  - 2. Associated with ocular abnormalities
    - a. Aniridia
    - b. Anterior chamber staphyloma
    - c. Axenfeld-Rieger syndrome
    - d. Congenital ectropion uveae
    - e. Congenital hereditary endothelial dystrophy
    - f. Congenital microcoria with myopia
    - g. Congenital ocular melanosis
    - h. Familial iris hypoplasia
    - i. Idiopathic or familial elevated episcleral venous pressure
    - j. Peters syndrome
    - k. Posterior polymorphous dystrophy
    - l. Sclerocornea

II. Secondary glaucoma
- A. Traumatic glaucoma
  - 1. Acute-onset
    - a. Angle concussion
    - b. Hyphema
  - 2. Late-onset with angle recession
  - 3. Arteriovenous fistula
- B. Glaucoma secondary to intraocular neoplasm
  - 1. Retinoblastoma
  - 2. Juvenile xanthogranuloma
  - 3. Leukemia
  - 4. Melanoma
  - 5. Melanocytoma
  - 6. Iris rhabdomyosarcoma
  - 7. Aggressive iris nevus
- C. Uveitic glaucoma
  - 1. Open-angle
  - 2. Angle closure
    - a. Synechial angle-closure
    - b. Iris bombé with pupillary block
- D. Lens-induced glaucoma
  - 1. Subluxation-dislocation and pupillary block
    - a. Marfan's syndrome
    - b. Homocystinuria
  - 2. Spherophakia and pupillary block
  - 3. Phacolytic
- E. Aphakic glaucoma after congenital cataract surgery
  - 1. Lens material blockage of trabecular meshwork
  - 2. Pupillary block
  - 3. Chronic open-angle
- F. Steroid-induced glaucoma
- G. Neovascular glaucoma
  - 1. Retinoblastoma
  - 2. Coats' disease
  - 3. Medulloepithelioma
  - 4. Familial exudative vitreoretinopathy
- H. Secondary angle-closure glaucoma
  - 1. Retinopathy of prematurity
  - 2. Microphthalmos
  - 3. Nanophthalmos
  - 4. Retinoblastoma
  - 5. Persistent hyperplastic primary vitreous
  - 6. Congenital pupillary iris-lens membrane
  - 7. Aniridia
  - 8. Iridoschisis
  - 9. Cornea plana
  - 10. Cystinosis
- I. Glaucoma with increased episcleral venous pressure
- J. Glaucoma secondary to intraocular infection
  - 1. Acute recurrent toxoplasmosis
  - 2. Acute herpetic iritis

Adapted from Walton DS: Glaucoma in infants and children. In: Pediatric Ophthalmology, 3rd ed. Edited by Nelson B, Calhoun JH, Harley RD: Philadelphia: WB Saunders, 1991.

DIFFERENTIAL DIAGNOSIS

The manifestations of epiphora, photophobia, and blepharospasm are not unique to infantile glaucoma, and also can occur as a result of nasolacrimal duct obstruction, ocular inflammation (uveitis), and corneal injury (e.g. abrasion). Corneal edema or opacification may occur in the setting of storage diseases (e.g. mucopolysaccharidoses, cystinosis), corneal dystrophies (e.g., congenital hereditary endothelial dystrophy or posterior polymorphous dystrophy), birth trauma (with resultant Descemet's tears), and congenital anomalies (e.g., sclerocornea, Peters' anomaly). Isolated corneal enlargement occurs in megalocornea and high axial myopia. Although other nonglaucomatous eye conditions may share one or more signs with childhood glaucoma, care must be taken to rule out glaucoma in each of these

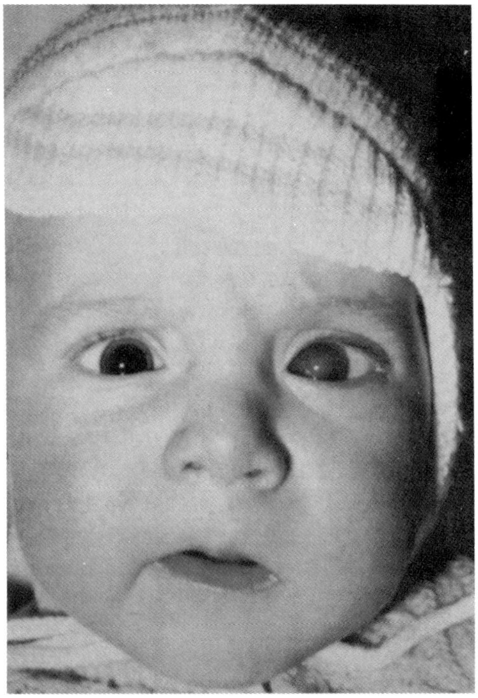

Figure 68.1. Unilateral corneal opacity and enlargement in an infant with glaucoma. (From Walton, DS. Primary congenital open-angle glaucoma. In: Chandler and Grant's Glaucoma, third ed. Edited by Epstein, DL. Philadelphia, Lea & Febiger, 1986.)

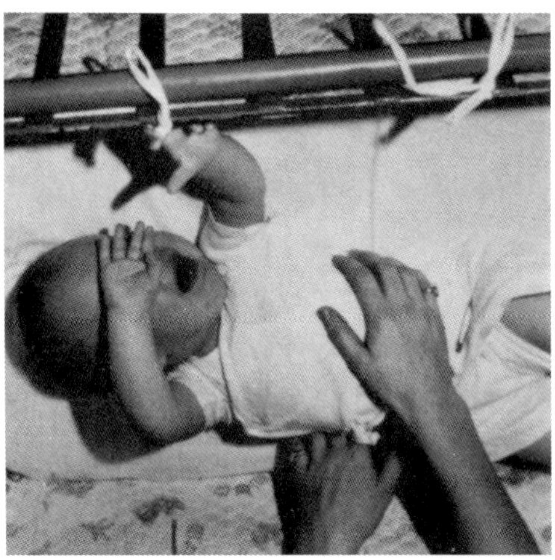

Figure 68.2. Photophobia in a patient with infantile glaucoma. (From Walton, DS. Primary congenital open-angle glaucoma. In: Chandler and Grant's Glaucoma, third ed. Edited by Epstein, DL. Philadelphia, Lea & Febiger, 1986.)

cases. For example, glaucoma may complicate uveitis, and has been reported in the setting of storage disease, corneal dystrophy, congenital anomalies such as Peter's anomaly, and megalocornea. Glaucoma may also occur coincident with congenital nasolacrimal duct obstruction (2).

Rarely, a child may present after infancy with findings suggestive of primary infantile glaucoma, yet have normal IOP. Spontaneous cure in cases of mild primary infantile glaucoma has been described (5,6,7) but remains a diagnosis of exclusion.

OCULAR EXPANSION

The neonatal globe is distensible, and enlarges in response to elevated intraocular pressure. Stretching may occur in all parts of the infant eye, including the cornea, anterior chamber angle structures, sclera, optic nerve, scleral canal, and lamina cribrosa (8). The normal horizontal corneal diameter at birth ranges from 9.5 to 10.5 mm (mean 10 mm), enlarging about 0.5 to 1.0 mm in the first year of life (Table 68.2) (9–11). **Under one year of age, diameters of 12 to 12.5 mm are suggestive of glaucoma, (9,11) and a measurement of 13mm or more at any time in childhood strongly suggests abnormality, as does asymmetry in corneal diameter between eyes in a child.** Whereas the cornea may enlarge because of elevated IOP until only the age of approximately three years, the sclera may deform in response to increased IOP until approximately ten years of age. **Progressive myopia and astigmatism are therefore often seen in older children with glaucoma** (8).

Elevated IOP stretches and sometimes breaks Descemet's membrane, resulting in acute localized corneal edema, followed by deposition of new basement membrane into hyaline ridges (called Haab's striae). These permanent striae are usually fairly horizontal and rarely occur in corneas less than 12.5 mm in horizontal diameter (8) or in children older than two years (Fig. 68.3). By contrast, breaks in Descemet's membrane arising from obstetrical trauma (usually involving use of forceps) tend to have a more vertical orientation, and to present at birth.

Ultrasonography has been used to record changes in the axial length of eyes in infants with infantile glaucoma (Table 68.2). Compared with corneal diameter, however, axial length seems less helpful in the evaluation of glaucomatous infant eyes (11).

OPTIC NERVE CUPPING

Optic nerve cupping occurs as a result of elevated IOP in childhood glaucoma, but its course (in infants and young children) may be quite different from that seen with adult glaucoma patients. In children with advanced glaucoma, as in adults, loss of neuroretinal rim tissue occurs, especially at the vertical poles of the disc, and the optic cup may extend to the disc margins (8). In very young patients, one more often sees generalized enlargement of the optic cup with preservation of an intact neuroretinal rim. This pattern of symmetric cupping has been attributed to stretching of the optic canal and backward bowing of the lamina cribrosa in these young patients (12). While this type of optic nerve cupping can occur early and quite rapidly in infants with glaucoma, **dramatic reversal of cup-**

HINTS OF POSSIBLE GLAUCOMA IN AN ASYMPTOMATIC CHILD

Sharon F. Freedman

Enlarged cornea(s)
Altered corneal clarity
Asymmetry in size between the eyes
Abnormality of pupil (shape) or iris (one or both eyes)
Opacity of lens (es)
High myopia
Optic nerve cupping (cup/disc ratio > 0.3 – 0.4)

Table 68.2
Corneal Diameter and Axial Length in Children: Normal and Glaucomatous Eyes*

Age	Corneal Diameter (horizontal, in mm) Normal	Corneal Diameter Suggestive of Glaucoma	Axial Length (by ultrasound, in mm) Normal	Axial Length Suggestive of Glaucoma
Term (newborn)	9.5–10.5	11.5	16–17	>20
One year	10–11.5	>12–12.5	~20	>22.5
Two years	11–12	>12.5	21	>23
Older child	12	>13	24	>25

* Data adapted from References 9–11.

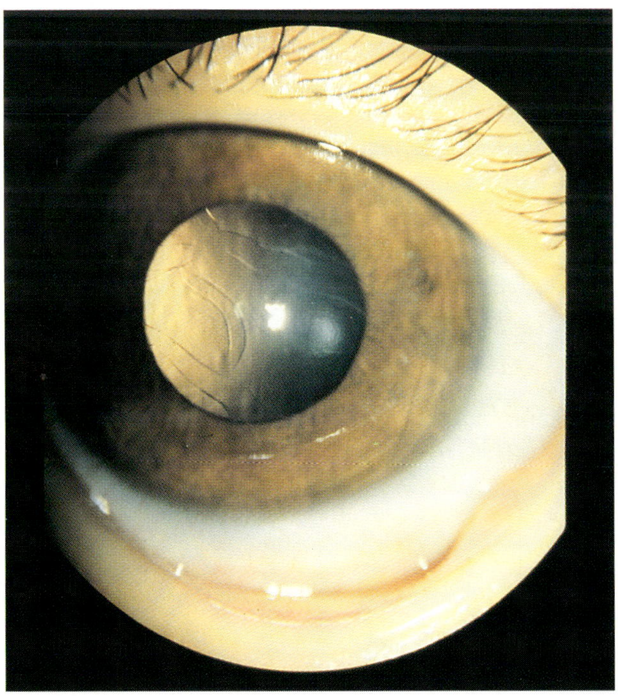

Figure 68.3. Haab's striae in infantile glaucoma.

ping may occur with normalization of IOP (Fig. 68.4) (8).

Large size of the optic nerve cup and asymmetry of cupping between fellow eyes is suggestive but not definite evidence of glaucoma. Illustratively, the cup/disc ratio exceeded 0.3 in 68% of 126 eyes with primary infantile glaucoma examined by Shaffer and Hetherington (13), but in only 2.6% of 936 normal newborn eyes examined by Richardson (12). Richardson also reported marked optic cup asymmetry in only 0.6% of normal eyes in his series, contrasted with 89% noted for infants with monocular glaucoma (12).

INTRAOCULAR PRESSURE ELEVATION

Intraocular pressure levels and measurement in children with glaucoma will be discussed below under "Diagnostic Examination."

THE DIAGNOSTIC EXAMINATION

The ophthalmic evaluation of the child with suspected glaucoma should address several specific objectives: a) confirming or excluding the diagnosis of glaucoma, b) determining the etiology of the glaucoma (if present), and c) obtaining additional medical information needed to plan for an examination under anesthesia. If one can confidently exclude the diagnosis of glaucoma, or if an older child with glaucoma is to undergo a trial of medical therapy, examination under anesthesia may not be indicated.

OFFICE EXAMINATION

History and Equipment

History taking from parents and caretakers can be especially valuable in evaluating patients too young to provide any useful verbal information. Information should be gathered regarding possible signs and symptoms of glaucoma, evidence of systemic abnormality, possible trauma, drug and medication exposure, and pertinent family history.

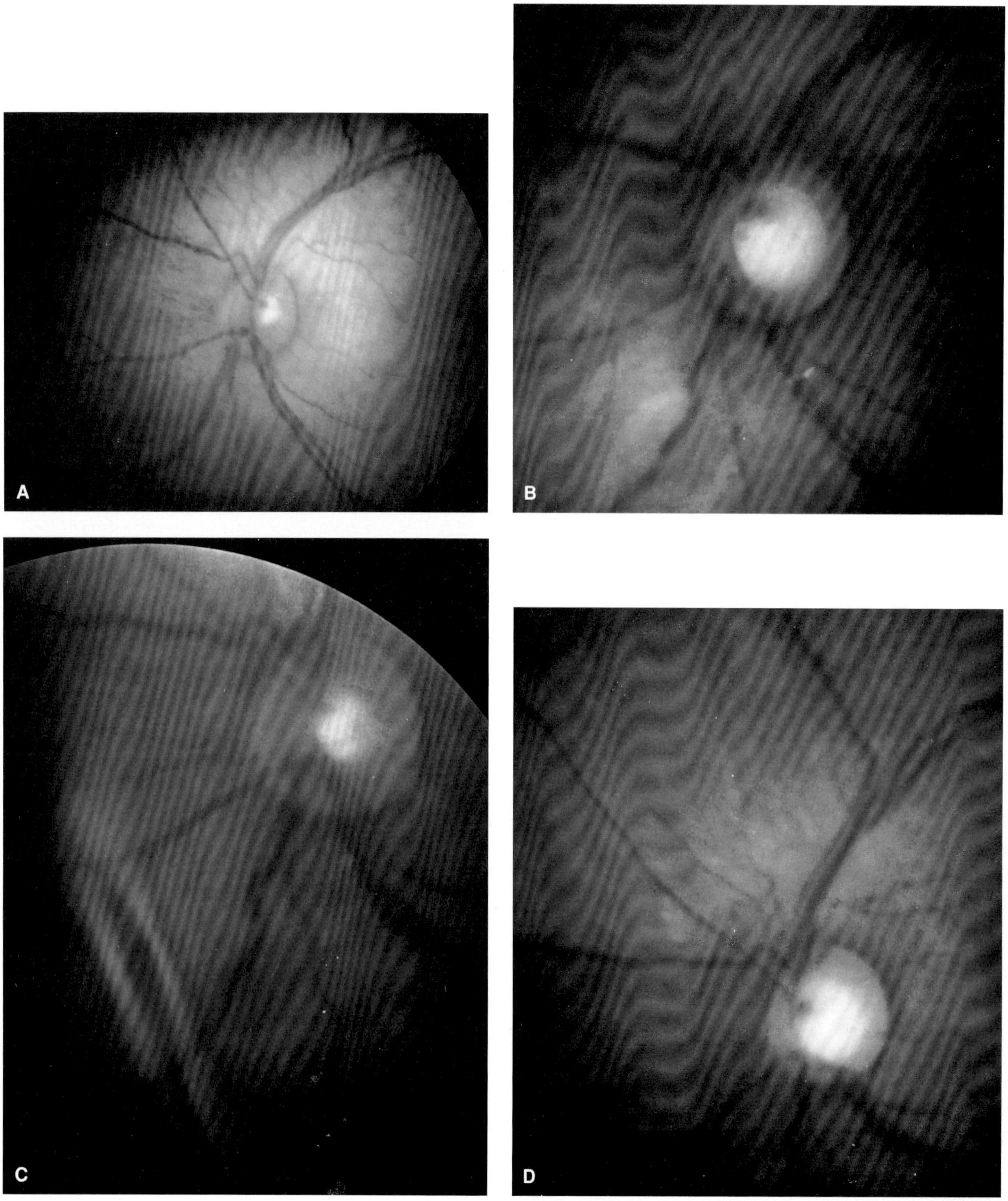

Figure 68.4. Reversible optic nerve cupping in the left eye of a child after lensectomy/vitrectomy for bilateral congenital cataracts. (A) Small optic nerve cup seen in the aphakic left eye of a six-month old child whose **fellow** eye developed angle closure glaucoma five months after uneventful lensectomy/vitrectomy. (B) Increased optic nerve cupping seen one year later in the setting of delayed angle closure glaucoma in the left eye (glaucoma in fellow eye cured after peripheral iridectomy). (C) Decreased cupping seen in the same (left) eye two weeks after initial synechialysis, peripheral iridectomy with IOP reduction to normal. (D) Cupping increased once again in this same (left) eye with loss of adequate IOP control after second angle surgery.

In addition to commonly used office equipment, the use of a portable slit lamp, millimeter ruler, Tono-Pen and/or Perkins tonometer, and Koeppe diagnostic gonioscopic lenses may be valuable (see below).

Assessment of Vision and Ocular Adnexa

Examination begins with an assessment of the general overall appearance and visual function. In infants, the ability to fix and follow well, and the absence of nystagmus suggest good visual function. Visual acuity and eventually visual fields can be evaluated in children older than about three years. The penlight and direct ophthalmoscope are useful instruments for inspecting the adnexa and corneas. (We often delay use of the portable slit lamp until after tonometry has been attempted, to maximize the opportunity for measuring IOP in an unanesthetized, undisturbed infant.) During the external examination one looks for abnormalities (e.g. lid malformations) to suggest congenital syndromes that may include glaucoma (Table 68.1) and for signs of lacrimal system obstruction that may explain epiphora.

Corneal Examination

The corneas are examined for possible edema and Haab's striae. In the presence of corneal epithelial edema, the corneal surface lacks its normal luster and produces an irregular penlight reflection off its bedewed surface. Since corneal opacification obscures details of the underlying pupil and iris, the relative visibility of these intraocular structures helps to quantify the degree of corneal haze or opacity and is well evaluated with the direct ophthalmoscope. In the worst cases, the cornea appears opaque white or pearly gray, and completely hides any view of the pupil. **In moderately severe cases, the cornea appears bluish, and allows visualization of the pupil but few iris details.** Corneal diameter can be estimated using a millimeter rule (4). The examiner may notice a difference in the overall size of one cornea compared to the other, even when corneal diameter measurements seem similar between the fellow eyes. Since the area of a circle varies as the square of its radius, it seems reasonable that the observer's eye may more easily note differences in area than in diameter of a patient's two corneas.

Tonometry and Intraocular Pressure

The best IOP measurements are those obtained on a cooperative patient using only topical anesthesia, since IOP may be falsely elevated in a struggling patient and often unpredictably altered by systemic sedatives and anesthetics (see below, under Examination Under Anesthesia). Sometimes tonometry can be achieved on a sleepy or hungry infant taking a bottle in his parent's arms (Fig. 68.5). Among various instruments used to measure IOP in children, the Perkins applanation tonometer and the Tono-Pen (a hand-held Mackay-Marg-type tonometer) rank highly in terms of accuracy and ease of use in these patients (14–17). The Pulsair, a hand-held noncontact tonometer, has also been successfully used to measure IOP in children (18,19). The slit lamp-mounted Goldmann applanation tonometer may be useful in older, cooperative children.

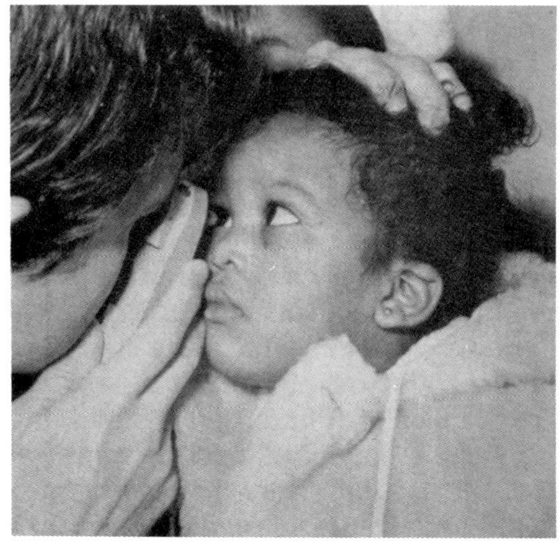

Figure 68.5. Office tonometry using the Perkins applanation tonometer. (From Walton, DS. Considerations peculiar to infants and children. In: Chandler and Grant's Glaucoma, third ed. Edited by Epstein, DL. Philadelphia, Lea & Febiger, 1986.)

Studies of IOP in unanesthetized infants and children suggest that normal values lie below the mean pressures for normal adults. Pensiero and colleagues (using a Pulsair noncontact tonometer) reported a mean IOP of 9.59 ± 2.3mm Hg in premature/newborn infants. They found that the mean IOP rose gradually with increasing age of the subjects, reaching 13.95 ± 2.49 mm Hg by age 7–8 years, and remaining essentially constant at that level through the middle teenage years (Fig. 68.6) (18). Speirer et al. noted a mean IOP of 10.11 ± 2.2 mm Hg in normal premature infants using a Pulsair tonometer (19). Using a Perkins applanation tonometer, Radtke and Cohen similarly found the mean IOP of unanesthetized newborns to be 11.24 ± 2.4 mm Hg (20). Others have reported mean IOP using the Perkins tonometer as low as 5.89 (21) and as high as 18 mm Hg (22) in infants and young children. Infants with primary infantile glaucoma commonly present with unanesthetized IOPs between 30 and 40 mm Hg, although occasionally values above or below this range occur. Often pressure measurements are confounded by a failure to cooperate, requiring measurement under anesthesia or sedation. The mean IOP in a group of struggling infants has been reported as 28.3 mm Hg by Perkins tonometry, more than twice the value (10.8 mm Hg) obtained in the same infants while quiet (20). Falsely elevated IOP measurements may either falsely alarm or falsely reassure the examiner. For example, measuring high IOP in both eyes of an intermittently struggling infant with unilateral glaucoma may obscure the

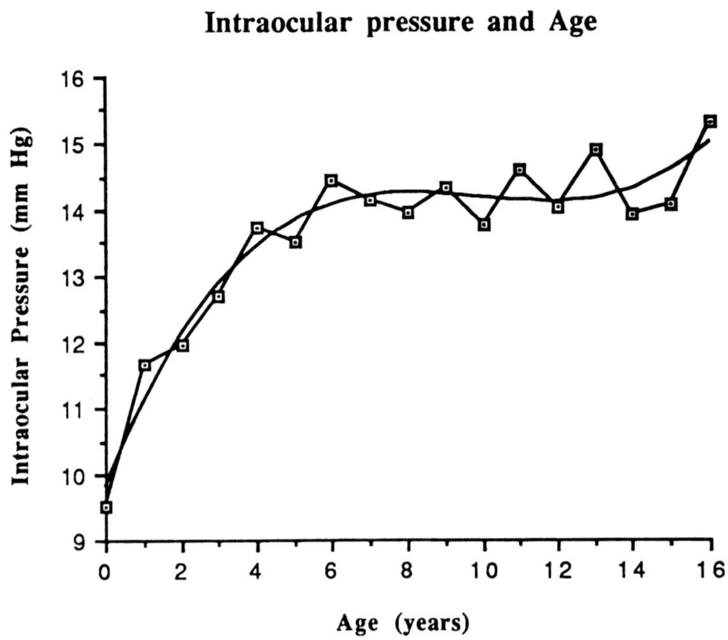

Figure 68.6. Normal IOP in children: variation with age. (Prepared using data from Pensiero, S, et al. Normal IOP in children. J Pediatr Ophthalmol Strabismus 29:79, 1992.)

actual IOP asymmetry between the eyes. The examiner might erroneously attach less importance to the elevated IOP in the glaucomatous eye, secure in the belief that it matched the falsely elevated IOP in the normal eye.

Anterior Segment Examination

Following tonometry (or attempts at it), use of the portable slit lamp allows more detailed inspection of the cornea and remainder of the anterior segment. An abnormally deep anterior chamber, or abnormalities of the iris may be additional clues to glaucoma in some cases (e.g. aniridia, Axenfeld-Rieger syndrome). Gonioscopy provides the most important anatomic information in the clinical examination regarding the mechanism of the glaucoma, and may sometimes be performed using Koeppe contact lenses and a portable slit lamp or loupes in the office (Fig. 68.7). Angle evaluation is then usually repeated in greater detail under anesthesia (unless glaucoma can be excluded from the office examination and findings). Gonioscopic findings are further discussed below.

Fundus Examination

Fundus examination centers on evaluation of the optic discs, although associated findings such as choroidal hemangioma (suggesting Sturge-Weber syndrome) can add useful information regarding the type of glaucoma present. If infant movements preclude direct ophthalmoscopic evaluation of the discs, indirect ophthalmoscopy using a 14 diopter lens can provide needed magnification. Recently described is a technique of posterior pole examination using a direct ophthalmoscope together with a 20 diopter condensing lens (23); this technique provides a view midway in magnification between that obtained with the direct and that obtained with the indirect ophthalmoscope and 20 diopter condensing lens. As with gonioscopy, disc examination should be repeated under anesthesia, unless normal findings and pressures have obviated this next step.

Refraction and Perimetry

Determination of refractive errors can be helpful, especially when they are asymmetric in the setting of probable unilateral glaucoma; in this case, **relative myopia of the affected eye supports the diagnosis of glaucoma.** Older

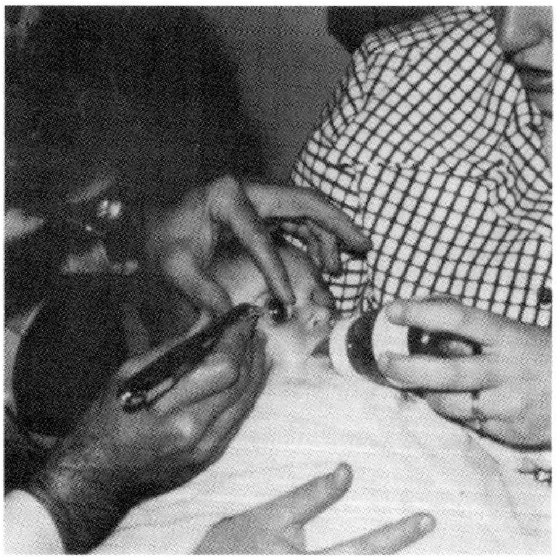

Figure 68.7. Office gonioscopy using Koeppe contact lens, hand-held slit lamp, and loupe magnifiers (From Walton, DS. Considerations peculiar to infants and children. In: Chandler and Grant's Glaucoma, third ed. Edited by Epstein, DL. Philadelphia, Lea & Febiger, 1986.)

children (beginning at six or seven years of age) can also undergo visual field examinations, allowing assessment of the extent of initial field loss, as well as stability of the remaining visual field over time (as one attempts to control the glaucoma). **Goldmann visual field testing is our choice for younger children**, since the tester may constantly encourage the patient, and may briefly suspend testing when fixation wanders or attention wanes. Teenage patients often perform well on standard automated perimetry programs, such as the Humphrey 24–2.

When one or more findings of the initial examination confirm or raise suspicions of childhood glaucoma, the administration of anesthesia is usually justified, both for a more complete examination as well as for probable surgical intervention.

EXAMINATION UNDER ANESTHESIA

General Anesthesia vs Sedation

General anesthesia in the operating room has advantages over sedation or anesthesia administered elsewhere, since it allows surgical intervention without further delay once the diagnosis of glaucoma is confirmed. An exception may be the use of chloral hydrate to facilitate office tonometry in the following patients: 1) patients felt unlikely actually to have glaucoma; 2) patients in whom the need for further surgical intervention seems unlikely, or in whom decision-making depends heavily upon obtaining IOP unaltered by inhaled anesthetics (see below).

Chloral Hydrate Sedation

Oral chloral hydrate sedation has been utilized by clinicians (pediatricians, pediatric ophthalmologists, radiologists and dentists) for many years, and may be particularly useful to the ophthalmologist when IOP determination is pivotal to decision-making in the office setting. **Chloral hydrate seems to minimally alter IOP recorded in children.** It has been stated that chloral hydrate is an effective short-term sedative that infrequently causes toxicity when administered orally at "appropriate dosages" (24) Jaafar and others have reported no serious systemic side effects with oral doses as high as 100 mg/kg for the first 10 kg, then 50 mg/kg for each additional kg body weight (25). **Recently, major medical centers have begun to formalize the setting under which "conscious sedation" may be performed (in compliance with JCAHO standards).** Key suggested guidelines include: 1) preprocedure evaluation of the patient by a physician prior to administration of medication; 2) informed consent to include risks of conscious sedation; 3) minimum of two personnel available (the operator, or physician performing the examination, as well as the monitor, or assistant trained to monitor the patient); 4) patient monitoring (and documentation on flowsheet) to include continuous pulse oximetry, as well as other vital signs and level of consciousness (recorded at least every 10 minutes); 5) minimum equipment available to include emergency airway equipment (e.g. oxygen and suction), pulse oximeter and blood pressure monitor, and cardiac arrest cart. Currently this policy at our institution limits oral chloral hydrate administration to 100 mg/kg, not to exceed a maximum dose of one gram.

Table 68.3
Examination Under General Anesthesia: Suggested Sequence

1. External examination (brief)
2. Tonometry (as early as possible after induction, and before intubation)
3. Corneal diameter measurement
4. Anterior segment examination
5. Koeppe gonioscopy
6. Fundus examination (optic disc)
7. (Optic disc photography)

Sequence of Examination Under Anesthesia

A logical sequence for examination under anesthesia (Table 68.3) begins with brief external examination, followed by IOP measurements. **Tonometry should be performed during the earliest possible moments after induction and before endotracheal intubation** (Fig. 68.8). One may then proceed with corneal diameter measurements (Fig. 68.9), followed by slit lamp examination of the anterior segment, and Koeppe gonioscopy and fundoscopy. Pupil dilation is performed only if results of the aforementioned examination are reassuring enough to obviate surgery. In this case, optic disc photography is also helpful in following children with glaucoma. Great care should be taken during administration of anesthesia and examination under anesthesia to avoid drying or damage to the corneal epithelium, as this may increase the difficulty and risk of subsequent surgical intervention (especially goniotomy).

Tonometry Under Anesthesia and Sedation

An unfortunate consequence of the anesthesia required for adequate examination is that IOP measurements are variably altered by sedatives, narcotics, and inhaled anesthetic agents (see Table 68.4). Jafaar and colleagues recently found no change in IOP recorded after high dose oral chloral hydrate (100 mg/kg for the first 10 kg, then 50 mg/kg for each additional kg body weight) was given to a group of 50 normal children under 6 years, as well as to a smaller group of children with glaucoma. **The mean IOP under chloral hydrate for normal eyes was 5.6 mm Hg by Perkins tonometry, and 14.7 mm Hg by Digilab pneumotonometry, while glaucomatous eyes measured 19.5 and 28.5 mm Hg, respectively** (25). Others have reported IOP in nonglaucomatous children under chloral hydrate ranging from 11–17 mm Hg by

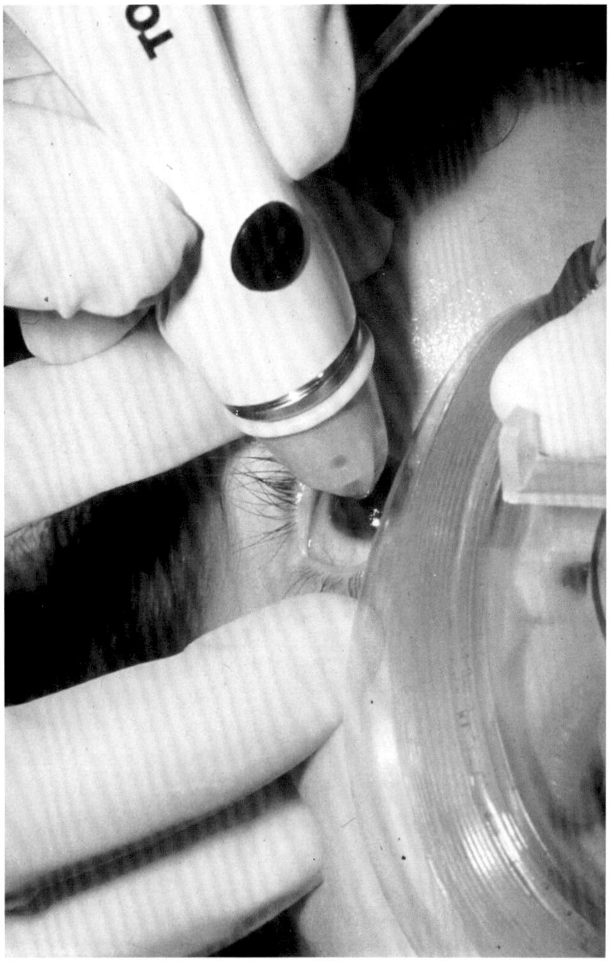

Figure 68.8. Measurement of IOP under anesthesia using the Tono-Pen tonometer.

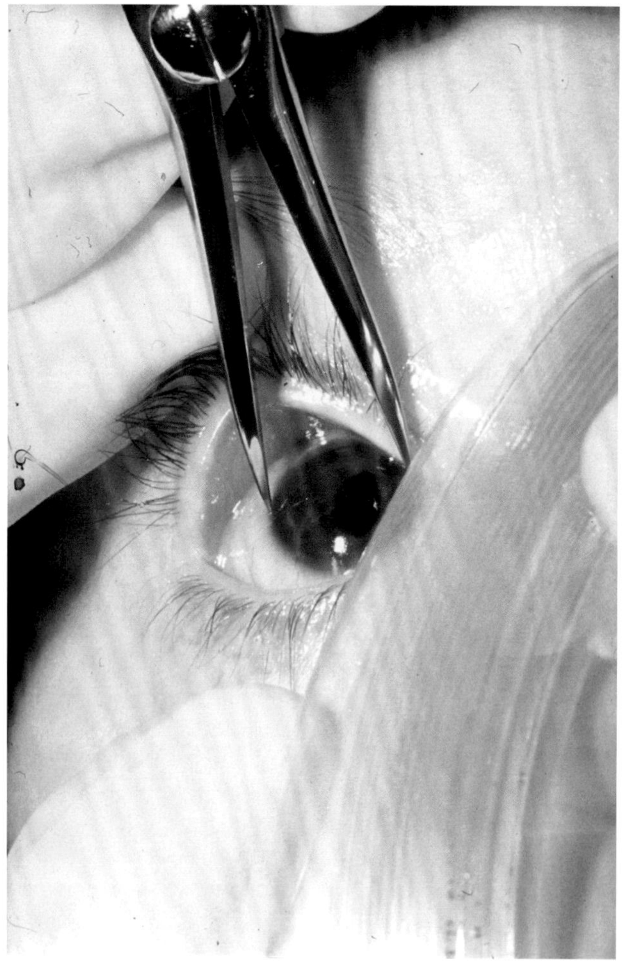

Figure 68.9. Measurement of horizontal corneal diameter under anesthesia using calipers.

Table 68.4
Intraocular Pressure and Sedatives/Anesthetics

Sedative/Anesthetic Agent	Route of Administration	Usual Effect on Intraocular Pressure
Chloral Hydrate	Oral or rectal	↔
Methohexital (Brevital)	Rectal, IM, IV	± ↓
Midazolam	Same as above	± ↓
Ketamine	Intramuscular	± ↑
Halothane (and similar agents)	Inhalation	↓ - ↓↓↓
Oxygen	Inhalation	↓
Nitrous Oxide/Oxygen	Inhalation	↓
Succinylcholine	IV	↑↑↑
Endotracheal Intubation		↑↑↑

Mackay-Marg tonometry (26). Ketamine has been variously reported to raise and to affect minimally the pressure in children (27,28).

Although there are conflicting reports, (29,30) **inhaled anesthetics (e.g., halothane and enflurane) are generally agreed to lower IOP measurements variably** (30). The normal IOP in an infant under halothane anesthesia is reported to be 9–10 mm Hg, with a pressure of 20 mm Hg or greater considered suspicious for glaucoma (31). IOP elevation is consistently reported after administration of succinylcholine, as well as with tracheal intubation (32). Even administration of 100% oxygen alone slightly lowers IOP (33), as does breathing nitrous oxide-oxygen mixtures (34).

Fortunately, although IOP measurements influenced by sedatives and anesthetics may vary greatly from true awake readings, high preanesthetic IOP usually remain in an abnormal range, even under anesthesia. **Asymmetric IOP measurements between fellow eyes more reliably indicate abnormality than do borderline IOP readings in both eyes taken under anesthesia.** IOP measurements under anesthesia should never be taken as the sole proof of glaucoma; if they are elevated in the setting of an otherwise negative glaucoma evaluation, conservative management and close observation are warranted. By contrast, when corneal and optic nerve abnormalities suggest glaucomatous damage, low IOP readings may be cause for repeat examination prior to surgical intervention, but should not provide false reassurance.

A comment about Schiotz indentation tonometry is worthwhile here, since many ophthalmologists may have ready access in the operating room to this instrument, but not to the Perkins applanation or Tono-Pen tonometers. While IOP measurement with Schiotz tonometry may be employed during examination under anesthesia, this technique has definite disadvantages. Because indentation tonometry is influenced by both scleral rigidity and corneal curvature and thickness (35), **IOP recorded in infants using Schiotz tonometry may differ significantly from that recorded by applanation**, depending upon the size and thickness of the cornea. For a given Schiotz pressure (1955 Calibration), the corresponding applanation IOP may be from five mm Hg higher to 7 mm Hg lower (David Walton, M.D., personal communication).

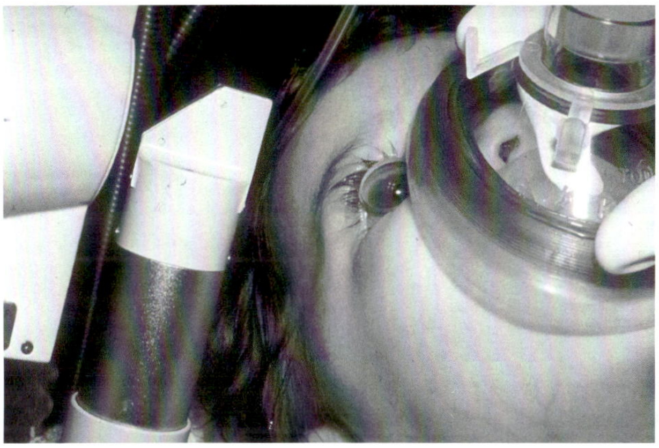

Figure 68.10. Gonioscopy under anesthesia using a Koeppe contact lens and a portable slit lamp.

Anterior Segment Examination

Corneal diameter measurements under anesthesia may be performed using a millimeter ruler held very close to the cornea; estimates of horizontal diameter to the nearest 0.25 mm may thus be made. Alternatively, a caliper (Fig. 68.9) ordinarily used for strabismus and other surgeries can be used for this purpose, with similar precision. Anterior segment examination with a portable slit lamp should be performed as described above for the office examination.

Gonioscopy Under Anesthesia

If the cornea is clear enough to permit it, gonioscopy should be performed using Koeppe gonioscopy lenses of proper size, together with a hand-held binocular microscope and Barkan focal illuminator, or a portable slit lamp (Fig. 68.10). Placing a Koeppe lens onto each eye at the

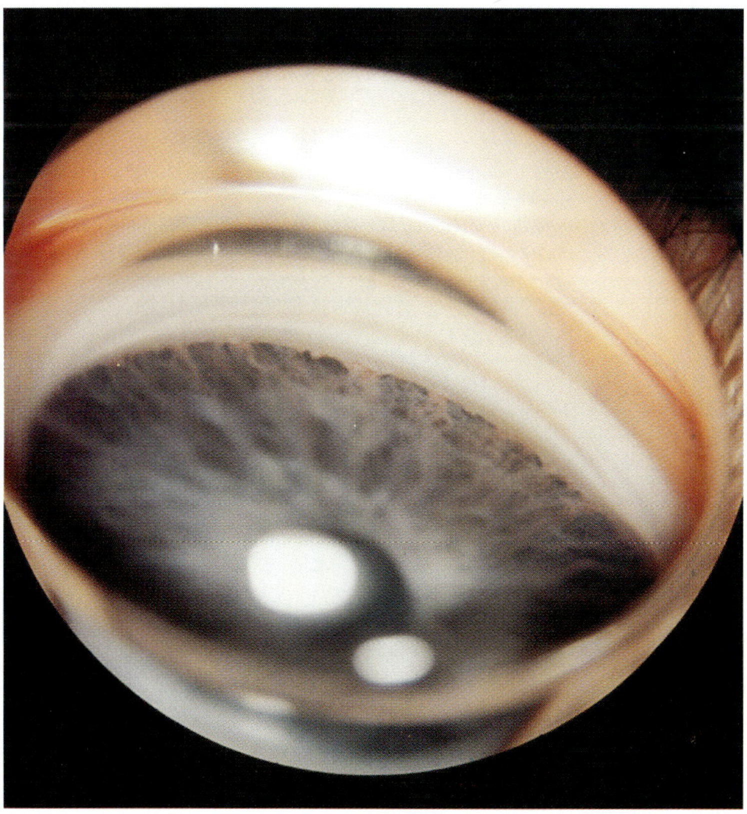

Figure 68.11. Gonioscopic view (through Koeppe gonioscopy lens) of an eye with infantile glaucoma.

same time facilitates comparison of the angle features in the fellow eyes.

Gonioscopic findings in normal infants and young children differ significantly from those of adults. Of the visible angle structures, the uveal meshwork (extending forward from peripheral iris onto corneoscleral meshwork) differs most greatly between the two age groups. In normal infants under one year of age the uveal meshwork is so delicate that the juncture of scleral spur and ciliary body band appears crisp and distinct. In later years, the uveal meshwork loses its early homogeneous, sheet-like appearance, and becomes a more coarse, lacy and open structure. In dark-eyed individuals, pigmentation of the uveal meshwork with increasing age increases visibility of this lacy structure.

The iris in infantile glaucoma often shows a more anterior insertion than that of the normal infant, with altered translucency of the angle face producing an indistinct ciliary body band, trabecular meshwork, and scleral spur (Fig. 68.11). The scalloped border of the iris pigment epithelium and the meshwork itself may be unusually prominent in infantile glaucoma, visible through the translucent peripheral iris stroma as if viewed through a "morning mist" (36,37). Juvenile open angle glaucoma patients (see Chapter 50) usually demonstrate a normal-appearing open angle, often with a prominent, lacy uveal meshwork.

Fundus Examination and Possible Surgery

After gonioscopy, direct ophthalmoscopy through a Koeppe lens (and undilated pupil) usually affords an excellent view of the optic nerves. At this point, if sufficient evidence suggests glaucoma, one may proceed directly to appropriate surgical intervention (see Chapters 69 and 70). Otherwise, if glaucoma is excluded, or conservative management indicated (as in the case of borderline pressures in the absence of suggestive corneal, angle, or optic nerve abnormalities), the pupils can be dilated. Pupil dilation facilitates photographic documentation of disc cupping, as well as cycloplegic refraction (although the latter can usually be performed with equal ease in the office setting, obviating prolonged anesthesia). Examination under anesthesia can often be accomplished entirely without endotracheal intubation in slightly older infants and children, until the need for surgical intervention has been confirmed in the operating room. If surgery is deferred, wake-up and recovery time for the patient may thereby be minimized.

References

1. Dickens CJ, Hoskins HD: Diagnosis and treatment of congenital glaucoma. In: The Glaucomas. Edited by Ritch R, Shields MB, Krupin T. St. Louis, C.V. Mosby Co., 1989.
2. Walton DS: Glaucoma in infants and children. In: Pediatric Ophthalmology. 3rd Ed. Edited by Nelson LB, Calhoun JH, Harley RD. Philadelphia, W.B. Saunders Company, 1991.
3. Scheie HG: Management of infantile glaucoma. Arch Ophthalmol 1959; 62:35.
4. Robin AL, et al: An analysis of visual acuity, visual fields, and disc cupping in childhood glaucoma. Am J Ophthalmol 1979;88:847.
5. Anderson JR: Hydrophthalmia or congenital glaucoma. London, Cambridge University Press, 1939.
6. Barkan O: Goniotomy. Trans Am Acad Ophthalmol 1955;59:322–332.
7. Scheie HG: Symposium on congenital glaucoma: diagnosis, clinical course and treatment other than goniotomy. Trans Am Acad Ophthalmol Otolaryngol 1955;59:309–321.
8. DeLuise VP, Anderson DR: Primary infantile glaucoma (Congenital glaucoma). Surv Ophthalmol 1983;28:1.
9. Sampaolesi R, Caruso R: Ocular echometry in the diagnosis of congenital glaucoma. Arch Ophthalmol 1982;100:54.
10. Becker B, Shaffer RN: Diagnosis and Therapy of the Glaucomas. St. Louis, C.V. Mosby, 1965.
11. Kiskis AA, Markowitz SN, Morin JD: Corneal diameter and axial length in congenital glaucoma. Can J Opththalmol 1985;20:93.
12. Richardson KT: Optic cup symmetry in normal newborn infants. Invest Ophthalmol 1968;7:137.
13. Shaffer RN, Hetherington J: Glaucomatous disc in infants. A suggested hypothesis for disc cupping. Trans Am Acad Ophthalmol Otolaryngol 1969;73:929.
14. Van Buskirk EM, Palmer EA: Office assessment of young children for glaucoma. Ann Ophthalmol 1979;11:1749.
15. Minckler DS, et al: Clinical evaluation of the Oculab Tono-Pen. Am J Ophthalmol 1987;104:168.
16. Mendelsohn AD, et al: Comparative tonometric measurements of eye bank eyes. Cornea 1987;6:219.
17. Armstrong TA: Evaluation of the Tono-Pen and the Pulsair tonometer. Am J Ophthalmol 1990;109:716.
18. Pensiero S, et al: Normal intraocular pressure in children. J Pediatr Ophthalmol Strabismus 1992;29:79.
19. Speirer A, Huna R, Hirsh A, et al: Normal intraocular pressure in premature infants. Am J Ophthalmol 1994;117:801.
20. Radtke ND, Cohen BF: Intraocular pressure measurement in the newborn. Am J Ophthalmol 1974;78:501.
21. Jaafar MS, Kazi GA: A comparative study of the Perkins applanation tonometer and the pneumotonometer. J Pediatr Ophthalmol Strabismus 1993;30:284.
22. Musarella MA, Morin JD: Anterior segment and intraocular pressure measurements of the unanesthetized premature infant. Metab Pediatr Syst Ophthalmol 1985;8:53.
23. Paysse EA, Helveston EM: Modified indirect opthalmoscopy for evaluation of the pediatric retina. Am Assoc Ped Ophthalmol Strabismus Abstract Book 1994;9.
24. American Academy of Pediatrics: Committee on Drugs and Committee on Environmental Health. Use of chloral hydrate for sedation in children. Pediatrics 1993;92:471.
25. Jaafar MS, Ghulamqadir AK: Effect of oral chloral hydrate sedation on the intraocular pressure measurement. J Ped Ophthalmol Strabismus 1993;30:372.
26. Judisch GF, Anderson S, Bell WE: Chloral hydrate sedation as a substitute for examination under anesthesia in pediatric ophthalmology. Am J Ophthalmol 1980;89:560–563.
27. Ausinsch B, Rayburn RL, Munson ES, et al: Ketamine and intraocular pressure in children. Anesth Analg 1976;55:773.
28. Yoshikawa K, Murai Y: The effect of ketamine on intraocular pressure in children. Anesth Analg 1971;50:199.
29. Watcha MF, Chu FC, Stevens JL, et al: Effects of halothane on intraocular pressure in anesthetized children. Anesth Analg 1990;71:181.
30. Murphy DF: Anesthesia and intraocular pressure. Anesth Analg 1985; 64:520.
31. Dominiguez A, et al: Intraocular pressure measurement in infants under general anesthesia. Am J Ophthalmol 1974;78:110.
32. Joshi C, Bruce DL: Thiopental and succinylcholine: action on intraocular pressure. Anesth Analg 1975;54:471.

33. Gallin-Cohen PF, Podos SM, Yablonski ME: Oxygen lowers intraocular pressure. Invest Opthalmol Vis Sci 1980;19:43.
34. Gunderson CA, et al: Nitrous oxide—effects on intraocular pressure. Invest Ophthalmol Vis Sci 1994;35 Suppl:2178.
35. Friedenwald JS: Some problems in the calibration of tonometers. Am J Ophthalmol 1948;31:935.
36. Barkan O: Pathogenesis of congenital glaucoma: gonioscopic and anatomic observation of the angle of the anterior chamber in the normal eye and in congenital glaucoma. Am J Ophthalmol 1955;40:1.
37. Worst JGF: The pathogenesis of congenital glaucoma. An embryological and goniosurgical study. Springfield, Ill, Charles C. Thomas, 1966.

Primary Congenital Open Angle Glaucoma 69

Edward G. Buckley

DEFINITION

Primary congenital open angle glaucoma (trabeculodysgenesis), commonly referred to as congenital glaucoma or infantile glaucoma, is a specific inherited developmental defect of the trabecular meshwork and anterior chamber angle in which the angle appears to be "open" in the sense that the iris and corneoscleral trabecular meshwork are separated (1). It is a significant cause of childhood blindness and is the most common type of glaucoma in infants. Characteristically it manifests itself in the neonatal or infantile period with clouding and enlargement of the cornea, buphthalmos, epiphora, photophobia, and blepharospasm (Fig. 69.1) (2–7). Because of its relative rarity, it is often misdiagnosed and confused with inflammatory or infectious processes affecting the conjunctiva, cornea, and lids (7). Approximately 25% of patients are diagnosed at birth, more than 60% are diagnosed by age 6 months, and greater than 80% will have their onset within the first year of life (3,5). Primary infantile glaucoma can occur in later childhood and then it is commonly termed "juvenile glaucoma." This type is usually not associated with buphthalmos and corneal enlargement, although these can continue to occur until ages 6–8 years (8).

Primary congenital glaucoma can be distinguished from secondary infantile glaucoma by the absence of easily recognizable congenital abnormalities of the iris (such as aniridia), obvious obstructions of the trabecular meshwork (such as iridocorneal dysgenesis), and other metabolic inflammatory or congenital diseases of the eye. A classification of childhood glaucoma is shown in Chapter 68.

DEMOGRAPHICS

Primary infantile glaucoma occurs in approximately .01% of children (1 out of 10,000 births) and results in blindness in 2–15% of individuals (Table 69.1) (9,10). **It is bilateral in 60–80% of patients and occurs more frequently in males (65%) than females (35%)** (9–11). There is no racial or geographic predilection.

INHERITANCE

Most cases of primary congenital glaucoma occur sporadically. However, an autosomal recessive form with variable expressivity has been described (7,12,13). A review of 64 families of patients with congenital glaucoma revealed three patients who had affected siblings and two families that had an affected parent (8). In two of these families glaucoma occurred in monozygotic twins. We and others have noted that in monozygotic twin pairs, both children appear to be affected whereas in dizygotic twin pairs only one child is usually affected (13–15). The fact that primary congenital glaucoma occurs in parent and sibling with approximate equal frequency, has an unequal distribution by sex, and occurs in multiple siblings of healthy parents supports an autosomal recessive inheritance pattern which is polygenic, multifactorial, and has variable penetrance (8,15).

Adult primary open angle glaucoma does not appear to be associated with primary infantile glaucoma. Steroid induced elevations of intraocular pressure (IOP), a risk factor for adult primary open angle glaucoma, occur no more frequently among parents of infants with primary infantile glaucoma than in the non-affected general population (7).

Hafez and co-workers (16) examined the correlation between human leucocyte antigen (HLA) and primary congenital glaucoma. Family studies revealed an autosomal recessive gene predisposing to congenital glaucoma with strong linkage to the HLA-B8 antigen.

Because of the known occurrence of primary congenital open angle glaucoma in siblings and in offspring of parents with childhood glaucoma, it is important to council parents about the probability of future offspring having the disease and to examine and follow the younger and older siblings of patients who have this glaucoma. **The chance of a second child having the disease is approximately 1–3%. If two children have the disease, the likelihood that subsequent children will be affected increases to as much as 25%** (7). Frequent examinations of these infants are important especially during the first six to twelve months of life. A single examination during the first month of life is inadequate.

PATHOGENESIS

The exact etiology of primary congenital glaucoma still remains obscure. Originally Barkan, and later Worst, proposed that an imperfect, thin "glass" membrane covered the anterior chamber angle and blocked aqueous outflow (17,18). To date, the presence of this membrane has not been established histopathologically. Most authorities now

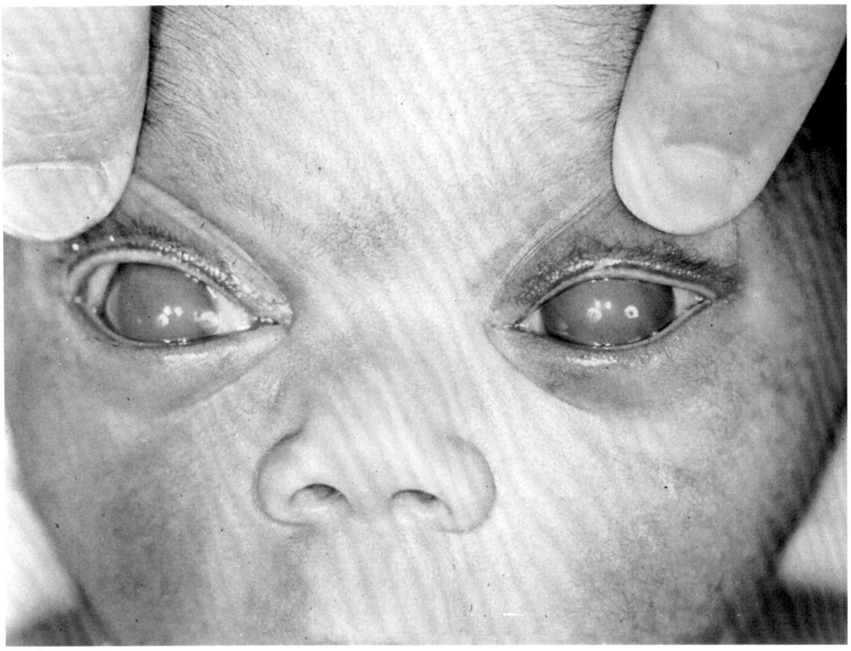

Figure 69.1. Seven day old infant with bilateral primary congenital glaucoma. Note marked corneal haze and enlargement. IOPs were 35 mm Hg OU. The patient required bilateral trabeculotomies.

Table 69.1.
Visual Loss in Primary Congenital Glaucoma

Amblyopia
Anisometropia
Strabismic
Corneal scarring
Myopic astigmatism
Cataracts
Optic nerve damage

believe that the site of obstruction is the trabecular meshwork rather than an overlying membrane (19,20).

A major obstacle to our understanding the etiology of primary infantile glaucoma is our lack of knowledge about the normal development of the anterior chamber angle. Allen, Burian, and Braley postulated that the anterior chamber angle normally forms by cleavage of mesoderm and that incomplete separation of the layers results in the formation of abnormal trabecular meshwork and, subsequently, infantile glaucoma (21). Mann postulated that the anterior chamber angle was formed by mesodermal atrophy rather than cleavage, and failure of this process resulted in retention of abnormal tissue in the trabecular meshwork that blocked aqueous outflow (6). Anderson concluded that the development of the anterior chamber does not occur by cleavage or atrophy, but by posterior sliding of uveal tissues in relation to the cornea and sclera (Fig. 69.2), and a repositioning of the various layers within the uveal tract along the inner side of the sclera (20). He suggested that premature or excessive formation of collagenous beams within the trabecular meshwork prevents the normal posterior sliding of the ciliary body and peripheral iris which results in an anterior insertion of the uvea into the trabecular meshwork with compression of the anterior trabecular spaces and blockage of aqueous outflow (20). His theory is consistent with the theory of Maumenee, who suggested that the abnormal insertion of the longitudinal ciliary muscle into the trabecular meshwork compresses the trabecular sheets when the muscle contracts (22). Shields has noted a similar microscopic appearance of the anterior chamber angle in eyes of patients with Axenfeld-Rieger's syndrome, although the ultrastructural appearance in these cases suggest that the compactness of the trabecular meshwork may be due to failure of the intertrabecular spaces to develop, rather than to subsequent mechanical compression (Fig. 69.3) (19).

The concept of a fundamental defect in cellular development was supported by Smelser and Ozanics (23) who proposed that normally there is a gradual rearrangement of mesodermal cells to form the anterior chamber angle and that failure of this process results in structural changes of the uveal meshwork which result in aqueous obstruction. The developmental process may be modulated by neural crest cells which appear to be the precursors to many of the anterior chamber structures. Kupfer has proposed that it is the faulty migration or differentiation of these cells that may result in the defects seen in the various types of congenital glaucoma (24). The occasional association of primary congenital glaucoma with other systemic anomalies may be explained in part by a common neural crest origin of the affected tissues.

It therefore appears that a true "Barkan's membrane" probably does not exist and that primary con-

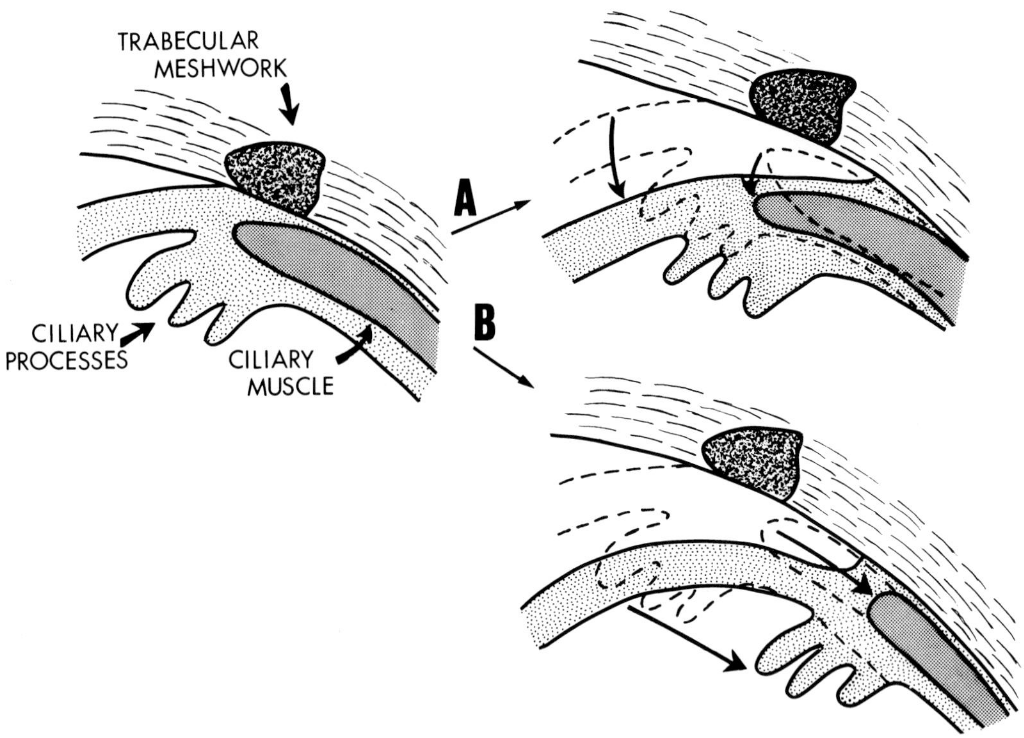

Figure 69.2. Process of exposing the trabecular meshwork to the anterior chamber during development. If the uveal tract simply splits away (A) by cleavage or by atrophy of tissue, the result would be an angle configuration in which the ciliary muscle extends into the iris and the ciliary processes are on the back of the iris. However, with slippage of the layers (B) due to differential growth rate, the ciliary muscle and the ciliary processes that initially overlapped the trabecular meshwork surface come to lie posteriorly. (Reprinted from Anderson DR: Trans Am Ophthal Soc 1981;79:461, with permission.)

genital glaucoma results from a developmental arrest of anterior chamber tissue derived from neural crest cells. Structurally this is manifested by the high insertion of ciliary body and iris into the posterior portion of the trabecular meshwork. The actual mechanism of aqueous outflow obstruction is uncertain and may result from compression of the trabecular beams, abnormal development of the trabecular meshwork or Schlemm's canal, or the persistence of some precursor material in the anterior chamber angle.

CLINICAL MANIFESTATIONS

The clinical appearance of an infant with primary congenital glaucoma is often striking. **The child normally presents during the first months of life with a history of epiphora, blepharospasm, and photophobia** (Fig. 69.4). **These findings are often initially confused with conjunctivitis or nasolacrimal duct obstruction and the child may have already been treated for these entities** (Fig. 69.5) (25). The most characteristic symptom is photophobia which causes the child to keep the eyes closed in light, to shy away from bright lights, and to blink excessively. This is often accompanied by moderate tearing, and, in older infants, by rubbing of the eyes. The photophobia appears to be related to corneal edema. The symptoms can be gradual in onset or occur suddenly as a result of rupturing of Descemet's membrane.

Although common, these symptoms are frequently not present. In a study by Seidman and co-workers, epiphora or photophobia were present in only half of the cases and the combination was present in approximately one third (26). **Parents were as likely to notice signs of glaucoma (corneal clouding and enlargement) as they were to notice symptoms.**

The classic signs (Table 69.2) of primary congenital glaucoma include corneal enlargement, enlargement of the globe, corneal clouding, and cupping of the optic disc. In children with bilateral enlarged corneas, particularly in the absence of visible corneal edema, recognition may be delayed as parents believe their baby's "big eyes" enhance his or her appearance (Fig. 69.6) (26). When local areas of corneal opacification are present, associated curvilinear breaks of Descemet's membrane, **Haab's striae,** are almost always found. The anterior chamber of an affected eye can be strikingly deep compared to the usual shallow infantile anterior chamber.

The severity of presenting signs and symptoms varies from patient to patient presumably because of differences in the elevation of IOP. Infants born with grey edematous and enlarged corneas (Fig. 69.1) presumably have had high IOP even before birth, while those infants in whom signs

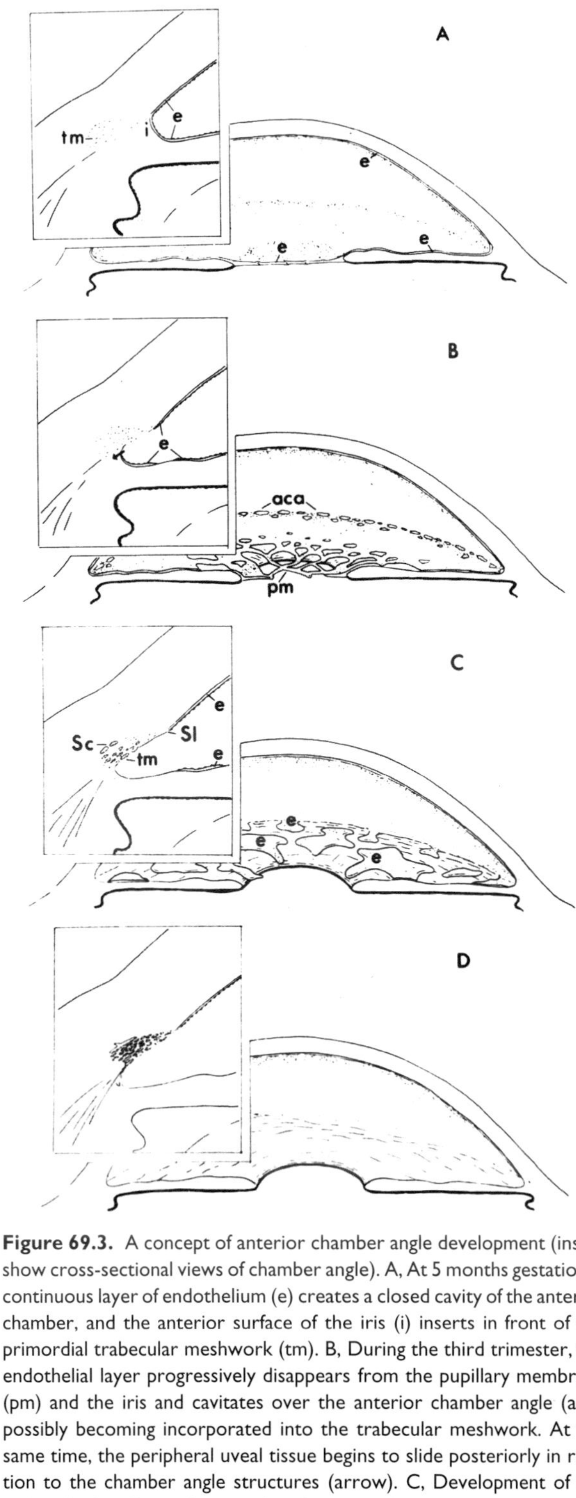

Figure 69.3. A concept of anterior chamber angle development (insets show cross-sectional views of chamber angle). A, At 5 months gestation, a continuous layer of endothelium (e) creates a closed cavity of the anterior chamber, and the anterior surface of the iris (i) inserts in front of the primordial trabecular meshwork (tm). B, During the third trimester, the endothelial layer progressively disappears from the pupillary membrane (pm) and the iris and cavitates over the anterior chamber angle (aca), possibly becoming incorporated into the trabecular meshwork. At the same time, the peripheral uveal tissue begins to slide posteriorly in relation to the chamber angle structures (arrow). C, Development of the trabecular lamellae and intertrabecular spaces begins in the inner, posterior aspect of the primordial tissue and progresses toward Schlemm's canal (Sc) and Schwalbe's line (Sl). D, The normal anterior chamber angle is not fully developed until 1 year of life. (Reprinted from Shields MB: Trans Am Ophthal Soc 1983;81:736 with permission.)

Table 69.2
Clinical Characteristics of Infants and Children with Primary Infantile Glaucoma

Clinical Characteristics	% of Infants and Children
Problems noted by parents	
Tearing	55
Photophobia	41
Tearing and photophobia	32
Corneal haze	41
Corneal enlargement	32
Signs noted by initial physician	
Corneal haze	83
Corneal/global enlargement	58
Corneal clouding and/or enlargement	92
Bilateral involvement	58
Male/Female	54/46

Reprinted from Seidman DJ, Nelson LB, Calhoun JH, et al: Signs and symptoms in the presentation of primary infantile glaucoma. Pediatrics 1986;77:399.

are present with minimal symptoms may have had a gradual rise in IOP after birth (Fig. 69.7). **In some cases of bilateral glaucoma the characteristic signs are much more evident in one eye than the other and, when the infant is initially examined, the diagnosis in the less affected eye may not be suspected.**

Nystagmus is seldom noted in primary congenital open angle glaucoma although it is common in aniridia and in glaucoma secondary to surgery for congenital cataracts. When nystagmus does occur in congenital glaucoma it is usually due to severe early loss of vision and is often pendular or searching in nature (8).

THE DIAGNOSTIC EXAMINATION

Some of the clinical findings in congenital glaucoma such as buphthalmos, enlarged corneal diameter, and corneal edema can be seen on gross inspection and do not require complicated examinations and techniques. The differential diagnosis of congenital glaucoma is listed in Table 69.3. Each of these conditions can be distinguished by means of a thorough ophthalmic evaluation which includes tonometry, measurement of corneal diameter, gonioscopy, and funduscopic examination. A very thorough explanation of these is given in Chapter 68.

It is important to note that determining the presence or absence of primary congenital glaucoma is not always easy. **There are equivocal cases in which some of the features may be missing and some of the evidence may be weak.** The correct diagnosis and further decision as to the proper form of treatment necessitate considering all the factors previously mentioned.

DIFFERENTIAL DIAGNOSIS

The diagnosis of primary congenital glaucoma is very straightforward when the classic triad of symptoms (epiphora, blepharospasm and photophobia) and signs (corneal

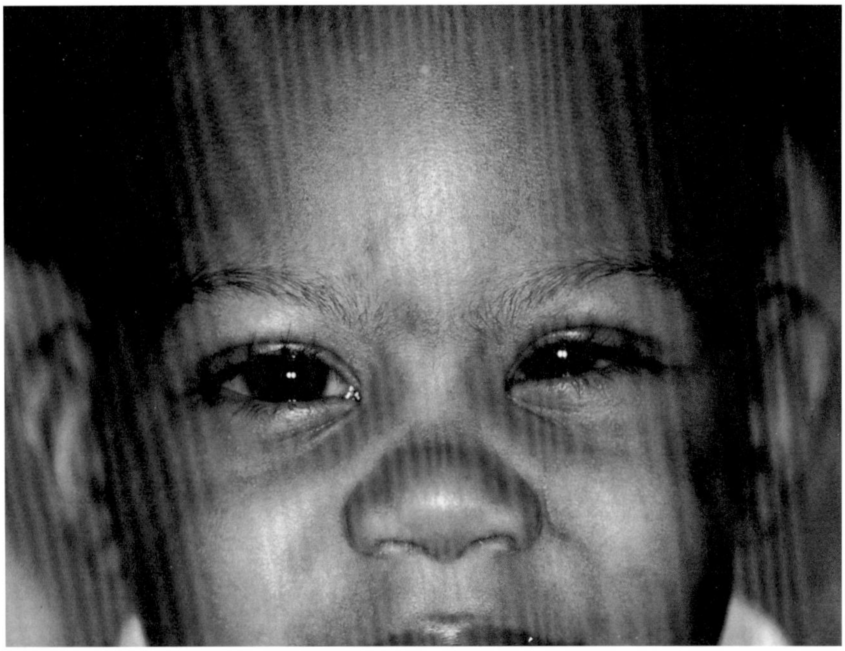

Figure 69.4. Patient demonstrating photophobia. Often patients with elevated IOP will be extremely sensitive to light. Squinting and tearing are important signs.

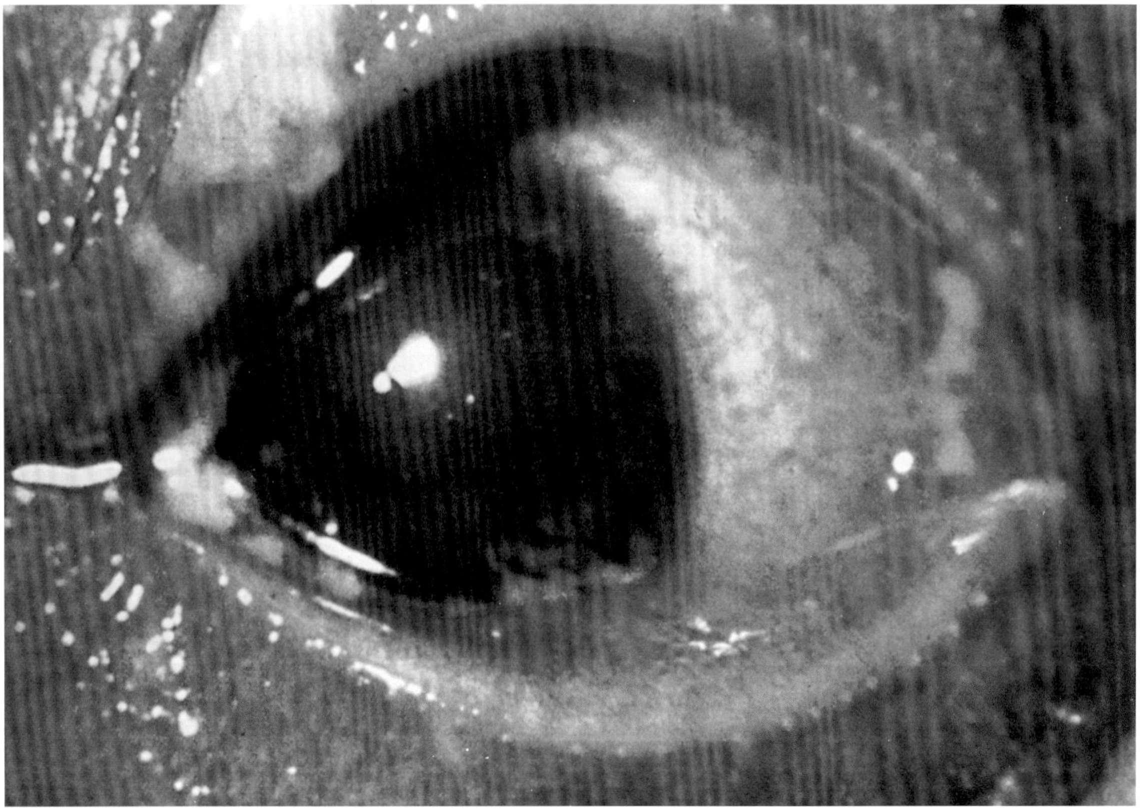

Figure 69.5. Patient with neonatal conjunctivitis. Presenting symptoms were photophobia, scleral injection, and discharge. The hallmark of an infection versus glaucoma is the presence of a purulent discharge.

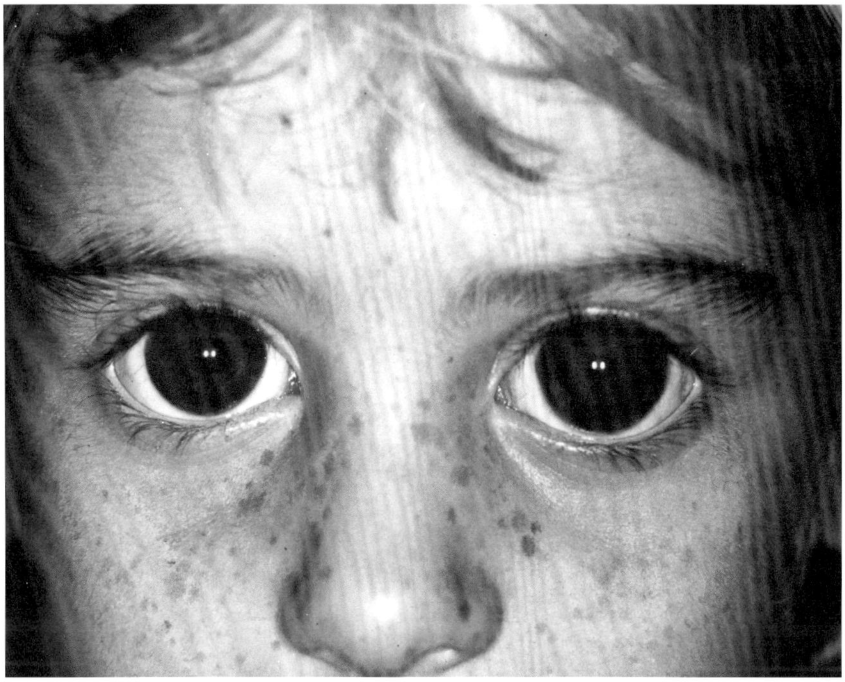

Figure 69.6. Patient with bilateral enlarged corneas and normal IOPs. The patient's refraction was +2.00 OD and +1.00 OS.

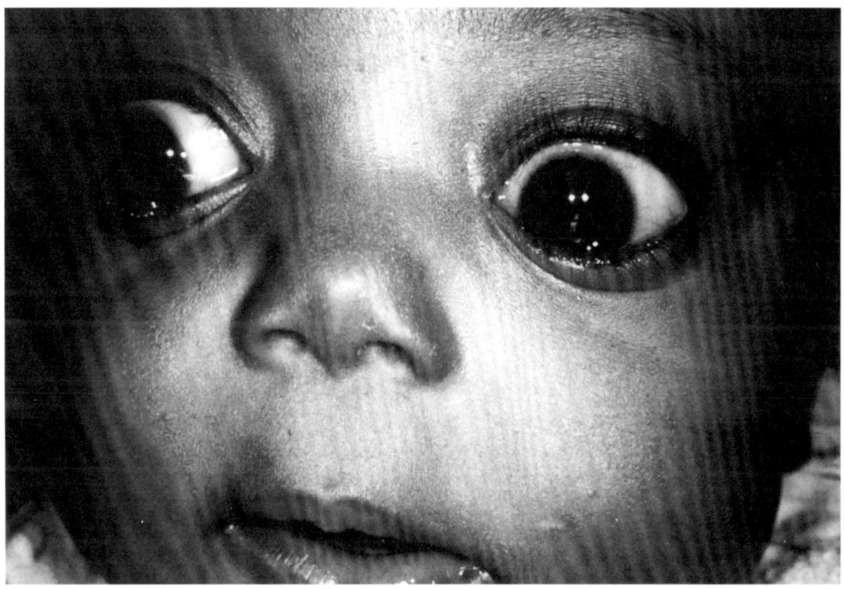

Figure 69.7. Bilateral buphthalmos. Note markedly enlarged globes with enlarged corneas. IOP was 25 mm Hg OU. Buphthalmos without corneal edema tends to occur with moderately elevated IOP. This patient responded well to goniotomies.

enlargement, corneal haze, and buphthalmos) are present. Interpretation of the child's eye problem with respect to glaucoma is more difficult in the absence of these pathognomic signs and other entities such as those listed in Table 69.3 should be considered (2,7,9).

In the absence of corneal haze or buphthalmos, abnormalities of the ocular surface or drainage system should be considered. Epiphora alone suggests nasolacrimal duct obstruction and a lacrimal duct probing should be entertained to confirm a diagnosis. A red eye plus epiphora and blepharospasm suggests an ocular infection or inflammation. In the absence of positive findings, a therapeutic trial or careful observation may be indicated.

Buphthalmos and corneal enlargement may be due to a congenital anomaly. **Megalocornea is a rare x-linked recessive condition of abnormal corneal enlargement, usually greater than 14 mm, with a deep anterior chamber, iridodonesis, normal IOP, absence of Haab's striae, and no optic nerve cupping** (7). Enlargement is practically always bilateral and symmetrical. Corneas may be thin but there is absence of photophobia, discomfort, edema, or clouding. Families have been reported in which

Table 69.3
Differential Diagnosis of Symptoms and Signs in Primary Infantile Glaucoma

I. Conditions sharing signs of epiphora and "red eye"
  A. Conjunctivitis
  B. Congenital nasolacrimal duct obstruction
  C. Corneal epithelial defect/abrasion
  D. Ocular inflammation (uveitis, trauma)
II. Conditions sharing signs of corneal edema or opacification
  A. Corneal dystrophy
    1. Congenital hereditary endothelial dystrophy
    2. Posterior polymorphous dystrophy
  B. Obstetrical birth trauma with Descemet's tears
  C. Storage disease
    1. Mucopolysaccharidoses
    2. Cystinosis
  D. Congenital anomalies
    1. Sclerocornea
    2. Peter's anomaly
  E. Keratitis
    1. Maternal rubella keratitis
    2. Herpetic
    3. Phlectenular
  F. Idiopathic (diagnosis of exclusion only)
III. Conditions sharing signs of corneal enlargement
  A. Axial myopia
  B. Megalocornea
IV. Conditions sharing sign of optic nerve cupping (real or apparent)
  A. Physiologic optic nerve cupping
  B. Optic nerve coloboma
  C. Optic atrophy
  D. Optic nerve hypoplasia
  E. Optic nerve malformation

some members have megalocornea and others have primary infantile glaucoma (5). Careful follow up is necessary to search for possible increased IOP changes indicative of primary infantile glaucoma (5,27).

Axial myopia can mimic a large buphthalmic eye and is commonly associated with corneal enlargement (Fig. 69.8). Funduscopic examination, however, is quite characteristic with a tilted insertion of the optic nerve, myopic crescent, and retinal pigmentary and choroidal abnormalities.

Corneal edema or opacities can be caused by breaks in Descemet's membrane, corneal dystrophies, or with abnormalities in metabolism such as storage diseases of mucopolysaccharides, gangliosides, or sphingomyelin. **Birth trauma may result in vertical breaks in Descemet's membrane with resultant corneal edema.** Obstetrical corneal trauma is usually unilateral (left greater than right because of the higher incidence of left occipital anterior presentation) and associated with signs of skin bruising as a result of the trauma. It is often stated that Descemet's membrane breaks from trauma are vertically oriented while those caused by increased IOP are horizontal. However, traumatic injuries can also be curvilinear and run diagonally across the cornea, but there is no corneal enlargement, and IOPs are normal.

Corneal dystrophic changes that most closely mimic primary congenital open angle glaucoma are severe infantile posterior polymorphous dystrophy (Fig. 69.9) and congenital hereditary endothelial dystrophy. In severe infantile posterior polymorphous dystrophy the patient often experiences a period of photophobia in the first year of life. A diffuse irregular thickening and opacification at the level of Descemet's membrane is found. The posterior surface of the cornea sometimes resembles "alligator skin" but the corneal diameters are normal. Some temporary elevation of IOP may occur, but the symptoms and disturbance of the corneas do not appear to be related to the IOP. It is an autosomal recessive condition.

Congenital hereditary endothelial dystrophy (CHED) is characterized by diffusely opacified and thickened corneal stroma. Abnormalities are seen clinically at the level of Descemet's membrane.

Metabolic diseases that produce corneal opacification are usually associated with obvious systemic abnormalities. Such entities as oculo-cerebral-renal syndrome of Lowe, mucopolysaccharidosis, cystinoses, and corneal lipidosis can produce corneal clouding, mimicking the corneal edema of primary infantile glaucoma.

It is important to remember that although primary congenital glaucoma is the most common form of glaucoma in early life, it is not the only form, and that the signs associated with this entity such as corneal enlargement, breaks in Descemet's membrane and edematous cornea, are abnormalities that can also be associated with the other types of glaucomas discussed in the following chapters.

TREATMENT

There are multiple treatment modalities available to aide in the control of IOP in primary congenital glaucoma. **The primary intervention is surgical and the initial procedure is usually a goniotomy or trabeculotomy** (Fig. 69.10). Pharmacologic agents, however, are often necessary to optimize pressure control. A complete explanation of the surgical procedures and medications used to control pediatric glaucoma can be found in Chapter 70.

Medical Treatment

INDICATIONS

Even though primary congenital glaucoma usually requires a surgical intervention, the role of pharmacological agents is significant. First, most patients are placed on some form of topical or oral medication to reduce IOP in preparation for surgery. In those patients who have significant corneal edema, preoperative management of the IOP has been advocated to clear the cornea which increases surgical safety and reduces complications. This is especially important if goniotomy is to be attempted. Secondly, medical therapy is often used as a temporizing measure to control IOP

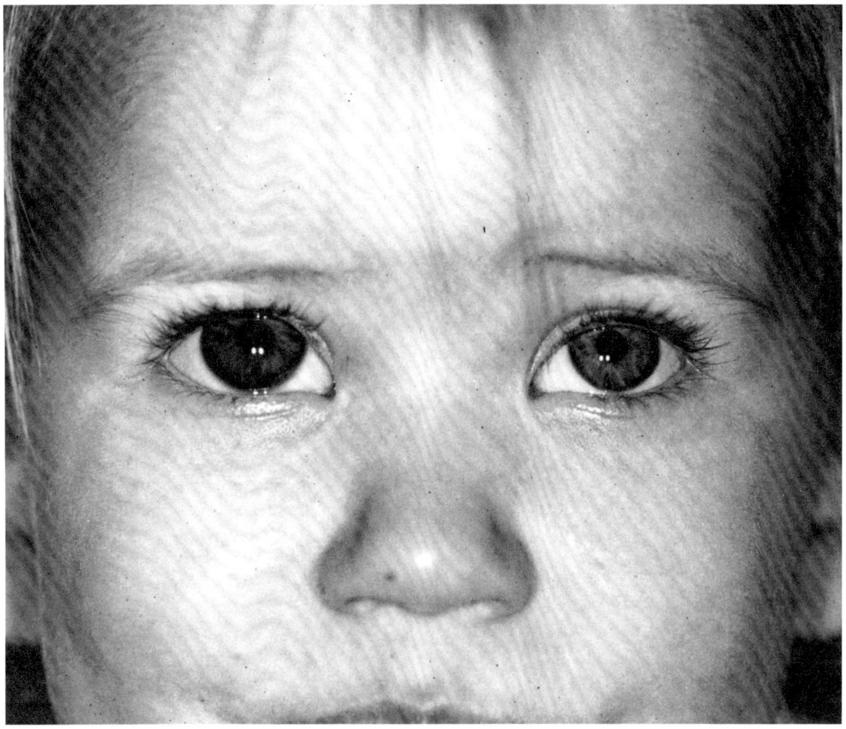

Figure 69.8. Patient with unilateral buphthalmos secondary to axial myopia. Refraction of the right eye is − 17 D. Aggressive rehabilitation is necessary to avoid visual loss from anisometropic amblyopia.

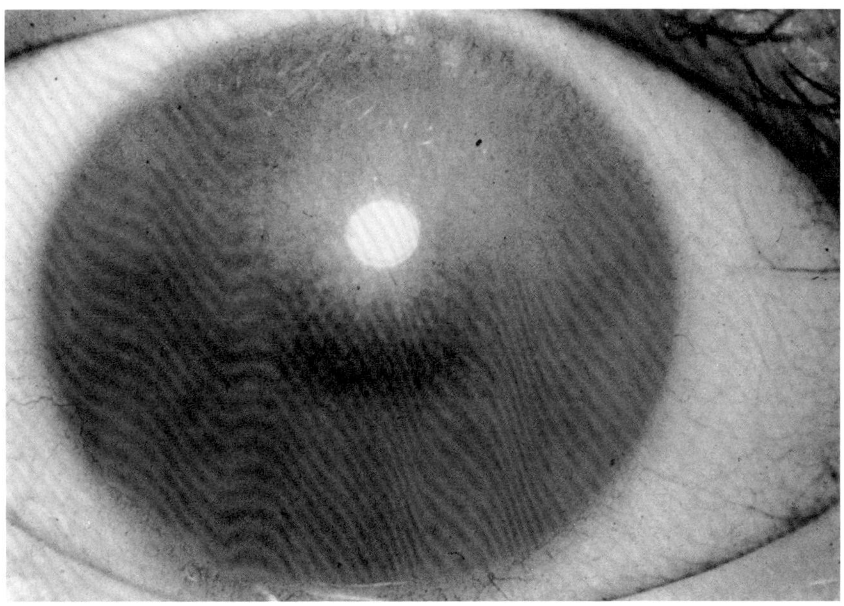

Figure 69.9. Posterior polymorphous corneal dystrophy. Note extensive corneal haze without corneal enlargement or elevated IOP.

between surgical procedures or to enhance control in those borderline situations where deferral of surgery is necessary. Lastly, in those patients with severe disease who have been unresponsive to surgical interventions, medications can be used to reduce IOP to the level which may preserve some visual function. Because surgery is performed in the vast majority of patients with primary infantile glaucoma, there are no long term studies using medical treatment alone (7).

TOPICAL MEDICATIONS

By far the most commonly used topical medication to reduce IOP in primary congenital glaucoma is a **beta blocker**, typically timolol (28,29). Timolol appears to be well tolerated in the pediatric population with minimal side effects in most patients. Beta blockers can exacerbate pre-existing asthma and may produce bradycardia; therefore, patients on this therapy should be closely followed

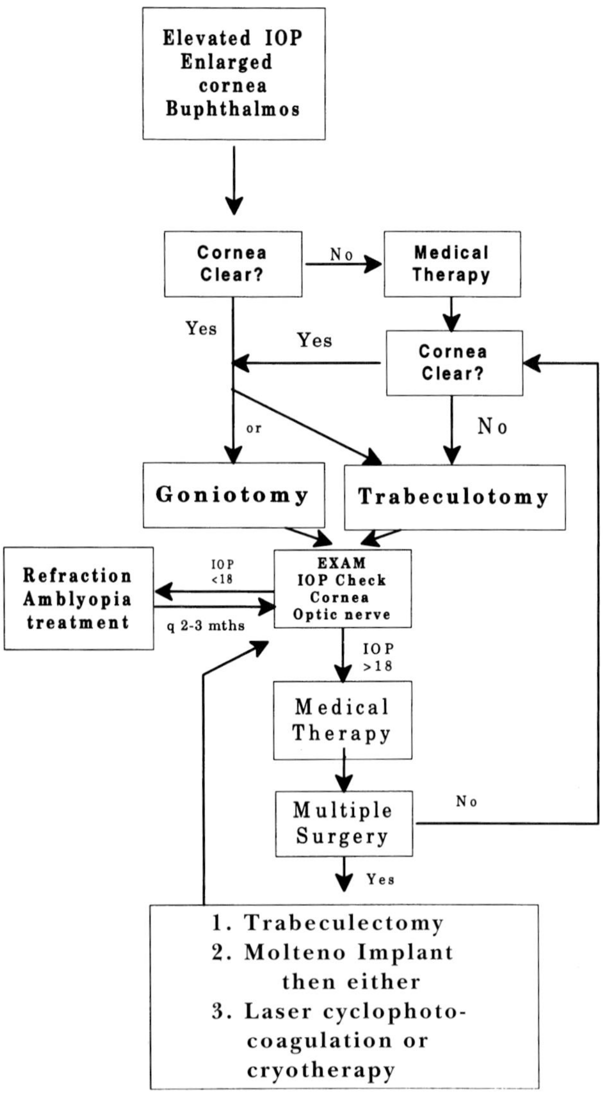

Figure 69.10. Flow charts demonstrating treatment options for primary congenital glaucoma. Cryotherapy can be entertained to clear the cornea or to control pressure prior to surgical intervention. Once pressure is controlled, frequent checks for reoccurrence and to manage refractive errors for amblyopia are important. In patients requiring multiple surgical procedures, secondary procedures may be necessary.

by a pediatrician. Due to small patient size and the corresponding volume of distribution, it is advisable to use the 0.25% concentration of timolol in the pediatric population. However, there is very little specific information about its effectiveness when used solely for primary congenital glaucoma. Boger and Walton found timolol to be effective in their patients and noted that this effect appeared to remain for over two years (28). Timolol also has an additive effect when combined with other topical or oral medications.

Other topical medications, while helpful in adult glaucoma, appear to be less effective in primary congenital glaucoma. **Miotics** such as pilocarpine or echothiophate

Table 69.4
Surgical Results in Congenital Glaucoma (age <1 year)

			Success (%)	
	Date	Eyes	1st	2nd
Goniotomy				
Barkan	1953	185	80	
Haas	1955	253	77	
Bietti	1966	321	82	
Shaffer	1967	100	85	
Morin	1980	171	56	76
Anderson	1982	16	81	100
McPherson	1983	24	33	83
Trabeculotomy				
Harms	1969	30	93	
Gregerson	1977	21	100	88
Anderson	1982	25	76	100
McPherson	1983	23	83	

Modified from deLuise and Anderson (7).

iodide (Phospholine Iodide) are usually not effective because of the abnormal insertion of the ciliary muscle into trabecular meshwork in congenital glaucoma. However, on occasion, echothiophate iodide can produce a significant pressure reduction in those patients who have been unresponsive to other topical medications. Epinephrine, theoretically, should be helpful in primary congenital glaucoma by improving aqueous outflow. Unfortunately, as in adult glaucoma, when used as an adjunct to a beta blocking agent, it results in little further reduction in IOP. There is no information available on its effectiveness as a solitary agent. There are no data available regarding the use of the alpha-2 agonist, apraclonidine (Iopidine). (See Chapter 70 for more detailed information on topical medications.)

ORAL MEDICATIONS

By far the most effective medication for the reduction of IOP in children with primary congenital glaucoma is acetazolamide (Diamox). When used in dosages of 5–15 mg per kg per day, acetazolamide can reduce IOP by as much as 10–15 mm Hg. In patients with extremely high IOP or who have significant corneal edema and buphthalmos, acetazolamide is quite effective in reducing the IOP until surgical intervention can be performed. In those patients who are unresponsive to surgical interventions, acetazolamide is often the only medication which is effective. Long-term use of this medication in the pediatric population appears to be safe. However, there have been several case reports of aplastic anemia developing in adult patients on acetazolamide therapy.

Surgical Treatment

The surgical procedures commonly used to treat primary congenital glaucoma are goniotomy and trabeculotomy ab externo (Table 69.4). There are proponents of each procedure and each has its merits. Hoskins (30) and Walton (8) favor goniotomy as the procedure of choice for primary congenital glaucoma. They argue that goniotomy specifically incises the internal layers of the trabecular meshwork thereby attacking the primary defect. They report excellent results with over 80% of the patients achieving control with one surgical procedure. McPherson and Quigley favor trabeculotomy (31,32). They felt that trabeculotomy eliminates the entire trabecular meshwork as an obstacle to aqueous outflow and therefore works in situations where multiple mechanisms exist such as impermeability of the inner wall or collapse of Schlemm's canal. Another advantage of a trabeculotomy is that it can be converted to a trabeculectomy to provide filtration from the anterior chamber into the subconjunctival space. This can be quite useful in situations where severe angle maldevelopment is discovered at surgery and Schlemm's canal cannot be located.

Anderson undertook the only published controlled study comparing the two procedures (Chapter 70). He performed goniotomy on one eye and trabeculotomy on the other in nine patients. He found no difference in the success or failure of either operation. When these data were combined with those from cases where trabeculotomy or goniotomy were performed bilaterally, he again found each procedure equally successful.

Thus, while each procedure may have its proponents, the overall success rate is quite similar (Table 69.4). It is important to note, however, that most studies indicate that goniotomy requires multiple procedures more often than trabeculotomy (7,31,33).

In addition to goniotomy and trabeculotomy, a variety of other interventions have been tried and all have achieved variable success. Trabeculectomy, which is the main surgical intervention in adult glaucoma, has not been as useful in primary congenital glaucoma. This is especially true in the very young patient and is thought to be due to the thick and active Tenon's capsule which heals rapidly. Cadera et al. reported an "acceptable control" of IOP in 71% of eyes treated with trabeculectomy (34). Recent advances in the use of anti-metabolites, especially mitomycin C, may result in better filtration in children and this technique is now being recommended as the second surgical choice in those patients who have failed goniotomy or trabeculotomy. (See Chapter 70)

Drainage devices (setons) such as the Molteno implant have been used successfully in primary congenital glaucoma (35,36). Unfortunately, there is little data about their long-term effectiveness. In one series of 14 pediatric patients, five who were considered to be primary congenital glaucoma, 54% of the patients were controlled with an implant (35).

Both cyclocryotherapy and laser cyclophotocoagulation have been successful in controlling IOP in patients who have failed surgical treatment. Multiple sessions are often necessary in order to achieve an acceptable result. Restraint is necessary, however, because treatment that is too vigorous can result in hypotony with subsequent phthisis bulbi.

PROGNOSIS

As a group, patients with primary congenital glaucoma respond well to therapy with more than 80% achieving reasonable IOP control. **The rate of success is related to the age of the patient at the initial diagnosis and surgery. If glaucoma was present at birth, the cure rate is only 55%. If, however, it presents later during the third or fourth month, the long-term success rate increases to almost 100%** (7). This favorable outlook con-

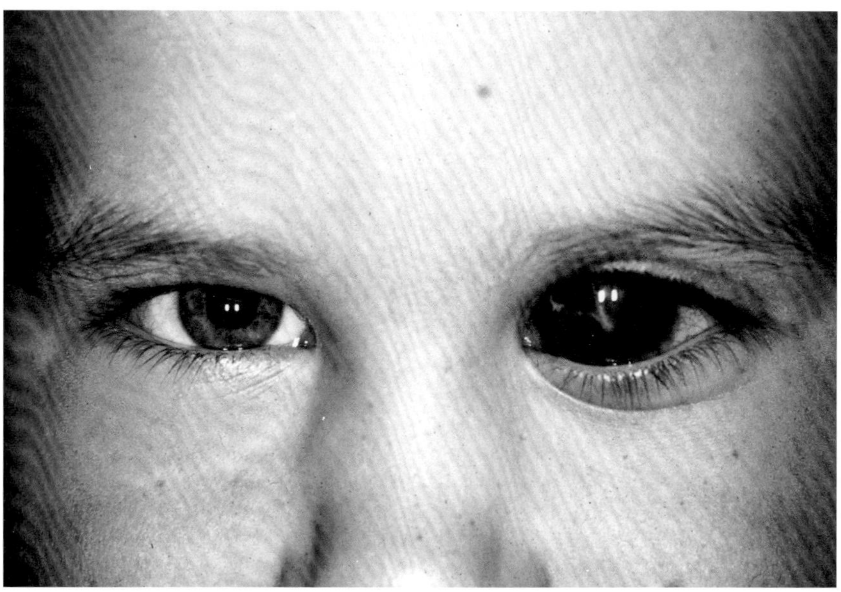

Figure 69.11. End stage unilateral *glaucoma.* Note marked buphthalmos with megalocornea. There are corneal defects. The patient's vision was light perception.

tinues for cases presenting within the first year of life. **Lifetime surveillance is warranted even in children whose glaucoma is cured after surgery; at least 10% of them will demonstrate a later recurrence of glaucoma** (7). The prognosis is poor for those who present after age two (Fig. 69.11).

The cornea can clear remarkably in eyes in which IOPs have been normalized. The faster the IOP is controlled the quicker the cornea will clear. Improved appearance, however, does not necessarily correlate with the return of normal vision. **Optical irregularities because of breaks in Descemet's membrane or persistent stromal haze can have profound effects on visual development.** The residual optical disturbance can often be appreciated on ophthalmoscopic and retinoscopic examination.

Glaucomatous cupping of the optic nerve can decrease in size when IOP is reduced early in life. It is not uncommon to see a striking reduction in depth and diameter of the optic cup in the immediate postoperative period after IOP is reduced to normal (see Fig. 68.4). In some eyes, the optic nerve heads have returned to completely physiologic form. Atrophy, however, when present, has been irreversible.

Myopia from enlargement of the globe usually is not reversible. **One of the major causes of visual loss in unilateral glaucoma is the anisometropic amblyopia which results.** This must be treated aggressively with frequent refractions and patching therapy to obtain the best visual outcome (37).

References

1. Walton DS: Primary congenital open angle glaucoma. A study of the anterior segment abnormalities. Trans Am Ophthalmol Soc 1979;77: 746–68.
2. Alkemade P: Dysgenesis mesodermalis of the iris and cornea. Springfield, Illinois, Charles C. Thomas, 1969.
3. Chandler PA, Grant WM: Lectures in glaucoma. Philadelphia, Lea and Febiger, 1965.
4. Chandler PA, Grant WM: Glaucoma. Philadelphia, Lea and Febiger, 1980.
5. Kolker AE, Hetherington J: Diagnosis and therapy of the glaucomas. St. Louis, CV Mosby, 1983;317–362.
6. Mann I: Developmental abnormalities of the eye. Philadelphia, JB Lippincott, 1957.
7. deLuise VP, Anderson DR: Primary infantile glaucoma (congenital glaucoma). Surv Ophthalmol 1983;28:1–19.
8. Walton DS: Primary congenital open angle glaucoma. In: Epstein DL, ed. Chandler and Grant's Glaucoma, 3rd ed. Philadelphia, Lea & Febiger, 1986.
9. Duke-Elder S: System of ophthalmology, Vol III, Pt. 2: Congenital deformities. St. Louis, CV Mosby, 1969;548–565.
10. Hoskins HD, Shaffer RN: Evaluation techniques for congenital glaucomas. J Ped Ophthalmol Strab 1971;8:81–87.
11. Moller PM: Goniotomy and congenital glaucoma. ACTA Ophthalmol 1977;55:436–442.
12. Miller SJA: Genetic aspects of glaucoma. Trans Ophthalmol Soc UK 1962;81:425–434.
13. Phelps CD, Podos SM: Glaucoma. In: Goldberg MF (ed). Genetic and Metabolic Eye Disease. Boston, Little Brown, 1974;252–253.
14. Freed K, Sachs P, Krakowsky D: Congenital glaucoma in only one of identical twins. Ophthalmologica 1977;174:185–187.
15. Waardenburg PJ, Franceschetti P, Klein D: Genetics and Ophthalmology. Vol I. Springfield, Charles Thomas, 1961.
16. Hafez M, Moustafa EE, Mokpel TH, et al: Evidence of HLA linked susceptibility gene (s) in primary congenital glaucoma. Disease Markers 1990;8:191–197.
17. Barkan O: Technique of goniotomy. Arch Ophthalmol 1938;19: 217–221.
18. Worst JGF: Congenital glaucoma. Remarks on the aspect of chamber angle: Ontogenic and pathogenic background and mode of action of goniotomy. Invest Ophthalmol 1968;7:127–134.
19. Shields MB: Textbook of glaucoma. Baltimore, Williams & Wilkins, 1992;220–223.
20. Anderson DR: The development of the trabecular meshwork and its abnormality in primary infantile glaucoma. Tran Am Ophthalmol Soc 1981;79:461.
21. Allen L, Burian HM, Braley AE: A new concept of the development of the anterior chamber angle. Its relationship to developmental glaucoma and other structural anomalies. Arch Ophthalmol 1955;53:783.
22. Maumenee AE: Further observations on the pathogenesis of congenital glaucoma. Am J Ophthalmol 1963;55:1165–1176.
23. Smelser GK, Ozanics V: The development of the trabecular meshwork in premature eyes. Am J Ophthalmol 1981;71:366–385.
24. Kupfer C, Kaiser-Kupfer MS: Observations on the development of the anterior chamber angle with reference to the pathogenesis of congenital glaucomas. Am J Ophthalmol 1979;88:424.
25. Buckley EG, Shields MB: Congenital glaucoma. In: Clinical Signs in Ophthalmology. St. Louis, CV Mosby, 1984;6:6.
26. Seidman DJ, Nelson LB, Calhoun JH, et al: Signs and symptoms in the presentation of primary infantile glaucoma. Pediatrics 1986;77:399.
27. Shaffer RN, Weiss DF: The congenital and pediatric glaucomas. St. Louis, CV Mosby, 1970.
28. Boger WP III: Timolol in childhood glaucoma. Surv Ophthalmol 1983; 28:259.
29. Zimmerman TJ, Kooner KS, Morgan KS: Safety and efficacy of timolol in pediatric glaucoma. Surv Ophthalmol 1983;28:262.
30. Hoskins DH, Jr, Shaffer RN, Hetherington J: Goniotomy vs trabeculotomy. J Pediatric Ophthalmol Strab 1984;21:153–158.
31. McPherson SD, Berry DP: Goniotomy vs external trabeculotomy for developmental glaucoma. Am J Ophthalmol 1983;95:427–431.
32. Quigley HA: Childhood glaucoma. Results with trabeculotomy and study of reversible cupping. Ophthalmology 1982;89:219–226.
33. Luntz MH: The advantages of trabeculotomy over goniotomy. J Ped Ophthalmol Strab 1984;21:150.
34. Cadera W, Pachtman MA, Cantor LB, et al: Filtering surgery in childhood glaucoma. Ophthalmic Surg 1984;15:319.
35. Minckler DS, Heuer DK, Hasty B, et al: Clinical experience with the single plate Molteno implant in complicated glaucoma. Ophthalmology 1988;95:1181.
36. Melamed S, Fiore P: Molteno implant surgery in refractory glaucoma. Surv Ophthalmol 1990;34:441.
37. Biglan AW, Hile DA: The visual results following infantile glaucoma surgery. J Pediatric Ophthalmol Strab 1979;16:377–381.

Medical and Surgical Treatments for Childhood Glaucomas

70

Sharon F. Freedman

Successful treatment of childhood glaucoma presents many challenges, with control of intraocular pressure (IOP) as the first, but not the only, priority. Although therapeutic options include the same medical, laser, and surgical choices available for treating adult glaucomas, optimal therapies for children often differ greatly from those for adults.

MEDICATIONS

Surgical intervention is the primary treatment for primary congenital glaucoma and most other childhood glaucomas, although medications have a supplemental but important role in controlling IOP. Preoperatively, medications may help clear the cornea to facilitate goniotomy, and postoperatively, they may help control IOP until the success of surgical intervention has been determined. Medical therapy is also indicated in managing difficult cases in which surgery poses particular risks or has incompletely controlled the glaucoma (1). Besides inadequate IOP control, multiple factors conspire against the success of long-term medical therapy in childhood glaucomas: the difficulties with long-term compliance, adequate ascertainment of drug-induced adverse effects, and potential adverse systemic effects of protracted therapy, among others.

Carbonic Anhydrase Inhibitors

Acetazolamide (Diamox) is usually well-tolerated by infants and children, and it often effectively lowers intaocular pressure in these patients when it is administered orally as 10–15 mg/kg/day, divided every 6–8 hours (1,2). Parents sometimes note diarrhea, diminished energy levels, and loss of appetite in their children on this therapy, thus requiring dosage adjustment or discontinuation. Metabolic acidosis has also been reported in infants, and it may be ameliorated with oral bicitra (1 meq/kg/day). In general, however, younger patients tolerate acetazolamide better than older ones: 77% of patients younger than 40 years were able to tolerate acetazolamide in Shrader's series (3).

Miotics

Historically, miotics have been of limited value in treating childhood glaucomas (4). In cases of congenital glaucoma, the abnormal insertion of the ciliary muscle into the trabecular meshwork (1,5) has been blamed for the poor response of IOP to miotics. Nonetheless, miotics have been useful in achieving miosis just before and after goniotomy (4,6). Whereas pilocarpine 2% every 6–8 hours has been used in treating congenital glaucoma (2,4), stronger miotics, such as Phospholine Iodide, have also been administered in infants, with less ocular irritation than that observed in adults (4). Phospholine Iodide therapy has sometimes been accompanied by diarrhea (4) and requires extreme care in the concurrent use of succinylcholine for general anesthesia. Older children often experience severe visual blurring attributable to myopia induced by even dilute miotics. If they are effective in treating the glaucoma, miotics in these children may be better tolerated when the induced myopia is rendered stable, so that it can be compensated by spectacles. To this end, higher concentrations (e.g., pilocarpine 2–4%) or longer-acting formulations (e.g., pilocarpine Ocusert) may be useful.

Beta-adrenergic Antagonists (Beta-Blockers)

Topical beta blockers have been available for the treatment of glaucoma since the introduction of timolol in 1978. Several studies have examined the role of timolol in treating uncontrolled childhood glaucomas, often after previous surgical intervention (7–10). In a study of 67 patients (100 eyes) with childhood glaucomas who began topical timolol before 18 years of age, 30 patients (40 eyes) experienced a mean IOP decrement of 21.3% and required no further surgery or medical therapy over a 2.5-year follow-up period. Most subjects who became stable on timolol did so on the 0.25% BID concentration, and all subjects with adverse reactions (10%) were using 0.5% timolol. Only two patients discontinued timolol because of side effects—one was a 10 year old who developed severe asthma, and the other was a 17 year old with symptomatic bradycardia (8).

In a series of 18 eyes of 11 patients who were mostly younger than 20 years old, Zimmerman noted that 72% were controlled without further surgery for up to 2 ½ years on regimens including timoptic 0.25% or 0.5% BID, with an overall IOP decline of 30.7% (7). Systemic side effects occurred in only 4% of the patients in this series. In earlier studies, the addition of timolol 0.25% or 0.5% to the regimen of young patients with severe uncontrolled glaucoma resulted in stabilization of glaucoma in about one-third of patients without further surgery, for up to 2½ years (9,10). Systemic adverse side effects were reported in none of 34 patients and 5 of 28 patients (18%), respectively, in these studies.

The most severe systemic adverse effects occurring in children on topical timolol therapy have included acute asthma attacks, bradycardia, (8,10) and apneic spells (the latter in neonates) (11,12). Plasma timolol levels measured in children on 0.25% timolol (ranging from 3.5 ng/ml in a five-year-old to 34 ng/ml in a three-week-old) vastly exceeded those in adults on 0.5% timolol (0.34 to 2.45 ng/ml) (12). The use of punctal occlusion in adults further lowered mean 1-hour plasma timolol levels by 40% in the adult patients in this study (from 1.34 to 0.9 ng/ml). The high plasma timolol levels in children may be explained by a child's volume of distribution for the drug, which is much smaller than that of an adult. For example, whereas the ocular volume of a neonate is about 50% that of an adult (reaching full size by about age 2 years), the average 3.5 kg newborn infant has a body mass only one-twentieth that of a small adult male (70 kg), with a blood volume relatively even smaller.

When timolol is used in small children, treatment should always begin with 0.25% drops, excluding those children with a history of asthma or bradycardia. **Topical beta blockers should be used with extreme caution in neonates, with particular attention paid to the possibility of apnea. It may be reasonable to observe children for adverse systemic effects for 1 to 2 hours in the office after an initial dose of beta blocker has been given,** before prescribing the beta blocker for outpatient use (7,12). Punctal occlusion, when feasible, should be performed by parents or caretakers (7).

Little data is available on the use of topical beta blockers other than timolol in the treatment of childhood glaucoma. Based on experience in adults, betaxolol, as a relatively beta 1-selective agent, may be less prone to precipitating acute asthma attacks (which may present as coughing) than the nonselective beta blockers. The remaining nonselective beta blockers should be approached in a fashion similar to timolol regarding risks and probable efficacy. As in adults, beta blockers used in children often have an additive effect to carbonic anhydrase inhibitors (acetazolamide) in treating children with glaucoma (9).

Adrenergic Agonists

Epinephrine compounds have been used in infants and children with glaucoma (4,13), but there is little published data to suggest optimal dosing schedules or the magnitude of the IOP decrement to be expected from these drugs. Furthermore, these drugs are relegated to secondary importance because of their potential for systemic toxicity (e.g., tachyarrhythmias, hypertension,) and for their ocular side effects (e.g., irritation, reactive hyperemia, epinephrine oxidation deposits), together with their limited effectiveness. Topical dipivefrin (Propine), as an epinephrine pro-drug, should theoretically have fewer systemic side effects in children than epinephrine. Based on adult studies, little additional pressure lowering effect would be expected with the use of Propine or epinephrine together with a nonselective beta blocker (14).

No data are available regarding the use of the alpha-2 agonist apraclonidine (Iopidine) in children with glaucoma. We have found this drug useful in the setting of goniotomy to minimize intraoperative hyphema (see Goniotomy later in this chapter).

SURGICAL THERAPY

Although surgical intervention provides the most definitive treatment for most forms of childhood glaucoma (Table 70.1), glaucoma surgery poses significant challenges, especially in young children. If the diagnosis of glaucoma has been secured in the office (which is not always the case), medical therapy (especially oral acetazolamide) can be used preoperatively to clear the cornea maximally for gonioscopy, fundus examination, and surgery. Anesthesia itself poses significant risks, especially in neonates. **The infant eye, with a smaller palpebral fissure, less rigid and often thinned sclera and limbal tissue (especially in buphthalmic eyes), behaves differently from an adult eye during surgery**. Postoperatively, difficulties may be encountered in protection of the operated eye from inadvertent injury, compliance with postoperative medications, and monitoring of the eye for possible surgical complications and response to surgery. **Family members should be informed preoperatively of the multiple visits and likely additional anesthesias that will be needed postoperatively**, as well as the likelihood that further surgery may be needed to control glaucoma. Often, the first examination under anesthesia can be followed immediately by the first indicated surgical procedure, thereby avoiding time delay in controlling IOP and avoiding at least one additional anesthesia.

Goniotomy

With the aim of incising the uveal trabecular meshwork under direct visualization, goniotomy is the surgical procedure of choice in most cases of primary congenital glaucoma. Trabeculotomy ab externo, covered later in this chapter, is an alternative procedure that is especially useful when corneal clouding prevents an optimal view of the angle structures by gonioscopy.

In 1893, the Italian ophthalmologist Carlo deVincentiis described a new operation that attempted to open

Table 70.1
Indications For Surgery in Childhood Glaucomas

I. Angle surgery
  A. Goniotomy (may repeat one or more times)
    1. Primary congenital/infantile open angle glaucoma
    2. Other primary glaucomas (generally poor success)
      a. Axenfeld-Rieger syndrome
      b. Lowe's syndrome
      c. Neurofibromatosis
      d. Sturge-Weber syndrome
      e. ?Other
    2. Selected secondary glaucomas
      a. Maternal rubella syndrome
      b. Open angle glaucoma after congenital cataract surgery
      c. Uveitic glaucoma (especially with juvenile rheumatoid arthritis)
    3. Prophylaxis against acquired glaucoma in aniridia*
    4. Early onset juvenile open angle glaucoma
  B. Trabeculotomy (may repeat one time)
    1. Same as for goniotomy, but preferred in the presence of corneal opacification.
    2. Performed by some surgeons after two goniotomies have failed
    3. May be combined with trabeculectomy (see IIIA. below)
II. Peripheral iridectomy
  (Secondary pupillary block glaucoma)
III. Filtration surgery
  A. Combined trabeculotomy/trabeculectomy
    1. When trabeculotomy cannot be completed (failure to cannulate Schlemm's canal)
    2. Failed previous angle surgery (2 goniotomies and/or trabeculotomies)
    3. Low likelihood of success with angle surgery alone (e.g. chronic aphakic glaucoma)
  B. Trabeculectomy (almost always with intraoperative mitomycin C)
    1. Any glaucoma in an eye with reasonable visual potential and unscarred conjunctiva after angle surgery has failed
    2. Low likelihood of success with angle surgery (would usually favor IIIA. above)
  C. Combined cataract removal/trabeculectomy
    1. Not usually recommended (suggest cataract first, then glaucoma surgery)
    2. Consider for older child with intact posterior capsule
IV. Drainage implant (seton) surgery
  A. Failed trabeculectomy with intraoperative mitomycin C and reasonable visual potential
  B. High risk for complications with filtration surgery (e.g., Sturge-Weber syndrome)
  C. High risk for failure with trabeculectomy from scarring (e.g. after multiple conjunctival surgeries)
V. Cyclodestructive procedures
  A. Laser cycloablation (Nd:YAG or diode)
    1. Failed angle surgery (or angle surgery not possible) and minimal visual potential
    2. Failed trabeculectomy and/or seton with poor central vision
    3. Anatomy precluding trabeculectomy or seton (e.g. disorganized anterior segment after trauma, sclerocornea)
    4. In patients who are gravely ill, or when followup and postoperative care cannot be assured, or prolonged intubation poses life-threatening risk
    5. High risk for complications with intraocular surgery (e.g. Sturge-Weber)
  B. Cyclocryotherapy
    1. Same as for cycloablation but in phakic patients with small or normal-sized eyes
    2. Repeat therapy in selected quadrants after previous cyclocryotherapy

*Should be performed only by surgeons very comfortable with goniotomy, given unprotected lens.

Schlemm's canal by incising the angle tissues (without visualization of the angle) (15). Because of a high complication rate and poor results in adults with open angle glaucoma, this operation was initially abandoned. With the advent of clinical gonioscopy, Otto Barkan modified the technique in 1938 as an operation for primary congenital glaucoma, dubbing it "goniotomy" (Gk. gonio = angle + tomein = to cut) (16). With this effective operation for congenital glaucoma, the dismal prognosis for this disease dramatically improved. The technique for performing goniotomy has remained essentially unaltered for more than 50 years—a testament to its importance and widespread use as the initial procedure for primary congenital glaucoma (1). Whereas the goal of goniotomy is to remove obstructing tissue and to open a route for aqueous humor to exit the anterior chamber into Schlemm's canal (1), the precise mechanism by which pressure reduction occurs remains obscure. Successful goniotomy does appear, however, to lower IOP as a result of improved facility of aqueous outflow (17).

Goniotomy enjoys its greatest success in the therapy of primary congenital glaucoma, but it may also be used in other primary developmental glaucomas, although with a lower success rate. Examples of these other primary glaucomas include those associated with Sturge-Weber syndrome, neurofibromatosis, Lowe's syndrome, Axenfeld-Rieger syndrome, and aniridia, among others. In addition, several secondary glaucomas may respond favorably to goniotomy in some cases. These include aphakic glaucoma presenting early after congenital cataract surgery, and glaucoma complicating chronic anterior uveitis. Goniotomy also deserves special consideration as a prophylactic procedure in congenital aniridia (17,18).

If the diagnosis of glaucoma has been confirmed before anesthesia, and if goniotomy is the preferred surgical procedure, oral acetazolamide therapy for at least several days preoperatively may help to maximize corneal clarity by lowering IOP. Topical antibiotics may also be used for 1–2 days preoperatively. **Pilocarpine 1% or 2% should be placed onto the eye(s) to be operated just before surgery to aid in protecting the crystalline lens from injury during surgery.** Miochol may be injected into the anterior chamber, if necessary, to promote further miosis.

Goniotomy is performed using a surgical goniolens and a goniotomy knife. There are several available goniolenses, in addition to the round-domed Barkan goniolens, including the Lister modification which includes irrigation, or the Swan-Jacobs lens, which incorporates a handle and facilitates use of a microscope. Several types of goniotomy knives are also available. A non-tapered Swan knife (or needle-knife) enters the anterior chamber easily, and cuts in either direction. Alternatively, a disposable 23- or 25-gauge needle attached to a syringe containing hyaluronic acid (Healon) may be used, allowing the anterior chamber to be deepened before incision, and to be maintained upon instrument removal (19). The author prefers the latter method, using only enough Healon to ensure chamber maintenance upon needle withdrawal. Enthusiastic use of Healon may acutely increase corneal edema by increasing IOP, thereby degrading the surgeon's view of the angle structures. Our patients old enough to cooperate for tonometry on the first postoperative day have not shown an IOP spike after goniotomy with the judicious use of Healon.

To perform goniotomy safely and effectively, the surgeon must ensure a degree of corneal clarity sufficient to allow an adequate view of the angle structures. If corneal epithelial (but not stromal) edema obscures an adequate angle view, the epithelium can be removed with the edge of a #15 Bard-Parker blade from a window of cornea nearest the surgeon (after sterile preparation of the eye and placement of a lid speculum has taken place). This cornea epithelial removal is best performed after applying topical proparacaine, followed by 70% isopropyl alcohol (on a swab) to the appropriate section of epithelium (17). Often, corneal stromal edema persists even after epithelial removal; in this setting, trabeculotomy may be preferred.

The surgeon may use a binocular operating loupe or operating microscope to view the angle for goniotomy. (We prefer the latter, which also affords the assistant a view of the angle structures.) The surgeon should be positioned opposite the portion of the angle to be operated (i.e., to the temporal side of the patient for nasal goniotomy), with the patient's head slightly rotated away from the surgeon. Elschnig-O'Connor or Moody locking fixation forceps are usually placed on the superior and inferior rectus muscles when a nasal or temporal goniotomy is planned. If the lids seem tight, a small lateral "single snip" canthotomy can be helpful. Apraclonidine 1% may be placed on the limbus overlying the angle to be operated, and then the operating goniolens is applied to the cornea. Healon may be helpful in preventing air bubble formation under the Barkan goniotomy lens, and the lens may be stabilized with a non-toothed fine forcep in the positioning holes of the lens.

The goniotomy knife or needle is placed through peripheral clear cornea 1 mm from the limbus, opposite the midpoint of the intended goniotomy, in a plane parallel to the iris. The knife or needle is guided over iris tissue (not pupil) to engage trabecular meshwork in its anterior third, just posterior to Schwalbe's line (Fig. 70.1A). A circumferential incision is then made (right to left for a right-handed surgeon) for about 4–5 clock hours (Fig. 70.1B), and the knife or needle is carefully and quickly withdrawn from the eye over iris tissue at all times. **The incision should be superficial, with no grating or scraping sensation noted. A deeper cleft, with exposure of whiter tissue may be noted in the wake of the incision, with a widening of the angle, and a posterior movement of peripheral iris in some cases.** The assistant may help the surgeon to extend the angle accessible to goniotomy, by rotating the eye clockwise and counterclockwise respectively at the surgeon's request. After knife withdrawal, blood often egresses from the angle incision, stopping when the chamber is refilled with balanced salt solution. A single suture of 9-0 or 10-0 vicryl (or 10-0 nylon in an older child, with the knot buried), secures the corneal wound if leakage occurs.

Postoperative treatment with a topical antibiotic-steroid (and miotic) are continued for one week. If bilateral goniotomies are needed, they may be performed during one anesthesia, provided that all instruments are sterilized, all drapes, gowns and gloves replaced, and the fellow eye reprepared and draped in sterile fashion following the first procedure (20).

Key points in the surgical technique of goniotomy are

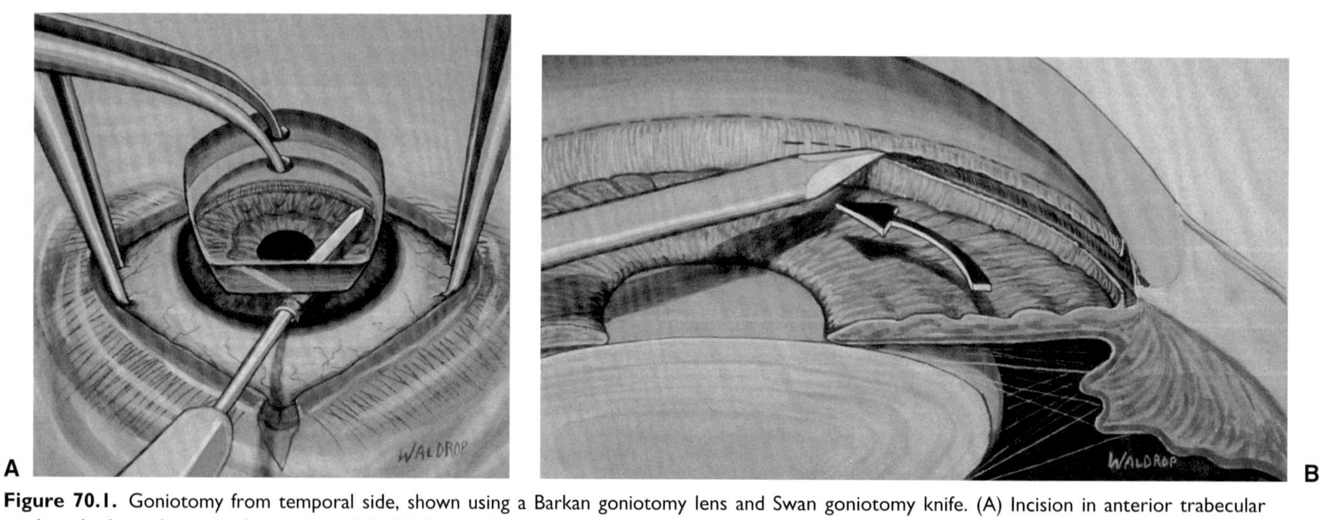

Figure 70.1. Goniotomy from temporal side, shown using a Barkan goniotomy lens and Swan goniotomy knife. (A) Incision in anterior trabecular meshwork, shown beginning from right to left. (B) Correct location and depth of the goniotomy incision. (From: Buckley, EG, Freedman, SF, and Shields, MB. Atlas of Ophthalmic Surgery Vol. 3: Strabismus and Glaucoma Surgery. St. Louis, Mosby Yearbook, Inc., 1995, with permission.)

Table 70.2
Goniotomy - Key Points in Surgical Technique

Key Point	Comment
Select patients with favorable surgical prognosis	Primary congenital glaucoma, aphakic glaucoma early after cataract surgery, uveitic glaucoma
Confirm adequate corneal clarity	Use medical therapy preoperatively, perform gonioscopy under anesthesia just before surgery
Position patient and surgeon for optimal access to surgical site	Easiest first goniotomy is nasal, with surgeon seated on temporal side, patient's head turned slightly away from the surgeon
Stabilize globe adequately for surgery	Place locking forceps on insertions of appropriate rectus muscle pair (usually superior and inferior recti)
Improve angle view if suboptimal	Consider scraping portion of corneal epithelium (glycerin marginally helpful); reposition eye, microscope, goniolens (Healon under lens helpful)
Make entry into anterior chamber	25-gauge needle on Healon syringe easiest; enter parallel to iris plane opposite angle to be operated; use miochol first if pupil not miotic
Guide needle (or knife) safely to engage angle tissue for incision	Pass over iris (not pupil), engaging angle tissue just below Schwalbe's line, in anterior-most uveal meshwork
Make angle incision smoothly and of adequate extent (4–5 clock hours)	Keep incision superficial, watch for cleft formation and posterior iris movement; have assistant rotate eye in same plane to gain access to additional angle
Remove needle (or knife) safely from eye	Keep instrument over iris tissue, move swiftly, inject Healon if needed to maintain anterior chamber
Refill chamber and close entry site	Balanced salt solution useful to deepen anterior chamber; single 10-0 vicryl adequate to close

Table 70.3
Goniotomy - Common Errors in Surgical Technique

Common Error	Consequence
Poor patient selection	Surgical success unlikely; time and effort of goniotomy could be better spent
Angle view suboptimal	Increased likelihood of damage to cornea, iris, or crystalline lens; decreased chance of incision in angle tissue
Globe position not stable	Same as above
Pupil not miotic	Increases danger of crystalline lens damage
Entry would too anterior	Angle tissue may be difficult to reach or incise; corneal endothelium may be injured
Entry wound too posterior	Needle (or knife) may engage iris upon entry; crystalline lens damage more likely; chamber may collapse as excessive lifting is needed to engage angle
Angle incision too anterior	Angle tissue may not be entered; surgery likely will be ineffective
Angle incision too posterior	Iridodialysis, cyclodialysis, and hyphema more likely to occur; angle tissue itself may not be incised
Anterior chamber collapse upon instrument withdrawal from eye	Needle (knife) more likely to injure cornea, iris, and crystalline lens; significant hyphema more likely to occur

summarized in Table 70.2. Common errors are listed in Table 70.3.

Mild to moderate hyphemas commonly occur after goniotomy, but almost always clear rapidly without sequelae over several days. Other complications following goniotomy are rare, and include iridodialysis, cyclodialysis, the appearance of small peripheral anterior synechias in the incised angle, damage to the crystalline lens, and retinal detachment in eyes with high myopia (18,21,22). Cardiopulmonary arrests (nonfatal) occurred during anesthesia in 1.8% of cases in a series of 401 goniotomies (21).

The results of goniotomy should be evaluated weekly in the immediate postoperative period and are often evident by 3–6 weeks. **Gonioscopy after successful goniotomy often reveals a widened angle in the previous incision site, with improved visibility of the ciliary band and scleral spur** (Fig. 70.2). This appearance suggests that an opening has been created in the uveal meshwork, with little injury to the underlying tissues. Scattered peripheral anterior synechias in the bed of the goniotomy may partially, or significantly obscure a view of the incised angle. Since 4–5 clock hours of angle tissue are incised with a single goniotomy, repeat procedures in untreated portions of the angle may enhance IOP control in selected

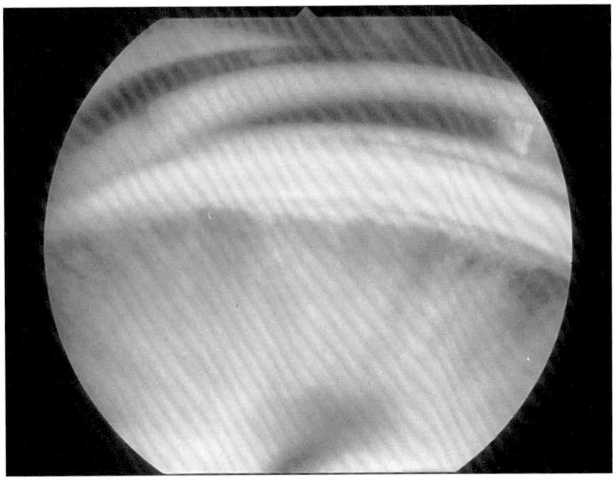

Figure 70.2. Cleft in angle after goniotomy, resulting in a widened angle to the right half of the gonioscopic view in a three-year-old with primary congenital glaucoma.

cases. Goniotomy may fail to control infantile glaucoma in some instances due to improper placement and depth of the angle incision, or the obliteration of the incision by peripheral synechias. Rarely, a third or even fourth goniotomy procedure may control glaucoma.

The success of goniotomy in controlling glaucoma varies with the etiology of the glaucoma. **The best results—80% to more than 90% success after 1 to 2 procedures—are achieved in infants with primary congenital glaucoma presenting between three months and one year of age** (1).

Procedures Related to Goniotomy

Scheie reported a modification of goniotomy termed goniopuncture, which involved passage of a goniotomy knife through the trabecular meshwork and sclera to the subconjunctival space following a standard goniotomy (22). However, scarring of the limbal incision limited the usefulness of goniopuncture.

The neodymium: YAG laser has been used to perform trabeculopuncture by directing laser energy gonioscopically at the trabecular meshwork, in order to penetrate through to Schlemm's canal. Success was reported with this procedure in six of eight eyes with juvenile glaucoma over a six month follow-up period (see Chapter 50) (23). A technique requiring a large limbal incision, direct goniotomy has also been described, but it has been superceded by trabeculotomy (24).

Trabeculodialysis, a modification of goniotomy in which the trabecular meshwork is scraped or retracted from the scleral sulcus after a standard goniotomy incision, has been effective in the treatment of children with glaucoma secondary to anterior uveitis (60% IOP control reported in a series of 23 such patients) (25). However, goniotomy alone is also effective in these patients (David Walton, personal communication, see Chapter 71).

Argon Laser Trabeculoplasty is not effective in the treatment of childhood glaucomas, nor is it possible to perform in young patients (26,27).

TRABECULOTOMY AB EXTERNO

Trabeculotomy ab externo, performed by cannulating Schlemm's canal from an external approach and then tearing through the trabecular meshwork into the anterior chamber, creates a direct communication between the anterior chamber and Schlemm's canal. Burian and Smith independently described trabeculotomy ab externo in 1960 as an alternative procedure to goniotomy (28,29). The technique was later modified by Harms, Dannheim, and McPherson (1). Success rates varying from 73–100% have been reported for this procedure in congenital glaucoma (1). In a series of 71 patients (most with primary infantile glaucoma), Akimoto et al recently reported total success probabilities of one or more trabeculotomies of 92.5% and 76.5%, at 5 and 10 years, resp (30). **Conjunctival scarring is the salient disadvantage of trabeculotomy.** As noted above, however, trabeculotomy's signal advantage is that it is little affected by an edematous or scarred cornea.

In the surgical technique described by McPherson, (31) a limbal-based conjunctival flap and a partial thickness triangular or rectangular scleral flap are created as for standard trabeculectomy (Chapter 62). Pilocarpine may be used preoperatively to induce miosis. We prefer a temporal approach for trabeculotomy, to spare the superior quadrants for possible later filtration surgery.

After a paracentesis (and injection into the anterior chamber of a small amount of viscoelastic), a radial scratch incision is made across the sclero-limbal junction in the bed of the scleral flap. This scratch incision is gradually deepened under high magnification until Schlemm's canal is visualized just anterior to the circumferential fibers of the scleral spur (near the posterior aspect of the limbal "gray zone"). Often a small amount of blood or aqueous humor will reflux through the cut ends of Schlemm's canal, and the internal wall of the canal will appear slightly pigmented. **To confirm the identity of the canal, a 5-0 or 6-0 nylon suture (with the needle removed) should thread easily to both the left and the right sides of the radial incision.** If resistance is met, the suture may need to be repositioned, the radial incision deepened, or a second parallel radial incision made beneath the same scleral flap to aid in locating Schlemm's canal. (The presence of the suture in Schlemm's canal may sometimes be confirmed by gonioscopy using a Zeiss four-mirror lens). Once the canal has been located, the internal arm of a trabeculotome should be passed gently into the canal (to the right side first for a right-handed surgeon) as far as possible without meeting resistance, and using the parallel

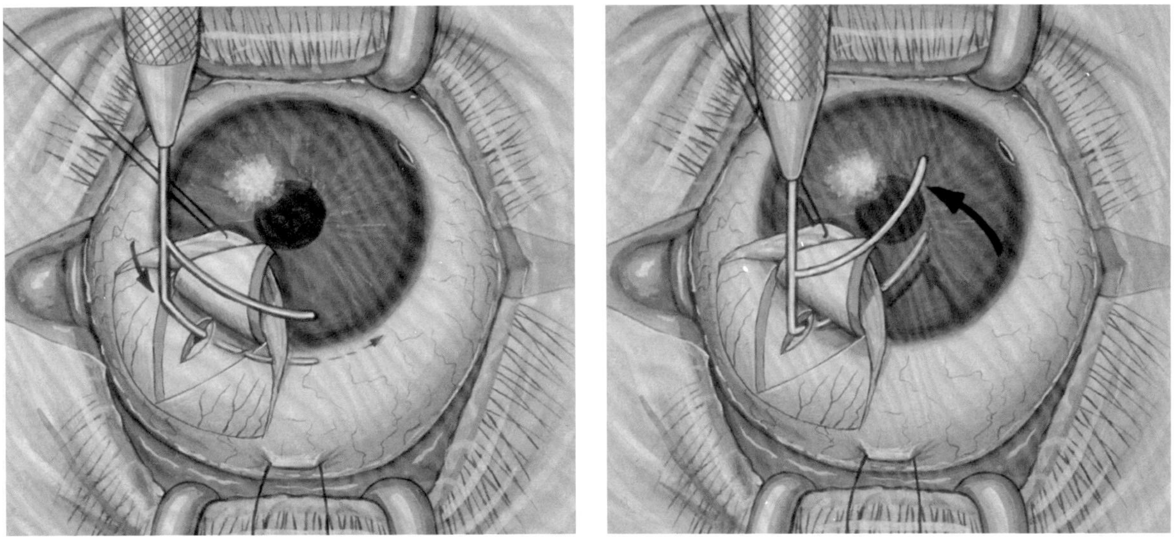

A

B

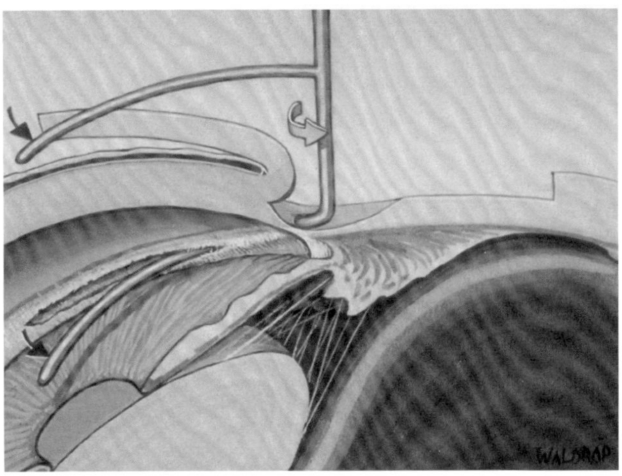

C

Figure 70.3. Trabeculotomy, under a limbus-based conjunctival and partial-thickness scleral flap. Superior approach is shown, using a traction suture to hold back the conjunctival and Tenon's layers. (A) Placement of trabeculotome into the cut end of Schlemm's canal to the right. (B) Rotation of the trabeculotome into the anterior chamber, tearing through the intervening trabecular meshwork. (C) View of internal arm of trabeculotome tearing through trabecular meshwork as the instrument is rotated into the anterior chamber. (From: Buckley, EG, Freedman, SF, and Shields, MB. Atlas of Ophthalmic Surgery Vol. 3: Strabismus and Glaucoma Surgery. St. Louis, Mosby Yearbook, Inc., 1995, with permission.)

external arm as a guide (Fig. 70.3A). The internal arm is then gently rotated into the anterior chamber, with care to avoid entry into peripheral cornea or beneath the iris plane (Fig. 70.3B). Rotation of the trabeculotome into the anterior chamber tears through the intervening trabecular meshwork (Fig. 70.3C), and requires very little force. Rotation should be halted once about 75–80% of the internal arm of the trabeculotome is visible in the anterior chamber. The anterior chamber may shallow slightly, and blood may egress from the torn trabecular meshwork, as the trabeculotome is removed from the eye along its path of entry. In similar fashion, the trabeculotome should be placed into the left side of the radial incision, and the procedure repeated to the left. By leaving a portion of intact trabecular meshwork underlying the radial incision into Schlemm's canal, one hopes to prevent prolapse of iris into the wound. The scleral flap is then sutured with 10-0 nylon, while the Tenon's capsule and conjunctival layers may be closed with a running suture of 8-0 or 10-0 vicryl, as for standard trabeculectomy (32).

Postoperatively, patients are treated with topical antibiotics and steroids, together with **low-dose pilocarpine** for 1–2 weeks. While hyphema occurs commonly after trabeculotomy, rarer complications include inadverent filtering blebs, choroidal detachment, iridotomy, damage to the lens, creation of a false passage into the anterior chamber or suprachoroidal space, and infection (1,32).

One proposed modification of trabeculotomy involves the use of a nylon or prolene suture to perform a 180-degree or 360-degree trabeculotomy at one surgery, using one or two external incisions into Schlemm's canal (33,34). Although intriguing, the early results of 360 degree trabeculotomy are similar to those reported for more conventional trabeculotomy procedures (which usually affect 100–120 degrees of the angle as described above).

The effects of trabeculotomy should be determined 3–4 weeks after surgery, usually under anesthesia. **Although trabeculotomy may be repeated in a different portion of the angle, it may be reasonable to combine the second procedure with a trabeculectomy if no beneficial effect was noted following the first trabeculotomy.** Key points in the surgical technique are listed in Table 70.4.

Table 70.4
Trabeculotomy - Key Points in Surgical Technique

Key Point	Comment	Related Complication
Select patient well	Same as for goniotomy, but may have opacified cornea	Surgical success unlikely, increased time to IOP control
Consider temporal approach	Spares superior conjunctiva for later filtration surgery	Superior scarring may predispose later filter to failure
Dissect conjunctival and scleral flap very anteriorly	Facilitates finding and cannulating Schlemm's canal	Schlemm's canal may not be found if dissection not carried well into limbal gray zone
Make paracentesis and inject Healon	Maintains anterior chamber access and facilitates second trabeculotome passage	Chamber may shallow and hyphema occur, precluding canal cannulation to the opposite side
Gradually deepen radial "scratch" incision	Transverse fibers of Schlemm's canal easier to see if exposed gradually without canal transection	Schlemms's canal may be transected and "missed" and anterior chamber entered if deep incision quickly made
Pass nylon suture to confirm canal	Facilitates confirmation of true Schlemm's canal, rather than false corneal or scleral passage	Metal trabeculotome may make false passage and canal can be missed altogether
Rotate trabeculotome gently into anterior chamber	Trabecular meshwork is delicate and easy to tear through	Excess force allows trabeculotome to rotate in incorrect plane into cornea or iris/ciliary body tissue
Prepare a parallel radial scratch incision if Schlemm's canal not found	Consider converting to trabeculectomy if Schlemm's canal not found after several attempts	Failure to facilitate aqueous outflow will prolong uncontrolled IOP

Combined Trabeculotomy-Trabeculectomy

If Schlemm's canal has not been successfully cannulated, and/or previous similar trabeculotomy procedures have failed to control IOP, the trabeculotomy can be combined with a trabeculectomy, by removal of a full-thickness block of limbal tissue in the bed of the scleral flap, followed by peripheral iridectomy as in standard trabeculectomy (20). If conversion to trabeculectomy seems likely, one may apply an antimetabolite such as mitomycin C to the sclera at the site of intended scleral flap formation, prior to dissection of the scleral flap (as described for adult trabeculectomy [Chapter 62]). If mitomycin C has been applied, we favor use of a rectangular partial thickness scleral flap with a rather secure closure, and a subsequent separate running closure of both Tenon's and conjunctival layers with 10-0 Dexon or Vicryl. Postoperatve care should be as for pediatric trabeculectomy in this case (see Trabeculectomy).

Goniotomy vs. Trabeculotomy

Each of these procedures has staunch advocates, who espouse the advantages of one technique over the other (35,36). Reported success has been similarily high with both procedures in favorable cases of glaucoma (e.g., previously unoperated eyes with primary congenital glaucoma, with onset postnatally, but before one year of life) (37).

If the cornea is clear, goniotomy has certain advantages over trabeculotomy: there is no conjunctival scarring, and the operating time is shorter with goniotomy than with trabeculotomy. On the other hand, the microsurgeon experienced in adult glaucoma surgery may find trabeculotomy a more familiar procedure than goniotomy.

Peripheral Iridectomy

Several types of pupillary block glaucoma occur in children (see Table 68.1). After cataract surgery, pupillary block glaucoma may respond to peripheral iridectomy (with or without anterior vitrectomy or synechialysis). Glaucoma associated with advanced cicatricial retinopathy of prematurity may similarly improve with iridectomy alone, or coupled with lens removal. In these cases, peripheral iridectomy should proceed essentially as described for adults (Chapter 67).

Filtering Surgery

Filtering surgery is usually employed when goniotomy and/or trabeculotomy either fails or, as is the case in many secondary glaucomas, are (is) very unlikely to succeed (see Chapter 71). Many such surgical procedures have been attempted over the years to treat children with glaucoma, including iridencleisis, cyclodiathermy, thermal sclerostomy (Scheie procedure), and standard trabeculectomy (1). Success rates were usually poor. For example, Cadera and colleagues reported a 52% success at IOP control (defined as IOP $<$ 22 mmHg) with thermal sclerostomy and trabe-

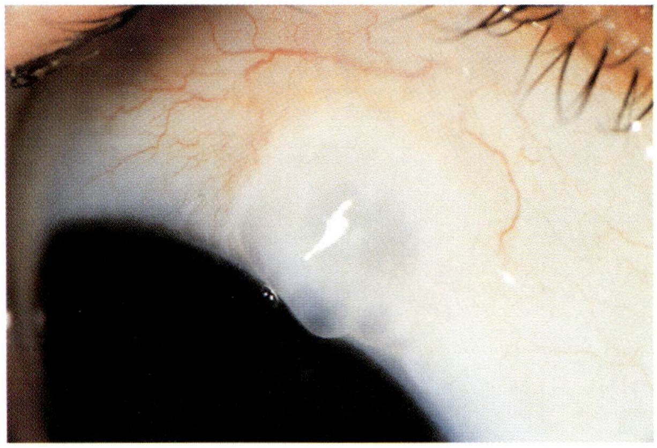

Figure 70.4. Functioning bleb seven months after trabeculectomy augmented with intraoperative mitomycin C and postoperative laser suture lysis in an eight-year-old African American girl with neglected primary congenital glaucoma after failed previous trabeculotomy in infancy. IOP is 11 mm Hg, without additional medications.

culectomy in a series of 24 children (average age 4 years) followed for several years (38). Scheie (39) and Beauchamp (40) reported similarly poor success with thermal sclerostomy (54% overall; 37% per surgery), and with trabeculectomy (50%), respectively. Beauchamp reported complications in 20% of trabeculectomies, including vitreous loss, scleral collapse, ectasia, retinal detachment, and endophthalmitis; no patients in this series achieved better than 20/200 vision (40).

Many factors contributed to poor outcome from trabeculectomy in children, including lower scleral rigidity, more rapid healing and exuberant scarring processes, and enlargement of glaucomatous eyes with thinning and distortion of intraocular anatomy. In addition to these physiologic considerations, there are difficulties in postoperative management in children, as well as visual loss from amblyopia even if glaucoma has been controlled.

In Britain, the use of intraoperative beta irradiation to the surgical site has improved the success of trabeculectomy. In a large retrospective series of 66 eyes (in patients less than 18 years old with congential glaucoma), IOP was controlled (IOP < 21 mmHg) in approximately 40% of eyes after standard trabeculectomy, compared with >65% after irriadiation-augmented trabeculectomy. No complications were attributed to the use of this low-dose beta irradiation (41).

Subconjunctival 5-fluorouracil has been administered postoperatively in children after trabeculectomy, resulting in successful filtration, but its administration usually requires multiple sequential anesthesias, and is limited by corneal epithelial toxicity, as in adults (42).

More recently, the intraoperative use of mitomycin C has greatly enhanced the success of trabeculectomy in controlling glaucoma in adults at high risk for surgical failure (see Chapter 62), (43,44) presumably by limiting postoperative scarring by Tenon's capsule and scleral fibroblasts. Early results of mitomycin C-augmented trabeculectomy in children are somewhat encouraging. Nguygen et al. reported successful control of IOP (IOP 21 mmHg) in 64% of eyes in a small series of 10 patients (less than 20 years old), with a short average follow-up of four months (45). Using 0.5 mg/ml mitomycin C for five minutes without major complications, Olivier and colleagues achieved IOP control (IOP < 21 mmHg) in 8/10 eyes in a series of eight patients with a mean age 4 years and an average 14 month follow-up (46). Noe, Lynch, and colleagues achieved a similar success rate of 75% using lower-dose mitomycin C (0.25 mg/ml) for 5 minutes in 24 young patients (mean age 6 years) over an average 11-month follow-up (47).

Because of a high incidence of hypotony, Lynch and colleagues developed a probe tip (a modified Hoskins lens) for the diode laser (Iris Medical) that allows postoperative laser suture lysis of scleral flap sutures, with the patient supine under anesthesia. Suture lysis is performed within 1 week after surgery to titrate IOP during the early healing phase after trabeculectomy (47). We have also used a similar probe with encouraging results after mitomycin C-augmented trabeculectomy in young patients (Fig. 70.4), although we prefer to delay laser suture lysis for 1–2 weeks after surgery. This delay allows patients to recover fully from anesthesia, allows us time to evaluate the eye's early response to the filtration surgery, and still seems effective in enhancing filtration in these patients. (The use of absorbable [e.g., 10-0 Vicryl] or releasable sutures [Chapter 62] in the trabeculectomy flap might also encourage the success of trabeculectomy in children.)

The response of very young children to mitomycin C-augmented trabeculectomy is extremely variable, with some patients scarring rapidly despite antifibrotic therapy, whereas others develop hypotony with large avascular filtration blebs.

In addition to postoperative laser suture lysis, postoperative subconjunctival 5-FU may be used after trabeculectomy with mitomycin C to further retard healing and enhance filtration. We have used suconjunctival 5-FU (5 mg) delivered in the quadrant adjacent to the bleb) periodically every 1–2 weeks for up to 2 months after trabeculectomy with mitomycin C in selected infants at high risk for failure. The use of mitomycin C seems to prolong the postoperative period during which laser suture lysis and 5-FU may be effective in enhancing filtration (48).

Hypotony, flat anterior chamber, choroidal detachment, and crystalline lens opacification are the most common complications noted after trabeculectomy with mitomycin C in recent series (49). In addition, we have encountered retinal and pre-retinal hemorrhages, which are sometimes impressive (Fig. 70.5), after mitomycin C-augmented trabeculectomy in children. Similar, "decompression" hemorrhages have been reported after stan-

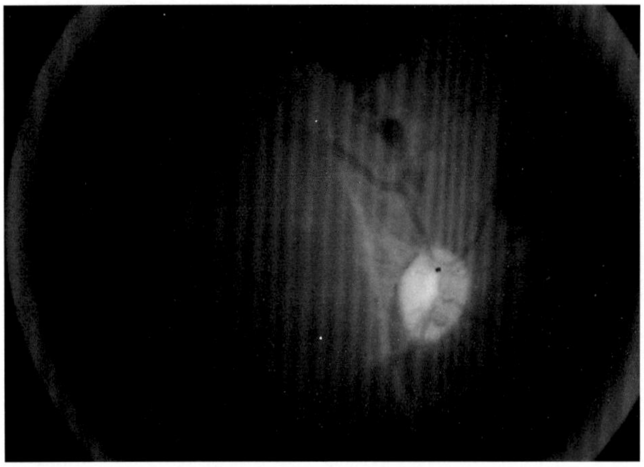

Figure 70.5. Massive retinal and preretinal hemorrhage shortly after trabeculectomy with mitomycin C for uncontrolled childhood glaucoma (same patient as shown in Figure 70.4). All hemorrhages resolved spontaneously without apparent sequelae.

dard trabeculectomy in young patients (50), and they usually resolve spontaneously without serious sequelae.

The use of intraoperative topical mitomycin C during filtering surgery may improve the overall success of this type of surgery in difficult cases of childhood glaucoma. Nevertheless, the application of even small amounts of this potent alkylating agent to a child's eye raises the theoretical concern of long term carcinogenicity (seen in rodents after systemic mitomycin C application) (51,52). Because mitomycin C has been administered mainly in the palliative therapy of cancers, no data exist regarding the risk of secondary malignancy in people after exposure to systemic mitomycin C. However, the total amount of mitomycin C applied topically to the sclera and Tenon's capsule before irrigation does not usually exceed 40–60 μg in most instances; this represents, at most, 0.3% of the chemo-therapeutic dose (for a single cycle of therapy) for a 70-kg adult (53). Evidence from trabeculectomy specimens further suggests at least a 48-fold dilution of mitomycin C concentration as it enters ocular tissue (54).

Despite the absence of prospective data, it seems reasonable to extrapolate from the oncologic literature that the ophthalmic administration of mitomycin C poses a small risk of systemic toxicity, both acute and delayed. The small risk may be justified by intraoperative mitomycin's potential for helping to preserve visual function in difficult glaucomas. Because we do not know the long term ocular sequelae of topical mitomycin C application to the sclera and Tenon's capsule of young children with glaucoma, caution is advised in repeating mitomycin C filters in children with glaucoma. One must weigh the potential and the as yet unknown long-term risks of mitomycin C against those of other alternative procedures.

Drainage Implant (Seton) Surgery

Despite improvements in trabeculectomy in children, this procedure still fails to control IOP in a number of difficult cases. Remaining surgical options include cyclodestructive and drainage implant (seton) procedures. Whereas the Molteno valve implant has been used in children for more than a decade, early experience is now also available for several other setons, including the Baerveldt and Ahmed valves. Reported success and complications rates vary widely (55–59).

Using a two-stage single-plate Molteno implant procedure, Molteno et al. reported a 95% success rate (IOP < 20 mmHg), with a low complication rate (10%), in patients with advanced childhood glaucomas (55). In his series of 83 eyes, average age at surgery was 11 years, with average 5-year follow-up, and all patients received systemic corticosteroids, fluphenamic acid, and colchicine. Billson and colleages subsequently reported 78% success (IOP < 21 mmHg) with the double-plate Molteno implant in a two-stage procedure in 23 eyes of 18 patients (age range 6 months to 46 years) with various childhood glaucomas (56). In this series, no added benefit of systemic antifibrosis therapy was noted.

Several studies have exclusively included younger children, with a lower reported success of IOP control. Lloyd et al. achieved a 56% success rate after placement of one or two single-plate Molteno implants in 16 children under 13 years old; most of these patients required concurrent anti-glaucoma medications (57). Hill et al. reported a 62% success (5 < IOP > 22 mmHg) after a two-stage one or two plate Molteno implant procedure in 70 eyes (patients younger than 21 years old) followed for at least 6 months; nonetheless, 83% of patients needed further glaucoma or other surgery, and complications were common (58). In another relatively large group of 49 children younger than 12 years old, Munoz et al. reported a similar 68% success at IOP control using a single-plate Molteno implant in one stage (59). In all of the aforementioned series, Molteno implants were used with ligation or other reversible partial blockade of the connecting tube if single-stage implantation was used. Some surgeons placed the Molteno tube under a host partial-thickness trabeculectomy-type scleral flap, whereas, more recently, many have favored using a full-thickness donor scleral graft.

Complications seen with Molteno implantation in children include not only those encountered after trabeculectomy in children, but also those specific to seton implantation (Chapter 65). Most common among the latter in many series were contact between the tube and corneal endothelium (tube-cornea touch), erosion of the tube externally through the conjunctiva, migration of the tube, and cataract formation or progression. Interestingly, motility disturbances, reported in adults after seton surgery, (60,61) have not yet been reported in children.

Netland and Walton recently reported results of Molteno and Baerveldt implants used to treat severe uncontrolled glaucoma in a series of 20 patients younger than 10 years (62). With a mean follow-up of 2 years, IOP control (IOP 21 mmHg without further surgery) was achieved in 80%, although 75% of these controlled patients also required glaucoma medical treatment. In addition to complications found in other series, chronic inflammation was noted in 20% of cases. Similarly high rates of success have been reported using the Baerveldt (86%) (63) and the Ahmed (85%) implants respectively (64).

Seton implantation can successfully control glaucoma in children, although many patients need postoperative glaucoma medications. Postoperative care of these patients is arduous, many complications occur, and long-term effects of drainage implants in the eyes of children are not yet known. Although many different seton designs and methods of implantation are available, published experience suggests that the Molteno, Baerveldt, and Ahmed implants can control IOP in children with difficult glaucomas (especially those with extensive scarring, or in whom trabeculectomy has failed) (62–64). The anticipated IOP decrement would be expected to increase with the surface area of the implant's reservoir. Hence the single-plate Molteno (135 square mm), Ahmed (185 square mm), and smallest Baerveldt (200 square mm) implants should have intermediate IOP-lowering ability, whereas the double-plate Molteno and larger Baerveldt setons might be reserved best for cases with exceedingly high preoperative pressures.

We recommend ligation of the Molteno and Baerveldt tubes for one-stage implantation; the Ahmed valve may be used without ligation. **In children with eyes scarred from previous surgeries, we prefer a fornix-based approach, securing the tube of the implant under a full-thickness donor scleral graft** (Fig. 70.6).

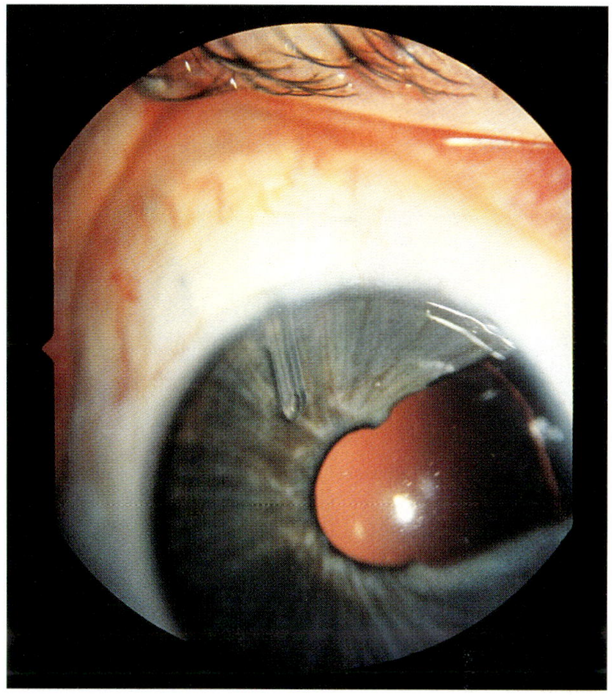

Figure 70.6. Ahmed valve in place under a donor scleral patch graft, in an 18-month-old patient with Sturge-Weber glaucoma, who failed goniotomy and mitomycin-augmented trabeculectomy, in addition to medical therapy for glaucoma.

Combined Filtration and Cataract Surgery

Although surgery for cataract removal in the setting of severe or uncontrolled glaucoma is relatively frequent in adults, the analogous situation in children is fortunately very rare. Children who present with primary congenital glaucoma usually have clear lenses, while those with congenital cataracts usually have normal IOP. Glaucoma most often arises in young children with cataracts some time after cataract surgery has been completed. Children do present with concurrent glaucoma and cataracts in several unusual settings: 1) with primary glaucoma and associated cataracts (i.e., Lowe syndrome), 2) with chronic uveitis and coexisting secondary glaucoma and cataract (i.e., as seen in juvenile rheumatoid arthritis), and 3) in other unusual cases of secondary glaucoma and cataract (e.g., post-traumatic or steroid-induced).

We do not favor combined cataract and glaucoma surgery in most children because of our personal experience with postoperative hypotony and ciliary body shutdown, secondary choroidal detachment, and subsequent bleb scarring and failure in these cases. In nonuveitic cases of cataract and glaucoma, we generally favor cataract surgery first, with subsequent filtration, implant placement, or cyclodestructive procedures (the latter as a last resort). In the rare instance of an older child with cataract and a quiet eye, one might consider extracapsular cataract removal with preservation of the posterior capsule and concurrent filtration surgery (with a tightly sutured scleral flap). In patients with uveitic glaucoma and cataract, in whom lensectomy and anterior or more extensive vitrectomy will be employed, we favor goniotomy (as the glaucoma procedure of choice) before cataract surgery. Although goniotomy can be effective even in children with uveitis who are aphakic (Chapter 71), postoperative hyphema may gain access to the vitreous cavity in aphakic but not phakic eyes. **If angle surgery has failed, and filtration surgery is needed, we recommend removal of the cataract first, followed by glaucoma surgery as a second procedure** (an adequate filtering bleb, arduous to achieve, may easily fail following cataract surgery).

Cyclodestructive Procedures

The surgical procedures previously described all share the goal of increasing facility of aqueous outflow from the eye, either through the angle structures or via a fistula or tube placed into the anterior chamber. By contrast, cyclodestructive procedures reduce the rate of aqueous production by injuring the ciliary processes; results are often unpredictable, and complications frequent. Cyclodestruction nonetheless constitutes a valid means of attempting control of otherwise vision-threatening glaucoma in children, once medical and other surgical means have been exhausted or have proven inadequate to the task.

Cyclocryotherapy (freezing the ciliary processes from an external approach) has been used as therapy for difficult childhood glaucomas for many years, and it is applied with a similar technique to that used in adults (Chapter 57). Unfortunately, overall success (IOP control without severe visual loss or phthisis) has been fairly poor (30% in a large series of children with advanced congenital glaucoma) (65). In children, cryotherapy should be applied to a maximum of 180 of the circumference of the eye at one session, using six or seven freezes (60 seconds each at −80 C) with a 2.5 mm diameter cryoprobe centered about 2.5 mm from the limbus (14). In retreatments, at least one quadrant of the ciliary body should be left untouched; no treatment is available if chronic postoperative hypotony or phthisis occurs (14). Aside from the risks of hypotony or phthisis, uveitis, cataract formation, and attendant visual loss are the major problems with cyclocryotherapy in children.

Transscleral cyclophotocoagulation with the Neodymium:YAG laser has recently reduced IOP in comparable fashion to cyclocryotherapy. With the continuous-wave Nd:YAG laser, Schuman et al. reported successful IOP control ($3 < IOP < 19$ mmHg) in 56% of adults with severe glaucoma after transscleral cyclophotocoagulation; phthisis or severe hypotony occured in 10% (66). This procedure is performed using a spherical-tipped probe, placed with its anterior edge 0.5 − 1.5 mm from the limbus and perpendicular to the eye; 32 to 40 applications of 7–9 watts for 0.5-0.7 seconds are applied for 360 often sparing the 3- and 9-o'clock positions (66).

Early experience with Nd:YAG contact transscleral cyclophotocoagulation in young children with advanced, uncontrolled glaucoma suggests effective IOP reduction in 50%, with a 70% retreatment rate (67). Significant advantages of Nd:YAG transscleral cyclophotocoagulation over cyclocryotherapy in adults (and likely also in children) include less transient IOP rise, a less exuberant uveitic response, and less pain postoperatively. Similar complications have nonetheless been reported with both procedures (15).

The Iris Medical G-Probe has recently been FDA-approved for use with the diode laser in performing transscleral cyclophotocoagulation. This procedure seems comparable to the contact Nd:YAG technique for cyclophotocoagulation in adults, with reported IOP reduction ($>20\%$ from baseline IOP) in 56% of subjects after two years (68). The technique in this series involved placement of 16 to 18 applications (of 2 seconds each) to three quadrants with the Iris G-probe, with variable power settings (mostly 1500–2000 mW). Using transillumination to guide diode transscleral cyclophotocoagulation in five buphthalmic eyes, Lehmann and colleagues reported at least a 25% IOP reduction in four of them after a minimum 6-month followup period (69). Further experience with this therapy in children may prove it a worthy alternative to cyclocryotherapy and Nd:YAG cyclophotocoagulation.

LONGTERM FOLLOWUP OF CHILDREN WITH GLAUCOMA

Even children whose glaucoma is well-controlled after surgical therapy (with or without adjunctive medical therapy) deserve lifetime followup. **Loss of IOP control may occur months or even decades after initial successful control with surgery, and may be asymptomatic in the older child/young adult.** In addition, young children with glaucoma often face vision-threatening difficulties such as corneal scarring, anisometropia, and resultant amblyopia even after IOP control has been achieved. Children with glaucoma which is controlled without medications should be followed at least every 6 months, and young children, or those with whom IOP has been controlled for less than 2 years, should probably be evaluated at least every 3 or 4 months. During these office examinations, the correlates of adequate IOP control include: 1) stable visual function, refractive error and optic nerve appearance, 2) corneas which are free of edema and stable in size, and 3) children who are free of epiphora, excessive photophobia and blepharospasm. By contrast, **even if the IOP is < 20 mm Hg, deteriorating vision, progressive myopia, and optic nerve cupping, and/or increases in corneal size, edema, or ocular symptomatology suggest that control of glaucoma may be inadequate for the longterm.**

Medical and surgical therapy for childhood glaucomas has challenged ophthalmologists for many years. Despite tremendous advances in medical, laser, and surgical technology over the past quarter century, we are still humbled by our inability to preserve sight in many children with glaucoma.

References

1. DeLuise VP, Anderson DR: Primary infantile glaucoma (congenital glaucoma). Surv Ophthalmol 1983;28:1.
2. Haas J: Principles and problems of treatment in congenital glaucoma. Invest Ophthalmol 1968;7:140.
3. Shrader CE, Thomas JV, Simmons RJ. Relationship of patient age and tolerance to carbonic anhydrase inhibitors. Am J Ophthalmol 1983;96: 730.
4. Becker B, Shaffer RN: Diagnosis and therapy of the glaucomas. St. Louis, C.V. Mosby, 1965.
5. Maumenee AE: Further observations on the pathogenesis of congenital glaucoma. Am J Ophthalmol 1963;55:1163.
6. Walton DS: Glaucoma in infants and children. In: Pediatric Ophthalmology. Edited by Nelson LB, Calhoun JH, Harley RD. Philadelphia, W.B. Saunders Company, 1983.

7. Zimmerman TJ, Kooner KS, Morgan KS: Safety and efficacy of timolol in pediatric glaucoma. Surv Ophthalmol 1983;28:262.
8. Hoskins HD, et al: Clinical experience with timolol in childhood glaucoma. Arch Opthalmol 1985;103:1163.
9. Boger WP, Walton DS: Timolol in uncontrolled childhood glaucomas. Ophthalmol 1981;88:253.
10. McMahon CD, Hetherington J, Hoskins HD, et al: Timolol and pediatric glaucomas. Ophthalmology 1981;88:249.
11. Olson RJ, Bromberg BB, Zimmerman TJ: Apneic spells associated with timolol therapy in a neonate. Am J Ophthalmol 1979;88:120.
12. Passo MS, Palmer EA, Van Buskirk EM: Plasma timolol in glaucoma patients. Ophthalmology 1984;91:1361.
13. Raab EL: Congenital glaucoma. Persp Ophthalmol 1978;2:35.
14. Shields MB: Textbook of glaucoma, 3rd Ed. Baltimore MD, Williams & Wilkins, 1992.
15. De Vincentiis C: Incisions dell angolo irideo nel glaucoma. Ann Ophthalmol 1893;22:540.
16. Barkan O: Technique of goniotomy. Arch Ophthalmol 1938;19:217.
17. Walton DS: Goniotomy. In: Glaucoma surgery. Edited by Thomas JV. St. Louis, C.V. Mosby, 1992.
18. Walton DS: Aniridic glaucoma: results of goniosurgery to prevent and treat this problem. Trans Am Ophthalmol Soc 1986;84:59.
19. Hodapp E, Heuer DK: A simple technique for goniotomy. Am J Ophthalmol 1986;102:537.
20. Buckley EG, Freedman SF, Shields MB: Atlas of ophthalmic surgery Vol. 3: Strabismus and glaucoma surgery. St. Louis, Mosby Yearbook, Inc., 1995.
21. Litinsky SM, Shaffer RN, Hetherington J, et al: Operative complications of goniotomy. Trans Am Acad Ophthalmol Otolaryngol 1977;83:78.
22. Scheie HG: Goniopuncture—a new filtering operation for glaucoma. Arch Ophthalmol 1950;44:761.
23. Melamed S, Latina MA, Epstein DL: Neodymium:YAG laser trabeculopuncture in juvenile open-angle glaucoma. Ophthalmology 1987;94:163.
24. Fernandez JL, Galin MA: Technique of direct goniotomy. Arch Ophthalmol 1973;90:305.
25. Kanski JJ, McAllister JA: Trabeculodialysis for inflammatory glaucoma in children and young adults. Ophthalmology 1985;92:927.
26. Safran MJ, Robin AL, Pollack IP: Trabeculoplasty in younger patients with primary open angle glaucoma. Am J Ophthalmol 1984;97:292.
27. Wilensky JT, Weinreb RN: Early and late failure of argon laser trabeculoplasty. Arch Ophthalmol 1983;101:895.
28. Smith R: A new technique for opening the canal of Schlemm. Br J Ophthalmol 1960;44:370.
29. Burian HM: A case of Marfan's syndrome with bilateral glaucoma with a description of a new type of operation for developmental glaucoma. Am J Ophthalmol 1960;50:1187.
30. Akimoto M, Tanihara H, Negi A, et al: Surgical results of trabeculotomy ab externo for developmental glaucoma. Arch Ophthalmol 1994;112:1540.
31. McPherson SDJ: Results of external trabeculotomy. Am J Ophthalmol 1973;76:918.
32. Shrader CE, Cibis GW: External trabeculotomy. In: Glaucoma surgery. Edited by Thomas JV. St. Louis, C.V. Mosby, 1992.
33. Beck AD, et al: Complete (360 degree) trabeculotomy as primary treatment for developmental glaucoma. Invest Ophthalmol Vis Sci 1994;35 Suppl:1914.
34. Smith R: Nylon filament trabeculotomy in glaucoma. Trans Ophth Soc UK 1963;82:439.
35. Hoskins HD, Shaffer RN, Hetherington J: Goniotomy vs. trabeculotomy. J Ped Ophthalmol Strabismus 1984;21:153.
36. Luntz MH: The advantages of trabeculotomy over goniotomy. J Ped Ophthalmol Strabismus 1984;21:150.
37. Anderson DR: Trabeculotomy compared to goniotomy for glaucoma in children. Ophthalmology 1983;90:805.
38. Cadera W, et al: Filtering surgery in childhood glaucoma. Ophth Surg 1984;15:319.
39. Scheie HG: Results of peripheral iridectomy with scleral cautery in congenital and juvenile glaucoma. Trans Am Ophthalmol Soc 1962;60:116.
40. Beauchamp GR, Parks MM: Filtering surgery in children: Barriers to success. Ophthalmology 1979;86:170.
41. Miller MH, Rice NSC: Beta-irradiation with trabeculectomy for congenital glaucoma. Br J Ophthalmol 1991;75:584.
42. Zalish M, Leiba H, Oliver M: Subconjunctival injection of 5-fluorouracil following trabeculectomy for congenital and infantile glaucoma. Ophthalmol Surg 1992;23:203.
43. Kitazawa Y, Kawase E, Matsushita H, et al: Trabeculectomy with mitomycin. A comparative study with fluorouracil. Arch Ophthalmol 1991;109:1693.
44. Palmer SS: Mitomycin as adjunct chemotherapy with trabeculectomy. Ophthalmology 1991;98:317.
45. Nguyen QH, et al: Trabeculectomy with mitomycin-C in pediatrics. Invest Ophthalmol Vis Sci 1993;34 Suppl:815.
46. Olivier MMG, et al: Trabeculectomy with adjunctive mitomycin C in pediatric patients. Invest Ophthalmol Vis Sci 1994;35 Suppl:1431.
47. Noe RL, Lynch MG, Beck D: Glaucoma filtering surgery with mitomycin-C in children. Invest Ophthalmol Vis Sci 1994;35 Suppl:1431.
48. Pappa KS, et al: Late argon laser suture lysis after mitomycin C trabeculectomy. Ophthalmology 1993;100:1268.
49. Kitazawa Y, Suemori-Matsushita H, Tamamoto T, et al: Low-dose and high-dose mitomycin trabeculectomy as an initial surgery in primary open-angle glaucoma. Ophthalmology 1993;100:1624.
50. Fechtner RD, et al: Complications of glaucoma surgery: ocular decompression retinopathy. Arch Ophthalmol 1992;110:965.
51. Crooke ST, Bradner WT: Mitomycin C: a review. Cancer Treat Rev 1976;3:121.
52. Glaubinger D, Ramu A: Antitumor antibiotics. In: Pharmacologic Principles of Cancer Treatment. Edited by Chabner BA. Phila, W.B. Saunders Co., 1982.
53. Calabresi P, Parks REJ: Antiproliferative agents and drugs used for immunosuppression. In: The Pharmacologic Basis of Therapeutics. Edited by Gilman AG, Goodman LS, Rall TW, Murad F. New York, MacMillan Publishing Co., 1985.
54. Kawase I, Matsushita H, Yamamato T, et al: Mitomycin concentration in rabbit and ocular tissues after topical administration. Ophthalmology 1992;99:203.
55. Molteno ACB, Ancker E, Van Biljon G: Surgical technique for advanced juvenile glaucoma. Arch Ophthalmol 1984;102:51.
56. Billson F, Thomas R, Aylward W: The use of two-stage Molteno implants in developmental glaucoma. J Ped Ophthalmol Strabismus 1989;26:3.
57. Lloyd MA, et al: Clinical experience with the single-plate Molteno implant in complicated glaucomas. Ophthalmology 1992;99:679.
58. Hill RA, et al: Molteno implantation for glaucoma in young patients. Ophthalmology 1991;98:1042.
59. Munoz M, Tomey KF, Traverso C, et al: Clinical experience with the Molteno implant in advanced infantile glaucoma. J Ped Ophthalmol Strabismus 1991;28:68.
60. Ball SF, Ellis GSJ, Herrington RG, et al: Brown's superior oblique tendon syndrome after Baerveldt glaucoma implant. Arch Ophthalmol 1992;110:1368.
61. Christmann LM, Wilson ME: Motility disturbances after Molteno implants. J Ped Ophthalmol Strabismus 1992;29:44.
62. Netland PA, Walton DS: Glaucoma drainage implants in pediatric patients. Ophthalmol Surg 1993;24:723.
63. Fellenbaum PS, et al: Experience with the Baerveldt implant in young patients with glaucoma. Invest Ophthalmol Vis Sci 1994;35Suppl:1424.
64. Smyth RJ, Tam MY, Coleman AL, et al: Pediatric glaucoma valve implantation. Invest Ophthalmol Vis Sci 1994;35 Suppl:1423.

65. Al Faran MF, Tomey KF, Al Mutlag FA: Cyclocryotherapy in selected cases of congenital glaucoma. Ophthalmol Surg 1990;21:794.
66. Schuman JS, et al: Contact transscleral Nd:YAG laser cyclophotocoagulation: midterm results. Ophthalmology 1992;99:1089.
67. Phelan MJ, Higginbotham EJ: Contact Transscleral Nd:YAG laser cyclophotocoagulation for the treatment of refractory pediatric glaucoma. Ophthalmic Surg Lasers 1995;26:401.
68. Kosoko O, et al: Long-term effect of the diode laser using the Iris G-probe on glaucoma patients. Invest Ophthalmol Vis Sci 1994;35 Suppl., 2173.
69. Lehmann OJ, et al: Diode laser transscleral cyclophotocoagulation in buphthalmic eyes: histological and clinical results. Invest Ophthalmol Vis Sci 1994;35 Suppl., 2172.

Unusual Pediatric Glaucomas

71

David S. Walton

PRIMARY GLAUCOMAS WITH SYSTEMIC OR OCULAR ABNORMALITIES

Childhood glaucoma may occur with defects confined to the filtration system, as seen in children with infantile open angle glaucoma and juvenile open angle glaucoma. In this section primary childhood glaucoma associated with systemic or ocular abnormalities will be described. See Table 68.1 for a complete listing of these types of childhood glaucoma.

PRIMARY CHILDHOOD GLAUCOMAS ASSOCIATED WITH SYSTEMIC CONDITIONS

Primary infantile glaucoma is associated with an astounding number of diverse systemic conditions (Table 68.1). While glaucoma associated with nevus flammeus is relatively common, each of the other listed causes is quite uncommon. Some conditions are nonhereditary (e.g., rubella syndrome, fetal alcohol syndrome), while others clearly are hereditary (e.g.., Lowe's syndrome, hepatocerebral renal syndrome, neurofibromatosis).

Congenital Rubella Syndrome

The diverse complications of the maternal rubella syndrome are well known and include ocular defects consisting of microphthalmia, cataracts, pigmentary retinitis, corneal opacification, and glaucoma (Fig. 71.1). Infantile glaucoma is probably the least common of these secondary ocular anomalies.

Congenital rubella infantile glaucoma is often detected in infancy secondary to corneal opacification and is usually bilateral. It must be differentiated from permanent rubella leucomas and transient corneal opacification seen in these affected infants. This glaucoma may be mild and not detected until later in life. In addition to corneal enlargement these children with glaucoma will possess diaphanous irides and pigmentary abnormalities in the posterior pole. Gonioscopy of children with rubella glaucoma reveals abnormalities similar to that seen in hereditary infantile glaucoma, characterized by increased opacification of the inner tissue of the filtration angle, making visualization of the scleral spur and ciliary body very difficult.

Treatment of this glaucoma by goniosurgery is often successful at all ages, providing an additional similarity to hereditary infantile glaucoma.

Nevus Flammeus of the Eyelids with Glaucoma

Nevus flammeus of the face is a well known component of the Sturge-Weber syndrome, Klippel-Trenaunay-Weber syndrome, and cutis marmorata telangiectasia congenita (Chapter 49). Childhood glaucoma commonly complicates Sturge-Weber syndrome and Klippel-Trenaunay-Weber syndrome and is seen infrequently with cutis marmorata telangiectasia congenita, possibly because of the latter condition's infrequent involvement of facial tissue.

In the Sturge-Weber syndrome, glaucoma is associated with a facial nevus flammeus and a leptomeningeal vascular defect. Usually, one side of the face is affected, but bilateral involvement also occurs. When the facial nevus is bilateral, glaucoma also is often bilateral. Apart from the Sturge-Weber syndrome children are seen with less widespread involvement, and without nevus flammeus of the upper eyelid. These patients seem to be at no risk for glaucoma. With intracranial involvement, seizures, hemiparesis, and hemianopsia may occur.

The glaucoma complicating the Sturge-Weber syndrome, Klippel-Trenaunay-Weber syndrome, and cutis marmorata telangiectasia congenita is usually of early onset and may often be congenital. In the absence of early intraocular pressure (IOP) measurements, enlargement of the cornea and globe indicates the presence of glaucoma during the first 2 years of life.

On examination of children with glaucoma associated with facial nevus flammeus (Fig. 71.2) the examiner is initially consumed by the patient's blood vessel anomalies. It is appropriate however to consider this entity to be a neurocristopathy and to remember the neural crest origin of components of the vascular system, meninges, pigmentation tissues, trabecular meshwork, iris as well as other tissues. Because of frequent unilateral involvement, the examiner should take advantage of the opportunity to compare affected and unaffected eyes.

Children seen with this type of glaucoma usually have moderately advanced glaucoma associated with decreased visual acuity, anisometropia, and disc abnormalities. The bulbar conjunctiva usually shows fine tortuous vessels. The episclera will show a more uniform grid of permanent vessels, abnormal by their number and size. The cornea is usually enlarged, but breaks in Descemet's membrane

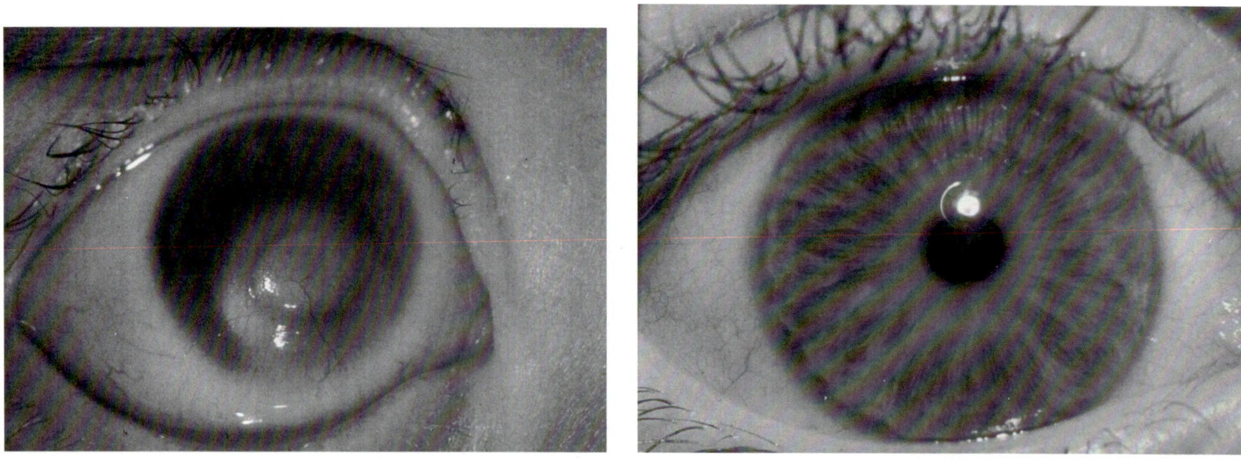

Figure 71.1. Maternal rubella syndrome. (A) Rubella keratopathy may be represented by diffuse edema or localized opacification with vascularization as seen in this infant patient. (B) The iris stroma of a 9-year-old girl with rubella glaucoma was porous and associated with a granular transillumination.

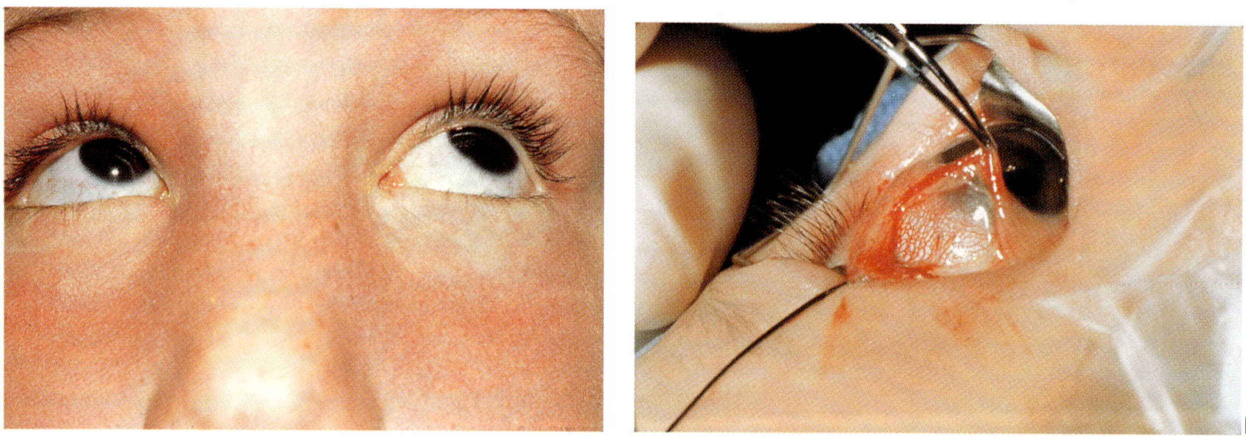

Figure 71.2. Sturge-Weber syndrome. In addition to signs of glaucoma, dark irides, abnormally tortuous conjunctival vessels and abnormal episcleral vessels are seen externally. (A) Note diffuse anastomotic episcleral blood vessels seen at surgery (B).

(Haab's striae) are infrequent. The anterior chamber is usually deep. The iris of the involved eye possesses a more compact and often more pigmented iris than seen in the contralateral normal eye. With bilateral occurrence the presence of bilateral iridal melanosis is less obvious than the heterochromia seen in unilateral cases. The lenses are clear. The fundi often appear diffusely red, suggesting the presence of an associated capillary hemangioma. Ultrasonography for choroidal thickness will show thickening of the choroid in the presence of a typical choroidal hemangioma in this condition. Blood vessel abnormalities of retinal vessels are not seen. If the IOP is excessive, glaucomatous cupping and atrophy develop, as in other glaucomas.

In 32 patients having nevus flammeus of the upper lid with glaucoma in whom we have performed gonioscopy, all have had open angles and have had little in the angle to suggest a vascular abnormality. In general when the glaucomatous eyes were compared with the contralateral normal eyes, except for peculiarities of Schlemm's canal, **the principal recognizable abnormality was similar to that which we believe is characteristic of ordinary congenital open angle glaucoma**. The ciliary band and scleral spur were indistinctly visible in the glaucomatous eyes, possibly due to veiling by overlying uveal meshwork, whereas in the contralateral normal eyes the ciliary band and scleral spur have been distinct with the overlying uveal meshwork thinner and more transparent than in glaucomatous eyes. The iris was commonly attached farther forward in the glaucomatous eyes than in the normal, but never hiding the scleral spur, and the level of attachment of the iris was variable, causing the insertion of the iris to appear wavy as one scanned circumferentially.

When blood has refluxed into Schlemm's canal during gonioscopy in some eyes having glaucoma with hemangioma, we have had the impression that the distribution in Schlemm's canal has been abnormal, and different from the ordinary congenital open angle glaucoma. In some eyes, no distinct line of blood, but only a diffuse reddish glow, was seen deep in the corneoscleral meshwork. **In eyes in which the blood in Schlemm's canal could be seen in more distinct lines, Schlemm's canal appeared to wander at a varying distance anterior to the scleral spur or to be broken up into multiple channels,** rather than to form a uniform discrete ring at a constant distance anterior to the scleral spur.

Measurements of episcleral venous pressure vessels in hemangioma of the lid with glaucoma show two categories of patients. One type has inconspicuous vessels on the globe, with normal pressure in them. The other type has elevated episcleral venous pressure, and the vessels appear abnormally prominent. According to tonography, there is obstruction to aqueous outflow in both types.

A noteworthy peculiarity about the IOP in this condition is that when the patient changes from sitting to recumbent position, the IOP undergoes a greater change than in other types of glaucoma or than in normal eyes. When the patient lies down, the IOP in the eye affected by hemangioma may increase by several mm Hg. However, if the patient remains in the recumbent position, the IOP drops again in 15 to 30 minutes, approaching what it was in the sitting position. Presumably the rise in IOP is due to a rapid distention of an intraocular hemangioma, probably in the choroid, after which the eye gradually returns to its steady-state IOP as a result of slow expulsion of an equal and compensatory volume of aqueous humor. When the eye is in a steady state, tonography indicates abnormal resistance to aqueous outflow to be responsible for the glaucoma.

Tonometry in childhood is always challenging. Crying raises the measured IOP. Resistance to tonometry in these conditions produces an exaggerated elevation of IOP which must be considered when the accuracy of an elevated IOP is being considered.

Glaucoma treatment should first be medical therapy, especially in young children who might be expected to have less good results with filtration surgery. Beta blockers, miotics, and carbonic anhydrase inhibitors are frequently helpful.

If medical control proves inadequate, then surgery must be attempted. Goniotomies performed during childhood in 6 patients by us have been uncomplicated, but unsuccessful in controlling this type of glaucoma. We support the general impression that **goniotomy performed once or several times offers little prospect of relief for this type of glaucoma.**

Filtration surgery, in light of the poor results that can be expected with a goniotomy procedure, must be considered in the presence of uncontrolled glaucoma in these patients, and filtration surgery is sometimes successful (Chapter 46). Trabeculectomy with use of intraoperative mitomycin C is the treatment of choice. Reasonably tight closure of the scleral flap with or without releasable sutures is appropriate, given the risk for rapid operative or postoperative uveal effusions. Consideration should be given to performing sclerotomy over the ciliary body at the time of surgery to allow immediate and postoperative choroidal drainage. The trabeculectomy surgeon will be impressed with the dense grid of episcleral vessels present at the flap and sclerostomy site (Fig. 71.2). These can be managed well with an underwater diathermy tip. In our experience with 5 young children with glaucoma associated with a nevus flammeus and who required trabeculectomy surgery with adjunctive use of mitomycin-C, successful control of the glaucoma was achieved without medication in each of these patients.

Our experience with cycloablative procedures, usually cyclocryotherapy, in a few patients suggests that it can also be helpful and that it is not more problematic in this glaucoma than in other types of glaucoma.

Iridocorneal Goniodysgenesis with Glaucoma

Under iridocorneal goniodysgenesis we include all congenital ocular abnormalities that tend to combine malformations of the cornea, iris, and filtration angle. The abnormality may be predominantly corneal (as in embryotoxon) or involve both cornea and iris (Axenfeld's anomaly and Peters' anomaly). In Rieger's anomaly the angle is involved, as well as the cornea and iris, and glaucoma is more likely. The pupils can be conspicuously abnormal. This eye condition also can be associated with systemic abnormalities, including abnormalities of the teeth, mid-face, hormonal system, cardiovascular system, genitalia, and umbilical skin (Rieger's syndrome). Dental anomalies are frequent and consist of hypodontia and microdontia.

Axenfeld-Rieger's syndrome is frequently transmitted as an autosomal dominant disorder. Cytogenetic studies have suggested that at least one of the genetic defects able to cause this syndrome is present on the long arm of the fourth chromosome.

Whether or not glaucoma develops in an eye with typical iridocorneal goniodysgenesis depends upon the degree of **obstruction of outflow of aqueous humor, either by iridocorneal tissue overlying the trabecular meshwork or apparently in certain cases by abnormalities in the outflow channels themselves** (Fig. 71.3). The conspicuous processes seen bridging the filtration angle face do not seem to contribute to the obstruction to outflow of aqueous humor. As expected, goniotomy surgery, which strips these processes, frequently does not treat the complicating glaucoma successfully.

For discussion, we have divided cases of iridocorneal dysgenesis into three groups, representing different degrees of severity. Actually, we think the conditions in the various categories probably are related in some instances. We know, for instance, that separating cases according to

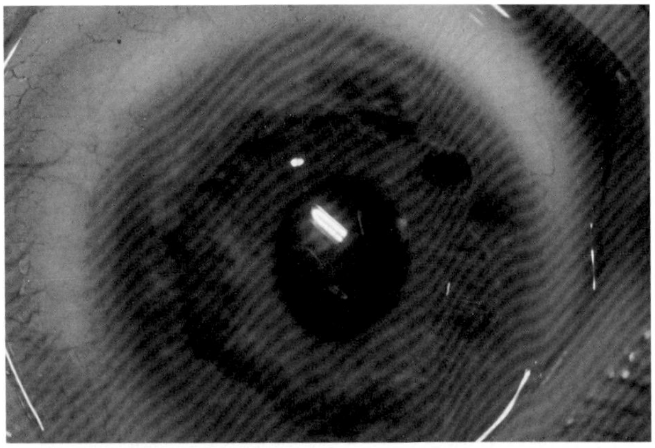

Figure 71.3. Iridocorneal goniodysgenesis. Forward attachment of iris stromal processes to a central displaced and prominent Schwalbe's line (posterior embryotoxon) is common with this anomaly.

whether or not the pupil is involved is artificial, since in 2 families we have seen pairs of individuals (mother and son, and a pair of sisters) with iridocorneal dysgenesis with glaucoma, but with the pupils normal in one and abnormal in the other member of each pair. The categories are for convenience in description.

EMBRYOTOXON WITHOUT ATTACHMENTS TO THE IRIS

Probably the mildest and most common abnormality one may consider under iridocorneal dysgenesis is simple embryotoxon, or marginal corneal dysplasia, occurring without other evident abnormality. Embryotoxon is an abnormal thickening of the peripheral rim of Descemet's membrane (Schwalbe's line). The thickening has a refractile glassy character. This thickening may be in the form of a uniform, circumferential, prominent ridge on the inner surface of the cornea, but more commonly it varies in thickness, and sometimes is abnormally prominent in only one sector. It often varies in thickness so much that it has a beaded appearance.

One can often see embryotoxon very well with the slit lamp biomicroscope through clear cornea adjacent to the limbus, but only by gonioscopy can one be sure whether there are associated structural abnormalities in the angle. Embryotoxon without other abnormality and without glaucoma is noted in adults as an incidental finding on routine examination and also in infants and children when slit lamp or gonioscopic examination is performed.

Slight degrees of what may be called embryotoxon are not rare in otherwise apparently normal eyes, and it is difficult to say at what stage it should be considered pathologic. **We have seen no eye in which we could relate embryotoxon to glaucoma, unless in addition to the embryotoxon there were congenital attachments across the angle between iris and cornea**, as we will next describe.

EMBRYOTOXON WITH CONGENITAL ATTACHMENTS BETWEEN PERIPHERAL IRIS AND CORNEA, BUT PUPIL NORMAL

In iridocorneal dysgenesis having these qualifications, the principal feature is congenital bridging of the angle between Schwalbe's line and peripheral iris by strands of tissue. The stroma of the iris may be normal, atrophic, or split, and the lens may or may not be cataractous, but the pupil is normal. The strands bridging the angle can usually be seen conclusively only by gonioscopy. These strands are variable in character: In some eyes they consist of refractile avascular material like ropes of Descemet's membrane. In other eyes they consist of avascular iris stroma, with or without pigmentation, and in still other eyes, of iris stroma together with iris blood vessels.

We have found congenital iridocorneal bridges of this sort with normal pupils in the following circumstances: 1) in adult or children's nonglaucomatous eyes, 2) in eyes having what seemed to be adult open angle glaucoma, and 3) in eyes having congenital or childhood glaucoma.

These anomalies are also seen in arteriohepatic dysplasia (Alagille's syndrome). In this syndrome posterior embryotoxon is a near constant abnormality and is frequently associated with multiple bridging angle processes and less frequent corectopia. This syndrome is an autosomal dominant condition with congenital cholestasis, facial defects, cardiovascular anomalies, and skeletal defects. The anterior segment anomalies are accompanied by other ocular defects including pigmentary retinopathy, but glaucoma does not seem to complicate this syndrome.

EMBRYOTOXON WITH CONGENITAL ATTACHMENTS BETWEEN PERIPHERAL IRIS AND CORNEA, PLUS ABNORMALITIES OF THE PUPIL

This combination of congenital abnormalities consists of a combination of posterior embryotoxon (posterior marginal dysplasia of the cornea), with attachments across the angle from iris to cornea and trabecular meshwork, often with hypoplasia of the stroma of the iris which may give the iris a dark appearance, plus a considerable variety of possible abnormalities of the pupil, including eccentric pupil (corectopia), pinpoint pupil, slit-like pupil, ectropion of the pigment layer of the iris at the pupil (ectropion uveae), and multiple holes in the iris, inaccurately called polycoria. (Eyes with "polycoria" may show progressive changes in the iris that may behave like essential atrophy of the iris.) If the angle face can be seen through the processes, it is usually not possible to define the trabecular meshwork, scleral spur, and ciliary body band. In their places a uniform plane of white tissue is typically seen. These malformations occasionally are associated with microphthalmia, or cataract.

This most conspicuous form of iridocorneal goniodysgenesis that involves the pupil and iris as well as the angle often has a hereditary basis, with similar conditions occurring in relatives, as seen in Rieger's syndrome.

Children with these associated defects of the pupil, iris, angle, and peripheral cornea are at significant risk for glaucoma which may be present in infancy or be acquired. Those patients with progressive anterior segment changes characterized by degeneration of the iris and associated blockage of the angle by peripheral iris tissue are especially at risk. These changes with development of glaucoma or worsening of glaucoma usually occur in the first 5 years of life.

When the anterior segment defects possess a dense central corneal opacification, the presence of Peters' anomaly should be considered. In this condition, which is often bilateral and may be hereditary, a dense central leucoma is present with the attachment of iris processes at the periphery of the opacity. A cataract may be present. The angle is usually open, but abnormal with scattered bridges of tissue from the iris root to the trabecular meshwork. These patients also are at risk for glaucoma. I have frequently seen moderate IOP elevations in infancy in this condition slowly improve over the first 5 years of life.

Treatment of children with glaucoma complicating iridocorneal goniodysgenesis should be initiated with medical therapy. Such treatment is more often helpful with cases of glaucoma that develop later in childhood. Beta blockers and carbonic anhydrase inhibitors have been helpful. When the glaucoma is present from infancy, medical therapy generally is inadequate for satisfactory IOP control, but may be useful before glaucoma surgery to decrease the IOP or as an adjunct to therapy after glaucoma surgery.

Goniosurgery should always be considered in these forms of trabecular dysgenesis, especially in infancy. Better control may be achieved with continued medical therapy for a period of time, but **in our experience definitive glaucoma control with goniosurgery is rarely achieved**. Best results with goniosurgery can be expected in those eyes with less severe defects, such as those with iris processes alone, unassociated with iris abnormalities. Failure of goniosurgery to help with one eye may be useful information in deciding against goniosurgery for a fellow eye.

Trabeculectomy with adjunctive use of mitomycin C has been helpful in these patients and now represents the surgical treatment of choice.

The Oculocerebrorenal (Lowe's) Syndrome

Lowe's syndrome is a rare X-linked (Xq24-q26) disease characterized by mental retardation, hypotonia, systemic acidosis, rickets, and ocular defects including glaucoma (Fig. 71.4). The most constant defect is cataracts which are characteristically bilateral, irregularly dense, thin, and are associated with extreme miosis. Glaucoma may occur less frequently than cataracts. However, each of five patients with this disorder cared for by the author had bilateral primary congenital glaucoma. (When patients are seen with glaucoma after cataract extraction it is difficult to be sure whether or not the glaucoma is primary or secondary.)

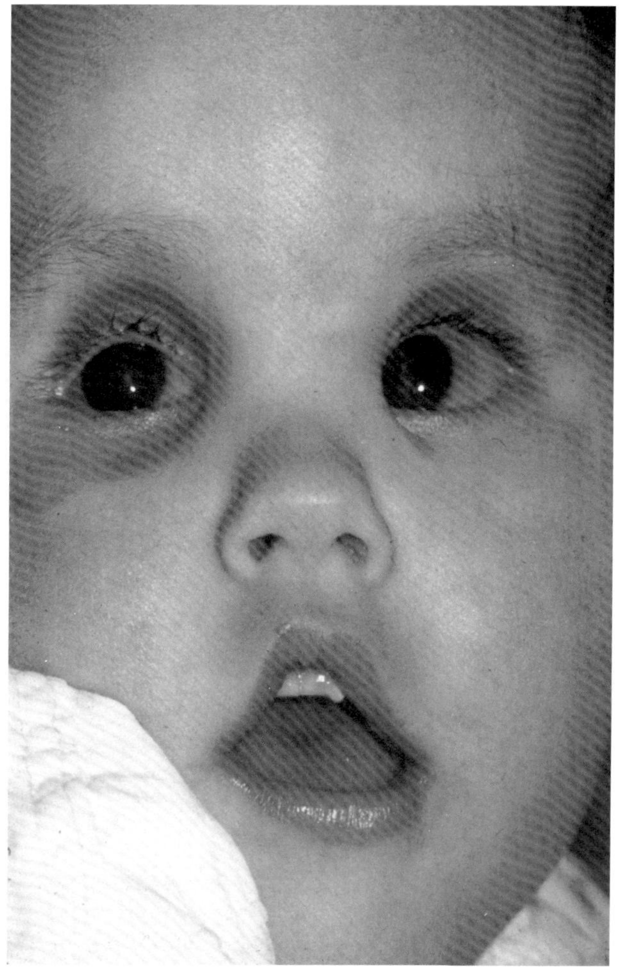

Figure 71.4. Lowe's syndrome. Ocular enlargement, glaucoma, cataracts, miosis and frontal bossing are common in this disorder.

Patients with Lowe's syndrome and glaucoma often possess extreme corneal enlargement. Gonioscopy reveals circumferential advanced failure of angle differentiation. Trabecular meshwork is usually visible and narrow, but scleral spur and ciliary body are typically difficult, if not impossible to define apart from other components of the filtration angle. Abnormal processes are not present.

Treatment of glaucoma associated with Lowe's syndrome is difficult. Goniotomy in my experience is most often unrewarding. It also has been associated with extensive postoperative bleeding. Before trying a goniotomy procedure on one eye, I would recommend medical therapy consisting of a beta blocker and a carbonic anhydrase inhibitor (CAI). There is an appropriate reluctance to recommend an oral CAI in the presence of a condition complicated already by systemic acidosis and rickets. Patients with Lowe's syndrome will be on supplemental base therapy (e.g., Bicitra/Polycitra-Baker Norton). The dose of this supplement usually can be increased to take into account the effect of the oral CAI to allow its use for this ocular indication. Consultation with the patient's pediatrician is recommended.

Neurofibromatosis

Neurofibromatosis type 1 (NF-1) is a multisystem disorder inherited by autosomal dominant transmission with its gene on chromosome 17 (17q11.2). NF-1 is one of the most common inherited disorders, and its systemic and ocular defects are well known including cafe-au-lait spots, optic nerve gliomas, and Lisch nodules. Childhood glaucoma may be one of the least common ocular complications of this disease, but when present it usually occurs as a congenital glaucoma.

An infant with NF-1 and glaucoma may show no non-ocular stigmata of this disease. Even cafe-au-lait spots, abundant later in childhood, may not be apparent before one year of age. **Glaucoma, however, almost always is associated with the development of a plexiform neuroma of the upper lid, producing a characteristic "S" curve deformity.** The glaucoma may be bilateral, but this is unusual. The globe is usually enlarged, as is the cornea, of the involved eye (Fig. 71.5). This enlargement may be striking and be associated with high myopia, even in the first months of life. The degree of enlargement often seems to be in excess of what would be expected secondary to the elevated IOP alone. On further examination abnormal pale subconjunctival tissue may be present suggesting a neurofibroma of the conjunctiva.

The iris of the affected eye typically possesses a uniform stroma. Though no Lisch nodules would be expected in early life, they also seem not to occur in the irides of eyes affected with glaucoma compared to fellow nonglaucoma eyes. An ectropion uveae, however, is a characteristic pupillary rim abnormality seen in these eyes. This abnormality is often considered to be congenital when, in point of fact, it is characteristically quite subtle in infants and not recognized easily unless suspected. Over the first year of life the width of the pigment layer will widen over the iris making it easily recognizable, especially when the iris is blue. Gonioscopy will reveal a striking deformity which has been seen in each of 6 eyes cared for by the author. The iris leaf appears straight rather than convex and inserts anteriorly on the trabecular meshwork. Scleral spur and the ciliary body band are typically not present. The exposed trabecular meshwork band is usually narrow.

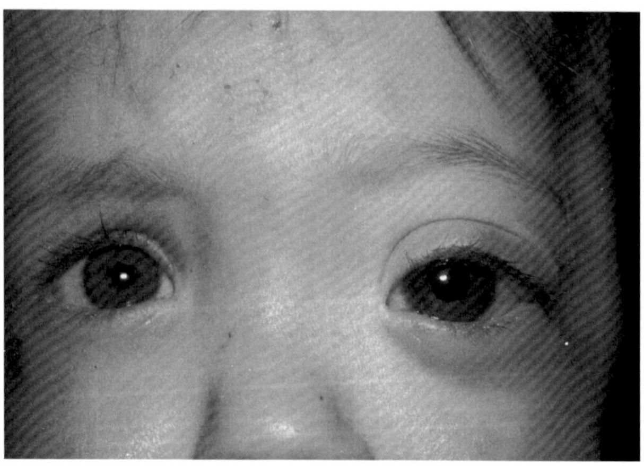

Figure 71.5. Neurofibromatosis. At age 17 months, congenital glaucoma is present with ocular enlargement *OS*. A uniform iris stroma with pupillary ectropion is also seen. The commonly associated plexiform neuroma was not evident until 3 years of age.

Treatment of infantile neurofibromatosis glaucoma should initially consist of a trial of medical therapy. The visual prognosis for these eyes may be poor if high myopia and glaucoma are present simultaneously. Short term use of oral carbonic anhydrase inhibitors seems appropriate. Goniosurgery characteristically fails to affect the IOP favorably.

Trabeculectomy with adjunct use of antimetabolites offers the best chance for successful surgery.

Stickler's, Rubinstein-Taybi Syndrome, and Marfan's Syndrome

Eyes with infantile glaucoma with Stickler's syndrome and the Rubinstein-Taybi syndrome resemble primary infantile glaucoma. Importantly, goniotomy is an effective treatment for glaucoma in these conditions. Stickler's syndrome also may be associated with an acquired juvenile open angle glaucoma which is less responsive to goniotomy than when the glaucoma is congenital. Infantile glaucoma is rarely seen with Marfan's syndrome. My experience with one child with these associated conditions suggests this condition also will do well with goniosurgery.

Hepatocerebrorenal Syndrome

Infantile glaucoma is seen in the hepatocerebrorenal syndrome. This autosomal recessive disorder is characterized by striking hypotonia, inability to feed, characteristic facies, and early death. Elevated very-long chain fatty acids (VLFA's) are indicative of the peroxisomal agenesis found in this condition. We have examined three patients with this disease. Glaucoma was present in one; gonioscopy revealed poor definition of the scleral spur and ciliary body band without abnormal processes. The posterior segment exam revealed typical equatorial black spots at the level of the retinal pigment epithelium which are possibly pathognomonic for this condition. No glaucoma therapy was administered, but medical therapy may be appropriate under some circumstances.

PRIMARY GLAUCOMA WITH OCULAR ABNORMALITIES

Childhood glaucoma is seen in the presence of other primary ocular disorders (Table 70.2). Congenital aniridia,

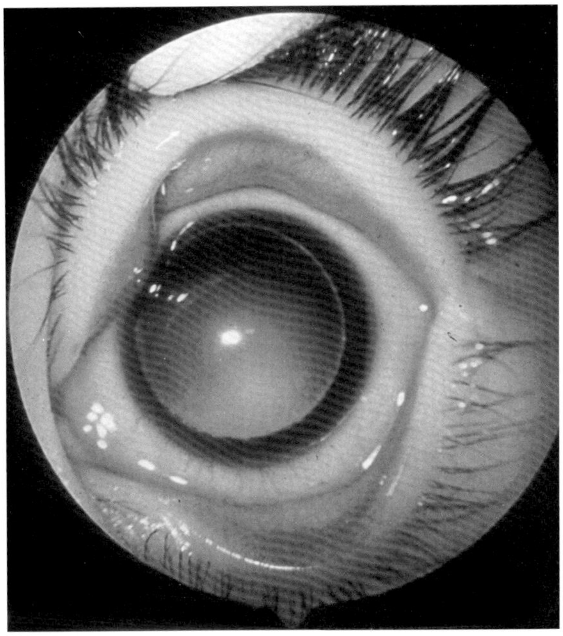

Figure 71.6. Aniridia. A young child with aniridia typically shows a clear cornea and lens and will rarely have glaucoma in infancy.

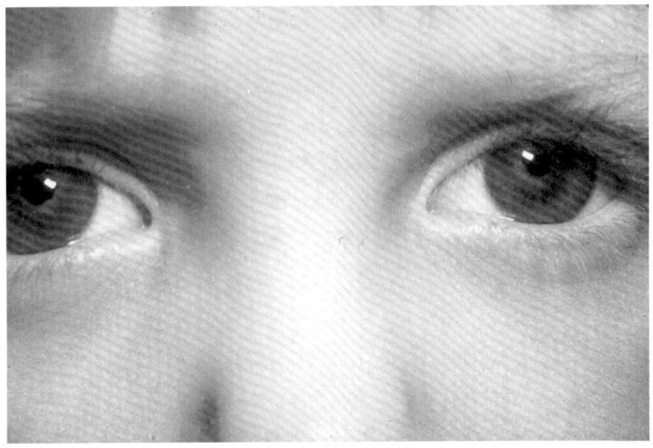

Figure 71.7. Aniridia. Atypically, some patients with aniridia have partial or complete irides; corectopia and defects in the stroma are present. Peripheral opacification of the cornea is important evidence of aniridia in such a patient.

congenital iris hypoplasia, and posterior polymorphous dystrophy are representative hereditary eye conditions complicated by childhood glaucoma. Congenital ectropion uveae is a nonhereditary ocular syndrome complicated by the occurrence of glaucoma.

Congenital Aniridia

Congenital aniridia is a hereditary disease of the eye with multiple congenital and acquired defects which become complicated by glaucoma in 50 to 75 percent of affected patients. Aniridia may occur sporadically or be familial. Offspring of affected parents are at 50 percent risk for aniridia related to autosomal dominant transmission. The molecular gene defect has been isolated to the PAX 6 region in the 14 band on the short arm of chromosome 11. When a chromosomal deletion occurs involving this region, detected by chromosome karyotype evaluation, aniridia occurs as the ocular component of a systemic syndrome consisting of retardation, genital anomalies, and a greatly increased risk for Wilms' tumor at a young age. Aniridia has also occurred in association with cerebellar ataxia. Extreme iridal hypoplasia resembling the ocular appearance of hereditary aniridia has also been seen in trisomy 13 and Meckel's syndrome.

Aniridia is usually represented by an obvious iris defect, decreased visual acuity with nystagmus, small corneas, cataracts, small discs, foveal hypoplasia, and frequent glaucoma (Fig. 71.6).

Near complete absence of the iris on slit lamp examination is characteristic; a narrow rim of iris, however, is often detectable. **On gonioscopy the iris stump becomes more obvious, is often of variable width, and presents circumferentially in a plane perpendicular to the visual axis.** A small percentage of patients will possess an intact iris, making the recognition of aniridia less certain; on examination, such irides are always abnormal (Fig. 71.7). The affected iris stroma is characteristically smooth and homogeneously lacking normal crypts, and furthermore, the collarette is usually absent or incomplete and located adjacent to the pupillary border. Mild corectopia is characteristic with symmetrical displacement in each eye. A partial ectropion uveae also is usually present, often located nasally or inferiorly.

The corneas in aniridia are small, often with horizontal diameters of 10.5 to 11.0 mm. The stromal and Descemet's membrane endothelial cell layers are normal. The epithelial layer is constantly abnormal. In young patients this defect is represented by an opacification of the peripheral cornea circumferentially, but usually more marked inferiorly. Fine subepithelial radial blood vessels are usually present in this opacity. This corneal opacity in aniridia is best located after applanation tonometry due to the bright fluorescein staining of the involved abnormal epithelium.

By ten years of age equatorial lens opacities are usually present which progress often to be visually significant by the late teenage years.

GLAUCOMA IN ANIRIDIA

We believe that glaucoma occurs in 50 percent to 75 percent of patients with aniridia. The presence or absence of glaucoma and its severity correlate well with the extent of gonioscopically visible obstruction of the filtration portion of the corneoscleral trabecular meshwork. **The filtration area is covered by the stump of the iris about in proportion to the severity of the glaucoma.** In some eyes only the stromal portion of the iris stump is forward and adherent, covering the ciliary band, scleral spur, and to a variable extent the trabecular meshwork, but in other eyes the whole thickness of the iris stump, including the pigment layer, is turned forward and is adherent to the angle wall. In those patients who do not have glaucoma, the trabecular meshwork is not so significantly covered by the stump of the iris, and the structures of the angle wall appear more normal.

Gonioscopy of more than 75 patients with aniridia has provided the following observations:

1. In aniridia in eyes without glaucoma, the filtration portion of the trabecular meshwork has very little or no covering by iris tissue in most of its circumference. If some covering is present, it is usually in the superior aspect of the angle. The ciliary band usually does show variable covering by iris tissue, but in nonglaucomatous eyes the ciliary body band usually appears wider than in eyes that have glaucoma. The scleral spur often can be seen in most of the circumference.

2. In aniridia in eyes with mild glaucoma, we have seen extensive blockage of less than half of the angle, as will be described in the next paragraph, but more commonly we have seen circumferential involvement of the angle. In this stage one sees multiple, thin sawtooth extensions of iris stroma reaching across the scleral spur and attaching on and anterior to the filtration area of the trabecular meshwork. These extensions are often in the form of a sheet in some areas and perforated in other areas; they usually possess little pigment. In young children these processes often have blood vessels that extend anteriorly in the sheet and can be seen to turn abruptly on the trabecular meshwork and run parallel to scleral spur and join other vessels from other similar extensions of iris stroma. These vessels do not characteristically branch and are less evident after early childhood. When these vessels are seen on the trabecular meshwork, mild glaucoma is usually present. In many areas the peripheral iris stroma appears to be pulled up onto the ciliary body band; a mild concavity of the anterior iris leaf may be present, and an inner separation of the iris stroma from the pigment epithelium may be seen.

3. In aniridia in eyes with moderate to severe glaucoma most of the filtration area of the trabecular meshwork is covered by forward attachment of the iris stroma tissue covering at least the posterior one-half of the trabecular meshwork in any meridian. Involvement superiorly again is most severe, usually with no recognizable trabecular meshwork in evidence. At this stage, the former anterior surface of the iris stroma now lies essentially parallel to the angle wall over much of its area. In meridians of most severe change, the former iris stromal stump is shifted completely onto the angle wall. At such sites the iris pigment epithelium may be left behind and is seen draped across the ciliary processes, remaining on a plane perpendicular to the visual axis. The anterior border of the iris tissue on the trabecular meshwork is often fairly uniform and wavy as one views around the circumference of the angle; the iris appears to have come to rest. Vessels are not in evidence at this stage.

Our observations on glaucoma associated with aniridia suggest that the IOP usually tends to become elevated later in childhood than is usual in ordinary congenital open angle glaucoma. What primarily suggests this is a fact already mentioned, that in glaucoma associated with aniridia the corneas are not usually enlarged. This is so different from what is frequently found in congenital glaucoma that one must conclude that the timing of the IOP elevation is significantly different. Generally, it is thought to be a normal characteristic of an infant's eye in the first year or two of life to be subject to stretching and enlargement, with attendant rupturing of Descemet's membrane, when the IOP is excessive. Since enlargement of the globe and ruptures of Descemet's membrane are seen in many types of glaucoma of early life, including secondary glaucomas, it is likely that the aniridic eye would behave in a similar fashion if significant glaucoma were present in early life, unless the aniridic eye possesses greater than usual resistance to such changes. **These observations support our belief that in most instances glaucoma in aniridia develops later in childhood, or even into the second decade of life,** consistent with what we have observed in aniridic patients followed since infancy. Among these patients it has been rare for glaucoma to occur during the first year of life and unusual for glaucoma to develop before 5 years of age.

In one aniridic child in whom glaucoma was present in his first year the trabecular meshwork was already completely blocked by iris tissue. In this patient and in one other patient with glaucoma before 18 months of age, enlargement of the cornea occurred from a baseline diameter that was somewhat smaller than normal, as is characteristic in aniridia patients. In other patients in whom glaucoma has been seen before five years of age the angle usually has not been blocked with iris stromal tissue but rather covered extensively by vascularized sheets extending from the iris. In one eye of one patient there was no visible trabecular meshwork obstruction at all.

The above clinical observations suggest that glaucoma is indeed unusual in young children with aniridia, but may occur. When it does occur, the angle abnormalities may be different than those seen in the more usual situation of glaucoma acquired in later childhood or in the teenage years. Most of our observations in aniridia are in patients during the first decade of life. Based on this selected population, it is our belief that the active stage of angle progression and development of glaucoma occurs during late childhood, rather than during the adult years.

The ciliary processes and the zonules of the lens are well exposed to view by gonioscopy in aniridia. In eyes that have not been subjected to surgery these structures as a rule appear normal.

Table 71-1
Management of Glaucoma in Aniridia

Stage of Aniridia	Treatment Considerations
Normal IOP, stable exam, no evidence of progressive angle closure	Frequent observation.
Normal IOP or early rise in IOP, progressive angle closure	Consider prophylactic goniotomy (refer to pediatric ophthalmologist); medical therapy for elevated IOP.
Glaucoma with advanced angle closure	Medical treatment with aqueous suppressants and miotics; trabeculectomy with adjuvant antimetabolites (mitomycin C).

TREATMENT OF ANIRIDIA

Treatment of glaucoma associated with aniridia is usually medical (Table 71.1). **Surgery has been resorted to only in those cases in which medical treatment has already proved inadequate.** The glaucoma associated with aniridia, unlike congenital glaucoma, does commonly respond to treatment with pilocarpine and other miotic drops. (Since there is no sphincter pupillae, it is assumed that in aniridia the miotic drops cause lowering of IOP by their effect on the ciliary muscle, inducing an improvement in facility of aqueous outflow through those portions of the trabecular meshwork that are unobstructed.)

Goniotomy procedures are disappointing in eyes with frank glaucoma. In 15 glaucomatous eyes in our series, we have found that, with a goniotomy knife under direct observation, the covering iris stroma, and an anterior veil that often precedes it, can be nicely dissected off the trabecular meshwork, exposing the scleral spur and ciliary body band, producing a permanent change in the angle. However, none of the eyes, even with multiple operations was cured by this goniosurgery. In some cases, a temporary improved response to miotic therapy has been obtained.

Trabeculectomy with use of mitomycin C has been successful in 3 of 4 eyes treated in our series of aniridia patients. A standard procedure is done; iridectomy is usually unnecessary. Because the lens and cornea are unprotected by an iris, careful postoperative observation is mandatory to prevent injury to these tissues that might occur from loss of the anterior chamber.

PROPHYLACTIC GONIOTOMY

Founded on our observations that suggest that the trabecular meshwork may be near normal in early childhood and then worsens when congenital synechias become impervious to aqueous humor, or more commonly when iris stroma becomes drawn up on the trabecular meshwork, we have attempted early preventive surgery. We speculate that removal of attachments early may prevent changes in the filtration tissue that appear not to be corrected by removal of the synechial iris attachments and stroma at a later stage. **Patients selected for this procedure have been young children who do not have glaucoma, but who on gonioscopy show extensive early bridging of synechial iris extensions across the scleral spur, and who usually have been observed to be undergoing a worsening of this angle abnormality.**

This preventive or **prophylactic goniosurgery** has been performed with a goniotomy knife under direct observation. The anterior border of the tissue extending onto the trabecular meshwork is engaged with the tip of the knife, and then, with movements of the knife parallel to the visual axis as well as circumferential, the tissue is stripped off the angle wall and a deep sulcus is created between the iris stump and the trabecular meshwork, leaving the latter appearing beautifully clean. Once a decision for surgery is made, two operations at separate hospitalizations are performed on a single eye to produce the desired change in more than one-half of the circumference of the angle.

The results of this procedure are encouraging. Sixty-three eyes in 34 patients have been operated upon in this way. This series includes one patient whose IOPs were beginning to rise. In each case an exposure of the trabecular meshwork, except for isolated strands, has been produced (Fig. 71.8). Postoperative follow up now ranges from less than one year to 26 years. IOPs above normal have developed in only two of these patients. One patient had glaucoma in one eye before prophylactic operation on the other eye. No postoperative complications have been encountered, except for the transient presence of blood in the anterior chamber in the immediate postoperative period.

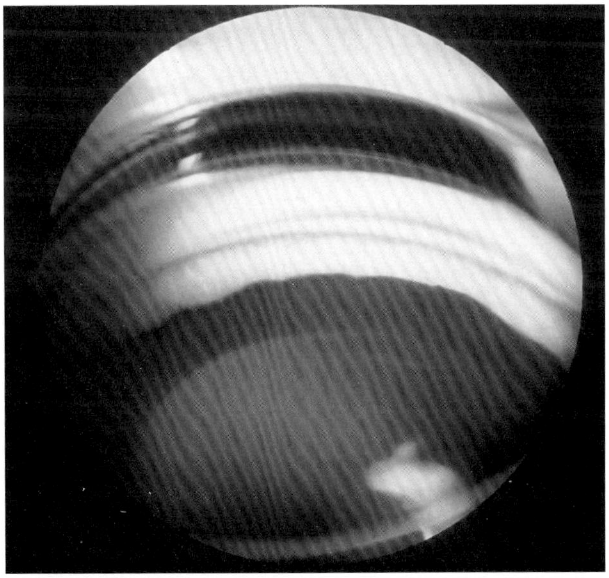

Figure 71.8. Aniridia. After prophylactic goniosurgery for aniridic glaucoma, the separation of the iris stump from the angle seen on gonioscopy is permanent.

Table 71.2
Developmental Disorders with Iris Abnormalities and Glaucoma

Axenfeld-Rieger's anomaly	Bilateral, autosomal dominant, variable degree of angle, iris, and pupil involvement.
Peter's anomaly	Bilateral, some cases inherited, attachment of iris processes to dense central leucoma.
Neurofibromatosis (NF-1)	Autosomal dominant, Lisch nodules, ectropion uveae.
Aniridia	Autosomal dominant or sporadic with deletion of chromosome 11, residual iris stump (variable), angle closure (progressive in some cases).
Congenital ectropion uveae (iridogoniodysgenesis)	Not inherited, unilateral with corneal enlargement, no systemic manifestations, affected iris smooth without crypts.
Familial (congenital) hypoplasia of the iris	Autosomal dominant, irides appear dark due to thin iris stroma, no polycoria or corectopia.

When considering this procedure, it is important to explain clearly to the child's parents that it is a preventive rather than therapeutic step, and, though results are encouraging, that its potential benefit still is unproved. Because of the small cornea in aniridia, with its peripheral zone of opacification, and because of the broad exposure of the clear lens in the anterior chamber in these children, we recommend that it be performed only by those surgeons who do goniotomy-type surgery regularly and who are familiar with the characteristics of angle changes in aniridia that are associated with glaucoma. Because of the shallowness of the anterior chamber in the first year of life, this surgery is best postponed until after this period. While considering whether a young child with aniridia is a candidate for this procedure, we usually perform gonioscopy at 6-month intervals under general anesthesia to evaluate what changes, if any, are occurring in the angle.

Weighing against the idea of early surgical intervention that is intended to be preventive is the knowledge that, when the glaucoma is mild, medical treatment may suffice for reasonable control. We do not yet know enough to be able to predict far in advance in which cases medical treatment ultimately will fail.

Glaucoma with Congenital Ectropion Uveae

A number of disorders which cause glaucoma in children are associated with iris abnormalities (Table 71.2). **The occurrence of glaucoma with a congenital ectropion uveae without neurofibromatosis is an important but unusual cause of childhood glaucoma** (Fig. 71.9). The development of an iris ectropion is also seen in patients with the Axenfeld-Rieger syndrome, ICE syndromes, partial aniridia, as well as in neurofibromatosis (NF-1). Glaucoma associated with a congenital ectropion of the iris, iridogoniodysgenesis, represents a recognizable cause of childhood glaucoma apart from entities considered within the Axenfeld-Rieger spectrum of disorders. This glaucoma is nonhereditary, unilateral, and unassociated with any systemic defects. The condition is usually recognized by an investigation of the abnormal pupil. The associated glaucoma is most often present in early childhood and persists, but it may also be acquired. Each of 5 patients with this entity cared for by the author had glaucoma at a young age, but none were examined until after the second year of life.

On examination corneal symmetry is typical without striking unilateral corneal enlargement as seen with other unilateral early onset glaucomas. Breaks in Descemet's membrane also are usually not present, suggesting further that IOP elevations in infancy are usually not great if present. The associated ptosis is mild. Striking abnormalities of the iris and filtration angle are present. The pupil is reactive but typically surrounded by an apparent ectropion uveae with the presence of dark iris pigment epithelium on the anterior surface of the iris. This defect is of variable width, may be partial, and in my experience has been stable. The unpigmented iris surface is smooth and without crypts or circumferential folds. It shares a similar color with the fellow eye, but the character of the stromal architecture differs greatly from the normal opposite eye. On gonioscopy the iris inserts anteriorly on the trabecular meshwork. The scleral spur and ciliary body band are not present. Some prominence of Schwalbe's line may be present. Pathological examination of iris and angle specimens from two of our patients has confirmed **endothelialization of the angle and anterior iris surface**.

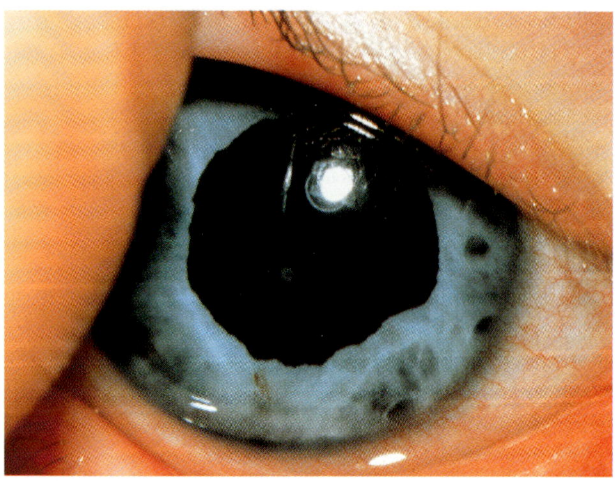

Figure 71.9. Glaucoma with congenital ectropion uveae. The unilateral abnormal iris stroma and pupillary ectropion are evident in this disorder. Gonioscopy revealed anterior insertion of the iris.

Treatment of children with this type of primary glaucoma should be initiated with medical therapy. However, in our experience this has not proven adequate. Goniosurgery has failed to provide improved control of the IOP following each of 6 operations performed by the author. Filtration surgery, in contrast, has been rewarding for these patients and is at present the initial glaucoma surgery of choice.

Familial Hypoplasia of the Iris with Glaucoma

Familial congenital hypoplasia of the iris with glaucoma is a rare cause of childhood glaucoma inherited by autosomal dominant transmission. A family history of glaucoma involving numerous family members is important early evidence of this type of glaucoma.

On examination striking corneal enlargement is not usually present. The anterior chamber is deep, and on further examination a low level of myopia may be found. The irides on inspection appear dark whether or not they are blue or brown. On slit lamp examination the iris stroma appears thin, allowing the appreciation of the more posterior iris pigment epithelium. Corectopia and iris hole formation do not occur. When brown, these irides appear rust colored and when blue appear gray. Gonioscopy is variable but always abnormal. Extra tissue obscuring the view of the scleral spur and ciliary body band may be present, or this tissue may seem to consist of fine processes directed from the iris root to the trabecular meshwork. The eye pressures are variable in this disease and may become progressively more elevated in childhood.

This entity must be distinguished from patients with an Axenfeld-Rieger's anomaly and from patients with congenital glaucoma associated with iris defects. While the former entity may share autosomal dominant inheritance, gonioscopy will show the expected array of abnormal processes characteristic of the Axenfeld anomaly. Patients with congenital glaucoma with iris defects are usually sporadic in occurrence, and the irides appear abnormal by their very uniform character and absence of crypts and by the near constant enlargement of the pupils and minor ectropion of the pupillary frill. Anterior segment enlargement also is present with this glaucoma which is severe early in life.

Treatment of children with glaucoma associated with congenital iris hypoplasia should be initiated with medical therapy. When surgery is necessary, goniotomy should be performed followed by filtration surgery when necessary.

Four young children with this entity cared for by the author have been controlled with topical beta blockers in two, while goniotomies with continued use of a beta blocker have been satisfactory for a third patient. The fourth patient required filtration surgery after failed goniotomies at 8 years of age.

JUVENILE OPEN ANGLE GLAUCOMA

Adult open angle glaucoma usually affects patients over 50 years of age. Phenotypically, juvenile open angle glaucoma (JOAG) is the occurrence of open angle glaucoma in children, often with the development of significant elevation of IOP by 10 years of age though, in some cases, IOP may not elevate until early adulthood. Clinically this glaucoma is often associated with moderate amounts of myopia. Transmission of this disease is by autosomal dominant inheritance, and the gene locus has been linked to the long arm of the first chromosome (1q21-q31).

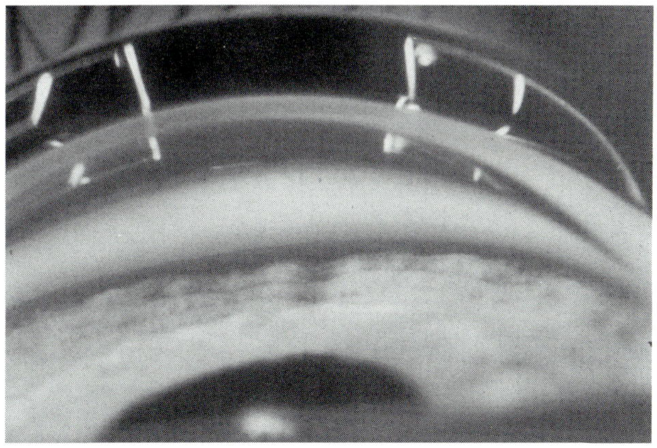

Figure 71.10. Juvenile glaucoma. On gonioscopy the angle structures appear normal. The ciliary body band is easily distinguished from the trabecular meshwork.

Candidate children who later develop glaucoma usually have normal IOP during the first 5 years of life, then develop a slow progression of IOP before 10 years of age. Anterior segment enlargement is not seen. On examination by slit lamp biomicroscopy and gonioscopy no abnormality is found (Fig. 71.10).

Children with JOAG must be differentiated from late recognized cases of congenital glaucoma and from sporadic cases of other types of juvenile glaucoma. Late recognized cases of congenital glaucoma are characterized by anterior segment enlargement, often associated with breaks in Descemet's membrane, suggesting the presence of glaucoma early in life. Other causes of juvenile glaucoma frequently demonstrate recognizable abnormalities on gonioscopy as well as frequent iris defects.

Treatment of JOAG is appropriately initiated with medical therapy. Miotics cause symptomatic blurring of vision and frequent headaches. A beta blocker and a carbonic anhydrase inhibitor will frequently, but temporarily, control the IOP in these patients. Goniotomy is the initial surgical glaucoma treatment of choice. If a second procedure does not produce adequate control, then trabeculectomy with adjunctive use of an antimetabolite in these young patients is indicated. Medical therapy followed by glaucoma surgery, if necessary, should be considered before the occurrence of disc damage and field loss, and when patients have been identified early and have developed uncontrolled IOP. See Chapter 50 for further information on this entity.

SECONDARY PEDIATRIC GLAUCOMA

The general ophthalmologist or pediatric ophthalmologist may infrequently see children with primary glaucoma, but can expect to see patients with a secondary glaucoma more frequently in the management of childhood ocular illness. Table 68.1 lists the diverse and multiple types of secondary pediatric glaucomas that collectively occur with significant frequency.

Traumatic Glaucoma

The principles that are understood in respect to adult traumatic glaucoma apply also to childhood (*see* Chapter 43). The most frequent cause of glaucoma after trauma in childhood is a recurrent hyphema. With such an occurrence children must be cared for aggressively to control the IOP to prevent corneal staining, iris atrophy, permanent mydriasis, and optic nerve injury.

Initial glaucoma treatment should include a beta blocker and carbonic anhydrase inhibitor. Early anterior chamber washout should be performed when IOP control is not achieved by medical therapy. When anterior chamber paracentesis and washout are performed, the surgeon should remember that complete clearing of the anterior chamber is unnecessary to achieve at least temporary IOP control. Following the initial release of blood from the anterior chamber an air injection aids the further evacuation of blood. Use of viscoelastics are not recommended. Consideration should be given to the use of tissue plasminogen activator (t-PA). Entry of instruments into the eye to assist evacuation of a resistant blood clot is risky and rarely helpful.

Following successful initial care of patients with glaucoma complicating a hyphema, careful follow up is indicated for potential recurrent glaucoma associated with further breakup of clots of blood, and in the long term related to permanent filtration angle defects.

Neoplastic Glaucoma

Glaucoma associated with a neoplasm in childhood is seen most frequently secondary to a retinoblastoma. Other causes are listed in Table 68.1 and include leukemia and juvenile xanthogranuloma of the iris.

Though retinoblastoma may occur with tumor cells in the anterior chamber, this is unusual. **The occurrence of glaucoma is most frequently secondary to rubeosis and closure of the angle**, but also may occur secondary to pupillary block when the lens is pushed forward by the posterior segment mass (Fig. 71.11).

Treatment of glaucoma is usually directed to the neoplasm present. Medical therapy for the glaucoma is appropriate when necessary.

Uveitic Glaucoma

Glaucoma is a common complication of anterior uveitis in children (see Chapter 42). It may be acute and seen with acute uveitis complicating herpetic uveitis and recurrent posterior segment toxoplasmosis. Chronic glaucoma is more common and occurs complicating chronic anterior uveitis as seen with juvenile rheumatoid arthritis, chronic cyclitis, and ocular sarcoidosis.

Children with chronic anterior uveitis require frequent reexamination including tonometry. Increasing inflammation may cause relative hypotony, while control of the inflammation may reveal increasing obstruction of

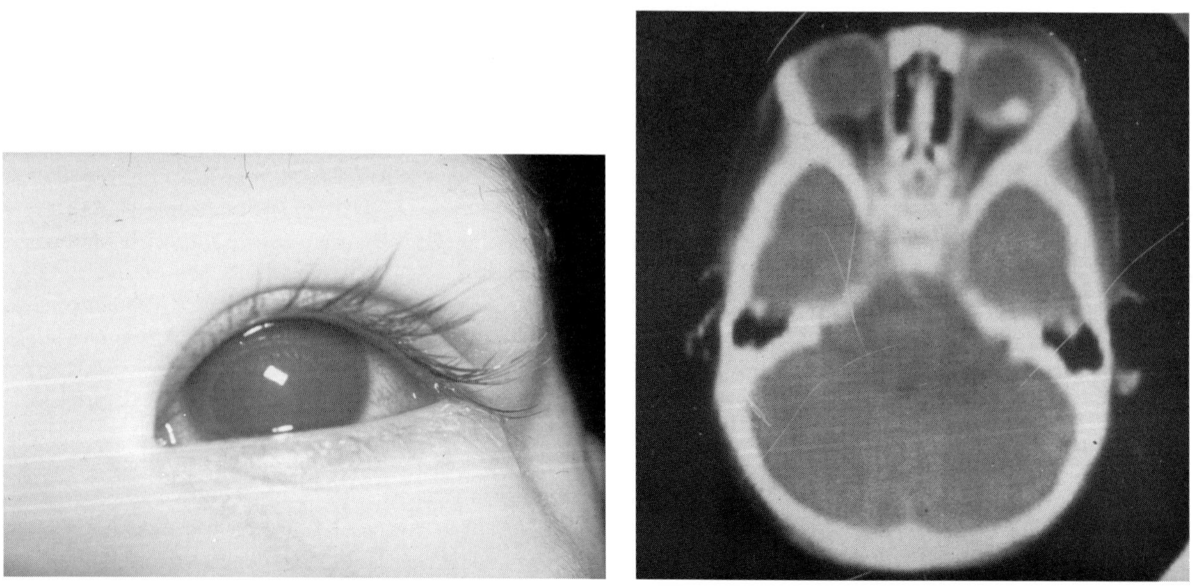

A B

Figure 71.11. Glaucoma with retinoblastoma. (A) This six month old boy presented with signs of glaucoma and intraocular hemorrhage. (B) CT scan suggested a retinoblastoma (intraocular calcification), which was confirmed on pathological examination.

aqueous outflow by the occurrence of an elevated IOP. Prevention of glaucoma by way of control of the intraocular inflammation is an important goal of treatment. When topical steroids are tapered, special caution must be exercised to be sure that recurrent episodes of increased inflammation do not occur. Correspondingly, when treatment is increased, the increased risk for glaucoma must be recognized. **Rarely can such patients be seen less frequently than every 6 weeks throughout childhood.**

When glaucoma occurs with chronic anterior uveitis, the inflammatory disease typically has been present for at least one or two years. If evidence of pupillary block is present, the mechanism causing the glaucoma is obvious and immediate iridectomy with or without goniosynechialysis is indicated as dictated by intraoperative gonioscopy.

When pupillary block is not present, the mechanism of the glaucoma is less obvious, and the potential risk of steroids causing an elevated IOP needs to be considered. Long term use of steroids before the development of glaucoma might be evidence against this etiology. However, it is often difficult to determine with certainty that steroids are not contributing to the glaucoma.

In most instances, the complicating glaucoma is an open angle type associated with recognizable angle defects. When these abnormalities are found, the causal role of steroids seems less likely. In most cases it will remain important to continue the steroid at an appropriate level for control of the inflammation.

On gonioscopy the angle in chronic anterior uveitis is typically found open, associated with unusual opacification of the trabecular meshwork and ciliary body band inferiorly. Scattered pigment dust may be seen along with a variable number of sawtoothed peripheral anterior synechias attaching the peripheral iris to the trabecular meshwork.

Treatment of the uveitic childhood glaucoma should be initiated with medical therapy consisting of a beta blocker and a carbonic anhydrase inhibitor when necessary. Strong miotics are contraindicated, but weak miotics (e.g., pilocarpine HCl ½%) may be helpful if used infrequently (e.g., bedtime daily).

Surgical treatment of childhood uveitic glaucoma is appropriately approached with caution. **For 23 eyes in 16 children treated with standard goniotomy by the author 83% achieved control of the IOP with a mean follow up of 5 years.** The procedure done was a standard goniotomy procedure without further manipulation of the trabecular tissue. Seven of the 23 eyes required an additional goniotomy procedure, usually within 2 months of the initial surgery, to achieve IOP control. The beneficial effect of goniotomy for this glaucoma is maintained even in the face of low grade persistent inflammation.

I would not favor initial seton implant surgery for glaucoma associated with uveitis because of the chronic intraocular inflammation associated with these devices. Filtration surgery with use of antimetabolites is an important surgery treatment for patients who are unresponsive to goniotomy.

Table 71.3
Acute Lens-induced Glaucomas of Childhood (Angle Closure)

Ectopia lentis Marfan's syndrome Homocystinuria Trauma	Pupillary block mechanism (particularly after pupillary dilation); perform iridectomy.
Following cataract surgery	Children operated prior to age 2 years at increased risk. Pupillary block from residual lens tissue. History of pupillary block post-operatively.

Lens Induced Glaucoma

The occurrence of glaucoma associated with the shape and position of the crystalline lens is an important cause of glaucoma in children. The glaucoma may develop acutely or be chronic (Table 71.3).

Typically with ectopia lentis complicating Marfan's syndrome or homocystinuria, flow through the pupil is obstructed by entry of the lens partway through the pupil. Pupillary block occurs with collapse of the anterior chamber and further repositioning of the lens against the back of the cornea. Acute glaucoma occurs abruptly which is painful and often associated with vomiting. Immediate care is necessary.

Glaucoma in these patients may be precipitated by a routine eye examination associated with pupillary dilation. Predisposed patients may best be examined during morning hours with instruction to avoid a face down position until normal pupil size returns. A free lens in the eye gravitates, causing entry into the pupil in a face down position.

Prevention of pupillary block in ectopia lentis can be successful by making these patients aware of the risks, using miotics selectively, and most importantly by creating a peripheral iridectomy. In the presence of a peripheral iridectomy, a patient will only be at risk for recurrence of pupillary block if the crystalline lens enters the anterior chamber. This event is much more frequent in patients with homocystinuria than in patients with Marfan's syndrome.

Treatment of the acute pupillary block glaucoma complicating ectopia lentis is challenging. Pain medication should be administered. Medical therapy consisting of a beta blocker, carbonic anhydrase inhibitor, and osmotic agents is appropriate but has typically little IOP benefit. **Effective treatment consists of relieving the pupillary block.**

The anterior segment must be examined carefully. The anterior chamber will be flat and the pupil will be dilated. If the pupillary border is visible, an attempt may be made with a muscle hook to break the pupillary block by pushing the crystalline lens posteriorly at one edge of the pupil. In spite of the elevated IOP, a surprising amount of indentation of cornea against the lens can be achieved. It is only necessary to move the lens away from the cornea a small amount for this maneuver to be successful. The cornea can be nicely protected by a soft contact lens. When the pupillary block is broken, aqueous will rush into the newly forming anterior chamber forcing the lens posteriorly. The aqueous will then dissect peripherally and separate the iris away from the peripheral cornea and eventually from the angle. Gonioscopic observation of these events is important to assure that the angle opens. Miotics and thymoxamine may accelerate this process.

Occasionally the iris may wrap itself around the equator of the lens circumferentially. On examination the eye with this arrangement may not appear very different. Careful inspection of the iris, however, will reveal a dilated pupil with no visible pigmentary frill, and examination of the anterior segment with a gonioscopy lens will reveal that the iris is wrapped around the equator of the lens. The lens in this position is in a fossa created by the iris and cannot be pushed posteriorly to break the pupillary block.

Large incisions into the eye in preparation for an anterior lensectomy would be expected to be complicated by prolapse of iris and other complications. To treat this problem I would suggest placement of a very beveled (long) paracentesis into the anterior chamber directed to the border of the iris against the lens. I have followed this entry with a smooth rounded spatula which I place between the lens and the iris directed posteriorly until the retrolenticular aqueous is reached. With slight rotation of the spatula away from the lens the pupillary block will be released followed by a rush of aqueous into the anterior chamber, soon followed by movement of the lens posteriorly.

Aphakic Glaucoma

Young children who have surgery for congenital cataracts are at significant risk for glaucoma. The mechanism of this glaucoma is secondary to pupillary block or secondary to chronic changes in the trabecular meshwork leading to an impairment of aqueous outflow.

Children who develop glaucoma after cataract surgery usually are those who require cataract surgery before 2 years of age. When occurring secondary to pupillary block the glaucoma usually occurs within 3 months following cataract surgery (Fig. 71.12). If a surgical iridectomy remains patent after cataract surgery, this type of complicating glaucoma does not occur.

In recent years with the use of vitreous cutting instruments the technique of childhood cataract surgery has evolved such that removal of the lens can be accomplished more completely and with more confidence. **In spite of these advances, young children remain at significant risk for glaucoma with an occurrence rate of approximately 20%.** Glaucoma is often not present until 1–2 years or more following the cataract surgery. On gonioscopy, abnormalities are consistently found in these patients with **open angles**. The abnormalities seen consist of an anterior insertion of the iris at the level of the posterior trabecular meshwork associated with fine peripheral anterior synechias and a variable fine pigment deposition on the trabecular meshwork. The residual exposed trabecular meshwork often appears glazed with loss of the silk screen appearance of the normal trabecular meshwork.

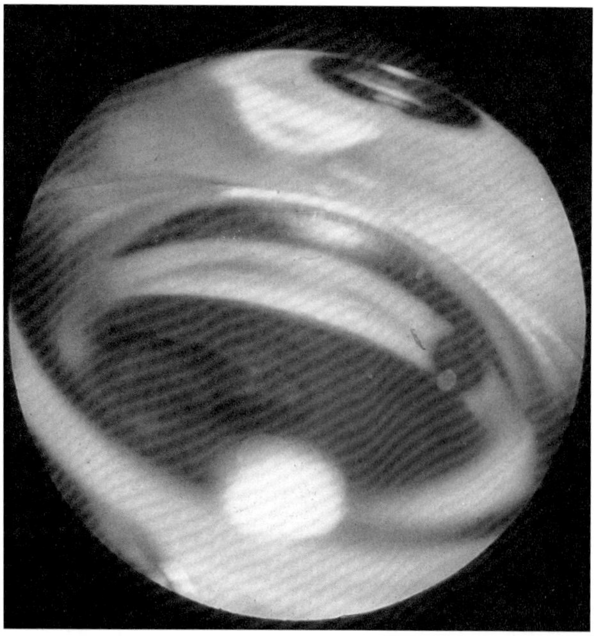

Figure 71.12. Aphakic glaucoma. On gonioscopy, abnormal synechial attachment of the iris anterior to the level of the posterior trabecular meshwork is seen and is typical of this glaucoma. Residual lens tissue is also present.

Young patients who develop open angle glaucoma following congenital cataract surgery more often have a history of secondary lens surgery for pupillary obstruction by residual lens tissue than those patients who don't develop this complication. Children who have congenital cataracts and who don't have lensectomy rarely develop glaucoma unless lens degeneration occurs. The mechanism of this glaucoma associated with a relatively open angle remains uncertain. Chronic inflammation following lens surgery may be a factor, but evidence of this inflammation on examination is not usually present. The release of lens proteins into the anterior chamber may be an additional provocative factor (Chapter 47). The presence and effect of cytokines produced by residual lens epithelial cells deserves continued study in an attempt to further understand the mechanism of this glaucoma.

Treatment of aphakic open angle glaucoma in young children is difficult. Medical therapy should be initiated with use of a beta blocker and carbonic anhydrase inhibitor.

Miotics do not seem to be helpful. I have tried goniotomy surgery for 13 eyes and have considered 11 to be failures. Trabeculectomy with use of mitomycin C has been helpful for 10 of 15 eyes. With failure of goniotomy and trabeculectomy surgery, seton implant surgery is indicated. Cycloablation has a role in an attempt to save some eyes when other procedures and therapies have failed.

Secondary Angle Closure Glaucoma in Children

Angle closure glaucoma is an important cause of secondary glaucoma in childhood. A review of the childhood secondary glaucomas listed in Table 68.1 reveals multiple causes for this mechanism of glaucoma. These include neoplasm, uveitic glaucoma, lens induced glaucoma, aphakic glaucoma, retinopathy of prematurity, and others.

GLAUCOMA ASSOCIATED WITH RETINOPATHY OF PREMATURITY

Retinopathy of prematurity (ROP) is of special importance because of the very frequent occurrence of glaucoma complicating cicatricial ROP and surgery for retinal detachment complicating ROP.

When ROP is complicated by glaucoma, it is usually angle closure glaucoma. In our experience, the age of onset of this complication ranges from 4 months to 22 years. Most cases occur after 1 year of age. Typically these eyes show advanced retinal abnormalities and possess variable amounts of equatorial perilenticular and retrolenticular membrane formation. The latter abnormality, if incomplete, is predictably more severe temporally and can be followed posteriorly to fuse with an organized mass of vitreous and retina. In some cases it may be so severe as to involve the whole retrolenticular space uniformly. The severity usually is asymmetric. The corneas are often small and steep. Myopia is a constant finding and more marked in the most severely affected eyes. The lenses are almost always clear and reveal the posterior abnormalities with brilliant clarity.

Of special importance to this discussion is the depth of the anterior chambers, which are almost always shallow in severely affected eyes. Careful inspection of the iris in these eyes may reveal noteworthy convexity of the iris leaf, greater than can be accounted for by the shape of the anterior lens surface, which is in fact relatively flat. When the trabecular meshwork and other angle structures can be seen, they usually appear normal in the absence of glaucoma.

The onset of the glaucoma may be acute with pain in the eye, nausea, and vomiting. We have known the glaucoma to be severe and to cause gray segmental atrophy of the stroma of the iris or even complete necrosis of the entire iris. Children with this condition are often treated as for an acute gastrointestinal disturbance because of the associated vomiting, or for a lid infection due to misinterpretation of lid swelling. Other children have presented with less acute symptoms consisting of eye rubbing, photophobia, and tearing.

We feel that embarrassment of the flow of aqueous humor between the lens and iris from the posterior chamber to the anterior chamber must be a significant factor in causing the angle to close, because in some cases this glaucoma has been cured by iridectomy. Presumably iridectomy works in these cases, as it does in ordinary angle closure glaucoma, by circumventing the obstruction at the pupil, and preventing abnormal accumulation of aqueous behind the iris. Whether the onset of embarrassment in the pupillary passage that causes angle closure glaucoma in association with ROP is due to growth of the crystalline lens, or due to change in retrolental membranes causing the lens to move farther forward, we do not know. In one instance we know that the precipitating factor that caused the angle finally to close was the use of mydriatic-cycloplegic drops for refraction. When iridectomy is performed in these eyes, the preoperative convexity of the iris is lost, and the iris conforms more closely to the lens surface and even takes on a concave curvature in its mid periphery. When synechias have not yet formed, the angle will appear strikingly more open.

The importance of an underlying anatomical or structural basis for angle closure glaucoma in ROP is indicated by the fact that in some patients in whom the ROP has been considerably more severe in one eye than in the other, the anterior chamber has become shallow and angle closure glaucoma has developed only in the eye with the more severe abnormality.

Because of the frequent acute onset of glaucoma in ROP and potential benefit of iridectomy in preventing its occurrence we have attempted to identify those patients who are at most risk for glaucoma. Severe posterior segment involvement, perilenticular membrane formation, shallow anterior chamber, narrow peripheral angle, iris leaf convexity, and most importantly progression of these anatomical findings are critical signs to be followed. We feel that **prophylactic iridectomy** should be seriously considered when these signs indicate a present and increasing risk of acute angle closure glaucoma.

In eyes in which acute glaucoma has not been treated early by iridectomy, the disease has taken various courses. In young children in whom the eye was essentially blind before the onset of glaucoma, pain has sometimes been controlled medically, with aspirin and acetazolamide, until the IOP has decreased and the globe has become atrophic and painless. Alternatively, the glaucoma may persist and be asymptomatic. If this occurs and enucleation is not necessary, there is sometimes later a remarkable spontaneous deepening of the anterior chamber, and the eye has become soft, despite permanent synechial closure of the angle.

The mechanism of the spontaneous variation in the depth of the anterior chamber that sometimes occurs in

ROP has not been apparent to us on clinical examination, but we suppose that the deepening might be explained by contraction of a retrolental membrane attached to the lens.

Rubeosis of the iris may be expected in a high percentage of eyes with chronic retinal detachment secondary to ROP. When such eyes become uncomfortable, treatment by enucleation must be considered.

Treatment of angle closure glaucoma associated with ROP is preferentially by iridectomy, with the same reasoning as in ordinary angle closure glaucoma, but additional medical treatment or other types of surgery, including goniosynechialysis may be indicated. This operation to open the angle after synechial closure has been surprisingly helpful even for eyes whose angles have been closed for an undetermined number of months.

We have observed a remarkable phenomenon after surgical peripheral iridectomies in ROP that we have not observed in any other condition in which this procedure has been performed. **Peripheral iridectomies in ROP eyes frequently have become closed as a result of gradual drawing of the coloboma into the angle where it has become obliterated in contact with the angle wall.** This necessitates reoperation. Because of this occurrence after initially successful peripheral iridectomy, we recommend that a large peripheral or a sector iridectomy be done, which may also facilitate posterior segment examination.

MICROPHTHALMOS

It is important to remember that the glaucoma mechanism that occurs complicating ROP can also be seen in any microphthalmic eye. We have seen angle closure in primary microphthalmos, microphthalmos associated with congenital diffuse choroiditis, and in microphthalmos associated with anterior displacement of the lens and high myopia, but we have most frequently observed this as a complication of ROP.

Special Considerations XI

Epidemiology of Glaucoma

72

Roy S. Wilson

DEFINITION

In its broadest interpretation, "epidemiology" encompasses a vast field and includes the following issues related to disease: 1) occurrence and distribution, 2) factors that influence that occurrence and distribution, and 3) health delivery and outcome measures. With respect to glaucoma, investigations related to epidemiology have been focused on determining occurrence and distribution and on investigating possible risk factors. The past decade has witnessed an explosion of knowledge in these areas. More recently, various outcome measures related to having glaucoma and to treating it have received increasing attention.

Knowledge derived from epidemiological studies contributes to a better understanding of the disease, assists in clinical decision-making, and allows a better appreciation of the individual and societal impact of having the disease. This chapter focuses on epidemiological aspects of primary open-angle glaucoma (POAG). Other types of glaucoma, e.g. pigmentary, exfoliation, and primary angle-closure, have distinguishing epidemiological features and are discussed elsewhere.

OCCURRENCE AND DISTRIBUTION

It is estimated that at least 2.25 million Americans 40 years of age and older have primary open-angle glaucoma and between 84,000 and 116,000 of these are believed to be bilaterally blind (visual acuity less than 20/200) from this disease (1). **Another 10 million are estimated to have elevated intraocular pressure (IOP) and are believed to be at increased risk for developing the disease** (2). The World Health Organization (WHO) has estimated the global population of people with POAG at 13,500,000, those with elevated IOP at 104,650,000, and those blinded by POAG at 3,000,000 (3).

Estimates of the prevalence of primary open angle glaucoma (POAG) can be relied upon with confidence only if standardized sampling methodology is used, if the diagnosis is based upon evidence of optic nerve and/or visual field damage, and if appropriate evaluations, including gonioscopy, are performed on a high proportion of subjects. In recent years, well designed population-based studies have been conducted to determine the prevalence of POAG in many areas of Europe, the United States, the Caribbean, and Asia. However, many regions of the world lack epidemiologically sound glaucoma prevalence data so the above global estimates of the numbers of people affected must be viewed with some caution. **The estimates of POAG in the United States were based on a prevalence rate of 1.7% for whites and other non-blacks and 5.5% for blacks.**

A prevalence of POAG between 1.1% and 2.1% has been consistently obtained by population-based studies performed in Baltimore, Maryland (1985–88) (4), Beaver Dam, Wisconsin (1987–88) (5), County Roscommon, Ireland (1988–90) (6), and Rotterdam, The Netherlands (1991–93) (7). These studies are particularly noteworthy for using highly standardized methodology and for defining glaucoma on the basis of optic nerve and/or visual field damage. Gonioscopy was performed as part of the evaluation in both the Baltimore and County Roscommon studies. An assessment of anterior chamber depth was made with a slit lamp in the Beaver Dam Study and with a penlight using the method of Van Herick in the Rotterdam Study, but gonioscopy was not performed. Without gonioscopy, cases of chronic angle closure glaucoma my be misclassified as open-angle glaucoma.

That prevalence of glaucoma increases with age has long been established (8–10). Prevalence estimates have generally been three to eight times higher in the oldest age groups compared with persons in their forties. A racial disparity in glaucoma prevalence also exists. The study in Baltimore (Baltimore Eye Survey) was performed in a racially mixed population and it found the prevalence of POAG among blacks to be three to four times higher than among whites (4). Also, higher prevalences have been reported among blacks in St. Lucia (11) and Barbados (12), West Indies than among blacks in Baltimore. **Prevalences of 8.8% were found among blacks 30 years of age and older in St. Lucia and 7.0% among blacks 40 years of age and older in Barbados.** Currently, we do not know whether the observed differences among blacks in the West Indies compared with blacks in Baltimore reflect an inherently higher rate of disease among the West Indians or are related to differences in design of the studies.

Data from Baltimore and from the West Indies suggest that there is a high prevalence among African blacks. A number of clinic-based studies and population-based general ophthalmology surveys have suggested a high prevalence among some African populations (13–15). However, these results have not been uniformly consistent, and it is likely that there are wide variations in prevalence of POAG and other types of glaucoma among the various regions of Africa.

Scant information is available on prevalence of POAG among Asians. Population-based general ophthalmology surveys and clinic-based data from various regions of Asia have indicated a high proportion of cases of glaucoma to be of the angle-closure variety (16). However, a nationwide glaucoma survey conducted in Japan found an open-angle glaucoma prevalence of 2.62% and only 0.34% for primary angle closure glaucoma (17). Thus, as is probably the situation in Africa, there are likely to be wide variations in both the prevalence of POAG and in the type of glaucoma that is predominant among the various Asian populations.

Although our knowledge of race-specific prevalence for POAG is less than complete, there is an even greater dearth of incidence data. Whereas "prevalence" reflects the number of cases in a given population at a given time, "incidence" reflects the number of new cases that develop in a given population within a given time frame. In a disease such as POAG, which is chronic and has a relatively low incidence, large cohorts and long follow-up periods are necessary to obtain a sufficient number of newly diagnosed cases to ensure valid estimates. Thus, only a few population-based studies to determine glaucoma incidence have been attempted. One such study performed in Dalby, Sweden found an incidence of between 0.19% to 0.24% per year (18). The previously mentioned survey performed in Barbados, West Indies was designed to yield incidence data but these results have not been reported to date (1996). A follow-up study to the Baltimore Eye Survey is currently being performed, and it is anticipated that incidence data will soon be available from this study.

Subjects believed to be at greater risk of developing glaucoma, i.e. subjects with elevated IOPs or family members of glaucomatous subjects, have been followed for variable time periods. The incidence in such an "enriched" population can be expected to be higher than in the general population. Yet, it is interesting to note that even in these subjects, visual field defects developed infrequently. For example, in the Collaborative Glaucoma Study, which was a prospective study conducted in five medical centers from 1959 to 1973 to identify factors that influence the development of glaucomatous visual field defects, the incidence was calculated to range from 0.25% to 0.54% per year (19).

FACTORS THAT INFLUENCE OCCURRENCE AND DISTRIBUTION OF POAG

It is well accepted that most diseases do not occur randomly throughout a population but that the frequency varies in different subgroups of people. It is important to understand what causes this uneven distribution. In so doing, risk factors for the disease can be identified (Table 72.1).

Table 72-1
Risk Factors for POAG

1. IOP
2. Age
3. Race (greater in black population)
4. Family history of POAG
5. Possible risk factors:
    - Myopia
    - Large cup to disc ratio
    - Systemic hypertension
    - Adult onset diabetes mellitus

Identifying risk factors is important because this information may lead to development of strategies for disease screening and prevention and may be useful for identifying persons for whom close medical supervision is indicated. Strictly defined, a factor can be considered a risk factor only if it truly predates disease occurrence. However, from a clinical perspective, it is often difficult to differentiate normal from very early disease. In fact, this determination is often dependent on how the disease is defined. Glaucoma is usually defined by the presence of characteristic visual field defects and sometimes, in the absence of visual field defects, by the appearance of optic nerve damage. How often this diagnosis is made in marginal cases is influenced by the sensitivity of available diagnostic tests. Thus, determining whether abnormalities in certain parameters—e.g., optic nerve parameters such as nerve fiber layer loss—are indicative of increased susceptibility to developing glaucoma or are signs of early disease may pose a dilemma. From a practical standpoint, the distinction is unimportant. Individuals manifesting such abnormalities must be closely monitored for signs of clinically significant disease development in either situation.

Current thinking regarding risk factors for glaucoma is influenced by data collected by ongoing studies. This entire area of inquiry is in a fluid state; what we believe today differs from what we believed only a few years ago and is likely to be modified yet again because of new information. **There is general agreement that IOP, age, race, and family history of glaucoma are risk factors for POAG.** The relevance of optic nerve parameters, refractive status, and various systemic factors such as diabetes, systemic hypertension, and arteriosclerotic and ischemic vascular diseases as factors that affect glaucoma risk, is less certain.

Elevated IOP is generally accepted as a risk factor for POAG. It is perhaps the most important of the risk factors in that it is the only factor for which a causal mechanism has been ascribed and is the only factor currently amenable to modification. A causal role of IOP in glaucoma is supported by considering examples of experimentally induced high IOP in animals that result in typical glaucomatous cupping (20,21), format examples of acute angle closure and unilateral secondary glaucoma in which glaucomatous damage occurs in the eye with elevated IOP, and examples of normal but asymmetric IOPs which result in asymmetrical cupping and visual field loss with greater damage on the side with the higher IOP (22,23). However, it must be recognized that a one-to-one relationship between elevated IOP and glaucoma does not exist. Glaucomatous damage may occur despite normal or even low IOP levels. The efficacy of lowering IOP in preventing progressive glaucomatous damage has not been clearly and unequivocally demonstrated in a controlled study. Thus belief in IOP as the primary causal factor in POAG is not without some contention.

As mentioned previously, population-based studies have clearly established that glaucoma prevalence increases with age (4–12). Although age-specific incidence rates of POAG in normal populations have not yet been adequately determined, the Collaborative Glaucoma Study found that visual field defects developed at a rate seven times higher in persons 60 years of age and older compared to persons younger than 40 years (19). The exact causal mechanisms responsible for increased susceptibility of older persons to POAG is not known. IOP tends to increase with age but this is not likely to be a primary explanation. The magnitude of the IOP increase with age is not great, and this age-related rise has not been consistently demonstrated among all populations. For example, among the Japanese, IOP apparently decreases with age whereas POAG increases with age (17).

As with age, race-specific incidence data are not yet available. Although there are theoretical reasons for why prevalence may not reflect incidence, the magnitude of the racial disparity in the prevalence data strongly suggests that blacks develop glaucoma at a higher rate than do whites. Among the hypotheses offered to explain this increased susceptibility among blacks are that blacks have higher intraocular pressures (24), larger cup to disc ratios (25,26), higher prevalences of diseases that may cause ischemia of the optic nervehead (27), and medical under-surveillance compared to whites (28,29). Data do not unequivocally support any of these hypotheses, and the exact biological, anatomical, or social factors that may be operational in placing blacks at greater risk of developing glaucoma are not yet known.

That family members of subjects with POAG have an underlying susceptibility to the development of the disease is well established. Exactly how much more at risk a family member is compared to the general population is not known with certainty. The Baltimore Eye Survey solicited information on history of glaucoma in relatives and reported age-adjusted associations with POAG subjects. Odds ratios for having a history of glaucoma were found to be 3.69 for siblings and 2.17 for parents (30). However, these estimates are susceptible to recall bias since persons with glaucoma are probably more likely to recall the disease or to attribute all vision disorders to glaucoma. A good family history study would require the standardized examination of a high proportion of relatives of subjects with POAG and relatives of an appropriate control group, but none is yet available.

The genetic basis for juvenile glaucoma is more firmly established than for POAG, and an autosomal dominant inheritance pattern has been documented in several large multi-generation families (31,32). A very exciting, new development in research has been that of identifying genes responsible for specific diseases, and a genetic marker associated with juvenile glaucoma has been isolated (33). The genetic factors influencing POAG appear to be far more complex than those for juvenile glaucoma. The search for genetic markers associated with POAG promises to be an intense area of investigation for the near future.

Data regarding the possible role of other factors in development of POAG are conflicting. Associations between myopia and POAG have been observed (34) but it is possible that these associations were influenced by selection bias since persons who have refractive errors are more likely to seek eye care and have a higher probability of being diagnosed as having glaucoma.

Various optic nerve parameters such as large cup to disc ratio (19,35,36), asymmetric cupping (37), disc hemorrhages (38), and loss of nerve fiber layer (39) have been declared risk factors for development of glaucoma. However, discs with large cup to disc ratios tend also to be larger with proportionately more neural rim tissue (40). An argument can thus be made that such discs may actually be less prone to glaucomatous damage. There is no clear consensus as to the relevance of a large cup to disc ratio in the pathogenesis of glaucoma. **In fact, in some cases, a large cup to disc ratio, as well as the other parameters listed above, may represent signs of early glaucoma.**

Positive associations between blood pressure and IOP (41) and between blood pressure and POAG have been reported (42). Although the evidence for systemic hypertension being a risk factor for glaucoma is not strong, the hypothesis that micro-circulatory effects on the optic disc may possibly lead to increased glaucoma susceptibility is biologically plausible. The Rotterdam Study reported an association of systemic hypertension with high-tension glaucoma but not with normal-tension glaucoma (43). The Baltimore Eye Survey reported modest, positive associations of systolic and diastolic blood pressure with POAG but the 95% confidence intervals of the odds ratios for these associations included 1.00, the value of no association (44). However, lower perfusion pressure (blood pressure − intraocular pressure) was strongly associated with an increased prevalence of POAG. Although not yet clearly documented, these results suggest that POAG may be associated with an alteration in factors related to ocular blood flow.

RISK FACTORS AND GENETIC LINKAGE ANALYSIS IN PRIMARY OPEN ANGLE GLAUCOMA

R. Rand Allingham

A positive family history is a major risk factor for the development of primary open angle glaucoma (POAG). Approximately 50% of affected individuals have an affected relative (1). A positive family history increases the risk of developing POAG 7–10 times that of the general population (2). The precise mechanism of inheritance is less clear. Families with autosomal dominant, autosomal recessive, and X-linked recessive modes of inheritance have been reported (3). However, formal segregation analysis has never been performed in studies on the inheritance of POAG.

A multifactorial or polygenic mode of inheritance was first proposed in the ophthalmic literature by Armaly in 1967 (4). The diagnosis of POAG is highly dependent on several measurable parameters. These include IOP, aqueous outflow facility, and cup/disc ratio. Interestingly, all three have been shown to have an inherited component (5). Race has also been demonstrated to have a significant impact on the prevalence of POAG. In one population based study the black population had a six-fold increased risk of developing POAG compared to the white population (6). Therefore, at a minimum there appear to be multiple inherited factors which may influence the risk of developing POAG.

POAG can best be described as a complex disorder. Complex disorders, such as diabetes mellitus, schizophrenia, and Alzheimer's disease lack a simple mode of inheritance; therefore a single underlying susceptibility gene can not be assumed. These diseases may involve more than one gene (polygenic), have a late or variable age of onset, demonstrate incomplete penetrance (meaning the disease may not develop even when the causative gene has been inherited), and may have significant environmental influences (e.g. steroid responsiveness in POAG).

It is now possible to identify the chromosomal location and ultimately the causative gene for inherited disorders by genetic linkage analysis without prior knowledge of the biochemical or pathophysiologic mechanism of the disease process. Genetic linkage analysis requires families where the disease is present, the presence of highly polymorphic genetic markers, and sophisticated statistical methodology.

The genetic map is the cornerstone of genetic linkage studies (7). Each gene has a locus, a specific location within a chromosome. Genes which occupy the same locus but contain different sequences are called alleles. The genes found in each chromosome have a specific order that is identical for all humans with few exceptions. Once a gene or marker is localized to a particular region on a chromosome it is placed on a map. Therefore, the genetic map depicts the order of genes, genetic markers, and other landmarks that compose the chromosomes of a particular organism.

An essential tool to successfully perform genetic linkage analysis is a group of genetic markers which have multiple alleles (polymorphic) and have a known locus. Markers are inherited in the same manner as genes (mendelian pattern) and therefore can be traced through pedigrees. The DNA sequence of each marker must be polymorphic (have multiple alleles) so that its maternal or paternal origin can be determined. The more alleles a marker has, the more likely it will be that the maternal or paternal genetic makeup will differ and therefore, the origin of a specific allele can be determined in the children. Markers with multiple alleles are more powerful (informative) for linkage analysis.

Genetic linkage is established when a chromosomal marker has a highly statistically significant association with a specific disease phenotype, in this case POAG. Once this has been demonstrated additional markers are analyzed until the position of the gene is well enough localized to begin the process of sequencing the gene. Once the gene is sequenced, the function of the gene can be examined and the disease causing mutation studied.

Genetic linkage analysis has been strikingly successful in identifying the location of genes for thousands of simple mendelian disorders including those associated with glaucoma such as juvenile open angle glaucoma (8) and Axenfeld-Rieger's syndrome (9). This powerful statistical methodology has now been successfully applied to complex disorders such as systemic hypertension (10) and Alzheimer's disease (11).

Alzheimer's disease has many parallels with POAG. Both diseases are complex disorders which are heterogeneic, occurring as both early and late onset disorders. The early onset disorders are highly penetrant autosomal dominant disorders, whereas the late onset disorders are characterized by a variable age of onset and incomplete penetrance. Using genetic analysis methods for complex diseases Pericak-Vance identified a region on chromosome 19 which was associated with late onset Alzheimer's disease. Shortly thereafter apolipoprotein E4 (APOE4) was determined to be the gene responsible for increased risk of developing Alzheimer's disease (12). Interestingly, APOE4 is one of three naturally occurring alleles of APOE, a major apolipoprotein in the nervous system. Individuals with homozygous APOE4 alleles (APOE4/4) develop Alzheimer's disease earlier than those who are heterozygous (e.g. APOE4/3). Those individuals with APOE4/3 develop Alzheimer's disease earlier than those with APOE3/3. Interestingly, the APOE2 allele has been shown to be protective for Alzheimer's disease. Therefore, the risk of developing Alzheimer's disease is proportional to the number of APOE4 alleles one has (13).

This discovery that relatively common alleles of a "housekeeping" gene such as APOE can exert major influence on the development of a late onset disorder such as Alzheimer's disease, represents a fundamental shift in thinking when compared to mendelian diseases which are characterized by rare genetic mutations and early onset. It is likely that many more examples of complex disorders caused by relatively common alleles which are "less efficient" or have some other long term detrimental effect will be discovered (13). As we live longer, the influence of these genes will become more apparent. This is highly relevant for POAG which shares many similarities with Alzheimer's disease.

Since POAG is a complex inherited disease with no known pathophysiologic mechanism, it is an excellent candidate for modern genetic linkage analysis. A number of ophthalmic institutions across the country are pursuing genetic linkage studies of POAG and other ocular complex disorders such as age-related macular degeneration. The single most important element of genetic linkage studies is the acquisition of well-ascertained families with the disease in question. POAG is a disease of exclusion. Therefore, families with exfoliation glaucoma, pigment dispersion syndrome, and other secondary forms of glaucoma must be excluded. Therefore, the practicing clinical ophthalmologist has the unparalleled opportunity to make a major contribution to this research by referring families with POAG or other ophthalmic disorders to centers where genetic linkage studies are being performed.

Identifying the gene(s) responsible for POAG will revolutionize our understanding of this disorder. In addition to major new therapies for POAG, it will be possible to better examine the basis for many known and suspected risk factors for POAG. For example, it will be possible to investigate the cause of increased IOP and its role in ganglion cell death; the relationship between POAG and steroid responsiveness; the cause of racial differences in the prevalence of POAG; the relationship, if any, with systemic hypertension, diabetes mellitus and other purported riskfactors; and the role of environmental factors in the pathophysiology of POAG.

Bibliography

1. Shin DH, Becker B, Kolker AE: Family history in primary open angle glaucoma. Arch Ophthalmol 1977;95:598.
2. Drance SM, Schulzer M, Thomas B, et al: Multivariate analysis in glaucoma: Use of discriminant analysis in predicting glaucomatous visual field damage. Arch Ophthalmol 1981;99:1019.
3. Jay B, Patterson B: The genetics of simple glaucoma. Trans Ophthalmol Soc UK 1970;90:161.
4. Armaly MF: The inheritance of dexamethasone hypertension and glaucoma. Arch Ophthalmol 1967;77:747.
5. Kass MA, Becker B: Genetics of primary open-angle glaucoma. Sight-Saving Rev 1978;48:21.
6. Sommer A, Tielsch JM, Katz, et al: Relationship between intraocular pressure and primary open angle glaucoma among white and black Americans. The Baltimore Eye Survey. Arch Ophthalmol 1991;109(8):1090.
7. Guyer MS, Collins FS: The human genome project and the future of medicine. AJDC 1993;147:1145.
8. Sheffield VC, Stone EM, Alward WLM, et al: Genetic linkage of familial open angle glaucoma to chromosome 1q21—q31. Nature Genetics 1993;336:164.
9. Vaux C, Sheffield L, Kieth CG, et al: Evidence that Rieger syndrome maps to 4q25 or 4q27. J Med Genetics 1992;29:256.
10. Jeunematre X, Soubrier F, Kotelevtsev YV, et al: Molecular basis of human hypertension: Role of angiotensinogen. Cell 1992;71:169.
11. Pericak-Vance MA, Bebout JL, Gaskell PC, et al: Linkage studies in familial Alzheimer's disease: Evidence for chromosome 19 linkage. Amer J Hum Genet 1991;48:1034.
12. Payami H, Kay J, Heston LL, et al: Apolipoprotein E genotype and Alzheimer's disease. Lancet 1993;342:738.
13. Roses AD: Alzheimer's disease as a model of molecular gerontology. J NIH Res 1995;7:51.

Diabetes has been widely reported to be a risk factor for POAG (45,46) but, as with myopia, self-selection into the health care system may also have influenced some of the associations found between diabetes and glaucoma. The possible role of arteriosclerotic and ischemic vascular diseases is also unclear. Migraine and peripheral vasospasm may be important in the development of some cases of glaucoma, particularly those with IOP in the normal or low range. Further study is needed to clarify the role of all of these factors in the development of glaucoma.

Data are conflicting as to whether POAG is more frequently associated with men or women (4,5,7,8,10,12). The possible relevance of general exposures such as diet, stress, alcohol consumption, and cigarette smoking has been inadequately studied and the scant data available are not convincing enough to warrant further consideration of any of these exposures at this time (10,47). It is interesting to note that IOP among the Japanese has not been found to increase with age as in Western populations studied (48). One hypothesis to explain this apparent discrepancy has been that IOP is related to body build, and that Japanese typically do not get obese with age as do many Americans and Europeans. Such an anthromorphologic consideration does not explain why glaucoma prevalence increases with age among the Japanese. Nonetheless, it suggests that anthromorphology may be an area worthy of further study.

HEALTH DELIVERY AND OUTCOME MEASURES

Because IOP is believed to be an important causal factor in glaucomatous damage, and because it is the factor most amenable to modification, the primary goal in treatment of glaucoma has traditionally been to lower the IOP. The efficacy of medications, laser treatments, and incisional surgeries in lowering IOP has been extensively documented. Most clinicians who take care of patients with glaucoma have had the unpleasant experience of witnessing the blinding sequelae of glaucoma left untreated. Understandably, clinicians have thus enthusiastically embraced the various modalities to lower IOP and undoubtedly, many patients will have been saved from blindness.

Despite the vast experience of many clinicians throughout the world and their overwhelming conviction that treating glaucoma by lowering IOP is beneficial, there has been a recent outcry for more evidence (49). With the tightening of the health care budget, the government, health insurers, and health provider organizations have begun the process of critically assessing the value of services provided. In this arena of health service research, the goal of glaucoma treatment has shifted from lowering IOP to stabilizing visual field loss and preserving vision.

Studies have certainly suggested that lowering IOP is beneficial in delaying onset of field loss in individuals with elevated IOPs and in decreasing the rate of field loss in individuals with manifest glaucoma (50–52). However, these results have not been uniformly and consistently obtained using study designs in which the potential for bias is minimized. Thus, the efficacy of lowering IOP has yet to be established to the satisfaction of skeptics.

In response to the demand for better evidence regarding the efficacy of lowering of IOP, two major clinical trials are currently underway (1995). The Ocular Hypertension Treatment Study is a multi-center clinical trial that is aimed at answering the question of whether medical treatment or no treatment of persons with only elevated IOP is more beneficial in delaying or preventing optic nerve damage and/or visual field loss. Another clinical trial, being performed in Sweden, is investigating the influence of medical treatment versus no treatment of manifest early open-angle glaucoma (including exfoliation glaucoma) with regard to progression of glaucoma. Results of these two clinical trials will have far-reaching implications, not only with regard to the optimal treatment, but to the pathogenesis of glaucoma.

Another outcome measure that is gaining increasing importance in studies of disease is that of quality of life. With glaucoma, there is a paucity of information related to having the disease or to treating it. For example, **depression may be a common element in persons with glaucoma, either because glaucoma is a chronic, potentially visually debilitating disease or because of the known depressive side effects of some of the medications used to treat the disease.** One study has analyzed determinants of serious falls among elderly glaucoma patients and has found that using topical medications was the greatest single factor (53). Undoubtedly, there are numerous other quality of life issues related to topical medication that have not yet been investigated.

An argument has been raised that optimal initial treatment of glaucoma should be surgical rather than medical. This viewpoint, though somewhat radical from the perspective of current training and practice, is supported by the generally favorable results obtained from early surgical intervention in clinical trials performed in Great Britain (54,55). There exists sufficient rationale to justify performing a study of initial medical versus surgical treatment of glaucoma. A multi-center clinical trial, the Collaborative Initial Glaucoma Treatment Study, is currently underway (1996). One of the important aspects of this trial is its emphasis on health-related quality of life outcomes associated with both treatments.

SUMMARY

The past decade has witnessed an explosion of information related to epidemiological aspects of glaucoma. Cross-sectional, population-based surveys have provided reliable age and race-specific prevalence data and have suggested factors that should be further investigated as potential risk factors. The next decade promises to be a particularly fruitful one for glaucoma epidemiology. Longitudinal studies are currently being performed from which estimates of glaucoma incidence, both in the general population and in persons with elevated IOP, can be made. Investigations of risk factors will be greatly facilitated and causal links will be better established by the availability of such longitudinal data. Factors that influence, not only glaucoma development, but also progression and other outcomes, will be better understood. The accumulation of such epidemiological data, in combination with contributions from the basic sciences and clinical practice, will bring us that much closer to the goal of designing intervention programs that can prevent, or at least control, the debilitating outcomes associated with glaucoma.

References

1. Tielsch JM, et al: Blindness and visual impairment in an American urban population: The Baltimore Eye Survey. Arch Ophthalmol 1990; 108:286.
2. Armaly MF: On the distribution of applanation pressure. I. Statistical features and the effect of age, sex, and the family history of glaucoma. Arch Ophthalmol 1965;73:11.
3. World Development Report 1993: Investing in Health. The International Bank for Reconstruction and Development/The World Bank. New York, N.Y. Oxford University Press, 1993.
4. Tielsch JM, et al: Racial variations in the prevalence of primary open-angle glaucoma: The Baltimore Eye Survey. JAMA 1991;226:369.

5. Klein BEK, et al: Prevalence of glaucoma: The Beaver Dam Eye Study. Ophthalmol 1992;99:1499.
6. Coffey M, et al: Prevalence of glaucoma in the West of Ireland. Br J Ophthalmol 1993;77:17.
7. Dielemans I, et al: The prevalence of primary open-angle glaucoma in a population-based study in the Netherlands. Ophthalmology 1994; 101:1851.
8. Bengtsson B: The prevalence of glaucoma. Br J Ophthalmol 1981;65: 46.
9. Hollows FC, Graham PA: Intraocular pressure, glaucoma, and glaucoma suspects in a defined population. Br J Ophthalmol 1986;50:570.
10. Kahn HA, Milton RC: Revised Framingham Eye Study: Prevalence of glaucoma and diabetic retinopathy. Am J Epidemiol 1989;111:769.
11. Mason RP, et al: National survey of the prevalence and risk factors of glaucoma in St. Lucia, West Indies. Part I: Prevalence findings. Ophthalmology 1989;65:1363.
12. Leske MC, et al: The Barbados Eye Study: Prevalence of open angle glaucoma. Arch Ophthalmol 1994;112:821.
13. Kragha Ikok: Prevalence of glaucoma in an eye hospital in Nigeria. Am J. Optom Physiol Opt 1987;64:617.
14. Neumann E, Zauberman H: Glaucoma Survey in Liberia. Am J Ophthalmol 1965;59:8–12.
15. Verrey JD, Foster A, Wormald R, et al: Chronic glaucoma in Northern Ghana. A retrospective study of 397 patients. Eye 1990;4:115.
16. Congdan N, Wang F, Tielsch JM: Issues in the epidemiology and population-based screening of primary angle-closure glaucoma. Surv Ophthalmol 1992;36:411.
17. Shiose Y, et al: Epidemiology of glaucoma in Japan: A nationwide glaucoma survey. Jpn J Ophthalmol 1991;35:133.
18. Bengtsson E: Incidence of manifest glaucoma. Br J Ophthalmol 1989; 73:483.
19. Armaly MF, et al: Biostatistical analysis of the Collaborative Glaucoma Study. I. Summary report of the risk factors for glaucomatous visual field defects. Arch Ophthalmol 1980;98:2163.
20. Quigley HA, Addicks EM: Chronic experimental glaucoma in primates: II. Effect of extended intraocular pressure elevation on optic nervehead and axonal transport. Invest Ophthalmol Vis Sci 1980;19:137.
21. Gaasterland O, Tanashima T, Kuwabara T: Axoplasmic flow during chronic experimental glaucoma. I. Light and electron microscopic studies of the monkey optic nervehead during development of glaucomatous cupping. Invest Ophthalmol Vis Sci 1978;17:838.
22. Cartwright MJ, Anderson DR: Correlation of asymmetric damage with asymmetric intraocular pressure in normal-tension glaucoma (low-tension glaucoma). Arch Ophthalmol 1988;106:898.
23. Crichton A, Drance SM, Douglas GR, et al: Unequal intraocular pressure and its relation to asymmetric visual field defects in low-tension glaucoma. Ophthalmology 1989;96:1312.
24. Coulehan JL, Helzlsouer KJ, Rogers KD, et al: Racial differences in intraocular tension and glaucoma surgery. Am J Epidemiol 1980;11: 759.
25. Beck RW, et al: Is there a racial difference in physiologic cup size? Ophthalmology 1985;92:873.
26. Chi T, et al: Racial differences in optic nervehead parameters. Arch Ophthalmol 1989;107:836.
27. Steinmann W, et al: A case-control study of the association of sickle cell trait and chronic open-angle glaucoma. Am J Epidemiol 1983;118: 288.
28. Javitt JC, et al: Undertreatment of glaucoma among black Americans. N Engl J Med 1991;325:1418.
29. Kahn KL, et al: Health care for black and poor hospitalized medicare patients. JAMA 1994;271:1169.
30. Tielsch JM, et al: Family history and risk of primary open-angle glaucoma: The Baltimore Eye Survey. Arch Ophthalmol 1994;112:69.
31. Johnson AT, et al: Clinical features and linkage analysis of a family with autosomal dominant juvenile glaucoma. Ophthalmology 1993;100:524.
32. Dorozynski A: Privacy rules blindside French glaucoma effort. Science 1991;252:369.
33. Richards JE, et al: Mapping of a gene for autosomal dominant juvenile-onset open-angle glaucoma to chromosome Iq. Am J Hum Gen 1994; 54:62.
34. Perkins ES, Phelps CS: Open angle glaucoma, ocular hypertension, low tension glaucoma, and refraction. Arch Ophthalmol 1982;100:1464.
35. Armaly MF: Cup/disc ratio in early open-angle glaucoma. Doc Ophthalmol 1969;26:526.
36. Hart WM Jr, et al: Multivariate analysis of the risk of glaucomatous visual field loss. Arch Ophthalmol 1979;97:1455.
37. Yablonski ME, Zimmerman TJ, Kass MA, et al: Prognostic significance of optic disc cupping in ocular hypertension patients. Am J Ophthalmol 1980;89:585.
38. Krakau T: Disc hemorrhages and the etiology of glaucoma. Acta Ophthalmol 1989;67:31.
39. Quigley HA, et al: An evaluation of optic disc and nerve fiber layer examinations in monitoring progression of early glaucoma damage. Ophthalmology 1992;99:19.
40. Quigley HA, Brown ME, Morrison JD, et al: The size and shape of the optic disc in normal human eyes. Arch Ophthalmol 1982;100:135.
41. Klein BEK, Klein R: Intraocular pressure and cardiovascular risk variables. Arch Ophthalmol 1981;99:837.
42. Leighton DA, Phillips CI: Systemic blood pressure in glaucoma. Br J Ophthalmol 1972;52:447.
43. Dielemans I, et al: Primary open-angle glaucoma, intraocular pressures, and systemic blood pressure in the general elderly population: The Rotterdam Study. Ophthalmology 1995;102:54.
44. Tielsch JM, et al: Hypertension, perfusion pressure, and primary open-angle glaucoma: A population-based assessment. Arch Ophthalmol 1995;113:216.
45. Nielsen NV: The prevalence of glaucoma and ocular hypertension in type 1 and type 2 diabetes mellitus. Acta Ophthalmol 1983;61:662.
46. Katz J, Sommer A: Risk factors for primary open-angle glaucoma. Am J Prev Med 1988;4:110.
47. Wilson MR, et al: A case-control study of risk factors in open-angle glaucoma. Arch Ophthalmol 1987;105:1066.
48. Shiose Y: Intraocular pressure: New perspectives. Surv Ophthalmol 1980;34:413.
49. Eddy DM, Billings J: The quality of medical evidence and medical practice. Report prepared for the National Leadership Commission on Health Care, 1988.
50. Quigley HA, Maumenee AE: Long-term follow-up of treated open-angle glaucoma. Am J Ophthalmol 1979;87:519.
51. Mao LK, Stewart WL, Shields MB: Correlation between intraocular pressure control and progressive glaucomatous damage in primary open-angle. Am J Ophthalmol 1991;111:51.
52. Stewart WC, Chorak RP, Hunt HH, et al: Factors associated with visual loss in patients with advanced glaucomatous changes in the optic nervehead. Am J Ophthalmol 1993;116:176.
53. Glynn RJ, et al: Falls in elderly patients with glaucoma. Arch Ophthalmol 1991;109:205.
54. Jay JL, Allan D: The benefit of early trabeculectomy versus conventional management in primary open-angle glaucoma relative to severity of disease. Eye 1989;3:528.
55. Midgal C, Hitchings R: Control of chronic simple glaucoma with primary medical, surgical, and laser treatment. Trans Ophthalmol Soc UK 1986;105:653.

Medico-Legal Issues In Glaucoma

73

Paul P. Lee

INTRODUCTION

It is a commentary on the evolution in medical practice within our society since the first edition of Chandler and Grant's *Lectures on Glaucoma* that there is sufficient material and interest to justify including a chapter on the medicolegal concerns associated with the care of patients with glaucoma. It is perhaps an even larger commentary that the potential area of discussion is even greater than that covered in brief in this chapter. Areas such as intellectual property rights in new glaucoma treatments (including on the part of patients whose tissues form the basis from which new products arise), the presence of a "right" to health care and to the care of glaucoma (for example, on the part of incarcerated prisoners), the ability of insurance companies to limit or deny coverage, the rules governing legal procedures and processes, the regulations covering the disposal of hazardous chemicals such as 5-FU and mitomycin C, and the right of patients to obtain experimental treatments (as has occurred with increasing regularity in cancer treatment) are not included here. Indeed, even those areas reviewed are summarized and are not meant as comprehensive guides to the legal rules that exist when the reader reviews this chapter. Instead, the objective is to acquaint the reader with the basic legal principles and the majority rules and trends that exist in 1996. The reader should consult with his or her attorney regarding any specific question that might arise.

One basic reason for this uncertainty is that our legal system is based on two major but very different elements: case law and statutory law. Statutory law is what most people think of when they think of legal rules—the laws enacted by local, state, and federal governments, as interpreted by the appropriate government agency, if needed. However, the vast majority of the rules that actually govern our standards and behaviors in providing health care today are based in case law. **Case law is those rules that are derived from court decisions resolving actual lawsuits between disputing parties.** Indeed, it is a truism that case law can significantly alter the effect of the statutory law, based on the judicial interpretation of such laws. As such, the applicable rules governing analogous or similar cases or situations are subject to change at any time that a case is decided; a court may decide to overturn prior rules or to disagree with other courts. Thus, two similar cases can reach very different results, even within the same legal jurisdiction, and even within the same time frame. **Thus, there are no certainties in legal cases, only probabilities** (as with medical care).

Clearly, a situation where courts could decide whatever they wished would be unworkably chaotic. Thus, a longstanding principle within the legal system is that of stare decisis, or of following the ruling of prior cases in the absence of a strong reason to the contrary. Second, there is a hierarchy of courts within a jurisdiction, so that lower level courts are obligated to follow the rules of higher level courts in subsequent decisions. However, the mechanism of change within the case law is for a lower court to rule in favor of a party in a lawsuit that is contrary to similar or higher courts and thus provide the higher court an opportunity to consider or reconsider its prior rules on appeal. While there are generally indicators that the legal system is interested in reviewing a given rule prior to it actually doing so (based on the opinions and rulings of prior cases or legal commentary), there is nothing to protect a given party who has relied upon a prior rule from being found responsible in the case which changes the prior rule(s). A common observation of today's court system is that they are being bound far less by stare decisis than courts in the past, increasing the uncertainty for interested parties.

A second reason for the uncertainty is that there are several different legal jurisdictions that may apply in a given case, each potentially with its own rules of procedures as well as substantive law. For example, negligence actions are typically brought in state courts, so that the procedures and the substantive law or rules vary from state to state. At the same time, claims that invoke discriminatory elements, such as an alleged refusal to treat an HIV patient, may be brought in federal or state courts, and parties may have to contend with state and federal statutory and case law. Thus, to reiterate, the law is in a constant state of flux and the flux can vary from state to state and from claim to claim. As such, matters of legal concern should be reviewed with an attorney familiar with the rules and procedures of the jurisdiction in question.

Despite this potential for uncertainty, there are certain basic principles that have been developed over the centuries that can provide useful information and understanding. Similarly, there are clearly perceptible trends in the law in specific areas, suggesting that parties may want to follow the trends even if their current jurisdiction currently clings to a more traditional standard. (Needless to say, virtually every trend is to impose greater liability and responsibility on the physician in medicolegal cases.)

This chapter will focus on traditional elements of medicolegal concern: malpractice allegations, claims of patient abandonment, and issues surrounding informed consent. In addition, because of new changes in the health delivery system, the chapter will also briefly review the effects of practice guidelines on malpractice actions, **the responsibility of physicians to advocate for their patients in a managed care system (or face legal liability),** and developing rules covering unapproved uses of drugs and devices.

TRADITIONAL MEDICOLEGAL CONCERNS

The case law has developed the concepts underlying the physician-patient relationship over many centuries: what is the obligation of the physician to the patient in providing care and in ending care. In determining the responsibilities related to the relationship, the law has clearly stated that a relationship must first exist between a patient and a physician in order for any duty or responsibility to arise. Thus, **the first issue for any legal inquiry is whether a relationship has been established**. Traditionally, the law has required that the patient seek care and that the physician agree to provide such care and actually do so by seeing the patient for the initial visit. Today, the relationship can be much more tenuous. The growing rule is that if a reasonable person would believe that the physician is acting primarily for the patient's benefit or that a reasonable person would rely on advice provided by the physician or physician's office of a medical nature, a relationship has been established. Thus, even telephone advice can be deemed sufficient in a growing number of states, even if the patient has never been seen in one's office. Merely making an appointment would not necessarily raise the contact to that of an established relationship today, but legal commentary suggests that even agreeing to see a patient may establish a relationship.

Malpractice

ELEMENTS OF MALPRACTICE

After establishing the first element of a patient-physician relationship, the patient must still prove three additional elements to succeed in a malpractice action or lawsuit for negligence in medical care. The patient must show that: 1) the physician breached the applicable standard of care for his or her case; 2) the patient suffered an injury; and 3) that the breach of the duty was the proximate cause of the injury. Over the last thirty years, each of these elements has undergone considerable change in the United States, again favoring the patient or plaintiff.

Standard of Care

In determining if a standard of care has been violated, the critical issue is determining what the standard of care is. There is no predetermined standard of care (except as noted below for practice guidelines in the state of Maine); **the standard of care is determined by expert testimony in every case**. The rules governing who may testify as to the standard of care and rules governing the procedures vary from state to state and are beyond the scope of this chapter. However, certain substantive issues have become clearer over time; courts are increasingly imposing higher standards through changes in the case law.

Physicians are responsible for the care provided by the average or typical practitioner in their defined geographic area. Increasingly, courts are expanding the traditional definition of applicable geographic area from the local community to local or like communities, to states, and thence to the nation. At this time, general physicians (including general ophthalmologists) are usually held to local or state standards. Specialists (including subspecialist ophthalmologists) are increasingly held to a national standard of care. The trend is clearly towards a larger and more national approach to what the standard of care is in each case.

The case law is also clear in holding physicians to that level of knowledge and expertise that existed at the time of the action in question. However, those physicians with specialized knowledge or special knowledge (including from their research), particularly if they led the patient to believe that they had such additional knowledge, may be held liable for applying or failing to apply such knowledge.

Physicians who use unorthodox approaches or non-mainstream therapies are protected from malpractice violations of the standard of care provided the therapy provided is deemed acceptable practice or care by a "respectable minority" or "significant minority" in most jurisdictions. As a practical matter, the "battle of experts" at trial often means that as long as some expert witnesses support the feasibility of a given treatment approach, the jury could find a given treatment as meeting a given community standard.

Injury

The case law requires that the patient suffer some form of injury from the alleged violation of the standard of care. Typically, in eye cases, the injury centers on loss of vision or of the eye. The rule in every state is that such a physical injury is sufficient grounds to meet the injury requirement. In dollar terms, the typical eye malpractice case adverse to the physician resulted in an award between $100,000 and $200,000 in the early 1990's.

Controversy exists in the legal commentary about the ability to sustain damages for emotional loss or pain and suffering. Short of statutory limits in a few states, such as

California, these damages can far exceed the dollar awards for the actual physical injury. The vast majority rule, and one that has continued to hold despite strong legal commentary from the plaintiff's bar, is that emotional damages cannot be sustained without the presence of a physical injury. Further, the physical injury generally must be permanent (or reasonably so) to support such emotional damages.

Proximate Cause

The final element in linking the three parts of a malpractice action is that the alleged breach of professional standards of care must "proximately" cause the injury being sued upon. While the cause-effect nature of most actions is intuitively obvious, this issue can arise in cases where, for example, the patient did not keep his or her scheduled follow-up appointments after surgery and then comes in weeks later with a complication that might have been successfully treated earlier. In this particular example, **the physician would be able to avoid or at least mitigate responsibility if he or she could demonstrate in the medical record that appropriate efforts were made to get the patient to come in for the follow-up and that the patient refused, even after being informed of the possible risks and outcomes.** Thus, the potential exists of disputing whether the action being complained of was in fact responsible for the injury.

Importance of Documentation

The most important practical consideration in determining whether non-obvious cases of negligence go forward to suit is the quality, extent, and legibility of the documentation in the medical record. The legal rule is that if it isn't written down, it probably wasn't done. When documentation doesn't exist, it becomes a choice for the jury between the word of the patient, who swears that he or she didn't have the given test done, or that of the physician. Clearly, if the test or measurement was made, it should be documented. Documentation is also important in situations where the patient is non-compliant, acts against medical advice, or refuses treatment. Documenting advice and recommended treatment is an antidote to patient claims that they were never properly informed of their treatment, of the importance of follow-up, or regular care. Indeed, having the patient sign (or even self-write) a statement of refusing offered treatment or medical advice, with the possible risks of doing so, in the chart itself would be ideal.

A second set of reasons to document in greater detail and frequency (discussed in greater detail below) is the rise of practice guidelines. Failure to document that the recommended steps were performed will raise the likelihood of an adverse outcome at trial, since the physician will have to justify deviations from the guideline. Finally, reimbursement for Medicare and other insurance sources are subject to audit, with certain levels of documentation needed to support certain visit intensity levels.

The importance of documentation extends to telephone calls for new or continuing patients. As noted in the section on establishing the physician-patient relationship, even a phone call may be enough to establish a relationship in a small number of jurisdictions. Thus, any telephone contact that goes beyond a mere scheduling call should be documented in the chart (continuing patient) or a phone log (new patient). Clearly, any advice, or even a significant rescheduling delay, should be noted in the chart, particularly if information of the risks of the delay or the risks and benefits of the advice are provided. Results of laboratory tests, follow-up to surgery on the first night, or any significant patient contact should be documented.

At the same time, documentation of financial disagreements should be filed in a separate part of the patient's overall record from the clinical record. Although there is no legal reason to do so, it is important to avoid the inadvertent appearance in the chart that financial considerations may influence the clinical care provided to the patient. Raising payment or other financial issues in the clinical record causes juries to wonder about this very concern.

The medical record per se belongs to the physician, but the patient has a right to the information contained therein. As such, the physician has the obligation to make copies of the record available to the patient or someone he or she has designated, though the physician may charge reasonable expenses for the process of providing copies (generally 10 cents to 50 cents per page). At the same time, the physician has an obligation NOT to release information without an authorization from the patient.

ENDING A DOCTOR-PATIENT RELATIONSHIP

The patient always has the right to terminate the physician-patient relationship. Issues of legal concern arise when the physician isn't sure whether the patient has done so (no-shows) or when the physician wishes to terminate the relationship for whatever reason. **The key concept is that the physician cannot abandon the patient who is in need of care.** For a chronic condition such as glaucoma, this effectively means that the physician cannot end the relationship or deem the relationship ended without notice to the patient and providing the patient an opportunity to find alternatives for care. As in malpractice, for a patient to prevail on an action for abandonment, the patient's reasonable expectations that care would be provided would not only have to be unfulfilled but also result in an injury to the patient.

For no-shows, the office should have a system for following up with patients to reschedule their visits

or to determine that they are no longer patients of the practice. One good method is to follow-up with either phone calls or reminder cards, much as a typical dentist or veterinarian does. In either case, the notice should be documented in the chart and the risks of failing to obtain regular care be mentioned. Even where the patient terminates the relationship, it is still good practice to confirm the termination and emphasize the need for regular follow-up care.

In the case of the physician wishing to end a relationship with a patient, whether for financial reasons or for non-compliance, the physician must let the patient know and must provide the patient an opportunity to locate and establish alternatives to care. In the written communication to the patient, the physician should, from a practical viewpoint, stay away from a specific financial reason (if that is the case) and refrain from judgmental statements. **The physician cannot, however, terminate a relationship solely because of HIV status, race, gender, disability status, or other protected classifications.**

The physician should have documentation in writing that the patient was sent notice, ideally by registered or certified mail. At the least, reasonable measures should include a phone call (documented) and regular mail, with a copy of the letter in the chart. The letter should state that the physician will be available for care for a specified period of time, but no longer, in order to provide the patient the opportunity to establish alternative care. Ideally, the letter should provide specific alternatives, such as the name and number of other appropriate physicians or the local university practice. In addition, the letter should let the patient know that his records will be made available to whoever the patient wishes; as a practical matter, it is generally wise to waive any copying fees in this particular situation.

If, after ending the relationship, the patient returns to the practice in an emergency, the patient should be seen until the emergency is stabilized. If the relationship is still not one desired by the physician, then a confirmation letter of the termination of the relationship would be appropriate.

INFORMED CONSENT

The third major action that has traditionally been of concern to physicians is the claim of battery for touching without the patient's permission. Unlike the actions of negligence and abandonment, patients need not show that the physician violated applicable community standards and can seek punitive damages (which generally are not covered by malpractice insurance) for any harm resulting from any act outside the scope of permission. Case law establishes that the patient has a right to refuse to consent to any recommended medical procedure and that, second, the patient has a right to sufficient information to make that decision. Inadequate information, as opposed to lack of consent in its entirety, can also be treated as an action in negligence for inadequate informed consent, where the patient alleges he or she would not have had the procedure which caused the harm if they were aware of such undisclosed risks.

Issues surrounding informed consent in glaucoma care can arise in virtually every arena; however, most questions center on: 1) the situations in which consent is needed, especially with systemic carbonic anhydrase inhibitors; 2) the amount of information that needs to be disclosed; and 3) how consent is documented.

When Consent is Needed

Consent is needed for any touching. Thus, even the physical exam requires consent. In the case of the physical exam, however, consent is deemed to be implied. In addition, **in many offices today, part of the paperwork of new patients includes permission for ordinary and reasonable examinations and procedures.** What requires explicit consent is, again, variable from state to state. The prevailing rule is that consent is needed if the applicable standard of care requires consent. Most invasive procedures require explicit consent, but phlebotomy and intravenous line insertion in most states do not. **As a general rule, any procedure with a risk of a significant adverse outcome should be consented.**

Controversy exists as to whether information should be given to patients regarding the side effects of prescription drugs. Since the prevailing practice is not to provide such information, most states with a prevailing practice standard do not impose a duty to disclose side effects to patients. Thus, the risks of systemic carbonic anhydrase inhibitors need not be disclosed in every case in every state. However, as prevailing practice changes, this rule will change. In other words, as more physicians tell patients about the risks of systemic carbonic anhydrase inhibitors, the rule will change to require disclosure. Further, the courts in more jurisdictions are changing the disclosure rule to what a reasonable person would want to know, therefore making it desirable for the physicians to disclose the risks. In effect, the standard will soon become in the vast majority of states that disclosure of the side effects of systemic carbonic anhydrase inhibitors will be needed.

Any specific question that the patient asks should be answered to the extent possible. **In situations where the law does not impose a duty to disclose, a specific patient question or request in that area acts to create a duty to disclose.** Thus, for example, if a patient were to ask about the side effects of a topical eye drop, the physician would have a duty to disclose the side effects, even though the case law would not have imposed such a responsibility in the absence of a patient request.

Amount of Information

How much needs to be disclosed is a second major issue area. The general rule as to the amount of information that should be disclosed is **what a reasonable person would want to know or in answer to a specific question by the patient.** The old rule of prevailing practice among physicians is a diminishing minority rule. The newest rule proposed by legal commentators would impose a patient specific standard, i.e., what that person would have wanted to know. Because of practical difficulties in using this standard (the ability to read into a patient's mind), no state so far has adopted this particular rule for all patients.

A rough yardstick for what a reasonable person would want to know is that all catastrophic occurrences, such as death, stroke, coma, blindness, or loss of the eye need to be disclosed. Case law clearly establishes that disclosure of death does NOT equate with consent to stroke or coma, since attorneys can make a cogent argument that life in a vegetative state is different and perhaps worse than death. Thus, these need to be explicitly mentioned. In addition, common complications or risks need to be disclosed; **a common rule is that any event occurring more often than once per 1000 patients should be disclosed.** Finally, knowledge of special or unique fears of the patient, especially if verbalized by the patient, may also require disclosure of applicable risks.

The level of detail of the disclosure is governed by the rule in that jurisdiction (prevailing practice or reasonable person). In the absence of a specific request by the patient for greater detail, exact numeric likelihood's are not generally required.

Documentation of Informed Consent

As noted earlier, the question of having performed a given service or procedure is a separate question from being able to prove years later that it was indeed done. Given research findings that patients remember less than 20% of what they are told, and virtually nothing if emotionally laden words or diagnoses such as cancer are used, even the most careful disclosure of facts will not be remembered by patients by the next visit, let alone months or years later when he or she decides to pursue legal action and the case finally comes to depositions and thence trial. Thus, being able to document that consent was obtained and that it was informed is vital.

At a minimum, there should be a notation in the medical record that the indications, risks/complications, benefits, and alternatives were discussed with the patient. Better would be a more explicit and standardized consent form. Ideal would be both a chart notation and a form. Detail in specifying the general areas covered, especially complications, is helpful. However, the more detailed the list, the greater the importance of completeness, since the presumption will be raised that anything not on a long, detailed list was probably not discussed, even if it really was.

Table 73-1
Distribution of Claims Made in Malpractice in Ophthalmology

Negligent diagnosis	38%
Negligent treatment	49%
Legal issues	16%

Table 73-2
Steps to Minimize Risk of Malpractice Claims

Maintain a supportive relationship with the patient and patient's family.
Acknowledge and explain treatment problems or unanticipated results.
Carefully document history and examinations at every visit.
Document discussions regarding risk and benefit of surgical procedures (informed consent).
When appropriate, offer a second opinion and document the offer.
Discuss difficult cases with colleagues and document discussions.
Terminate therapeutic relationship with patient properly.

If the patient allows, having a family member present during the discussion and sign as a witness to the consent and the process is useful, since some suits are caused by disgruntled family members and an otherwise accepting patient going along to preserve family harmony. In addition, there may be a benefit to the patient in having a loved and trusted family member help remember some of the details of the discussion. Some of these points are highlighted in Tables 73.1 and 73.2.

NEW "TWISTS" ON TRADITIONAL CONCERNS

The underlying concepts and practical aspects of medicolegal analysis for today's new issues arise from the same roots as noted in the prior section on malpractice/negligence, abandonment, and informed consent. The same sources of law, the same vitality and unpredictability of case law, and the same common sense responses still apply. This section concentrates on three distinct issue areas of increasing concern to physicians as we enter the 21st century in the United States: 1) non-FDA approved therapies; 2) practice guidelines; and 3) denial of services by an insurance company or health care plan. In each area, the same legal principles outlined in the prior section exist; what is different is how they interact with statutory law and their recent emergence.

Unapproved Therapies

Regulation of drugs and devices by the federal government has occurred only since the Food, Drug & Cosmetic Act of 1938. Before and since, the vast majority of medical practice by physicians has not been regulated or restricted except by the case law. There is still, for example, no regulation of medical procedures or of surgical operations by state or federal governments. Thus, at its roots, physicians' major concern with unorthodox therapies should center on whether such practices might represent negligence or malpractice and whether adequate informed consent was obtained.

At the same time, there is heightened sensitivity to the requirements of the federal government in our increasingly technology-dependent age and to the appearance of impropriety and possible negligence by choosing a treatment that is "not approved by the Food and Drug Administration (FDA)." The FDA has jurisdiction over the marketing, sale, and distribution of medical drugs and devices, not over the use of such drugs and devices by physicians or others who are not manufacturers, distributors, or those engaged in selling or marketing such drugs and devices. As such, physicians cannot be in violation of FDA rules or regulations by merely using drugs and devices.

Current concern over drugs and devices deal with using approved drugs and devices for unapproved uses (as was the case with 5-FU for glaucoma filtration surgery) and with the use of unapproved drugs for investigation or compassionate use purposes (for example, topical carbonic anhydrase inhibitors prior to their approval). In the first instance, **once a drug is approved for any use, physicians can choose to use the drug for any other use or indication. The FDA only bans the marketing or sale of the drug for such "unlabeled" uses. The only practical restraint on physicians is the potential liability for either negligence or a lack of informed consent for the experimental or investigational use of such a drug or device.**

The area of never-approved drugs and devices is subject to greater control by the FDA. Specific steps are laid out by the FDA to obtain experimental drugs and devices for compassionate use and even more stringent steps for the conduct of clinical trials of new drugs or devices. Again, in these situations, caution should be exercised to avoid negligence or lack of a valid informed consent, since drug or device use in these circumstances would certainly have to be considered investigational. Case law clearly requires a much higher duty and extent of disclosure of any pertinent information for "experimental" or investigational purposes. In addition, the federal government has specified what adequate informed consent is under these circumstances.

Government regulation of therapies thus extends only to the marketing and sale of drugs and devices that physicians utilize in treating patients. The use per se of the drugs and devices is not regulated by the FDA. For physicians, the greatest legal concerns with unapproved drugs and devices are with negligence and lack of informed consent. There is no regulation of surgical procedures per se; the FDA would regulate only the drugs and devices used in such surgical procedures.

Role of Practice Guidelines

Practice guidelines have increasingly been accepted by health policy analysts and physicians alike. Within ophthalmology, the American Academy of Ophthalmology has promulgated several guidelines dealing with various eye conditions, including primary open-angle glaucoma, primary angle-closure glaucoma, and glaucoma suspect. Preliminary study has found these guidelines not only to be easily usable but also followed to a large degree. **The impact of these guidelines on malpractice actions is thus likely to be high, since they are promulgated by an authoritative organization, designed to improve patient care, written in a specific (or able to be made specific with minimal difficulty) manner, designed scientifically, and supported by most ophthalmologists.**

In a malpractice action, practice guidelines may speak authoritatively to what the applicable standard of care is in a community. For subspecialists in glaucoma, they may be even more pertinent, since the Academy's preferred practice patterns are a national approach to the national standard to which subspecialists are generally held. The absence of competing guidelines makes the Academy's patterns even more influential in this regard.

The impact is not definitive, however, since guidelines can only help establish a plausible standard of care. Only in Maine does following a guideline result in immunity from negligence. In many other states, practice guidelines have been used against physicians who have not followed the guidelines and who have not documented reasons why guideline recommendations were not appropriate or were not utilized. Understanding what the Academy's guidelines state and reacting to them by following them or documenting reasons for not following them will become more important, as the acceptance and usefulness of the guidelines grow. Finally, the continued revision and updating of the Academy guidelines will only serve to enhance their authoritativeness and importance to physicians and the medico-legal system.

Physician Responsibility and Payor or Health Plan Denial of Services

With the growth of prepaid health plans and of heightened review and approval processes by all third party payors, situations where the plan or insurance company refuses coverage for a recommended treatment or visit interval have become more common. By law, all plans and payors must have appeals processes for denial of coverage. Physicians generally assist patients in this process to maximize the chances of obtaining needed approval. At the same time, however, physicians are coming under closer scrutiny in terms of their resource utilization, particularly under prepaid health care plans. More and more insurance companies and plans have clearly stated that continued participation of a physician in a given plan or policy network is dependent in part on their cost efficiency in caring for patients. The result is a growing conflict for physicians about the vigor with which to pursue patient appeals for denial of services or coverage.

Case law in at least one state (California) clearly lets the physician know that he or she has to continue to be the patient's advocate. In other words, **the physician must make reasonable and diligent efforts to protect the patient's interests during any process relating to the denial of services or coverage.** Failure to do so will make the physician liable as well as the health plan for denial of services or coverage. Since juries tend to take a dim view of organizations and parties that deny services to a sick or dying patient, this places the physician at substantial risk for failing to meet his or her legal (and ethical) obligations.

As a practical matter, there should be documentation of such efforts within the medical record. Records and notes of telephone calls should be kept, and one or more written communications with the plan or payor should also be retained. The communications would ideally include the risks of not performing the procedure or service in an explicit fashion, so that the health plan could not argue that it was not appropriately informed of the urgency or importance by the physician.

Suggested Reading

Albrecht K, Lee PP: Conformance with Preferred Practice Patterns in caring for patients with glaucoma. Ophthalmology 1994;101: 1668–1671.

Epstein R: Legal liability for medical innovation. Cardozo Law Review 1987;8:1139–59.

Frantz LB: Modern status of views as to general measure of physician's duty to inform patient of risks of proposed treatment. ALR 1989;88: 1008.

Kessler DA: The regulation of investigational drugs. N Engl J Med 1989; 320:281–88.

Kraushar MF, Robb JH. Ophthalmic malpractice lawsuits with large monetary awards. Arch Ophthalmol 1996;114:333–337.

Kraushar MF, Turner M. Medical malpractice litigation in ophthalmology: the New Jersey experience. Ophthalmic Surg 1986;17:671–674.

Lee PP: The effect of preferred practice patterns on malpractice actions. J Glaucoma 1992;1:286–89.

Lee PP, Yang JC, Schachat AP: Is informed consent needed for fluorescein angiography? Arch Ophthalmol 1993;111:327–30.

Tietz GF: Informed consent in the prescription drug context: the special case. Wash Law Rev 1986;61:367–417.

Index

Note: Page numbers in italics indicate figures; those followed by t indicate tables.